"Outstanding Reference Source."
—American Library Association

"Best of the Home Health Books."
—Changing Times

"One of the simplest and most thorough guides ever put together on the subject."
—United Press International

**"This is just what patients want and need to know—
and you've made it easy to find."**
—Louis A. Morris of the U.S. Food and Drug Administration

"Comprehensive, easy to use and informative."
—The Los Angeles Times

Tucson, Arizona
October, 1989

Dear Readers:

We are very pleased to present the 7th edition of our
Complete Guide to Prescription & Non-Prescription Drugs.

With this new edition, we strengthen our commitment to
improved patient/physician understanding and the free
exchange of vital, accurate information regarding your
health. Each annual edition presents special challenges to
us. For example, we add hundreds and sometimes
thousands of NEW brand names after the annual update of
our data bases. Similarly, generic entries grow each year.

As you might imagine, it takes a lot of hard work to make
this book so easy to use. For this ongoing effort, I must
thank Anne Olson, my project coordinator here in Tucson.
There are surely many others involved to whom I also
extend my deepest appreciation.

My greatest thanks, as always, is reserved for you, the
health-conscious individual. We hope we can continue to
justify your trust and confidence in our medical reference
books, and we hope you will continue to use them in
robust health.

Sincerely,

H. Winter Griffith, M.D.

H. Winter Griffith, M.D.

COMPLETE GUIDE TO PRESCRIPTION & NON-PRESCRIPTION

DRUGS

By H. WINTER GRIFFITH, M.D.

Technical consultants:
John D. Palmer, M.D., Ph.D.
William N. Jones, B.S., M.S.

NEW!
Revised for 1990
Over 5000 Brand Names
Over 700 Generic Names

❧ **THE BODY PRESS**
a division of
PRICE STERN SLOAN
Los Angeles

Published by The Body Press, a division of Price Stern Sloan, Inc.
360 N. La Cienega Boulevard, Los Angeles, California 90048
Printed in U.S.A.
9 8 7 6 5 4 3 2 1
Seventh Edition

Notice: The information in this book is true and complete to the best of our knowledge. The book is intended only as a guide to drugs used for medical treatment. It is not intended as a replacement for sound medical advice from a doctor. Only a doctor can include the variables of an individual's age, sex and past medical history needed for wise drug prescription. This book does not contain every possible side effect, adverse reaction or interaction with other drugs or substances. Final decision about a drug's safety or effectiveness must be made by the individual and his doctor. All recommendations herein are made without guarantees on the part of the author or the publisher. The author and publisher disclaim all liability in connection with the use of this information.

CONTENTS

ABOUT THE AUTHOR

H. Winter Griffith has authored many medical books, including the *Complete Guide to Symptoms, Illness & Surgery* and *Complete Guide to Sports Injuries,* both published by The Body Press. Others include *Instructions for Patients; Drug Information for Patients; Instructions for Dental Patients; Information and Instructions for Pediatric Patients; Vitamins, Minerals and Supplements;* and *Medical Tests—Doctor Ordered and Do-It-Yourself.* Dr. Griffith received his medical degree from Emory University in 1953. After 20 years in private practice, he established a basic medical-science program at Florida State University. He then became an associate professor of family and community medicine at the University of Arizona College of Medicine. Dr. Griffith now devotes all of his time and attention to his writing.

Technical Consultants

John D. Palmer, M.D., Ph.D.
  Associate professor of pharmacology, University of Arizona College of Medicine
  Associate professor of medicine (clinical pharmacology), University of Arizona
    College of Medicine

William N. Jones, Pharmacist, B.S., M.S.
  Clinical pharmacy coordinator, Veterans Administration Medical Center, Tucson,
    Arizona
  Adjunct assistant professor, Department of Pharmacy Practice, College of
    Pharmacy, University of Arizona

DRUGS AND YOU

My first day of pharmacology class in medical school started with a jolt. The professor began by writing on the blackboard, "Drugs are poisons."

I thought the statement was extreme. New drug discoveries promised to solve medical problems that had baffled men for centuries. The medical community was intrigued with new possibilities for drugs.

In the 30 years since then, many drug "miracles" have lived up to those early expectations. But the years have also shown the damage drugs can cause when they are misused or not fully understood. As a family doctor and teacher, I have developed a healthy respect for what drugs can and can't do. I now appreciate my professor's warning.

A drug cannot "cure." It aids the body's natural defenses to promote recovery. Likewise, a manufacturer or doctor cannot guarantee a drug will be useful for everyone. The complexity of the human body, individual responses in different people and in the same person under different circumstances, past and present health, age and sex influence how well a drug works.

All effective drugs produce desirable changes in the body, but a drug can also cause undesirable adverse reactions or side effects in some people. Despite uncertainties, the drug discoveries of the last 40 years have given us tools to save lives and reduce discomfort. Before you decide whether to take a drug, you or your doctor must ask, "Will the benefits outweigh the risks?"

The purpose of this book is to give you enough information about the most widely used drugs so you can make a wise decision. The information will alert you to potential or preventable problems. You can learn what to do if problems arise.

The information is derived from several expert sources. Every effort has been made to ensure accuracy and completeness. Where information from different sources conflicts, I have used the majority's opinion, coupled with my clinical judgment and that of my technical consultants. Drug information changes with continuing observations by clinicians and users.

Information in this book applies to generic drugs in both the United States and Canada. Generic names do not vary in these countries, but brand names do.

BE SAFE! TELL YOUR DOCTOR

Some suggestions for wise drug use apply to all drugs. Always give the following information to your physician, dentist or other health-care professional. They must have complete information to prescribe drugs safely for you. This information includes your medical history, your medical plans and progress while under medication.

MEDICAL HISTORY

Tell the important facts of your medical history dealing with drugs. Include allergic or adverse reactions you have had to any medicine in the past. Name the allergic symptoms you have, such as hay fever, asthma, eye watering and itching, throat irritation and reactions to food. People who have allergies to common substances are more likely to develop drug allergies.

List all drugs you take. Don't forget vitamin and mineral supplements; skin, rectal or vaginal medicines; antacids; antihistamines; cold and cough remedies; aspirin, aspirin combinations or other pain relievers; motion sickness remedies; weight-loss aids; salt and sugar substitutes; caffeine; oral contraceptives; sleeping pills or "tonics."

FUTURE MEDICAL PLANS
Discuss plans for elective surgery, pregnancy and breastfeeding.

QUESTIONS
Don't hesitate to ask questions about a drug. Your doctor, nurse or pharmacist may be able to provide more information if they are familiar with you and your medical history.

YOUR ROLE

Learn the generic names and brand names of all your medicines. Write them down to help you remember. If a drug is a mixture, learn the names of its generic ingredients.

TAKING A DRUG
Never take medicine in the dark! Recheck the label before each use. You could be taking the *wrong* drug! Tell your doctor about any unexpected new symptoms you have while taking medicine. You may need to change medicines or have a dose adjustment.

STORAGE
Keep all medicines out of children's reach. Store drugs in a cool, dry place, such as a kitchen cabinet or bedroom. Avoid medicine cabinets in bathrooms. They get too moist and warm at times.

Keep medicine in its original container, tightly closed. Don't remove the label! If directions call for refrigeration, don't freeze.

DISCARDING
Don't save leftover medicine to use later. Discard it on the expiration date shown on the container. Dispose safely to protect children and pets.

REFILLS
All refills must be ordered by your doctor or dentist, either in the first prescription or later. Only the pharmacy that originally filled the prescription can refill it without checking with your doctor or previous pharmacy. If you go to a *new* pharmacy, you must have a new prescription, or the new pharmacist must call your doctor or original pharmacy to see if a refill is authorized. Pharmacies don't usually transfer prescriptions.

If you need a refill, call your pharmacist and order your refill by number and name.

Use one pharmacy for the whole family if you can. The pharmacist then has a record of all of your drugs and can communicate effectively with your doctor. If you have questions about your drugs, ask the pharmacist.

LEARN ABOUT DRUGS
Study the information in this book's charts regarding your medications. Read each chart completely. Because of space limitations, most information that fits more than one category appears only once.

Take care of yourself. You are the most important member of your health-care team.

GUIDE TO DRUG CHARTS

The drug information in this book is organized in condensed, easy-to-read charts. Each drug is described in a two-page format, as shown in the sample chart below and opposite. Charts are arranged alphabetically by drug generic names, and in a few instances, such as *ADRENOCORTICOIDS, TOPICAL*, by drug class name.

A *generic name* is the official chemical name for a drug. A *brand name* is a drug manufacturer's registered trademark for a generic drug. Brand names listed on the charts

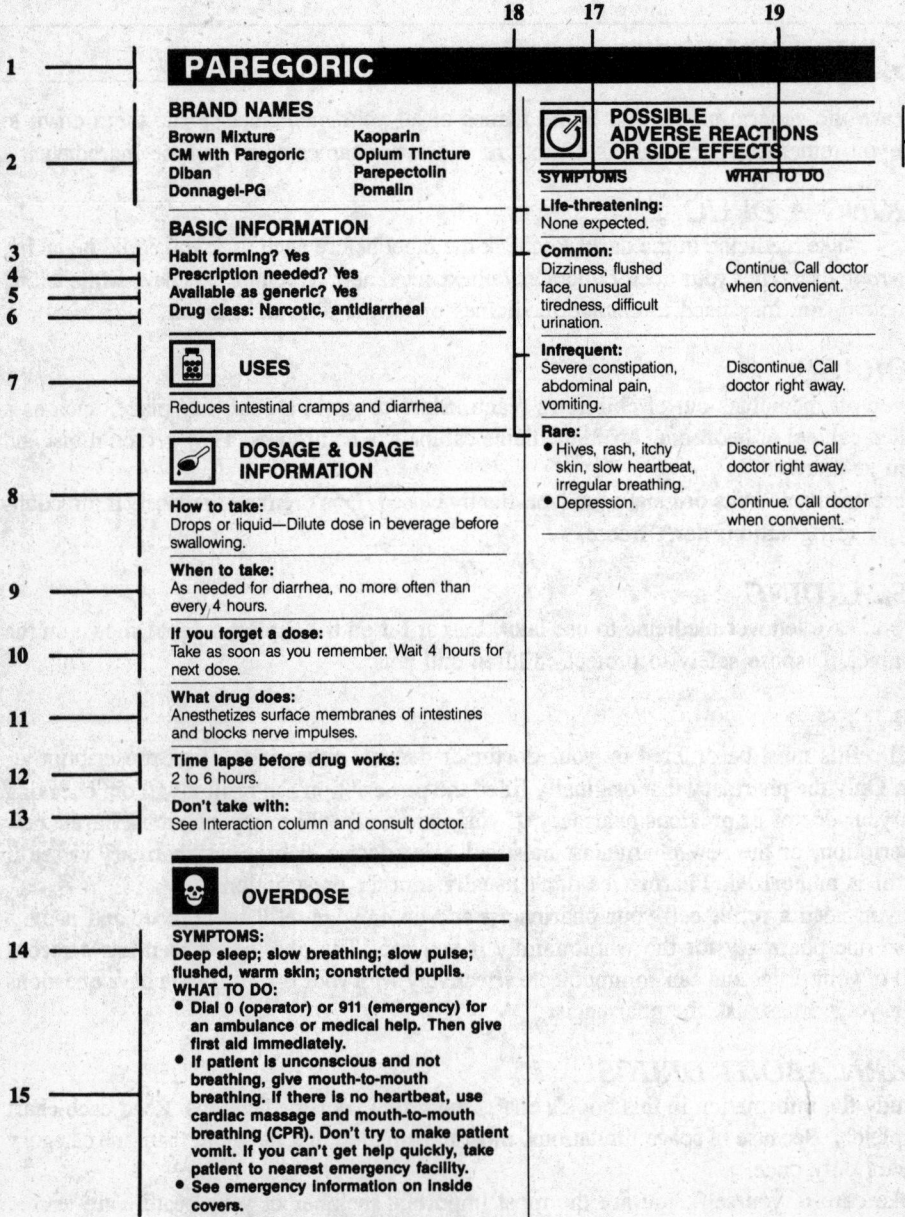

18   **17**   **19**

1

PAREGORIC

2

BRAND NAMES

Brown Mixture	Kaoparin
CM with Paregoric	Opium Tincture
Diban	Parepectolin
Donnagel-PG	Pomalin

BASIC INFORMATION

3 Habit forming? Yes
4 Prescription needed? Yes
5 Available as generic? Yes
6 Drug class: Narcotic, antidiarrheal

7 ### USES

Reduces intestinal cramps and diarrhea.

DOSAGE & USAGE INFORMATION

8 **How to take:**
Drops or liquid—Dilute dose in beverage before swallowing.

9 **When to take:**
As needed for diarrhea, no more often than every 4 hours.

10 **If you forget a dose:**
Take as soon as you remember. Wait 4 hours for next dose.

11 **What drug does:**
Anesthetizes surface membranes of intestines and blocks nerve impulses.

12 **Time lapse before drug works:**
2 to 6 hours.

13 **Don't take with:**
See Interaction column and consult doctor.

OVERDOSE

14 **SYMPTOMS:**
Deep sleep; slow breathing; slow pulse; flushed, warm skin; constricted pupils.
WHAT TO DO:
15
- Dial 0 (operator) or 911 (emergency) for an ambulance or medical help. Then give first aid immediately.
- If patient is unconscious and not breathing, give mouth-to-mouth breathing. If there is no heartbeat, use cardiac massage and mouth-to-mouth breathing (CPR). Don't try to make patient vomit. If you can't get help quickly, take patient to nearest emergency facility.
- See emergency information on inside covers.

POSSIBLE ADVERSE REACTIONS OR SIDE EFFECTS

16

SYMPTOMS	WHAT TO DO
Life-threatening: None expected.	
Common: Dizziness, flushed face, unusual tiredness, difficult urination.	Continue. Call doctor when convenient.
Infrequent: Severe constipation, abdominal pain, vomiting.	Discontinue. Call doctor right away.
Rare: • Hives, rash, itchy skin, slow heartbeat, irregular breathing.	Discontinue. Call doctor right away.
• Depression.	Continue. Call doctor when convenient.

include those from the United States and Canada. A generic drug may have one or many brand names.

To find information about a generic drug, look it up in the alphabetical charts. To learn about a brand name, check the index first, where brand names are followed by their generic ingredients and chart page numbers.

The chart design is the same for every drug. When you are familiar with the chart, you can quickly find information you want to know about a drug.

On the next few pages, each of the numbered chart sections below is explained. This information will guide you in reading and understanding the charts that begin on page 2.

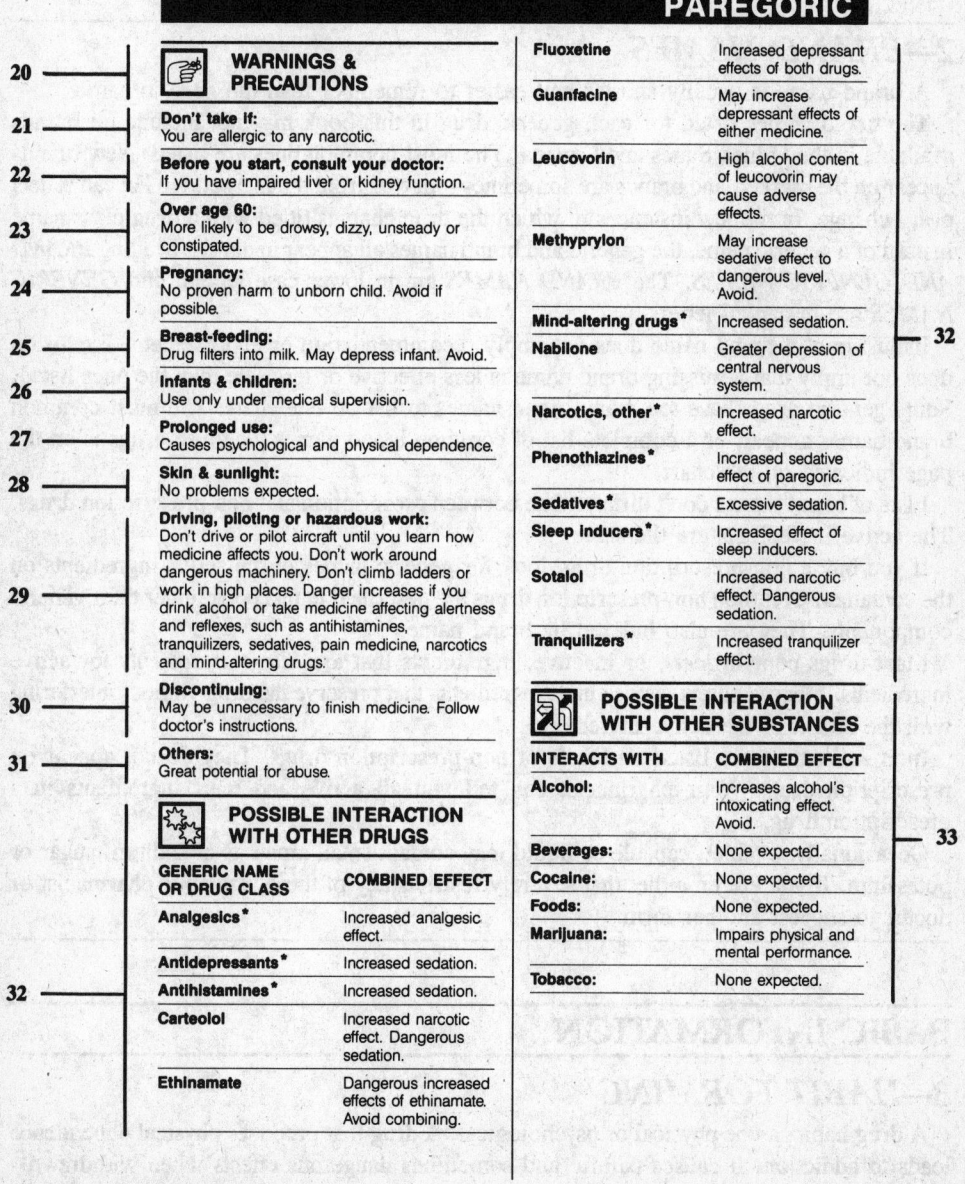

PAREGORIC

20 —
⌲ **WARNINGS & PRECAUTIONS**

21 — **Don't take if:**
You are allergic to any narcotic.

22 — **Before you start, consult your doctor:**
If you have impaired liver or kidney function.

23 — **Over age 60:**
More likely to be drowsy, dizzy, unsteady or constipated.

24 — **Pregnancy:**
No proven harm to unborn child. Avoid if possible.

25 — **Breast-feeding:**
Drug filters into milk. May depress infant. Avoid.

26 — **Infants & children:**
Use only under medical supervision.

27 — **Prolonged use:**
Causes psychological and physical dependence.

28 — **Skin & sunlight:**
No problems expected.

29 — **Driving, piloting or hazardous work:**
Don't drive or pilot aircraft until you learn how medicine affects you. Don't work around dangerous machinery. Don't climb ladders or work in high places. Danger increases if you drink alcohol or take medicine affecting alertness and reflexes, such as antihistamines, tranquilizers, sedatives, pain medicine, narcotics and mind-altering drugs.

30 — **Discontinuing:**
May be unnecessary to finish medicine. Follow doctor's instructions.

31 — **Others:**
Great potential for abuse.

⚕ **POSSIBLE INTERACTION WITH OTHER DRUGS**

GENERIC NAME OR DRUG CLASS	COMBINED EFFECT
Analgesics*	Increased analgesic effect.
Antidepressants*	Increased sedation.
Antihistamines*	Increased sedation.
Carteolol	Increased narcotic effect. Dangerous sedation.
Ethinamate	Dangerous increased effects of ethinamate. Avoid combining.

32 —

Fluoxetine	Increased depressant effects of both drugs.
Guanfacine	May increase depressant effects of either medicine.
Leucovorin	High alcohol content of leucovorin may cause adverse effects.
Methyprylon	May increase sedative effect to dangerous level. Avoid.
Mind-altering drugs*	Increased sedation.
Nabilone	Greater depression of central nervous system.
Narcotics, other*	Increased narcotic effect.
Phenothiazines*	Increased sedative effect of paregoric.
Sedatives*	Excessive sedation.
Sleep inducers*	Increased effect of sleep inducers.
Sotalol	Increased narcotic effect. Dangerous sedation.
Tranquilizers*	Increased tranquilizer effect.

— **32**

⚕ **POSSIBLE INTERACTION WITH OTHER SUBSTANCES**

INTERACTS WITH	COMBINED EFFECT
Alcohol:	Increases alcohol's intoxicating effect. Avoid.
Beverages:	None expected.
Cocaine:	None expected.
Foods:	None expected.
Marijuana:	Impairs physical and mental performance.
Tobacco:	None expected.

— **33**

*See Glossary

1—GENERIC NAME

Each drug chart is titled by generic name, or in a few instances, by the name of the drug class, such as *DIGITALIS PREPARATIONS*.

Sometimes a drug is known by more than one generic name. The chart is titled by the most common one. Less-common generic names appear in parentheses following the first. For example, vitamin C is also known as ascorbic acid. Its chart title is *VITAMIN C (ASCORBIC ACID)*. The index will include a reference for each name.

Your drug container may show a generic name, a brand name or both. If you have only a brand name, use the index to find the drug's generic name and chart.

If your drug container shows no name, ask your doctor or pharmacist for the name.

2—BRAND NAMES

A brand name is usually shorter and easier to remember than the generic name.

The brand names listed for each generic drug in this book may not include all brands available in the United States and Canada. The most-common ones are listed. New brands appear on the market, and brands are sometimes removed from the market. No list can reflect every change. In the few instances in which the drug chart is titled with a drug class name instead of a generic name, the generic and brand names all appear under the heading *BRAND AND GENERIC NAMES*. The *BRAND NAMES* are in lower case letters, and *GENERIC NAMES* are in capital letters.

Inclusion of a brand name does not imply recommendation or endorsement. Exclusion does not imply that a missing brand name is less effective or less safe than the ones listed. Some generic drugs have too many brand names to list on one chart. The most common brand names appear, or a complete list of common brand names for those drugs is on the page indicated on the chart.

Lists of brand names don't differentiate between prescription and non-prescription drugs. The active ingredients are the same.

If you buy a non-prescription drug, look for generic names of the active ingredients on the container. Common non-prescription drugs are described in this book under their generic components. They are also indexed by brand name.

Most drugs contain *inert*, or inactive, ingredients that are *fillers* or *solvents* for active ingredients. Manufacturers choose inert ingredients that preserve the drug without interfering with the action of the active ingredients.

Inert substances are listed on labels of non-prescription drugs. They do not appear on prescription drugs. Your pharmacist can tell you all active and inert ingredients in a prescription drug.

Occasionally, a tablet, capsule or liquid may contain small amounts of sodium, sugar or potassium. If you are on a diet that severely restricts any of these, ask your pharmacist or doctor to suggest another form.

BASIC INFORMATION

3—HABIT FORMING

A drug habit can be physical or psychological. A drug that produces physical dependence leads to addiction. It causes painful and sometimes dangerous effects when withdrawn.

Psychological dependence does not cause dangerous withdrawal effects. It may cause stress and unwanted behavior changes until the habit is broken.

4—PRESCRIPTION NEEDED?

"Yes" means a doctor must prescribe the drug for you. "No" means you can buy this drug without prescription. Sometimes low strengths of a drug are available without prescription, while high strengths require prescription.

The information about the generic drug applies whether it requires prescription or not. If the generic ingredients are the same, non-prescription drugs have the same dangers, warnings, precautions and interactions as prescribed drugs.

5—AVAILABLE AS GENERIC?

Some generic drugs have copyright restrictions that protect the manufacturer or distributor of that drug. These drugs may be purchased only by brand name.

In recent years, drug manufacturers have marketed more drugs under generic names. Drugs purchased by generic name sometimes are less expensive than brand names.

Some states allow pharmacists to fill prescriptions by brand names or generic names. This allows patients to buy the least expensive form of a drug.

A doctor may specify a brand name because he or she trusts a known source more than an unknown manufacturer of generic drugs. You and your doctor should decide whether you should buy a medicine by generic or brand name.

Generic drugs manufactured in other countries are not subject to regulation by the U.S. Food and Drug Administration. Drugs manufactured in the United States are subject to regulation.

6—DRUG CLASS

Drugs that possess similar chemical structure and similar therapeutic effects are grouped into classes. Most drugs within a class produce similar benefits, side effects, adverse reactions and interactions with other drugs and substances. For example, there are 15 generic drugs in the narcotic drug class. All have similar effects on the body.

Some information on the charts applies to all drugs in a class. For example, a reference may be made to narcotics. The index lists the class—narcotics—and lists drugs in that class.

Drug classes are not standardized, so classes listed in other references may vary from the classes in this book.

7—USES

This section lists the disease or disorder for which a drug is prescribed.

Most uses listed are approved by the U.S. Food and Drug Administration. Some uses are listed if experiments and clinical trials indicate effectiveness and safety. Still, other uses are included that may not be officially sanctioned, but for which doctors commonly prescribe the drug.

The use for which your doctor prescribes the drug may not appear. You and your doctor should discuss the reason for any prescription medicine you take. You alone will probably decide whether to take a non-prescription drug. This section may help you make a decision.

DOSAGE & USAGE INFORMATION

8—HOW TO TAKE

Drugs are available in tablets, capsules, liquids, suppositories, injections, transdermal patches (See Glossary), aerosol inhalers and topical forms such as drops, sprays, creams, ointments and lotions. This section gives general instructions for taking each form.

This information supplements drug-label information. If your doctor's instructions differ from the suggestions, follow your *doctor's* instructions.

Instructions are left out for how *much* to take. Dose amounts can't be generalized. They must be individualized for you by your doctor, or you must read the drug label.

9—WHEN TO TAKE

Dose schedules vary for medicines and for patients.

Drugs prescribed on a schedule should usually be taken at approximately the same times each day. Some *must* be taken at regular intervals to maintain a steady level of the drug in the body. If the schedule interferes with your sleep, consult with your doctor.

Instructions to take on an empty stomach mean the drug is absorbed best in your body this way. Many drugs must be taken with liquid or food because they irritate the stomach.

Instructions for other dose schedules are usually on the label. Variations in standard dose schedules may apply because some medicines interact with others if you take them at the same time.

10—IF YOU FORGET A DOSE

Suggestions in this section vary from drug to drug. Most tell you when to resume taking the medicine if you forget a scheduled dose.

Establish habits so you won't forget doses. Forgotten doses decrease a drug's therapeutic effect.

11—WHAT DRUG DOES

This is a simple description of the drug's action in the body. The wording is generalized and may not be a complete explanation of the complex chemical process that takes place.

12—TIME LAPSE BEFORE DRUG WORKS

The times given are approximations. Times vary a great deal from person to person, and from time to time in the same person. The figures give you some idea of when to expect improvement.

13—DON'T TAKE WITH

Some drugs create problems when taken in combination with other substances. Most problems are detailed in the Interaction column of each chart. This section mentions substances that don't appear in the Interaction column.

Occasionally, an interaction is singled out if the combination is particularly harmful.

OVERDOSE

14—SYMPTOMS

The symptoms listed are most likely to develop with accidental or purposeful overdose. An overdose patient may not show all symptoms listed. Sometimes symptoms are identical to ones listed as side effects. The difference is intensity and severity. You will have to judge. Consult a doctor or poison-control center if you have any doubt.

15—WHAT TO DO

If you suspect an overdose, whether symptoms are apparent or not, follow instructions in this section. Expanded instructions for emergency treatment for overdose are on the inside cover.

16—POSSIBLE ADVERSE REACTIONS OR SIDE EFFECTS

Adverse reactions or side effects are symptoms that may occur when you take a drug. They are effects on the body other than the desired therapeutic effect.

The term *side effect* implies expected and usually unavoidable effects of a drug. Side effects have nothing to do with the drug's intended use.

For example, the generic drug paregoric reduces intestinal cramps and vomiting. It also often causes a flushed face. The flushing is a side effect that is harmless and does not affect the drug's therapeutic potential.

The term *adverse reaction* is more significant. For example, paregoric can cause serious adverse allergic reaction in some people. This reaction can include hives, rash and severe itch.

Some adverse reactions can be prevented, which is one reason this information is included in the book. Most adverse reactions are minor and last only a short time. With many drugs, adverse reactions that might occur will frequently diminish in intensity as time passes.

The majority of drugs used properly for valid reasons offer benefits that outweigh potential hazards.

17—SYMPTOMS

Symptoms are grouped by various body systems. Symptoms that don't naturally apply to these body systems or which overlap systems are listed under "Others."

18—FREQUENCY

This is an estimation of how often symptoms occur in persons who take the drug. The four most common categories of frequency can be found under the **SYMPTOMS** heading and are as follows. **Life-threatening** means exactly what it says: Seek emergency treatment immediately. **Common** means these symptoms are expected and sometimes inevitable. **Infrequent** means the symptoms occur in approximately 1% to 10% of patients. **Rare** means symptoms occur in less than 1%.

19—WHAT TO DO

Carefully follow the instructions provided opposite the symptoms that apply to you.

20—WARNINGS AND PRECAUTIONS

Read these entries to determine special information that applies to you.

21—DON'T TAKE IF

This section lists circumstances that indicate the use of a drug may not be safe. On some drug labels and in formal medical literature, these circumstances are called *contraindications*.

22—BEFORE YOU START, CONSULT YOUR DOCTOR

This section lists conditions under which a drug should be used with caution.

23—OVER AGE 60

As a person ages, physical changes occur that require special consideration in drug use. Liver and kidney functions decrease, metabolism slows and the prostate gland enlarges in men.

Most drugs are metabolized or excreted at a rate dependent on kidney and liver functions. Small doses or longer intervals between doses may be necessary to prevent unhealthy concentration of a drug. Toxic effects and adverse reactions occur more frequently and cause more serious problems in this age group.

24—PREGNANCY

The best rule to follow during pregnancy is to avoid all drugs, including tobacco and alcohol. Any medicine—prescription or non-prescription—requires medical advice and supervision.

This section will alert you if there is evidence that a drug harms the unborn child. Lack of evidence does not guarantee a drug's safety. If safety is undetermined, and reasonable doubt exists, "No proven problems" is indicated.

25—BREAST-FEEDING

Many drugs filter into a mother's milk. Some drugs have dangerous or unwanted effects on the nursing infant. This section suggests ways to minimize harm to the child.

26—INFANTS & CHILDREN

Many drugs carry special warnings and precautions for children because of a child's size and immaturity. In medical terminology, *newborns* are babies up to 2 weeks old, *infants* are 2 weeks to 1 year, and *children* are 1 to 12 years.

27—PROLONGED USE

Most drugs produce no ill effects during short periods of treatment. However, relatively safe drugs taken for long periods may produce unwanted effects. These are listed. Drugs should be taken in the smallest dose and for the shortest time possible. Nevertheless, some diseases and conditions require an indefinite period of treatment. Your doctor may want to change drugs occasionally or alter your treatment regimen to minimize problems.

The words "functional dependence" sometimes appear in this section. This does not mean *physical* or *psychological addiction*. Sometimes a body function ceases to work naturally because it has been replaced or interfered with by the drug. The body then becomes dependent on the drug to continue the function.

28—SKIN & SUNLIGHT

Many drugs cause *photosensitivity*, which means increased skin sensitivity to ultraviolet rays from sunlight or artificial rays from a sunlamp. This section will alert you to this potential problem.

29—DRIVING, PILOTING OR HAZARDOUS WORK

Any drug that decreases alertness, muscular coordination or reflexes may make these activities hazardous. The effects may not appear in all people, or they may disappear after a short exposure to the drug. If this section contains a warning, use caution until you determine how a new drug affects you.

30—DISCONTINUING

Some patients stop taking a drug when symptoms begin to go away, although complete recovery may require longer treatment.

Other patients continue taking a drug when it is no longer needed. This section will tell you when you may safely discontinue a drug.

Some drugs cause symptoms days or weeks after discontinuing. This section warns you so the symptoms won't puzzle you if they occur.

31—OTHERS

Warnings and precautions appear here if they don't fit into the other categories. This section includes storage instructions, how to dispose of outdated drugs, weather influences on drug effect, changes in blood and urine tests, warnings to persons with chronic illness and other information.

32—POSSIBLE INTERACTION WITH OTHER DRUGS

Drugs interact in your body with other drugs, whether prescription or non-prescription. Interactions affect absorption, elimination or distribution of either drug. The chart lists interactions by generic name or drug class. An asterisk (*) beside drug class names in this column reminds you to "See Glossary" in the back of the book, where that drug class is described and where generic drug names for that class are listed.

If a drug class appears, the generic drug interacts with any drug in that class. Drugs in each class that are included in the book are listed in the index.

Interactions are sometimes beneficial. You may not be able to determine from the chart which interactions are good and which are bad. Don't guess! Consult your doctor if you take drugs that interact. Some combinations are fatal!

Occasionally, drugs appear in the Interaction column that are not included in this book. These drugs are listed under Interactions for your safety.

Some drugs have too many interactions to list on one chart. The additional interactions appear on the page indicated at the bottom of the list.

33—POSSIBLE INTERACTION WITH OTHER SUBSTANCES

The substances listed here are repeated on every drug chart. All people eat food and drink beverages. Many adults consume alcohol. Many people use cocaine and smoke tobacco or marijuana. This section shows possible interactions between these substances and each drug.

DRUGS OF ABUSE

Each of the drug charts beginning on page 2 contains a section listing the interactions of alcohol, marijuana and cocaine with the therapeutic drug in the bloodstream. These three drugs are singled out because of their widespread use and abuse. The information is factual, not judgmental.

The long-term effects of alcohol and tobacco abuse are numerous. They have been well-publicized and information is provided here as a reminder of the inherent dangers of these drugs.

Drugs of potential abuse include those that are addictive and harmful. They usually produce a temporary, false sense of wellbeing. The long-term effects, however, are harmful and can be devastating to the body and psyche of the addict.

Refresh your memory frequently about the potential harm from prolonged use of *any* drugs or substances you take. Avoid unwise use of habit-forming drugs.

These are the most common drugs of abuse:

TOBACCO (NICOTINE)

What it does: Tobacco smoke contains noxious and cancer-producing ingredients. They include nicotine, carbon monoxide, ammonia, and a variety of harmful tars. Carcinogens in smoke probably come from the tars. Most are present in chewing tobacco and snuff as well as smoke from cigarettes, cigars, and pipes. Tobacco smoke interferes with the immune mechanisms of the body.

Short-term effects of average amount: Relaxation of mood if you are a steady smoker. Constriction of blood vessels.

Short terms effects of large amount inhaled: Headache, appetite loss, nausea.

Long term effects: Greatly enhanced chances of developing lung cancer. Impaired breathing and chronic lung disease (asthma, emphysema, bronchiectasis, lung abscess and others) much more likely. Heart and blood vessel disease more frequent and more severe when they happen. These include myocardial infarction (heart attack), coronary artery disease, heart beat irregularities, generalized atherosclerosis (hardening of the arteries making brain, heart, and kidney more vulnerable to disease), peripheral vascular disease such as intermittent claudication, Buerger's disease and others. Tobacco and nicotine lead to an increased incidence of abortion and significantly reduce the birth weight of children brought to term and delivered of women who smoke during pregnancy. Tobacco smoking causes higher frequency not only of lung cancer, but also increases the likelihood of developing cancer of the throat, larynx, mouth, esophagus, bladder, and pancreas.

Cigarette smoking has been linked to this many deaths per year in the U.S. alone:
    80,000 lung cancer
    22,000 other cancer
    15,000 chronic lung disease
    225,000 cardiovascular disease
    346,000 TOTAL

ALCOHOL

What it does:

- **Central Nervous System**

Depresses, does *not* stimulate, the action of all parts of the central nervous system, including the depression of normal mental activity and normal muscle function. Short term effects of an average amount: relaxation, breakdown of inhibitions, euphoria, decreased alertness. Short term effects of large amounts: nausea, stupor, hangover, unconsciousness, even death.

- **Gastrointestinal System**

Increases stomach acid, poisons liver function. Chronic alcoholism frequently leads to permanent damage to the liver.

- **Heart and Blood Vessels**

Decreased normal function, leading to heart diseases such as cardiomyopathy and disorders of the blood vessels and kidney such as high blood pressure. Bleeding from the esophagus and stomach frequently accompany chronic alcoholism.

- **Unborn Fetus (teratogenicity)**

Alcoholism in the mother carrying a fetus causes *fetal alcohol syndrome (FAS)*, which includes the production of mental deficiency, facial abnormalities, slow growth and other major and minor malformations in the newborn.

Signs of Use:

Early signs: Prominent smell of alcohol on the breath, behavior changes (aggressive; passive; sexually uninhibited; poor judgment; outbursts of uncontrolled emotion, such as rage or tearfulness).

Intoxication signs: Unsteady gait, slurred speech, poor performance of any brain or muscle function, stupor or coma in *severe* alcoholic intoxication with slow, noisy breathing, cold and clammy skin, heartbeat faster than usual.

Long term effects:

Addiction: Compulsive use of alcohol. Persons addicted to alcohol have severe withdrawal symptoms when alcohol is unavailable. Even with successful treatment, addiction to alcohol (and other drugs that cause addiction) has a high tendency to relapse. (Memory of euphoric feelings plus family, social, emotional, psychological, and genetic factors probably are all important factors in producing the addiction.)

Liver disease: Usually cirrhosis; also, deleterious effects on the unborn child of an alcoholic mother.

Loss of sexual function: Impotence, erectile dysfunction, loss of libido.

Increased incidence of cancer: Mouth, pharynx, larynx, esophagus, liver, and lung.

Changes in blood: Makes it less likely for blood to clot efficiently.

Heart disease: Decreased normal function leading to possible damage and disease.

Stomach and intestinal problems: Increased production of stomach acid.

Interference with expected or normal actions of many medications: Detailed on every chart in this book, drugs such as sedatives, pain killers, narcotics, antihistamines, anticonvulsants, anticoagulants, and others.

MARIJUANA (CANNABIS, HASHISH)

What they do: Heighten perception, cause mood swings, relax mind and body.
Signs of use: Red eyes, lethargy, uncoordinated body movements.
Long-term effects: Decreased motivation. Possible brain, heart, lung and reproductive system damage.

AMPHETAMINES

What they do: Speed up physical and mental processes to cause a false sense of energy and excitement. The moods are temporary and unreal.
Signs of use: Dilated pupils, insomnia, trembling.
Long-term effects: Violent behavior, paranoia, possible death from overdose.

BARBITURATES

What they do: Produce drowsiness and lethargy.
Signs of use: Confused speech, lack of coordination and balance.
Long-term effects: Disrupts normal sleep pattern. Possible death from overdose, especially in combination with alcohol.

COCAINE

What it does: Stimulates the nervous system, heightens sensations and may produce hallucinations.

Signs of use: Trembling, intoxication, dilated pupils, constant sniffling.

Long-term effects: Ulceration of nasal passages where sniffed. Itching all over body, sometimes with open sores. Possible brain damage. Possible death from overdose.

OPIATES (CODEINE, HEROIN, METHADONE, MORPHINE, OPIUM)

What they do: Relieve pain, create temporary and false sense of well-being.

Signs of use: Constricted pupils, mood swings, slurred speech, sore eyes, lethargy, weight loss, sweating.

Long-term effects: Malnutrition, extreme susceptibility to infection, the need to increase drug amount to produce the same effects. Possible death from overdose.

PSYCHEDELIC DRUGS (LSD, MESCALINE)

What they do: Produce hallucinations, either pleasant or frightening.

Signs of use: Dilated pupils, sweating, trembling, fever, chills.

Long-term effects: Lack of motivation, unpredictable behavior, narcissism, recurrent hallucinations without drug use ("flashbacks"). Possible death from overdose.

VOLATILE SUBSTANCES (GLUE, SOLVENTS)

What they do: Produce hallucinations, temporary, false sense of well-being and possible unconsciousness.

Signs of use: Dilated pupils, flushed face, confusion.

Long-term effects: Permanent brain, liver, kidney damage. Possible death from overdose.

CHECKLIST FOR SAFER DRUG USE

- Tell your doctor about *any* drug you take (even aspirin, allergy pills, laxatives, vitamins, etc.) *before* you take *any* new drug.

- Learn all you can about drugs you may take *before* you take them. Information sources are your doctor, your nurse, your pharmacist, this book and other books in your public library.

- Don't take drugs prescribed for someone else—even if your symptoms are the same.

- Keep your prescription drugs to yourself. Your drugs may be harmful to someone else.

- Tell your doctor about any symptoms you believe are caused by a drug—prescription or non-prescription—that you take.

- Take only medicines that are *necessary*. Avoid taking non-prescription drugs while taking prescription drugs for a medical problem.

- Before your doctor prescribes for you, tell him about your previous experiences with any drug—beneficial results, side effects, adverse reactions or allergies.

- Take medicine in good light after you have identified it. If you wear glasses to read, put them on to check drug labels. It is easy to take the wrong drug at the wrong time.

- Don't keep any drugs that change mood, alertness or judgment—such as sedatives, narcotics or tranquilizers—by your bedside. These cause many accidental deaths by overdose. You may unknowingly repeat a dose when you are half asleep or confused.

- Know the names of your medicines. These include the generic name, the brand name and the generic names of all ingredients in a drug mixture. Your doctor, nurse or pharmacist can give you this information.

- Study the labels on all non-prescription drugs. If the information is incomplete or if you have questions, ask the pharmacist for more details.

- If you must deviate from your prescribed dose schedule, tell your doctor.

- Shake liquid medicines before taking.

- Store all medicines away from moisture and heat. Bathroom medicine cabinets are usually unsuitable.

- If a drug needs refrigeration, don't freeze.

- Obtain a standard measuring spoon from your pharmacy for liquid medicines. Kitchen teaspoons and tablespoons are not accurate enough.

- Follow diet instructions when you take medicines. Some work better on a full stomach, others on an empty stomach. Some drugs are more useful with special diets. For example, medicine for high blood pressure is more effective if accompanied by a sodium-restricted diet.

- Tell your doctor about any allergies you have. A previous allergy to a drug may make it dangerous to prescribe again. People with other allergies, such as eczema, hay fever, asthma, bronchitis and food allergies, are more likely to be allergic to drugs.

- Prior to surgery, tell your doctor, anesthesiologist or dentist about any drug you have taken in the past few weeks. Advise them of any cortisone drugs you have taken within two years.

- If you become pregnant while taking any medicine, including birth-control pills, tell your doctor immediately.

- Avoid *all* drugs while you are pregnant, if possible. If you must take drugs during pregnancy, record names, amounts, dates and reasons.

- If you see more than one doctor, tell each one about drugs others have prescribed.

- When you use non-prescription drugs, report it so the information is on your medical record.

- Store all drugs away from the reach of children.

- Note the expiration date on each drug label. Discard outdated ones safely. If no expiration date appears and it has been at least one year since taking the medication, it may be best to discard it.

- Pay attention to the information in the charts about safety while driving, piloting or working in dangerous places.

- Alcohol, cocaine, marijuana or other mood-altering drugs as well as tobacco—mixed with some drugs—can cause a life-threatening interaction, prevent your medicine from being effective or delay your return to health. Common sense dictates that you avoid them during illness.

DRUG CHARTS

ACEBUTOLOL

BRAND NAMES

Monitan   Sectral

BASIC INFORMATION

Habit forming? No
Prescription needed? Yes
Available as generic? No
Drug class: Beta-adrenergic blocker

USES

- Reduces frequency and severity of angina attacks.
- Stabilizes irregular heartbeat.
- Lowers blood pressure.
- Reduces frequency of migraine headaches. (Does not relieve headache pain.)

DOSAGE & USAGE INFORMATION

How to take:
Capsule—Swallow with liquid. If you can't swallow whole, open capsule and take with liquid or food.

When to take:
With meals or immediately after.

If you forget a dose:
Take as soon as you remember. Return to regular schedule, but allow 3 hours between doses.

What drug does:
- Blocks actions of sympathetic nervous system.
- Lowers heart's oxygen requirements.
- Slows nerve impulses through heart.
- Reduces blood-vessel contraction in several major organs and glands.

Time lapse before drug works:
1 to 4 hours.

Continued next column

OVERDOSE

SYMPTOMS:
Weakness, slow or weak pulse, blood-pressure drop, difficulty breathing, fainting, convulsions, cold and sweaty skin.
WHAT TO DO:
- Dial 0 (operator) or 911 (emergency) for an ambulance or medical help. Then give first aid immediately.
- See emergency information on inside covers.

Don't take with:
Non-prescription drugs or drugs in interaction column without consulting doctor.

POSSIBLE ADVERSE REACTIONS OR SIDE EFFECTS

SYMPTOMS	WHAT TO DO
Life-threatening: None expected.	
Common:	
• Drowsiness, numbness or tingling in fingers and toes, dizziness, diarrhea, nausea, fatigue, weakness.	Continue. Call doctor when convenient.
• Pulse slower than 50 beats per minute.	Discontinue. Call doctor right away.
• Cold hands and feet; dry mouth, skin or eyes.	Continue. Tell doctor at next visit.
Infrequent:	
• Hallucinations, nightmares, anxiety, insomnia, headache, difficulty breathing.	Discontinue. Call doctor right away.
• Confusion, reduced alertness, depression.	Continue. Call doctor when convenient.
• Constipation.	Continue. Tell doctor at next visit.
Rare:	
• Sore throat, fever, rash.	Discontinue. Call doctor right away.
• Impotence, unexplained bleeding and bruising.	Continue. Call doctor when convenient.

WARNINGS & PRECAUTIONS

Don't take if:
- You are allergic to any beta-adrenergic blocker.
- You have asthma.
- You have hay-fever symptoms.
- You have taken MAO inhibitors in past 2 weeks.

Before you start, consult your doctor:
- If you have heart disease or poor circulation to extremities.
- If you have hay fever, asthma, chronic bronchitis or emphysema.
- If you have overactive thyroid function.
- If you have impaired liver or kidney function.
- If you will have surgery within 2 months, including dental surgery, requiring general or spinal anesthesia.
- If you have diabetes or hypoglycemia.

Over age 60:
Adverse reactions and side effects may be more frequent and severe than in younger persons.

Pregnancy:
Risk to unborn child outweighs drug benefits. Don't use.

Breast-feeding:
Drug passes into milk. Avoid drug or discontinue nursing until you finish medicine. Consult doctor for advice on maintaining milk supply.

Infants & children:
Not recommended. Safety and dosage have not been established.

Prolonged use:
Weakens heart-muscle contractions.

Skin & sunlight:
No problems expected.

Driving, piloting or hazardous work:
Don't drive or pilot aircraft until you learn how medicine affects you. Don't work around dangerous machinery. Don't climb ladders or work in high places. Danger increases if you drink alcohol or take medicine affecting alertness and reflexes.

Discontinuing:
Don't discontinue without consulting doctor. Dose may require gradual reduction if you have taken drug for a long time. Doses of other drugs may also require adjustment.

Others:
May mask hypoglycemia.

POSSIBLE INTERACTION WITH OTHER DRUGS

GENERIC NAME OR DRUG CLASS	COMBINED EFFECT
ACE inhibitors: captopril, enalapril, lisinopril*	Increased antihypertensive effect. Dosage of each may require adjustment.
Anesthetics used in surgery	Increased antihypertensive effect.
Antidiabetics*	May make blood sugar more difficult to control.
Antihypertensives*	Increased antihypertensive effect.
Betaxolol eyedrops	Possible increased acebutolol effect.
Calcium-channel blockers*	May worsen congestive heart failure.
Clonidine	Possible blood-pressure rise when clonidine is discontinued.

Digitalis preparations*	Increased or decreased heart rate. Improves irregular heartbeat.
Diuretics*	Increased antihypertensive effect.
Insulin	Hypoglycemic effect of insulin may be prolonged.
Ketoprofen	Decreased antihypertensive effect of acebutolol.
Levobunolol eyedrops	Possible increased acebutolol effect.
Molindone	Increased tranquilizer effect.
MAO inhibitors*	Possible excessive blood-pressure rise when MAO inhibitor is discontinued.
Nicardipine	Possible irregular heartbeat and congestive heart failure.
Nitrates*	Possible decreased blood pressure.
Non-steroidal anti-inflammatory drugs (NSAIDs)*	Decreased antihypertensive effect.
Pentoxifylline	Increased antihypertensive effect.
Reserpine	Possible excessively low blood pressure and slow heartbeat.
Rifampin	Decreased propranolol effect.
Sympathomimetics*	Decreased effects of both drugs.

Continued page 1074

POSSIBLE INTERACTION WITH OTHER SUBSTANCES

INTERACTS WITH	COMBINED EFFECT
Alcohol:	Excessive blood-pressure drop. Avoid.
Beverages:	None expected.
Cocaine:	Irregular heartbeat. Avoid.
Foods:	None expected.
Marijuana:	Daily use—Impaired circulation to hands and feet.
Tobacco:	Possible irregular heartbeat.

*See Glossary

ACETAMINOPHEN

BRAND NAMES

See complete list of brand names in the *Brand Name Directory*, page 1052.

BASIC INFORMATION

Habit forming? No
Prescription needed? No
Available as generic? Yes
Drug class: Analgesic, fever-reducer

 ## USES

Treatment of mild to moderate pain and fever. Acetaminophen does not relieve redness, stiffness or swelling of joints or tissue inflammation. Use aspirin or other drugs for inflammation.

 ## DOSAGE & USAGE INFORMATION

How to take:
- Tablet or capsule—Swallow with liquid.
- Effervescent granules—Dissolve granules in 4 oz. of cool water. Drink all the water.
- Elixir—Swallow with liquid.
- Suppositories—Remove wrapper and moisten suppository with water. Gently insert larger end into rectum. Push well into rectum with finger.

When to take:
As needed, no more often than every 3 hours.

If you forget a dose:
Take as soon as you remember. Wait 3 hours for next dose.

What drug does:
May affect hypothalamus—part of brain that helps regulate body heat and receives body's pain messages.

Time lapse before drug works:
15 to 30 minutes. May last 4 hours.

Continued next column

 ## OVERDOSE

SYMPTOMS:
Stomach upset, irritability, sweating, anorexia, convulsions, coma.
WHAT TO DO:
- **Call your doctor or poison-control center for advice if you suspect overdose, even if not sure. Symptoms may not appear until damage has occurred.**
- **See emergency information on inside covers.**

Don't take with:
- Other drugs with acetaminophen. Too much acetaminophen can damage liver and kidneys.
- See Interaction column and consult doctor.

 ## POSSIBLE ADVERSE REACTIONS OR SIDE EFFECTS

SYMPTOMS	WHAT TO DO
Life-threatening: None expected.	
Common: Lightheadedness.	Continue. Call doctor when convenient.
Infrequent: Trembling.	Continue. Call doctor when convenient.
Rare: • Extreme fatigue; rash, itch, hives; sore throat and fever after taking regularly a few days; unexplained bleeding or bruising; blood in urine; painful or frequent urination; jaundice; anemia.	Discontinue. Call doctor right away.
• Decreased volume of urine output.	Continue. Call doctor when convenient.

WARNINGS & PRECAUTIONS

Don't take if:
- You are allergic to acetaminophen.
- Your symptoms don't improve after 2 days use. Call your doctor.

Before you start, consult your doctor:
If you have kidney disease or liver damage.

Over age 60:
Don't exceed recommended dose. You can't eliminate drug as efficiently as younger persons.

Pregnancy:
No proven harm to unborn child. Avoid if possible.

Breast-feeding:
No proven harm to nursing infant.

Infants & children:
Use only under medical supervision.

Prolonged use:
May affect blood system and cause anemia. Limit use to 5 days for children 12 and under, and 10 days for adults.

Skin & sunlight:
No problems expected.

Driving, piloting or hazardous work:
Avoid if you feel drowsy. Otherwise, no restrictions.

Discontinuing:
Discontinue in 2 days if symptoms don't improve.

Others:
No problems expected.

POSSIBLE INTERACTION WITH OTHER DRUGS

GENERIC NAME OR DRUG CLASS	COMBINED EFFECT
Anticoagulants, oral*	May increase anticoagulant effect. If combined frequently, prothrombin time should be monitored.
Phenobarbital	Quicker elimination of and decreased effect of acetaminophen.
Zidovudine (AZT)	Increased toxic effect of zidovudine.

POSSIBLE INTERACTION WITH OTHER SUBSTANCES

INTERACTS WITH	COMBINED EFFECT
Alcohol:	Drowsiness, long-term use may cause toxic effect in liver.
Beverages:	None expected.
Cocaine:	None expected. However, cocaine may slow body's recovery. Avoid.
Foods:	None expected.
Marijuana:	Increased pain relief. However, marijuana may slow body's recovery. Avoid.
Tobacco:	None expected.

ACETAMINOPHEN & SALICYLATES

BRAND NAMES

See complete list of brand names in the *Brand Name Directory*, page 1052.

BASIC INFORMATION

Habit forming? No
Prescription needed?
 High strength: Yes
 Low strength: No
 Yes, for some combinations
Available as generic? No
Drug class: Analgesic, fever-reducer (acetaminophen and salicylates), non-steroidal anti-inflammatory (salicylates)

 USES

- Treatment of mild pain and fever.
- Salicylates are useful in the treatment of inflammatory conditions such as stiffness, swelling, joint pain of arthritis or rheumatism. For long term use for inflammatory problems, separate drugs instead of this combination may be safer and more effective.

 DOSAGE & USAGE INFORMATION

How to take:
- Tablet or capsule—swallow with liquid.
- Effervescent granules—dissolve granules in 4 oz. of cool water.

When to take:
As needed, no more often than every 3 hours or as prescribed by your doctor.

If you forget a dose:
Take as soon as you remember. Wait 3 hours for next dose.

What drug does:
- May affect hypothalamus, the part of the brain that helps regulate body heat and receives body's pain messages.

Continued next column

 OVERDOSE

SYMPTOMS:
Ringing in ears; nausea; vomiting; dizziness; fever; deep, rapid breathing; hallucinations; coma; unusual sweating; blood in urine.
WHAT TO DO:
- **Dial 0 (operator) or 911 (emergency) for an ambulance or medical help. Then give first aid immediately.**
- **See emergency information on inside covers.**

- May affect production of prostaglandins to reduce inflammation.

Time lapse before drug works:
15 to 30 minutes. May last 4 hours.

Don't take with:
- Other drugs with acetaminophen or aspirin or other salicylates. Too much can cause damage to liver, kidneys and peripheral nerves.
- Any laxative containing cellulose.
- If medicine you take has a buffering agent added, don't take with tetracyclines.

 POSSIBLE ADVERSE REACTIONS OR SIDE EFFECTS

SYMPTOMS	WHAT TO DO
Life-threatening:	
Wheezing and marked shortness of breath.	Seek emergency treatment immediately.
Common:	
• Jaundice, vomiting blood, black stools, cloudy urine, nausea and vomiting, unexplained tiredness, discomfort on urinating.	Discontinue. Call doctor right away.
• Indigestion or heartburn.	Continue. Call doctor when convenient.
Infrequent:	
Shortness of breath; wheezing (for medicines containing aspirin); decreased urine volume; feet swelling; black or tarry stools; pain on urinating; nausea and vomiting; skin rash, hives; sore throat, fever; easy bruising.	Discontinue. Call doctor right away.
Rare:	
• While taking medicine: Sudden decrease in urine volume.	Discontinue. Call doctor right away.
• After discontinuing medicine: Swelling of feet; rapid weight gain; bloating or puffiness; any urinary problems, such as painful, cloudy or bloody urine.	Check with doctor immediately.

WARNINGS & PRECAUTIONS

Don't take if:
- You are allergic to acetaminophen or any salicylates. *
- Your symptoms don't improve after 3 days use.
- You take a buffered form and need to restrict sodium in your diet.
- You have a peptic ulcer.
- You have a bleeding disorder.

Before you start, consult your doctor:
- If you have ever had peptic ulcers.
- If you have had gout.
- If you have asthma or nasal polyps.
- If you have kidney disease or liver damage.

Over age 60:
Don't exceed recommended dose. More likely to be harmful to kidney and liver or cause hidden bleeding in stomach or intestines. Watch for black stools or decreased urine output.

Pregnancy:
Risk to unborn child outweighs drug benefits. Don't use.

Breast-feeding:
Drug passes into milk. Avoid drug or discontinue nursing until you finish medicine. Consult doctor on maintaining milk supply.

Infants & children:
Overdose frequent and severe. Keep bottles out of children's reach. Consult doctor before giving to persons under age 18 who have fever and discomfort of viral illness, especially chicken pox and influenza. Probably increases risk of Reye's syndrome*.

Prolonged use:
High doses for severe inflammatory conditions taken for long periods may increase likelihood of kidney damage.

Skin & sunlight:
Aspirin combined with sunscreen may decrease sunburn.

Driving, piloting or hazardous work:
No problems expected unless you feel drowsy.

Discontinuing:
No problems expected.

Others:
- Children up to 12 years—Don't take more than 5 doses per day for more than 5 consecutive days.
- Adults—Don't take for more than 10 consecutive days.
- Urine test for sugar may be inaccurate.
- Don't take if container has a strong vinegar-like odor.

POSSIBLE INTERACTION WITH OTHER DRUGS

GENERIC NAME OR DRUG CLASS	COMBINED EFFECT
Antacids*	Decreased acetaminophen and salicylates effect.
Anticoagulants*	Increased anticoagulant effect. Abnormal bleeding.
Antidiabetics, oral*	Low blood sugar.
Aspirin and other salicylates*	Likely toxicity.
Carteolol	Decreased antihypertensive effect of carteolol.
Cortisone drugs*	Increased cortisone effect. Risk of ulcers and stomach bleeding.
Furosemide	Possible salicylate toxicity, decreased furosemide effect.
Indomethacin	Risk of stomach bleeding and ulcers.
Lisinopril	Decreased lisinopril effect.
Methotrexate	Increased methotrexate effect.
Non-steroidal anti-inflammatory drugs (NSAIDs)*	Risk of stomach bleeding and ulcers.

Continued page 1074

POSSIBLE INTERACTION WITH OTHER SUBSTANCES

INTERACTS WITH	COMBINED EFFECT
Alcohol:	Increased chance of stomach irritation and bleeding.
Beverages:	None expected.
Cocaine:	None expected. However, cocaine may deter body's recovery. Avoid.
Foods:	None expected.
Marijuana:	Possible increased pain relief, but marijuana may deter body's recovery. Avoid.
Tobacco:	None expected.

*See Glossary

ACETOHEXAMIDE

BRAND NAMES

Dimelor   Dymelor

BASIC INFORMATION

Habit forming? No
Prescription needed? Yes
Available as generic? No
Drug class: Antidiabetic (oral), sulfonurea

USES

Treatment for diabetes in adults who can't control blood sugar by diet, weight loss and exercise.

DOSAGE & USAGE INFORMATION

How to take:
Tablet—Swallow with liquid or food to lessen stomach irritation. If you can't swallow whole, crumble tablet and take with liquid or food.

When to take:
At the same times each day.

If you forget a dose:
Take as soon as you remember up to 2 hours late. If more than 2 hours, wait for next scheduled dose (don't double this dose).

What drug does:
Stimulates pancreas to produce more insulin. Insulin in blood forces cells to use sugar in blood.

Time lapse before drug works:
3 to 4 hours. May require 2 weeks for maximum benefit.

Don't take with:
See Interaction column and consult doctor.

OVERDOSE

SYMPTOMS:
Excessive hunger, nausea, anxiety, cool skin, cold sweats, drowsiness, rapid heartbeat, weakness, unconsciousness, coma.
WHAT TO DO:
- Dial 0 (operator) or 911 (emergency) for an ambulance or medical help. Then give first aid immediately.
- See emergency information on inside covers.

POSSIBLE ADVERSE REACTIONS OR SIDE EFFECTS

SYMPTOMS	WHAT TO DO
Life-threatening: Low blood sugar (hunger, anxiety, cold sweats, rapid pulse).	Seek emergency treatment immediately.
Common: • Dizziness.	Discontinue. Call doctor right away.
• Diarrhea, appetite loss, nausea, stomach pain, heartburn.	Continue. Call doctor when convenient.
Infrequent: • Fatigue, itching or rash, ringing in ears.	Discontinue. Call doctor right away.
Rare: • Sore throat, fever, unusual bleeding or bruising, jaundice.	Discontinue. Call doctor right away.

WARNINGS & PRECAUTIONS

Don't take if:
- You are allergic to any sulfonurea.
- You have impaired kidney or liver function.

Before you start, consult your doctor:
- If you have a severe infection.
- If you have thyroid disease.
- If you take insulin.
- If you have heart disease.

Over age 60:
Dose usually smaller than for younger adults. Avoid "low-blood-sugar" episodes because repeated ones can damage brain permanently.

Pregnancy:
No proven harm to unborn child. Avoid if possible.

Breast-feeding:
Drug filters into milk. May lower baby's blood sugar. Avoid.

Infants & children:
Don't give to infants or children.

Prolonged use:
None expected.

Skin & sunlight:
May cause rash or intensify sunburn in areas exposed to sun or sunlamp.

Driving, piloting or hazardous work:
No problems expected unless you develop hypoglycemia (low blood sugar). If so, avoid driving or hazardous activity.

Discontinuing:
Don't discontinue without consulting doctor. Dose may require gradual reduction if you have taken drug for a long time. Doses of other drugs may also require adjustment.

Others:
Don't exceed recommended dose. Hypoglycemia (low blood sugar) may occur, even with proper dose schedule. You must balance medicine, diet and exercise.

POSSIBLE INTERACTION WITH OTHER DRUGS

GENERIC NAME OR DRUG CLASS	COMBINED EFFECT
Anticoagulants, oral*	Unpredictable prothrombin times.
Anticonvulsants, hydantoin*	Decreased acetohexamide effect.
Aspirin	Increased acetohexamide effect.
Beta-adrenergic blockers*	Increased acetohexamide effect. May make blood sugar more difficult to control.
Bismuth subsalicylate	Increased insulin effect. May require dosage adjustment.
Carteolol	Increased antidiabetic effect.
Chloramphenicol	Increased acetohexamide effect.
Cimetidine	Increased acetohexamide effect.
Clofibrate	Increased acetohexamide effect.
Contraceptives, oral*	Decreased acetohexamide effect.
Cortisone drugs*	Decreased acetohexamide effect.
Diuretics, thiazide*	Decreased acetohexamide effect.
Epinephrine	Decreased acetohexamide effect.
Estrogens*	Increased acetohexamide effect.

Guanethidine	Unpredictable acetohexamide effect.
Isoniazid	Decreased acetohexamide effect.
Labetalol	Increased antidiabetic effect, may mask hypoglycemia.
MAO inhibitors*	Increased acetohexamide effect.
Non-steroidal anti-inflammatory drugs (NSAIDs)*	Increased acetohexamide effect.
Oxyphenbutazone	Increased acetohexamide effect.
Phenylbutazone	Increased acetohexamide effect.
Phenyramidol	Increased acetohexamide effect.
Probenecid	Increased acetohexamide effect.
Pyrazinamide	Decreased acetohexamide effect.
Sotalol	Increased antidiabetic effect.
Sulfa drugs*	Increased acetohexamide effect.
Sulfaphenazole	Increased acetohexamide effect.
Thyroid hormones*	Decreased acetohexamide effect.

POSSIBLE INTERACTION WITH OTHER SUBSTANCES

INTERACTS WITH	COMBINED EFFECT
Alcohol:	Disulfiram reaction.* Avoid.
Beverages:	None expected.
Cocaine:	No proven problems.
Foods:	None expected.
Marijuana:	Decreased acetohexamide effect. Avoid.
Tobacco:	None expected.

*See Glossary

ACETOHYDROXAMIC ACID (AHA)

BRAND NAMES

Lithostat

BASIC INFORMATION

Habit forming? No
Prescription needed? Yes
Available as generic? No
Drug class: Antibacterial, antiurolithic

USES

- Treatment for chronic urinary-tract infections.
- Prevents formation of urinary-tract stones. Will not dissolve stones already present.

DOSAGE & USAGE INFORMATION

How to take:
Tablet—Swallow with liquid. If you can't swallow whole, crumble tablet and take with liquid or food.

When to take:
At the same time each day, according to instructions on prescription label.

If you forget a dose:
Take as soon as you remember up to 2 hours late. If more than 2 hours, wait for next scheduled dose (don't double this dose).

What drug does:
Stops enzyme action that makes urine too alkaline. Alkaline urine favors bacterial growth and stone formation and growth.

Time lapse before drug works:
1 to 3 weeks.

Don't take with:
Alcohol or iron. See Interaction column and consult doctor.

OVERDOSE

SYMPTOMS:
Loss of appetite, tremor, nausea, vomiting.
WHAT TO DO:
Overdose unlikely to threaten life. If person takes much larger amount than prescribed, call doctor, poison-control center or hospital emergency room for instructions.

POSSIBLE ADVERSE REACTIONS OR SIDE EFFECTS

SYMPTOMS	WHAT TO DO
Life-threatening: None expected.	
Common:	
• Appetite loss, nausea, vomiting.	Discontinue. Seek emergency treatment.
• Anxiety, depression, mild headache, unusual tiredness.	Continue. Call doctor when convenient.
Infrequent:	
• Loss of coordination, slurred speech, severe headache, sudden change in vision, shortness of breath, clot or pain over a blood vessel, sudden chest pain, leg pain in calf (deep vein blood clot).	Discontinue. Seek emergency treatment.
• Rash on arms and face.	Discontinue. Call doctor right away.
Rare:	
• Sore throat, fever, unusual bleeding, bruising.	Discontinue. Call right away.
• Hair loss.	Continue. Call doctor when convenient.

WARNINGS & PRECAUTIONS

Don't take if:
You have severe chronic kidney disease.

Before you start, consult your doctor:
- If you are anemic.
- If you have or have had phlebitis or thrombophlebitis.

Over age 60:
Adverse reactions and side effects may be more frequent and severe than in younger persons.

Pregnancy:
Studies inconclusive on harm to unborn child. Animal studies show fetal abnormalities. Decide with your doctor whether drug benefits justify risk to unborn child.

Breast-feeding:
No proven problems. Avoid if possible.

Infants & children:
Not recommended. Safety and dosage have not been established.

Prolonged use:
No problems expected.

Skin & sunlight:
No problems expected.

Driving, piloting or hazardous work:
Don't drive or pilot aircraft until you learn how medicine affects you. Don't work around dangerous machinery. Don't climb ladders or work in high places. Danger increases if you drink alcohol or take medicine affecting alertness and reflexes, such as antihistamines, tranquilizers, sedatives, pain medicines, narcotics and mind-altering drugs.

Discontinuing:
Don't discontinue without consulting doctor. Dose may require gradual reduction if you have taken drug for a long time. Doses of other drugs may also require adjustment.

Others:
No problems expected.

POSSIBLE INTERACTION WITH OTHER DRUGS

GENERIC NAME OR DRUG CLASS	COMBINED EFFECT
Iron	Decreased effects of both drugs.

POSSIBLE INTERACTION WITH OTHER SUBSTANCES

INTERACTS WITH	COMBINED EFFECT
Alcohol:	Severe skin rash common in many patients within 30 to 45 minutes after drinking alcohol.
Beverages:	None expected.
Cocaine:	None expected.
Foods:	None expected.
Marijuana:	None expected.
Tobacco:	None expected.

ACETOPHENAZINE

BRAND NAMES

Tindal

BASIC INFORMATION

Habit forming? No
Prescription needed? Yes
Available as generic? No
Drug class: Tranquilizer, antiemetic (phenothiazine)

 ## USES

- Stops nausea, vomiting.
- Reduces anxiety, agitation.

 ## DOSAGE & USAGE INFORMATION

How to take:
- Tablet—Swallow with liquid or food to lessen stomach irritation.

When to take:
- Nervous and mental disorders—Take at the same times each day.
- Nausea and vomiting—Take as needed, no more often than every 4 hours.

If you forget a dose:
- Nervous and mental disorders—Take up to 2 hours late. If more than 2 hours, wait for next scheduled dose (don't double this dose).
- Nausea and vomiting—Take as soon as you remember. Wait 4 hours for next dose.

What drug does:
- Suppresses brain's vomiting center.
- Suppresses brain centers that control abnormal emotions and behavior.

Continued next column

 ## OVERDOSE

SYMPTOMS:
Stupor, convulsions, coma.
WHAT TO DO:
- Dial 0 (operator) or 911 (emergency) for an ambulance or medical help. Then give first aid immediately.
- See emergency information on inside covers.

Time lapse before drug works:
- Nausea and vomiting—1 hour or less.
- Nervous and mental disorders—4-6 weeks.

Don't take with:
- Antacid or medicine for diarrhea.
- Non-prescription drug for cough, cold or allergy.
- See Interaction column and consult doctor.

 ## POSSIBLE ADVERSE REACTIONS OR SIDE EFFECTS

SYMPTOMS	WHAT TO DO
Life-threatening: None expected.	
Common:	
• Muscle spasms of face and neck, unsteady gait.	Discontinue. Seek emergency treatment.
• Restlessness, tremor, drowsiness.	Discontinue. Call doctor right away.
• Decreased sweating, dry mouth, stuffy nose, constipation.	Continue. Call doctor when convenient.
Infrequent:	
• Fainting, fever, body rigidity.	Discontinue. Seek emergency treatment.
• Rash.	Discontinue. Call doctor right away.
• Difficult or painful urination, diminished sex drive, swollen breasts, menstrual irregularities, dizziness.	Continue. Call doctor when convenient.
Rare:	
Change in vision, sore throat and fever, jaundice.	Discontinue. Call doctor right away.

12

WARNINGS & PRECAUTIONS

Don't take if:
- You are allergic to any phenothiazine.
- You have a blood or bone-marrow disease.

Before you start, consult your doctor:
- If you will have surgery within 2 months, including dental surgery, requiring general or spinal anesthesia.
- If you have asthma, emphysema or other lung disorder.
- If you take non-prescription ulcer medicine, asthma medicine or amphetamines.

Over age 60:
Adverse reactions and side effects may be more frequent and severe than in younger persons. More likely to develop involuntary movement of jaws, lips, tongue, chewing. Report this to your doctor immediately. Early treatment can help.

Pregnancy:
Risk to unborn child outweighs drug benefits. Don't use.

Breast-feeding:
Drug passes into milk. Avoid drug or discontinue nursing until you finish medicine. Consult doctor for advice on maintaining milk supply.

Infants & children:
Don't give to children younger than 2.

Prolonged use:
May lead to tardive dyskinesia (involuntary movement of jaws, lips, tongue, chewing).

Skin & sunlight:
May cause rash or intensify sunburn in areas exposed to sun or sunlamp. Skin may remain sensitive for 3 months after discontinuing.

Driving, piloting or hazardous work:
Don't drive or pilot aircraft until you learn how medicine affects you. Don't work around dangerous machinery. Don't climb ladders or work in high places. Danger increases if you drink alcohol or take medicine affecting alertness and reflexes.

Discontinuing:
- Nervous and mental disorders—Don't discontinue without doctor's advice until you complete prescribed dose, even though symptoms diminish or disappear.
- Nausea and vomiting—May be unnecessary to finish medicine. Follow doctor's instructions.

POSSIBLE INTERACTION WITH OTHER DRUGS

GENERIC NAME OR DRUG CLASS	COMBINED EFFECT
Anticholinergics*	Increased anti-cholinergic effect.
Antidepressants, tricyclic (TCA)*	Increased aceto-phenazine effect.
Antihistamines*	Increased antihistamine effect. Possible oversedation.
Appetite suppressants*	Decreased suppressant effect.
Dronabinol	Increased effects of both drugs. Avoid.
Levodopa	Decreased levodopa effect.
Mind-altering drugs*	Increased effect of mind-altering drugs.
Molindone	Increased tranquilizer effect.
Nabilone	Greater depression of central nervous system.
Narcotics*	Increased narcotic effect.
Phenytoin	Increased phenytoin effect.
Quinidine	Impaired heart function. Dangerous mixture.
Sedatives*	Increased sedation.
Tranquilizers, other*	Increased tranquilizer effect.

POSSIBLE INTERACTION WITH OTHER SUBSTANCES

INTERACTS WITH	COMBINED EFFECT
Alcohol:	Dangerous oversedation.
Beverages:	Effect of acetophenazine may be reduced if taken chronically with caffeine.
Cocaine:	Decreased acetophenazine effect. Avoid.
Foods:	None expected.
Marijuana:	Drowsiness. May increase antinausea effect.
Tobacco:	None expected.

ACRISORCIN (Topical)

BRAND NAMES

Acrisorcin Cream

BASIC INFORMATION

Habit forming? No
Prescription needed? Yes
Available as generic? No
Drug class: Antifungal (topical)

USES

- Used on skin to treat tinea versicolor, a yeast infection that changes the color of skin it affects. Sometimes called "sun fungus," it's more common in adolescents and adults and more likely to occur with exposure to heat and high humidity.
- Acrisorcin is not useful for other fungus or yeast skin infections.

DOSAGE & USAGE INFORMATION

How to use:
- Cream, lotion, ointment—Bathe and dry area before use. Apply small amount and rub gently.
- After using, wash hands with soap to prevent medicine from getting in eyes.

When to use:
Apply at night.

If you forget a dose:
Take as soon as you remember.

What drug does:
Unknown. Probably removes outer layer of skin to remove the infecting fungus.

Time lapse before drug works:
2 to 3 weeks.

Don't use with:
See Interaction column and consult doctor.

OVERDOSE

SYMPTOMS:
None expected.
WHAT TO DO:
Not for internal use. If child accidentally swallows, call poison-control center.

POSSIBLE ADVERSE REACTIONS OR SIDE EFFECTS

SYMPTOMS	WHAT TO DO
Life-threatening:	None expected.
Common:	None expected.
Infrequent: Redness, itching, blistering, hives, new skin rash.	Discontinue. Call doctor right away.
Rare:	None expected.

**WARNINGS &
PRECAUTIONS**

Don't use if:
You are allergic to acrisorcin.

Before you start, consult your doctor:
If you are allergic to any substance such as dyes or preservatives.

Over age 60:
No problems expected.

Pregnancy:
No problems expected, but check with doctor.

Breast-feeding:
No problems expected.

Infants & children:
Use only under close medical supervision.

Prolonged use:
May lead to skin sensitivity.

Skin & sunlight:
May cause itching.

Driving, piloting or hazardous work:
No problems expected.

Discontinuing:
No problems expected.

Others:
- Check with doctor if no improvement in 6 weeks.
- Do not apply plastic wraps over treated skin.

 **POSSIBLE INTERACTION
WITH OTHER DRUGS**

GENERIC NAME OR DRUG CLASS	COMBINED EFFECT
None expected.	

 **POSSIBLE INTERACTION
WITH OTHER SUBSTANCES**

INTERACTS WITH	COMBINED EFFECT
Alcohol:	None expected.
Beverages:	None expected.
Cocaine:	None expected.
Foods:	None expected.
Marijuana:	None expected.
Tobacco:	None expected.

ACYCLOVIR (Oral & Topical)

BRAND NAMES

Zovirax   Zovirax Ointment

BASIC INFORMATION

Habit forming? No
Prescription needed? Yes
Available as generic? No
Drug class: Antiviral

 ## USES

- Treatment of severe herpes infections of genitals occurring for first time in special cases.
- Treatment of severe herpes infections on mucous membrane of mouth and lips in special cases.
- Used (although not yet approved by FDA) for shingles (herpes zoster) and chicken pox (varicella) in special cases.

 ## DOSAGE & USAGE INFORMATION

How to take:
- Capsule—Swallow with liquid.
- Ointment—Apply to skin and mucous membranes every 3 hours (6 times a day) for 7 days. Use rubber glove when applying. Apply 1/2-inch strip to each sore or blister. Wash before using.

When to use:
As directed on label.

If you forget a dose:
Take as soon as you remember up to 2 hours late. If more than 2 hours, wait for next scheduled dose (don't double this dose).

What drug does:
- Inhibits reproduction of virus in cells without killing normal cells.
- Does not cure. Herpes may recur.

Continued next column

 ## OVERDOSE

SYMPTOMS:
Hallucinations, seizures, kidney shutdown.
WHAT TO DO:
- **Dial 0 (operator) or 911 (emergency) for an ambulance or medical help. Then give first aid immediately.**
- **See emergency information on inside covers.**

Time lapse before drug works:
2 hours.

Don't take with:
See Interaction column and consult doctor.

 ## POSSIBLE ADVERSE REACTIONS OR SIDE EFFECTS

SYMPTOMS	WHAT TO DO
Life-threatening: None expected.	
Common: Rash, hives, itch, mild pain, burning or stinging of skin, lightheadedness, headache.	Continue. Call doctor when convenient.
Infrequent: Confusion, hallucinations, trembling.	Discontinue. Call doctor right away.
Rare: Abdominal pain, decreased appetite, nausea, vomiting, breathing difficulty, blood in urine, decreased urine volume.	Discontinue. Call doctor right away.

WARNINGS & PRECAUTIONS

Don't take if:
You are allergic to acyclovir.

Before you start, consult your doctor:
- If pregnant or plan pregnancy.
- If breast-feeding.
- If you have kidney disease.
- If you have any nerve disorder.

Over age 60:
Adverse reactions and side effects may be more frequent and severe than in younger persons.

Pregnancy:
Risk to unborn child outweighs drug benefits. Don't use.

Breast-feeding:
Drug passes into milk. Avoid drug or discontinue nursing until you finish medicine. Consult doctor for advice on maintaining milk supply.

Infants & children:
Use only under special medical supervision by experienced clinician.

Prolonged use:
Don't use longer than prescribed time.

Skin & sunlight:
No problems expected.

Driving, piloting or hazardous work:
No problems expected.

Discontinuing:
May be unnecessary to finish medicine. Follow doctor's instructions.

Others:
- Women: Get Pap smear every 6 months because those with herpes infections are more likely to develop cancer of cervix. Avoid sexual activity until all blisters or sores heal. Don't get medicine in eyes.
- Protect from freezing.
- Check with doctor if no improvement in 1 week.

POSSIBLE INTERACTION WITH OTHER DRUGS

GENERIC NAME OR DRUG CLASS	COMBINED EFFECT
Interferon	Neurological abnormalities. Avoid.
Methotrexate	Neurological abnormalities. Avoid.
Other medications that can cause toxic effects on kidneys: amikacin amphotericin B capreomycin colistimethate colistin cyclosporine gentamycin kanamycin neomycin netilmicin polymixin B probenecid streptomycin tobramycin vancomycin	Possible increased kidney toxicity.

POSSIBLE INTERACTION WITH OTHER SUBSTANCES

INTERACTS WITH	COMBINED EFFECT
Alcohol:	Increased chance of brain and nervous system adverse reaction. Avoid.
Beverages:	No problems expected.
Cocaine:	Increased chance of brain and nervous system adverse reaction. Avoid.
Foods:	No problems expected.
Marijuana:	Increased chance of brain and nervous system adverse reaction. Avoid.
Tobacco:	No problems expected.

*See Glossary

ADRENOCORTICOIDS (Topical)

BRAND NAMES

Some of these brand names are available as oral medicine. Look under specific generic name for each brand. See complete list of brand names in the *Brand Name Directory,* page 1053.

BASIC INFORMATION

Habit forming? No
Prescription needed? For some
Available as generic? Yes
Drug class: Adrenocorticoid (topical)

 ## USES

Relieves redness, swelling, itching, skin discomfort of hemorrhoids, insect bites, poison ivy, oak, sumac, soaps, cosmetics and jewelry.

 ## DOSAGE & USAGE INFORMATION

How to use:
- Cream, lotion, ointment, gel—Apply small amount and rub in gently.
- Topical aerosol—Follow directions on container. Don't breathe vapors.

When to use:
When needed or as directed. Don't use more often than directions allow.

If you forget an application:
Use as soon as you remember.

What drug does:
Reduces inflammation by affecting enzymes that produce inflammation.

Time lapse before drug works:
15 to 20 minutes.

Don't use with:
See Interaction column and consult doctor.

 ## OVERDOSE

SYMPTOMS:
None expected.
WHAT TO DO:
If person swallows or inhales drug, call doctor, poison-control center or hospital emergency room for instructions.

 ## POSSIBLE ADVERSE REACTIONS OR SIDE EFFECTS

SYMPTOMS	WHAT TO DO
Life-threatening: None expected.	
Common: None expected.	
Infrequent: Infection on skin with pain, redness, blisters, pus; skin irritation with burning, itching, blistering or peeling; acne-like skin eruptions.	Continue. Call doctor when convenient.
Rare: None expected.	

WARNINGS & PRECAUTIONS

Don't take if:
You are allergic to any topical adrenocorticoid (cortisone) preparation.

Before you start, consult your doctor:
- If you plan pregnancy within medication period.
- If you have diabetes.
- If you have infection at treatment site.
- If you have stomach ulcer.
- If you have tuberculosis.

Over age 60:
Adverse reactions and side effects may be more frequent and severe than in younger persons, especially thinning of the skin.

Pregnancy:
Risk to unborn child outweighs drug benefits. Don't use.

Breast-feeding:
No problems expected.

Infants & children:
- Use only under medical supervision. Too much for too long can be absorbed into bloodstream through skin and retard growth.
- For infants in diapers, avoid plastic pants or tight diapers.

Prolonged use:
- Increases chance of absorption into bloodstream to cause side effects of oral cortisone drugs.
- May thin skin where used.

Skin & sunlight:
No problems expected.

Driving, piloting or hazardous work:
No problems expected.

Discontinuing:
May be unnecessary to finish medicine. Follow doctor's instructions.

Others:
- Don't use a plastic dressing longer than 2 weeks.
- Aerosol spray—Store in cool place. Don't use near heat or open flame or while smoking. Don't puncture, break or burn container.

POSSIBLE INTERACTION WITH OTHER DRUGS

GENERIC NAME OR DRUG CLASS	COMBINED EFFECT
Antibiotics* (topical)	Decreased antibiotic effects.
Antifungals* (topical)	Decreased antifungal effect.

POSSIBLE INTERACTION WITH OTHER SUBSTANCES

INTERACTS WITH	COMBINED EFFECT
Alcohol:	None expected.
Beverages:	None expected.
Cocaine:	None expected.
Foods:	None expected.
Marijuana:	None expected.
Tobacco:	None expected.

*See Glossary

ALBUTEROL

BRAND AND GENERIC NAMES

ALBUTEROL   **Salbutamol**
Novosalmol   **Ventolin**
Proventil

BASIC INFORMATION

Habit forming? No
Prescription needed? Yes
Available as generic? No
Drug class: Bronchodilator,
  sympathomimetic

USES

- Relieves wheezing and shortness of breath in bronchial asthma attacks, allergies, bronchitis, emphysema or other conditions that cause spasm of the bronchial tubes.
- Temporarily increases blood pressure.

DOSAGE & USAGE INFORMATION

How to take:
- Oral liquid or tablet—Swallow with liquid or food to lessen stomach irritation.
- Inhaler—Follow instructions on package.

When to take:
When needed according to doctor's instructions. Don't take more than 2 doses 1 hour apart.

If you forget a dose:
Take when you remember. Wait 2 hours before next dose.

What drug does:
Relaxes smooth muscles to relieve constriction of bronchial tubes.

Continued next column

OVERDOSE

SYMPTOMS:
Chest pain, irregular heartbeat, convulsions, coma.
WHAT TO DO:
- **Dial 0 (operator) or 911 (emergency) for an ambulance or medical help. Then give first aid immediately.**
- **If patient is unconscious and not breathing, give mouth-to-mouth breathing.**
- **If there is no heartbeat, use cardiac massage and mouth-to-mouth breathing (CPR). Don't try to make patient vomit. If you can't get help quickly, take patient to nearest emergency facility.**
- **See emergency information on inside covers.**

Time lapse before drug works:
5 to 30 minutes.

Don't take with:
See Interaction column and consult doctor.

POSSIBLE ADVERSE REACTIONS OR SIDE EFFECTS

SYMPTOMS	WHAT TO DO
Life-threatening: Severe chest pain, extremely rapid heart-beat (200/min. or more).	Seek emergency treatment immediately.
Common: Dizziness, lightheadedness, headache, nausea or vomiting, large pupils, blurred vision.	Discontinue. Call doctor right away.
Infrequent: Difficult or painful urination, muscle cramps in legs, dry mouth.	Continue. Call doctor when convenient.
Rare: Light chest pain, hallucinations, mood changes.	Discontinue. Call doctor right away.

ALBUTEROL

WARNINGS & PRECAUTIONS

Don't take if:
You are allergic to any sympathomimetic.

Before you start, consult your doctor:
- If you have irregular or rapid heartbeat, congestive heart failure, coronary-artery disease or high blood pressure.
- If you have diabetes.
- If you have overactive thyroid.

Over age 60:
Adverse reactions and side affects may be more frequent and severe than in younger persons.

Pregnancy:
Risk to unborn child outweights drug benefits. Don't use.

Breast-feeding:
Drug passes into milk. Avoid drug or discontinue nursing until you finish medicine. Consult doctor for advice on maintaining milk supply.

Infants & children:
Use only under medical supervision.

Prolonged use:
No problems expected.

Skin & sunlight:
No problems expected.

Driving, piloting or hazardous work:
Don't drive or pilot aircraft until you learn how medicine affects you. Don't work around dangerous machinery. Don't climb ladders or work in high places. Danger increases if you drink alcohol or take medicine affecting alertness and reflexes, such as antihistamines, tranquilizers, sedatives, pain medicine, narcotics and mind-altering drugs.

Discontinuing:
No problems expected.

Others:
- May change blood glucose laboratory determinations (increased).
- May increase serum lactic acid concentrations.

POSSIBLE INTERACTION WITH OTHER DRUGS

GENERIC NAME OR DRUG CLASS	COMBINED EFFECT
Antidepressants, tricyclic (TCA)*	Increased effect of both drugs.
Beta-adrenergic blockers*	Decreased albuterol effect and beta-adrenergic blocker effect.
Carteolol	Decreased beta-agonist effect.
Digitalis preparations*	Increased risk of heartbeat irregularity.
Levodopa	Increased risk of heartbeat irregularity.
Reserpine	May reduce effectiveness of albuterol.
Sotalol	Decreased beta-agonist effect.
Sympathomimetics, others*	Increased effects of both drugs, especially harmful side effects.
Terazosin	Decreases effectiveness of terazosin.

POSSIBLE INTERACTION WITH OTHER SUBSTANCES

INTERACTS WITH	COMBINED EFFECT
Alcohol:	Decreased albuterol effect.
Beverages:	None expected.
Cocaine:	High risk of heartbeat irregularities and high blood pressure.
Foods:	None expected.
Marijuana:	Overstimulation. Avoid.
Tobacco:	No proven problems.

ALLOPURINOL

BRAND NAMES

Alloprin	Purinol
Aluline	Roucol
Apo-Allopurinol	Zurinol
Caplenal	Zyloprim
Lopurin	Zyloric
Novopurol	

BASIC INFORMATION

Habit forming? No
Prescription needed? Yes
Available as generic? Yes
Drug class: Antigout

 USES

- Treatment for chronic gout.
- Prevention of kidney stones caused by uric acid.

 DOSAGE & USAGE INFORMATION

How to take:
Tablet—Swallow with liquid or food to lessen stomach irritation.

When to take:
At the same times each day.

If you forget a dose:
- 1 dose per day—Take as soon as you remember up to 6 hours late. If more than 6 hours, wait for next scheduled dose (don't double this dose).
- More than 1 dose per day—Take as soon as you remember up to 3 hours late. If more than 3 hours, wait for next scheduled dose (don't double this dose).

What drug does:
Slows formation of uric acid by inhibiting enzyme (xanthine oxidase) activity.

Time lapse before drug works:
Reduces blood uric acid in 1 to 3 weeks. May require 6 months to prevent acute gout attacks.

Continued next column

 OVERDOSE

SYMPTOMS:
None expected.
WHAT TO DO:
Overdose unlikely to threaten life. If person takes much larger amount than prescribed, call doctor, poison-control center or hospital emergency room for instructions.

Don't take with:
See Interaction column and consult doctor.

 POSSIBLE ADVERSE REACTIONS OR SIDE EFFECTS

SYMPTOMS	WHAT TO DO
Life-threatening: None expected.	
Common: Rash, hives, itch.	Discontinue. Call doctor right away.
Infrequent: • Jaundice.	Discontinue. Call doctor right away.
• Drowsiness, diarrhea, stomach pain, nausea, vomiting, headache.	Continue. Call doctor when convenient.
Rare: • Sore throat, fever, unusual bleeding or bruising.	Discontinue. Call doctor right away.
• Numbness, tingling, pain in hands or feet.	Continue. Call doctor when convenient.

 WARNINGS & PRECAUTIONS

Don't take if:
You are allergic to allopurinol.

Before you start, consult your doctor:
If you have had liver or kidney problems.

Over age 60:
Adverse reactions and side effects may be more frequent and severe than in younger persons.

Pregnancy:
Studies inconclusive on harm to unborn child. Animal studies show fetal abnormalities. Decide with your doctor whether drug benefits justify risk to unborn child.

Breast-feeding:
Drug passes into milk. Avoid drug or discontinue nursing.

Infants & children:
Not recommended.

Prolonged use:
No problems expected.

Skin & sunlight:
No problems expected.

Driving, piloting or hazardous work:
Avoid if you feel drowsy. Use may disqualify you for piloting aircraft.

Discontinuing:
Don't discontinue without doctor's advice until you complete prescribed dose, even though symptoms diminish or disappear.

Others:
Acute gout attacks may increase during first weeks of use. If so, consult doctor about additional medicine.

POSSIBLE INTERACTION WITH OTHER DRUGS

GENERIC NAME OR DRUG CLASS	COMBINED EFFECT
Ampicillin	Likely skin rash.
Anticoagulants, oral*	May increase anticoagulant effect.
Antidiabetics, oral*	Increased uric-acid elimination.
Azathioprine	Increased azathioprine effect.
Chlorpropamide	May increase chlorpropamide effect.
Chlorthalidone	Decreased allopurinol effect.
Cyclophosphamide	Increased cyclophosphamide toxicity.
Diuretics, thiazide*	Decreased allopurinol effect.
Ethacrynic acid	Decreased allopurinol effect.
Furosemide	Decreased allopurinol effect.
Indapamide	Decreased allopurinol effect.
Iron supplements*	Excessive accumulation of iron in tissues.
Mercaptopurine	Increased mercaptopurine effect.
Metolazone	Decreased allopurinol effect.
Probenecid	Increased allopurinol effect.
Theophylline	May increase theophylline effect.

POSSIBLE INTERACTION WITH OTHER SUBSTANCES

INTERACTS WITH	COMBINED EFFECT
Alcohol:	None expected, but may impair management of gout.
Beverages:	Caffeine drinks. Decreased allopurinol effect.
Cocaine:	Decreased allopurinol effect. Avoid.
Foods:	None expected. Low-purine diet* recommended.
Marijuana:	Occasional use—None expected. Daily use—Possible increase in uric-acid level.
Tobacco:	None expected.

*See Glossary

ALPRAZOLAM

BRAND NAMES

Xanax

BASIC INFORMATION

Habit forming? Yes
Prescription needed? Yes
Available as generic? No
Drug class: Tranquilizer (benzodiazepine)

 ## USES

Treatment for nervousness or tension and depression.

 ## DOSAGE & USAGE INFORMATION

How to take:
Tablet—Swallow with liquid. If you can't swallow whole, crumble tablet and take with liquid or food.

When to take:
At the same time each day, according to instructions on prescription label.

If you forget a dose:
Take as soon as you remember up to 2 hours late. If more than 2 hours, wait for next scheduled dose (don't double this dose).

What drug does:
Affects limbic system of brain—part that controls emotions.

Time lapse before drug works:
2 hours. May take 6 weeks for full benefit.

Don't take with:
See Interaction column and consult doctor.

 ## OVERDOSE

SYMPTOMS:
Drowsiness, weakness, tremor, stupor, coma.
WHAT TO DO:
- Dial 0 (operator) or 911 (emergency) for an ambulance or medical help. Then give first aid immediately.
- If patient is unconscious and not breathing, give mouth-to-mouth breathing. If there is no heartbeat, use cardiac massage and mouth-to-mouth breathing (CPR). Don't try to make patient vomit. If you can't get help quickly, take patient to nearest emergency facility.
- See emergency information on inside covers.

 ## POSSIBLE ADVERSE REACTIONS OR SIDE EFFECTS

SYMPTOMS	WHAT TO DO
Life-threatening: None expected.	
Common: Clumsiness, drowsiness, dizziness.	Continue. Call doctor when convenient.
Infrequent: • Hallucinations, confusion, depression, irritability, rash, itch, vision changes.	Discontinue. Call doctor right away.
• Constipation or diarrhea, nausea, vomiting, difficult or painful urination.	Continue. Call doctor when convenient.
Rare: • Slow heartbeat, breathing difficulty.	Discontinue. Seek emergency treatment.
• Mouth or throat ulcers, jaundice.	Discontinue. Call doctor right away.

 ## WARNINGS & PRECAUTIONS

Don't take if:
- You are allergic to any benzodiazepine.
- You have myasthenia gravis.
- You are active or recovering alcoholic.
- Patient is younger than 6 months.

Before you start, consult your doctor:
- If you have liver, kidney or lung disease.
- If you have diabetes, epilepsy or porphyria.

Over age 60:
Adverse reactions and side effects may be more frequent and severe than in younger persons. You need smaller doses for shorter periods of time. May develop agitation, rage or "hangover" effect.

Pregnancy:
Risk to unborn child outweighs drug benefits. Don't use.

Breast-feeding:
Drug passes into milk. Avoid drug or discontinue nursing until you finish medicine. Consult doctor for advice on maintaining milk supply.

Infants & children:
Use only under medical supervision for children older than 6 months.

Prolonged use:
May impair liver function.

Skin & sunlight:
No problems expected.

Driving, piloting or hazardous work:
Don't drive or pilot aircraft until you learn how medicine affects you. Don't work around dangerous machinery. Don't climb ladders or work in high places. Danger increases if you drink alcohol or take medicine affecting alertness and reflexes.

Discontinuing:
Don't discontinue without consulting doctor. Dose may require gradual reduction if you have taken drug for a long time. Doses of other drugs may also require adjustment.

Others:
- Hot weather, heavy exercise and profuse sweat may reduce excretion and cause overdose.
- Blood sugar may rise in diabetics, requiring insulin adjustment.

POSSIBLE INTERACTION WITH OTHER DRUGS

GENERIC NAME OR DRUG CLASS	COMBINED EFFECT
Anticonvulsants*	Change in seizure frequency or severity.
Antidepressants*	Increased sedative effect of both drugs.
Antihistamines*	Increased sedative effect of both drugs.
Antihypertensives*	Excessively low blood pressure.
Cimetidine	Excess sedation.
Disulfiram	Increased alprazolam effect.
Dronabinol	Increased effects of both drugs. Avoid.
Ketoconazole	May increase sedative effect.
MAO inhibitors*	Convulsions, deep sedation, rage.
Molindone	Increased tranquilizer effect.
Nabilone	Greater depression of the central nervous system.
Narcotics*	Increased sedative effect of both drugs.

Nizatidine	Increased effect and toxicity of alprazolam.
Rifampin	Decreased alprazolam effect.
Sedatives*	Increased sedative effect of both drugs.
Sleep inducers*	Increased sedative effect of both drugs.
Tranquilizers*	Increased sedative effect of both drugs.

POSSIBLE INTERACTION WITH OTHER SUBSTANCES

INTERACTS WITH	COMBINED EFFECT
Alcohol:	Heavy sedation. Avoid.
Beverages:	None expected.
Cocaine:	Decreased alprazolam effect.
Foods:	None expected.
Marijuana:	Heavy sedation. Avoid.
Tobacco:	Decreased alprazolam effect.

*See Glossary

ALUMINUM, CALCIUM & MAGNESIUM ANTACIDS

BRAND NAMES

Camalox

BASIC INFORMATION

Habit forming? No
Prescription needed? No
Available as generic? No
Drug class: Antacids

 USES

- Binds excess phosphate in intestine.
- Treatment for hyperacidity in upper gastrointestinal tract, including stomach and esophagus. Symptoms may be heartburn or acid indigestion. Diseases include peptic ulcer, gastritis, esophagitis, hiatal hernia.
- Constipation relief.

 DOSAGE & USAGE INFORMATION

How to take:
- Chewable tablets—Chew well before swallowing with liquid.
- Liquid—Shake well and take undiluted.

When to take:
1 to 3 hours after meals and at bedtime unless directed otherwise by your doctor.

If you forget a dose:
Take as soon as you remember, but not simultaneously with any other medicine.

What drug does:
- Neutralizes some of the hydrochloric acid in the stomach.
- Reduces action of pepsin, a digestive enzyme.
- Stimulates muscles in lower bowel wall.

Continued next column

 OVERDOSE

SYMPTOMS:
Dry mouth, diarrhea, shallow breathing, weakness, fatigue, stupor.
WHAT TO DO:
- **Dial 0 (operator) or 911 (emergency) for an ambulance or medical help. Then give first aid immediately.**
- **See emergency information on inside covers.**

Time lapse before drug works:
15 minutes.

Don't take with:
Other medicines at the same time. Decreases absorption of other drugs. Wait 2 hours between doses.

 POSSIBLE ADVERSE REACTIONS OR SIDE EFFECTS

SYMPTOMS	WHAT TO DO
Life-threatening: Heartbeat irregularity in patient with heart disease.	Discontinue. Seek emergency treatment.
Common: • Constipation, headache, appetite loss, distended stomach.	Discontinue. Call doctor right away.
• Unpleasant taste in mouth, abdominal pain, laxative effect, belching.	Continue. Call doctor when convenient.
Infrequent: Bone pain, frequent urination, dizziness, urgent urination, muscle weakness or pain, nausea.	Discontinue. Call doctor right away.
Rare: Mood changes, headache, vomiting, nervousness, swollen feet and ankles.	Discontinue. Call doctor right away.

 WARNINGS & PRECAUTIONS

Don't take if:
- You are allergic to any antacid.
- You have a high blood-calcium level.

Before you start, consult your doctor:
- If you have kidney disease.
- If you have chronic constipation, colitis or diarrhea.
- If you have symptoms of appendicitis.
- If you have stomach or intestinal bleeding.
- If you have irregular heartbeat.

Over age 60:
Adverse reactions and side effects may be more frequent and severe than in younger persons. Diarrhea or constipation particularly likely.

Pregnancy:
Risk to unborn child outweighs drug benefits. Don't use.

Breast-feeding:
Drug passes into milk. Avoid drug or discontinue nursing until you finish medicine. Consult doctor for advice on maintaining milk supply.

Infants & children:
Use only under medical supervision.

Prolonged use:
- Decreased phosphate level in blood weakens bones.
- High blood level of calcium which disturbs electrolyte balance.
- Kidney stones, impaired kidney function.

Skin & sunlight:
No problems expected.

Driving, piloting or hazardous work:
No problems expected.

Discontinuing:
May be unnecessary to finish medicine. Follow doctor's instructions.

Others:
Don't take longer than 2 weeks unless under medical supervision.

 POSSIBLE INTERACTION WITH OTHER DRUGS

GENERIC NAME OR DRUG CLASS	COMBINED EFFECT
Anticoagulants*	Decreased anti-coagulant effect.
Calcitonin	Decreased calcitonin effect.
Chlorpromazine	Decreased chlor-promazine effect.
Ciprofloxacin	May cause kidney dysfunction.
Digitalis preparations*	Decreased digitalis effect.
Diuretics*	Increased calcium in blood.
Iron supplements*	Decreased iron effect.
Isoniazid	Decreased isoniazid effect.
Levodopa	Increased levodopa effect.
Meperidine	Increased meperidine effect.
Nalidixic acid	Decreased effect of nalidixic acid.
Nizatidine	Decreased nizatidine absorption.
Norfloxacin	Decreased norfloxacin effect.
Oxyphenbutazone	Decreased oxyphen-butazone effect.
Para-aminosalicylic acid (PAS)	Decreased PAS effect.
Penicillins*	Decreased penicillin effect.
Pentobarbital	Decreased pento-barbital effect.
Phenylbutazone	Decreased phenyl-butazone effect.
Pseudoephedrine	Increased pseudo-ephedrine effect.
Quinidine	Increased quinidine effect.
Salicylates*	Increased salicylate effect.
Sulfa drugs*	Decreased sulfa effect.
Tetracyclines*	Decreased tetracycline effect.
Ursodiol	Decreased absorption ursodiol.
Vitamins A and C	Decreased vitamin effect.
Vitamin D	Too much calcium in blood.

 POSSIBLE INTERACTION WITH OTHER SUBSTANCES

INTERACTS WITH	COMBINED EFFECT
Alcohol:	Decreased antacid effect.
Beverages:	No proven problems.
Cocaine:	No proven problems.
Foods:	Decreased antacid effect. Wait 1 hour after eating.
Marijuana:	No proven problems.
Tobacco:	Decreased antacid effect.

*See Glossary

ALUMINUM HYDROXIDE

BRAND NAMES

See complete list of brand names in the *Brand Name Directory*, page 1053.

BASIC INFORMATION

Habit forming? No
Prescription needed? No
Available as generic? Yes
Drug class: Antacid, antidiarrheal

 ## USES

- Binds excess phosphate in intestine.
- Treatment for hyperacidity in upper gastrointestinal tract, including stomach and esophagus. Symptoms may be heartburn or acid indigestion. Diseases include peptic ulcer, gastritis, esophagitis, hiatal hernia.
- Treatment for diarrhea.

 ## DOSAGE & USAGE INFORMATION

How to take:
- Tablet or capsule—Swallow with liquid.
- Chewable tablets or wafers—Chew well before swallowing.
- Liquid—Shake well and take undiluted.

When to take:
1 to 3 hours after meals unless directed otherwise by your doctor.

If you forget a dose:
Take as soon as you remember, but not simultaneously with any other medicine.

What drug does:
- Neutralizes some of the hydrochloric acid in the stomach.
- Reduces action of pepsin, a digestive enzyme.

Time lapse before drug works:
15 minutes.

Continued next column

 ## OVERDOSE

SYMPTOMS:
Weakness, fatigue, dizziness.
WHAT TO DO:
Overdose unlikely to threaten life. If person takes much larger amount than prescribed, call doctor, poison-control center or hospital emergency room for instructions.

Don't take with:
Other medicines at the same time. Decreases absorption of other drugs. Wait 2 hours between doses.

 ## POSSIBLE ADVERSE REACTIONS OR SIDE EFFECTS

SYMPTOMS	WHAT TO DO
Life-threatening: None expected.	
Common: Constipation, appetite loss.	Continue. Call doctor when convenient.
Infrequent:	
• Lower abdominal pain and swelling, bone pain, muscle weakness, swollen wrists or ankles.	Discontinue. Call doctor right away.
• Mood changes, nausea, vomiting, weight loss.	Continue. Call doctor when convenient.
Rare: None expected.	

WARNINGS & PRECAUTIONS

Don't take if:
You are allergic to any antacid.

Before you start, consult your doctor:
- If you have kidney disease.
- If you have chronic constipation, colitis or diarrhea.
- If you have symptoms of appendicitis.
- If you have have stomach or intestinal bleeding.

Over age 60:
Adverse reactions and side effects may be more frequent and severe than in younger persons. Diarrhea or constipation particularly likely.

Pregnancy:
Risk to unborn child outweighs drug benefits. Don't use.

Breast-feeding:
Drug passes into milk. Avoid drug or discontinue nursing until you finish medicine. Consult doctor for advice on maintaining milk supply.

Infants & children:
Use only under medical supervision.

Prolonged use:
Decreased phosphate level in blood weakens bones.

Skin & sunlight:
No problems expected.

Driving, piloting or hazardous work:
No problems expected.

Discontinuing:
May be unnecessary to finish medicine. Follow doctor's instructions.

Others:
Don't take longer than 2 weeks unless under medical supervision.

POSSIBLE INTERACTION WITH OTHER DRUGS

GENERIC NAME OR DRUG CLASS	COMBINED EFFECT
Anticoagulants*	Decreased anticoagulant effect.
Chlorpromazine	Decreased chlorpromazine effect.
Ciprofloxacin	May cause kidney dysfunction.
Digitalis preparations*	Decreased digitalis effect.
Iron supplements*	Decreased iron effect.
Meperidine	Increased meperidine effect.
Nalidixic acid	Decreased effect of nalidixic acid.
Nizatidine	Decreased nizatidine absorption.
Norfloxacin	Decreased norfloxacin effect.
Oxyphenbutazone	Decreased oxyphenbutazone effect.
Para-aminosalicylic acid (PAS)	Decreased PAS effect.
Penicillins*	Decreased penicillin effect.
Pentobarbital	Decreased pentobarbital effect.
Phenylbutazone	Decreased phenylbutazone effect.
Pseudoephedrine	Increased pseudoephedrine effect.
Sulfa drugs*	Decreased sulfa effect.
Tetracyclines*	Decreased tetracycline effect.
Ursodiol	Decreased absorption of ursodiol.
Vitamins A and C	Decreased vitamin effect.

POSSIBLE INTERACTION WITH OTHER SUBSTANCES

INTERACTS WITH	COMBINED EFFECT
Alcohol:	Decreased antacid effect.
Beverages:	No proven problems.
Cocaine:	No proven problems.
Foods:	Decreased antacid effect. Wait 1 hour after eating.
Marijuana:	No proven problems.
Tobacco:	Decreased antacid effect.

*See Glossary

ALUMINUM & MAGNESIUM ANTACIDS

BRAND NAMES

See complete list of brand names in the *Brand Name Directory,* page 1054.

BASIC INFORMATION

Habit forming? No
Prescription needed? No
Available as generic? Yes
Drug class: Antacids

 ## USES

- Binds excess phosphate in intestine.
- Treatment for hyperacidity in upper gastrointestinal tract, including stomach and esophagus. Symptoms may be heartburn or acid indigestion. Diseases include peptic ulcer, gastritis, esophagitis, hiatal hernia.
- Constipation relief.

 ## DOSAGE & USAGE INFORMATION

How to take:
- Tablet or capsule—Swallow with liquid.
- Chewable tablets or wafers—Chew well before swallowing with liquid.
- Liquid—Shake well and take undiluted.

When to take:
1 to 3 hours after meals unless directed otherwise by your doctor.

If you forget a dose:
Take as soon as you remember, but not simultaneously with any other medicine.

What drug does:
- Neutralizes some of the hydrochloric acid in the stomach.
- Reduces action of pepsin, a digestive enzyme.
- Stimulates muscles in lower bowel wall.

Time lapse before drug works:
15 minutes for acid relief.

Continued next column

 ## OVERDOSE

SYMPTOMS:
Weakness, fatigue, dizziness, dry mouth, diarrhea, shallow breathing, stupor.
WHAT TO DO:
- **Dial 0 (operator) or 911 (emergency) for an ambulance or medical help. Then give first aid immediately.**
- **See emergency information on inside covers.**

Don't take with:
Other medicines at the same time. Decreases absorption of other drugs. Wait 2 hours between doses.

 ## POSSIBLE ADVERSE REACTIONS OR SIDE EFFECTS

SYMPTOMS	WHAT TO DO
Life-threatening:	
Heartbeat irregularity in patient with heart disease.	Discontinue. Seek emergency treatment.
Common:	
• Constipation, headache, appetite loss, distended stomach.	Discontinue. Call doctor right away.
• Unpleasant taste in mouth, abdominal pain, laxative effect, belching.	Continue. Call doctor when convenient.
Infrequent:	
Bone pain, frequent or urgent urination, dizziness, muscle weakness or pain, nausea.	Discontinue. Call doctor right away.
Rare:	
Mood changes, vomiting, nervousness, swollen feet and ankles.	Discontinue. Call doctor right away.

ALUMINUM & MAGNESIUM ANTACIDS

WARNINGS & PRECAUTIONS

Don't take if:
You are allergic to any antacid.

Before you start, consult your doctor:
If you have kidney disease, chronic constipation, colitis, diarrhea, symptoms of appendicitis, stomach or intestinal bleeding.

Over age 60:
Adverse reactions and side effects may be more frequent and severe than in younger persons. Diarrhea or constipation particularly likely.

Pregnancy:
Risk to unborn child outweighs drug benefits. Don't use.

Breast-feeding:
Drug passes into milk. Avoid drug or discontinue nursing until you finish medicine. Consult doctor for advice on maintaining milk supply.

Infants & children:
Use only under medical supervision.

Prolonged use:
Decreased phosphate level in blood weakens bones.

Skin & sunlight:
No problems expected.

Driving, piloting or hazardous work:
No problems expected.

Discontinuing:
May be unnecessary to finish medicine. Follow doctor's instructions.

Others:
Don't take longer than 2 weeks unless under medical supervision.

POSSIBLE INTERACTION WITH OTHER DRUGS

GENERIC NAME OR DRUG CLASS	COMBINED EFFECT
Anticoagulants, oral*	Decreased anticoagulant effect.
Chlorpromazine	Decreased chlorpromazine effect.
Ciprofloxacin	May cause kidney dysfunction.
Digitalis preparations*	Decreased digitalis effect.
Iron supplements*	Decreased iron effect.
Isoniazid	Decreased isoniazid effect.
Levodopa	Increased levodopa effect.
Meperidine	Increased meperidine effect.
Nalidixic acid	Decreased effect of nalidixic acid.
Nizatidine	Decreased nizatidine absorption.
Norfloxacin	Decreased norfloxacin effect.
Oxyphenbutazone	Decreased oxyphenbutazone effect.
Para-aminosalicylic acid (PAS)	Decreased PAS effect.
Penicillins*	Decreased penicillin effect.
Pentobarbital	Decreased pentobarbital effect.
Phenylbutazone	Decreased phenylbutazone effect.
Pseudoephedrine	Increased pseudoephedrine effect.
Sulfa drugs*	Decreased sulfa effect.
Tetracyclines*	Decreased tetracycline effect.
Ursodiol	Decreased absorption of ursodiol.

POSSIBLE INTERACTION WITH OTHER SUBSTANCES

INTERACTS WITH	COMBINED EFFECT
Alcohol:	Decreased antacid effect.
Beverages:	No proven problems.
Cocaine:	No proven problems.
Foods:	Decreased antacid effect. Wait 1 hour after eating.
Marijuana:	No proven problems.
Tobacco:	Decreased antacid effect.

*See Glossary

31

ALUMINUM, MAGNESIUM, MAGALDRATE & SIMETHICONE ANTACIDS

BRAND NAMES

See complete list of brand names in the *Brand Name Directory*, page 1054.

BASIC INFORMATION

Habit forming? No
Prescription needed? No
Available as generic? No
Drug class: Antacid, antiflatulent

USES

- Treatment for hyperacidity in upper gastrointestinal tract, including stomach and esophagus. Symptoms may be heartburn or acid indigestion. Diseases include peptic ulcer, gastritis, esophagitis, hiatal hernia.
- Relief of constipation or diarrhea (sometimes).
- Treatment for retention of abdominal gas.
- Used prior to x-ray of abdomen to reduce gas shadows.

DOSAGE & USAGE INFORMATION

How to take:
- Tablet—Swallow with liquid.
- Liquid—Dissolve in water. Drink complete dose.
- Chewable tablets—Chew completely. Don't swallow whole, follow with liquid.

When to take:
1 to 3 hours after meals unless directed otherwise by your doctor.

If you forget a dose:
Take as soon as you remember, but not simultaneously with any other medicine.

Continued next column

OVERDOSE

SYMPTOMS:
Dry mouth, shallow breathing, diarrhea, weakness, fatigue, dizziness, stupor.
WHAT TO DO:
- **Dial 0 (operator) or 911 (emergency) for an ambulance or medical help. Then give first aid immediately.**
- **See emergency information on inside covers.**

What drug does:
- Neutralizes some of the hydrochloric acid in the stomach.
- Reduces action of pepsin, a digestive enzyme.
- Stimulates muscles in lower bowel wall.

Time lapse before drug works:
15 minutes.

Don't take with:
Other medicines at the same time. Decreases absorption of other drugs. Wait 2 hours between doses.

POSSIBLE ADVERSE REACTIONS OR SIDE EFFECTS

SYMPTOMS	WHAT TO DO
Life-threatening:	
Heartbeat irregularity in patient with heart disease.	Discontinue. Seek emergency treatment.
Common:	
• Constipation, headache, appetite loss, distended stomach.	Discontinue. Call doctor right away.
• Unpleasant taste in mouth, abdominal pain, laxative effect, belching.	Continue. Call doctor when convenient.
Infrequent:	
Bone pain, frequent urination, dizziness, urgent urination, muscle weakness or pain, nausea.	Discontinue. Call doctor right away.
Rare:	
Mood changes, vomiting, nervousness, swollen feet and ankles.	Discontinue. Call doctor right away.

WARNINGS & PRECAUTIONS

Don't take if:
You are allergic to any antacid or simethicone.

Before you start, consult your doctor:
If you have kidney disease, chronic constipation, colitis, diarrhea, symptoms of appendicitis, stomach or intestinal bleeding.

Over age 60:
Adverse reactions and side effects may be more frequent and severe than in younger persons. Diarrhea or constipation particularly likely.

ALUMINUM, MAGNESIUM, MAGALDRATE & SIMETHICONE ANTACIDS

Pregnancy:
Risk to unborn child outweighs drug benefits. Don't use.

Breast-feeding:
Drug passes into milk. Avoid drug or discontinue nursing until you finish medicine. Consult doctor for advice on maintaining milk supply.

Infants & children:
Use only under medical supervision.

Prolonged use:
Decreased phosphate level in blood weakens bones.

Skin & sunlight:
No problems expected.

Driving, piloting or hazardous work:
No problems expected.

Discontinuing:
May be unnecessary to finish medicine. Follow doctor's instructions.

Others:
Don't take longer than 2 weeks unless under medical supervision.

 ## POSSIBLE INTERACTION WITH OTHER DRUGS

GENERIC NAME OR DRUG CLASS	COMBINED EFFECT
Anticoagulants, oral*	Decreased anticoagulant effect.
Chlorpromazine	Decreased chlorpromazine effect.
Ciprofloxacin	May cause kidney dysfunction.
Digitalis preparations*	Decreased digitalis effect.
Iron supplements*	Decreased iron effect.
Isoniazid	Decreased isoniazid effect.
Levodopa	Increased levodopa effect.
Meperidine	Increased meperidine effect.
Nalidixic acid	Decreased effect of nalidixic acid.
Nizatidine	Decreased nizatidine absorption.
Norfloxacin	Decreased norfloxacin effect.
Oxyphenbutazone	Decreased oxyphenbutazone effect.
Para-aminosalicylic acid (PAS)	Decreased PAS effect.
Penicillins*	Decreased penicillin effect.
Pentobarbital	Decreased pentobarbital effect.
Phenylbutazone	Decreased phenylbutazone effect.
Pseudoephedrine	Increased pseudoephedrine effect.
Sulfa drugs*	Decreased sulfa effect.
Tetracyclines*	Decreased tetracycline effect.
Ursodiol	Decreased absorption of ursodiol.
Vitamins A and C	Decreased vitamin effect.

 ## POSSIBLE INTERACTION WITH OTHER SUBSTANCES

INTERACTS WITH	COMBINED EFFECT
Alcohol:	Decreased antacid effect.
Beverages:	No proven problems.
Cocaine:	No proven problems.
Foods:	Decreased antacid effect. Wait 1 hour after eating.
Marijuana:	No proven problems.
Tobacco:	Decreased antacid effect.

ALUMINUM, MAGNESIUM & SODIUM BICARBONATE ANTACIDS

BRAND NAMES

Gas-Is-Gon   Triconsil

BASIC INFORMATION

Habit forming? No
Prescription needed? No
Available as generic? No
Drug class: Antacid, antiflatulent

USES

- Binds excess phosphate in intestine.
- Treatment for hyperacidity in upper gastrointestinal tract, including stomach and esophagus. Symptoms may be heartburn or acid indigestion. Diseases include peptic ulcer, gastritis, esophagitis, hiatal hernia.
- Relief of constipation or diarrhea (sometimes).

DOSAGE & USAGE INFORMATION

How to take:
Chewable tablets—Chew completely. Don't swallow whole, follow with liquid.

When to take:
1 to 3 hours after meals unless directed otherwise by your doctor.

If you forget a dose:
Take as soon as you remember, but not simultaneously with any other medicine.

Continued next column

OVERDOSE

SYMPTOMS:
Dry mouth, shallow breathing, diarrhea, weakness, fatigue, dizziness, stupor.
WHAT TO DO:
- Overdose unlikely to threaten life. Depending on severity of symptoms and amount taken, call doctor, poison-control center or hospital emergency room for instructions.
- Dial 0 (operator) or 911 (emergency) for an ambulance or medical help. Then give first aid immediately.
- See emergency information on inside covers.

What drug does:
- Neutralizes some of the hydrochloric acid in the stomach.
- Reduces action of pepsin, a digestive enzyme.
- Stimulates muscles in lower bowel wall.

Time lapse before drug works:
15 minutes.

Don't take with:
Other medicines at the same time. Decreases absorption of other drugs. Wait 2 hours between doses.

POSSIBLE ADVERSE REACTIONS OR SIDE EFFECTS

SYMPTOMS	WHAT TO DO
Life-threatening:	
Heartbeat irregularity in patient with heart disease.	Discontinue. Seek emergency treatment.
Common:	
• Constipation, headache, appetite loss, distended stomach.	Discontinue. Call doctor right away.
• Unpleasant taste in mouth, abdominal pain, laxative effect, belching.	Continue. Call doctor when convenient.
Infrequent:	
Bone pain, frequent or urgent urination, dizziness, muscle weakness or pain, nausea, weight gain.	Discontinue. Call doctor right away.
Rare:	
Mood changes, vomiting, nervousness, swollen feet and ankles.	Discontinue. Call doctor right away.

ALUMINUM, MAGNESIUM & SODIUM BICARBONATE ANTACIDS

WARNINGS & PRECAUTIONS

Don't take if:
You are allergic to any antacid.

Before you start, consult your doctor:
If you have kidney or liver disease, high blood pressure, congestive heart failure, chronic constipation, colitis, diarrhea, symptoms of appendicitis, stomach or intestinal bleeding.

Over age 60:
Adverse reactions and side effects may be more frequent and severe than in younger persons. Diarrhea or constipation particularly likely.

Pregnancy:
Risk to unborn child outweighs drug benefits. Don't use.

Breast-feeding:
Drug passes into milk. Avoid drug or discontinue nursing until you finish medicine. Consult doctor for advice on maintaining milk supply.

Infants & children:
Use only under medical supervision.

Prolonged use:
Decreased phosphate level in blood weakens bones.

Skin & sunlight:
No problems expected.

Driving, piloting or hazardous work:
No problems expected.

Discontinuing:
May be unnecessary to finish medicine. Follow doctor's instructions.

Others:
Don't take longer than 2 weeks unless under medical supervision.

POSSIBLE INTERACTION WITH OTHER DRUGS

GENERIC NAME OR DRUG CLASS	COMBINED EFFECT
Anticoagulants, oral*	Decreased anti-coagulant effect.
Chlorpromazine	Decreased chlor-promazine effect.
Ciprofloxacin	May cause kidney dysfunction.
Digitalis preparations*	Decreased digitalis effect.
Iron supplements*	Decreased iron effect.
Isoniazid	Decreased isoniazid effect.
Levodopa	Increased levodopa effect.
Meperidine	Increased meperidine effect.
Nalidixic acid	Decreased effect of nalidixic acid.
Nizatidine	Decreased nizatidine absorption.
Norfloxacin	Decreased norfloxacin effect.
Oxyphenbutazone	Decreased oxyphen-butazone effect.
Para-aminosalicylic acid (PAS)	Decreased PAS effect.
Penicillins*	Decreased penicillin effect.
Pentobarbital	Decreased pento-barbital effect.
Phenylbutazone	Decreased phenyl-butazone effect.
Pseudoephedrine	Increased pseudo-ephedrine effect.
Sulfa drugs*	Decreased sulfa effect.
Tetracyclines*	Decreased tetracycline effect.
Ursodiol	Decreased absorption of ursodiol.
Vitamins A and C	Decreased vitamin effect.

POSSIBLE INTERACTION WITH OTHER SUBSTANCES

INTERACTS WITH	COMBINED EFFECT
Alcohol:	Decreased antacid effect.
Beverages:	No proven problems.
Cocaine:	No proven problems.
Foods:	Decreased antacid effect. Wait 1 hour after eating.
Marijuana:	Decreased antacid effect.
Tobacco:	No proven problems.

*See Glossary

35

AMANTADINE

BRAND NAMES

Symadine   Symmetrel

BASIC INFORMATION

Habit forming? No
Prescription needed? Yes
Available as generic? Yes
Drug class: Antiviral, antiparkinsonism

USES

- Treatment for Type-A flu infections.
- Relief for symptoms of Parkinson's disease.

DOSAGE & USAGE INFORMATION

How to take:
- Capsule—Swallow with liquid or food to lessen stomach irritation.
- Syrup—Dilute dose in beverage before swallowing.

When to take:
At the same times each day. For Type-A flu it is especially important to take regular doses as prescribed.

If you forget a dose:
Take as soon as you remember. Wait 4 hours for next dose. Return to schedule.

What drug does:
- Type-A flu—May block penetration of tissue cells by infectious material from virus cells.
- Parkinson's disease—Improves muscular condition and coordination.

Time lapse before drug works:
- Type-A flu—48 hours.
- Parkinson's disease—2 days to 2 weeks.

Don't take with:
- Alcohol
- See Interaction column and consult doctor.

OVERDOSE

SYMPTOMS:
Heart-rhythm disturbances, blood-pressure drop, convulsions, toxic psychosis.
WHAT TO DO:
- Dial 0 (operator) or 911 (emergency) for an ambulance or medical help. Then give first aid immediately.
- See emergency information on inside covers.

POSSIBLE ADVERSE REACTIONS OR SIDE EFFECTS

SYMPTOMS	WHAT TO DO
Life-threatening: None expected.	
Common:	
• Hallucinations, confusion, lightheadedness.	Continue. Call doctor when convenient.
• Dizziness, headache, purple blotches, appetite loss, nausea.	Continue. Tell doctor at next visit.
• Dry mouth.	No action necessary.
Infrequent:	
• Fainting, slurred speech.	Discontinue. Call doctor right away.
• Difficult or painful urination.	Continue. Call doctor when convenient.
Rare:	
• Rash, uncontrollable rolling of eyes, irregular heartbeats, blurred vision, sore throat, fever.	Discontinue. Call doctor right away.
• Vomiting.	Continue. Call doctor when convenient.
• Constipation.	Continue. Tell doctor at next visit.

WARNINGS & PRECAUTIONS

Don't take if:
You are allergic to amantadine.

Before you start, consult your doctor:
- If you have had epilepsy or other seizures.
- If you have had heart disease or heart failure.
- If you have had liver or kidney disease.
- If you have had peptic ulcers.
- If you have had eczema or skin rashes.
- If you have had emotional or mental disorders or taken drugs for them.

Over age 60:
Adverse reactions and side effects may be more frequent and severe than in younger persons.

Pregnancy:
Studies inconclusive on harm to unborn child. Animal studies show fetal abnormalities. Decide with your doctor whether benefits justify risk to unborn child.

Breast-feeding:
Drug passes into milk. Avoid drug or discontinue nursing until you finish medicine. Consult doctor for advice on maintaining milk supply.

Infants & children:
Use only under medical supervision.

Prolonged use:
Skin splotches, feet swelling, rapid weight gain, shortness of breath. Consult doctor.

Skin & sunlight:
No problems expected.

Driving, piloting or hazardous work:
Don't drive or pilot aircraft until you learn how medicine affects you. Don't work around dangerous machinery. Don't climb ladders or work in high places. Danger increases if you drink alcohol or take medicine affecting alertness and reflexes.

Discontinuing:
- Parkinson's disease—Don't discontinue without doctor's advice until you complete prescribed dose, even though symptoms diminish or disappear.
- Type-A flu—Discontinue 48 hours after symptoms disappear.

Others:
- Parkinson's disease—May lose effectiveness in 3 to 6 months. Consult doctor.
- Amantadine may increase susceptibility to German measles.

 ## POSSIBLE INTERACTION WITH OTHER DRUGS

GENERIC NAME OR DRUG CLASS	COMBINED EFFECT
Amphetamines*	Increased amantadine effect. Possible excessive stimulation and agitation.
Anticholinergics*	Increased benefit, but excessive anticholinergic dose produces mental confusion, hallucinations, delirium.
Appetite suppressants*	Increased amantadine effect. Possible excessive stimulation and agitation.
Guanfacine	Increased effect of both drugs.
Levodopa	Increased benefit of levodopa. Can cause agitation.
Sympathomimetics*	Increased amantadine effect. Possible excessive stimulation and agitation.

 ## POSSIBLE INTERACTION WITH OTHER SUBSTANCES

INTERACTS WITH	COMBINED EFFECT
Alcohol:	Increased alcohol effect. Possible fainting.
Beverages:	None expected.
Cocaine:	Dangerous overstimulation.
Foods:	None expected.
Marijuana:	None expected.
Tobacco:	None expected.

AMBENONIUM

BRAND NAMES

Mytelase

BASIC INFORMATION

Habit forming? No
Prescription needed? Yes
Available as generic? No
Drug class: Cholinergic (anticholinesterase)

 USES

- Treatment of myasthenia gravis.
- Treatment of urinary retention and abdominal distention.

 DOSAGE & USAGE INFORMATION

How to take:
Tablet—Swallow with liquid or food to lessen stomach irritation.

When to take:
As directed, usually 3 or 4 times a day.

If you forget a dose:
Take as soon as you remember up to 2 hours late. If more than 2 hours, wait for next scheduled dose (don't double this dose).

What drug does:
Inhibits the chemical activity of an enzyme (cholinesterase) so nerve impulses can cross the junction of nerves and muscles.

Time lapse before drug works:
3 hours.

Don't take with:
See Interaction column and consult doctor.

 OVERDOSE

SYMPTOMS:
Muscle weakness, cramps, twitching or clumsiness; severe diarrhea, nausea, vomiting, stomach cramps or pain; breathing difficulty; confusion, irritability, nervousness, restlessness, fear; unusually slow heartbeat; seizures.
WHAT TO DO:
- **Dial 0 (operator) or 911 (emergency) for an ambulance or medical help. Then give first aid immediately.**
- **See emergency information on inside covers.**

 POSSIBLE ADVERSE REACTIONS OR SIDE EFFECTS

SYMPTOMS	WHAT TO DO
Life-threatening:	
None expected.	
Common:	
• Mild diarrhea, nausea, vomiting, stomach cramps or pain.	Discontinue. Call doctor right away.
• Excess saliva, unusual sweating.	Continue. Call doctor when convenient.
Infrequent:	
• Confusion, irritability.	Discontinue. Seek emergency treatment.
• Constricted pupils, watery eyes, lung congestion, urgent or frequent urination.	Continue. Call doctor when convenient.
Rare:	
None expected.	

WARNINGS & PRECAUTIONS

Don't take if:
- You are allergic to any cholinergic or bromide.
- You take mecamylamine.

Before you start, consult your doctor:
- If you plan to become pregnant within medication period.
- If you have bronchial asthma.
- If you have heartbeat irregularities.
- If you have urinary obstruction or urinary-tract infection.

Over age 60:
Adverse reactions and side effects may be more frequent and severe than in younger persons.

Pregnancy:
No proven harm to unborn child. Avoid if possible. May increase uterus contractions close to delivery.

Breast-feeding:
No problems expected, but consult doctor.

Infants & children:
Not recommended.

Prolonged use:
Medication may lose effectiveness. Discontinuing for a few days may restore effect.

Skin & sunlight:
No problems expected.

Driving, piloting or hazardous work:
Don't drive or pilot aircraft until you learn how medicine affects you. Don't work around dangerous machinery. Don't climb ladders or work in high places. Danger increases if you drink alcohol or take medicine affecting alertness and reflexes, such as antihistamines, tranquilizers, sedatives, pain medicine, narcotics and mind-altering drugs.

Discontinuing:
Don't discontinue without doctor's advice until you complete prescribed dose, even though symptoms diminish or disappear.

Others:
No problems expected.

POSSIBLE INTERACTION WITH OTHER DRUGS

GENERIC NAME OR DRUG CLASS	COMBINED EFFECT
Anesthetics, local or general*	Decreased ambenonium effect.
Antiarrhythmics*	Decreased ambenonium effect.
Antibiotics*	Decreased ambenonium effect.
Anticholinergics*	Decreased ambenonium effect. May mask severe side effects.
Cholinergics, other*	Reduced intestinal-tract function. Possible brain and nervous-system toxicity.
Mecamylamine	Decreased ambenonium effect.
Nitrates*	Decreased ambenonium effect.
Quinidine	Decreased ambenonium effect.

POSSIBLE INTERACTION WITH OTHER SUBSTANCES

INTERACTS WITH	COMBINED EFFECT
Alcohol:	No proven problems with small doses.
Beverages:	None expected.
Cocaine:	Decreased ambenonium effect. Avoid.
Foods:	None expected.
Marijuana:	No proven problems.
Tobacco:	No proven problems.

AMILORIDE

BRAND NAMES

Midamor

BASIC INFORMATION

Habit forming? No
Prescription needed? Yes
Available as generic? Yes
Drug class: Diuretic

USES

Treatment for high blood pressure and congestive heart failure. Decreases fluid retention and prevents potassium loss.

DOSAGE & USAGE INFORMATION

How to take:
Tablet—Swallow with liquid.

When to take:
At the same time each day, preferably in the morning. May interfere with sleep if taken after 6 p.m.

If you forget a dose:
Take as soon as you remember up to 8 hours late. If more than 8 hours, wait for next scheduled dose (don't double this dose).

What drug does:
Blocks exchange of certain chemicals in the kidney so sodium is excreted. Conserves potassium.

Continued next column

OVERDOSE

SYMPTOMS:
Rapid, irregular heartbeat; confusion; shortness of breath; nervousness; extreme weakness.
WHAT TO DO:
- **Dial 0 (operator) or 911 (emergency) for an ambulance or medical help. Then give first aid immediately.**
- **If patient is unconscious and not breathing, give mouth-to-mouth breathing. If there is no heartbeat, use cardiac massage and mouth-to-mouth breathing (CPR). Don't try to make patient vomit. If you can't get help quickly, take patient to nearest emergency facility.**
- **See emergency information on inside covers.**

Time lapse before drug works:
2 hours.

Don't take with:
See Interaction column and consult doctor.

POSSIBLE ADVERSE REACTIONS OR SIDE EFFECTS

SYMPTOMS	WHAT TO DO
Life-threatening: None expected.	
Common: Headache, nausea, appetite loss, vomiting, diarrhea.	Continue. Call doctor when convenient.
Infrequent: • Cough, shortness of breath.	Discontinue. Call doctor right away.
• Dizziness, constipation, pain, bloating, muscle cramps.	Continue. Call doctor when convenient.
Rare: None expected.	

WARNINGS & PRECAUTIONS

Don't take if:
- You are allergic to amiloride.
- Your serum potassium level is high.

Before you start, consult your doctor:
- If you plan to become pregnant within medication period.
- If you have diabetes.
- If you have heart disease.
- If you have kidney or liver disease.

Over age 60:
Adverse reactions and side effects may be more frequent and severe than in younger persons. More likely to exceed safe potassium blood levels.

Pregnancy:
No proven harm to unborn child. Avoid if possible.

Breast-feeding:
No problems expected, but consult doctor.

Infants & children:
Not recommended.

Prolonged use:
No problems expected.

Skin & sunlight:
No problems expected.

Driving, piloting or hazardous work:
Don't drive or pilot aircraft until you learn how medicine affects you. Don't work around dangerous machinery. Don't climb ladders or work in high places. Danger increases if you drink alcohol or take medicine affecting alertness and reflexes, such as antihistamines, tranquilizers, sedatives, pain medicine, narcotics and mind-altering drugs.

Discontinuing:
Don't discontinue without doctor's advice until you complete prescribed dose, even though symptoms diminish or disappear.

Others:
Periodic physical checkups and potassium-level tests recommended.

POSSIBLE INTERACTION WITH OTHER DRUGS

GENERIC NAME OR DRUG CLASS	COMBINED EFFECT
Acebutolol	Increased antihypertensive effect. Dosages may require adjustment.
ACE inhibitors: captopril, enalapril, lisinopril*	Possible excessive potassium in blood.
Amiodarone	Increased risk of heartbeat irregularity due to low potassium.
Antihypertensives*	Increased effect of both drugs.
Blood-bank blood	Increased potassium levels.
Calcium supplements*	Increased calcium in blood.
Diuretics, other*	Increased effect of both drugs.
Labetalol	Increased antihypertensive effects.
Lithium	Possible lithium toxicity.
Nicardipine	Dangerous blood-pressure drop. Dosages may require adjustment.
Nitrates*	Excessive blood-pressure drop.
Oxprenolol	Increased antihypertensive effect. Dosages may require adjustment.
Potassium supplements*	Increased potassium levels.
Sodium bicarbonate	Decreased potassium levels.

POSSIBLE INTERACTION WITH OTHER SUBSTANCES

INTERACTS WITH	COMBINED EFFECT
Alcohol:	Increased blood-pressure drop. Avoid.
Beverages: Low-salt milk.	Possible excess potassium levels. Low-salt milk has extra potassium.
Cocaine:	Blood-pressure rise. Avoid.
Foods: Salt substitutes.	Possible excess potassium levels.
Marijuana:	None expected.
Tobacco:	None expected.

AMILORIDE & HYDROCHLOROTHIAZIDE

BRAND NAMES

Moduret   Moduretic

BASIC INFORMATION

Habit forming? No
Prescription needed? Yes
Available as generic? Yes
Drug class: Diuretic (thiazide),
    antihypertensive

USES

- Controls, but doesn't cure, high blood pressure.
- Reduces fluid retention (edema), decreasing likelihood of congestive heart failure.

DOSAGE & USAGE INFORMATION

How to take:
Tablet—Swallow with liquid. If you can't swallow whole, crumble tablet and take with liquid or food.

When to take:
At the same time each day, no later than 6 p.m.

If you forget a dose:
Take as soon as you remember up to 2 hours late. If more than 2 hours, wait for next scheduled dose (don't double this dose).

What drug does:
- Forces sodium and water excretion, conserves potassium, reducing body fluid.
- Relaxes muscle cells of small arteries.
- Reduced body fluid and relaxed arteries lower blood pressure.

Time lapse before drug works:
2-6 hours. May require several weeks to lower blood pressure.

Continued next column

OVERDOSE

SYMPTOMS:
Cramps, weakness, drowsiness, weak pulse, coma, rapid, irregular heartbeat.
WHAT TO DO:
- Dial 0 (operator) or 911 (emergency) for an ambulance or medical help. Then give first aid immediately.
- See emergency information on inside covers.

Don't take with:
- See Interaction column and consult doctor.
- Non-prescription drugs without consulting doctor.

POSSIBLE ADVERSE REACTIONS OR SIDE EFFECTS

SYMPTOMS	WHAT TO DO
Life-threatening: None expected.	
Common: • Increased thirst, irregular heartbeat, cramps in muscles, numbness and tingling in hands and feet, thready pulse, shortness of breath.	Discontinue. Call doctor right away.
• Tiredness, weakness, dry mouth, diarrhea, headache, appetite loss, nausea.	Continue. Call doctor when convenient.
Infrequent: Mood changes, constipation, decreased sex function, dizziness, lightheadedness.	Continue. Call doctor when convenient.
Rare: Jaundice; unusual bleeding or bruising; abdominal pain with nausea and vomiting; sore throat, fever, sores in mouth; hives, skin rash; joint pain.	Discontinue. Seek emergency treatment.

AMILORIDE & HYDROCHLOROTHIAZIDE

WARNINGS & PRECAUTIONS

Don't take if:
You are allergic to amiloride or any thiazide diuretic drug.

Before you start, consult your doctor:
- If you are allergic to any sulfa drug.
- If you have gout, diabetes, heart disease.
- If you have liver, pancreas or kidney disorder.

Over age 60:
Adverse reactions and side effects may be more frequent and severe than in younger persons, especially dizziness and excessive potassium loss.

Pregnancy:
Risk to unborn child outweighs drug benefits. Don't use.

Breast-feeding:
Drug passes into milk. Avoid drug or discontinue nursing until you finish medicine.

Infants & children:
Not recommended unless closely supervised.

Prolonged use:
You may need medicine to treat high blood pressure for the rest of your life.

Skin & sunlight:
May cause rash or intensify sunburn in areas exposed to sun or sunlamp. Avoid overexposure.

Driving, piloting or hazardous work:
Don't drive or pilot aircraft until you learn how medicine affects you. Don't work around dangerous machinery. Don't climb ladders or work in high places. Danger increases if you drink alcohol or take medicine affecting alertness and reflexes, such as antihistamines, tranquilizers, sedatives, pain medicine, narcotics and mind-altering drugs.

Discontinuing:
Don't discontinue without medical advice.

Others:
- Hot weather and fever may cause dehydration and drop in blood pressure. Dose may require temporary adjustment. Weigh daily and report any unexpected weight decreases to your doctor.
- May cause rise in uric acid, leading to gout.
- May cause blood-sugar rise in diabetics.
- Get periodic check-ups and potassium-level laboratory tests.

POSSIBLE INTERACTION WITH OTHER DRUGS

GENERIC NAME OR DRUG CLASS	COMBINED EFFECT
Allopurinol	Decreased allopurinol effect.
Antidepressants, tricyclic (TCA)*	Dangerous drop in blood pressure. Avoid combination unless under medical supervision.
Antihypertensives, other*	Increased effect of both drugs.
Barbiturates*	Increased hydro-chlorothiazide effect.
Beta-adrenergic blockers*	Increased antihyper-tensive effect. Dosages of both drugs may require adjustments.
Blood-bank blood	Increased potassium levels.
Carteolol	Increased antihyper-tensive effect.
Cortisone drugs*	Excessive potassium loss that causes dangerous heart rhythms.

Continued page 1074

POSSIBLE INTERACTION WITH OTHER SUBSTANCES

INTERACTS WITH	COMBINED EFFECT
Alcohol:	Dangerous blood-pressure drop.
Beverages: Low-salt milk.	Possible excess potassium levels. Low-salt milk has extra potassium.
Cocaine:	Increased risk of heart block and high blood pressure.
Foods: Salt substitutes.	Possible excess potassium levels.
Marijuana:	May increase blood pressure.
Tobacco:	None expected.

*See Glossary

AMINOBENZOATE POTASSIUM

BRAND NAMES

KPAB
Potaba
Potassium
  Aminobenzoate
Potassium
Para-
  aminobenzoate

BASIC INFORMATION

Habit forming? No
Prescription needed? Yes
Available as generic? No
Drug class: Antifibrosis

USES

Reduces inflammation and relieves contractions in tissues lying under the skin that have become tight from such disorders as dermatomyositis, Peyronie's disease, scleroderma, pemphigus, morphea.

DOSAGE & USAGE INFORMATION

How to take:
- Tablets—Dissolve in liquid or take with food to prevent stomach upset.
- Capsules—Take with full glass of liquid.
- Oral solution—Swallow with liquid to lessen stomach upset.
- Powder—Mix with liquid.

When to take:
At the same times each day, according to instructions on prescription label. Usually taken with meals and at bedtime with a snack.

If you forget a dose:
Take as soon as you remember up to 2 hours late. If more than 2 hours, wait for next scheduled dose (don't double this dose).

What drug does:
May increase ability of diseased tissues to use oxygen.

Time lapse before drug works:
May require 3 to 10 months for improvement to begin.

Don't take with:
See Interaction column and consult doctor.

OVERDOSE

SYMPTOMS:
Nausea, vomiting.
WHAT TO DO:
Overdose unlikely to threaten life. If person takes much larger amount than prescribed, call doctor, poison-control center or hospital emergency room for instructions.

POSSIBLE ADVERSE REACTIONS OR SIDE EFFECTS

SYMPTOMS	WHAT TO DO
Life-threatening: None expected.	
Common: Appetite loss, nausea, rash, fever.	Continue. Call doctor when convenient.
Infrequent: • Low blood sugar (hunger, anxiety, cold sweats, rapid pulse).	Discontinue. Seek emergency treatment. (Note: Take sugar or honey on the way to emergency room.)
• Sore throat.	Discontinue. Call doctor right away.
Rare: None expected.	

WARNINGS & PRECAUTIONS

Don't take if:
You are allergic to aminobenzoate potassium or aminobenzoic acid (PABA).

Before you start, consult your doctor:
- If you have low blood sugar.
- If you have diabetes mellitus.
- If you have kidney disease.

Over age 60:
Adverse reactions and side effects may be more frequent and severe than in younger persons, particularly low blood sugar.

Pregnancy:
Safety not established.

Breast-feeding:
Drug passes into milk. Avoid drug or discontinue nursing.

Infants & children:
Not recommended. Safety and dosage have not been established.

Prolonged use:
No problems expected.

Skin & sunlight:
No problems expected.

Driving, piloting or hazardous work:
No problems expected.

Discontinuing:
No problems expected.

Others:
If you become acutely ill and cannot eat well for even a short while, tell your doctor. These circumstances can lead to low blood sugar, and dosage may need adjustment.

POSSIBLE INTERACTION WITH OTHER DRUGS

GENERIC NAME OR DRUG CLASS	COMBINED EFFECT
Dapsone	Decreased dapsone effect.
Methotrexate	Increased methotrexate effect and toxicity.
Salicylates*	May increase salicylate blood level.
Sulfa drugs* (sulfonamides)	Decreased sulfa effect.

POSSIBLE INTERACTION WITH OTHER SUBSTANCES

INTERACTS WITH	COMBINED EFFECT
Alcohol:	None expected.
Beverages:	None expected.
Cocaine:	None expected.
Foods:	None expected.
Marijuana:	None expected.
Tobacco:	None expected.

AMIODARONE

BRAND NAMES

Cordarone

BASIC INFORMATION

Habit forming? No
Prescription needed? Yes
Available as generic? No
Drug class: Antiarrhythmic

 ## USES

Prevents and treats life-threatening heartbeat irregularities involving both the large chambers of the heart (auricles and ventricles).

 ## DOSAGE & USAGE INFORMATION

How to take:
Tablets—Swallow whole with liquid or food to lessen stomach irritation. If you can't swallow whole, crumble tablet and take with liquid or food.

When to take:
According to prescription instructions.

If you forget a dose:
Skip this dose and resume regular schedule. Do not double the next dose. If you forget 2 doses or more, consult your doctor.

What drug does:
- Slows nerve impulses in the heart.
- Makes heart muscle fibers less responsive to abnormal electrical impulses arising in the electrical regulatory system of the heart.

Continued next column

 ## OVERDOSE

SYMPTOMS:
Irregular heartbeat, loss of consciousness, seizures.
WHAT TO DO:
- **Dial 0 (operator) or 911 (emergency) for an ambulance or medical help. Then give first aid immediately.**
- **If patient is unconscious and not breathing, give mouth-to-mouth breathing. If there is no heartbeat, use cardiac massage and mouth-to-mouth breathing (CPR). Don't try to make patient vomit. If you can't get help quickly, take patient to nearest emergency facility.**
- **See emergency information on inside covers.**

Time lapse before drug works:
2 to 3 days to 2 to 3 months.

Don't take with:
See Interaction column and consult doctor.

 ## POSSIBLE ADVERSE REACTIONS OR SIDE EFFECTS

SYMPTOMS	WHAT TO DO
Life-threatening:	
Shortness of breath, difficulty breathing, cough (not uncommon).	Discontinue. Seek emergency treatment.
Common:	
• Walking difficulty, fever, numbness or tingling in hands or feet, shakiness, weakness in arms and legs.	Discontinue. Call doctor right away.
• Constipation, headache, appetite loss, nausea, vomiting.	Continue. Call doctor when convenient.
Infrequent:	
• Skin color change to blue-gray, blurred vision, cold feeling, dry eyes, nervousness, scrotum swelling or pain, insomnia, swollen feet and ankles, fast or slow heartbeat, eyes hurt in light, weight gain or loss.	Discontinue. Call doctor right away.
• Bitter or metallic taste, diminished sex drive, dizziness, flushed face.	Continue. Call doctor when convenient.
Rare:	
Jaundice, skin rash.	Discontinue. Call doctor right away.

WARNINGS & PRECAUTIONS

Don't take if:
You are allergic to amiodarone.

Before you start, consult your doctor:
- If you have liver, kidney or thyroid disease.
- If you have heart disease other than coronary artery disease.

Over age 60:
- Adverse reactions and side effects may be more frequent and severe than in younger persons. Ask about smaller doses.
- Pain in legs (while walking) considerably more likely.

Pregnancy:
Safety to unborn child unestablished. Thyroid abnormalities possible in fetus. Avoid if possible.

Breast-feeding:
Drug passes into milk. Avoid drug or discontinue nursing until you finish medicine. Consult doctor for advice on maintaining milk supply.

Infants & children:
Safety not established. Use only under close medical supervision.

Prolonged use:
- Blue-gray discoloration of skin may appear.
- Don't discontinue without consulting doctor. Dose may require gradual reduction if you have taken drug for a long time. Doses of other drugs may also require adjustment.

Skin & sunlight:
May cause rash or intensify sunburn in areas exposed to sun or sunlamp. Avoid undue exposure, use sunscreens.

Driving, piloting or hazardous work:
Avoid if you feel dizzy or lightheaded. Otherwise, no problems expected.

Discontinuing:
- Don't discontinue without consulting doctor. Dose may require gradual reduction if you have taken drug for a long time. Doses of other drugs may also require adjustment.
- Notify doctor if cough, fever, breathing difficulty or shortness of breath occur after discontinuing medicine.

Others:
Learn to check your own pulse. If it drops to lower than 50 or rises to higher than 100 beats per minute, don't take amiodarone until you consult your doctor.

POSSIBLE INTERACTION WITH OTHER DRUGS

GENERIC NAME OR DRUG CLASS	COMBINED EFFECT
Anticoagulants*	Increased anticoagulant effect.
Antiarrhythmics, other*	Increased likelihood of heartbeat irregularity.
Beta-adrenergic blockers*	Increased likelihood of slow heartbeat.
Cholestyramine	May decrease amiodarone blood levels.
Digitalis	Increased digitalis effect.
Diltiazem	Increased likelihood of slow heartbeat.
Diuretics*	Increased risk of heartbeat irregularity due to low potassium level.
Encainide	Increased effect of toxicity on the heart muscle.
Flecainide	Increased flecainide effect.
Nicardipine	Possible increased effect and toxicity of each drug.
Nifedipine	Increased likelihood of slow heartbeat.
Phenytoin	Increased effect of phenytoin.
Procainamide	Increased procainamide effect.
Quinidine	Increased quinidine effect.
Verapamil	Increased likelihood of slow heartbeat.

POSSIBLE INTERACTION WITH OTHER SUBSTANCES

INTERACTS WITH	COMBINED EFFECT
Alcohol:	Increased risk of heartbeat irregularity. Avoid.
Beverages:	None expected.
Cocaine:	Increased risk of heartbeat irregularity. Avoid.
Foods:	None expected.
Marijuana:	Possible irregular heartbeat. Avoid.
Tobacco:	Possible irregular heartbeat. Avoid.

*See Glossary

AMOBARBITAL

BRAND NAMES

Amytal
Dexamyl
Isobec

Novamobarb
Tuinal

BASIC INFORMATION

Habit forming? Yes
Prescription needed? Yes
Available as generic? Yes
Drug class: Sedative, hypnotic (barbiturate)

USES

- Reduces anxiety or nervous tension (low dose).
- Relieves insomnia (higher bedtime dose).

DOSAGE & USAGE INFORMATION

How to take:
Tablet, capsule or powder—Swallow with food or liquid to lessen stomach irritation. If you can't swallow whole, crumble tablet or open capsule and take with liquid or food.

When to take:
At the same times each day.

If you forget a dose:
Take as soon as you remember up to 2 hours late. If more than 2 hours, wait for next scheduled dose (don't double this dose).

What drug does:
May partially block nerve impulses at nerve-cell connections.

Time lapse before drug works:
60 minutes.

Continued next column

OVERDOSE

SYMPTOMS:
Deep sleep, weak pulse, coma.
WHAT TO DO:
- Dial 0 (operator) or 911 (emergency) for an ambulance or medical help. Then give first aid immediately.
- If patient is unconscious and not breathing, give mouth-to-mouth breathing. If there is no heartbeat use cardiac massage and mouth-to-mouth breathing (CPR). Don't try to make patient vomit. If you can't help quickly, take patient to nearest emergency facility.
- See emergency information on inside covers.

Don't take with:
- Non-prescription drugs without consulting doctor.
- See Interaction column and consult doctor.

POSSIBLE ADVERSE REACTIONS OR SIDE EFFECTS

SYMPTOMS	WHAT TO DO
Life-threatening: None expected.	
Common: Dizziness, drowsiness, "hangover" effect.	Continue. Call doctor when convenient.
Infrequent: • Rash or hives; swollen face, lips, eyelids; sore throat, fever.	Discontinue. Call doctor right away.
• Depression, confusion, slurred speech, nausea, vomiting, joint or muscle pain.	Continue. Call doctor when convenient.
Rare: • Agitation, slow heartbeat, breathing difficulty, jaundice.	Discontinue. Call doctor right away.
• Unexplained bleeding or bruising.	Continue. Call doctor when convenient.

WARNINGS & PRECAUTIONS

Don't take if:
- You are allergic to any barbiturate.
- You have porphyria.

Before you start, consult your doctor:
- If you have epilepsy, kidney or liver damage, asthma, anemia, chronic pain.
- If you will have surgery within 2 months, including dental surgery, requiring general or spinal anesthesia.

Over age 60:
Adverse reactions and side effects may be more frequent and severe than in younger persons. Use small doses.

Pregnancy:
Risk to unborn child outweighs drug benefits. Don't use.

Breast-feeding:
Drug passes into milk. Avoid drug or discontinue nursing until you finish medicine. Consult doctor for advice on maintaining milk supply.

Infants & children:
May cause irritability. Use only under doctor's supervision.

Prolonged use:
- May cause addiction, anemia, chronic intoxication.
- May lower body temperature, making exposure to cold temperatures hazardous.

Skin & sunlight:
May cause rash or intensify sunburn in areas exposed to sun or sunlamp.

Driving, piloting or hazardous work:
Don't drive or pilot aircraft until you learn how medicine affects you. Don't work around dangerous machinery. Don't climb ladders or work in high places. Danger increases if you drink alcohol or take medicine affecting alertness and reflexes.

Discontinuing:
May be unnecessary to finish medicine. Follow doctor's instructions. If you develop withdrawal symptoms of hallucinations, agitation or sleeplessness after discontinuing, call doctor right away.

Others:
Great potential for abuse.

 POSSIBLE INTERACTION WITH OTHER DRUGS

GENERIC NAME OR DRUG CLASS	COMBINED EFFECT
Anticoagulants, oral*	Decreased anti-coagulant effect.
Anticonvulsants*	Changed seizure patterns.
Antidepressants, tricyclics (TCA)*	Decreased antidepressant effect. Possible dangerous oversedation.
Antidiabetics, oral*	Increased amobarbital effect.
Antihistamines*	Dangerous sedation. Avoid.
Aspirin	Decreased aspirin effect.
Beta-adrenergic blockers*	Decreased effect of beta-adrenergic blocker.
Carteolol	Increased barbiturate effect. Dangerous sedation.

Contraceptives, oral*	Decreased contraceptive effect.
Cortisone drugs*	Decreased cortisone effect.
Digitoxin	Decreased digitoxin effect.
Doxycycline	Decreased doxycycline effect.
Dronabinol	Increased effects of both drugs. Avoid.
Griseofulvin	Decreased griseofulvin effect.
Indapamide	Increased indapamide effect.
MAO inhibitors*	Increased amobarbital effect.
Metronidazole	May decrease metronidazole effect.
Mind-altering drugs*	Dangerous sedation. Avoid.
Nabilone	Greater depression of the central nervous system.
Narcotics*	Dangerous sedation. Avoid.
Non-steroidal anti-inflammatory drugs (NSAIDs)*	Decreased anti-inflammatory effect.
Pain relievers*	Dangerous sedation. Avoid.
Rifampin	Decreased amobarbital effect.
Sedatives*	Dangerous sedation. Avoid.

Continued page 1075

POSSIBLE INTERACTION WITH OTHER SUBSTANCES

INTERACTS WITH	COMBINED EFFECT
Alcohol:	Possible fatal oversedation. Avoid.
Beverages:	None expected.
Cocaine:	Decreased amobarbital effect.
Foods:	None expected.
Marijuana:	Excessive sedation. Avoid.
Tobacco:	None expected.

*See Glossary

AMOXICILLIN

BRAND NAMES

Amoxil	Penamox
Apo-Amoxi	Polymox
Augmentin	Robamox
Clavulin	Sumox
Larotid	Trimox
Moxilean	Utimox
Novamoxin	Wymox

BASIC INFORMATION

Habit forming? No
Prescription needed? Yes
Available as generic? Yes
Drug class: Antibiotic (penicillin)

USES

Treatment of bacterial infections that are susceptible to amoxicillin.

DOSAGE & USAGE INFORMATION

How to take:
- Tablet or capsule—Swallow with liquid on an empty stomach 1 hour before or 2 hours after eating.
- Chewable tablets—Chew well before swallowing.
- Liquid—Take with cold beverage. Liquid form is perishable and effective for only 7 days at room temperature. Effective for 14 days if stored in refrigerator. Don't freeze.

When to take:
Follow instructions on prescription label or side of package. Doses should be evenly spaced. For example, 4 times a day means before meals and bedtime.

If you forget a dose:
Take as soon as you remember. Continue regular schedule.

What drug does:
Destroys susceptible bacteria. Does not kill viruses.

Continued next column

OVERDOSE

SYMPTOMS:
Severe diarrhea, nausea or vomiting.
WHAT TO DO:
Overdose unlikely to threaten life. If person takes much larger amount than prescribed, call doctor, poison-control center or hospital emergency room for instructions.

Time lapse before drug works:
May be several days before medicine affects infection.

Don't take with:
See Interaction column and consult doctor.

POSSIBLE ADVERSE REACTIONS OR SIDE EFFECTS

SYMPTOMS	WHAT TO DO
Life-threatening:	
Hives, rash, intense itching, faintness soon after a dose (anaphylaxis); difficulty breathing.	Seek emergency treatment immediately.
Common:	
Dark or discolored tongue.	Continue. Tell doctor at next visit.
Infrequent:	
Mild nausea, vomiting, diarrhea.	Continue. Call doctor when convenient.
Rare:	
Unexplained bleeding, weakness, sore throat.	Discontinue. Call doctor right away.

WARNINGS & PRECAUTIONS

Don't take if:
You are allergic to amoxicillin, cephalosporin antibiotics, other penicillins. Life-threatening reaction may occur.

Before you start, consult your doctor:
If you are allergic to any substance or drug.

Over age 60:
You may have skin reactions, particularly around genitals and anus.

Pregnancy:
Studies inconclusive on harm to unborn child. Animal studies show fetal abnormalities. Decide with your doctor whether drug benefits justify risk to unborn child.

Breast-feeding:
Drug passes into milk. Child may become sensitive to penicillins and have allergic reactions to penicillin drugs. Avoid amoxicillin or discontinue nursing until you finish medicine. Consult doctor for advice on maintaining milk supply.

Infants & children:
No problems expected.

Prolonged use:
You may become more susceptible to infections caused by germs not responsive to amoxicillin. Super infection also a potential.

Skin & sunlight:
No problems expected.

Driving, piloting or hazardous work:
Usually not dangerous. Most hazardous reactions likely to occur a few minutes after taking amoxicillin.

Discontinuing:
Don't discontinue without doctor's advice until you complete prescribed dose, even though symptoms diminish or disappear.

Others:
No problems expected.

POSSIBLE INTERACTION WITH OTHER DRUGS

GENERIC NAME OR DRUG CLASS	COMBINED EFFECT
Beta-adrenergic blockers*	Increased chance of anaphylaxis (see emergency information on inside front cover).
Chloramphenicol	Decreased effect of both drugs.
Erythromycins*	Decreased effect of both drugs.
Loperamide	Decreased amoxicillin effect.
Paromomycin	Decreased effect of both drugs.
Tetracyclines*	Decreased effect of both drugs.
Troleandomycin	Decreased effect of both drugs.

POSSIBLE INTERACTION WITH OTHER SUBSTANCES

INTERACTS WITH	COMBINED EFFECT
Alcohol:	Occasional stomach irritation.
Beverages:	None expected.
Cocaine:	No proven problems.
Foods:	None expected.
Marijuana:	No proven problems.
Tobacco:	None expected.

*See Glossary

AMPHETAMINE

BRAND NAMES

Amphaplex 10 & 20	Biphetamine
Benzedrine	Declobese
Bexedrine	Obetrol 10 & 20

BASIC INFORMATION

Habit forming? Yes
Prescription needed? Yes
Available as generic? Yes
Drug class: Central-nervous-system
stimulant (amphetamine)

 ## USES

- Prevents narcolepsy (attacks of uncontrollable sleepiness).
- Controls hyperactivity in children.

 ## DOSAGE & USAGE INFORMATION

How to take:
Tablet—Swallow with liquid.

When to take:
- At the same times each day.
- Short-acting form—Don't take later than 6 hours before bedtime.
- Long-acting form—Take on awakening.

If you forget a dose:
- Short-acting form—Take up to 2 hours late. If more than 2 hours, wait for next dose (don't double this dose).
- Long-acting form—Take as soon as you remember. Wait 20 hours for next dose.

Continued next column

 ## OVERDOSE

SYMPTOMS:
Rapid heartbeat, hyperactivity, high fever, hallucinations, suicidal or homicidal feelings, convulsions, coma.
WHAT TO DO:
- Dial 0 (operator) or 911 (emergency) for an ambulance or medical help. Then give first aid immediately.
- See emergency information on inside covers.

What drug does:
- Narcolepsy—Apparently affects brain centers to decrease fatigue or sleepiness and increase alertness and motor activity.
- Hyperactive children—Calms children, opposite to effect on narcoleptic adults.

Time lapse before drug works:
15 to 30 minutes.

Don't take with:
See Interaction column and consult doctor.

 ## POSSIBLE ADVERSE REACTIONS OR SIDE EFFECTS

SYMPTOMS	WHAT TO DO
Life-threatening:	
None expected.	
Common:	
• Irritability, nervousness, insomnia.	Continue. Call doctor when convenient.
• Dry mouth.	Continue. Tell doctor at next visit.
Infrequent:	
• Dizziness; reduced alertness; blurred vision; fast, pounding heartbeat; unusual sweating.	Discontinue. Call doctor right away.
• Headache.	Continue. Call doctor when convenient.
• Diarrhea or constipation, appetite loss, stomach pain, nausea, vomiting, weight loss, diminished sex drive, impotence.	Continue. Tell doctor at next visit.
Rare:	
• Rash, hives; chest pain or irregular heartbeat; uncontrollable movements of head, neck, arms, legs.	Discontinue. Call doctor right away.
• Mood changes, swollen breasts.	Continue. Call doctor when convenient.

WARNINGS & PRECAUTIONS

Don't take if:
- You are allergic to any amphetamine.
- You will have surgery within 2 months, including dental surgery, requiring general or spinal anesthesia.

Before you start, consult your doctor:
- If you plan to become pregnant within medication period.
- If you have glaucoma.
- If you have heart or blood-vessel disease, or high blood pressure.
- If you have overactive thyroid, anxiety or tension.
- If you have a severe mental illness (especially children).

Over age 60:
Adverse reactions and side effects may be more frequent and severe than in younger persons.

Pregnancy:
Risk to unborn child outweighs drug benefits. Don't use.

Breast-feeding:
Drug passes into milk. Avoid drug or discontinue nursing.

Infants & children:
Not recommended for children under 12.

Prolonged use:
Habit forming.

Skin & sunlight:
No problems expected.

Driving, piloting or hazardous work:
Don't drive or pilot aircraft until you learn how medicine affects you. Don't work around dangerous machinery. Don't climb ladders or work in high places. Danger increases if you drink alcohol or take medicine affecting alertness and reflexes.

Discontinuing:
May be unnecessary to finish medicine. Follow doctor's instructions.

Others:
- This is a dangerous drug and must be closely supervised. Don't use for appetite control or depression. Potential for damage and abuse.
- During withdrawal phase, may cause prolonged sleep of several days.

POSSIBLE INTERACTION WITH OTHER DRUGS

GENERIC NAME OR DRUG CLASS	COMBINED EFFECT
Acetazolamide	Increased amphetamine effect.
Anesthesias, general*	Irregular heartbeat.
Antidepressants, tricyclic (TCA)*	Decreased amphetamine effect.
Antihypertensives*	Decreased antihypertensive effect.
Carbonic anhydrase inhibitors*	Increased amphetamine effect.
Guanethidine	Decreased guanethidine effect.
Haloperidol	Decreased amphetamine effect.
MAO inhibitors*	May severely increase blood pressure.
Nabilone	Greater depression of the central nervous system.
Phenothiazines*	Decreased amphetamine effect.
Sodium bicarbonate	Increased amphetamine effect.

POSSIBLE INTERACTION WITH OTHER SUBSTANCES

INTERACTS WITH	COMBINED EFFECT
Alcohol:	Decreased amphetamine effect. Avoid.
Beverages: Caffeine drinks.	Overstimulation. Avoid.
Cocaine:	Dangerous stimulation of nervous system. Avoid.
Foods:	None expected.
Marijuana:	Frequent use— Severely impaired mental function.
Tobacco:	None expected.

AMPICILLIN

BRAND NAMES

Alpen	Penbritin
Amcill	Polycillin
Ampicin	Polycillin-N
Ampilean	Prinicipen
Apo-Ampi	SK-Ampicillin
NaMpiCIL	Supen
Novo-Ampicillin	Totacillin
Omnipen	Totacillin-N
Omnipen-N	

BASIC INFORMATION

Habit forming? No
Prescription needed? Yes
Available as generic? Yes
Drug class: Antibiotic (penicillin)

 ## USES

Treatment of bacterial infections that are susceptible to ampicillin.

 ## DOSAGE & USAGE INFORMATION

How to take:
- Capsules—Swallow with liquid on an empty stomach 1 hour before or 2 hours after eating.
- Chewable tablets—Chew well before swallowing.
- Liquid—Take with cold beverage. Liquid form is perishable and effective for only 7 days at room temperature. Effective for 14 days if stored in refrigerator. Don't freeze.

When to take:
Follow instructions on prescription label or side of package. Doses should be evenly spaced. For example, 4 times a day means before meals and at bedtime.

If you forget a dose:
Take as soon as you remember. Continue regular schedule.

Continued next column

 ## OVERDOSE

SYMPTOMS:
Severe diarrhea, nausea or vomiting.
WHAT TO DO:
Overdose unlikely to threaten life. If person takes much larger amount than prescribed, call doctor, poison-control center or hospital emergency room for instructions.

What drug does:
Destroys susceptible bacteria. Does not kill viruses.

Time lapse before drug works:
May be several days before medicine affects infection.

Don't take with:
See Interaction column and consult doctor.

 ## POSSIBLE ADVERSE REACTIONS OR SIDE EFFECTS

SYMPTOMS	WHAT TO DO
Life-threatening:	
Hives, rash, intense itching, faintness soon after a dose (anaphylaxis); difficulty breathing.	Seek emergency treatment immediately.
Common:	
Dark or discolored tongue.	Continue. Tell doctor at next visit.
Infrequent:	
Mild nausea, vomiting, diarrhea.	Continue. Call doctor when convenient.
Rare:	
Unexplained bleeding, weakness, sore throat.	Discontinue. Call doctor right away.

WARNINGS & PRECAUTIONS

Don't take if:
You are allergic to ampicillin, cephalosporin antibiotics, other penicillins. Life-threatening reaction may occur.

Before you start, consult your doctor:
If you are allergic to any substance or drug.

Over age 60:
You may have skin reactions, particularly around genitals and anus.

Pregnancy:
Studies inconclusive on harm to unborn child. Animal studies show fetal abnormalities. Decide with your doctor whether drug benefits justify risk to unborn child.

Breast-feeding:
Drug passes into milk. Child may become sensitive to penicillins and have allergic reactions to penicillin drugs. Avoid ampicillin or discontinue nursing until you finish medicine. Consult doctor for advice on maintaining milk supply.

Infants & children:
No problems expected.

Prolonged use:
You may become more susceptible to infections caused by germs not responsive to ampicillin. Super-infection also a potential.

Skin & sunlight:
No problems expected.

Driving, piloting or hazardous work:
Usually not dangerous. Most hazardous reactions likely to occur a few minutes after taking ampicillin.

Discontinuing:
Don't discontinue without doctor's advice until you complete prescribed dose, even though symptoms diminish or disappear.

Others:
Urine sugar test for diabetes may show false positive result.

POSSIBLE INTERACTION WITH OTHER DRUGS

GENERIC NAME OR DRUG CLASS	COMBINED EFFECT
Beta-adrenergic blockers*	Increased chance of anaphylaxis (see emergency information on inside front cover).
Chloramphenicol	Decreased effect of both drugs.
Contraceptives, oral*	Occasionally impairs contraceptive efficiency.
Erythromycins*	Decreased effect of both drugs.
Loperamide	Decreased ampicillin effect.
Paromomycin	Decreased effect of both drugs.
Tetracyclines*	Decreased effect of both drugs.
Troleandomycin	Decreased effect of both drugs.

POSSIBLE INTERACTION WITH OTHER SUBSTANCES

INTERACTS WITH	COMBINED EFFECT
Alcohol:	Occasional stomach irritation.
Beverages:	None expected.
Cocaine:	No proven problems.
Foods:	None expected.
Marijuana:	No proven problems.
Tobacco:	None expected.

*See Glossary

ANALGESICS (Topical-Otic)

BRAND AND GENERIC NAMES

ANTIPYRINE AND
  BENZOCAINE
Auralgan

Aurodex
Auromid
Oto

BASIC INFORMATION

Habit forming? No
Prescription needed? Yes
Available as generic? No
Drug class: Analgesic-anesthetic (otic)

USES

Relieves pain of middle ear infections (otitis media). It does not treat the infection itself.

DOSAGE & USAGE INFORMATION

How to use:
- Warm ear drops under running water around the unopened bottle.
- Lie down with affected ear up.
- Adults—Pull ear lobe back and up.
- Children—Pull ear lobe down and back.
- Drop medicine into ear canal until canal is full.
- Stay lying down for 2 minutes.
- Gently insert cotton plug into ear to prevent leaking.

When to use:
Every 1 to 2 hours for 4 hours, then 4 times a day when needed for pain.

If you forget a dose:
Use as soon as you remember.

What drug does:
Functions as a topical anesthetic/analgesic on the eardrum.

Time lapse before drug works:
10 minutes.

Don't use with:
Other topical ear medicines without consulting your doctor.

OVERDOSE

SYMPTOMS:
None expected.
WHAT TO DO:
Not intended for internal use. If child accidentally swallows, call poison-control center.

POSSIBLE ADVERSE REACTIONS OR SIDE EFFECTS

SYMPTOMS	WHAT TO DO
Life-threatening: None expected.	
Common: None expected.	
Infrequent: Itching or burning in ear (probably represents allergic reaction).	Discontinue. Call doctor right away.
Rare: None expected.	

WARNINGS & PRECAUTIONS

Don't use if:
You are allergic to any local anesthetic (name usually ends with 'caine').

Before you start, consult your doctor:
If eardrum is ruptured.

Over age 60:
No problems expected.

Pregnancy:
No problems expected.

Breast-feeding:
No problems expected.

Infants & children:
No problems expected.

Prolonged use:
Not intended for prolonged use.

Skin & sunlight:
No problems expected.

Driving, piloting or hazardous work:
No problems expected.

Discontinuing:
No problems expected.

Others:
- Keep cool, but don't freeze.
- Don't touch tip of dropper to any other surface.
- Don't rinse the dropper, wipe with clean cloth and close tightly.

POSSIBLE INTERACTION WITH OTHER DRUGS

GENERIC NAME OR DRUG CLASS	COMBINED EFFECT
None expected.	

POSSIBLE INTERACTION WITH OTHER SUBSTANCES

INTERACTS WITH	COMBINED EFFECT
Alcohol:	None expected.
Beverages:	None expected.
Cocaine:	None expected.
Foods:	None expected.
Marijuana:	None expected.
Tobacco:	None expected.

ANDROGENS

BRAND AND GENERIC NAMES

See complete list of brand names in the *Brand Name Directory*, page 1054.

BASIC INFORMATION

Habit forming? No
Available as generic? Yes
Prescription needed? Yes
Drug class: Androgens

 USES

- Corrects male hormone deficiency.
- Reduces "male menopause" symptoms (loss of sex drive, depression, anxiety).
- Decreases calcium loss of osteoporosis (softened bones).
- Blocks growth of breast-cancer cells in females.
- Corrects undescended testicles in male children.
- Reduces breast pain and fullness following childbirth.
- Augments treatment of aplastic anemia.
- Stimulates weight gain after illness, injury or for chronically underweight persons.
- Stimulates growth in treatment of dwarfism.

 DOSAGE & USAGE INFORMATION

How to take:
- Tablets or capsules—With food to lessen stomach irritation.
- Injection—Once or twice a month.

When to take:
At the same time each day.

If you forget a dose:
Take as soon as you remember up to 2 hours late. If more than 2 hours, wait for next scheduled dose (don't double this dose).

Continued next column

 OVERDOSE

SYMPTOMS:
None expected.
WHAT TO DO:
Overdose unlikely to threaten life. If person takes much larger amount than prescribed, call doctor, poison-control center or hospital emergency room for instructions.

What drug does:
- Stimulates cells that produce male sex characteristics.
- Replaces hormone deficiencies.
- Stimulates red-blood-cell production.
- Suppresses production of estrogen (female sex hormone).

Time lapse before drug works:
Varies with problems treated. May require 2 or 3 months of regular use for desired effects.

Don't take with:
See Interaction column and consult doctor.

 POSSIBLE ADVERSE REACTIONS OR SIDE EFFECTS

SYMPTOMS	WHAT TO DO
Life-threatening:	
Intense itching, weakness, loss of consciousness.	Seek emergency treatment immediately.
Common:	
• Acne or oily skin in females, deep voice, enlarged clitoris, frequent erections, swollen breasts in men.	Continue. Call doctor when convenient.
• Sore mouth, higher sex drive.	Continue. Tell doctor at next visit.
Infrequent:	
• Jaundice.	Discontinue. Seek emergency treatment.
• Depression or confusion, flushed face, rash or itch, nausea, vomiting, diarrhea, swollen feet or legs, vaginal bleeding.	Discontinue. Call doctor right away.
Rare:	
• Hives, black stool.	Discontinue. Seek emergency treatment.
• Sore throat, fever, abdominal pain.	Discontinue. Call doctor right away.

WARNINGS & PRECAUTIONS

Don't take if:
You are allergic to any male hormone.

Before you start, consult your doctor:
- If you might be pregnant.
- If you have cancer of prostate.
- If you have heart disease or arteriosclerosis.
- If you have kidney or liver disease.
- If you have breast cancer (males).
- If you have high blood pressure.
- If you have migraine attacks.
- If you have high level of blood calcium.
- If you have epilepsy.

Over age 60:
- May stimulate sexual activity.
- Can make high blood pressure or heart disease worse.
- Can enlarge prostate and cause urinary retention.

Pregnancy:
Risk to unborn child outweighs drug benefits. Don't use.

Breast-feeding:
Drug passes into milk. Avoid drug or discontinue nursing until you finish medicine. Consult doctor for advice on maintaining milk supply.

Infants & children:
Don't give to children younger than 2. Use with older children only under medical supervision.

Prolonged use:
- Reduces sperm count and volume of semen.
- Possible kidney stones.
- Unnatural hair growth and deep voice in women.

Skin & sunlight:
No problems expected.

Driving, piloting or hazardous work:
No problems expected.

Discontinuing:
No problems expected.

Others:
- May cause atrophy of testicles.
- Will not increase strength in athletes.

POSSIBLE INTERACTION WITH OTHER DRUGS

GENERIC NAME OR DRUG CLASS	COMBINED EFFECT
Anticoagulants*	Increased anticoagulant effect.
Antidiabetics, oral*	Increased antidiabetic effect.
Chlorzoxazone	Decreased androgen effect.
Insulin	Increased antidiabetic effect.
Oxyphenbutazone	Decreased androgen effect.
Phenobarbital	Decreased androgen effect.
Phenylbutazone	Decreased androgen effect.

POSSIBLE INTERACTION WITH OTHER SUBSTANCES

INTERACTS WITH	COMBINED EFFECT
Alcohol:	None expected.
Beverages:	None expected.
Cocaine:	No proven problems.
Foods: Salt.	Excessive fluid retention (edema). Decrease salt intake while taking male hormones.
Marijuana:	Decreased blood levels of androgens.
Tobacco:	No proven problems.

ANESTHETICS (Rectal)

BRAND AND GENERIC NAMES

Americaine
BENZOCAINE
DIBUCAINE
Ethyl Aminobenzoate
Fleet Relief
Nupercainal
Pontocaine Cream
Pontocaine Ointment

Preparation "H"
Proctofoam
TETRACAINE
TETRACAINE
  AND MENTHOL
Tronolane
Tronothane

BASIC INFORMATION

Habit forming? No
Prescription needed? Yes
Available as generic? Yes, Dibucaine. No others, but most brands are available without prescription.
Drug class: Anesthetic (rectal)

USES

- Relieves pain, itching and swelling of hemorrhoids (piles).
- Relieves pain of rectal fissures (breaks in lining membrane of the anus).

DOSAGE & USAGE INFORMATION

How to use:
- Rectal cream or ointment—Apply to surface of rectum with fingers. Insert applicator into rectum no farther than 1/2 and apply inside. Wash applicator with warm soapy water or discard.
- Aerosol foam—Read patient instructions. Don't insert in rectum. Use the special applicator and wash carefully after using.

When to use:
- As directed.
- Suppository—Remove wrapper and moisten with water. Lie on side. Push blunt end of suppository into rectum with finger. If suppository is too soft, run cold water over or put in refrigerator for 15 to 45 minutes before using wrapper.

Continued next column

OVERDOSE

SYMPTOMS:
None expected.
WHAT TO DO:
Not intended for internal use. If child accidentally swallows, call poison-control center.

If you forget a dose:
Use as soon as you remember.

What drug does:
Deadens nerve endings to pain and touch.

Time lapse before drug works:
5 to 15 minutes.

Don't use with:
Any other topical or rectal medicine without consulting your doctor.

POSSIBLE ADVERSE REACTIONS OR SIDE EFFECTS

SYMPTOMS	WHAT TO DO
Life-threatening None expected.	
Common None expected.	
Infrequent	
• Nervousness, trembling, hives, rash, itch, inflammation or tenderness not present before application, slow heartbeat.	Discontinue. Call doctor right away.
• Dizziness, blurred vision, swollen feet.	Continue. Call doctor when convenient.
Rare	
• Blood in urine.	Discontinue. Call doctor right away.
• Increased or painful urination.	Continue. Call doctor when convenient.

WARNINGS & PRECAUTIONS

Don't use if:
You are allergic to any topical anesthetic.

Before you start, consult your doctor:
- If you have skin infection at site of treatment.
- If you have had severe or extensive skin disorders such as eczema or psoriasis.
- If you have bleeding hemorrhoids.

Over age 60:
Adverse reactions and side effects may be more frequent and severe than in younger persons.

Pregnancy:
No proven harm to unborn child. Avoid if possible.

Breast-feeding:
No problems expected.

Infants & children:
Use caution. More likely to be absorbed through skin and cause adverse reactions.

Prolonged use:
Possible excess absorption. Don't use longer than 3 days for any one problem.

Skin & sunlight:
No problems expected.

Driving, piloting or hazardous work:
No problems expected.

Discontinuing:
May be unnecessary to finish medicine. Follow doctor's instructions.

Others:
- Report any rectal bleeding to your doctor.
- Keep cool, but don't freeze.

POSSIBLE INTERACTION WITH OTHER DRUGS

GENERIC NAME OR DRUG CLASS	COMBINED EFFECT
Sulfa drugs*	Decreased anti-infective effect of sulfa drugs.

POSSIBLE INTERACTION WITH OTHER SUBSTANCES

INTERACTS WITH	COMBINED EFFECT
Alcohol:	None expected.
Beverages:	None expected.
Cocaine:	Possible nervous-system toxicity. Avoid.
Foods:	None expected.
Marijuana:	None expected.
Tobacco:	None expected.

ANESTHETICS (Topical)

BRAND NAMES

See complete list of brand names in the *Brand Name Directory*, page 1054.

BASIC INFORMATION

Habit forming? No
Prescription needed?
  High strength: Yes
  Low strength: No
Available as generic? Yes
Drug class: Anesthetic (topical)

USES

- Relieves pain and itch of sunburn, insect bites, scratches and other minor skin irritations.
- Relieves discomfort and itch of hemorrhoids and other disorders of anus and rectum.

DOSAGE & USAGE INFORMATION

How to use:
- Suppositories—Remove wrapper and moisten suppository with water. Gently insert larger end into rectum. Push well into rectum with finger.
- All other forms—Use only enough to cover irritated area. Follow instructions on label.

When to use:
When needed for discomfort, no more often than every hour.

If you forget an application:
Use as needed.

What drug does:
Blocks pain impulses from skin to brain.

Time lapse before drug works:
3 to 15 minutes.

Don't take with:
See Interaction column and consult doctor.

OVERDOSE

SYMPTOMS:
If swallowed or inhaled—Dizziness, nervousness, trembling, seizures.
WHAT TO DO:
- **Dial 0 (operator) or 911 (emergency) for an ambulance or medical help. Then give first aid immediately.**
- **See emergency information on inside covers.**

POSSIBLE ADVERSE REACTIONS OR SIDE EFFECTS

SYMPTOMS	WHAT TO DO
Life-threatening:	
None expected.	
Common:	
None expected.	
Infrequent:	
• Nervousness; trembling; hives, rash, itch; inflammation or tenderness not present before application; slow heartbeat.	Discontinue. Call doctor right away.
• Dizziness, blurred vision, swollen feet.	Continue. Call doctor when convenient.
Rare:	
• Blood in urine.	Discontinue. Call doctor right away.
• Increased or painful urination.	Continue. Call doctor when convenient.

WARNINGS & PRECAUTIONS

Don't use if:
You are allergic to any topical anesthetic.

Before you start, consult your doctor:
- If you have skin infection at site of treatment.
- If you have had severe or extensive skin disorders such as eczema or psoriasis.
- If you have bleeding hemorrhoids.

Over age 60:
Adverse reactions and side effects may be more frequent and severe than in younger persons.

Pregnancy:
No proven harm to unborn child. Avoid if possible.

Breast-feeding:
No problems expected.

Infants & children:
Use caution. More likely to be absorbed through skin and cause adverse reactions.

Prolonged use:
Possible excess absorption. Don't use longer than 3 days for any one problem.

Skin & sunlight:
No problems expected.

Driving, piloting or hazardous work:
No problems expected.

Discontinuing:
May be unnecessary to finish medicine. Follow doctor's instructions.

Others:
No problems expected.

POSSIBLE INTERACTION WITH OTHER DRUGS

GENERIC NAME OR DRUG CLASS	COMBINED EFFECT
Sulfa drugs*	Decreased effect of sulfa drugs for infection.

POSSIBLE INTERACTION WITH OTHER SUBSTANCES

INTERACTS WITH	COMBINED EFFECT
Alcohol:	None expected.
Beverages:	None expected.
Cocaine:	Possible nervous-system toxicity. Avoid.
Foods:	None expected.
Marijuana:	None expected.
Tobacco:	None expected.

*See Glossary

ANESTHETICS (Topical-Rectal)

BRAND NAMES

Anusol-H.C.

BASIC INFORMATION

Habit forming? No
Prescription needed? Yes
Available as generic? No
Drug class: Rectal adrenocorticoid emollient

 USES

Disorders of the anus and rectum including hemorrhoids, anal fissures, postoperative anal pain, proctitis, itching skin around anus.

 DOSAGE & USAGE INFORMATION

How to use:
- Rectal suppositories—Remove wrapper and moisten suppository with water. Gently insert into rectum, large end first. If suppository is too soft, chill in refrigerator or cool water before removing wrapper.
- Rectal cream—Attach plastic applicator, insert tip into rectum, gently squeeze the tube. Wash tip after emoving.
- Cream—Bathe and dry area before use. Apply small amount and rub gently.

When to use:
As directed.

If you forget a dose:
Use as soon as you remember.

What drug does:
Reduces inflammation by affecting enzymes that produce inflammation.

Time lapse before drug works:
15 to 20 minutes.

Don't use with:
See Interaction column and consult doctor.

 OVERDOSE

SYMPTOMS:
None expected.
WHAT TO DO:
Not for internal use. If child accidentally swallows, call poison-control center.

 POSSIBLE ADVERSE REACTIONS OR SIDE EFFECTS

SYMPTOMS	WHAT TO DO
Life-threatening: None expected.	
Common: None expected.	
Infrequent: Signs of infection— fever, redness, increased tenderness.	Discontinue. Call doctor right away.
Rare: Rectal bleeding, pain or burning; itching not present before beginning.	Discontinue. Call doctor right away.

WARNINGS & PRECAUTIONS

Don't use if:
You are allergic to any topical adrenocorticoid (cortisone) preparation.

Before you start, consult your doctor:
- If you plan pregnancy within medication period.
- If you have diabetes.
- If you have infection at treatment site.
- If you have stomach ulcer.
- If you have tuberculosis.

Over age 60:
Adverse reactions and side effects may be more frequent and severe than in younger persons, especially thinning of the skin.

Pregnancy:
Risk to unborn child outweighs drug benefits. Don't use.

Breast-feeding:
No problems expected, but check with doctor.

Infants & children:
- Use only under close medical supervision. Too much for too long can be absorbed into bloodstream through skin and retard growth.
- For infants in diapers, avoid plastic pants or tight diapers.

Prolonged use:
- Increases chance of absorption into bloodstream to cause side effects of oral cortisone drugs.
- May thin skin where used.

Skin & sunlight:
No problems expected.

Driving, piloting or hazardous work:
No problems expected.

Discontinuing:
May be unnecessary to finish medicine. Follow doctor's instructions.

Others:
- Store in cool place, but don't freeze.
- Wash with household detergents to remove stains from clothing.

POSSIBLE INTERACTION WITH OTHER DRUGS

GENERIC NAME OR DRUG CLASS	COMBINED EFFECT
Antibiotics* (topical)	Decreased antibiotic effects.
Antifungals* (topical)	Decreased antifungal effect.

POSSIBLE INTERACTION WITH OTHER SUBSTANCES

INTERACTS WITH	COMBINED EFFECT
Alcohol:	None expected.
Beverages:	None expected.
Cocaine:	None expected.
Foods:	None expected.
Marijuana:	None expected.
Tobacco:	None expected.

ANESTHETICS, DENTAL (Topical)

BRAND AND GENERIC NAMES

BENZOCAINE
BUTACAINE
LIDOCAINE
Americaine
Ethyl aminobenzoate
Hurricaine
Orabase with
  Benzocaine

Orajel
Butyn
Xylocaine
Xylocaine viscous
Triamcinolone in
  Orabase

BASIC INFORMATION

Habit forming? No
Prescription needed? Yes
Available as generic? Yes for Lidocaine, no
** for others**
Drug class: Anesthetic (topical)

 USES

Relieves pain or irritation in mouth caused by
toothache, teething, mouth sores, dentures,
braces, dental appliances. Also relieves pain of
sore throat for short periods of time.

 DOSAGE & USAGE
INFORMATION

How to use:
- For mouth problems—Apply to sore places
  with cotton-tipped applicator. Don't swallow.
- For throat—Gargle, but don't swallow.
- For aerosol spray—Don't inhale.

When to use:
As directed by physician or label on package.

If you forget a dose:
Use as soon as you remember.

What drug does:
Blocks pain impulses from the injection site to
the brain.

Continued next column

 OVERDOSE

SYMPTOMS:
Overabsorption by body—Dizziness, blurred
vision, seizures, drowsiness.
WHAT TO DO:
- **Dial 0 (operator) or 911 (emergency) for**
  an ambulance or medical help. Then give
  first aid immediately.
- **Not for internal use. If child accidentally**
  swallows, call poison-control center.
- **See emergency information on inside covers.**

Time lapse before drug works:
Immediately.

Don't use with:
See Interaction column and consult doctor.

 POSSIBLE
ADVERSE REACTIONS
OR SIDE EFFECTS

SYMPTOMS	WHAT TO DO
Life-threatening: Unusual anxiety, excitement, nervousness, irregular or slow heartbeat.	Discontinue. Seek emergency treatment.
Common: Ringing or buzzing in ears.	Discontinue. Call doctor right away.
Infrequent: Redness, irritation, sores not present before treatment, rash, itchy skin, hives.	Discontinue. Call doctor right away.
Rare: Paleness, sweating.	Discontinue. Call doctor right away.

WARNINGS & PRECAUTIONS

Don't use if:
You are allergic to any of the products listed.

Before you start, consult your doctor:
- If you are allergic to anything.
- If you have infection, canker sores or other sores in your mouth.
- If you take medicine for myasthenia gravis, eye drops for glaucoma or any sulfa medicine.

Over age 60:
Adverse reactions and side effects may be more frequent and severe than in younger persons. Ask doctor about smaller doses.

Pregnancy:
No problems expected, but check with doctor.

Breast-feeding:
No problems expected, but check with doctor.

Infants & children:
No problems expected, but check with doctor.

Prolonged use:
Not intended for prolonged use.

Skin & sunlight:
No problems expected.

Driving, piloting or hazardous work:
Wait to see if causes dizziness, sweating, drowsiness or blurred vision. If not, no problems expected.

Discontinuing:
No problems expected.

Others:
- Keep cool, but don't freeze.
- Don't puncture, break or burn aerosol containers.
- Don't eat, drink or chew gum for 1 hour after use.
- Heat and moisture in bathroom medicine cabinet can cause breakdown of medicine. Store someplace else.
- Before anesthesia, tell dentist about any medicines you take or use.

POSSIBLE INTERACTION WITH OTHER DRUGS

GENERIC NAME OR DRUG CLASS	COMBINED EFFECT
So remote, they are not considered clinically significant.	

POSSIBLE INTERACTION WITH OTHER SUBSTANCES

INTERACTS WITH	COMBINED EFFECT
Alcohol:	Adverse reactions more common.
Beverages:	None expected.
Cocaine:	May cause too much nervousness and trembling. Avoid.
Foods:	None expected.
Marijuana:	None expected.
Tobacco:	Avoid. Tobacco makes mouth problems worse.

ANESTHETICS, LOCAL (Ophthalmic)

BRAND AND GENERIC NAMES

Ak-Taine
Alcaine
Kainaire
Ocu-Caine
Ophthaine

Ophthetic
Pontocaine
PROPARACAINE
TETRACAINE

BASIC INFORMATION

Habit forming? No
Prescription needed? Yes
Available as generic? Yes
Drug class: Anesthetic, local (ophthalmic)

 ## USES

Eliminates pain in eye temporarily to measure pressure in eye to check for glaucoma, remove foreign bodies and stitches and corneal scraping for diagnostic procedures.

 ## DOSAGE & USAGE INFORMATION

How to use:
Eye drops
- Wash hands.
- Apply pressure to inside corner of eye with middle finger.
- Continue pressure for 1 minute after placing medicine in eye.
- Tilt head backward. Pull lower lid away from eye with index finger of the same hand.
- Drop eye drops into pouch and close eye. Don't blink.
- Keep eyes closed for 1 to 2 minutes.
Eye ointment
- Wash hands.
- Pull lower lid down from eye to form a pouch.
- Squeeze tube to apply thin strip of ointment into pouch.
- Close eye for 1 to 2 minutes.
- Don't touch applicator tip to any surface (including the eye). If you accidentally touch tip, clean with warm soap and water.
- Keep container tightly closed.
- Keep cool, but don't freeze.
- Wash hands immediately after using.

Continued next column

 ## OVERDOSE

SYMPTOMS:
None expected.
WHAT TO DO:
Not intended for internal use. If child accidentally swallows, call poison-control center.

When to use:
As directed on label.

If you forget a dose:
Use as soon as you remember.

What drug does:
Blocks conduction of pain impulses.

Time lapse before drug works:
13-15 seconds.

Don't use with:
Other drops in eyes such as antiglaucoma eye drops.

 ## POSSIBLE ADVERSE REACTIONS OR SIDE EFFECTS

SYMPTOMS	WHAT TO DO
Life-threatening: None-expected.	
Common: Mild stinging and burning.	Continue. Tell doctor at next visit.
Infrequent: Allergic reaction symptoms—itching, pain, redness, swelling, watery eyes.	Discontinue. Call doctor right away.
Rare (extremely): Symptoms of excess medicine absorbed by body—Weakness, increased sweating, nervousness, difficult breathing, vomiting, nausea, muscle spasms, irregular heartbeat, dizziness, drowsiness.	Discontinue. Call doctor right away.

WARNINGS & PRECAUTIONS

Don't use if:
You are allergic to any eye anesthetic.

Before you start, consult your doctor:
* If you have ever had an allergic reaction to any local anesthetic applied to skin, ears, mucous membranes or injected, such as benzocaine, butacaine, butamben, chloroprocaine, procaine, propoxycaine.
* If you have had an allergic reaction to sunscreens.

Over age 60:
No problems expected.

Pregnancy:
No problems expected, but check with doctor.

Breast-feeding:
No problems expected, but check with doctor.

Infants & children:
Use only under close medical supervision.

Prolonged use:
May retard healing. Avoid if possible.

Skin & sunlight:
No problems expected.

Driving, piloting or hazardous work:
No problems expected.

Discontinuing:
No problems expected.

Others:
* Don't rub or wipe eye until anesthetic has worn off (usually about 20 minutes) or until normal feeling in eye returns.
* Keep cool, but don't freeze.

POSSIBLE INTERACTION WITH OTHER DRUGS

GENERIC NAME OR DRUG CLASS	COMBINED EFFECT
Clinically significant interactions with oral or injected medicines unlikely.	

POSSIBLE INTERACTION WITH OTHER SUBSTANCES

INTERACTS WITH	COMBINED EFFECT
Alcohol:	None expected.
Beverages:	None expected.
Cocaine:	None expected.
Foods:	None expected.
Marijuana:	None expected.
Tobacco:	None expected.

ANTHRALIN (Topical)

BRAND NAMES

Anthra-Derm	Drithocreme HP
Anthraforte	Lasan
Anthranol	Lasan HP
Dithranol	Lasan Pomade
Drithocreme	Lasan Unguent

BASIC INFORMATION

Habit forming? No
Prescription needed? Yes
Available as generic? No
Drug class: Antipsoriasis; hair growth stimulant

USES

- Treats quiescent or chronic psoriasis.
- Stimulates hair growth in some people (not an approved use by the FDA).

DOSAGE & USAGE INFORMATION

How to use:
- Wear plastic gloves for all applications.
- If directed, apply at night.
- Cream, lotion, ointment—Bathe and dry area before use. Apply small amount and rub gently.
- If for short contact, same as above for cream.
- Leave on 20 to 30 minutes. Then remove medicine by bathing or shampooing.
- If for scalp overnight—Shampoo before use to remove scales or medicine. Dry hair. Part hair several times and apply to scalp. Wear plastic cap on head. Clean off next morning with petroleum, then shampoo.

When to use:
As directed.

If you forget a dose:
Use as soon as you remember.

What drug does:
Reduces growth activity within abnormal cells by inhibiting enzymes.

Continued next column

OVERDOSE

SYMPTOMS:
None expected.
WHAT TO DO:
Not for internal use. If child accidentally swallows, call poison-control center.

Time lapse before drug works:
May require several weeks or more.

Don't use with:
See Interaction column and consult doctor.

POSSIBLE ADVERSE REACTIONS OR SIDE EFFECTS

SYMPTOMS	WHAT TO DO
Life-threatening: None expected.	
Common: None expected.	
Infrequent: Redness or irritation of skin not present before application, rash.	Discontinue. Call doctor right away.
Rare: None expected.	

WARNINGS & PRECAUTIONS

Don't use if:
- You are allergic to anthralin.
- You have infected skin.

Before you start, consult your doctor:
- If you have chronic kidney disease.
- If you are allergic to anything.

Over age 60:
No problems expected, but check with doctor.

Pregnancy:
No problems expected, but check with doctor.

Breast-feeding:
No problems expected, but check with doctor.

Infants & children:
No problems expected, but check with doctor.

Prolonged use:
No problems expected, but check with doctor.

Skin & sunlight:
May cause rash or intensify sunburn in areas exposed to sun or sunlamp. Avoid undue exposure.

Driving, piloting or hazardous work:
No problems expected.

Discontinuing:
No problems expected.

Others:
- Keep cool, but don't freeze.
- Apply petroleum jelly to normal skin or scalp to protect areas not being treated.
- Will stain hair, clothing, shower, bathtub or sheets. Wash as soon as possible.
- Heat and moisture in bathroom medicine cabinet can cause breakdown of medicine. Store someplace else.

POSSIBLE INTERACTION WITH OTHER DRUGS

GENERIC NAME OR DRUG CLASS	COMBINED EFFECT
Antidiabetic agents*	Increased sensitivity to sun exposure.
Coal tar preparations*	Increased sensitivity to sun exposure.
Diuretics, thiazide*	Increased sensitivity to sun exposure.
Griseofulvin	Increased sensitivity to sun exposure.
Methosalen	Increased sensitivity to sun exposure.
Nalidixic acid	Increased sensitivity to sun exposure.
Phenothiazines*	Increased sensitivity to sun exposure.
Sulfa medicine	Increased sensitivity to sun exposure.
Tetracyclines*	Increased sensitivity to sun exposure.
Trioxsalen	Increased sensitivity to sun exposure.

POSSIBLE INTERACTION WITH OTHER SUBSTANCES

INTERACTS WITH	COMBINED EFFECT
Alcohol:	None expected.
Beverages:	None expected.
Cocaine:	None expected.
Foods:	None expected.
Marijuana:	None expected.
Tobacco:	None expected.

BRAND AND GENERIC NAMES

Acne Aid
ALCOHOL
 AND ACETONE
ALCOHOL
 AND SULFUR
Liquimat
Portacne
Seba-Nil

Sebasum
SULFURATED LIME
Transact
Tyrosum
Vlem-Dome
Vlemasque
Vlemickz's solution
Xerac

BASIC INFORMATION

Habit forming? No
Prescription needed? Yes
Available as generic? No
Drug class: Anti-acne agent, cleansing
 agent

 ## USES

Treats acne or oily skin.

 ## DOSAGE & USAGE INFORMATION

How to use:
Lotion, gel or pledget—Start with small amount
and wipe over face to remove dirt and surface
oil. Don't apply to wounds or burns. Don't rinse
with water and avoid contact with eyes. Skin
may be more sensitive in dry or cold climates.

When to use:
As directed. May increase frequency up to 3 or
more times daily as tolerated. Warm, humid
weather may allow more frequent use.

If you forget a dose:
Use as soon as you remember and then go
back to regular schedule.

What drug does:
Helps remove oil from skin's surface.

Time lapse before drug works:
Works immediately.

Continued next column

 ## OVERDOSE

SYMPTOMS:
None expected.
WHAT TO DO:
- Not for internal use. If child accidentally
 swallows, call poison-control center.
- Dial 0 (operator) or 911 (emergency) for
 an ambulance or medical help. Then give
 first aid immediately.
- See emergency information on inside
 covers.

Don't use with:
- Other topical acne treatments unless directed
 by doctor.
- See Interaction column and consult doctor.

 ## POSSIBLE ADVERSE REACTIONS OR SIDE EFFECTS

SYMPTOMS	WHAT TO DO
Life-threatening None expected.	
Common None expected.	
Infrequent Skin infection, pustules or rash; unusual pain, swelling or redness of treated skin; burning or stinging of skin.	Discontinue. Call doctor right away.
Rare None expected.	

WARNINGS & PRECAUTIONS

Don't use if:
You have to apply over a wounded or burned area.

Before you start, consult your doctor:
If you use benzoyl peroxide, resorcinol, salicylic acid, sulfur or tretinoin (vitamin A acid).

Over age 60:
No problems expected.

Pregnancy:
No problems expected, but check with doctor.

Breast-feeding:
No problems expected, but check with doctor.

Infants & children:
No problems expected, but check with doctor. Use only under close medical supervision.

Prolonged use:
Excessive drying of skin.

Skin & sunlight:
No problems expected, but check with doctor.

Driving, piloting or hazardous work:
No problems expected, but check with doctor.

Discontinuing:
No problems expected, but check with doctor.

Others:
Some antiacne agents are flammable. Don't use near fire or while smoking.

POSSIBLE INTERACTION WITH OTHER DRUGS

GENERIC NAME OR DRUG CLASS	COMBINED EFFECT
Abrasive or medicated soaps	Irritation or too much drying.
Other topical acne preparations	Irritation or too much drying.
After-shave lotions	Irritation or too much drying.
Perfumed toilet water	Irritation or too much drying.
Drying cosmetic soaps	Irritation or too much drying.
Isoretinoin	Irritation or too much drying.
"Cover-up" cosmetics	Irritation or too much drying.
Preparations containing skin peeling agents such as benzoyl peroxide, esorcinol, salicylic acid, sulfur, tretinoin	Irritation or too much drying.
Mercury compounds	May stain skin black and smell bad.

POSSIBLE INTERACTION WITH OTHER SUBSTANCES

INTERACTS WITH	COMBINED EFFECT
Alcohol:	None expected.
Beverages:	None expected.
Cocaine:	None expected.
Foods:	None expected.
Marijuana:	None expected.
Tobacco:	None expected.

ANTI-ACNE (Topical)

BRAND NAMES

See complete list of brand names in the *Brand Name Directory*, page 1055.

BASIC INFORMATION

Habit forming? No
Prescription needed? Yes
Available as generic? Yes
Drug class: Antiacne (topical)

 ## USES

Treatment for acne, psoriasis, ichthyosis, keratosis, folliculitis, flat warts.

 ## DOSAGE & USAGE INFORMATION

How to use:
- Wash skin with non-medicated soap, pat dry, wait 20 minutes before applying.
- Cream or gel—Apply to affected areas with fingertips and rub in gently.
- Solution—Apply to affected areas with gauze pad or cotton swab. Avoid getting too wet so medicine doesn't drip into eyes, mouth, lips or inside nose.
- Follow manufacturer's directions on container.

When to use:
At the same time each day.

If you forget an application:
Use as soon as you remember.

What drug does:
Increases skin-cell turnover so skin layer peels off more easily.

Time lapse before drug works:
2 to 3 weeks. May require 6 weeks for maximum improvement.

Don't use with:
- Benzoyl peroxide. Apply 12 hours apart.
- See Interaction column and consult doctor.

 ## OVERDOSE

SYMPTOMS:
None expected.
WHAT TO DO:
If person swallows drug, call doctor, poison-control center or hospital emergency room for instructions.

 ## POSSIBLE ADVERSE REACTIONS OR SIDE EFFECTS

SYMPTOMS	WHAT TO DO
Life-threatening	
None expected.	
Common	
• Pigment change in treated area, warmth or stinging, peeling.	Continue. Tell doctor at next visit.
• Senstivity to wind or cold.	No action necessary.
Infrequent	
Blistering crusting, severe burning, swelling.	Discontinue. Call doctor right away.
Rare	
None expected.	

WARNINGS & PRECAUTIONS

Don't take if:
- You are allergic to tretinoin.
- You are sunburned, windburned or have an open skin wound.

Before you start, consult your doctor:
If you have eczema.

Over age 60:
Not recommended.

Pregnancy:
No proven harm to unborn child. Avoid if possible.

Breast-feeding:
No problems expected.

Infants & children:
Not recommended.

Prolonged use:
No problems expected.

Skin & sunlight:
- May cause rash or intensify sunburn in areas exposed to sun or sunlamp.
- In some animal studies, tretinoin caused skin tumors to develop faster when treated area was exposed to ultraviolet light (sunlight or sunlamp). No proven similar effects in humans.

Driving, piloting or hazardous work:
No problems expected.

Discontinuing:
Don't discontinue without doctor's advice until you complete prescribed dose, even though symptoms diminish or disappear.

Others:
Acne may get worse before improvement starts in 2 or 3 weeks. Don't wash face more than 2 or 3 times daily.

POSSIBLE INTERACTION WITH OTHER DRUGS

GENERIC NAME OR DRUG CLASS	COMBINED EFFECT
Anti-acne topical preparations (other)	Severe skin irritation.
Cosmetics (medicated)	Severe skin irritation.
Skin preparations with alcohol	Severe skin irritation.
Soaps or cleansers (abrasive)	Severe skin irritation.

POSSIBLE INTERACTION WITH OTHER SUBSTANCES

INTERACTS WITH	COMBINED EFFECT
Alcohol:	None expected.
Beverages:	None expected.
Cocaine:	None expected.
Foods:	None expected.
Marijuana:	None expected.
Tobacco:	None expected.

ANTIBACTERIALS (Ophthalmic)

BRAND NAMES

See complete list of brand names in the *Brand Name Directory*, page 1055.

BASIC INFORMATION

Habit forming? No
Prescription needed? Yes
Available as generic? Yes, for some
Drug class: Antibacterial (ophthalmic)

 USES

Helps body overcome eye infections on surface tissues of the eye.

 DOSAGE & USAGE INFORMATION

How to use:
Eye drops
- Wash hands.
- Apply pressure to inside corner of eye with middle finger.
- Continue pressure for 1 minute after placing medicine in eye.
- Tilt head backward. Pull lower lid away from eye with index finger of the same hand.
- Drop eye drops into pouch and close eye. Don't blink.
- Keep eyes closed for 1 to 2 minutes.

Eye ointment
- Wash hands.
- Pull lower lid down from eye to form a pouch.
- Squeeze tube to apply thin strip of ointment into pouch.
- Close eye for 1 to 2 minutes.
- Don't touch applicator tip to any surface (including the eye). If you accidentally touch tip, clean with warm soap and water.
- Keep container tightly closed.
- Keep cool, but don't freeze.
- Wash hands immediately after using.

When to use:
As directed. Don't miss doses.

If you forget a dose:
Use as soon as you remember.

 OVERDOSE

SYMPTOMS:
None expected.
WHAT TO DO:
Not intended for internal use. If child accidentally swallows, call poison-control center.

What drug does:
Penetrates bacterial cell membrane and prevents cells from multiplying.

Time lapse before drug works:
Begins in 1 hour. May require 7 to 10 days to control infection.

Don't use with:
Any other eye drops or ointment without checking with your ophthalmologist.

 POSSIBLE ADVERSE REACTIONS OR SIDE EFFECTS

SYMPTOMS	WHAT TO DO
Life-threatening: None expected.	
Common: Ointments cause blurred vision for a few minutes.	Continue. Tell doctor at next visit.
Infrequent: None expected.	
Rare: None expected.	

WARNINGS & PRECAUTIONS

Don't use if:
You are allergic to any antibiotic used on skin, ears, vagina or rectum.

Before you start, consult your doctor:
If you have had an allergic reaction to any medicine, food or other substances.

Over age 60:
No problems expected.

Pregnancy:
No problems expected, but check with doctor.

Breast-feeding:
No problems expected, but check with doctor.

Infants & children:
No problems expected.

Prolonged use:
Sensitivity reaction may develop.

Skin & sunlight:
No problems expected.

Driving, piloting or hazardous work:
No problems expected.

Discontinuing:
No problems expected.

Others:
- Notify doctor if symptoms fail to improve in 2 to 4 days.
- Keep cool, but don't freeze.

POSSIBLE INTERACTION WITH OTHER DRUGS

GENERIC NAME OR DRUG CLASS	COMBINED EFFECT
Clinically significant interactions with oral or injected medicines unlikely.	

POSSIBLE INTERACTION WITH OTHER SUBSTANCES

INTERACTS WITH	COMBINED EFFECT
Alcohol:	None expected.
Beverages:	None expected.
Cocaine:	None expected.
Foods:	None expected.
Marijuana:	None expected.
Tobacco:	None expected.

ANTIBACTERIALS (Otic)

BRAND AND GENERIC NAMES

CHLORAMPHENICOL
Chloromycetin
Colistin
Neomycin and
  Hydrocortisone
Coly-Mycin S
Cortisporin
Desonide and
  Acetic Acid
Garamycin
Genoptic

GENTAMICIN
HYDROCORTISONE
  AND ACETIC ACID
NEOMYCIN,
  POLYMIXIN B AND
  HYDRO-
    CORTISONE
Otobione
Tridesilon Solution
VoSol HC

BASIC INFORMATION

Habit forming? No
Prescription needed? Yes
Available as generic? No
Drug class: Antibacterial, otic

USES

Ear infections in external ear canal (not middle ear) caused by susceptible germs (bacteria, virus, fungus).

DOSAGE & USAGE INFORMATION

How to use:
Ear drops
- Warm ear drops under running water around the unopened bottle.
- Lie down with affected ear up.
- Adults—Pull ear lobe back and up.
- Children—Pull ear lobe down and back.
- Drop medicine into ear canal until canal is full.
- Stay lying down for 2 minutes.
- Gently insert cotton plug into ear to prevent leaking.

Ear ointment
- Apply small amount to skin just inside the ear canal.
- Use finger or piece of sterile gauze.
- Don't use cotton-tipped applicators.

Continued next column

OVERDOSE

SYMPTOMS:
None expected.
WHAT TO DO:
Not intended for internal use. If child accidentally swallows, call poison-control center.

When to use:
As directed on label.

If you forget a dose:
Use as soon as you remember.

What drug does:
Kills germs that infect the skin of the external ear canal.

Time lapse before drug works:
15 minutes.

Don't use with:
Other ear medications unless directed by your doctor.

POSSIBLE ADVERSE REACTIONS OR SIDE EFFECTS

SYMPTOMS	WHAT TO DO
Life-threatening None expected.	
Common None expected.	
Infrequent Itching, burning, redness, swelling.	Discontinue. Call doctor right away.
Rare None expected.	

WARNINGS & PRECAUTIONS

Don't use if:
You are allergic to any of the medicines listed.

Before you start, consult your doctor:
If eardrum is punctured.

Over age 60:
No problems expected.

Pregnancy:
No problems expected.

Breast-feeding:
No problems expected.

Infants & children:
No problems expected.

Prolonged use:
Not intended for prolonged use.

Skin & sunlight:
Skin sensitivity more likely.

Driving, piloting or hazardous work:
No problems expected.

Discontinuing:
No problems expected.

Others:
Keep cool, but don't freeze.

POSSIBLE INTERACTION WITH OTHER DRUGS

GENERIC NAME OR DRUG CLASS	COMBINED EFFECT
None expected.	

POSSIBLE INTERACTION WITH OTHER SUBSTANCES

INTERACTS WITH	COMBINED EFFECT
Alcohol:	None expected.
Beverages:	None expected.
Cocaine:	None expected.
Foods:	None expected.
Marijuana:	None expected.
Tobacco:	None expected.

ANTIBACTERIALS (Topical)

BRAND AND GENERIC NAMES

See complete list of brand and generic names in the *Brand & Generic Name Directory*, page 1055.

BASIC INFORMATION

Habit forming? No
Prescription needed? Yes
Available as generic? Yes
Drug class: Antibacterial (topical)

USES

Treats skin infections that may accompany burns, superficial boils, insect bites or stings, skin ulcers, minor surgical wounds.

DOSAGE & USAGE INFORMATION

How to use:
- Cream, lotion, ointment—Bathe and dry area before use. Apply small amount and rub gently.
- May cover with gauze or bandage if desired.

When to use:
3 or 4 times daily, or as directed by doctor.

If you forget a dose:
Use as soon as you remember.

What drug does:
Kills susceptible bacteria by interfering with bacterial DNA and RNA.

Time lapse before drug works:
Begins first day. May require treatment for a week or longer to cure infection.

Don't use with:
See Interaction column and consult doctor.

OVERDOSE

SYMPTOMS:
None expected.
WHAT TO DO:
- Not for internal use. If child accidentally swallows, call poison-control center.
- Dial 0 (operator) or 911 (emergency) for an ambulance or medical help. Then give first aid immediately.
- See emergency information on inside covers.

POSSIBLE ADVERSE REACTIONS OR SIDE EFFECTS

SYMPTOMS	WHAT TO DO
Life-threatening: None expected.	
Common: None expected.	
Infrequent: Itching, swollen, red skin.	Discontinue. Call doctor right away.
Rare: None expected.	

WARNINGS & PRECAUTIONS

Don't use if:
You are allergic to gentamycin or any topical medication.

Before you start, consult your doctor:
If any of the lesions on the skin are open sores.

Over age 60:
No problems expected.

Pregnancy:
No problems expected, but check with doctor.

Breast-feeding:
No problems expected, but check with doctor.

Infants & children:
No problems expected, but check with doctor.

Prolonged use:
No problems expected, but check with doctor.

Skin & sunlight:
No problems expected, but check with doctor.

Driving, piloting or hazardous work:
No problems expected, but check with doctor.

Discontinuing:
No problems expected, but check with doctor.

Others:
- Heat and moisture in bathroom medicine cabinet can cause breakdown of medicine. Store someplace else.
- Keep cool, but don't freeze.

POSSIBLE INTERACTION WITH OTHER DRUGS

GENERIC NAME OR DRUG CLASS	COMBINED EFFECT
Any other topical medication	Hypersensitivity reactions more likely to occur.

POSSIBLE INTERACTION WITH OTHER SUBSTANCES

INTERACTS WITH	COMBINED EFFECT
Alcohol:	None expected.
Beverages:	None expected.
Cocaine:	None expected.
Foods:	None expected.
Marijuana:	None expected.
Tobacco:	None expected.

BRAND NAMES

See complete list of brand names in the *Brand Name Directory*, page 1055.

BASIC INFORMATION

Habit forming? No
Prescription needed? Yes
Available as generic? Yes, some are
Drug class: Topical antibacterial, topical antifungal

USES

Treats eczema, other inflammatory skin conditions, athlete's foot, skin infections.

DOSAGE & USAGE INFORMATION

How to use:
- Cream, lotion, ointment—Bathe and dry area before use. Apply small amount and rub gently.
- Keep away from eyes.

When to use:
2 to 4 times a day.

If you forget a dose:
Use as soon as you remember.

What drug does:
Kills some types of fungus and bacteria on contact.

Time lapse before drug works:
2 to 4 weeks, sometimes longer.

Don't use with:
Other ointments, creams or lotions without consulting doctor.

OVERDOSE

SYMPTOMS:
Severe nausea, vomiting, diarrhea.
WHAT TO DO:
- **Not for internal use. If child accidentally swallows, call poison-control center.**
- **Dial 0 (operator) or 911 (emergency) for an ambulance or medical help. Then give first aid immediately.**
- **See emergency information on inside covers.**

POSSIBLE ADVERSE REACTIONS OR SIDE EFFECTS

SYMPTOMS	WHAT TO DO
Life-threatening: None expected.	
Common: May stain skin around nails.	Continue. Tell doctor at next visit.
Infrequent: Stomach cramps; hives; itching, burning, peeling, red, stinging, swelling skin.	Discontinue. Call doctor right away.
Rare: None expected.	

ANTIBACTERIALS, ANTIFUNGALS (Topical)

 WARNINGS & PRECAUTIONS

Don't use if:
You are allergic to clioquinol, iodine or any iodine-containing preparation.

Before you start, consult your doctor:
If you are allergic to anything that touches your skin.

Over age 60:
No problems expected.

Pregnancy:
No problems expected, but check with doctor.

Breast-feeding:
No problems expected, but check with doctor.

Infants & children:
No problems expected, but check with doctor.

Prolonged use:
No problems expected, but check with doctor.

Skin & sunlight:
No problems expected, but check with doctor.

Driving, piloting or hazardous work:
No problems expected, but check with doctor.

Discontinuing:
No problems expected, but check with doctor.

Others:
- If not improved in 2 weeks, check with doctor.
- May stain clothing or bed linens.
- May stain hair, skin and nails yellow.
- If accidentally gets into eyes, flush with clear water immediately.
- Tests of thyroid function may yield inaccurate results if you use clioquinol within 1 month before testing.

 POSSIBLE INTERACTION WITH OTHER DRUGS

GENERIC NAME OR DRUG CLASS	COMBINED EFFECT
None expected.	

 POSSIBLE INTERACTION WITH OTHER SUBSTANCES

INTERACTS WITH	COMBINED EFFECT
Alcohol:	None expected.
Beverages:	None expected.
Cocaine:	None expected.
Foods:	None expected.
Marijuana:	None expected.
Tobacco:	None expected.

ANTIBACTERIALS FOR ACNE (Topical)

BRAND AND GENERIC NAMES

Achromycin
Akne-mycin
A/T/S
Aureomycin
CHLORTETRA-
  CYCLINE
CLINDAMYCIN
  SOLUTION
Cleocin T
EryDerm
Erycette
Erymax

ERYTHROMYCIN
  OINTMENT,
  PLEDGETS,
  SOLUTION
Meclan
MECLOCYCLINE
Sansac
Staticin
T-Stat
TETRACYCLINE
Topicycline

BASIC INFORMATION

Habit forming? No
Prescription needed? Yes
Available as generic? No
Drug class: Antibacterial (topical)

 ## USES

Treats acne by killing skin bacteria that may be part of the cause of acne.

 ## DOSAGE & USAGE INFORMATION

How to use:
- Pledgets and solutions are flammable. Use away from flame or heat.
- Apply medication to entire area, not just to pimples.
- If you use other acne medicines on skin, wait an hour after using erythromycin before applying other medicine.
- Cream, lotion, ointment—Bathe and dry area before use. Apply small amount and rub gently.

When to use:
2 times a day, morning and evening, or as directed by your doctor.

If you forget a dose:
Use as soon as you remember.

What drug does:
Kills bacteria on skin, skin glands or in hair follicles.

Continued next column

 ## OVERDOSE

SYMPTOMS:
None expected.
WHAT TO DO:
Not for internal use. If child accidentally swallows, call poison-control center.

Time lapse before drug works:
3 to 4 weeks to begin improvement.

Don't use with:
- Other skin medicine without telling your doctor.
- See Interaction column and consult doctor.

 ## POSSIBLE ADVERSE REACTIONS OR SIDE EFFECTS

SYMPTOMS	WHAT TO DO
Life-threatening: None expected.	
Common: Stinging or burning of skin for a few minutes after application.	Continue. Tell doctor at next visit.
Infrequent: Red, peeling, itching, irritated skin.	Continue. Call doctor when convenient.
Rare: (Extremely; only when overuse leads to absorption into bloodstream) Abdominal pain, diarrhea, fever, nausea, vomiting, thirst, weakness, weight loss.	Discontinue. Call doctor right away.

WARNINGS & PRECAUTIONS

Don't use if:
You are allergic to erythromycin.

Before you start, consult your doctor:
- If you are allergic to any substance that touches your skin.
- If you use benzoyl peroxide, resorcinol, salicylic acid, sulfur or tretinoin (vitamin A acid).

Over age 60:
No problems expected.

Pregnancy:
No problems expected, but check with doctor.

Breast-feeding:
No problems expected, but check with doctor.

Infants & children:
No problems expected, but check with doctor.

Prolonged use:
Excess irritation to skin.

Skin & sunlight:
No problems expected, but check with doctor.

Driving, piloting or hazardous work:
No problems expected, but check with doctor.

Discontinuing:
No problems expected, but check with doctor.

Others:
- Use water-base cosmetics.
- Keep medicine away from mouth or eyes.
- If accidentally gets into eyes, flush immediately with clear water.
- Keep away from heat or flame.
- Keep cool, but don't freeze.

POSSIBLE INTERACTION WITH OTHER DRUGS

GENERIC NAME OR DRUG CLASS	COMBINED EFFECT
Abrasive or medicated soaps	Irritation or too much drying.
Other topical acne preparations	Irritation or too much drying.
After-shave lotions	Irritation or too much drying.
Perfumed toilet water	Irritation or too much drying.
Drying cosmetic soaps	Irritation or too much drying.
Isoretinoin	Irritation or too much drying.
"Cover-up" cosmetics	Irritation or too much drying.
Preparations containing skin peeling agents such as benzoyl peroxide, esorcinol, salicylic acid, sulfur, tretinoin	Irritation or too much drying.
Mercury compounds	May stain skin black and smell bad.

POSSIBLE INTERACTION WITH OTHER SUBSTANCES

INTERACTS WITH	COMBINED EFFECT
Alcohol:	None expected.
Beverages:	None expected.
Cocaine:	None expected.
Foods:	None expected.
Marijuana:	None expected.
Tobacco:	None expected.

BRAND AND GENERIC NAMES

ANISINDIONE
Anthrombin-K
Coumadin
Danilone
DICUMAROL
Dufalone
Hedulin
Liquamar
Marcumar
Marevan
Melitoxin

Miradon
Panwarfin
PHENINDIONE
PHENPROCOUMON
Sofarin
WARFARIN
   POTASSIUM
WARFARIN SODIUM
Warfilone
Warnerin

BASIC INFORMATION

Habit forming? No
Prescription needed? Yes
Available as generic? Yes
Drug class: Anticoagulant

USES

Reduces blood clots. Used for abnormal clotting inside blood vessels.

DOSAGE & USAGE INFORMATION

How to take:
Tablet—Swallow with liquid. If you can't swallow whole, crumble tablet and take with liquid or food.

When to take:
At the same time each day.

If you forget a dose:
Take as soon as you remember up to 12 hours late. If more than 12 hours, wait for next scheduled dose (don't double this dose). Inform your doctor of any missed doses.

What drug does:
Blocks action of vitamin K necessary for blood clotting.

Time lapse before drug works:
36 to 48 hours.

Continued next column

OVERDOSE

SYMPTOMS:
Bloody vomit and bloody or black stools, red urine.
WHAT TO DO:
- **Dial 0 (operator) or 911 (emergency) for an ambulance or medical help. Then give first aid immediately.**
- **See emergency information on inside covers.**

Don't take with:
See Interaction column and consult doctor.

POSSIBLE ADVERSE REACTIONS OR SIDE EFFECTS

SYMPTOMS	WHAT TO DO
Life-threatening: None expected.	
Common: Bloating, gas.	Continue. Tell doctor at next visit.
Infrequent: • Black stools or bloody vomit, coughing up blood.	Discontinue. Seek emergency treatment.
• Rash, hives, itch, blurred vision, sore throat, easy bruising, bleeding, cloudy or red urine, back pain, jaundice, fever, chills, fatigue, weakness.	Discontinue. Call doctor right away.
• Diarrhea, cramps, nausea, vomiting, swollen feet or legs, hair loss.	Continue. Call doctor when convenient.
Rare: • Necrosis of skin	Discontinue. Seek emergency treatment
• Dizziness, headache, mouth sores.	Discontinue. Call doctor right away.

WARNINGS & PRECAUTIONS

Don't take if:
- You have been allergic to any oral anticoagulant.
- You have a bleeding disorder.
- You have an active peptic ulcer.
- You have ulcerative colitis.

Before you start, consult your doctor:
- If you take any other drugs, including non-prescription drugs.
- If you have high blood pressure.
- If you have heavy or prolonged menstrual periods.
- If you have diabetes.
- If you have a bladder catheter.
- If you have serious liver or kidney disease.
- If you will have surgery within 2 months, including dental surgery, requiring general or spinal anesthesia.

Over age 60:
Adverse reactions and side effects may be more frequent and severe than in younger persons.

Pregnancy:
Risk to unborn child outweighs drug benefits.
Don't use.

Breast-feeding:
Drug filters into milk. May harm child. Avoid.

Infants & children:
Use only under doctor's supervision.

Prolonged use:
No problems expected.

Skin & sunlight:
No problems expected.

Driving, piloting or hazardous work:
- Avoid hazardous activities that could cause injury.
- Don't drive if you feel dizzy or have blurred vision.

Discontinuing:
Don't discontinue without consulting doctor.
Dose may require gradual reduction if you have
taken drug for a long time. Doses of other drugs
may also require adjustment.

Others:
Carry identification to state you take anticoagulants.

 POSSIBLE INTERACTION WITH OTHER DRUGS

GENERIC NAME OR DRUG CLASS	COMBINED EFFECT
Acetaminophen	Increased effect of anticoagulant.
Allopurinol	Increased effect of anticoagulant.
Amiodarone	Increased effect of anticoagulant.
Androgens*	Increased effect of anticoagulant.
Antacids* (large doses)	Decreased effect of anticoagulant.
Antibiotics*	Increased effect of anticoagulant.
Anticonvulsants, hydantoin*	Increased effect of both drugs.
Antidepressants, tricyclic (TCA)*	Increased effect of anticoagulant.
Antidiabetics, oral*	Increased effect of anticoagulant.
Antihistamines*	Unpredictable increased or decreased effect of anticoagulant.
Aspirin	Possible spontaneous bleeding.
Barbiturates*	Decreased effect of anticoagulant.
Benzodiazepines*	Unpredictable increased or decreased anticoagulant effect.
Bismuth subsalicylate	Increased risk of bleeding.
Calcium supplements*	Decreased anticoagulant effect.
Carbamazepine	Decreased effect of anticoagulant.
Diclofenac	Increased risk of bleeding.
Fluoxetine	May cause confusion, agitation, convulsions and high blood pressure. Avoid combining.
Griseofulvin	Decreased effect of anticoagulant.
Nicardipine	Possible increased anticoagulant effect.
Nizatidine	Increased anticoagulant effect.
Non-steroidal anti-inflammatory drugs (NSAIDs)*	Increased risk of bleeding.
Phenytoin	Decreased phenytoin levels.
Rifampin	Decreased effect of anticoagulant.
Suprofen	Increased risk of bleeding.
Vitamin K	Decreased effect of anticoagulant.

 POSSIBLE INTERACTION WITH OTHER SUBSTANCES

INTERACTS WITH	COMBINED EFFECT
Alcohol:	Can increase or decrease effect of anticoagulant. Use with caution.
Beverages:	None expected.
Cocaine:	None expected.
Foods: High in vitamin K such as fish, liver, spinach, cabbage.	May decrease anticoagulant effect.
Marijuana:	None expected.
Tobacco:	None expected.

*See Glossary

BRAND AND GENERIC NAMES

PARAMETHADIONE   TRIMETHADIONE
Paradione   Tridione

BASIC INFORMATION

Habit forming? No
Prescription needed? Yes
Available as generic? No
Drug class: Anticonvulsant (Dione-type)

USES

Controls but does not cure petit mal seizures (absence seizures).

DOSAGE & USAGE INFORMATION

How to take:
Tablets, capsules or liquid: Take with food or milk to lessen stomach irritation.

When to take:
At the same time each day.

If you forget a dose:
Take as soon as you remember up to 2 hours late. If more than 2 hours, wait for next scheduled dose (don't double this dose).

What drug does:
Raises threshold of seizures in cerebral cortex. Does not alter seizure pattern.

Time lapse before drug works:
1 to 3 hours.

Don't take with:
See Interaction column and consult doctor.

OVERDOSE

SYMPTOMS:
Bleeding, nausea, drowsiness, ataxia, coma.
WHAT TO DO:
- **Dial 0 (operator) or 911 (emergency) for an ambulance or medical help. Then give first aid immediately.**
- **If patient is unconscious and not breathing, give mouth-to-mouth breathing. If there is no heartbeat, use cardiac massage and mouth-to-mouth breathing (CPR). Don't try to make patient vomit. If you can't get help quickly, take patient to nearest emergency facility.**
- **See emergency information on inside covers.**

POSSIBLE ADVERSE REACTIONS OR SIDE EFFECTS

SYMPTOMS	WHAT TO DO
Life-threatening: None expected.	
Common: Dizziness, drowsiness, headache, rash.	Continue. Call doctor when convenient.
Infrequent: Itching, nausea, vomiting.	Continue. Call doctor when convenient.
Rare:	
• Changes in vision; sore throat with fever and mouth sores; bleeding gums; easy bleeding or bruising; smoky or bloody urine; jaundice; puffed hands, face, feet or legs; swollen lymph glands; unusual weakness and fatigue.	Discontinue. Call doctor right away.
• Sensitivity to light.	Continue. Call doctor when convenient.

ANTICONVULSANTS, DIONE-TYPE

WARNINGS & PRECAUTIONS

Don't take if:
You are allergic to this drug or any anticonvulsant.

Before you start, consult your doctor:
- If you are pregnant or plan pregnancy.
- If you have blood disease.
- If you have liver or kidney disease.
- If you have disease of optic nerve or eye.
- If you will have surgery within 2 months, including dental surgery, requiring general or spinal anesthesia.

Over age 60:
Adverse reactions and side effects may be more frequent and severe than in younger persons.

Pregnancy:
Risk to unborn child outweighs drug benefits. Don't use.

Breast-feeding:
No problems proven. Avoid if possible. Consult doctor.

Infants & children:
Use only under close medical supervision of clinician experienced in convulsive disorders.

Prolonged use:
Have regular checkups, especially during early months of treatment.

Skin & sunlight:
Increased sensitivity to sunlight or sun lamp. Avoid overexposure.

Driving, piloting or hazardous work:
Don't drive or pilot aircraft until you learn how medicine affects you. Don't work around dangerous machinery. Don't climb ladders or work in high places. Danger increases if you drink alcohol or take medicine affecting alertness and reflexes, such as antihistamines, tranquilizers, sedatives, pain medicine, narcotics and mind-altering drugs. Be especially careful driving at night because medicine can affect vision.

Discontinuing:
Don't discontinue without consulting doctor. Dose may require gradual reduction if you have taken drug for a long time. Doses of other drugs may also require adjustment.

Others:
Arrange for eye exams every 6 months as well as blood counts and kidney-function studies.

POSSIBLE INTERACTION WITH OTHER DRUGS

GENERIC NAME OR DRUG CLASS	COMBINED EFFECT
Antidepressants, tricyclic (TCA)*	Greater likelihood of seizures.
Antipsychotic medicines*	Greater likelihood of seizures.
Anticonvulsants*	Increased chance of blood toxicity.
Ethinamate	Dangerous increased effects of ethinamate. Avoid combining.
Fluoxetine	Increased depressant effects of both drugs.
Guanfacine	May increase depressant effects of either drug.
Leucovorin	High alcohol content of leucovorin may cause adverse effects.
Methyprylon	Increased sedative effect, perhaps to dangerous level. Avoid.
Sedatives, sleeping pills, alcohol, pain medicine, antihistamines, tranquilizers, narcotics, mind-altering drugs.	Extreme drowsiness. Avoid.

POSSIBLE INTERACTION WITH OTHER SUBSTANCES

INTERACTS WITH	COMBINED EFFECT
Alcohol:	Increased chance of seizures and liver damage. Avoid.
Beverages: Caffeine drinks.	May decrease anticonvulsant effect.
Cocaine:	Increased chance of seizures. Avoid.
Foods:	No problems expected.
Marijuana:	Increased chance of seizures. Avoid.
Tobacco:	Decreased absorption of medicine leading to uneven control of disease.

*See Glossary

BRAND AND GENERIC NAMES

Amicar
Aminocaproic Acid
Cyclokapron

Epsikapron
TRANEXAMIC ACID

BASIC INFORMATION

Habit forming? No
Prescription needed? Yes
Available as generic? Yes
Drug class: Antifibrinolytic, antihemorrhagic

 ## USES

- Treats serious bleeding, especially occurring after surgery, dental or otherwise.
- Sometimes used before surgery in hopes of preventing excessive bleeding in patients with disorders that increase the chance of serious bleeding.

 ## DOSAGE & USAGE INFORMATION

How to take:
- Tablet—Swallow with liquid or food to lessen stomach irritation. If you can't swallow whole, crumble tablet and take with liquid or food.
- Syrup—Take as directed on label.

When to take:
As directed by your doctor.

If you forget a dose:
Take as soon as you remember. Don't double this dose.

What drug does:
Inhibits activation of plasminogen to cause blood clots to disintegrate.

Time lapse before drug works:
Within 2 hours.

Don't take with:
- Thrombolytic chemicals such as streptokinase, urokinase.
- See Interaction column and consult doctor.

 ## OVERDOSE

SYMPTOMS:
None expected for oral forms. Injectable forms may cause drop in blood pressure or slow heartbeat.
WHAT TO DO:
Follow doctor's instructions.

 ## POSSIBLE ADVERSE REACTIONS OR SIDE EFFECTS

SYMPTOMS	WHAT TO DO
Life-threatening: None expected.	
Common: None expected.	
Infrequent: Dizziness; headache; muscular pain and weakness; red eyes; ringing in ears; skin rash; abdominal pain; irregular heartbeat; stuffy nose; decreased urine; swelling of feet, face, legs; weight gain.	Discontinue. Call doctor right away.
Rare: • Unusual tiredness.	Discontinue. Call doctor right away.
• Diarrhea, nausea, clotting of menstrual flow.	Continue. Call doctor when convenient.

WARNINGS & PRECAUTIONS

Don't take if:
- You are allergic to aminocaproic acid or tranexamic acid.
- You have a diagnosis of disseminated intravascular coagulation (DIC).

Before you start, consult your doctor:
- If you have heart disease.
- If you have bleeding from the kidney.
- If you have had impaired liver function.
- If you have had kidney disease or urination difficulty.
- If you have blood clots in parts of the body.

Over age 60:
No changes from other age groups expected.

Pregnancy:
Animal studies show fetal abnormalities. Decide with your doctor whether drug benefits justify risk to unborn child.

Breast-feeding:
No problems documented.

Infants & children:
Use for children only under doctor's supervision.

Prolonged use:
Unusual tiredness.

Skin & sunlight:
No problems expected.

Driving, piloting or hazardous work:
Don't drive or pilot aircraft until you learn how medicine affects you. Don't work around dangerous machinery. Don't climb ladders or work in high places. Danger increases if you drink alcohol or take medicine affecting alertness and reflexes, such as antihistamines, tranquilizers, sedatives, pain medicine, narcotics and mind-altering drugs.

Discontinuing:
Don't discontinue without consulting doctor. Dose may require gradual reduction if you have taken drug for a long time. Doses of other drugs may also require adjustment.

Others:
Should not be used in patients with disseminated intravascular coagulation.

POSSIBLE INTERACTION WITH OTHER DRUGS

GENERIC NAME OR DRUG CLASS	COMBINED EFFECT
Contraceptives, oral*	Increased possibility of blood clotting.
Estrogens*	Increased possibility of blood clotting.
Thrombolytic agents* (alteplase, streptokinase, urokinase)	Decreased effects of both drugs.

POSSIBLE INTERACTION WITH OTHER SUBSTANCES

INTERACTS WITH	COMBINED EFFECT
Alcohol:	Decreases effectiveness of thrombolytic agents.
Beverages:	No problems expected.
Cocaine:	Combined effect unknown. Avoid.
Foods:	No problems expected.
Marijuana:	Combined effect unknown. Avoid.
Tobacco:	Combined effect unknown. Avoid.

*See Glossary

ANTIFUNGALS (Topical)

BRAND NAMES

See complete list of brand names in the *Brand Name Directory*, page 1056.

BASIC INFORMATION

Habit forming? No
Prescription needed? Yes, for some
Available as generic? No
Drug class: Antifungal

USES

Fights fungus infections such as ringworm of the scalp, athlete's foot, jockey itch, "sun fungus," nail fungus and others.

DOSAGE & USAGE INFORMATION

How to use:
- Cream, lotion, ointment—Bathe and dry area before use. Apply small amount and rub gently.
- Powder—Apply lightly to skin.
- Don't bandage or cover treated areas with plastic wrap.
- Follow other instructions from manufacturer listed on label.

When to use:
Twice a day, morning and evening, unless otherwise directed by your doctor.

If you forget a dose:
Use as soon as you remember.

What drug does:
Kills fungi by damaging the fungal cell wall.

Time lapse before drug works:
May require 6 to 8 weeks for cure.

Don't use with:
Other skin medicines without telling your doctor.

OVERDOSE

SYMPTOMS:
None expected.
WHAT TO DO:
- Not for internal use. If child accidentally swallows, call poison-control center.
- Dial 0 (operator) or 911 (emergency) for an ambulance or medical help. Then give first aid immediately.
- See emergency information on inside covers.

POSSIBLE ADVERSE REACTIONS OR SIDE EFFECTS

SYMPTOMS	WHAT TO DO
Life-threatening None expected.	
Common None expected.	
Infrequent Itching, redness, swelling of treated skin not present before treatment.	Discontinue. Call doctor right away.
Rare None expected.	

WARNINGS & PRECAUTIONS

Don't use if:
You are allergic to any topical antifungal medicine listed.

Before you start, consult your doctor:
If you are allergic to anything that touches your skin.

Over age 60:
No problems expected.

Pregnancy:
No problems expected, but check with doctor.

Breast-feeding:
No problems expected, but check with doctor.

Infants & children:
No problems expected, but check with doctor.

Prolonged use:
No problems expected, but check with doctor.

Skin & sunlight:
No problems expected, but check with doctor.

Driving, piloting or hazardous work:
No problems expected, but check with doctor.

Discontinuing:
No problems expected, but check with doctor.

Others:
- Avoid contact with eyes.
- Heat and moisture in bathroom medicine cabinet can cause breakdown of medicine. Store someplace else.
- Keep cool, but don't freeze.
- Store away from heat or sunlight.
- Don't use on other members of the family without consulting your doctor.
- If using for jock itch, avoid wearing tight underwear.
- If using for athlete's foot, dry feet carefully after bathing, wear clean cotton socks with sandals or well-ventilated shoes.

POSSIBLE INTERACTION WITH OTHER DRUGS

GENERIC NAME OR DRUG CLASS	COMBINED EFFECT
None expected.	

POSSIBLE INTERACTION WITH OTHER SUBSTANCES

INTERACTS WITH	COMBINED EFFECT
Alcohol:	None expected.
Beverages:	None expected.
Cocaine:	None expected.
Foods:	None expected.
Marijuana:	None expected.
Tobacco:	None expected.

ANTIFUNGALS (Vaginal)

BRAND AND GENERIC NAMES

See complete list of brand names in the *Brand Name Directory*, page 1056.

BASIC INFORMATION

Habit forming? No
Prescription needed? Yes
Available as generic? Yes, some
Drug class: Antifungal (vaginal)

 ## USES

Treats fungus infections of the vagina.

 ## DOSAGE & USAGE INFORMATION

How to use:
- Vaginal creams—Insert into vagina with applicator as illustrated in patient instructions that comes with prescription.
- Vaginal tablets—Insert with applicator as illustrated.

When to use:
According to instructions. Usually once or twice daily.

If you forget a dose:
Use as soon as you remember.

What drug does:
Destroys fungus cells membrane causing loss of essential elements to sustain fungus cell life.

Time lapse before drug works:
Begins immediately. May require 2 weeks of treatment to cure vaginal fungus infections. Recurrence common.

Don't use with:
Other vaginal preparations or douches unless otherwise instructed by your doctor.

 ## OVERDOSE

SYMPTOMS:
None expected.
WHAT TO DO:
Overdose unlikely to threaten life.

 ## POSSIBLE ADVERSE REACTIONS OR SIDE EFFECTS

SYMPTOMS	WHAT TO DO
Life-threatening	
None expected.	
Common	
None expected.	
Infrequent	
Vaginal burning, itching, irriation, swelling of labia, redness, increased discharge (not present before starting medicine).	Discontinue. Call doctor right away.
Rare	
Skin rash, hives, irritation of sex partner's penis.	Discontinue. Call doctor right away.

WARNINGS & PRECAUTIONS

Don't use if:
- You are allergic to any of the products listed.
- You have pre-existing liver disease.

Before you start, consult your doctor:
If you are pregnant.

Over age 60:
No problems expected.

Pregnancy:
No problems expected, but check with doctor.

Breast-feeding:
No problems expected.

Infants & children:
Use only under close medical supervision.

Prolonged use:
No problems expected.

Skin & sunlight:
No problems expected.

Driving, piloting or hazardous work:
No problems expected.

Discontinuing:
Recurrence likely if you stop before time suggested.

Others:
- Gentian Violet and some of the other products can stain clothing. Sanitary napkins may protect against staining.
- Keep the genital area clean. Use plain unscented soap.
- Take showers rather than tub baths.
- Wear cotton panties or pantyhose with a cotton crotch. Avoid panties made from non-ventilating materials. Wear freshly laundered underwear.
- Don't sit around in wet clothing—especially a wet bathing suit.
- If you will take antibiotics in the future, ask your doctor about eating yogurt, sour cream, buttermilk or taking acidophilus tablets.
- After urination or bowel movements, cleanse by wiping or washing from front to back (vagina to anus).
- Don't douche unless your doctor recommends it.
- If urinating causes burning, urinate through a tubular device, such as a toilet-paper roll or plastic cup with the end cut out.

POSSIBLE INTERACTION WITH OTHER DRUGS

GENERIC NAME OR DRUG CLASS	COMBINED EFFECT
Clinically significant interactions with oral or injected medicines unlikely.	

POSSIBLE INTERACTION WITH OTHER SUBSTANCES

INTERACTS WITH	COMBINED EFFECT
Alcohol:	None expected.
Beverages:	None expected.
Cocaine:	None expected.
Foods:	None expected.
Marijuana:	None expected.
Tobacco:	None expected.

ANTIGLAUCOMA, LONG-ACTING (Ophthalmic)

BRAND AND GENERIC NAMES

DEMECARIUM   Floropryl
ECHOTHIOPHATE   Humorsol
ISOFLUROPHATE   Phospholine Iodide

BASIC INFORMATION

Habit forming? No
Prescription needed? Yes
Available as generic? No
Drug class: Antiglaucoma (ophthalmic)

USES

Treats glaucoma (open-angle type), glaucoma after some forms of eye surgery and a few other eye disorders.

DOSAGE & USAGE INFORMATION

How to use:
Eye drops
- Wash hands.
- Apply pressure to inside corner of eye with middle finger.
- Continue pressure for 1 minute after placing medicine in eye.
- Tilt head backward. Pull lower lid away from eye with index finger of the same hand.
- Drop eye drops into pouch and close eye. Don't blink.
- Keep eyes closed for 1 to 2 minutes.
- Press finger to tear duct in corner of eye for 2 minutes to prevent possible absorption by body.

Eye ointment
- Wash hands.
- Pull lower lid down from eye to form a pouch.
- Squeeze tube to apply thin strip of ointment into pouch.
- Close eye for 1 to 2 minutes.
- Don't touch applicator tip to any surface (including the eye). If you accidentally touch tip, clean with warm soap and water.
- Keep container tightly closed.
- Keep cool, but don't freeze.

Continued next column

OVERDOSE

SYMPTOMS:
None expected.
WHAT TO DO:
Not intended for internal use. If child accidentally swallows, call poison-control center.

- Wash hands immediately after using.
- Press finger to tear duct in corner of eye for 2 minutes to prevent possible absorption by body.

When to use:
As directed on label.

If you forget a dose:
Use as soon as you remember.

What drug does:
Inactivates an enzyme to reduce pressure inside the eye.

Time lapse before drug works:
5 to 60 minutes.

Don't use with:
Any other eye medicine without consulting your doctor.

POSSIBLE ADVERSE REACTIONS OR SIDE EFFECTS

SYMPTOMS	WHAT TO DO
Life-threatening: None expected.	
Common: Pupils become small.	No action necessary.
Infrequent: Blurred vision, change in vision, eye pain, eyelids twitch, headache, watery eyes.	Discontinue. Call doctor right away.
Rare: Decreased vision with veil or curtain appearing, loss of bladder control, slow heartbeat, increased sweating, weakness, difficult breathing, vomiting, nausea, diarrhea.	Discontinue. Call doctor right away.

WARNINGS & PRECAUTIONS

Don't use if:
You are allergic to demecarium, echothiophate, isoflurophate.

Before you start, consult your doctor:
- If you have a history of retinal detachment.
- If you plan surgery under general or local anesthesia.
- If you have asthma, epilepsy, Down's syndrome, eye infection or other eye disease, heart disease, Parkinson's disease, ulcer in stomach or duodenum.

Over age 60:
No problems expected.

Pregnancy:
No problems expected, but check with doctor.

Breast-feeding:
No problems expected, but check with doctor.

Infants & children:
Use under medical supervision only.

Prolonged use:
No problems expected.

Skin & sunlight:
No problems expected.

Driving, piloting or hazardous work:
Don't drive or pilot aircraft until you learn how medicine affects you. Don't work around dangerous machinery. Don't climb ladders or work in high places. Danger increases if you drink alcohol or take medicine affecting alertness and reflexes, such as antihistamines, tranquilizers, sedatives, pain medicine, narcotics and mind-altering drugs.

Discontinuing:
- Discontinue 2 to 3 weeks prior to eye surgery.
- Otherwise, don't discontinue without consulting your doctor. Dose may require gradual reduction if you have used drug for a long time. Doses of other drugs may also require adjustment.

Others:
- Keep appointments for regular eye examinations to measure pressure in the eye.
- Keep cool, but don't freeze.
- Eyeglass prescription may need changing.

POSSIBLE INTERACTION WITH OTHER DRUGS

GENERIC NAME OR DRUG CLASS	COMBINED EFFECT
Atropine (ophthalmic)	May not be safe. Check with doctor.
Cyclopentolate (ophthalmic)	Reduces effect of antiglaucoma eye medicines.
Insecticides or pesticides with organic phosphates	Increased toxic absorption of pesticides.
Medicines to treat myasthenia gravis	Additive toxicity.
Physostigmine (ophthalmic)	Shortens action of antiglaucoma medicines.
Topical anesthetics	Increased risk of toxic effects of antiglaucoma eye medicines.

POSSIBLE INTERACTION WITH OTHER SUBSTANCES

INTERACTS WITH	COMBINED EFFECT
Alcohol:	None expected.
Beverages:	None expected.
Cocaine:	None expected.
Foods:	None expected.
Marijuana:	None expected.
Tobacco:	None expected.

ANTIGLAUCOMA, SHORT-ACTING (Ophthalmic)

BRAND AND GENERIC NAMES

CARBACHOL
DIPIVEFRIN
Epifrin
Epinal
EPINEPHRINE
Epitrate
Eppy/N

Eserine
Glaucon
Isopto Carbachol
Isopto Eserine
Miostate
Mytrate
PHYSOSTIGMINE

BASIC INFORMATION

Habit forming? No
Prescription needed? Yes
Available as generic? Yes, some are
Drug class: Antiglaucoma, miotic

USES

Treats glaucoma (open-angle, secondary, angle-closure during or after eye surgery).

DOSAGE & USAGE INFORMATION

How to use:
Eye drops
- Wash hands.
- Apply pressure to inside corner of eye with middle finger.
- Continue pressure for 1 minute after placing medicine in eye.
- Tilt head backward. Pull lower lid away from eye with index finger of the same hand.
- Drop eye drops into pouch and close eye. Don't blink.
- Keep eyes closed for 1 to 2 minutes.

Eye ointment
- Wash hands.
- Pull lower lid down from eye to form a pouch.
- Squeeze tube to apply thin strip of ointment into pouch.
- Close eye for 1 to 2 minutes.
- Don't touch applicator tip to any surface (including the eye). If you accidentally touch tip, clean with warm soap and water.

Continued next column

OVERDOSE

SYMPTOMS:
None expected.
WHAT TO DO:
Not intended for internal use. If child accidentally swallows, call poison-control center.

- Keep container tightly closed.
- Keep cool, but don't freeze.
- Wash hands immediately after using.

When to use:
As directed on label.

If you forget a dose:
Use as soon as you remember.

What drug does:
Inactivates enzyme and facilitates movement of fluid (aquemous humor) into and out of the eye.

Time lapse before drug works:
10-30 minutes.

Don't use with:
Any other eye medicine without consulting your doctor.

POSSIBLE ADVERSE REACTIONS OR SIDE EFFECTS

SYMPTOMS	WHAT TO DO
Life-threatening None expected.	
Common Headache, stinging, burning, watery eyes.	Continue. Call doctor when convenient.
Infrequent Eye pain, changes in vision, blurred vision.	Discontinue. Call doctor right away.
Rare Faintness, increased sweating, irregular or fast heartbeat, paleness.	Discontinue. Call doctor right away.

WARNINGS & PRECAUTIONS

Don't use if:
You are allergic to any eye medicine for glaucoma.

Before you start, consult your doctor:
- If you plan to have eye or dental surgery.
- If you have any eye disease.
- If you have heart problems or high blood pressure.
- If you have diabetes.

Over age 60:
Adverse reactions and side effects may be more frequent and severe than in younger persons. Ask doctor about smaller doses.

Pregnancy:
Safety to unborn child unestablished. Avoid if possible.

Breast-feeding:
Safety unestablished. Avoid if possible.

Infants & children:
Use only under close medical supervision.

Prolonged use:
May be necessary.

Skin & sunlight:
No problems expected.

Driving, piloting or hazardous work:
Don't drive or pilot aircraft until you learn how medicine affects you. Don't work around dangerous machinery. Don't climb ladders or work in high places. Danger increases if you drink alcohol or take medicine affecting alertness and reflexes, such as antihistamines, tranquilizers, sedatives, pain medicine, narcotics and mind-altering drugs.

Discontinuing:
Don't discontinue without consulting your doctor. Dose may require gradual reduction if you have used drug for a long time. Doses of other drugs may also require adjustment.

Others:
- Most normal physical activities, including swimming or other exercise, are okay while you use this medicine.
- Keep cool, but don't freeze.
- Keep appointments for regular eye examinations to measure pressure in the eye.

POSSIBLE INTERACTION WITH OTHER DRUGS

GENERIC NAME OR DRUG CLASS	COMBINED EFFECT
Clinically significant interactions with oral or injected medicines unlikely.	

POSSIBLE INTERACTION WITH OTHER SUBSTANCES

INTERACTS WITH	COMBINED EFFECT
Alcohol:	None expected.
Beverages:	None expected.
Cocaine:	None expected.
Foods:	None expected.
Marijuana:	None expected.
Tobacco:	None expected.

ANTI-INFLAMMATORY (Otic)

BRAND AND GENERIC NAMES

BETAMETHASONE
Betnesol
Cortamed
Cortisol
Decadron

DECAMETHASONE
HYDROCORTISONE
Metroton
PREDNISOLONE

BASIC INFORMATION

Habit forming? No
Prescription needed? Yes
Available as generic? No
Drug class: Anti-inflammatory, otic;
adrenocorticoid, otic

USES

- Treats allergic conditions involving external ear.
- Used together with antibiotics to treat ear infections.
- Treats seborrheic and eczematoid dermatitis involving the ear.

DOSAGE & USAGE INFORMATION

How to use:
Ear drops
- Warm ear drops under running water around the unopened bottle.
- Lie down with affected ear up.
- Adults—Pull ear lobe back and up.
- Children—Pull ear lobe down and back.
- Drop medicine into ear canal until canal is full.
- Stay lying down for 2 minutes.
- Gently insert cotton plug into ear to prevent leaking.

Ear ointment
- Apply small amount to skin just inside the ear canal.
- Use finger or piece of sterile gauze.
- Don't use cotton-tipped applicators.

When to use:
As directed by your doctor.

If you forget a dose:
Use as soon as you remember.

Continued next column

OVERDOSE

SYMPTOMS:
None expected.
WHAT TO DO:
Not intended for internal use. If child accidentally swallows, call poison-control center.

What drug does:
Decreases tissue inflammation, decreases scarring.

Time lapse before drug works:
15 minutes.

Don't use with:
Other ear medications unless directed by your doctor.

POSSIBLE ADVERSE REACTIONS OR SIDE EFFECTS

SYMPTOMS	WHAT TO DO
Life-threatening: None expected.	
Common: None expected.	
Infrequent: Itching, burning, redness, swelling.	Discontinue. Call doctor right away.
Rare: None expected.	

WARNINGS & PRECAUTIONS

Don't use if:
You are allergic to any of the antibiotics listed.

Before you start, consult your doctor:
If eardrum is punctured.

Over age 60:
No problems expected.

Pregnancy:
No problems expected.

Breast-feeding:
No problems expected.

Infants & children:
Use small amounts only.

Prolonged use:
Not intended for prolonged use.

Skin & sunlight:
No problems expected.

Driving, piloting or hazardous work:
No problems expected.

Discontinuing:
No problems expected.

Others:
Keep cool, but don't freeze.

POSSIBLE INTERACTION WITH OTHER DRUGS

GENERIC NAME OR DRUG CLASS	COMBINED EFFECT
None expected.	

POSSIBLE INTERACTION WITH OTHER SUBSTANCES

INTERACTS WITH	COMBINED EFFECT
Alcohol:	None expected.
Beverages:	None expected.
Cocaine:	None expected.
Foods:	None expected.
Marijuana:	None expected.
Tobacco:	None expected.

ANTI-INFLAMMATORY, STEROIDAL (Ophthalmic)

BRAND NAMES

See complete list of brand names in the *Brand Name Directory*, page 1056.

BASIC INFORMATION

Habit forming? No
Prescription needed? Yes
Available as generic? Yes
Drug class: Adrenocorticoid (ophthalmic), anti-inflammatory steroidal (ophthalmic)

USES

- Relieves redness and irritation due to allergies or other irritants.
- Prevents damage to eye.

DOSAGE & USAGE INFORMATION

How to use:
Eye drops
- Wash hands.
- Apply pressure to inside corner of eye with middle finger.
- Continue pressure for 1 minute after placing medicine in eye.
- Tilt head backward. Pull lower lid away from eye with index finger of the same hand.
- Drop eye drops into pouch and close eye. Don't blink.
- Keep eyes closed for 1 to 2 minutes.

Eye ointment
- Wash hands.
- Pull lower lid down from eye to form a pouch.
- Squeeze tube to apply thin strip of ointment into pouch.
- Close eye for 1 to 2 minutes.
- Don't touch applicator tip to any surface (including the eye). If you accidentally touch tip, clean with warm soap and water.
- Keep container tightly closed.
- Keep cool, but don't freeze.
- Wash hands immediately after using.

Continued next column

OVERDOSE

SYMPTOMS:
None expected.
WHAT TO DO:
Not intended for internal use. If child accidentally swallows, call poison-control center.

When to use:
As directed.

If you forget a dose:
Use as soon as you remember.

What drug does:
Affects cell membranes and decreases response to irritating substances.

Time lapse before drug works:
Immediately.

Don't use with:
Medicines for abdominal cramps or glaucoma without first consulting doctor.

POSSIBLE ADVERSE REACTIONS OR SIDE EFFECTS

SYMPTOMS	WHAT TO DO
Life-threatening None expected.	
Common None expected.	
Infrequent Watery, stinging, burning eyes.	Continue. Call doctor when convenient.
Rare (extremely) Eye pain, blurred vision, eyelid droops, halos around lights, enlarged pupils.	Discontinue. Call doctor right away.

ANTI-INFLAMMATORY, STEROIDAL
(Ophthalmic)

 ## WARNINGS & PRECAUTIONS

Don't use if:
You are allergic to any cortisone medicine.

Before you start, consult your doctor:
If you have or ever have had any eye infection, glaucoma, virus (herpes) infection of the eye, tuberculosis of the eye.

Over age 60:
No problems expected.

Pregnancy:
Safety to unborn child unestablished. Avoid if possible.

Breast-feeding:
Safety unestablished. Avoid if possible.

Infants & children:
Use for short periods of time only.

Prolonged use:
Recheck with eye doctor at regular intervals.

Skin & sunlight:
No problems expected.

Driving, piloting or hazardous work:
No problems expected.

Discontinuing:
No problems expected.

Others:
- Cortisone eye medicines should not be used for bacterial, viral, fungal or tubercular infections.
- Keep cool, but don't freeze.
- Notify doctor if condition doesn't improve within 3 days.

 ## POSSIBLE INTERACTION WITH OTHER DRUGS

GENERIC NAME OR DRUG CLASS	COMBINED EFFECT
Clinically significant interactions with oral or injected medicines unlikely.	

 ## POSSIBLE INTERACTION WITH OTHER SUBSTANCES

INTERACTS WITH	COMBINED EFFECT
Alcohol:	None expected.
Beverages:	None expected.
Cocaine:	None expected.
Foods:	None expected.
Marijuana:	None expected.
Tobacco:	None expected.

ANTISEBORRHEIC (Topical)

BRAND AND GENERIC NAMES

Buf-Bar
Capitrol
DHS Zinc
Danex
Excel
Head and Shoulders
PYRITHIONE
SALICYLIC ACID,
  SULFUR AND
  COAL TAR

Sebex-T
Sebutone
SELENIUM
SULFIDE
Selsun
Selsun Blue
Sul-Blue
SULFUR
Vanseb-T
Zincon

BASIC INFORMATION

Habit forming? No
Prescription needed? Yes
Available as generic? No
Drug class: Antiseborrheic

USES

Treats dandruff or seborrheic dermatitis of scalp.

DOSAGE & USAGE INFORMATION

How to use:
- Wet hair and scalp.
- Apply enough medicine to form lather.
- Rub in well. Keep away from eyes.
- Allow to remain on scalp 3 to 5 minutes then rinse.
- Repeat above steps once.

When to use:
As directed by doctor. Twice a week for shampoo is average.

If you forget a dose:
Use as soon as you remember.

What drug does:
Slows cell growth in scales on scalp.

Continued next column

OVERDOSE

SYMPTOMS:
None expected.
WHAT TO DO:
- Not for internal use. If child accidentally swallows, call poison-control center.
- Dial 0 (operator) or 911 (emergency) for an ambulance or medical help. Then give first aid immediately.
- See emergency information on inside covers.

Time lapse before drug works:
Varies a great deal. If no improvement in 2 weeks, notify doctor.

Don't use with:
- Other scalp preparations without notifying doctor.
- See Interaction column and consult doctor.

POSSIBLE ADVERSE REACTIONS OR SIDE EFFECTS

SYMPTOMS	WHAT TO DO
Life-threatening None expected.	
Common None expected.	
Infrequent • Irritation not present before using, rash.	Discontinue. Call doctor right away.
• Dryness or itching scalp.	Continue. Call doctor when convenient.
Rare None expected.	

ANTISEBORRHEIC (Topical)

WARNINGS & PRECAUTIONS

Don't use if:
- You have had an allergic reaction to chloroxine, clioquinol (iodochlorhydroxyquin), iodoquinol (diiodohydroxyquin) or edate sodium.
- Scalp is blistered or infected with oozing or raw areas.

Before you start, consult your doctor:
If you are allergic to anything.

Over age 60:
No problems expected.

Pregnancy:
No problems expected, but check with doctor.

Breast-feeding:
No problems expected, but check with doctor.

Infants & children:
No problems expected, but check with doctor.

Prolonged use:
No problems expected, but check with doctor.

Skin & sunlight:
No problems expected, but check with doctor.

Driving, piloting or hazardous work:
No problems expected, but check with doctor.

Discontinuing:
No problems expected, but check with doctor.

Others:
- If medicine accidentally gets into eyes, flush them immediately with cool water.
- Heat and moisture in bathroom medicine cabinet can cause breakdown of medicine. Store someplace else.
- Keep cool, but don't freeze.

POSSIBLE INTERACTION WITH OTHER DRUGS

GENERIC NAME OR DRUG CLASS	COMBINED EFFECT
Other medical shampoos	May accentuate adverse reactions of each medicine.

POSSIBLE INTERACTION WITH OTHER SUBSTANCES

INTERACTS WITH	COMBINED EFFECT
Alcohol:	None expected.
Beverages:	None expected.
Cocaine:	None expected.
Foods:	None expected.
Marijuana:	None expected.
Tobacco:	None expected.

ANTITHYROID

BRAND AND GENERIC NAMES

METHIMAZOLE   Tapazole
PROPYLTHIOURACIL   Thiamazole
Propyl-Thyracil

BASIC INFORMATION

Habit forming? No
Prescription needed? Yes
Available as generic? Yes
Drug class: Antihyperthyroid

 ## USES

- Treatment of overactive thyroid (hyperthyroidism).
- Treatment of angina in patients who have overactive thyroid.

 ## DOSAGE & USAGE INFORMATION

How to take:
Tablet—Swallow with liquid or food to lessen stomach irritation. If you can't swallow whole, crumble tablet and take with liquid or food.

When to take:
At the same times each day.

If you forget a dose:
Take as soon as you remember up to 2 hours late. If more than 2 hours, wait for next scheduled dose (don't double this dose).

What drug does:
Prevents thyroid gland from producing excess thyroid hormone.

Time lapse before drug works:
10 to 20 days.

Don't take with:
- Anticoagulants
- See Interaction column and consult doctor.

 ## OVERDOSE

SYMPTOMS:
Bleeding, spots on skin, jaundice (yellow eyes and skin), loss of consciousness.
WHAT TO DO:
Overdose unlikely to threaten life. If person takes much larger amount than prescribed, call doctor, poison-control center or hospital emergency room for instructions.

 ## POSSIBLE ADVERSE REACTIONS OR SIDE EFFECTS

SYMPTOMS	WHAT TO DO
Life-threatening: None expected.	
Common: Skin rash, itching, dryness.	Discontinue. Call doctor right away.
Infrequent: Dizziness, taste loss, sore throat with chills and fever, abdominal pain, constipation, diarrhea.	Discontinue. Call doctor right away.
Rare: Headache; enlarged lymph glands; irregular or rapid heartbeat; unusual bruising or bleeding; backache; numbness or tingling in toes, fingers or face; joint pain; muscle aches; menstrual irregularities; jaundice; tired, weak, sleepy, listless; swollen eyes or feet.	Discontinue. Call doctor right away.

WARNINGS & PRECAUTIONS

Don't take if:
You are allergic to antithyroid medicines.

Before you start, consult your doctor:
- If you have liver disease.
- If you have blood disease.
- If you have an infection.
- If you take anticoagulants.

Over age 60:
Adverse reactions and side effects may be more frequent and severe than in younger persons.

Pregnancy:
Risk to unborn child outweighs drug benefits. Don't use.

Breast-feeding:
Drug filters into milk. May harm child. Don't use.

Infants & children:
Use only under special medical supervision by experienced clinician.

Prolonged use:
Adverse reactions and side effects more common.

Skin & sunlight:
No problems expected.

Driving, piloting or hazardous work:
Don't drive or pilot aircraft until you learn how medicine affects you. Don't work around dangerous machinery. Don't climb ladders or work in high places. Danger increases if you drink alcohol or take medicine affecting alertness and reflexes, such as antihistamines, tranquilizers, sedatives, pain medicine, narcotics and mind-altering drugs.

Discontinuing:
Don't discontinue without consulting doctor. Dose may require gradual reduction if you have taken drug for a long time. Doses of other drugs may also require adjustment.

Others:
No problems expected.

POSSIBLE INTERACTION WITH OTHER DRUGS

GENERIC NAME OR DRUG CLASS	COMBINED EFFECT
Anticoagulants*	Increased effect of anticoagulants.
Antineoplastic drugs*	Increased chance to suppress bone marrow.
Chloramphenicol	Increased chance to suppress bone marrow.

POSSIBLE INTERACTION WITH OTHER SUBSTANCES

INTERACTS WITH	COMBINED EFFECT
Alcohol:	Increased possibility of liver toxicity. Avoid.
Beverages:	No problems expected.
Cocaine:	Increased toxicity potential of medicines. Avoid.
Foods:	No problems expected.
Marijuana:	Increased rapid or irregular heartbeat. Avoid.
Tobacco:	Increased chance of rapid heartbeat. Avoid.

ANTIVIRALS (Ophthalmic)

BRAND AND GENERIC NAMES

Herplex Eye Drops
IDOXURIDINE DROPS
& OINTMENT

Stoxil Eye Ointment
Viroptic

BASIC INFORMATION

Habit forming? No
Prescription needed? Yes
Available as generic? No
Drug class: Antiviral (ophthalmic)

 ## USES

Treats virus infections of the eye (usually herpes simplex virus)

 ## DOSAGE & USAGE INFORMATION

How to use:
Eye drops
- Wash hands.
- Apply pressure to inside corner of eye with middle finger.
- Continue pressure for 1 minute after placing medicine in eye.
- Tilt head backward. Pull lower lid away from eye with index finger of the same hand.
- Drop eye drops into pouch and close eye. Don't blink.
- Keep eyes closed for 1 to 2 minutes.

Eye ointment
- Wash hands.
- Pull lower lid down from eye to form a pouch.
- Squeeze tube to apply thin strip of ointment into pouch.
- Close eye for 1 to 2 minutes.
- Don't touch applicator tip to any surface (including the eye). If you accidentally touch tip, clean with warm soap and water.
- Keep container tightly closed.
- Keep cool, but don't freeze.
- Wash hands immediately after using.

When to use:
As directed. Usually 1 drop every 2 hours up to maximum of 9 drops daily.

Continued next column

 ## OVERDOSE

SYMPTOMS:
None expected.
WHAT TO DO:
Not intended for internal use. If child accidentally swallows, call poison-control center.

If you forget a dose:
Use as soon as you remember.

What drug does:
Destroys reproductive capacity of virus.

Time lapse before drug works:
Begins work immediately. Usual course of treatment is 7 days.

Don't use with:
Other eye drops, boric acid or ointment without consulting doctor.

 ## POSSIBLE ADVERSE REACTIONS OR SIDE EFFECTS

SYMPTOMS	WHAT TO DO
Life-threatening None expected.	
Common Stinging or burning eyes.	Continue. Tell doctor at next visit.
Infrequent None expected.	
Rare Itchy, red eyes, swollen eyelid or eye, excess flow of tears.	Discontinue. Call doctor right away.

WARNINGS & PRECAUTIONS

Don't use if:
You are allergic to trifluridine.

Before you start, consult your doctor:
- If you have had any other eye problems.
- If you use eye drops for glaucoma.

Over age 60:
No problems expected.

Pregnancy:
No problems expected, but safety not established.

Breast-feeding:
No problems expected, but safety not established.

Infants & children:
Use only under close medical supervision.

Prolonged use:
Avoid unless directed by your eye doctor.

Skin & sunlight:
No problems expected.

Driving, piloting or hazardous work:
No problems expected.

Discontinuing:
Don't discontinue without consulting doctor.

Others:
- Don't use more often or longer than prescribed.
- Keep cool, but don't freeze.
- If problem doesn't improve within a week, notify your doctor.

 ## POSSIBLE INTERACTION WITH OTHER DRUGS

GENERIC NAME OR DRUG CLASS	COMBINED EFFECT
Clinically significant interactions with oral or injected medicines unlikely.	

 ## POSSIBLE INTERACTION WITH OTHER SUBSTANCES

INTERACTS WITH	COMBINED EFFECT
Alcohol:	None expected.
Beverages:	None expected.
Cocaine:	None expected.
Foods:	None expected.
Marijuana:	None expected.
Tobacco:	None expected.

APPETITE SUPPRESSANTS

BRAND AND GENERIC NAMES

See complete list of brand names in the *Brand Name Directory*, page 1056.

BASIC INFORMATION

Habit forming? Yes
Prescription needed? Yes
Available as generic? Yes
Drug class: Appetite suppressant

 ## USES

Suppresses appetite.

 ## DOSAGE & USAGE INFORMATION

How to take:
- Tablet or capsule—Swallow with liquid. You may chew or crush tablet.
- Extended-release tablets or capsules— Swallow each dose whole with liquid; do not crush.
- Elixir—Swallow with liquid.

When to take:
- Long-acting forms—10 to 14 hours before bedtime.
- Short-acting forms—1 hour before meals. Last dose no later than 4 to 6 hours before bedtime.

If you forget a dose:
- Long-acting form—Take as soon as you remember up to 2 hours late. If more than 2 hours, wait for next scheduled dose (don't double this dose).
- Short-acting form—Wait for next scheduled dose. Don't double this dose.

What drug does:
Apparently stimulates brain's appetite-control center.

Continued next column

 ## OVERDOSE

SYMPTOMS:
Irritability, overactivity, trembling, insomnia, mood changes, fever, rapid heartbeat, confusion, disorientation, hallucinations, convulsions, coma.
WHAT TO DO:
- **Dial 0 (operator) or 911 (emergency) for an ambulance or medical help. Then give first aid immediately.**
- **See emergency information on inside covers.**

Time lapse before drug works:
Begins in 1 hour. Short-acting form lasts 4 hours. Long-acting form lasts 14 hours.

Don't take with:
- Non-prescription drugs without consulting doctor.
- See Interaction column and consult doctor.

 ## POSSIBLE ADVERSE REACTIONS OR SIDE EFFECTS

SYMPTOMS	WHAT TO DO
Life-threatening: None expected.	
Common: Irritability, nervousness, insomnia, false sense of well-being.	Continue. Call doctor when convenient.
Infrequent: • Irregular or pounding heartbeat, urgent or difficult urination.	Discontinue. Call doctor right away.
• Blurred vision, unpleasant taste or dry mouth, constipation or diarrhea, nausea, vomiting, cramps, changes in sex drive, increased sweating.	Continue. Call doctor when convenient.
Rare: • Mood changes, rash or hives, breathing difficulty.	Discontinue. Call doctor right away.
• Hair loss.	Continue. Call doctor when convenient.

110

WARNINGS & PRECAUTIONS

Don't take if:
- You are allergic to any sympathomimetic or phenylpropanolamine.
- You have glaucoma.
- You have taken MAO inhibitors within 2 weeks.
- You plan to become pregnant within medication period.
- You have a history of drug abuse.
- You have irregular or rapid heartbeat.

Before you start, consult your doctor:
- If you have high blood pressure or heart disease.
- If you have an overactive thyroid, nervous tension or "anxiety."
- If you have epilepsy.
- If you will have surgery within 2 months, including dental surgery, requiring general or spinal anesthesia.

Over age 60:
Adverse reactions and side effects may be more frequent and severe than in younger persons.

Pregnancy:
Safety not established. Avoid.

Breast-feeding:
Safety not established. Consult doctor.

Infants & children:
Don't give to children younger than 12.

Prolonged use:
Loses effectiveness. Avoid.

Skin & sunlight:
No problems expected.

Driving, piloting or hazardous work:
Don't drive or pilot aircraft until you learn how medicine affects you. Don't work around dangerous machinery. Don't climb ladders or work in high places. Danger increases if you drink alcohol or take medicine affecting alertness and reflexes, such as antihistamines, tranquilizers, sedatives, pain medicine, narcotics and mind-altering drugs.

Discontinuing:
Don't discontinue without consulting doctor. Dose may require gradual reduction if you have taken drug for a long time. Doses of other drugs may also require adjustment.

Others:
Don't increase dose.

POSSIBLE INTERACTION WITH OTHER DRUGS

GENERIC NAME OR DRUG CLASS	COMBINED EFFECT
Antihypertensives*	Decreased antihypertensive effect.
Appetite suppressants, other*	Dangerous overstimulation.
Caffeine	Increased stimulant effect of phentermine.
Guanethidine	Decreased guanethidine effect.
Hydralazine	Decreased hydralazine effect.
MAO inhibitors*	Dangerous blood-pressure rise.
Methyldopa	Decreased methyldopa effect.
Molindone	Decreased suppressant effect.
Phenothiazines*	Decreased appetite suppressant effect.
Rauwolfia alkaloids*	Decreased effect of rauwolfia alkaloids.
Sodium bicarbonate	Increased action of amphetamines.

POSSIBLE INTERACTION WITH OTHER SUBSTANCES

INTERACTS WITH	COMBINED EFFECT
Alcohol: Beer, chianti wines, vermouth.	Dangerous blood-pressure rise.
Beverages: • Caffeine drinks. • Drinks containing tyramine.*	Excessive stimulation. Blood-pressure rise.
Cocaine	Convulsions or excessive nervousness.
Foods: Foods containing tyramine.*	Blood-pressure rise.
Marijuana:	Frequent use— Irregular heartbeat.
Tobacco:	None expected.

ASPIRIN

BRAND NAMES

See complete list of brand names in the *Brand Name Directory*, page 1057.

BASIC INFORMATION

Habit forming? No
Prescription needed? No
Available as generic? Yes
Drug class: Analgesic, anti-inflammatory (salicylate)

 ## USES

- Reduces pain, fever, inflammation.
- Relieves swelling, stiffness, joint pain of arthritis or rheumatism.
- Antiplatelet effect.

 ## DOSAGE & USAGE INFORMATION

How to take:
- Tablet or capsule—Swallow with liquid.
- Extended-release tablets or capsules—Swallow each dose whole.
- Effervescent tablets—Dissolve in water.
- Chewing gum tablets—Chew completely. Don't swallow whole.
- Suppositories—Remove wrapper and moisten suppository with water. Gently insert into rectum, large end first.

When to take:
Pain, fever, inflammation—As needed, no more often than every 4 hours.

If you forget a dose:
- Pain, fever—Take as soon as you remember. Wait 4 hours for next dose.
- Arthritis—Take as soon as you remember up to 2 hours late. Return to regular schedule.

What drug does:
- Affects hypothalamus, the part of the brain which regulates temperature by dilating small blood vessels in skin.

Continued next column

 ## OVERDOSE

SYMPTOMS:
Ringing in ears; nausea; vomiting; dizziness; fever; deep, rapid breathing; hallucinations; convulsions; coma.
WHAT TO DO:
- **Dial 0 (operator) or 911 (emergency) for an ambulance or medical help. Then give first aid immediately.**
- **See emergency information on inside covers.**

- Prevents clumping of platelets (small blood cells) so blood vessels remain open.
- Decreases prostaglandin effect.
- Suppresses body's pain messages.

Time lapse before drug works:
30 minutes for pain, fever, arthritis.

Don't take with:
- Tetracyclines. Space doses 1 hour apart.
- See Interaction column and consult doctor.

 ## POSSIBLE ADVERSE REACTIONS OR SIDE EFFECTS

SYMPTOMS	WHAT TO DO
Life-threatening:	
Black or bloody vomit; blood in urine; difficulty breathing; hives, rash, intense itching, faintness soon after a dose (anaphylaxis).	Seek emergency treatment immediately.
Common:	
• Nausea, vomiting.	Discontinue. Seek emergency treatment.
• Heartburn, indigestion.	Continue. Call doctor when convenient.
• Ringing in ears.	Continue. Tell doctor at next visit.
Infrequent:	
None expected.	
Rare:	
• Black stools, unexplained fever.	Discontinue. Seek emergency treatment.
• Rash, hives, itch, diminished vision, shortness of breath, wheezing, jaundice, mental confusion.	Discontinue. Call doctor right away.
• Drowsiness.	Continue. Call doctor when convenient.

 ## WARNINGS & PRECAUTIONS

Don't take if:
- You need to restrict sodium in your diet. Buffered effervescent tablets and sodium salicylate are high in sodium.
- You are sensitive to aspirin or aspirin has a strong vinegar-like odor, which means it has decomposed.
- You have a peptic ulcer of stomach or duodenum or a bleeding disorder.

Before you start, consult your doctor:
- If you have had stomach or duodenal ulcers.
- If you have had gout.
- If you have asthma or nasal polyps.

Over age 60:
More likely to cause hidden bleeding in stomach or intestines. Watch for dark stools.

Pregnancy:
Risk to unborn child outweighs drug benefits. Don't use.

Breast-feeding:
Drug passes into milk. Avoid drug or discontinue nursing until you finish medicine. Consult doctor for advice on maintaining milk supply.

Infants & children:
- Overdose frequent and severe. Keep bottles out of children's reach.
- Consult doctor before giving to persons under age 18 who have fever and discomfort of viral illness, especially chicken pox and influenza. Probably increases risk of Reye's syndrome.

Prolonged use:
Kidney damage. Periodic kidney-function test recommended.

Skin & sunlight:
Aspirin combined with sunscreen may decrease sunburn.

Driving, piloting or hazardous work:
No restrictions unless you feel drowsy.

Discontinuing:
For chronic illness—Don't discontinue without doctor's advice until you complete prescribed dose, even though symptoms diminish or disappear.

Others:
- Aspirin can complicate surgery, pregnancy, labor and delivery, and illness.
- For arthritis—Don't change dose without consulting doctor.
- Urine tests for blood sugar may be inaccurate.

 ## POSSIBLE INTERACTION WITH OTHER DRUGS

GENERIC NAME OR DRUG CLASS	COMBINED EFFECT
Acebutolol	Decreased anti-hypertensive effect of acebutolol.
ACE inhibitors: captopril, enalapril, lisinopril*	Decreased ACE inhibitor effect.
Allopurinol	Decreased allopurinol effect.
Antacids*	Decreased aspirin effect.
Anticoagulants*	Increased anticoagulant effect. Abnormal bleeding.

Antidiabetics, oral*	Low blood sugar.
Aspirin, other	Likely aspirin toxicity.
Bumetanide	Possible aspirin toxicity.
Carteolol	Decreased anti-hypertensive effect of carteolol.
Cortisone drugs*	Increased cortisone effect. Risk of ulcers and stomach bleeding.
Diclofenac	Increased risk of stomach ulcer.
Ethacrynic acid	Possible aspirin toxicity.
Furosemide	Possible aspirin toxicity. May decrease furosemide effect.
Gold compounds*	Increased likelihood of kidney damage.
Indomethacin	Risk of stomach bleeding and ulcers.
Ketoprofen	Increased risk of stomach ulcer.
Methotrexate	Increased methotrexate effect.
Minoxidil	Decreased minoxidil effect.
Non-steroidal anti-inflammatory drugs (NSAIDs)*	Risk of stomach bleeding and ulcers.
Oxprenolol	Decreased antihyper-tensive effect of oxprenolol.

Continued page 1075

 ## POSSIBLE INTERACTION WITH OTHER SUBSTANCES

INTERACTS WITH	COMBINED EFFECT
Alcohol:	Possible stomach irritation and bleeding. Avoid.
Beverages:	None expected.
Cocaine:	None expected.
Foods:	None expected.
Marijuana:	Possible increased pain relief, but marijuana may slow body's recovery. Avoid.
Tobacco:	None expected.

*See Glossary

ATENOLOL

BRAND NAMES

Tenormin

BASIC INFORMATION

Habit forming? No
Prescription needed? Yes
Available as generic? No
Drug class: Beta-adrenergic blocker

 ## USES

- Reduces angina attacks.
- Stabilizes irregular heartbeat.
- Lowers blood pressure.
- Reduces frequency of migraine headaches. (Does not relieve headache pain.)
- Other uses prescribed by your doctor.

 ## DOSAGE & USAGE INFORMATION

How to take:
Tablet—Swallow with liquid. If you can't swallow whole, crumble tablet and take with liquid or food.

When to take:
With meals or immediately after.

If you forget a dose:
Take as soon as you remember. Return to regular schedule, but allow 3 hours between doses.

What drug does:
- Blocks certain actions of sympathetic nervous system.
- Lowers heart's oxygen requirements.
- Slows nerve impulses through heart.
- Reduces blood vessel contraction in heart, scalp and other body parts.

Time lapse before drug works:
1 to 4 hours.

Continued next column

 ## OVERDOSE

SYMPTOMS:
Weakness, slow or weak pulse, blood pressure drop, fainting, convulsions, cold and sweaty skin, coma.
WHAT TO DO:
- **Dial 0 (operator) or 911 (emergency) for an ambulance or medical help. Then give first aid immediately.**
- **See emergency information on inside covers.**

Don't take with:
Non-prescription drugs or drugs in Interaction column without consulting doctor.

 ## POSSIBLE ADVERSE REACTIONS OR SIDE EFFECTS

SYMPTOMS	WHAT TO DO
Life-threatening: None expected.	
Common:	
• Pulse slower than 50 beats per minute.	Discontinue. Call doctor right away.
• Drowsiness, fatigue, numbness or tingling in fingers or toes, dizziness, diarrhea, nausea, weakness.	Continue. Call doctor when convenient.
• Cold hands or feet; dry mouth, eyes, skin.	Continue. Tell doctor at next visit.
Infrequent:	
• Hallucinations, nightmares, insomnia, headache, breathing difficulty, joint pain, abdominal pain.	Discontinue. Call doctor right away.
• Confusion, reduced alertness, depression.	Continue. Call doctor when convenient.
• Constipation.	Continue. Tell doctor at next visit.
Rare:	
• Rash, sore throat, fever.	Discontinue. Call doctor right away.
• Unusual bleeding or bruising, impotence.	Continue. Call doctor when convenient.

 ## WARNINGS & PRECAUTIONS

Don't take if:
- You are allergic to any beta-adrenergic blocker.
- You have asthma or hay fever symptoms.
- You have taken MAO inhibitors in past 2 weeks.

Before you start, consult your doctor:
- If you have heart disease or poor circulation to the extremities.
- If you have hay fever, asthma, chronic bronchitis, emphysema.
- If you have overactive thyroid function, diabetes, hypoglycemia, impaired liver or kidney function.
- If you will have surgery within 2 months, including dental surgery, requiring general or spinal anesthesia.

Over age 60:
Adverse reactions and side effects may be more frequent and severe than in younger persons.

Pregnancy:
Risk to unborn child outweighs drug benefits. Don't use.

Breast-feeding:
Drug passes into milk. Avoid drug or discontinue nursing until you finish medicine. Consult doctor for advice on maintaining milk supply.

Infants & children:
Not recommended.

Prolonged use:
No problems expected.

Skin & sunlight:
No problems expected.

Driving, piloting or hazardous work:
Don't drive or pilot aircraft until you learn how medicine affects you. Don't work around dangerous machinery. Don't climb ladders or work in high places. Danger increases if you drink alcohol or take medicine affecting alertness and reflexes.

Discontinuing:
Don't discontinue without consulting doctor. Dose may require gradual reduction if you have taken drug for a long time. Doses of other drugs may also require adjustment.

Others:
May mask hypoglycemia symptoms.

POSSIBLE INTERACTION WITH OTHER DRUGS

GENERIC NAME OR DRUG CLASS	COMBINED EFFECT
ACE inhibitors: captopril, enalapril, lisinopril *	Possible excessive potassium in blood.
Albuterol	Decreased albuterol effect and beta-adrenergic blocking effect.
Antidiabetics *	Increased antidiabetic effect.
Antihistamines *	Decreased antihistamine effect.
Antihypertensives *	Increased effect of antihypertensive.
Barbiturates *	Increased barbiturate effect. Oversedation.
Beta-adrenergic blockers *	Increased antihypertensive effects of both drugs.
Digitalis preparations *	Increased or decreased heart rate. Improves irregular heartbeat.

Diltiazem	May worsen congestive heart failure
Encainide	Increased effect of toxicity on the heart muscle.
Indomethacin	Decreased atenolol effect.
Metaproterenol	Decreased effect of metaproterenol.
Narcotics *	Increased narcotic effect. Oversedation.
Nicardipine	Possible irregular heartbeat and congestive heart failure.
Nifedipine	May worsen congestive heart failure.
Nitrates *	Possible excessive blood-pressure drop.
Non-steroidal anti-inflammatory drugs (NSAIDs) *	Decreased effect of anti-inflammatory.
Pentoxifylline	Increased antihypertensive effect.
Phenytoin	Increased atenolol effect.
Quinidine	Slows heart excessively.
Reserpine	Increased reserpine effect. Excessive sedation and depression.
Theophylline	Decreased theophylline effect.
Tocainide	May worsen congestive heart failure.
Verapamil	May worsen congestive heart failure.

POSSIBLE INTERACTION WITH OTHER SUBSTANCES

INTERACTS WITH	COMBINED EFFECT
Alcohol:	Excessive blood pressure drop. Avoid.
Beverages:	None expected.
Cocaine:	Irregular heartbeat.
Foods:	None expected.
Marijuana:	Daily use—Impaired circulation to hands and feet.
Tobacco:	Possible irregular heartbeat.

*See Glossary

ATROPINE

BRAND NAMES

See complete list of brand names in the *Brand Name Directory*, page 1057.

BASIC INFORMATION

Habit forming? No
Prescription needed?
  Low strength: No
  High strength: Yes
Available as generic? Yes
Drug class: Antispasmodic, anticholinergic

 USES

- Reduces spasms of digestive system, bladder and urethra.
- Treatment of bronchial spasms.

 DOSAGE & USAGE INFORMATION

How to take:
- Tablet—Swallow with liquid or food to lessen stomach irritation.
- Aerosol—Dilute in saline and inhale as nebulizer.

When to take:
30 minutes before meals (unless directed otherwise by doctor).

If you forget a dose:
Take as soon as you remember up to 2 hours late. If more than 2 hours, wait for next scheduled dose (don't double this dose).

What drug does:
Blocks nerve impulses at parasympathetic nerve endings, preventing muscle contractions and gland secretions of organs involved.

Time lapse before drug works:
15 to 30 minutes.

Don't take with:
See Interaction column and consult doctor.

 OVERDOSE

SYMPTOMS:
Dilated pupils, rapid pulse and breathing, dizziness, fever, hallucinations, confusion, slurred speech, agitation, flushed face, convulsions, coma.
WHAT TO DO:
- **Dial 0 (operator) or 911 (emergency) for an ambulance or medical help. Then give first aid immediately.**
- **See emergency information on inside covers.**

 POSSIBLE ADVERSE REACTIONS OR SIDE EFFECTS

SYMPTOMS	WHAT TO DO
Life-threatening: None expected.	
Common:	
• Confusion, delirium, rapid heartbeat.	Discontinue. Call doctor right away.
• Nausea, vomiting, decreased sweating,	Continue. Call doctor when convenient.
• Constipation.	Continue. Tell doctor at next visit.
• Dryness in ears, nose, throat.	No action necessary.
Infrequent: Headache, difficult or painful urination.	Continue. Call doctor when convenient.
Rare: Rash or hives, pain, blurred vision, fever.	Discontinue. Call doctor right away.

 WARNINGS & PRECAUTIONS

Don't take if:
- You are allergic to any anticholinergic.
- You have trouble with stomach bloating.
- You have difficulty emptying your bladder completely.
- You have narrow-angle glaucoma.
- You have severe ulcerative colitis.

Before you start, consult your doctor:
- If you have open-angle glaucoma.
- If you have angina.
- If you have chronic bronchitis or asthma.
- If you have liver disease.
- If you have hiatal hernia.
- If you have enlarged prostate.
- If you have myasthenia gravis.
- If you have peptic ulcer.
- If you will have surgery within 2 months, including dental surgery, requiring general or spinal anesthesia.

Over age 60:
Adverse reactions and side effects may be more frequent and severe than in younger persons.

Pregnancy:
Studies inconclusive on harm to unborn child. Animal studies show fetal abnormalities. Decide with your doctor whether drug benefits justify risk to unborn child.

Breast-feeding:
Drug passes into milk and decreases milk flow. Avoid drug or discontinue nursing until you finish medicine. Consult doctor for advice on maintaining milk supply.

Infants & children:
Use only under medical supervision.

Prolonged use:
Chronic constipation, possible fecal impaction. Consult doctor immediately.

Skin & sunlight:
No problems expected.

Driving, piloting or hazardous work:
Use disqualifies you for piloting aircraft. Otherwise, no problems expected.

Discontinuing:
May be unnecessary to finish medicine. Follow doctor's instructions.

Others:
No problems expected.

POSSIBLE INTERACTION WITH OTHER DRUGS

GENERIC NAME OR DRUG CLASS	COMBINED EFFECT
Amantadine	Increased atropine effect.
Anticholinergics, other*	Increased atropine effect.
Antidepressants, tricyclic (TCA)*	Increased atropine effect. Increased sedation.
Antihistamines*	Increased atropine effect.
Cortisone drugs*	Increased internal-eye pressure.
Disopyramide	Increased atropine effect.
Haloperidol	Increased internal-eye pressure.
MAO inhibitors*	Increased atropine effect.
Meperidine	Increased atropine effect.
Methylphenidate	Increased atropine effect.
Molindone	Increased anticholinergic effect.
Nitrates*	Increased internal-eye pressure.

Nizatidine	Increased nizatidine effect.
Orphenadrine	Increased atropine effect.
Phenothiazines*	Increased atropine effect.
Pilocarpine	Loss of pilocarpine effect in glaucoma treatment.
Potassium supplements*	Possible intestinal ulcers with oral potassium tablets.
Quinidine	Increased atropine effect.
Vitamin C	Decreased atropine effect. Avoid large doses of vitamin C.

POSSIBLE INTERACTION WITH OTHER SUBSTANCES

INTERACTS WITH	COMBINED EFFECT
Alcohol:	None expected.
Beverages:	None expected.
Cocaine:	Excessively rapid heartbeat. Avoid.
Foods:	None expected.
Marijuana:	Drowsiness and dry mouth.
Tobacco:	None expected.

*See Glossary

ATROPINE, HYOSCYAMINE, METHENAMINE, METHYLENE BLUE, PHENYLSALICYLATE & BENZOIC ACID

BRAND NAMES

Doised	Urinary
Hexalol	Antiseptic No. 2
Prosed	Urised
Trac Tabs	Urisep
U-Tract	Uritab
UAA	Urithol
Uramine	Uritin
Uridon Modified	Uroblue
Urimed	Uro-Ves

BASIC INFORMATION

Habit forming? No
Prescription needed? Yes
Available as generic? No
Drug class: Urinary tract analgesic, antispasmodic, anti-infective

 ## USES

A combination medicine to control infection, spasms and pain caused by urinary tract infections.

 ## DOSAGE & USAGE INFORMATION

How to take:
Tablet—Swallow with liquid or food to lessen stomach irritation.

When to take:
30 minutes before meals (unless directed otherwise by doctor).

If you forget a dose:
Take as soon as you remember up to 2 hours late. If more than 2 hours, wait for next scheduled dose (don't double this dose).

Continued next column

 ## OVERDOSE

SYMPTOMS:
Dilated pupils, rapid pulse and breathing, dizziness, fever, hallucinations, confusion, slurred speech, agitation, flushed face, convulsions, coma.
WHAT TO DO:
- **Dial 0 (operator) or 911 (emergency) for an ambulance or medical help. Then give first aid immediately.**
- **See emergency information on inside covers.**

What drug does:
Makes urine acid. Blocks nerve impulses at parasympathetic nerve endings, preventing muscle contractions and gland secretions of organs involved. Methenamine destroys some germs.

Time lapse before drug works:
15 to 30 minutes.

Don't take with:
See Interaction column and consult doctor.

 ## POSSIBLE ADVERSE REACTIONS OR SIDE EFFECTS

SYMPTOMS	WHAT TO DO
Life-threatening:	
Heartbeat irregularity, shortness of breath or difficulty breathing.	Seek emergency treatment immediately.
Common:	
Dry mouth, throat.	Continue. Call doctor when convenient.
Infrequent:	
Flushed, red face; drowsiness; difficult urination; nausea and vomiting; abdominal pain; ringing or buzzing in ears; severe drowsiness; back pain.	Discontinue. Call doctor right away.
Rare:	
Blurred vision; pain in eyes; skin rash, hives.	Discontinue. Seek emergency treatment.

 ## WARNINGS & PRECAUTIONS

Don't take if:
- You are allergic to any of the ingredients or aspirin.
- Brain damage in child.
- You have glaucoma.

Before you start, consult your doctor:
- If you are on any special diet such as low-sodium.
- If you have had a hiatal hernia, bronchitis, asthma, liver disease, stomach or duodenal ulcers.
- If you have asthma, nasal polyps, bleeding disorder or enlarged prostate.
- If you will have any surgery within 2 months.

ATROPINE, HYOSCYAMINE, METHENAMINE, METHYLENE BLUE, PHENYLSALICYLATE & BENZOIC ACID

Over age 60:
- Adverse reactions and side effects may be more frequent and severe than in younger persons.
- More likely to cause hidden bleeding in stomach or intestines. Watch for dark stools.

Pregnancy:
Risk to unborn child outweighs benefits. Don't use.

Breast-feeding:
Drug passes into milk. Avoid or discontinue nursing until you finish medicine.

Infants & children:
Side effects more likely. Not recommended in children under 12.

Prolonged use:
May lead to constipation or kidney damage. Request lab studies to monitor effects of prolonged use.

Skin & sunlight:
No problems expected.

Driving, piloting or hazardous work:
May disqualify for piloting aircraft during time you take medicine.

Discontinuing:
May be unnecessary to finish medicine. Follow your symptoms and doctor's advice.

Others:
- Salicylates can complicate surgery, pregnancy, labor and delivery, and illness.
- Urine tests for blood sugar may be inaccurate.
- Drink cranberry juice or eat prunes or plums to help make urine more acid.

 POSSIBLE INTERACTION WITH OTHER DRUGS

GENERIC NAME OR DRUG CLASS	COMBINED EFFECT
Allopurinol	Decreased allopurinol effect.
Amantadine	Increased atropine and belladonna effect.
Antacids*	Decreased salicylate and methenamine effect.
Anticoagulants*	Increased anticoagulant effect. Abnormal bleeding.
Anticholinergics, other*	Increased atropine and belladonna effect.
Antidepressants, other*	Increased hyoscyamine and belladonna effect. Increased sedation.
Antidiabetics, oral*	Low blood sugar.
Antihistamines*	Increased atropine and hyoscyamine effect.
Aspirin	Likely salicylate toxicity.
Beta-adrenergic blockers*	Decreased antihypertensive effect.
Carbonic anhydrase inhibitors*	Decreased methenamine effect.
Cortisone drugs*	Increased internal-eye pressure, increased cortisone effect. Risk of ulcers and stomach bleeding.
Diuretics, thiazide*	Decreased urine acidity.
Furosemide	Possible salicylate toxicity.
Gold compounds*	Increased likelihood of kidney damage.
Haloperidol	Increased internal-eye pressure.
Indomethacin	Risk of stomach bleeding and ulcers.
MAO inhibitors*	Increased belladonna and atropine effect.

Continued page 1075

 POSSIBLE INTERACTION WITH OTHER SUBSTANCES

INTERACTS WITH	COMBINED EFFECT
Alcohol:	Excessive sedation. Possible stomach irritation and bleeding. Avoid.
Beverages:	None expected.
Cocaine:	Excessively rapid heartbeat. Avoid.
Foods:	None expected.
Marijuana:	Drowsiness and dry mouth. May slow body's recovery.
Tobacco:	Dry mouth.

*See Glossary

119

AZATADINE

BRAND NAMES

Optimine   **Trinalin Repetabs**

BASIC INFORMATION

Habit forming? No
Prescription needed? Yes
Available as generic? No
Drug class: Antihistamine

USES

- Reduces allergic symptoms such as hay fever, hives, rash or itching.
- Induces sleep.

DOSAGE & USAGE INFORMATION

How to take:
Tablet—Swallow with liquid or food to lessen stomach irritation.

When to take:
Varies with form. Follow label directions.

If you forget a dose:
Take as soon as you remember up to 2 hours late. If more than 2 hours, wait for next scheduled dose (don't double this dose).

What drug does:
Blocks action of histamine after an allergic response triggers histamine release in sensitive cells.

Time lapse before drug works:
30 minutes.

Don't take with:
See Interaction column and consult doctor.

OVERDOSE

SYMPTOMS:
Convulsions, red face, hallucinations, coma.
WHAT TO DO:
- **Dial 0 (operator) or 911 (emergency) for an ambulance or medical help. Then give first aid immediately.**
- **If patient is unconscious and not breathing, give mouth-to-mouth breathing. If there is no heartbeat, use cardiac massage and mouth-to-mouth breathing (CPR). Don't try to make patient vomit. If you can't get help quickly, take patient to nearest emergency facility.**
- **See emergency information on inside covers.**

POSSIBLE ADVERSE REACTIONS OR SIDE EFFECTS

SYMPTOMS	WHAT TO DO
Life-threatening: None expected.	
Common: Drowsiness; dizziness; dry mouth, nose, throat; nausea.	Continue. Tell doctor at next visit.
Infrequent:	
• Changes in vision.	Discontinue. Call doctor right away.
• Less tolerance for contact lenses, difficult urination.	Continue. Call doctor when convenient.
• Appetite loss, gastric discomfort.	Continue. Tell doctor at next visit.
Rare: Nightmares, agitation, irritability, sore throat, fever, rapid or slow heartbeat, unusual bleeding or bruising, fatigue, weakness, decreased libido, impotence.	Discontinue. Call doctor right away.

WARNINGS & PRECAUTIONS

Don't take if:
You are allergic to any antihistamine.

Before you start, consult your doctor:
- If you have glaucoma.
- If you have enlarged prostate.
- If you have asthma.
- If you have kidney disease.
- If you have peptic ulcer.
- If you will have surgery within 2 months, including dental surgery, requiring general or spinal anesthesia.

Over age 60:
Don't exceed recommended dose. Adverse reactions and side effects may be more frequent and severe than in younger persons, especially urination difficulty, diminished alertness and other brain and nervous-system symptoms.

Pregnancy:
Unknown effect on unborn child. Avoid if possible.

Breast-feeding:
Drug passes into milk. Avoid drug or discontinue nursing until you finish medicine. Consult doctor for advice on maintaining milk supply.

Infants & children:
Not recommended for premature or newborn infants. Otherwise, no problems expected.

Prolonged use:
Avoid. May damage bone-marrow and nerve cells.

Skin & sunlight:
May cause rash or intensify sunburn in areas exposed to sun or sunlamp.

Driving, piloting or hazardous work:
Don't drive or pilot aircraft until you learn how medicine affects you. Don't work around dangerous machinery. Don't climb ladders or work in high places. Danger increases if you drink alcohol or take medicine affecting alertness and reflexes, such as antihistamines, tranquilizers, sedatives, pain medicine, narcotics and mind-altering drugs.

Discontinuing:
No problems expected.

Others:
May mask symptoms of hearing damage from aspirin, other salicylates, cisplatin, paromomycin, vancomycin or anticonvulsants. Consult doctor if you use these.

POSSIBLE INTERACTION WITH OTHER DRUGS

GENERIC NAME OR DRUG CLASS	COMBINED EFFECT
Anticholinergics*	Increased anticholinergic effect.
Anticoagulants, oral*	Possible decreased anticoagulant effect.
Antidepressants*	Excess sedation. Avoid.
Antihistamines, other*	Excess sedation. Avoid.
Carteolol	Decreased antihistamine effect.
Dronabinol	Increased effects of both drugs. Avoid.
Hypnotics*	Excess sedation. Avoid.
MAO inhibitors*	Increased azatadine effect.
Mind-altering drugs*	Excess sedation. Avoid.
Molindone	Increased antihistamine effect.
Nabilone	Greater depression of the central nervous system.
Narcotics*	Excess sedation. Avoid.
Sedatives*	Excess sedation. Avoid.
Sleep inducers*	Excess sedation. Avoid.
Sotalol	Increased antihistamine effect.
Tranquilizers*	Excess sedation. Avoid.

POSSIBLE INTERACTION WITH OTHER SUBSTANCES

INTERACTS WITH	COMBINED EFFECT
Alcohol:	Excess sedation. Avoid.
Beverages: Caffeine drinks.	Less azatadine sedation.
Cocaine:	Decreased azatadine effect. Avoid.
Foods:	None expected.
Marijuana:	Excess sedation. Avoid.
Tobacco:	None expected.

BACAMPICILLIN

BRAND NAMES

Penglobe   Spectrobid

BASIC INFORMATION

Habit forming? No
Prescription needed? Yes
Available as generic? No
Drug class: Antibiotic (penicillin)

 USES

Treatment of bacterial infections that are
susceptible to bacampicillin.

 DOSAGE & USAGE INFORMATION

How to take:
- Capsules—Swallow with liquid on an empty
  stomach 1 hour before meals or 2 hours after
  eating.
- Chewable tablets—Chew well before
  swallowing.
- Liquid—Take with cold beverage. Liquid form
  is perishable and effective for only 7 days at
  room temperature. Effective for 14 days if
  stored in refrigerator. Don't freeze.

When to take:
Follow instructions on prescription label or side
of package. Doses should be evenly spaced.
For example, 4 times a day means before meals
at bedtime.

If you forget a dose:
Take as soon as you remember. Continue
regular schedule.

What drug does:
Destroys susceptible bacteria. Does not kill
viruses.

Time lapse before drug works:
May be several days before medicine affects
infection.

Don't take with:
See Interaction column and consult doctor.

 OVERDOSE

SYMPTOMS:
Severe diarrhea, nausea or vomiting.
WHAT TO DO:
Overdose unlikely to threaten life. If person
takes much larger amount than prescribed,
call doctor, poison-control center or hospital
emergency room for specific instructions.

 POSSIBLE ADVERSE REACTIONS OR SIDE EFFECTS

SYMPTOMS	WHAT TO DO
Life-threatening:	
Hives, rash, intense itching, faintness soon after a dose (anaphylaxis); difficulty breathing.	Seek emergency treatment immediately.
Common:	
Dark or discolored tongue.	Continue. Tell doctor at next visit.
Infrequent:	
Mild nausea, vomiting, diarrhea.	Continue. Call doctor when convenient.
Rare:	
Unexplained bleeding, weakness, sore throat.	Discontinue. Call doctor right away.

WARNINGS & PRECAUTIONS

Don't take if:
You are allergic to bacampicillin, cephalosporin antibiotics, or other penicillins. Life-threatening reaction may occur.

Before you start, consult your doctor:
If you are allergic to any substance or drug.

Over age 60:
You may have skin reactions, particularly around genitals and anus.

Pregnancy:
Studies inconclusive on harm to unborn child. Animal studies show fetal abnormalities. Decide with your doctor whether drug benefits justify risk to unborn child.

Breast-feeding:
Drug passes into milk. Child may become sensitive to this and all penicillins. Avoid bacampicillin or discontinue nursing until you finish medicine. Consult doctor for advice on maintaining milk supply.

Infants & children:
No problems expected.

Prolonged use:
You may become more susceptible to infections caused by germs not responsive to bacampicillin. Super-infection also a potential.

Skin & sunlight:
No problems expected.

Driving, piloting, or hazardous work:
Usually not dangerous. Most hazardous reactions likely to occur a few minutes after taking bacampicillin.

Discontinuing:
Don't discontinue without doctor's advice until you complete prescribed dose, even though symptoms diminish or disappear.

Others:
Urine sugar test for diabetes may show false positive result.

POSSIBLE INTERACTION WITH OTHER DRUGS

GENERIC NAME OR DRUG CLASS	COMBINED EFFECT
Beta-adrenergic blockers*	Increased chance of anaphylaxis (see emergency information on inside front cover).
Chloramphenicol	Decreased effect of both drugs.
Erythromycins*	Decreased effect of both drugs.
Loperamide	Decreased bacampicillin effect.
Paromomycin	Decreased effect of both drugs.
Tetracyclines*	Decreased effect of both drugs.
Troleandomycin	Decreased effect of both drugs.

POSSIBLE INTERACTION WITH OTHER SUBSTANCES

INTERACTS WITH	COMBINED EFFECT
Alcohol:	Occasional stomach irritation.
Beverages:	None expected.
Cocaine:	No proven problems.
Foods:	None expected.
Marijuana:	No proven problems.
Tobacco:	None expected.

BACLOFEN

BRAND NAMES

Lioresal

BASIC INFORMATION

Habit forming? No
Prescription needed? Yes
Available as generic? No
Drug class: Muscle relaxant in multiple sclerosis

USES

- Relieves spasms, cramps and spasticity of muscles caused by medical problems, including multiple sclerosis and spine injuries.
- Reduces number and severity of trigeminal neuralgia attacks.

DOSAGE & USAGE INFORMATION

How to take:
Tablet—Swallow with liquid or food to lessen stomach irritation.

When to take:
3 or 4 times daily as directed.

If you forget a dose:
Take as soon as you remember up to 2 hours late. If more than 2 hours, wait for next scheduled dose (don't double this dose).

What drug does:
Blocks body's pain and reflex messages to brain.

Time lapse before drug works:
Variable. Few hours to weeks.

Continued next column

OVERDOSE

SYMPTOMS:
Blurred vision, blindness, difficult breathing, vomiting, drowsiness, muscle weakness, convulsive seizures.
WHAT TO DO:
- **Dial 0 (operator) or 911 (emergency) for an ambulance or medical help. Then give first aid immediately.**
- **If patient is unconscious and not breathing, give mouth-to-mouth breathing. If there is no heartbeat, use cardiac massage and mouth-to-mouth breathing (CPR). Don't try to make patient vomit. If you can't get help quickly, take patient to nearest emergency facility.**
- **See emergency information on inside covers.**

Don't take with:
See Interaction column and consult doctor.

POSSIBLE ADVERSE REACTIONS OR SIDE EFFECTS

SYMPTOMS	WHAT TO DO
Life-threatening: None expected.	
Common: Dizziness, lightheadedness, confusion, insomnia, drowsiness, nausea.	Continue. Call doctor when convenient.
Infrequent: • Rash with itching, numbness or tingling in hands or feet.	Discontinue. Call doctor right away.
• Headache, abdominal pain, diarrhea or constipation, appetite loss, muscle weakness, difficult or painful urination, male sex problems, nasal congestion.	Continue. Call doctor when convenient.
Rare: • Fainting, weakness, hallucinations, depression, chest pain, muscle pain.	Discontinue. Call doctor right away.
• Ringing in ears, lowered blood pressure, pounding heartbeat, dry mouth, taste disturbance.	Continue. Call doctor when convenient.

WARNINGS & PRECAUTIONS

Don't take if:
- You are allergic to any muscle relaxant.
- Muscle spasm due to strain or sprain.

Before you start, consult your doctor:
- If you have Parkinson's disease.
- If you have cerebral palsy.
- If you have had a recent stroke.
- If you have had a recent head injury.
- If you have arthritis.
- If you have diabetes.
- If you have epilepsy.
- If you have psychosis.
- If you have kidney disease.
- If you will have surgery within 2 months, including dental surgery, requiring general or spinal anesthesia.

Over age 60:
Adverse reactions and side effects may be more frequent and severe than in younger persons.

Pregnancy:
Risk to unborn child outweighs drug benefits. Don't use.

Breast-feeding:
Avoid nursing or discontinue until you finish medicine.

Infants & children:
Not recommended.

Prolonged use:
Epileptic patients should be monitored with EEGs. Diabetics should more closely monitor blood sugar levels. Obtain periodic liver function tests.

Skin & sunlight:
No problems expected.

Driving, piloting or hazardous work:
Don't drive or pilot aircraft until you learn how medicine affects you. Don't work around dangerous machinery. Don't climb ladders or work in high places. Danger increases if you drink alcohol or take medicine affecting alertness and reflexes, such as antihistamines, tranquilizers, sedatives, pain medicine, narcotics and mind-altering drugs.

Discontinuing:
Don't discontinue without consulting doctor. Dose may require gradual reduction if you have taken drug for a long time. Doses of other drugs may also require adjustment.

Others:
No problems expected.

POSSIBLE INTERACTION WITH OTHER DRUGS

GENERIC NAME OR DRUG CLASS	COMBINED EFFECT
Anesthetics, general*	Increased sedation. Low blood pressure. Avoid.
CNS depressants* (antidepressants,* antihistamines,* narcotics,* other muscle relaxants,* sedatives,* sleeping pills,* tranquilizers*)	Increased sedation. Low blood pressure. Avoid.
Ethinamate	Dangerous increased effects of ethinamate. Avoid combining.
Fluoxetine	Increased depressant effects of both drugs.
Guanfacine	May increase depressant effects of either drug.
Insulin or oral antidiabetic drugs*	Need to adjust diabetes medicine dosage.
Leucovorin	High alcohol content of leucovorin may cause adverse effects.
Methyprylon	Increased sedative effect, perhaps to dangerous level. Avoid.
Nabilone	Greater depression of the central nervous system.

POSSIBLE INTERACTION WITH OTHER SUBSTANCES

INTERACTS WITH	COMBINED EFFECT
Alcohol:	Increased sedation. Low blood pressure. Avoid.
Beverages:	No problems expected.
Cocaine:	Increased spasticity. Avoid.
Foods:	No problems expected.
Marijuana:	Increased spasticity. Avoid.
Tobacco:	May interfere with absorption of medicine.

*See Glossary

BECLOMETHASONE

BRAND NAMES

Beclovent
Beclovent Rotacaps
Beconase Inhaler
Becotide

Propaderm
Vancenase Inhaler
Vanceril

BASIC INFORMATION

Habit forming? No
Prescription needed? Yes
Available as generic? No
Drug class: Cortisone drug (adrenal
corticosteroid), antiasthmatic

USES

Prevents attacks of bronchial asthma and allergic
hay fever. Does not stop an active asthma
attack.

DOSAGE & USAGE INFORMATION

How to take:
- Aerosol—Follow package instructions. Don't
  inhale more than 4 times twice a day. Rinse
  mouth after use to prevent hoarseness, throat
  irritation and mouth infection. Wait at least 1
  minute between inhalations.
- Use other inhaled asthma drugs before
  beclomethasone.

When to take:
Regularly at the same times each day.

If you forget a dose:
Take as soon as you remember up to 2 hours
late. If more than 2 hours, wait for next
scheduled dose (don't double this dose).

What drug does:
Reduces inflammation in bronchial tubes.

Time lapse before drug works:
1 to 4 weeks.

Don't take with:
See Interaction column and consult doctor.

OVERDOSE

SYMPTOMS:
Fluid retention, flushed face, nervousness,
stomach irritation.
WHAT TO DO:
Overdose unlikely to threaten life. If person
inhales much larger amount than
prescribed, call doctor, poison-control
center or hospital emergency room for
instructions.

POSSIBLE ADVERSE REACTIONS OR SIDE EFFECTS

SYMPTOMS	WHAT TO DO
Life-threatening: None expected.	
Common: Fungus infection with white patches in mouth, dryness, sore throat.	Continue. Call doctor when convenient.
Infrequent: • Rash.	Discontinue. Call doctor right away.
• Lung inflammation, spasm of bronchial tubes.	Continue. Call doctor when convenient.
Rare: None expected.	

BECLOMETHASONE

WARNINGS & PRECAUTIONS

Don't take if:
- You are allergic to beclomethasone.
- You have had tuberculosis/systemic fungal infection.
- You are having an asthma attack.

Before you start, consult your doctor:
- If you take other cortisone drugs.
- If you have an infection.

Over age 60:
More likely to develop lung infections.

Pregnancy:
Risk to unborn child outweighs drug benefits. Don't use.

Breast-feeding:
Drug passes into milk. Avoid drug or discontinue nursing.

Infants & children:
Use only under medical supervision.

Prolonged use:
No problems expected.

Skin & sunlight:
No problems expected.

Driving, piloting or hazardous work:
No problems expected.

Discontinuing:
Don't discontinue without doctor's advice until you complete prescribed dose, even though symptoms diminish or disappear.

Others:
- Unrelated illness or injury may require cortisone drugs by mouth or injection. Notify your doctor.
- Consult doctor as soon as possible if your asthma returns while using beclamethasone as a preventive.
- Drug can reactivate tuberculosis or lung fungal infection.
- Consult doctor frequently if changing from oral cortisone drug to beclomethasone inhaler.

POSSIBLE INTERACTION WITH OTHER DRUGS

GENERIC NAME OR DRUG CLASS	COMBINED EFFECT
Albuterol	Increased beclomethasone effect.
Antiasthmatics, other*	Increased anti-asthmatic effect.
Bitolerol	Increased beclomethasone effect.
Ephedrine	Increased beclomethasone effect.
Epinephrine	Increased beclomethasone effect.
Indapamide	Possible excessive potassium loss, causing dangerous heartbeat irregularity.
Isoetharine	Increased beclomethasone effect.
Isoproterenol	Increased beclomethasone effect.
Metaproterenol	Increased beclomethasone effect.
Potassium supplements*	Decreased potassium effect.
Terbutaline	Increased beclomethasone effect.
Theophylline	Increased beclomethasone effect.

POSSIBLE INTERACTION WITH OTHER SUBSTANCES

INTERACTS WITH	COMBINED EFFECT
Alcohol:	None expected.
Beverages:	None expected.
Cocaine:	None expected.
Foods:	None expected.
Marijuana:	Decreased beclomethasone effect.
Tobacco:	Decreased beclomethasone effect.

*See Glossary

BELLADONNA

BRAND NAMES

See complete list of brand names in the *Brand Name Directory*, page 1058.

BASIC INFORMATION

Habit forming? No
Prescription needed?
  Low strength: No
  High strength: Yes
Available as generic? Yes
Drug class: Antispasmodic, anticholinergic

USES

Reduces spasms of digestive system, bladder and urethra.

DOSAGE & USAGE INFORMATION

How to take:
- Tablet, elixir or capsule—Swallow with liquid or food to lessen stomach irritation.
- Drops—Dilute dose in beverage before swallowing.

When to take:
30 minutes before meals (unless directed otherwise by doctor).

If you forget a dose:
Take as soon as you remember up to 2 hours late. If more than 2 hours, wait for next scheduled dose (don't double this dose).

What drug does:
Blocks nerve impulses at parasympathetic nerve endings, preventing muscle contractions and gland secretions of organs involved.

Time lapse before drug works:
15 to 30 minutes.

Don't take with:
See Interaction column and consult doctor.

OVERDOSE

SYMPTOMS:
Dilated pupils, rapid pulse and breathing, dizziness, fever, hallucinations, confusion, slurred speech, agitation, flushed face, convulsions, coma.
WHAT TO DO:
- **Dial 0 (operator) or 911 (emergency) for an ambulance or medical help. Then give first aid immediately.**
- **See emergency information on inside covers.**

POSSIBLE ADVERSE REACTIONS OR SIDE EFFECTS

SYMPTOMS	WHAT TO DO
Life-threatening:	
None expected.	
Common:	
• Confusion, delirium, rapid heartbeat.	Discontinue. Call doctor right away.
• Nausea, vomiting, decreased sweating,	Continue. Call doctor when convenient.
• Constipation.	Continue. Tell doctor at next visit.
• Dryness in ears, nose, throat.	No action necessary.
Infrequent:	
Headache, difficult urination.	Continue. Call doctor when convenient.
Rare:	
Rash or hives, pain, blurred vision.	Discontinue. Call doctor right away.

WARNINGS & PRECAUTIONS

Don't take if:
- You are allergic to any anticholinergic.
- You have trouble with stomach bloating.
- You have difficulty emptying your bladder completely.
- You have narrow-angle glaucoma.
- You have severe ulcerative colitis.

Before you start, consult your doctor:
- If you have open-angle glaucoma.
- If you have angina or fast heartbeat.
- If you have chronic bronchitis or asthma.
- If you have hiatal hernia, liver disease, enlarged prostate or myasthenia gravis.
- If you will have surgery within 2 months, including dental surgery, requiring general or spinal anesthesia.

Over age 60:
Adverse reactions and side effects may be more frequent and severe than in younger persons.

Pregnancy:
Safety not established. Studies inconclusive on harm to unborn child. Animal studies show fetal abnormalities. Decide with your doctor whether drug benefits justify risk to unborn child. May cause bleeding in neonate.

Breast-feeding:
Drug passes into milk and decreases milk flow. Avoid drug or discontinue nursing until you finish medicine. Consult doctor for advice on maintaining milk supply.

Infants & children:
Use only under medical supervision. Do not use if under 6 months of age.

Prolonged use:
Chronic constipation, possible fecal impaction. Consult doctor immediately.

Skin & sunlight:
No problems expected.

Driving, piloting or hazardous work:
Use disqualifies you for piloting aircraft. Otherwise, no problems expected.

Discontinuing:
May be unnecessary to finish medicine. Follow doctor's instructions.

Others:
No problems expected.

 ## POSSIBLE INTERACTION WITH OTHER DRUGS

GENERIC NAME OR DRUG CLASS	COMBINED EFFECT
Amantadine	Increased belladonna effect.
Anticholinergics, other*	Increased belladonna effect.
Antidepressants, tricyclic (TCA)*	Increased belladonna effect. Increased sedation.
Antihistamines*	Increased belladonna effect.
Cortisone drugs*	Increased internal-eye pressure.
Guanethidine	Decreased belladonna effect.
Haloperidol	Increased internal-eye pressure.
MAO inhibitors*	Increased belladonna effect.
Meperidine	Increased belladonna effect.
Methylphenidate	Increased belladonna effect.
Metoclopramide	May decrease metoclopramide effect.
Molindone	Increased anticholinergic effect.
Nitrates*	Increased internal-eye pressure.
Nizatidine	Increased nizatidine effect.
Orphenadrine	Increased belladonna effect.
Phenothiazines*	Increased belladonna effect.
Quinidine	Increased belladonna effect.
Reserpine	Decreased belladonna effect.
Pilocarpine	Loss of pilocarpine effect in glaucoma treatment.
Potassium supplements*	Possible intestinal ulcers with oral potassium tablets.
Vitamin C	Decreased belladonna effect. Avoid large doses of vitamin C.

 ## POSSIBLE INTERACTION WITH OTHER SUBSTANCES

INTERACTS WITH	COMBINED EFFECT
Alcohol:	None expected.
Beverages:	None expected.
Cocaine:	Excessively rapid heartbeat. Avoid.
Foods:	None expected.
Marijuana:	Drowsiness and dry mouth.
Tobacco:	None expected.

*See Glossary

BELLADONNA ALKALOIDS & BARBITURATES

BRAND NAMES
See complete list of brand names in the *Brand Name Directory*, page 1058.

BASIC INFORMATION

Habit forming? Yes
Prescription needed? Yes
Available as generic? Some yes, some no
Drug class: Antispasmodic, anticholinergic, sedative

 ## USES

- Reduces spasms of digestive system, bladder and urethra.
- Reduces anxiety or nervous tension (low dose).
- Relieves insomnia (higher bedtime dose).

 ## DOSAGE & USAGE INFORMATION

How to take:
- Tablet, liquid or capsule—Swallow with liquid or food to lessen stomach irritation. If you can't swallow whole, crumble tablet or open capsule and take with liquid or food.
- Extended-release tablets or capsules—Swallow each dose whole.
- Chewable tablets—Chew well before swallowing.
- Drops—Dilute dose in beverage before swallowing.

When to take:
At the same times each day.

If you forget a dose:
Take as soon as you remember up to 2 hours late. If more than 2 hours, wait for next scheduled dose (don't double this dose).

Continued next column

 ## OVERDOSE

SYMPTOMS:
Blurred vision, confusion, convulsions, irregular heartbeat, hallucinations, coma.
WHAT TO DO:
- **Dial 0 (operator) or 911 (emergency) for an ambulance or medical help. Then give first aid immediately.**
- **See emergency information on inside covers.**

What drug does:
- May partially block nerve impulses at nerve-cell connections.
- Blocks nerve impulses at parasympathetic nerve endings, preventing muscle contractions and gland secretions of organs involved.

Time lapse before drug works:
15 to 30 minutes.

Don't take with:
See Interaction column and consult doctor.

 ## POSSIBLE ADVERSE REACTIONS OR SIDE EFFECTS

SYMPTOMS	WHAT TO DO
Life-threatening:	
Unusual excitement, restlessness, fast heartbeat, breathing difficulty.	Seek emergency treatment immediately.
Common:	
• Dry mouth, throat, nose; drowsiness; constipation; dizziness; nausea; vomiting; "hangover" effect; depression; confusion.	Discontinue. Call doctor right away.
• Reduced sweating, slurred speech, agitation.	Continue. Call doctor when convenient.
Infrequent:	
Difficult urination; difficult swallowing; rash or hives; face, lip or eyelid swelling; joint or muscle pain.	Discontinue. Call doctor right away.
Rare:	
Jaundice; unusual bruising or bleeding; hives, skin rash; pain in eyes; blurred vision; sore throat, fever, mouth sores; unexplained bleeding or bruising.	Discontinue. Call doctor right away.

WARNINGS & PRECAUTIONS

Don't take if:
- You are allergic to any barbiturate or any anticholinergic.
- You have porphyria, trouble with stomach bloating, difficulty emptying your bladder completely, narrow-angle glaucoma, severe ulcerative colitis.

Before you start, consult your doctor:
- If you have open-angle glaucoma, angina, chronic bronchitis or asthma, hiatal hernia, liver disease, enlarged prostate, myasthenia gravis, peptic ulcer, epilepsy, kidney or liver damage, anemia, chronic pain.
- If you will have surgery within 2 months, including dental surgery, requiring general or spinal anesthesia.

Over age 60:
Adverse reactions and side effects may be more frequent and severe than in younger persons. Ask your doctor about small doses.

Pregnancy:
Risk to unborn child outweighs drug benefits. Don't use.

Breast-feeding:
Drug passes into milk. Avoid drug or discontinue nursing until you finish medicine.

Infants & children:
Use only under doctor's supervision.

Prolonged use:
- May cause addiction, anemia, chronic intoxication.
- May lower body temperature, making exposure to cold temperatures hazardous.

Skin & sunlight:
May cause rash or intensify sunburn in areas exposed to sun or sunlamp.

Driving, piloting or hazardous work:
Don't drive or pilot aircraft until you learn how medicine affects you. Don't work around dangerous machinery. Don't climb ladders or work in high places. Danger increases if you drink alcohol or take medicine affecting alertness and reflexes.

Discontinuing:
May be unnecessary to finish medicine. Follow doctor's instructions. If you develop withdrawal symptoms of hallucinations, agitation or sleeplessness after discontinuing, call doctor right away.

Others:
Great potential for abuse.

 ## POSSIBLE INTERACTION WITH OTHER DRUGS

GENERIC NAME OR DRUG CLASS	COMBINED EFFECT
Acetaminophen	Possible decreased barbiturate effect.
Amantadine	Increased belladonna effect.
Anticoagulants, oral*	Decreased anti-coagulant effect.
Anticholinergics, other*	Increased belladonna effect.
Anticonvulsants*	Changed seizure patterns.
Antidepressants, tricyclics (TCA)*	Possible dangerous oversedation. Avoid.
Antidiabetics, oral*	Increased barbiturate effect.
Antihistamines*	Dangerous sedation. Avoid.
Aspirin	Decreased aspirin effect.
Beta-adrenergic blockers*	Decreased effects of beta-adrenergic blocker.
Carteolol	Increased barbiturate effect. Dangerous sedation.
Contraceptives, oral*	Decreased contra-ceptive effect.

Continued page 1076

 ## POSSIBLE INTERACTION WITH OTHER SUBSTANCES

INTERACTS WITH	COMBINED EFFECT
Alcohol:	Possible fatal oversedation. Avoid.
Beverages:	None expected.
Cocaine:	Excessively rapid heartbeat. Avoid.
Foods:	None expected.
Marijuana:	Drowsiness and dry mouth. Avoid.
Tobacco:	Decreased effect-iveness of acid reduction in stomach.

BENDROFLUMETHIAZIDE

BRAND NAMES

Corzide   Rauzide
Naturetin

BASIC INFORMATION

Habit forming? No
Prescription needed? Yes
Available as generic? No
Drug class: Antihypertensive, diuretic
(thiazide)

USES

- Controls, but doesn't cure, high blood pressure.
- Reduces fluid retention (edema) caused by conditions such as heart disorders and liver disease.

DOSAGE & USAGE INFORMATION

How to take:
Tablet—Swallow with liquid. If you can't swallow whole, crumble tablet and take with liquid or food. Don't exceed dose.

When to take:
At the same time each day.

If you forget a dose:
Take as soon as you remember up to 2 hours late. If more than 2 hours, wait for next scheduled dose (don't double this dose).

What drug does:
- Forces sodium and water excretion, reducing body fluid.
- Relaxes muscle cells of small arteries.
- Reduced body fluid and relaxed arteries lower blood pressure.

Time lapse before drug works:
4 to 6 hours. May require several weeks to lower blood pressure.

Continued next column

OVERDOSE

SYMPTOMS:
Cramps, weakness, confusion, drowsiness, weak pulse, coma.
WHAT TO DO:
- Dial 0 (operator) or 911 (emergency) for an ambulance or medical help. Then give first aid immediately.
- See emergency information on inside covers.

Don't take with:
- See Interaction column and consult doctor.
- Non-prescription drugs without consulting doctor.

POSSIBLE ADVERSE REACTIONS OR SIDE EFFECTS

SYMPTOMS	WHAT TO DO
Life-threatening: None expected.	
Common: None expected.	
Infrequent:	
• Blurred vision, severe abdominal pain, nausea, vomiting, irregular heartbeat, weak pulse.	Discontinue. Call doctor right away.
• Dizziness, mood changes, headaches, weakness, tiredness, weight changes.	Continue. Call doctor when convenient.
• Dry mouth, thirst.	Continue. Tell doctor at next visit.
Rare:	
• Rash or hives.	Discontinue. Seek emergency treatment.
• Sore throat, fever, jaundice.	Discontinue. Call doctor right away.

WARNINGS & PRECAUTIONS

Don't take if:
You are allergic to any thiazide diuretic drug.

Before you start, consult your doctor:
- If you are allergic to any sulfa drug or tartrazine dye.
- If you have gout, diabetes, liver, pancreas or kidney disorder, systemic lupus erythematosus.

Over age 60:
Adverse reactions and side effects may be more frequent and severe than in younger persons, especially dizziness and excessive potassium loss.

Pregnancy:
Risk to unborn child outweighs drug benefits. Don't use.

Breast-feeding:
Drug passes into milk. Avoid this medicine or discontinue nursing.

Infants & children:
No problems expected.

Prolonged use:
You may need medicine to treat high blood pressure for the rest of your life.

Skin & sunlight:
May cause rash or intensify sunburn in areas exposed to sun or sunlamp.

Driving, piloting or hazardous work:
Don't drive or pilot aircraft until you learn how medicine affects you. Don't work around dangerous machinery. Don't climb ladders or work in high places. Danger increases if you drink alcohol or take medicine affecting alertness and reflexes, such as antihistamines, tranquilizers, sedatives, pain medicine, narcotics and mind-altering drugs.

Discontinuing:
Don't discontinue without medical advice.

Others:
- Hot weather and fever may cause dehydration and drop in blood pressure. Dose may require temporary adjustment. Weigh daily and report any unexpected weight decreases to your doctor.
- May cause rise in uric acid, leading to gout.
- May cause blood-sugar rise in diabetics.

 ## POSSIBLE INTERACTION WITH OTHER DRUGS

GENERIC NAME OR DRUG CLASS	COMBINED EFFECT
Amiodarone (and other anti-arrhythmics*)	Increased risk of heartbeat irregularity due to low potassium.
Antidepressants, tricyclic (TCA)*	Dangerous drop in blood pressure. Avoid combination unless under medical supervision.
Antihypertensives*	Increased bendro-flumethiazide effect or decreased blood pressure.
Beta-adrenergic blockers*	Increased antihypertensive effect. Dosages of both drugs may require adjustments.
Bumetanide	Increased diuretic effect.
Calcium supplements*	May decrease calcium in blood.
Carteolol	Increased antihypertensive effect.
Cholestyramine	Decreased bendro-flumethiazide effect.
Colestipol	Decreased bendro-flumethiazide effect.

Cortisone drugs*	Excessive potassium loss that causes dangerous heart rhythms.
Digitalis preparations*	Excessive potassium loss that causes dangerous heart rhythms.
Diuretics, thiazide*	Increased effect of other thiazide diuretics.
Ethacrynic acid	Increased diuretic effect.
Furosemide	Increased diuretic effect.
Indapamide	Increased diuretic effect.
Indomethacin	Decreased bendro-flumethiazide effect.
Insulin (oral)	Decreased ability to lower blood glucose.
Labetalol	Increased antihypertensive effects.
Lisinopril	Increased antihypertensive effect. Dosage of each may require adjustment.
Lithium	Increased effect of lithium.
MAO inhibitors*	Increased bendro-flumethiazide effect.
Metolazone	Increased diuretic effect.

Continued page 1077

 ## POSSIBLE INTERACTION WITH OTHER SUBSTANCES

INTERACTS WITH	COMBINED EFFECT
Alcohol:	Dangerous blood-pressure drop.
Beverages:	None expected.
Cocaine	Increased risk of heart block and high blood pressure.
Foods: Licorice.	Excessive potassium loss that causes dangerous heart rhythms.
Marijuana:	May increase blood pressure.
Tobacco:	None expected.

*See Glossary

BENZOYL PEROXIDE

BRAND NAMES

See complete list of brand names in the *Brand Name Directory*, page 1058.

BASIC INFORMATION

Habit forming? No
Prescription needed? No
Available as generic? Yes
Drug class: Antiacne (topical)

USES

- Treatment for acne.
- Decreases wrinkles in face.

DOSAGE & USAGE INFORMATION

How to use:
Cream, gel, pads, sticks, lotion, cleansing bar or facial mask—Wash affected area with plain soap and water. Dry gently with towel. Rub medicine into affected areas. Keep away from eyes, nose, mouth.

When to use:
Apply 1 or more times daily. If you have a fair complexion, start with single application at bedtime.

If you forget an application:
Use as soon as you remember.

What drug does:
Slowly releases oxygen from skin, which controls some skin bacteria. Also causes peeling and drying, helping control blackheads and whiteheads.

Time lapse before drug works:
1 to 2 weeks.

Don't use with:
See Interaction column and consult doctor.

OVERDOSE

SYMPTOMS:
None expected.
WHAT TO DO:
- **If person swallows drug, call doctor, poison-control center or hospital emergency room for instructions.**
- **See emergency information on inside covers.**

POSSIBLE ADVERSE REACTIONS OR SIDE EFFECTS

SYMPTOMS	WHAT TO DO
Life-threatening: None expected.	
Common: None expected.	
Infrequent:	
• Rash, excessive dryness.	Discontinue. Call doctor right away.
• Painful skin irritation.	Continue. Call doctor when convenient.
Rare: None expected.	

WARNINGS & PRECAUTIONS

Don't take if:
You are allergic to benzoyl peroxide.

Before you start, consult your doctor:
- If you plan to become pregnant within medication period.
- If you take oral contraceptives.

Over age 60:
No problems expected.

Pregnancy:
No proven problems. Consult doctor.

Breast-feeding:
No proven problems. Consult doctor.

Infants & children:
Not recommended.

Prolonged use:
Permanent rash or scarring.

Skin & sunlight:
No problems expected.

Driving, piloting or hazardous work:
No problems expected.

Discontinuing:
- May be unnecessary to finish medicine. Discontinue when acne improves.
- If acne doesn't improve in 2 weeks, call doctor.

Others:
- Keep away from hair and clothing. May bleach.
- Store away from heat in cool, dry place.
- Avoid contact with eyes, lips, nose and sensitive areas of the neck.

 ## POSSIBLE INTERACTION WITH OTHER DRUGS

GENERIC NAME OR DRUG CLASS	COMBINED EFFECT
Antiacne topical preparations, other	Excessive skin irritation.
Skin-peeling agents (salicylic acid, sulfur, resorcinol, tretinoin)	Excessive skin irritation.

 ## POSSIBLE INTERACTION WITH OTHER SUBSTANCES

INTERACTS WITH	COMBINED EFFECT
Alcohol:	None expected.
Beverages:	None expected.
Cocaine:	None expected.
Foods: Cinnamon, foods with benzoic acid.	Skin rash.
Marijuana:	None expected.
Tobacco:	None expected.

BENZTHIAZIDE

BRAND NAMES

Aquastat   Exna
Aquatag   Hydrex

BASIC INFORMATION

Habit forming? No
Prescription needed? Yes
Available as generic? Yes
Drug class: Antihypertensive, diuretic (thiazide)

 USES

- Controls, but doesn't cure, high blood pressure.
- Reduces fluid retention (edema) caused by conditions such as heart disorders and liver disease.

 DOSAGE & USAGE INFORMATION

How to take:
Tablet —Swallow with liquid. If you can't swallow whole, crumble tablet and take with liquid or food. Don't exceed dose.

When to take:
At the same time each day.

If you forget a dose:
Take as soon as you remember up to 2 hours late. If more than 2 hours, wait for next scheduled dose (don't double this dose).

What drug does:
- Forces sodium and water excretion, reducing body fluid.
- Relaxes muscle cells of small arteries.
- Reduced body fluid and relaxed arteries lower blood pressure.

Time lapse before drug works:
4 to 6 hours. May require several weeks to lower blood pressure.

Continued next column

 OVERDOSE

SYMPTOMS:
Cramps, weakness, confusion, drowsiness, weak pulse, coma.
WHAT TO DO:
- Dial 0 (operator) or 911 (emergency) for an ambulance or medical help. Then give first aid immediately.
- See emergency information on inside covers.

Don't take with:
- See Interaction column and consult doctor.
- Non-prescription drugs without consulting doctor.

 POSSIBLE ADVERSE REACTIONS OR SIDE EFFECTS

SYMPTOMS	WHAT TO DO
Life-threatening: None expected.	
Common: None expected.	
Infrequent:	
• Blurred vision, severe abdominal pain, nausea, vomiting, irregular heartbeat, weak pulse.	Discontinue. Call doctor right away.
• Dizziness, mood changes, headaches, weakness, tiredness, weight changes.	Continue. Call doctor when convenient.
• Dry mouth, thirst.	Continue. Tell doctor at next visit.
Rare:	
• Rash or hives.	Discontinue. Seek emergency treatment.
• Sore throat, fever, jaundice.	Discontinue. Call doctor right away.

 WARNINGS & PRECAUTIONS

Don't take if:
You are allergic to any thiazide diuretic drug.

Before you start, consult your doctor:
- If you are allergic to any sulfa drug or tartrazine dye.
- If you have gout, diabetes, liver, pancreas or kidney disorder, systemic lupus erythematosus.

Over age 60:
Adverse reactions and side effects may be more frequent and severe than in younger persons, especially dizziness and excessive potassium loss.

Pregnancy:
Risk to unborn child outweighs drug benefits. Don't use.

Breast-feeding:
Drug passes into milk. Avoid drug or discontinue nursing.

Infants & children:
No problems expected.

Prolonged use:
You may need medicine to treat high blood pressure for the rest of your life.

Skin & sunlight:
May cause rash or intensify sunburn in areas exposed to sun or sunlamp.

Driving, piloting or hazardous work:
Don't drive or pilot aircraft until you learn how medicine affects you. Don't work around dangerous machinery. Don't climb ladders or work in high places. Danger increases if you drink alcohol or take medicine affecting alertness and reflexes, such as antihistamines, tranquilizers, sedatives, pain medicine, narcotics and mind-altering drugs.

Discontinuing:
Don't discontinue without medical advice.

Others:
- Hot weather and fever may cause dehydration and drop in blood pressure. Dose may require temporary adjustment. Weigh daily and report any unexpected weight decreases to your doctor.
- May cause rise in uric acid, leading to gout.
- May cause blood-sugar rise in diabetics.

POSSIBLE INTERACTION WITH OTHER DRUGS

GENERIC NAME OR DRUG CLASS	COMBINED EFFECT
Amiodarone (and other anti-arrhythmics)*	Increased risk of heartbeat irregularity due to low potassium.
Antihypertensives*	Increased benzthiazide effect or decreased blood pressure.
Antidepressants, tricyclic (TCA)*	Dangerous drop in blood pressure. Avoid combination unless under medical supervision.
Beta-adrenergic blockers*	Increased antihypertensive effect. Dosages of both drugs may require adjustments.
Bumetanide	Increased diuretic effect.
Calcium supplements*	May increase calcium in blood.
Carteolol	Increased antihypertensive effect.
Cholestyramine	Decreased benzthiazide effect.
Colestipol	Decreased benzthiazide effect.
Cortisone drugs*	Excessive potassium loss that causes dangerous heart rhythms.
Digitalis preparations*	Excessive potassium loss that causes dangerous heart rhythms.
Diuretics, thiazide*	Increased effect of other thiazide diuretics.
Ethacrynic acid	Increased benzthiazide effect.
Furosemide	Increased diuretic effect.
Indapamide	Increased diuretic effect.
Indomethacin	Decreased benzthiazide effect.
Insulin, oral	Decreased ability to lower blood glucose.
Labetalol	Increased antihypertensive effects.
Lisinopril	Increased antihypertensive effect. Dosage of each may require adjustment.
Lithium	Increased effect of lithium.
MAO inhibitors*	Increased benzthiazide effect.
Metolazone	Increased diuretic effect.

Continued page 1077

POSSIBLE INTERACTION WITH OTHER SUBSTANCES

INTERACTS WITH	COMBINED EFFECT
Alcohol:	Dangerous blood-pressure drop.
Beverages:	None expected.
Cocaine	Increased risk of heart block and high blood pressure.
Foods: Licorice.	Excessive potassium loss that causes dangerous heart rhythms.
Marijuana:	May increase blood pressure.
Tobacco:	None expected.

*See Glossary

BENZTROPINE

BRAND NAMES

Apo-Benztropine
Bensylate

Cogentin
PMS-Benztropine

BASIC INFORMATION

Habit forming? No
Prescription needed? Yes
Available as generic? Yes
Drug class: Antidyskinetic, antiparkinsonism

USES

- Treatment of Parkinson's disease.
- Treatment of adverse effects of phenothiazines.

DOSAGE & USAGE INFORMATION

How to take:
Tablets—Take with food to lessen stomach irritation.

When to take:
At the same times each day.

If you forget a dose:
Take as soon as you remember up to 2 hours late. If more than 2 hours, wait for next scheduled dose (don't double this dose).

What drug does:
- Balances chemical reactions necessary to send nerve impulses within base of brain.
- Improves muscle control and reduces stiffness.

Time lapse before drug works:
1 to 2 hours.

Continued next column

OVERDOSE

SYMPTOMS:
Agitation, dilated pupils, hallucinations, dry mouth, rapid heartbeat, sleepiness.
WHAT TO DO:
- Dial 0 (operator) or 911 (emergency) for an ambulance or medical help. Then give first aid immediately.
- If patient is unconscious and not breathing, give mouth-to-mouth breathing. If there is no heartbeat, use cardiac massage and mouth-to-mouth breathing (CPR). Don't try to make patient vomit. If you can't get help quickly, take patient to nearest emergency facility.
- See emergency information on inside covers.

Don't take with:
- Non-prescription drugs for colds, cough or allergy.
- See Interaction column and consult doctor.

POSSIBLE ADVERSE REACTIONS OR SIDE EFFECTS

SYMPTOMS	WHAT TO DO
Life-threatening: None expected.	
Common: • Blurred vision, light sensitivity, constipation, nausea, vomiting.	Continue. Call doctor when convenient.
• Difficult or painful urination, dry mouth.	Continue. Tell doctor at next visit.
Infrequent: None expected.	
Rare: • Rash, pain in eyes.	Discontinue. Call doctor right away.
• Confusion, dizziness, sore mouth or tongue, muscle cramps, numbness or weakness in hands or feet.	Continue. Call doctor when convenient.

BENZTROPINE

WARNINGS & PRECAUTIONS

Don't take if:
You are allergic to any antidyskinetic.

Before you start, consult your doctor:
- If you have had glaucoma.
- If you have had high blood pressure or heart disease.
- If you have had impaired liver function.
- If you have had prostate trouble.
- If you have had myasthenia gravis.
- If you have had kidney disease, urination difficulty or ulcers.

Over age 60:
More sensitive to drug. Aggravates symptoms of enlarged prostate. Causes impaired thinking, hallucinations, nightmares. Consult doctor about any of these.

Pregnancy:
Studies inconclusive on harm to unborn child. Animal studies show fetal abnormalities. Decide with your doctor whether drug benefits justify risk to unborn child.

Breast-feeding:
May inhibit lactation. Avoid if possible.

Infants & children:
Not recommended for children 3 and younger. Use for older children only under doctor's supervision.

Prolonged use:
Possible glaucoma.

Skin & sunlight:
No problems expected.

Driving, piloting or hazardous work:
Don't drive or pilot aircraft until you learn how medicine affects you. Don't work around dangerous machinery. Don't climb ladders or work in high places. Danger increases if you drink alcohol or take medicine affecting alertness and reflexes, such as antihistamines, tranquilizers, sedatives, pain medicine, narcotics and mind-altering drugs.

Discontinuing:
Don't discontinue without consulting doctor. Dose may require gradual reduction if you have taken drug for a long time. Doses of other drugs may also require adjustment.

Others:
- Internal eye pressure should be measured regularly.
- Avoid becoming overheated.

POSSIBLE INTERACTION WITH OTHER DRUGS

GENERIC NAME OR DRUG CLASS	COMBINED EFFECT
Amantadine	Increased amantadine effect.
Antidepressants, tricyclic (TCA)*	Increased benztropine effect. May cause glaucoma.
Antihistamines*	Increased benztropine effect.
Digoxin	May increase digoxin effect.
Levodopa	May decrease or increase levodopa effect. Improved results in treating Parkinson's disease.
Meperidine	Increased benztropine effect.
MAO inhibitors*	Increased benztropine effect.
Narcotics*	Increased benztropine effect.
Nabilone	Greater depression of the central nervous system.
Orphenadrine	Increased benztropine effect.
Phenothiazines*	Behavior changes.
Primidone	Excessive sedation.
Procainamide	Increased procainamide effect.
Quinidine	Increased benztropine effect.
Tranquilizers*	Excessive sedation.

POSSIBLE INTERACTION WITH OTHER SUBSTANCES

INTERACTS WITH	COMBINED EFFECT
Alcohol:	None expected.
Beverages:	None expected.
Cocaine:	Decreased benztropine effect. Avoid.
Foods:	None expected.
Marijuana:	None expected.
Tobacco:	None expected.

*See Glossary

BETA-ADRENERGIC BLOCKING AGENTS & THIAZIDE DIURETICS

BRAND AND GENERIC NAMES

ATENOLOL &
   CHLORTHALIDONE
Co-Betaloc
Corzide
Inderide
Inderide LA
Lopressor HCT
METOPROLOL &
   HYDROCHLORO-
   THIAZIDE
NADOLOL &
   BENDROFLUME-
   THIAZIDE
Normozide

PINDOLOL &
   HYDROCHLORO-
   THIAZIDE
PROPRANOLOL &
   HYDROCHLORO-
   THIAZIDE
Tenoretic
Timolide
TIMOLOL &
   HYDROCHLORO-
   THIAZIDE
Trandate HCT
Viskazide

BASIC INFORMATION

Habit forming? No
Prescription needed? Yes
Available as generic? Yes
Drug class: Beta-adrenergic blocker, thiazide
   diuretic

USES

- Controls, but doesn't cure, high blood pressure.
- Reduces fluid retention (edema).
- Reduces angina attacks.
- Stabilizes irregular heartbeat.
- Lowers blood pressure.
- Reduces frequency of migraine headaches. (Does not relieve headache pain.)
- Other uses prescribed by your doctor.

DOSAGE & USAGE INFORMATION

How to take:
Extended-release capsules—Swallow with liquid.
If you can't swallow whole, open capsule and
take with liquid or food.

When to take:
At the same time each day.

Continued next column

OVERDOSE

SYMPTOMS:
Irregular heartbeat (usually too slow),
confusion, fainting, convulsions, coma.
WHAT TO DO:
- Dial 0 (operator) or 911 (emergency) for an ambulance or medical help. Then give first aid immediately.
- See emergency information on inside covers.

If you forget a dose:
Take as soon as you remember up to 4 hours
late. If more than 4 hours, wait for next
scheduled dose (don't double this dose).

What drug does:
- Forces sodium and water excretion, reducing body fluid.
- Relaxes muscle cells of small arteries.
- Reduced body fluid and relaxed arteries lower blood pressure.
- Blocks some of the actions of sympathetic nervous system.
- Lowers heart's oxygen requirements.
- Slows nerve impulses through heart.
- Reduces blood vessel contraction in heart, scalp and other body parts.

Time lapse before drug works:
- 1 to 4 hours for beta-blocker effect.
- May require several weeks to lower blood pressure.

Don't take with:
Any other medicines, even OTC drugs such as
cough/cold medicines, diet pills, nose drops,
caffeine, without consulting your doctor.

POSSIBLE ADVERSE REACTIONS OR SIDE EFFECTS

SYMPTOMS	WHAT TO DO
Life-threatening:	
Wheezing, chest pain, irregular heartbeat.	Seek emergency treatment immediately.
Common:	
• Dry mouth, weak pulse, vomiting, muscle cramps, increased thirst, mood changes.	Discontinue. Call doctor right away.
• Weakness, tiredness, dizziness, mental depression, diminished sex drive, constipation, nightmares, insomnia.	Continue. Call doctor when convenient.
Infrequent:	
Cold feet and hands, chest pain, breathing difficulty, anxiety, nervousness, headache, appetite loss, abdominal pain, numbness and tingling in fingers and toes.	Discontinue. Call doctor right away.
Rare:	
• Hives, skin rash; joint pain; jaundice; fever, sore throat, mouth ulcers.	Discontinue. Call doctor right away.
• Impotence.	Continue. Call doctor when convenient.

BETA-ADRENERGIC BLOCKING AGENTS & THIAZIDE DIURETICS

WARNINGS & PRECAUTIONS

Don't take if:
- You are allergic to any beta-adrenergic blocker or any thiazide diuretic drug.
- You have asthma or hay fever symptoms.
- You have taken MAO inhibitors in past two weeks.

Before you start, consult your doctor:
- If you have heart disease or poor circulation to the extremities.
- If you have hay fever, asthma, chronic bronchitis, emphysema, overactive thyroid function, impaired liver or kidney function, gout, diabetes, hypoglycemia, pancreas disorder, systemic lupus erythematosus.
- If you are allergic to any sulfa drug or tartrazine dye.
- If you will have surgery within 2 months, including dental surgery, requiring general or spinal anesthesia.

Over age 60:
Adverse reactions and side effects may be more frequent and severe than in younger persons, especially dizziness and excessive potassium loss.

Pregnancy:
Risk to unborn child outweighs drug benefits. Don't use.

Breast-feeding:
Drug passes into milk. Avoid drug or discontinue nursing until you finish medicine. Consult doctor for advice on maintaining milk supply.

Infants & children:
Not recommended.

Prolonged use:
- Weakens heart muscle contractions.
- You may need medicine to treat high blood pressure for the rest of your life.

Skin & sunlight:
May cause rash or intensify sunburn in areas exposed to sun or sunlamp.

Driving, piloting or hazardous work:
Don't drive or pilot aircraft until you learn how medicine affects you. Don't work around dangerous machinery. Don't climb ladders or work in high places. Danger increases if you drink alcohol or take medicine affecting alertness and reflexes, such as antihistamines, tranquilizers, sedatives, pain medicine, narcotics and mind-altering drugs.

Discontinuing:
Don't discontinue without consulting doctor. Dose may require gradual reduction if you have taken drug for a long time. Doses of other drugs may also require adjustment.

Others:
- May mask hypoglycemia symptoms.
- Hot weather and fever may cause dehydration and drop in blood pressure. Dose may require temporary adjustment. Weigh daily and report any unexpected weight decreases to your doctor.
- May cause rise in uric acid, leading to gout.
- May cause blood-sugar rise in diabetics.

POSSIBLE INTERACTION WITH OTHER DRUGS

GENERIC NAME OR DRUG CLASS	COMBINED EFFECT
Allopurinol	Decreased allopurinol effect.
Antidepressants, tricyclic (TCA)*	Dangerous drop in blood pressure. Avoid combination unless under medical supervision.
Antidiabetics*	Increased antidiabetic effect.
Antihistamines*	Decreased antihistamine effect.

Continued page 1077

POSSIBLE INTERACTION WITH OTHER SUBSTANCES

INTERACTS WITH	COMBINED EFFECT
Alcohol:	Dangerous blood-pressure drop. Avoid.
Beverages:	None expected.
Cocaine:	Irregular heartbeat. Avoid.
Foods: Licorice.	Excessive potassium loss that causes dangerous heart rhythms.
Marijuana:	May increase blood pressure.
Tobacco:	May increase blood pressure and make heart work harder. Avoid.

*See Glossary

BETAMETHASONE

BRAND NAMES

See complete list of brand names in the *Brand Name Directory*, page 1058.

BASIC INFORMATION

Habit forming? No
Prescription needed? Yes
Available as generic? Yes
Drug class: Cortisone drug (adrenal corticosteroid)

USES

- Reduces inflammation caused by many different medical problems.
- Treatment for some allergic diseases, blood disorders, kidney diseases, asthma and emphysema.
- Replaces corticosteroid deficiencies.

DOSAGE & USAGE INFORMATION

How to take:
- Tablet, extended-release tablet, syrup or liquid—Swallow with liquid or food to lessen stomach irritation. If you can't swallow whole, crumble tablet and take with liquid or food.
- Inhaler—Follow label instructions.

When to take:
At the same times each day. Take once-a-day or once-every-other-day doses in mornings.

If you forget a dose:
- Several-doses-per-day prescription—Take as soon as you remember up to 2 hours late. If more than 2 hours, wait for next scheduled dose (don't double this dose).
- Once-a-day dose or less—Wait for next dose. Double this dose.

What drug does:
Decreases inflammatory responses.

Time lapse before drug works:
2 to 4 days.

Don't take with:
See Interaction column and consult doctor.

OVERDOSE

SYMPTOMS:
Headache, convulsions, heart failure.
WHAT TO DO:
- **Dial 0 (operator) or 911 (emergency) for an ambulance or medical help. Then give first aid immediately.**
- **See emergency information on inside covers.**

POSSIBLE ADVERSE REACTIONS OR SIDE EFFECTS

SYMPTOMS	WHAT TO DO
Life-threatening: Difficulty breathing.	Discontinue. Seek emergency treatment.
Common: Acne, poor wound healing, thirst, indigestion, nausea, vomiting.	Continue. Call doctor when convenient.
Infrequent: • Bloody or black, tarry stool.	Discontinue. Seek emergency treatment.
• Blurred vision, halos around lights, sore throat, fever, abdominal pain.	Discontinue. Call doctor right away.
• Mood changes, insomnia, fatigue, restlessness, frequent urination, weight gain, round face, weakness, TB recurrence, menstrual irregularities.	Continue. Call doctor when convenient.
Rare: • Irregular heartbeat.	Discontinue. Seek emergency treatment.
• Rash.	Discontinue. Call doctor right away.

WARNINGS & PRECAUTIONS

Don't take if:
- You are allergic to any cortisone drug.
- You have tuberculosis or fungus infection.
- You have herpes infection of eyes, lips or genitals.

Before you start, consult your doctor:
- If you have had tuberculosis.
- If you have an infection, congestive heart failure, diabetes, peptic ulcer, glaucoma, underactive thyroid, high blood pressure, myasthenia gravis, blood clots in legs or lungs.

Over age 60:
Adverse reactions and side effects may be more frequent and severe than in younger persons. Likely to aggravate edema, diabetes or ulcers. Likely to cause cataracts and osteoporosis (softening of the bones).

Pregnancy:
Risk to unborn child outweighs drug benefits. Don't use.

Breast-feeding:
Drug passes into milk. Avoid drug or discontinue nursing until you finish medicine. Consult doctor for advice on maintaining milk supply.

Infants & children:
Use only under medical supervision.

Prolonged use:
- Retards growth in children.
- Possible glaucoma, cataracts, diabetes, fragile bones and thin skin.
- Functional dependence.

Skin & sunlight:
No problems expected.

Driving, piloting or hazardous work:
No problems expected.

Discontinuing:
- Don't discontinue without doctor's advice until you complete prescribed dose, even though symptoms diminish or disappear.
- Drug affects your response to surgery, illness, injury or stress for up to 2 years after discontinuing. Inform doctor.

Others:
Avoid immunizations if possible.

 ## POSSIBLE INTERACTION WITH OTHER DRUGS

GENERIC NAME OR DRUG CLASS	COMBINED EFFECT
Amphotericin B	Potassium depletion.
Anticholinergics*	Possible glaucoma.
Anticoagulants, oral*	Decreased anticoagulant effect.
Anticonvulsants, hydantoin*	Decreased betamethasone effect.
Antidiabetics, oral*	Decreased antidiabetic effect.
Antihistamines*	Decreased betamethasone effect.
Aspirin	Increased betamethasone effect.
Barbiturates*	Decreased betamethasone effect. Oversedation.
Beta-adrenergic blockers*	Decreased betamethasone effect.
Butmetanide	Potassium depletion.
Chloral hydrate	Decreased betamethasone effect.
Chlorthalidone	Potassium depletion.

Cholestyramine	Decreased betamethasone effect.
Cholinergics*	Decreased cholinergic effect.
Colestipol	Decreased betamethasone effect.
Contraceptives, oral*	Increased betamethasone effect.
Cyclosporin	May increase cyclosporin effect.
Digitalis preparations*	Dangerous potassium depletion. Possible digitalis toxicity.
Diuretics thiazide*	Potassium depletion.
Ephedrine	Decreased betamethasone effect.
Estrogens*	Increased betamethasone effect.
Ethacrynic acid	Potassium depletion.
Furosemide	Potassium depletion.
Glutethimide	Decreased betamethasone effect.
Indapamide	Possible excessive potassium loss, causing dangerous heartbeat irregularity.
Indomethacin	Increased betamethasone effect.
Insulin	Decreased insulin effect.
Isoniazid	Decreased isoniazid effect.
Oxyphenbutazone	Possible ulcers.
Phenylbutazone	Possible ulcers.
Phenytoin	Decreased betamethasone effect.

Continued page 1078

 ## POSSIBLE INTERACTION WITH OTHER SUBSTANCES

INTERACTS WITH	COMBINED EFFECT
Alcohol:	Risk of stomach ulcers.
Beverages:	No proven problems.
Cocaine:	Overstimulation. Avoid.
Foods:	No proven problems.
Marijuana:	Decreased immunity.
Tobacco:	Increased betamethasone effect. Possible toxicity.

*See Glossary

BETHANECHOL

BRAND NAMES

Duvoid   Urecholine
Myotonachol

BASIC INFORMATION

Habit forming? No
Prescription needed? Yes
Available as generic? Yes
Drug class: Cholinergic

 ## USES

- Helps initiate urination following surgery, or for persons with urinary infections or enlarged prostate.
- Treats reflux esophagitis.

 ## DOSAGE & USAGE INFORMATION

How to take:
Tablet—Swallow with liquid, 1 hour before or 2 hours after eating.

When to take:
At the same times each day.

If you forget a dose:
Take as soon as you remember up to 2 hours late. If more than 2 hours, wait for next scheduled dose (don't double this dose).

What drug does:
Affects chemical reactions in the body that strengthen bladder muscles.

Time lapse before drug works:
30 to 90 minutes.

Don't take with:
See Interaction column and consult doctor.

 ## OVERDOSE

SYMPTOMS:
Shortness of breath, wheezing or chest tightness, unconsciousness, coma.
WHAT TO DO:
- Dial 0 (operator) or 911 (emergency) for an ambulance or medical help. Then give first aid immediately.
- If patient is unconscious and not breathing, give mouth-to-mouth breathing. If there is no heartbeat, use cardiac massage and mouth-to-mouth breathing (CPR). Don't try to make patient vomit. If you can't get help quickly, take patient to nearest emergency facility.
- See emergency information on inside covers.

 ## POSSIBLE ADVERSE REACTIONS OR SIDE EFFECTS

SYMPTOMS	WHAT TO DO
Life-threatening: None expected.	
Common: None expected.	
Infrequent: Dizziness, headache, faintness, blurred or changed vision, diarrhea, nausea, vomiting, stomach discomfort, belching, excessive urge to urinate.	Continue. Call doctor when convenient.
Rare: Shortness of breath, wheezing, tightness in chest.	Discontinue. Call doctor right away.

WARNINGS & PRECAUTIONS

Don't take if:
You are allergic to any cholinergic.

Before you start, consult your doctor:
- If you plan to become pregnant within medication period.
- If you have asthma.
- If you have epilepsy.
- If you have heart or blood-vessel disease.
- If you have high or low blood pressure.
- If you have overactive thyroid.
- If you have intestinal blockage.
- If you have Parkinson's disease.
- If you have stomach problems (including ulcer).
- If you have had bladder or intestinal surgery within 1 month.

Over age 60:
Adverse reactions and side effects may be more frequent and severe than in younger persons.

Pregnancy:
Risk to unborn child outweighs drug benefits. Don't use.

Breast-feeding:
Drug filters into milk. May harm child. Avoid.

Infants & children:
Use only under medical supervision.

Prolonged use:
No problems expected.

Skin & sunlight:
No problems expected.

Driving, piloting or hazardous work:
Don't drive or pilot aircraft until you learn how medicine affects you. Don't work around dangerous machinery. Don't climb ladders or work in high places. Danger increases if you drink alcohol or take medicine affecting alertness and reflexes, such as antihistamines, tranquilizers, sedatives, pain medicine, narcotics and mind-altering drugs.

Discontinuing:
May be unnecessary to finish medicine. Follow doctor's instructions.

Others:
- Be cautious about standing up suddenly.
- Interferes with laboratory studies of liver and pancreas function.
- Side effects more likely with injections.

POSSIBLE INTERACTION WITH OTHER DRUGS

GENERIC NAME OR DRUG CLASS	COMBINED EFFECT
Cholinergics, other*	Increased effect of both drugs. Possible toxicity.
Ganglionic blockers*	Decreased blood pressure.
Nitrates*	Decreased bethanechol effect.
Procainamide	Decreased bethanechol effect.
Quinidine	Decreased bethanechol effect.

POSSIBLE INTERACTION WITH OTHER SUBSTANCES

INTERACTS WITH	COMBINED EFFECT
Alcohol:	None expected.
Beverages:	None expected.
Cocaine:	None expected.
Foods:	None expected.
Marijuana:	None expected.
Tobacco:	None expected.

*See Glossary

BIPERIDEN

BRAND NAMES

Akineton

BASIC INFORMATION

Habit forming? No
Prescription needed? Yes
Available as generic? No
Drug class: Antidyskinetic, antiparkinsonism

 USES

- Treatment of Parkinson's disease.
- Treatment of adverse effects of phenothiazines.

 DOSAGE & USAGE INFORMATION

How to take:
Tablet—Take with food to lessen stomach irritation.

When to take:
At the same times each day.

If you forget a dose:
Take as soon as you remember up to 2 hours late. If more than 2 hours, wait for next scheduled dose (don't double this dose).

What drug does:
- Balances chemical reactions necessary to send nerve impulses within base of brain.
- Improves muscle control and reduces stiffness.

Time lapse before drug works:
1 to 2 hours.

Continued next column

 OVERDOSE

SYMPTOMS:
Agitation, dilated pupils, hallucinations, dry mouth, rapid heartbeat, sleepiness.
WHAT TO DO:
- Dial 0 (operator) or 911 (emergency) for an ambulance or medical help. Then give first aid immediately.
- If patient is unconscious and not breathing, give mouth-to-mouth breathing. If there is no heartbeat, use cardiac massage and mouth-to-mouth breathing (CPR). Don't try to make patient vomit. If you can't get help quickly, take patient to nearest emergency facility.
- See emergency information on inside covers.

Don't take with:
- Non-prescription drugs for colds, cough or allergy.
- See Interaction column and consult doctor.

 POSSIBLE ADVERSE REACTIONS OR SIDE EFFECTS

SYMPTOMS	WHAT TO DO
Life-threatening: None expected.	
Common:	
• Blurred vision, light sensitivity, constipation, nausea, vomiting.	Continue. Call doctor when convenient.
• Difficult or painful urination, dry mouth.	Continue. Tell doctor at next visit.
Infrequent: None expected.	
Rare:	
• Rash, pain in eyes.	Discontinue. Call doctor right away.
• Confusion, dizziness, sore mouth or tongue, muscle cramps, numbness or weakness in hands or feet.	Continue. Call doctor when convenient.

WARNINGS & PRECAUTIONS

Don't take if:
You are allergic to any antidyskinetic.

Before you start, consult your doctor:
- If you have had glaucoma.
- If you have had high blood pressure or heart disease.
- If you have had impaired liver function.
- If you have had myasthenia gravis.
- If you have had kidney disease, urination difficulty, ulcers or prostate trouble.

Over age 60:
More sensitive to drug. Aggravates symptoms of enlarged prostate. Causes impaired thinking, hallucinations, nightmares. Consult doctor about any of these.

Pregnancy:
Studies inconclusive on harm to unborn child. Animal studies show fetal abnormalities. Decide with your doctor whether drug benefits justify risk to unborn child.

Breast-feeding:
May inhibit milk secretion. Avoid if possible.

Infants & children:
Not recommended for children 3 and younger. Use for older children only under doctor's supervision.

Prolonged use:
Possible glaucoma.

Skin & sunlight:
No problems expected.

Driving, piloting or hazardous work:
Don't drive or pilot aircraft until you learn how medicine affects you. Don't work around dangerous machinery. Don't climb ladders or work in high places. Danger increases if you drink alcohol or take medicine affecting alertness and reflexes, such as antihistamines, tranquilizers, sedatives, pain medicine, narcotics and mind-altering drugs.

Discontinuing:
Don't discontinue without consulting doctor. Dose may require gradual reduction if you have taken drug for a long time. Doses of other drugs may also require adjustment.

Others:
- Internal eye pressure should be measured regularly.
- Avoid becoming overheated.

POSSIBLE INTERACTION WITH OTHER DRUGS

GENERIC NAME OR DRUG CLASS	COMBINED EFFECT
Amantadine	Increased amantadine effect.
Antidepressants, tricyclic (TCA)*	Increased biperiden effect. May cause glaucoma.
Antihistamines*	Increased biperiden effect.
Digoxin	May increase digoxin effect.
Levodopa	May decrease or increase levodopa effect. Improved results in treating Parkinson's disease.
Meperidine	Increased biperiden effect.
MAO inhibitors*	Increased biperiden effect.
Narcotics*	Increased biperiden effect.
Nabilone	Greater depression of the central nervous system.
Orphenadrine	Increased biperiden effect.
Phenothiazines*	Behavior changes.
Primidone	Excessive sedation.
Procainamide	Increased procainamide effect.
Quinidine	Increased biperiden effect.
Tranquilizers*	Excessive sedation.

POSSIBLE INTERACTION WITH OTHER SUBSTANCES

INTERACTS WITH	COMBINED EFFECT
Alcohol:	None expected.
Beverages:	None expected.
Cocaine:	Decreased biperiden effect. Avoid.
Foods:	None expected.
Marijuana:	None expected.
Tobacco:	None expected.

*See Glossary

BISACODYL

BRAND NAMES

Apo-Bisacodyl
Bisco-Lax
Carter's Little Pills
Cenalax
Clysodrast
Codylax
Dacodyl
Deficol

Dulcolax
Evac-Q-Kwik
Fleet Bisacodyl
Fleet Bisacodyl Prep
Fleet Enema
Nulac
Theralax

BASIC INFORMATION

Habit forming? No
Prescription needed? No
Available as generic? Yes
Drug class: Laxative (stimulant)

 ## USES

Constipation relief.

 ## DOSAGE & USAGE INFORMATION

How to take:
- Tablet—Swallow with liquid, do not crush.
- Suppository—Remove wrapper and moisten suppository with water. Gently insert larger end into rectum. Push well into rectum with finger. Retain in rectum 20-30 minutes.

When to take:
Usually at bedtime with a snack, unless directed otherwise.

If you forget a dose:
Take as soon as you remember.

What drug does:
Acts on smooth muscles of intestine wall to cause vigorous bowel movement.

Time lapse before drug works:
6 to 10 hours.

Don't take with:
- See Interaction column and consult doctor.
- Don't take within 2 hours of taking another medicine. Laxative interferes with medicine absorption.

 ## OVERDOSE

SYMPTOMS:
Vomiting, electrolyte depletion.
WHAT TO DO:
Overdose unlikely to threaten life. If person takes much larger amount than prescribed, call doctor, poison-control center or hospital emergency room for instructions.

 ## POSSIBLE ADVERSE REACTIONS OR SIDE EFFECTS

SYMPTOMS	WHAT TO DO
Life-threatening: None expected.	
Common: Rectal irritation.	Continue. Call doctor when convenient.
Infrequent:	
• Dangerous potassium loss.	Discontinue. Call doctor right away.
• Belching, cramps, nausea.	Continue. Call doctor when convenient.
Rare:	
• Irritability, headache, confusion, rash, breathing difficulty, irregular heartbeat, muscle cramps, unusual tiredness or weakness.	Discontinue. Call doctor right away.
• Burning on urination.	Continue. Call doctor when convenient.

148

WARNINGS & PRECAUTIONS

Don't take if:
- You have symptoms of appendicitis, inflamed bowel or intestinal blockage.
- You are allergic to a stimulant laxative.
- You have missed a bowel movement for only 1 or 2 days.

Before you start, consult your doctor:
- If you have a colostomy or ileostomy.
- If you have congestive heart disease.
- If you have diabetes.
- If you have high blood pressure.
- If you have a laxative habit.
- If you have rectal bleeding.
- If you take other laxatives.

Over age 60:
Adverse reactions and side effects may be more frequent and severe than in younger persons.

Pregnancy:
Risk to mother and unborn child outweighs drug benefits. Don't use.

Breast-feeding:
Drug passes into milk. Avoid drug or discontinue nursing until you finish medicine. Consult doctor for advice on maintaining milk supply.

Infants & children:
Use only under medical supervision.

Prolonged use:
Don't take for more than 1 week unless under doctor's supervision. May cause laxative dependence.

Skin & sunlight:
No problems expected.

Driving, piloting or hazardous work:
No problems expected.

Discontinuing:
May be unnecessary to finish medicine. Follow doctor's instructions.

Others:
Don't take to "flush out" your system or as a "tonic."

POSSIBLE INTERACTION WITH OTHER DRUGS

GENERIC NAME OR DRUG CLASS	COMBINED EFFECT
Antacids*	Tablet coating may dissolve too rapidly, irritating stomach or bowel.
Antihypertensives*	May cause dangerous low potassium level.
Cimetidine	Stomach or bowel irritation.
Diuretics*	May cause dangerous low potassium level.
Famotidine	Stomach or bowel irritation.
Ranitidine	Stomach or bowel irritation.

POSSIBLE INTERACTION WITH OTHER SUBSTANCES

INTERACTS WITH	COMBINED EFFECT
Alcohol:	None expected.
Beverages:	None expected.
Cocaine:	None expected.
Foods:	None expected.
Marijuana:	None expected.
Tobacco:	None expected.

*See Glossary

BISMUTH SUBSALICYLATE

BRAND NAMES

Pepto-Bismol

BASIC INFORMATION

Habit forming? No
Prescription needed? No
Available as generic? No
Drug class: Antidiarrheal; antacid

 ## USES

- Treats symptoms of diarrhea, heartburn, nausea, acid indigestion.
- Helps prevent traveler's diarrhea.

 ## DOSAGE & USAGE INFORMATION

How to take:
- Chewable tablets—Chew well before swallowing.
- Liquid—Dilute dose in beverage before swallowing.

When to take:
As directed on label or by your doctor.

If you forget a dose:
Take as soon as you remember. Don't double this dose.

What drug does:
- Binds toxin of some bacteria.
- Stimulates absorption of fluid and electrolytes across the intestinal wall.
- Decreases inflammation and increased motility of the intestinal muscles and lining.

Time lapse before drug works:
30 minutes to 1 hour.

Don't take with:
See Interaction column and consult doctor.

 ## OVERDOSE

SYMPTOMS:
Anxiety, confusion, speech difficulty, severe headache, muscle spasms, depression, trembling.
WHAT TO DO:
- **Dial 0 (operator) or 911 (emergency) for an ambulance or medical help. Then give first aid immediately.**
- **See emergency information on inside covers.**

 ## POSSIBLE ADVERSE REACTIONS OR SIDE EFFECTS

SYMPTOMS	WHAT TO DO
Life-threatening: None likely for short course of therapy (see Overdose).	
Common: Black stools, dark tongue. (These symptoms are normal and medically insignificant.)	No action necessary.
Infrequent: • Hearing loss, confusion, dizziness, fast breathing, headache, increased thirst, ringing or buzzing in ears, vision problems.	Discontinue. Call doctor right away.
• Constipation.	Continue. Call doctor when convenient.
Rare: See Overdose.	

150

BISMUTH SUBSALICYLATE

WARNINGS & PRECAUTIONS

Don't take if:
- You are allergic to aspirin, salicylates or other non-steroidal anti-inflammatory drugs.
- You have stomach ulcers that have ever bled.
- The patient is a child with fever.

Before you start, consult your doctor:
- If you are on a low-sodium, low-sugar or other special diet.
- If you have had diarrhea for more than 24 hours. This is especially applicable to infants, children and those over 60.
- If you have had kidney disease.

Over age 60:
- Consult doctor before using.
- May cause severe constipation.

Pregnancy:
- Don't use during last 3 months of pregnancy.
- Studies inconclusive on harm to unborn child. Decide with your doctor whether drug benefits justify risk to unborn child.

Breast-feeding:
- Drug passes into milk. Avoid or discontinue nursing until you finish medicine.
- May harm baby if mother takes large amounts.

Infants & children:
Not recommended for children 3 and younger. May cause constipation.

Prolonged use:
May cause constipation.

Skin & sunlight:
No problems expected.

Driving, piloting or hazardous work:
Don't drive or pilot aircraft if you take high or prolonged dose until you learn how medicine affects you. Don't work around dangerous machinery. Don't climb ladders or work in high places. Danger increases if you drink alcohol or take medicine affecting alertness and reflexes, such as antihistamines, tranquilizers, sedatives, pain medicine, narcotics and mind-altering drugs.

Discontinuing:
No problems expected.

Others:
- Pepto-Bismol contains salicylates. When given to children with flu or chickenpox, salicylates may cause a serious illness called Reye's syndrome. An overdose in children can cause the same problems as aspirin poisoning.
- May cause false urine sugar tests.

POSSIBLE INTERACTION WITH OTHER DRUGS

GENERIC NAME OR DRUG CLASS	COMBINED EFFECT
Anticoagulants*	Increased risk of bleeding.
Insulin or oral antidiabetic drugs*	Increased insulin effect. May require dosage adjustment.
Probenecid	Decreased effect of probenecid.
Salicylates, other*	Increased risk of salicylate toxicity.
Sulfinpyrazone	Decreased effect of sulfinpyrazone.
Tetracylines*	Decreased absorption of tetracycline.
Thrombolytic agents*	Increased risk of bleeding.

POSSIBLE INTERACTION WITH OTHER SUBSTANCES

INTERACTS WITH	COMBINED EFFECT
Alcohol:	None expected.
Beverages:	None expected.
Cocaine:	Decreased Pepto-bismol effect. Avoid.
Foods:	None expected.
Marijuana:	None expected.
Tobacco:	None expected.

BROMOCRIPTINE

BRAND NAMES

Parlodel .

BASIC INFORMATION

Habit forming? No
Prescription needed? Yes
Available as generic? No
Drug class: Antiparkinsonism

 USES

- Controls Parkinson's disease symptoms such as rigidity, tremors and unsteady gait.
- Treats female infertility.
- Prevents lactation.
- Treats acromegaly.

 DOSAGE & USAGE INFORMATION

How to take:
Tablet or capsule—Swallow with liquid or food to lessen stomach irritation. If you can't swallow whole, crumble tablet or open capsule and take with liquid or food.

When to take:
At the same times each day.

If you forget a dose:
Take as soon as you remember up to 2 hours late. If more than 2 hours, wait for next scheduled dose (don't double this dose).

Continued next column

 OVERDOSE

SYMPTOMS:
Muscle twitch, spastic eyelid closure, nausea, vomiting, diarrhea, irregular and rapid pulse, weakness, fainting, confusion, agitation, hallucination, coma.
WHAT TO DO:
- **Dial 0 (operator) or 911 (emergency) for an ambulance or medical help. Then give first aid immediately.**
- **If patient is unconscious and not breathing, give mouth-to-mouth breathing. If there is no heartbeat, use cardiac massage and mouth-to-mouth breathing (CPR). Don't try to make patient vomit. If you can't get help quickly, take patient to nearest emergency facility.**
- **See emergency information on inside covers.**

What drug does:
Restores chemical balance necessary for normal nerve impulses.

Time lapse before drug works:
2 to 3 weeks to improve; 6 weeks or longer for maximum benefit.

Don't take with:
See Interaction column and consult doctor.

 POSSIBLE ADVERSE REACTIONS OR SIDE EFFECTS

SYMPTOMS	WHAT TO DO
Life-threatening: None expected.	
Common:	
• Mood changes, uncontrollable body movements, diarrhea, nausea.	Continue. Call doctor when convenient.
• Dry mouth, body odor.	No action necessary.
Infrequent:	
• Fainting, severe dizziness, headache, insomnia, nightmares, rash, itch, vomiting, irregular heartbeat.	Discontinue. Call doctor right away.
• Flushed face, blurred vision, muscle twitching, discolored or dark urine, difficult urination.	Continue. Call doctor when convenient.
• Constipation, tiredness.	Continue. Tell doctor at next visit.
Rare:	
• High blood pressure, hallucinations, psychosis.	Discontinue. Call doctor right away.
• Anemia, duodenal ulcer.	Continue. Call doctor when convenient.
• Hair loss.	Continue. Tell doctor at next visit.

BROMOCRIPTINE

WARNINGS & PRECAUTIONS

Don't take if:
- You are allergic to bromocriptine or ergotamine.
- You have taken MAO inhibitors in past 2 weeks.
- You have glaucoma (narrow-angle type).

Before you start, consult your doctor:
- If you have diabetes or epilepsy.
- If you have had high blood pressure, heart or lung disease.
- If you have had liver or kidney disease.
- If you have a peptic ulcer.
- If you will have surgery within 2 months, including dental surgery, requiring general or spinal anesthesia.

Over age 60:
Adverse reactions and side effects may be more frequent and severe than in younger persons.

Pregnancy:
Risk to unborn child outweighs drug benefits. Don't use.

Breast-feeding:
Drug filters into milk. May harm child. Avoid.

Infants & children:
Not recommended if under 15 years old.

Prolonged use:
May lead to uncontrolled movements of head, face, mouth, tongue, arms or legs.

Skin & sunlight:
No problems expected.

Driving, piloting or hazardous work:
Don't drive or pilot aircraft until you learn how medicine affects you. Don't work around dangerous machinery. Don't climb ladders or work in high places. Danger increases if you drink alcohol or take medicine affecting alertness and reflexes, such as antihistamines, tranquilizers, sedatives, pain medicine, narcotics and mind-altering drugs.

Discontinuing:
Don't discontinue without doctor's advice until you complete prescribed dose, even though symptoms diminish or disappear.

Others:
Expect to start with small doses and increase gradually to lessen frequency and severity of adverse reactions.

POSSIBLE INTERACTION WITH OTHER DRUGS

GENERIC NAME OR DRUG CLASS	COMBINED EFFECT
Antihypertensives*	May decrease blood pressure.
Antiparkinsonism drugs, other*	Increased bromocriptine effect.
Contraceptives, oral*	Decreased bromocriptine effect.
Guanfacine	Increased effect of both drugs.
Haloperidol	Decreased bromocriptine effect.
Levodopa	Decreased antiparkinson effect.
MAO inhibitors*	Dangerous rise in blood pressure.
Methyldopa	Decreased bromocriptine effect.
Papaverine	Decreased bromocriptine effect.
Phenothiazines*	Decreased bromocriptine effect.
Pyridoxine (Vitamin B-6)	Decreased bromocriptine effect.
Rauwolfia alkaloids*	Decreased bromocriptine effect.

POSSIBLE INTERACTION WITH OTHER SUBSTANCES

INTERACTS WITH	COMBINED EFFECT
Alcohol:	Decreased alcohol tolerance.
Beverages:	None expected.
Cocaine:	Decreased bromocriptine effect. Avoid.
Foods:	None expected.
Marijuana:	Increased fatigue, lethargy, fainting. Avoid.
Tobacco:	Interferes with absorption. Avoid.

BROMODIPHENHYDRAMINE

BRAND NAMES

Ambenyl Expectorant   Ambodryl

BASIC INFORMATION

Habit forming? No
Prescription needed? Yes
Available as generic? No
Drug class: Antihistamine

 USES

- Reduces allergic symptoms such as hay fever, hives, rash or itching.
- Induces sleep.

 DOSAGE & USAGE INFORMATION

How to take:
Liquid—Swallow with liquid or food to lessen stomach irritation.

When to take:
Follow label directions.

If you forget a dose:
Take as soon as you remember up to 2 hours late. If more than 2 hours, wait for next scheduled dose (don't double this dose).

What drug does:
Blocks action of histamine after an allergic response triggers histamine release in sensitive cells.

Time lapse before drug works:
30 minutes.

Don't take with:
See Interaction column and consult doctor.

 OVERDOSE

SYMPTOMS:
Convulsions, red face, hallucinations, coma.
WHAT TO DO:
- Dial 0 (operator) or 911 (emergency) for an ambulance or medical help. Then give first aid immediately.
- If patient is unconscious and not breathing, give mouth-to-mouth breathing. If there is no heartbeat, use cardiac massage and mouth-to-mouth breathing (CPR). Don't try to make patient vomit. If you can't get help quickly, take patient to nearest emergency facility.
- See emergency information on inside covers.

 POSSIBLE ADVERSE REACTIONS OR SIDE EFFECTS

SYMPTOMS	WHAT TO DO
Life-threatening: Difficulty breating.	Discontinue. Seek emergency treatment.
Common: Drowsiness, dizziness, dry mouth or throat, nausea.	Continue. Tell doctor at next visit.
Infrequent: • Vision changes.	Discontinue. Call doctor right away.
• Less tolerance for contact lenses, difficult or painful urination.	Continue. Call doctor when convenient.
• Appetite loss.	Continue. Tell doctor at next visit.
Rare: Nightmares, agitation, irritability, sore throat, fever, rapid heartbeat, unusual bleeding or bruising, fatigue, weakness.	Discontinue. Call doctor right away.

BROMODIPHENHYDRAMINE

 ## WARNINGS & PRECAUTIONS

Don't take if:
You are allergic to any antihistamine.

Before you start, consult your doctor:
- If you have glaucoma.
- If you have enlarged prostate.
- If you have asthma.
- If you have kidney disease.
- If you have peptic ulcer.
- If you will have surgery within 2 months, including dental surgery, requiring general or spinal anesthesia.

Over age 60:
Don't exceed recommended dose. Adverse reactions and side effects may be more frequent and severe than in younger persons, especially urination difficulty, diminished alertness and other brain and nervous-system symptoms.

Pregnancy:
Safety not established. Avoid if possible.

Breast-feeding:
Drug passes into milk. Avoid drug or discontinue nursing until you finish medicine. Consult doctor for advice on maintaining milk supply.

Infants & children:
Not recommended for premature or newborn infants. Otherwise, no problems expected.

Prolonged use:
Avoid. May damage bone-marrow and nerve cells.

Skin & sunlight:
May cause rash or intensify sunburn in areas exposed to sun or sunlamp.

Driving, piloting or hazardous work:
Don't drive or pilot aircraft until you learn how medicine affects you. Don't work around dangerous machinery. Don't climb ladders or work in high places. Danger increases if you drink alcohol or take medicine affecting alertness and reflexes, such as antihistamines, tranquilizers, sedatives, pain medicine, narcotics and mind-altering drugs.

Discontinuing:
No problems expected.

Others:
May mask symptoms of hearing damage from aspirin, other salicylates, cisplatin, paromomycin, vancomycin or anticonvulsants. Consult doctor if you use these.

 ## POSSIBLE INTERACTION WITH OTHER DRUGS

GENERIC NAME OR DRUG CLASS	COMBINED EFFECT
Anticholinergics*	Increased anticholinergic effect.
Anticoagulants, oral*	May decrease anticoagulant effect.
Antidepressants*	Excess sedation. Avoid.
Antihistamines, other*	Excess sedation. Avoid.
Carteolol	Decreased antihistamine effect.
Dronabinol	Increased effects of both drugs. Avoid.
Hypnotics*	Excess sedation. Avoid.
MAO inhibitors*	Increased bromodiphenhydramine effect.
Mind-altering drugs*	Excess sedation. Avoid.
Nabilone	Greater depression of the central nervous system.
Narcotics*	Excess sedation. Avoid.
Sedatives*	Excess sedation. Avoid.
Sleep inducers*	Excess sedation. Avoid.
Sotalol	Increased antihistamine effect.
Tranquilizers*	Excess sedation. Avoid.

 ## POSSIBLE INTERACTION WITH OTHER SUBSTANCES

INTERACTS WITH	COMBINED EFFECT
Alcohol:	Excess sedation. Avoid.
Beverages: Caffeine drinks.	Less bromodiphenhydramine sedation.
Cocaine:	Decreased bromodiphenhydramine effect. Avoid.
Foods:	None expected.
Marijuana:	Excess sedation. Avoid.
Tobacco:	None expected.

BROMPHENIRAMINE

BRAND NAMES

See complete list of brand names in the *Brand Name Directory*, page 1059.

BASIC INFORMATION

Habit forming? No
Prescription needed? Yes
Available as generic? Yes
Drug class: Antihistamine

 ## USES

- Reduces allergic symptoms such as hay fever, hives, rash or itching.
- Induces sleep.

 ## DOSAGE & USAGE INFORMATION

How to take:
- Tablet or elixir—Swallow with liquid or food to lessen stomach irritation.
- Extended-release tablets—Swallow each dose whole.

When to take:
Varies with form. Follow label directions.

If you forget a dose:
Take as soon as you remember up to 2 hours late. If more than 2 hours, wait for next scheduled dose (don't double this dose).

What drug does:
Blocks action of histamine after an allergic response triggers histamine release in sensitive cells.

Time lapse before drug works:
30 minutes.

Don't take with:
See Interaction column and consult doctor.

 ## OVERDOSE

SYMPTOMS:
Convulsions, red face, hallucinations, coma.
WHAT TO DO:
- **Dial 0 (operator) or 911 (emergency) for an ambulance or medical help. Then give first aid immediately.**
- **See emergency information on inside covers.**

 ## POSSIBLE ADVERSE REACTIONS OR SIDE EFFECTS

SYMPTOMS	WHAT TO DO
Life-threatening: Difficulty breathing.	Discontinue. Seek emergency treatment.
Common: Drowsiness; dizziness; dry mouth, nose or throat; nausea.	Continue. Tell doctor at next visit.
Infrequent:	
• Vision changes.	Discontinue. Call doctor right away.
• Less tolerance for contact lenses, difficult or painful urination.	Continue. Call doctor when convenient.
• Appetite loss.	Continue. Tell doctor at next visit.
Rare: Nightmares, agitation, irritability, sore throat, fever, rapid heartbeat, unusual bleeding or bruising, fatigue, weakness.	Discontinue. Call doctor right away.

WARNINGS & PRECAUTIONS

Don't take if:
You are allergic to any antihistamine.

Before you start, consult your doctor:
- If you have glaucoma.
- If you have enlarged prostate.
- If you have asthma.
- If you have kidney disease.
- If you have peptic ulcer.
- If you will have surgery within 2 months, including dental surgery, requiring general or spinal anesthesia.

Over age 60:
Don't exceed recommended dose. Adverse reactions and side effects may be more frequent and severe than in younger persons, especially urination difficulty, diminished alertness and other brain and nervous-system symptoms.

Pregnancy:
Safety not established. Avoid if possible.

Breast-feeding:
Drug passes into milk. Avoid drug or discontinue nursing until you finish medicine. Consult doctor for advice on maintaining milk supply.

Infants & children:
Not recommended for premature or newborn infants. Otherwise, no problems expected.

Prolonged use:
Avoid. May damage bone marrow and nerve cells.

Skin & sunlight:
May cause rash or intensify sunburn in areas exposed to sun or sunlamp.

Driving, piloting or hazardous work:
Don't drive or pilot aircraft until you learn how medicine affects you. Don't work around dangerous machinery. Don't climb ladders or work in high places. Danger increases if you drink alcohol or take medicine affecting alertness and reflexes, such as antihistamines, tranquilizers, sedatives, pain medicine, narcotics and mind-altering drugs.

Discontinuing:
No problems expected.

Others:
May mask symptoms of hearing damage from aspirin, other salicylates, cisplatin, paromomycin, vancomycin or anticonvulsants. Consult doctor if you use these.

POSSIBLE INTERACTION WITH OTHER DRUGS

GENERIC NAME OR DRUG CLASS	COMBINED EFFECT
Anticholinergics*	Increased anticholinergic effect.
Anticoagulants, oral*	May decrease anticoagulant effect.
Antidepressants*	Excess sedation. Avoid.
Antihistamines, other*	Excess sedation. Avoid.
Carteolol	Decreased antihistamine effect.
Dronabinol	Increased effects of both drugs. Avoid.
Hypnotics*	Excess sedation. Avoid.
MAO inhibitors*	Increased brompheniramine effect.
Mind-altering drugs*	Excess sedation. Avoid.
Molindone	Increased antihistamine effect.
Nabilone	Greater depression of central nervous system.
Narcotics*	Excess sedation. Avoid.
Sedatives*	Excess sedation. Avoid.
Sleep inducers*	Excess sedation. Avoid.
Sotalol	Increased antihistamine effect.
Tranquilizers*	Excess sedation. Avoid.

POSSIBLE INTERACTION WITH OTHER SUBSTANCES

INTERACTS WITH	COMBINED EFFECT
Alcohol:	Excess sedation. Avoid.
Beverages: Caffeine drinks.	Less brompheniramine sedation.
Cocaine:	Decreased brompheniramine effect. Avoid.
Foods:	None expected.
Marijuana:	Excess sedation. Avoid.
Tobacco:	None expected.

BUCLIZINE

BRAND NAMES

Bucladin-S

BASIC INFORMATION

Habit forming? No
Prescription needed?
  U.S.: No
  Canada: Yes
Available as generic? No
Drug class: Antihistamine, antiemetic

 USES

Prevents motion sickness.

 DOSAGE & USAGE INFORMATION

How to take:
Tablet—Swallow with liquid or food to lessen stomach irritation. If you can't swallow whole, crumble tablet and chew or take with liquid or food.

When to take:
30 minutes to 1 hour before traveling.

If you forget a dose:
Take as soon as you remember. Wait 4 hours for next dose.

What drug does:
Reduces sensitivity of nerve endings in inner ear, blocking messages to brain's vomiting center.

Time lapse before drug works:
30 to 60 minutes.

Don't take with:
See Interaction column and consult doctor.

 OVERDOSE

SYMPTOMS:
Drowsiness, confusion, incoordination, stupor, coma, weak pulse, shallow breathing, hallucinations.
WHAT TO DO:
- **Dial 0 (operator) or 911 (emergency) for an ambulance or medical help. Then give first aid immediately.**
- **See emergency information on inside covers.**

 POSSIBLE ADVERSE REACTIONS OR SIDE EFFECTS

SYMPTOMS	WHAT TO DO
Life-threatening: None expected.	
Common: Drowsiness.	Continue. Tell doctor at next visit.
Infrequent:	
• Headache, diarrhea or constipation, fast heartbeat.	Continue. Call doctor when convenient.
• Dry mouth, nose, throat.	Continue. Tell doctor at next visit.
Rare:	
• Rash or hives.	Discontinue. Call doctor right away.
• Restlessness, excitement, insomnia, blurred vision, frequent urination, difficult urination, hallucinations.	Continue. Call doctor when convenient.
• Appetite loss, nausea.	Continue. Tell doctor at next visit.

 WARNINGS & PRECAUTIONS

Don't take if:
- You are allergic to meclizine, buclizine or cyclizine.
- You have taken MAO inhibitors in the past 2 weeks.

Before you start, consult your doctor:
- If you have glaucoma.
- If you have prostate enlargement.
- If you have reacted badly to any antihistamine.

Over age 60:
Adverse reactions and side effects may be more frequent and severe than in younger persons, especially impaired urination from enlarged prostate gland.

Pregnancy:
Studies inconclusive on harm to unborn child. Animal studies show fetal abnormalities. Decide with your doctor whether drug benefits justify risk to unborn child.

Breast-feeding:
Drug passes into milk. Avoid drug or discontinue nursing until you finish medicine. Consult doctor for advice on maintaining milk supply.

Infants & children:
Safety not established. Avoid if less than 12 years old.

Prolonged use:
No problems expected.

Skin & sunlight:
No problems expected.

Driving, piloting or hazardous work:
Don't fly aircraft. Don't drive until you learn how medicine affects you. Don't work around dangerous machinery. Don't climb ladders or work in high places. Danger increases if you drink alcohol or take medicine affecting alertness and reflexes, such as antihistamines, tranquilizers, sedatives, pain medicine, narcotics and mind-altering drugs.

Discontinuing:
No problems expected.

Others:
Buclizine contains tartrazine dye. Avoid if allergic (especially aspirin hypersensitivity).

 POSSIBLE INTERACTION WITH OTHER DRUGS

GENERIC NAME OR DRUG CLASS	COMBINED EFFECT
Amphetamines*	May decrease drowsiness caused by buclizine.
Anticholinergics*	Increased effect of both drugs.
Antidepressants, tricyclic (TCA)*	Increased effect of both drugs.
Carteolol	Decreased anti-histamine effect.
Dronabinol	Increases effect of buclizine.
Ethinamate	Dangerous increased effects of ethinamate. Avoid combining.
Fluoxetine	Increased depressant effects of both drugs.
Guanfacine	May increase depressant effects of either drug.
MAO inhibitors*	Increased buclizine effect.
Methyprylon	Increased sedative effect, perhaps to dangerous level. Avoid.
Nabilone	Greater depression of central nervous system.
Narcotics*	Increased effect of both drugs.
Pain relievers*	Increased effect of both drugs.
Sedatives*	Increased effect of both drugs.
Sleep inducers*	Increased effect of both drugs.
Sotalol	Increased antihistamine effect.
Tranquilizers*	Increased effect of both drugs.

 POSSIBLE INTERACTION WITH OTHER SUBSTANCES

INTERACTS WITH	COMBINED EFFECT
Alcohol:	Increased sedation. Avoid.
Beverages: Caffeine drinks.	May decrease drowsiness.
Cocaine:	None expected.
Foods:	None expected.
Marijuana:	Increased drowsiness, dry mouth.
Tobacco:	None expected.

BUMETANIDE

BRAND NAMES

Bumex

BASIC INFORMATION

Habit forming? No
Prescription needed? Yes
Available as generic? No
Drug class: Diuretic

USES

Decreases fluid retention.

DOSAGE & USAGE INFORMATION

How to take:
Tablet—Swallow with liquid or food to lessen stomach irritation. If you can't swallow whole, crumble tablet and take with liquid or food.

When to take:
- 1 dose a day—Take after breakfast.
- More than 1 dose a day—Take last dose no later than 6 p.m. unless otherwise directed.

If you forget a dose:
- 1 dose a day—Take as soon as you remember up to 12 hours late. If more than 12 hours, wait for next scheduled dose (don't double this dose).
- More than 1 dose a day—Take as soon as you remember up to 2 hours late. If more than 2 hours, wait for next scheduled dose (don't double this dose).

What drug does:
Increases elimination of sodium and water from body. Decreased body fluid reduces blood pressure.

Time lapse before drug works:
1 hour to increase water loss.

Don't take with:
See Interaction column and consult doctor.

OVERDOSE

SYMPTOMS:
Weakness, lethargy, dizziness, confusion, nausea, vomiting, leg-muscle cramps, thirst, stupor, deep sleep, weak and rapid pulse, cardiac arrest.
WHAT TO DO:
- **Dial 0 (operator) or 911 (emergency) for an ambulance or medical help. Then give first aid immediately.**
- **See emergency information on inside covers.**

POSSIBLE ADVERSE REACTIONS OR SIDE EFFECTS

SYMPTOMS	WHAT TO DO
Life-threatening: None expected.	
Common: Dizziness.	Continue. Call doctor when convenient.
Infrequent: Mood changes, fatigue, appetite loss, watery diarrhea, irregular heartbeat, muscle cramps, weakness, abdominal pain, low blood pressure.	Discontinue. Call doctor right away.
Rare: Rash or hives; yellow vision; ringing in ears; hearing loss; sore throat, fever; dry mouth; thirst; side or stomach pain; nausea; vomiting; unusual bleeding or bruising; joint pain; numbness or tingling in hands or feet, jaundice.	Discontinue. Call doctor right away.

WARNINGS & PRECAUTIONS

Don't take if:
You are allergic to bumetanide.

Before you start, consult your doctor:
- If you have liver or kidney disease.
- If you have gout.
- If you have diabetes.
- If you are allergic to sulfa.
- If you have impaired hearing.
- If you will have surgery within 2 months, including dental surgery, requiring general or spinal anesthesia.

Over age 60:
Adverse reactions and side effects may be more frequent and severe than in younger persons.

Pregnancy:
Risk to unborn child outweighs drug benefits. Don't use.

Breast-feeding:
Drug filters into milk. May harm child. Avoid.

Infants & children:
Use only under medical supervision.

Prolonged use:
- Impaired balance of water, salt and potassium in blood and body tissues. Request periodic laboratory studies of electrolytes in blood.
- Possible diabetes.

Skin & sunlight:
May cause rash or intensify sunburn in areas exposed to sun or sunlamp.

Driving, piloting or hazardous work:
No problems expected.

Discontinuing:
Don't discontinue without doctor's advice until you complete prescribed dose, even though symptoms diminish or disappear.

Others:
Frequent laboratory studies to monitor potassium level in blood recommended. Eat foods rich in potassium or take potassium supplements. Consult doctor.

POSSIBLE INTERACTION WITH OTHER DRUGS

GENERIC NAME OR DRUG CLASS	COMBINED EFFECT
ACE inhibitors: captopril, enalapril, lisinopril*	Possible excessive potassium in blood.
Amiodarone	Increased risk of heartbeat irregularity due to low potassium.
Amikain, gentamycin, kanamycin, streptomycin, tobramycin, cisplatin, ethacrynic acid, furosemide, mercaptopurine, polymixins vancomycin.	Increased possibility of hearing loss.
Amitriptyline	Increased amitriptyline effect.
Anticoagulants, oral*	Possible increased anticoagulant effect.
Antihypertensives*	Increased blood-pressure drop. Dosages may require adjustment.
Beta-adrenergic blockers*	Increased antihypertensive effect. Dosages may require adjustment.
Calcium supplements*	Decreased calcium in blood.
Corticosteroids*	Decreased potassium.
Digoxin	Increased possibility of digitalis toxicity because bumetanide can cause lowered potassium levels.
Diuretics, other*	Increased diuretic effect.
Indomethacin	Decreased effect of bumetanide.
Labetalol	Increased anti-hypertensive effects.
Lithium	Increased possibility of lithium toxicity.
Nicardipine	Dangerous blood-pressure drop. Dosages may require adjustment.
Nitrates*	Excessive blood-pressure drop.
Non-steroidal anti-inflammatory drugs (NSAIDs)*	Decreased effect of bumetanide
Phenytoin	Decreased bumetanide effect.
Potassium supplements*	Decreased potassium effect.
Probenecid	Decreased effect of bumetanide.

POSSIBLE INTERACTION WITH OTHER SUBSTANCES

INTERACTS WITH	COMBINED EFFECT
Alcohol:	Blood-pressure drop. Avoid.
Beverages: Caffeine.	Decreased bumetanide effect.
Cocaine:	Dangerous blood-pressure drop. Avoid.
Foods:	None expected.
Marijuana:	Increased thirst and urinary frequency, fainting.
Tobacco:	Decreased bumetanide effect.

BUSPIRONE

BRAND NAMES

BuSpar

BASIC INFORMATION

Habit forming? Unknown
Prescription needed? Yes
Available as generic? No
Drug class: Anti-anxiety (tranquilizer)

 ## USES

Treats anxiety disorders with nervousness or tension. Not intended for treatment of ordinary stress of daily living. Causes less sedation than some anti-anxiety drugs.

 ## DOSAGE & USAGE INFORMATION

How to take:
Tablets—Take with a glass of liquid.

When to take:
As directed. Usually 3 times daily. Food does not interfere with absorption.

If you forget a dose:
Take as soon as you remember, but skip this dose and don't double the next dose if it is almost time for the next dose.

What drug does:
Chemical family azaspirodecanedione; *not* a benzodiazepine. Probably has an effect on neurotransmitter systems.

Time lapse before drug works:
1 or 2 weeks before beneficial effects may be observed.

Don't take with:
Alcohol, other tranquilizers, antihistamines, muscle relaxants, sedatives or narcotics.

 ## OVERDOSE

SYMPTOMS:
Severe drowsiness or nausea, vomiting, small pupils, unconsciousness.
WHAT TO DO:
- **Dial 0 (operator) or 911 (emergency) for an ambulance or medical help. Then give first aid immediately.**
- **See emergency information on inside covers.**

 ## POSSIBLE ADVERSE REACTIONS OR SIDE EFFECTS

SYMPTOMS	WHAT TO DO
Life-threatening:	
Chest pain; pounding, fast heartbeat (rare).	Discontinue. Seek emergency treatment.
Common:	
Lightheadedness, headache, nausea, restlessness, dizziness.	Discontinue. Call doctor right away.
Infrequent:	
Drowsiness, dry mouth, ringing in ears, nightmares or vivid dreams, unusual fatigue.	Continue. Call doctor when convenient.
Rare:	
Numbness or tingling in feet or hands; sore throat; fever; depression or confusion; uncontrollable movements of tongue, lips, arms and legs; slurred speech; psychosis; dream disturbance.	Discontinue. Call doctor right away.

WARNINGS & PRECAUTIONS

Don't take if:
If you are allergic to buspirone.

Before you start, consult your doctor:
* If you have ever been addicted to any substance.
* If you have chronic kidney or liver disease.
* If you are already taking *any* medicine.

Over age 60:
Adverse reactions and side effects may be more frequent and severe than in younger persons.

Pregnancy:
No problems expected, but better to avoid if possible.

Breast-feeding:
Buspirone passes into milk of lactating experimental animals. Avoid if possible.

Infants & children:
Safety and efficacy not established for under 18 years old.

Prolonged use:
Not recommended for prolonged use. Adverse side effects more likely.

Skin & sunlight:
No problems expected.

Driving, piloting or hazardous work:
Don't drive or pilot aircraft until you learn how medicine affects you. Don't work around dangerous machinery. Don't climb ladders or work in high places. Danger increases if you drink alcohol or take medicine affecting alertness and reflexes, such as antihistamines, tranquilizers, sedatives, pain medicine, narcotics and mind-altering drugs.

Discontinuing:
No problems expected.

Others:
Before elective surgery requiring local or general anesthesia, tell your dentist, surgeon or anesthesiologist that you take buspirone.

POSSIBLE INTERACTION WITH OTHER DRUGS

GENERIC NAME OR DRUG CLASS	COMBINED EFFECT
Antihistamines*	Excessive sedation. Sedative effect of both drugs may be increased.
Barbiturates*	Excessive sedation. Sedative effect of both drugs may be increased.
MAO inhibitors*	May increase blood pressure.
Muscle relaxants*	Excessive sedation. Sedative effect of both drugs may be increased.
Narcotics*	Excessive sedation. Sedative effect of both drugs may be increased.
Sedatives*	Excessive sedation. Sedative effect of both drugs may be increased.
Tranquilizers, other*	Excessive sedation. Sedative effect of both drugs may be increased.

POSSIBLE INTERACTION WITH OTHER SUBSTANCES

INTERACTS WITH	COMBINED EFFECT
Alcohol:	Excess sedation. Avoid.
Beverages: Caffeine-containing drinks.	Avoid. Decreased anti-anxiety effect of busiprone.
Cocaine:	Avoid. Decreased anti-anxiety effect of busiprone.
Foods:	None expected.
Marijuana:	Avoid. Decreased anti-anxiety effect of busiprone.
Tobacco:	Avoid. Decreased antianxiety effect of busiprone.

BUSULFAN

BRAND NAMES

Myleran

BASIC INFORMATION

Habit forming? No
Prescription needed? Yes
Available as generic? No
Drug class: Antineoplastic,
  Immunosuppressant

 USES

- Treatment for some kinds of cancer.
- Suppresses immune response after transplant and in immune disorders.

 DOSAGE & USAGE INFORMATION

How to take:
Tablet—Swallow with liquid after light meal. Don't drink fluids with meals. Drink extra fluids between meals. Avoid sweet or fatty foods.

When to take:
At the same time each day.

If you forget a dose:
Take as soon as you remember. Don't ever double dose.

What drug does:
Inhibits abnormal cell reproduction. May suppress immune system.

Time lapse before drug works:
Up to 6 weeks for full effect.

Don't take with:
See Interaction column and consult doctor.

 OVERDOSE

SYMPTOMS:
Bleeding, chills, fever, collapse, stupor, seizure.
WHAT TO DO:
- Dial 0 (operator) or 911 (emergency) for an ambulance or medical help. Then give first aid immediately.
- If patient is unconscious and not breathing, give mouth-to-mouth breathing. If there is no heartbeat, use cardiac massage and mouth-to-mouth breathing (CPR). Don't try to make patient vomit. If you can't get help quickly, take patient to nearest emergency facility.
- See emergency information on inside covers.

 POSSIBLE ADVERSE REACTIONS OR SIDE EFFECTS

SYMPTOMS	WHAT TO DO
Life-threatening: None expected.	
Common: • Unusual bleeding or bruising, mouth sores with sore throat, chills and fever, black stools, lip sores, menstrual irregularities.	Discontinue. Call doctor right away.
• Hair loss, joint pain.	Continue. Call doctor when convenient.
• Nausea, vomiting, diarrhea (unavoidable), tiredness, weakness.	Continue. Tell doctor at next visit.
Infrequent: • Mental confusion, shortness of breath, may increase chance of developing leukemia.	Continue. Call doctor when convenient.
• Cough.	Continue. Tell doctor at next visit.
Rare: • Jaundice, cataracts, symptoms of myasthenia gravis.*	Discontinue. Call doctor right away.
• Swollen breasts.	Continue. Call doctor when convenient.

164

WARNINGS & PRECAUTIONS

Don't take if:
- You have had hypersensitivity to alkylating antineoplastic drugs.
- Your physician has not explained the serious nature of your medical problem and risks of taking this medicine.

Before you start, consult your doctor:
- If you have gout.
- If you have had kidney stones.
- If you have active infection.
- If you have impaired kidney or liver function.
- If you have taken other antineoplastic drugs or had radiation treatment in last 3 weeks.

Over age 60:
Adverse reactions and side effects may be more frequent and severe than in younger persons.

Pregnancy:
Consult doctor. Risk to child is significant.

Breast-feeding:
Drug passes into milk. Don't nurse.

Infants & children:
Use only under care of medical supervisors who are experienced in anticancer drugs.

Prolonged use:
Adverse reactions more likely the longer drug is required.

Skin & sunlight:
No problems expected.

Driving, piloting or hazardous work:
No problems expected.

Discontinuing:
Don't discontinue without doctor's advice until you complete prescribed dose, even though symptoms diminish or disappear. Some side effects may follow discontinuing. Report to doctor blurred vision, convulsions, confusion, persistent headache.

Others:
May cause sterility.

POSSIBLE INTERACTION WITH OTHER DRUGS

GENERIC NAME OR DRUG CLASS	COMBINED EFFECT
Antigout drugs*	Decreased antigout effect.
Antineoplastic drugs, other*	Increased effect of all drugs (may be beneficial).
Chloramphenicol	Increased likelihood of toxic effects of both drugs.
Lovastatin	Increased heart and kidney damage.

POSSIBLE INTERACTION WITH OTHER SUBSTANCES

INTERACTS WITH	COMBINED EFFECT
Alcohol:	May increase chance of intestinal bleeding.
Beverages:	No problems expected.
Cocaine:	Increases chance of toxicity.
Foods:	Reduces irritation in stomach.
Marijuana:	No problems expected.
Tobacco:	Increases lung toxicity.

*See Glossary

BUTABARBITAL

BRAND NAMES

See complete list of brand names in the
Brand Name Directory, page 1059.

BASIC INFORMATION

Habit forming? Yes
Prescription needed? Yes
Available as generic? Yes
Drug class: Sedative, hypnotic (barbiturate)

 ## USES

- Reduces anxiety or nervous tension (low dose).
- Relieves insomnia (higher bedtime dose).

 ## DOSAGE & USAGE INFORMATION

How to take:
Tablet, capsule or liquid—Swallow with food or liquid to lessen stomach irritation. If you can't swallow whole, crumble tablet or open capsule and take with liquid or food.

When to take:
At the same times each day.

If you forget a dose:
Take as soon as you remember up to 2 hours late. If more than 2 hours, wait for next scheduled dose (don't double this dose).

What drug does:
May partially block nerve impulses at nerve-cell connections.

Time lapse before drug works:
60 minutes.

Don't take with:
- Non-prescription drugs without consulting doctor.
- See Interaction column and consult doctor.

 ## OVERDOSE

SYMPTOMS:
Deep sleep, weak pulse, coma.
WHAT TO DO:
- **Dial 0 (operator) or 911 (emergency) for an ambulance or medical help. Then give first aid immediately.**
- **See emergency information on inside covers.**

 ## POSSIBLE ADVERSE REACTIONS OR SIDE EFFECTS

SYMPTOMS	WHAT TO DO
Life-threatening: None expected.	
Common: Dizziness, drowsiness, "hangover" effect.	Continue. Call doctor when convenient.
Infrequent: • Rash or hives; swollen lips, face or eyelids; sore throat, fever.	Discontinue. Call doctor right away.
• Depression, confusion, slurred speech, diarrhea, nausea, vomiting, joint or muscle pain.	Continue. Call doctor when convenient.
Rare: • Agitation, slow heartbeat, breathing difficulty, jaundice.	Discontinue. Call doctor right away.
• Unexplained bleeding or bruising.	Continue. Call doctor when convenient.

 ## WARNINGS & PRECAUTIONS

Don't take if:
- You are allergic to any barbiturate.
- You have porphyria.

Before you start, consult your doctor:
- If you have epilepsy.
- If you have kidney or liver damage.
- If you have asthma.
- If you have anemia.
- If you have chronic pain.
- If you will have surgery within 2 months, including dental surgery, requiring general or spinal anesthesia.

Over age 60:
Adverse reactions and side effects may be more frequent and severe than in younger persons. Use small doses.

Pregnancy:
Risk to unborn child outweighs drug benefits. Don't use.

Breast-feeding:
Drug passes into milk. Avoid drug or discontinue nursing until you finish medicine. Consult doctor for advice on maintaining milk supply.

Infants & children:
Use only under doctor's supervision.

Prolonged use:
- May cause addiction, anemia, chronic intoxication.
- May lower body temperature, making exposure to cold temperatures hazardous.

Skin & sunlight:
May cause rash or intensify sunburn in areas exposed to sun or sunlamp.

Driving, piloting or hazardous work:
Don't drive or pilot aircraft until you learn how medicine affects you. Don't work around dangerous machinery. Don't climb ladders or work in high places. Danger increases if you drink alcohol or take medicine affecting alertness and reflexes.

Discontinuing:
May be unnecessary to finish medicine. Follow doctor's instructions. If you develop withdrawal symptoms of hallucinations, agitation or sleeplessness after discontinuing, call doctor right away.

Others:
High potential for abuse.

 POSSIBLE INTERACTION WITH OTHER DRUGS

GENERIC NAME OR DRUG CLASS	COMBINED EFFECT
Anticoagulants, oral*	Decreased anticoagulant effect.
Anticonvulsants*	Changed seizure patterns.
Antidepressants, tricyclics (TCA)*	Decreased antidepressant effect. Possible dangerous oversedation.
Antidiabetics, oral*	Increased butabarbital effect.
Antihistamines*	Dangerous sedation. Avoid.
Aspirin	Decreased aspirin effect.
Beta-adrenergic blockers*	Decreased effect of beta-adrenergic blocker.
Carteolol	Increased barbiturate effect. Dangerous sedation.
Contraceptives, oral*	Decreased contraceptive effect.
Cortisone drugs*	Decreased cortisone effect.
Digitoxin	Decreased digitoxin effect.
Doxycycline	Decreased doxycycline effect.
Dronabinol	Increased effects of both drugs. Avoid.
Griseofulvin	Decreased griseofulvin effect.
Indapamide	Increased indapamide effect.
MAO inhibitors*	Increased butabarbital effect.
Mind-altering drugs*	Dangerous sedation. Avoid.
Molindone	Increased sedative effect.
Nabilone	Greater depression of central nervous system.
Narcotics*	Dangerous sedation. Avoid.
Non-steroidal anti-inflammatory drugs (NSAIDs)*	Decreased anti-inflammatory effect.
Pain relievers*	Dangerous sedation. Avoid.
Rifampin	May decrease butabarbital effect.
Sedatives*	Dangerous sedation. Avoid.
Sleep inducers*	Dangerous sedation. Avoid.
Sotalol	Increased barbiturate effect. Dangerous sedation.
Tranquilizers*	Dangerous sedation. Avoid.
Valproic acid	Increased butabarbital effect.

 POSSIBLE INTERACTION WITH OTHER SUBSTANCES

INTERACTS WITH	COMBINED EFFECT
Alcohol:	Possible fatal oversedation. Avoid.
Beverages:	None expected.
Cocaine:	Decreased butabarbital effect.
Foods:	None expected.
Marijuana:	Excessive sedation. Avoid.
Tobacco:	None expected.

BUTALBITAL & ASPIRIN
(Also contains caffeine)

BRAND AND GENERIC NAMES

Axotal
B-A-C
Buff-A-Comp
Butalbital A-C
BUTALBITAL,
  ASPIRIN &
  CAFFEINE
Butal Compound

Fiorgen PF
Fiorinal
Isollyl (Improved)
Lanorinal
Marnal
Protension
Tenstan

BASIC INFORMATION

Habit forming? Yes
Prescription needed? Yes
Available as generic? Yes
Drug class: Analgesic, anti-inflammatory,
  sedative

 ## USES

- Reduces anxiety or nervous tension (low
  dose).
- Reduces pain, fever, inflammation.

 ## DOSAGE & USAGE
INFORMATION

How to take:
- Tablet or capsule—Swallow with liquid or food
  to lessen stomach irritation. If you can't
  swallow whole, crumble tablet or open
  capsule and take with liquid or food.
- Suppositories—Remove wrapper and moisten
  suppository with water. Gently insert into
  rectum, large end first.

When to take:
At the same times each day. No more often than
every 4 hours.

Continued next column

 ## OVERDOSE

SYMPTOMS:
**Deep sleep, weak pulse, ringing in ears,
nausea, vomiting, dizziness, fever, deep and
rapid breathing, hallucinations, convulsions,
coma.**
WHAT TO DO:
- **Dial 0 (operator) or 911 (emergency) for
  an ambulance or medical help. Then give
  first aid immediately.**
- **See emergency information on inside
  covers.**

If you forget a dose:
Take as soon as you remember up to 2 hours
late. If more than 2 hours, wait for next
scheduled dose (don't double this dose).

What drug does:
- May partially block nerve impulses at nerve-
  cell connections.
- Affects hypothalamus, the part of the brain
  which regulates temperature by dilating small
  blood vessels in skin.
- Prevents clumping of platelets (small blood
  cells) so blood vessels remain open.
- Decreases prostaglandin effect.
- Suppresses body's pain messages.

Time lapse before drug works:
30 minutes.

Don't take with:
- Non-prescription drugs without consulting
  doctor.
- See Interaction column and consult doctor.

 ## POSSIBLE
ADVERSE REACTIONS
OR SIDE EFFECTS

SYMPTOMS	WHAT TO DO
Life-threatening: Hives, rash, intense itching, faintness soon after a dose (anaphylaxis); wheezing; tightness in chest; black or bloody vomit; black stools; shortness of breath.	Seek emergency treatment immediately.
Common: Dizziness, drowsiness, heartburn.	Continue. Call doctor when convenient.
Infrequent: Jaundice; vomiting blood; easy bruising; skin rash, hives; confusion; depression; sore throat, fever, mouth sores; hearing loss; slurred speech; decreased vision.	Discontinue. Call doctor right away.
Rare: • Diminished vision, blood in urine, unexplained fever.	Discontinue. Call doctor right away.
• Insomnia, nightmares, constipation, headache, jaundice, nervousness.	Continue. Call doctor when convenient.

BUTALBITAL & ASPIRIN
(Also contains caffeine)

WARNINGS & PRECAUTIONS

Don't take if:
- You are allergic to any barbiturate or aspirin.
- You have a peptic ulcer of stomach or duodenum, bleeding disorder, porphyria.

Before you start, consult your doctor:
- If you have had stomach or duodenal ulcers.
- If you have asthma, nasal polyps, epilepsy, kidney or liver damage, anemia, chronic pain.
- If you will have surgery within 2 months, including dental surgery, requiring general or spinal anesthesia.

Over age 60:
- Adverse reactions and side effects may be more frequent and severe than in younger persons.
- More likely to cause hidden bleeding in stomach or intestines. Watch for dark stools.

Pregnancy:
Risk to unborn child outweighs drug benefits. Don't use.

Breast-feeding:
Drug passes into milk. Avoid drug or discontinue nursing until you finish medicine. Consult doctor for advice on maintaining milk supply.

Infants & children:
- Overdose frequent and severe. Keep bottles out of children's reach.
- Use only under doctor's supervision.

Prolonged use:
- Kidney damage. Periodic kidney-function test recommended.
- May cause addiction, anemia, chronic intoxication.
- May lower body temperature, making exposure to cold temperatures hazardous.

Skin & sunlight:
May cause rash or intensify sunburn in areas exposed to sun or sunlamp.

Driving, piloting or hazardous work:
Don't drive or pilot aircraft until you learn how medicine affects you. Don't work around dangerous machinery. Don't climb ladders or work in high places. Danger increases if you drink alcohol or take medicine affecting alertness and reflexes, such as antihistamines, tranquilizers, sedatives, pain medicine, narcotics and mind-altering drugs.

Discontinuing:
May be unnecessary to finish medicine. Follow doctor's instructions. If you develop withdrawal symptoms of hallucinations, agitation or sleeplessness after discontinuing, call doctor right away.

Others:
- Aspirin can complicate surgery; illness; pregnancy, labor and delivery.
- For arthritis—Don't change dose without consulting doctor.
- Urine tests for blood sugar may be inaccurate.
- Great potential for abuse.

POSSIBLE INTERACTION WITH OTHER DRUGS

GENERIC NAME OR DRUG CLASS	COMBINED EFFECT
Allopurinol	Decreased allopurinol effect.
Antacids*	Decreased aspirin effect.
Anticoagulants, oral*	Increased anticoagulant effect. Abnormal bleeding.
Anticonvulsants*	Changed seizure patterns.
Antidepressants*	Decreased antidepressant effect. Possible dangerous oversedation.
Antidiabetics, oral*	Increased butalbital effect. Low blood sugar.
Antihistamines*	Dangerous sedation. Avoid.

Continued page 1078

POSSIBLE INTERACTION WITH OTHER SUBSTANCES

INTERACTS WITH	COMBINED EFFECT
Alcohol:	Possible stomach irritation and bleeding, possible fatal oversedation. Avoid.
Beverages:	None expected.
Cocaine:	Decreased butalbital effect.
Foods:	None expected.
Marijuana:	Possible increased pain relief, but marijuana may slow body's recovery. Avoid.
Tobacco:	None expected.

---

*See Glossary

BUTALBITAL, ASPIRIN & CODEINE
(Also contains caffeine)

BRAND NAMES

ABC Compound
  with Codeine
B-A-C with Codeine
Buff-A-Comp –3
Fiorgen
  with Codeine

Fiorinal
  with Codeine
Isollyl with Codeine

BASIC INFORMATION

Habit forming? Yes
Prescription needed? Yes
Available as generic? No
Drug class: Narcotic, analgesic

USES

- Reduces anxiety or nervous tension (low dose).
- Reduces pain, fever, inflammation.

DOSAGE & USAGE INFORMATION

How to take:
- Tablet or capsule—Swallow with liquid or food to lessen stomach irritation. If you can't swallow whole, crumble tablet or open capsule and take with liquid or food.
- Extended-release tablets or capsules— Swallow each dose whole.

When to take:
When needed. No more often than every 4 hours.

Continued next column

OVERDOSE

SYMPTOMS:
Deep sleep, slow and weak pulse, ringing in ears, nausea, vomiting, dizziness, fever, deep and rapid breathing, hallucinations, convulsions, coma.
WHAT TO DO:
- **Dial 0 (operator) or 911 (emergency) for an ambulance or medical help. Then give first aid immediately.**
- **If patient is unconscious and not breathing, give mouth-to-mouth breathing. If there is no heartbeat, use cardiac massage and mouth-to-mouth breathing (CPR). Don't try to make patient vomit. If you can't get help quickly, take patient to nearest emergency facility.**
- **See emergency information on inside covers.**

If you forget a dose:
Take as soon as you remember. Wait 4 hours for next dose.

What drug does:
- May partially block nerve impulses at nerve-cell connections.
- Affects hypothalamus, the part of the brain which regulates temperature by dilating small blood vessels in skin.
- Prevents clumping of platelets (small blood cells) so blood vessels remain open.
- Decreases prostaglandin effect.
- Blocks pain messages to brain and spinal cord.
- Reduces sensitivity of brain's cough-control center.

Time lapse before drug works:
30 minutes.

Don't take with:
- Non-prescription drugs without consulting doctor.
- See Interaction column and consult doctor.

POSSIBLE ADVERSE REACTIONS OR SIDE EFFECTS

SYMPTOMS	WHAT TO DO
Life-threatening:	
Wheezing, tightness in chest, pinpoint pupils.	Seek emergency treatment immediately.
Common:	
Dizziness, drowsiness, heartburn, flushed face, depression, false sense of well-being, increased urination.	Continue. Call doctor when convenient.
Infrequent:	
Jaundice; vomiting blood; easy bruising; skin rash, hives; confusion; depression; sore throat, fever, mouth sores; difficult urination; hearing loss; slurred speech; blood in urine; decreased vision.	Discontinue. Call doctor right away.
Rare:	
Insomnia, nightmares, constipation, headache, nervousness, flushed face, increased sweating, unusual tiredness.	Continue. Call doctor when convenient.

BUTALBITAL, ASPIRIN & CODEINE
(Also contains caffeine)

 WARNINGS & PRECAUTIONS

Don't take if:
- You are allergic to any barbiturate or narcotic.
- You have a peptic ulcer of stomach or duodenum, bleeding disorder, porphyria.

Before you start, consult your doctor:
- If you have had stomach or duodenal ulcers.
- If you have asthma, epilepsy, kidney or liver damage, anemia, chronic pain, gout.
- If you will have surgery within 2 months, including dental surgery, requiring general or spinal anesthesia.

Over age 60:
- Adverse reactions and side effects may be more frequent and severe than in younger persons.
- More likely to cause hidden bleeding in stomach or intestines. Watch for dark stools.
- More likely to be drowsy, dizzy, unsteady or constipated. Use only if absolutely necessary.

Pregnancy:
Risk to unborn child outweighs drug benefits. Don't use.

Breast-feeding:
Drug passes into milk. Avoid drug or discontinue nursing until you finish medicine. Consult doctor for advice on maintaining milk supply.

Infants & children:
- Overdose frequent and severe. Keep bottles out of children's reach.
- Use only under doctor's supervision.
- Consult doctor before giving to persons under age 18 who have fever and discomfort of viral illness, especially chicken pox and influenza. Probably increases risk of Reye's syndrome.

Prolonged use:
- Kidney damage. Periodic kidney-function test recommended.
- May cause addiction, anemia, chronic intoxication.
- May lower body temperature, making exposure to cold temperatures hazardous.

Skin & sunlight:
May cause rash or intensify sunburn in areas exposed to sun or sunlamp.

Driving, piloting or hazardous work:
Don't drive or pilot aircraft until you learn how medicine affects you. Don't work around dangerous machinery. Don't climb ladders or work in high places. Danger increases if you drink alcohol or take medicine affecting alertness and reflexes, such as antihistamines, tranquilizers, sedatives, pain medicine, narcotics and mind-altering drugs.

Discontinuing:
May be unnecessary to finish medicine. Follow doctor's instructions. If you develop withdrawal symptoms of hallucinations, agitation or sleeplessness after discontinuing, call doctor right away.

Others:
- Aspirin can complicate surgery; illness; pregnancy, labor and delivery.
- For arthritis—Don't change dose without consulting doctor.
- Urine tests for blood sugar may be inaccurate.
- Great potential for abuse.

 POSSIBLE INTERACTION WITH OTHER DRUGS

GENERIC NAME OR DRUG CLASS	COMBINED EFFECT
Allopurinol	Decreased allopurinol effect.
Analgesics, other*	Increased analgesic effect.
Antacids*	Decreased aspirin effect.
Anticoagulants, oral*	Increased anticoagulant effect. Abnormal bleeding.
Anticonvulsants*	Changed seizure patterns.

Continued page 1079

 POSSIBLE INTERACTION WITH OTHER SUBSTANCES

INTERACTS WITH	COMBINED EFFECT
Alcohol:	Possible stomach irritation and bleeding, possible fatal oversedation. Avoid.
Beverages:	None expected.
Cocaine:	Increased cocaine toxic effects. Avoid.
Foods:	None expected.
Marijuana:	Possible increased pain relief, but marijuana may slow body's recovery. Impairs physical and mental performance. Avoid.
Tobacco:	None expected.

*See Glossary

CAFFEINE

BRAND NAMES

See complete list of brand names in the *Brand Name Directory*, page 1059.

BASIC INFORMATION

Habit forming? Yes
Prescription needed? No
Available as generic? Yes
**Drug class: Stimulant (xanthine),
   vasoconstrictor**

USES

- Treatment for drowsiness and fatigue.
- Treatment for migraine and other vascular headaches in combination with ergot.

DOSAGE & USAGE INFORMATION

How to take:
- Tablet or liquid—Swallow with liquid or food to lessen stomach irritation. If you can't swallow whole, crumble tablet and take with liquid or food.
- Extended-release capsules—Swallow whole with liquid.

When to take:
At the same times each day.

If you forget a dose:
Take as soon as you remember up to 2 hours late. If more than 2 hours, wait for next scheduled dose (don't double this dose).

What drug does:
- Constricts blood-vessel walls.
- Stimulates central nervous system.

Time lapse before drug works:
30 minutes.

Continued next column

OVERDOSE

SYMPTOMS:
**Excitement, insomnia, rapid heartbeat
(infants can have slow heartbeat),
hallucinations, convulsions, coma.**
WHAT TO DO:
- **Dial 0 (operator) or 911 (emergency) for an ambulance or medical help. Then give first aid immediately.**
- **See emergency information on inside covers.**

Don't take with:
- Non-prescription drugs without consulting doctor.
- See Interaction column and consult doctor.

POSSIBLE ADVERSE REACTIONS OR SIDE EFFECTS

SYMPTOMS	WHAT TO DO
Life-threatening: None expected.	
Common:	
• Rapid heartbeat, low blood sugar (hunger, anxiety, cold sweats, rapid pulse) with tremor, irritability.	Continue. Call doctor when convenient.
• Nervousness, insomnia.	Continue. Tell doctor at next visit.
• Increased urination.	No action necessary.
Infrequent:	
• Confusion, irritability.	Discontinue. Call doctor right away.
• Nausea, indigestion, burning feeling in stomach.	Continue. Call doctor when convenient.
Rare: None expected.	

WARNINGS & PRECAUTIONS

Don't take if:
- You are allergic to any stimulant.
- You have heart disease.
- You have active peptic ulcer of stomach or duodenum.

Before you start, consult your doctor:
- If you have irregular heartbeat.
- If you have hypoglycemia (low blood sugar).
- If you have epilepsy.

Over age 60:
Adverse reactions and side effects may be more frequent and severe than in younger persons.

Pregnancy:
Risk to unborn child outweighs drug benefits. Don't use.

Breast-feeding:
Drug passes into milk. Avoid drug or discontinue nursing until you finish medicine. Consult doctor for advice on maintaining milk supply.

Infants & children:
Not recommended.

Prolonged use:
Stomach ulcers.

Skin & sunlight:
No problems expected.

Driving, piloting or hazardous work:
No problems expected.

Discontinuing:
Will cause withdrawal symptoms of headache, irritability, drowsiness. Discontinue gradually if you use caffeine for a month or more.

Others:
May produce or aggravate fibrocystic disease of the breast in women.

POSSIBLE INTERACTION WITH OTHER DRUGS

GENERIC NAME OR DRUG CLASS	COMBINED EFFECT
Cimetidine	Increased caffeine effect.
Contraceptives, oral*	Increased caffeine effect.
Isoniazid	Increased caffeine effect.
MAO inhibitors*	Dangerous blood-pressure rise.
Sedatives*	Decreased sedative effect.
Sleep inducers*	Decreased sedative effect.
Sympathomimetics*	Overstimulation.
Thyroid hormones*	Increased thyroid effect.
Tranquilizers*	Decreased tranquilizer effect.

POSSIBLE INTERACTION WITH OTHER SUBSTANCES

INTERACTS WITH	COMBINED EFFECT
Alcohol:	Decreased alcohol effect.
Beverages: Caffeine drinks.	Increased caffeine effect.
Cocaine	Convulsions or excessive nervousness.
Foods:	No proven problems.
Marijuana:	Increased effect of both drugs. May lead to dangerous, rapid heartbeat. Avoid.
Tobacco:	Increased heartbeat. Avoid. Decreased caffeine effect.

CALCIUM CARBONATE

BRAND NAMES

See complete list of brand names in the *Brand Name Directory*, page 1059.

BASIC INFORMATION

Habit forming? No
Prescription needed? No
Available as generic? Yes
Drug class: Antacid, dietary replacement

 ## USES

- Treatment for hyperacidity in upper gastro-intestinal tract, including stomach and esophagus. Symptoms may be heartburn or acid indigestion. Diseases include peptic ulcer, gastritis, esophagitis, hiatal hernia.
- Dietary supplement when calcium ingestion is insufficient or there is a deficiency such as osteomalacia or rickets.

 ## DOSAGE & USAGE INFORMATION

How to take:
- Tablet—Swallow with liquid.
- Chewable tablets or wafers—Chew well before swallowing.
- Suspension—Swallow with liquid or food to lessen stomach irritation.

When to take:
1 to 3 hours after meals unless directed otherwise by your doctor.

If you forget a dose:
Take as soon as you remember.

What drug does:
- Neutralizes some of the hydrochloric acid in the stomach.
- Reduces action of pepsin, a digestive enzyme.
- Provides calcium necessary for bone, nerve function.

Time lapse before drug works:
15 minutes.

Continued next column

 ## OVERDOSE

SYMPTOMS:
Weakness, fatigue, dizziness, confusion.
WHAT TO DO:
Overdose unlikely to threaten life. If person takes much larger amount than prescribed, call doctor, poison-control center or hospital emergency room for instructions.

Don't take with:
Other medicines at the same time. Decreases absorption of other drugs.

 ## POSSIBLE ADVERSE REACTIONS OR SIDE EFFECTS

SYMPTOMS	WHAT TO DO
Life-threatening: None expected.	
Common: Constipation, appetite loss.	Continue. Call doctor when convenient.
Infrequent:	
• Lower abdominal pain and swelling, bone pain, muscle weakness, swollen wrists or ankles.	Discontinue. Call doctor right away.
• Mood changes, nausea, vomiting, weight loss.	Continue. Call doctor when convenient.
Rare: Difficult or painful urination, unusual tiredness or weakness.	Discontinue. Call doctor right away.

 ## WARNINGS & PRECAUTIONS

Don't take if:
- You are allergic to any antacid.
- You have a high blood-calcium level.

Before you start, consult your doctor:
- If you have kidney disease.
- If you have chronic constipation, colitis or diarrhea.
- If you have symptoms of appendicitis.
- If you have stomach or intestinal bleeding.
- If you have irregular heartbeat.

Over age 60:
Adverse reactions and side effects may be more frequent and severe than in younger persons. Diarrhea or constipation particularly likely.

Pregnancy:
Risk to unborn child outweighs drug benefits. Don't use.

Breast-feeding:
Drug passes into milk. Avoid drug or discontinue nursing until you finish medicine. Consult doctor for advice on maintaining milk supply.

Infants & children:
Use only under medical supervision.

Prolonged use:
- High blood level of calcium which disturbs electrolyte balance.
- Kidney stones, impaired kidney function.

Skin & sunlight:
No problems expected.

Driving, piloting or hazardous work:
No problems expected.

Discontinuing:
May be unnecessary to finish medicine. Follow doctor's instructions.

Others:
Don't take longer than 2 weeks unless under medical supervision.

POSSIBLE INTERACTION WITH OTHER DRUGS

GENERIC NAME OR DRUG CLASS	COMBINED EFFECT
Anticoagulants*	Decreased anticoagulant effect.
Calcitonin	Decreased calcitonin effect.
Chlorpromazine	Decreased chlorpromazine effect.
Ciprofloxacin	May cause kidney dysfunction.
Corticosteroids*	Decreased calcium absorption effect.
Digitalis preparations*	Decreased digitalis effect.
Diuretics thiazide*	Increased calcium in blood.
Iron supplements*	Decreased iron effect.
Meperidine	Increased meperidine effect.
Mexiletine	May slow elimination of mexiletine and cause need to adjust dosage.
Nalidixic acid	Decreased effect of nalidixic acid.
Nicardipine	Possible decreased nicardipine effect.
Nizatidine	Decreased nizatidine absorption.
Oxyphenbutazone	Decreased oxyphenbutazone effect.
Para-aminosalicylic acid (PAS)	Decreased PAS effect.
Penicillins*	Decreased penicillin effect.
Pentobarbital	Decreased pentobarbital effect.
Phenylbutazone	Decreased phenylbutazone effect.
Phenytoin	Decreased phenytoin absorption.
Pseudoephedrine	Increased pseudoephedrine effect.
Quinidine	Decreased quinidine effect.
Salicylates*	Decreased salicylate effect.
Sulfa drugs*	Decreased sulfa effect.
Tetracyclines*	Decreased tetracycline effect.
Vitamin A	Decreased vitamin effect.
Vitamin D (large doses)	Excessive absorption of calcium.

POSSIBLE INTERACTION WITH OTHER SUBSTANCES

INTERACTS WITH	COMBINED EFFECT
Alcohol:	Decreased antacid effect.
Beverages:	No proven problems.
Cocaine:	No proven problems.
Foods:	Decreased antacid effect if taken with food. Wait 1 hour after eating.
Marijuana:	No proven problems.
Tobacco:	Decreased antacid effect.

CALCIUM & MAGNESIUM ANTACIDS

BRAND AND GENERIC NAMES

Advanced Formula
  DI-gel
Alkets
Bisodol
Calcitrel
CALCIUM &
  MAGNESIUM
  CARBONATES
CALCIUM &
  MAGNESIUM
  CARBONATES &
  MAGNESIUM OXIDE

CALCIUM
  CARBONATE &
  MAGNESIA
Marblen
Noralac
Ratio
Spastosed

BASIC INFORMATION

Habit forming? No
Prescription needed? No
Available as generic? Yes
Drug class: Antacid

USES

- Treatment for hyperacidity in upper gastrointestinal tract, including stomach and esophagus. Symptoms may be heartburn or acid indigestion. Diseases include peptic ulcer, gastritis, esophagitis, hiatal hernia.
- Constipation relief.

DOSAGE & USAGE INFORMATION

How to take:
- Tablet—Swallow with liquid.
- Chewable tablets or wafers—Chew well before swallowing.
- Liquid—Shake well and take undiluted.

Continued next column

OVERDOSE

SYMPTOMS:
Dry mouth, shallow breathing, diarrhea, weakness, fatigue, stupor.
WHAT TO DO:
- **Overdose unlikely to threaten life. Depending on severity of symptoms and amount taken, call doctor, poison-control center or hospital emergency room for instructions.**
- **Dial 0 (operator) or 911 (emergency) for an ambulance or medical help. Then give first aid immediately.**
- **See emergency information on inside covers.**

When to take:
1 to 3 hours after meals unless directed otherwise by your doctor.

If you forget a dose:
Take as soon as you remember, but not simultaneously with any other medicine.

What drug does:
- Neutralizes some of the hydrochloric acid in the stomach.
- Reduces action of pepsin, a digestive enzyme.
- Stimulates muscles in lower bowel wall.

Time lapse before drug works:
15 minutes for antacid effect.

Don't take with:
Other medicines at the same time. Decreases absorption of other drugs. Wait 2 hours between doses.

POSSIBLE ADVERSE REACTIONS OR SIDE EFFECTS

SYMPTOMS	WHAT TO DO
Life-threatening: Heartbeat irregularity in patient with heart disease.	Discontinue. Seek emergency treatment.
Common: • Constipation, headache, appetite loss, distended stomach.	Discontinue. Call doctor right away.
• Unpleasant taste in mouth, abdominal pain, laxative effect, belching.	Continue. Call doctor when convenient.
Infrequent: Bone pain, frequent urination, dizziness, urgent urination, muscle weakness or pain, nausea, weight gain.	Discontinue. Call doctor right away.
Rare: Mood changes, vomiting, nervousness, swollen feet and ankles.	Discontinue. Call doctor right away.

WARNINGS & PRECAUTIONS

Don't take if:
- You are allergic to any antacid.
- You have a high blood-calcium level.

Before you start, consult your doctor:
If you have kidney disease, chronic constipation, colitis, diarrhea, symptoms of appendicitis, stomach or intestinal bleeding, irregular heartbeat.

Over age 60:
Adverse reactions and side effects may be more frequent and severe than in younger persons. Diarrhea or constipation particularly likely.

Pregnancy:
Risk to unborn child outweighs drug benefits. Don't use.

Breast-feeding:
Drug passes into milk. Avoid drug or discontinue nursing until you finish medicine. Consult doctor for advice on maintaining milk supply.

Infants & children:
Use only under medical supervision.

Prolonged use:
- High blood level of calcium which disturbs electrolyte balance.
- Kidney stones, impaired kidney function.

Skin & sunlight:
No problems expected.

Driving, piloting or hazardous work:
No problems expected.

Discontinuing:
May be unnecessary to finish medicine. Follow doctor's instructions.

Others:
Don't take longer than 2 weeks unless under medical supervision.

POSSIBLE INTERACTION WITH OTHER DRUGS

GENERIC NAME OR DRUG CLASS	COMBINED EFFECT
Anticoagulants, oral*	Decreased anti-coagulant effect.
Calcitonin	Decreased calcitonin effect.
Chlorpromazine	Decreased chlorpromazine effect.
Ciprofloxacin	May cause kidney dysfunction.
Digitalis preparations*	Decreased digitalis effect.
Iron supplements*	Decreased iron effect.
Isoniazid	Decreased isoniazid effect.
Levodopa	Increased levodopa effect.
Meperidine	Increased meperidine effect.
Nalidixic acid	Decreased nalidixic acid effect.
Nicardipine	Possible decreased nicardipine effect.
Nizatidine	Decreased nizatidine absorption.
Oxyphenbutazone	Decreased oxyphenbutazone effect.
Para-aminosalicylic acid (PAS)	Decreased PAS effect.
Penicillins*	Decreased penicillin effect.
Pentobarbital	Decreased pentobarbital effect.
Phenylbutazone	Decreased phenylbutazone effect.
Pseudoephedrine	Increased pseudoephedrine effect.
Quinidine	Increased quinidine effect.
Salicylates*	Increased salicylate effect.
Sulfa drugs*	Decreased sulfa effect.

POSSIBLE INTERACTION WITH OTHER SUBSTANCES

INTERACTS WITH	COMBINED EFFECT
Alcohol:	Decreased antacid effect.
Beverages:	No proven problems.
Cocaine:	No proven problems.
Foods:	Decreased antacid effect. Wait 1 hour after eating.
Marijuana:	Decreased antacid effect.
Tobacco:	Decreased antacid effect.

*See Glossary

CALCIUM SUPPLEMENTS

BRAND NAMES

See complete list of brand names in the *Brand Name Directory*, page 1059.

BASIC INFORMATION

Habit forming? No
Prescription needed? For some
Available as generic? Yes
Drug class: Antihypocalcemic, dietary replacement

 USES

- Treats or prevents osteoporosis (thin, porous, easily fractured bones). Frequently prescribed with estrogen beginning at menopause.
- Helps heart, muscle and nervous system to work properly.
- Dietary supplement when calcium ingestion is insufficient or there is a deficiency such as osteomalacia or rickets.

 DOSAGE & USAGE INFORMATION

How to take:

- Take in addition to foods high in calcium (milk, yogurt, sardines, cheese, canned salmon, turnip greens, broccoli, shrimp, tofu).
- Tablet—Swallow with liquid or food to lessen stomach irritation. If you can't swallow whole, crumble tablet and take with food or liquid.
- Syrup—Take before meals.
- Suspension—Swallow with liquid or food to lessen stomach irritation.

When to take:

As directed. Don't take within 2 hours of any other medicine you take by mouth.

If you forget a dose:

Use as soon as you remember.

Continued next column

 OVERDOSE

SYMPTOMS:
Confusion, irregular heartbeat, depression, bone pain, coma.
WHAT TO DO:

- **Dial 0 (operator) or 911 (emergency) for an ambulance or medical help. Then give first aid immediately.**
- **See emergency information on inside covers.**

What drug does:

- Participates in metabolism of all activities essential for normal life and function of cells.
- Provides calcium necessary for bone, nerve function.

Time lapse before drug works:
15 to 30 minutes.

Don't take with:

- Any other medicine until 2 hours have passed since taking calcium.
- See Interaction column and consult doctor.

 POSSIBLE ADVERSE REACTIONS OR SIDE EFFECTS

SYMPTOMS	WHAT TO DO
Life-threatening: Irregular or very slow heart rate.	Discontinue. Seek emergency treatment.
Common: None expected.	
Infrequent: Constipation, diarrhea, drowsiness, headache, appetite loss, dry mouth, weakness.	Discontinue. Call doctor right away.
Rare: Frequent, painful or difficult urination; increased thirst; nausea, vomiting; rash; urine frequency increased and volume larger; confusion; high blood pressure; eyes sensitive to light.	Discontinue. Call doctor right away.

 WARNINGS & PRECAUTIONS

Don't take if:

- You are allergic to calcium.
- You have a high blood-calcium level.

Before you start, consult your doctor:
If you have diarrhea, heart disease, kidney stones, kidney disease, sarcoidosis, malabsorption.

Over age 60:
No problems expected.

Pregnancy:
No problems expected, but ask your doctor.

Breast-feeding:
No problems expected.

Infants & children:
Use only under close medical supervision.

Prolonged use:
Side effects more likely.

Skin & sunlight:
No problems expected.

Driving, piloting or hazardous work:
No problems expected.

Discontinuing:
No problems expected.

Others:
- Exercise, along with vitamin D from sunshine and calcium, helps prevent osteoporosis.
- Don't use bone meal or dolomite as a source for calcium supplement (they may contain lead).

POSSIBLE INTERACTION WITH OTHER DRUGS

GENERIC NAME OR DRUG CLASS	COMBINED EFFECT
Anticoagulants, oral*	Decreased anti-coagulant effect.
Calcitonin	Decreased calcitonin effect.
Chlorpromazine	Decreased chlorpromazine effect.
Corticosteroids*	Decreased calcium absorption and effect.
Digitalis preparations*	Decreased digitalis effect.
Diuretics, thiazide*	Increased calcium in blood.
Estrogens and birth control pills*	May increase absorption of calcium—frequently a desirable combined effect.
Iron supplements*	Decreased iron effect.
Meperidine	Increased meperidine effect.
Mexiletine	May slow elimination of mexiletine and cause need to adjust dosage.
Nalidixic acid	Decreased effect of nalidixic acid.
Nicardipine	Possible decreased nicardipine effect.
Oxyphenbutazone	Decreased oxyphenbutazone effect.
Para-aminosalicylic acid (PAS)	Decreased PAS effect.

Penicillins*	Decreased penicillin effect.
Pentobarbital	Decreased pentobarbital effect.
Phenylbutazone	Decreased phenylbutazone effect.
Phenytoin	Decreased phenytoin absorption.
Pseudoephedrine	Increased pseudoephedrine effect.
Quinidine	Increased quinidine effect.
Salicylates*	Increased salicylate effect.
Sulfa drugs*	Decreased sulfa effect.
Tetracyclines*	Decreased tetracycline effect.
Vitamins A and C	Decreased vitamin effect.
Vitamin D	Increased vitamin absorption, sometimes excessively.

POSSIBLE INTERACTION WITH OTHER SUBSTANCES

INTERACTS WITH	COMBINED EFFECT
Alcohol:	Decreased absorption of calcium.
Beverages:	No problems expected.
Cocaine:	No proven problems.
Foods: Don't take within 1 or 2 hours of food.	Decreased absorption of calcium.
Marijuana:	Decreased absorption of calcium.
Tobacco:	Decreased absorption of calcium.

CAPTOPRIL

BRAND NAMES

Capoten

BASIC INFORMATION

Habit forming? No
Prescription needed? Yes
Available as generic? No
Drug class: Antihypertensive, ACE inhibitor*

USES

Treatment for high blood pressure and congestive heart failure.

DOSAGE & USAGE INFORMATION

How to take:
Tablet—Swallow with liquid. Instructions to take on empty stomach mean 1 hour before or 2 hours after eating.

When to take:
At the same times each day, usually 2-3 times daily. Take first dose at bedtime and lie down immediately.

If you forget a dose:
Take as soon as you remember up to 2 hours late. If more than 2 hours, wait for next scheduled dose (don't double this dose).

What drug does:
• Reduces resistance in arteries.
• Strengthens heartbeat.

Time lapse before drug works:
60 to 90 minutes.

Don't take with:
See Interaction column and consult doctor.

OVERDOSE

SYMPTOMS:
Low blood pressure.
WHAT TO DO:
• **Dial 0 (operator) or 911 (emergency) for an ambulance or medical help. Then give first aid immediately.**
• **See emergency information on inside covers.**

POSSIBLE ADVERSE REACTIONS OR SIDE EFFECTS

SYMPTOMS	WHAT TO DO
Life-threatening:	
Hives, rash, intense itching, faintness soon after a dose (anaphylaxis); difficulty breathing.	Seek emergency treatment immediately.
Common:	
Rash, loss of taste.	Discontinue. Call doctor right away.
Infrequent:	
• Swelling of mouth, face, hands or feet.	Discontinue. Seek emergency treatment.
• Dizziness, fainting, chest pain, fast or irregular heartbeat, coughing.	Discontinue. Call doctor right away.
Rare:	
• Sore throat, cloudy urine, fever, chills.	Discontinue. Call doctor right away.
• Nausea, vomiting, indigestion, abdominal pain.	Continue. Call doctor when convenient.

WARNINGS & PRECAUTIONS

Don't take if:
• You are allergic to captopril.
• You have any autoimmune disease, including AIDS or lupus.
• You are receiving blood from a blood bank.
• You take drugs for cancer.
• You will have surgery within 2 months, including dental surgery, requiring general or spinal anesthesia.

Before you start, consult your doctor:
• If you have had a stroke.
• If you have angina or heart or blood-vessel disease.
• If you have high level of potassium in blood.
• If you have kidney disease.
• If you are on severe salt-restricted diet.
• If you have lupus.

Over age 60:
Adverse reactions and side effects may be more frequent and severe than in younger persons.

Pregnancy:
Risk to unborn child outweighs drug benefits. Don't use.

Breast-feeding:
Drug passes into milk. Avoid drug or discontinue nursing.

Infants & children:
Not recommended.

Prolonged use:
May decrease white cells in blood or cause protein loss in urine. Request periodic laboratory blood counts and urine tests.

Skin & sunlight:
No problems expected.

Driving, piloting or hazardous work:
Avoid if you become dizzy or faint. Otherwise, no problems expected.

Discontinuing:
Don't discontinue without consulting doctor. Dose may require gradual reduction if you have taken drug for a long time. Doses of other drugs may also require adjustment.

Others:
- Stop taking diuretics or increase salt intake 1 week before starting captopril.
- Avoid exercising in hot weather.

POSSIBLE INTERACTION WITH OTHER DRUGS

GENERIC NAME OR DRUG CLASS	COMBINED EFFECT
Amiloride	Possible excessive potassium in blood.
Antihypertensives, other*	Increased antihypertensive effect. Dosage of each may require adjustment.
Beta-adrenergic blockers*	Increased antihypertensive effect. Dosage of each may require adjustment.
Carteolol	Increased antihypertensive effects of both drugs. Dosages may require adjustment.
Chloramphenicol	Possible blood disorders.
Diuretics*	Possible severe blood-pressure drop with first dose.
Diclofenac	May decrease ACE inhibitor effect.
Enalapril	Possible excessive blood-pressure drop.
Guanfacine	Increased effect of both drugs.
Lisinopril	Increased antihypertensive effect. Dosage of each may require adjustment.
Nicardipine	Possible excessive potassium in blood. Dosages may require adjustment.
Nitrates*	Possible excessive blood-pressure drop.
Non-steroidal anti-inflammatory drugs (NSAIDs)*	Decreased captopril effect.
Pentoxifylline	Increased antihypertensive effect.
Potassium supplements*	Possible increased potassium in blood.
Sotalol	Increased antihypertensive effects of both drugs. Dosages may require adjustment.
Spironolactone	Possible excessive potassium in blood.
Terazosin	Decreases effectiveness of terazosin.
Triamterene	Possible excessive potassium in blood.

POSSIBLE INTERACTION WITH OTHER SUBSTANCES

INTERACTS WITH	COMBINED EFFECT
Alcohol:	Possible excessive blood-pressure drop.
Beverages: Low-salt milk.	Possible excessive potassium in blood.
Cocaine	Increased risk of heart block and high blood pressure.
Foods: Salt substitutes.	Possible excessive potassium.
Marijuana:	Increased dizziness.
Tobacco:	May decrease captopril effect.

*See Glossary

CAPTOPRIL & HYDROCHLOROTHIAZIDE

BRAND NAMES

Capozide

BASIC INFORMATION

Habit forming? No
Prescription needed? Yes
Available as generic? No
Drug class: Antihypertensive, diuretic
(thiazide), ACE inhibitor*

 USES

- Treatment for high blood pressure and congestive heart failure.
- Reduces fluid retention.

 DOSAGE & USAGE INFORMATION

How to take:
Tablet—Swallow with liquid. Instructions to take on empty stomach mean 1 hour before or 2 hours after eating.

When to take:
At the same times each day, usually 2 to 3 times daily. Take first dose at bedtime and lie down immediately.

If you forget a dose:
Take as soon as you remember up to 2 hours late. If more than 2 hours, wait for next scheduled dose (don't double this dose).

What drug does:
- Forces sodium and water excretion, reducing body fluid.
- Relaxes muscle cells of small arteries.
- Reduced body fluid and relaxed arteries lower blood pressure.
- Reduces resistance in arteries.
- Strengthens heartbeat.

Continued next column

 OVERDOSE

SYMPTOMS:
Cramps, weakness, drowsiness, weak pulse, low blood pressure.
WHAT TO DO:
- Dial 0 (operator) or 911 (emergency) for an ambulance or medical help. Then give first aid immediately.
- See emergency information on inside covers.

Time lapse before drug works:
4 to 6 hours. May require several weeks to lower blood pressure.

Don't take with:
- Non-prescription drugs without consulting doctor.
- See Interaction column and consult doctor.

 POSSIBLE ADVERSE REACTIONS OR SIDE EFFECTS

SYMPTOMS	WHAT TO DO
Life-threatening:	
Irregular heartbeat (fast or uneven); hives, rash, intense itching, faintness soon after a dose (anaphylaxis).	Discontinue. Seek emergency treatment.
Common:	
• Dry mouth, thirst, tiredness, weakness, muscle cramps, vomiting, chest pain, skin rash, coughing.	Discontinue. Call doctor right away.
• Taste loss, dizziness.	Continue. Call doctor when convenient.
Infrequent:	
• Face, mouth, hands swell.	Discontinue. Call doctor right away.
• Nausea, diarrhea.	Continue. Call doctor when convenient.
Rare:	
None expected.	

 WARNINGS & PRECAUTIONS

Don't take if:
- You are allergic to captopril, or any thiazide diuretic drug.
- You have any autoimmune disease, including AIDS or lupus.
- You are receiving blood from a blood bank.
- You take drugs for cancer.
- If you will have surgery within 2 months, including dental surgery, requiring general or spinal anesthesia.

Before you start, consult your doctor:
- If you have had a stroke.
- If you have angina, heart or blood-vessel disease, a high level of potassium in blood, lupus, gout, liver, pancreas or kidney disorder.
- If you are on severe salt-restricted diet.
- If you are allergic to any sulfa drug.

CAPTOPRIL & HYDROCHLOROTHIAZIDE

Over age 60:
Adverse reactions and side effects may be more frequent and severe than in younger persons, especially dizziness and excessive potassium loss.

Pregnancy:
Risk to unborn child outweighs drug benefits. Don't use.

Breast-feeding:
Drug passes into milk. Avoid drug or discontinue nursing until you finish medicine. Consult doctor for advice on maintaining milk supply.

Infants & children:
Not recommended.

Prolonged use:
May decrease white cells in blood or cause protein loss in urine. Request periodic laboratory blood counts and urine tests.

Skin & sunlight:
May cause rash or intensify sunburn in areas exposed to sun or sunlamp.

Driving, piloting or hazardous work:
Don't drive or pilot aircraft until you learn how medicine affects you. Don't work around dangerous machinery. Don't climb ladders or work in high places. Danger increases if you drink alcohol or take medicine affecting alertness and reflexes, such as antihistamines, tranquilizers, sedatives, pain medicine, narcotics and mind-altering drugs.

Discontinuing:
Don't discontinue without consulting doctor. Dose may require gradual reduction if you have taken drug for a long time. Doses of other drugs may also require adjustment.

Others:
- Hot weather and fever may cause dehydration and drop in blood pressure. Dose may require temporary adjustment. Weigh daily and report any unexpected weight decreases to your doctor.
- May cause rise in uric acid, leading to gout.
- May cause blood-sugar rise in diabetics.

 POSSIBLE INTERACTION WITH OTHER DRUGS

GENERIC NAME OR DRUG CLASS	COMBINED EFFECT
Allopurinol	Decreased allopurinol effect.
Amiloride	Possible excessive potassium in blood.
Antidepressants, tricyclic (TCA)*	Dangerous drop in blood pressure. Avoid combination unless under medical supervision.
Antihypertensives, other*	Increased antihypertensive effect. Dosage of each may require adjustment.
Barbiturates*	Increased hydrochlorothiazide effect.
Beta-adrenergic blockers*	Increased antihypertensive effect. Dosage of each may require adjustments.
Carteolol	Increased antihypertensive effects of both drugs. Dosages may require adjustment.
Chloramphenicol	Possible blood disorders.
Cholestyramine	Decreased hydrochlorothiazide effect.
Cortisone drugs*	Excessive potassium loss that causes dangerous heart rhythms.
Digitalis preparations*	Excessive potassium loss that causes dangerous heart rhythms.
Diuretics*	Decreased blood pressure.
Lisinopril	Increased antihypertensive effect. Dosage of each may require adjustment.

Continued page 1080

 POSSIBLE INTERACTION WITH OTHER SUBSTANCES

INTERACTS WITH	COMBINED EFFECT
Alcohol:	Dangerous blood-pressure drop. Avoid.
Beverages: Low-salt milk.	Possible excessive potassium in blood.
Cocaine	Increased risk of heart block and high blood pressure.
Foods: Salt substitutes.	Possible excessive potassium.
Marijuana:	Increased dizziness, may increase blood pressure.
Tobacco:	May decrease captopril effect.

*See Glossary

CARBAMAZEPINE

BRAND NAMES

Apo-Carbamazepine   Mazepine
Epitol   Tegretol

BASIC INFORMATION

Habit forming? No
Prescription needed? Yes
Available as generic? Yes
Drug class: Analgesic, anticonvulsant

USES

- Decreased frequency, severity and duration of attacks of tic douloureaux.*
- Prevents seizures.

DOSAGE & USAGE INFORMATION

How to take:
Regular or chewable tablet—Swallow with liquid or food to lessen stomach irritation.

When to take:
At the same times each day.

If you forget a dose:
Take as soon as you remember up to 2 hours late. If more than 2 hours, wait for next scheduled dose (don't double this dose).

What drug does:
- Reduces transmission of pain messages at certain nerve terminals.
- Reduces excitability of nerve fibers in brain, thus inhibiting repetitive spread of nerve impulses.

Continued next column

OVERDOSE

SYMPTOMS:
Involuntary movements, irregular bleeding, decreased urination, decreased blood pressure, dilated pupils, flushed skin, stupor, coma.
WHAT TO DO:
- **Dial 0 (operator) or 911 (emergency) for an ambulance or medical help. Then give first aid immediately.**
- **If patient is unconscious and not breathing, give mouth-to-mouth breathing. If there is no heartbeat, use cardiac massage and mouth-to-mouth breathing (CPR). Don't try to make patient vomit. If you can't get help quickly, take patient to nearest emergency facility.**
- **See emergency information on inside covers.**

Time lapse before drug works:
- Tic douloureaux—24 to 72 hours.
- Seizures—1 to 2 weeks.

Don't take with:
See Interaction column and consult doctor.

POSSIBLE ADVERSE REACTIONS OR SIDE EFFECTS

SYMPTOMS	WHAT TO DO
Life-threatening: None expected.	
Common: Blurred vision.	Continue. Call doctor when convenient.
Infrequent:	
• Confusion, slurred speech, fainting, depression, headache, hallucinations, hives, rash, mouth sores, sore throat, fever, unusual bleeding or bruising, unusual fatigue, jaundice.	Discontinue. Call doctor right away.
• Diarrhea, nausea, vomiting, constipation, dry mouth.	Continue. Call doctor when convenient.
Rare:	
• Back-and-forth eye movements; breathing difficulty; irregular, pounding or slow heartbeat; chest pain; uncontrollable body jerks; numbness, weakness or tingling in hands and feet; tender, bluish legs or feet; less urine; swollen lymph glands.	Discontinue. Call doctor right away.
• Frequent urination. muscle pains, joint aches.	Continue. Call doctor when convenient.

WARNINGS & PRECAUTIONS

Don't take if:
- You are allergic to carbamazepine.
- You have had liver or bone-marrow disease.
- You have taken MAO inhibitors in the past 2 weeks.

Before you start, consult your doctor:
- If you have high blood pressure, thrombophlebitis or heart disease.
- If you have glaucoma.
- If you have emotional or mental problems.
- If you have liver or kidney disease.
- If you drink more than 2 alcoholic drinks per day.

Over age 60:
Adverse reactions and side effects may be more frequent and severe than in younger persons.

Pregnancy:
Studies inconclusive on harm to unborn child. Animal studies show fetal abnormalities. Decide with your doctor whether drug benefits justify risk to unborn child.

Breast-feeding:
Drug passes into milk. Avoid drug or discontinue nursing until you finish medicine. Consult doctor for advice on maintaining milk supply.

Infants & children:
Not recommended.

Prolonged use:
- Jaundice and liver damage.
- Hair loss.
- Ringing in ears.
- Lower sex drive.

Skin & sunlight:
May cause rash or intensify sunburn in areas exposed to sun or sunlamp.

Driving, piloting or hazardous work:
Don't drive or pilot aircraft until you learn how medicine affects you. Don't work around dangerous machinery. Don't climb ladders or work in high places. Danger increases if you drink alcohol or take medicine affecting alertness and reflexes.

Discontinuing:
Don't discontinue without doctor's advice until you complete prescribed dose, even though symptoms diminish or disappear.

Others:
- Use only if less-hazardous drugs are not effective. Stay under medical supervision.
- Periodic blood tests are needed.

POSSIBLE INTERACTION WITH OTHER DRUGS

GENERIC NAME OR DRUG CLASS	COMBINED EFFECT
Anticoagulants, oral*	Decreased anticoagulant effect.
Anticonvulsants, hydantoin*	Decreased effect of both drugs.
Antidepressants, tricyclic (TCA)*	Confusion. Possible psychosis.
Cimetidine	Increased carbamazepine effect.
Contraceptives, oral*	Reduced contraceptive protection. Use another birth-control method.
Digitalis preparations*	Excess slowing of heart.
Doxycycline	Decreased doxycycline effect.
Erythromycin	Increased carbamazepine effect.
Ethinamate	Dangerous increased effects of ethinamate. Avoid combining.
Fluoxetine	Increased depressant effects of both drugs.
Guanfacine	May increase depressant effects of either drug.
Isonicotinic hydrazide (INH)	May increase carbamazepine effect.

Continued page 1080

POSSIBLE INTERACTION WITH OTHER SUBSTANCES

INTERACTS WITH	COMBINED EFFECT
Alcohol:	Increased sedative effect of alcohol. Avoid.
Beverages:	None expected.
Cocaine:	Increased adverse effects of carbamazepine. Avoid.
Foods:	None expected.
Marijuana:	Increased adverse effects of carbamazepine. Avoid.
Tobacco:	None expected.

*See Glossary

CARBENICILLIN

BRAND NAMES

Geocillin
Geopen

Geopen Oral
Pyopen

BASIC INFORMATION

Habit forming? No
Prescription needed? Yes
Available as generic? No
Drug class: Antibiotic (penicillin)

USES

Treatment of bacterial urinary tract infections that are susceptible to carbenicillin.

DOSAGE & USAGE INFORMATION

How to take:
Tablet—Swallow with liquid on an empty stomach 1 hour before or 2 hours after eating.

When to take:
Follow instructions on prescription label or side of package. Doses should be evenly spaced. For example, 4 times a day means every 6 hours.

If you forget a dose:
Take as soon as you remember. Continue regular schedule.

What drug does:
Destroys susceptible bacteria. Does not kill viruses.

Time lapse before drug works:
May be several days before medicine affects infection.

Don't take with:
See Interaction column and consult doctor.

OVERDOSE

SYMPTOMS:
Severe diarrhea, nausea or vomiting.
WHAT TO DO:
Overdose unlikely to threaten life. If person takes much larger amount than prescribed, call doctor, poison-control center or hospital emergency room for instructions.

POSSIBLE ADVERSE REACTIONS OR SIDE EFFECTS

SYMPTOMS	WHAT TO DO
Life-threatening: Hives, rash, intense itching, faintness soon after a dose (anaphylaxis).	Seek emergency treatment immediately.
Common: Dark or discolored tongue.	Continue. Tell doctor at next visit.
Infrequent: Mild nausea, vomiting, diarrhea.	Continue. Call doctor when convenient.
Rare: Unexplained bleeding.	Discontinue. Call doctor right away.

WARNINGS & PRECAUTIONS

Don't take if:
You are allergic to carbenicillin, cephalosporin antibiotics, or other penicillins. Life-threatening reaction may occur.

Before you start, consult your doctor:
If you are allergic to any substance or drug.

Over age 60:
You may have skin reactions, particularly around genitals and anus.

Pregnancy:
Studies inconclusive on harm to unborn child. Animal studies show fetal abnormalities. Decide with your doctor whether drug benefits justify risk to unborn child.

Breast-feeding:
Drug passes into milk. Child may become sensitive to penicillins and have allergic reactions to penicillin drugs. Avoid carbenicillin or discontinue nursing until you finish medicine. Consult doctor for advice on maintaining milk supply.

Infants & children:
No problems expected.

Prolonged use:
You may become more susceptible to infections caused by germs not responsive to carbenicillin.

Skin & sunlight:
No problems expected.

Driving, piloting or hazardous work:
Usually not dangerous. Most hazardous reactions likely to occur a few minutes after taking carbenicillin.

Discontinuing:
Don't discontinue without doctor's advice until you complete prescribed dose, even though symptoms diminish or disappear.

Others:
Injection forms may cause fluid retention (edema) with weakness and low potassium in the blood.

POSSIBLE INTERACTION WITH OTHER DRUGS

GENERIC NAME OR DRUG CLASS	COMBINED EFFECT
Beta-adrenergic blockers*	Increased chance of anaphylaxis (see emergency information on inside front cover).
Chloramphenicol	Decreased effect of both drugs.
Cholestyramine	May decrease carbenicillin effect.
Colestipol	May decrease carbenicillin effect.
Contraceptives, oral*	Possible decreased contraceptive effect.
Erythromycins*	Decreased effect of both drugs.
Paromomycin	Decreased effect of both drugs.
Probenecid	Possible carbenicillin effect.
Tetracyclines*	Decreased effect of both drugs.
Troleandomycin	Decreased effect of both drugs.

POSSIBLE INTERACTION WITH OTHER SUBSTANCES

INTERACTS WITH	COMBINED EFFECT
Alcohol:	Occasional stomach irritation.
Beverages:	None expected.
Cocaine:	No proven problems.
Foods:	Decreased effect of oral carbenicillin.
Marijuana:	No proven problems.
Tobacco:	None expected.

*See Glossary

CARBIDOPA & LEVODOPA

BRAND NAMES

Dopar   Sinemet
Larodopa

BASIC INFORMATION

Habit forming? No
Prescription needed? Yes
Available as generic? No
Drug class: Antiparkinsonism

 ## USES

Controls Parkinson's disease symptoms such as rigidity, tremor and unsteady gait.

 ## DOSAGE & USAGE INFORMATION

How to take:
Tablet—Swallow with liquid or food to lessen stomach irritation. If you can't swallow whole, crumble tablet and take with liquid or food.

When to take:
At the same times each day.

If you forget a dose:
Take as soon as you remember up to 2 hours late. If more than 2 hours, wait for next scheduled dose (don't double this dose).

What drug does:
Restores chemical balance necessary for normal nerve impulses.

Continued next column

 ## OVERDOSE

SYMPTOMS:
Muscle twitch, spastic eyelid closure, nausea, vomiting, diarrhea, irregular and rapid pulse, weakness, fainting, confusion, agitation, hallucination, coma.

WHAT TO DO:
- Dial 0 (operator) or 911 (emergency) for an ambulance or medical help. Then give first aid immediately.
- If patient is unconscious and not breathing, give mouth-to-mouth breathing. If there is no heartbeat, use cardiac massage and mouth-to-mouth breathing (CPR). Don't try to make patient vomit. If you can't get help quickly, take patient to nearest emergency facility.
- See emergency information on inside covers.

Time lapse before drug works:
2 to 3 weeks to improve; 6 weeks or longer for maximum benefit.

Don't take with:
See Interaction column and consult doctor.

 ## POSSIBLE ADVERSE REACTIONS OR SIDE EFFECTS

SYMPTOMS	WHAT TO DO
Life-threatening:	
None expected.	
Common:	
• Mood changes, uncontrollable body movements, diarrhea.	Continue. Call doctor when convenient.
• Dry mouth, body odor.	No action necessary.
Infrequent:	
• Fainting, severe dizziness, headache, insomnia, nightmares, rash, itch, nausea, vomiting, irregular heartbeat.	Discontinue. Call doctor right away.
• Flushed face, blurred vision, muscle twitching, discolored or dark urine, difficult urination.	Continue. Call doctor when convenient.
• Constipation, tiredness.	Continue. Tell doctor at next visit.
Rare:	
• High blood pressure.	Discontinue. Call doctor right away.
• Duodenal ulcer, anemia.	Continue. Call doctor when convenient.

WARNINGS & PRECAUTIONS

Don't take if:
- You are allergic to levodopa or carbidopa.
- You have taken MAO inhibitors in past 2 weeks.
- You have glaucoma (narrow-angle type).

Before you start, consult your doctor:
- You have diabetes or epilepsy.
- If you have had high blood pressure, heart or lung disease.
- If you have had liver or kidney disease.
- If you have a peptic ulcer.
- If you have malignant melanoma.
- If you will have surgery within 2 months, including dental surgery, requiring general or spinal anesthesia.

Over age 60:
Adverse reactions and side effects may be more frequent and severe than in younger persons.

Pregnancy:
Risk to unborn child outweighs drug benefits. Don't use.

Breast-feeding:
Drug filters into milk. May harm child. Avoid.

Infants & children:
Not recommended.

Prolonged use:
May lead to uncontrolled movements of head, face, mouth, tongue, arms or legs.

Skin & sunlight:
No problems expected.

Driving, piloting or hazardous work:
Don't drive or pilot aircraft until you learn how medicine affects you. Don't work around dangerous machinery. Don't climb ladders or work in high places. Danger increases if you drink alcohol or take medicine affecting alertness and reflexes, such as antihistamines, tranquilizers, sedatives, pain medicine, narcotics and mind-altering drugs.

Discontinuing:
Don't discontinue without doctor's advice until you complete prescribed dose, even though symptoms diminish or disappear.

Others:
Expect to start with small dose and increase gradually to lessen frequency and severity of adverse reactions.

POSSIBLE INTERACTION WITH OTHER DRUGS

GENERIC NAME OR DRUG CLASS	COMBINED EFFECT
Antidepressants, other*	Weakness or faintness when arising from bed or chair.
Antihypertensives*	Decreased blood pressure and effect of carbidopa and levodopa.
Antiparkinsonism drugs, other*	Increased effect of carbidopa and levodopa.
Haloperidol	Decreased effect of carbidopa and levodopa.
MAO inhibitors*	Dangerous rise in blood pressure.
Methyldopa	Decreased effect of carbidopa and levodopa.
Papaverine	Decreased effect of carbidopa and levodopa.
Phenothiazines*	Decreased effect of carbidopa and levodopa.
Phenytoin	Decreased levodopa effect.
Pyridoxine (Vitamin B-6)	Decreased effect of carbidopa and levodopa.
Rauwolfia alkaloids*	Decreased effect of carbidopa and levodopa.

POSSIBLE INTERACTION WITH OTHER SUBSTANCES

INTERACTS WITH	COMBINED EFFECT
Alcohol:	None expected.
Beverages:	None expected.
Cocaine:	Decreased carbidopa and levodopa effect.
Foods:	None expected.
Marijuana:	Increased fatigue, lethargy, fainting.
Tobacco:	None expected.

*See Glossary

CARBINOXAMINE

BRAND NAMES

Clistin   Clistin R-A

BASIC INFORMATION

Habit forming? No
Prescription needed? Yes
Available as generic? No
Drug class: Antihistamine

 USES

Reduces allergic symptoms such as hay fever, hives, rash or itching.

 DOSAGE & USAGE INFORMATION

How to take:
Tablet—Swallow with liquid or food to lessen stomach irritation.

When to take:
Varies with form. Follow label directions.

If you forget a dose:
Take as soon as you remember up to 2 hours late. If more than 2 hours, wait for next scheduled dose (don't double this dose).

What drug does:
Blocks action of histamine after an allergic response triggers histamine release in sensitive cells.

Time lapse before drug works:
30 minutes.

Don't take with:
See Interaction column and consult doctor.

 OVERDOSE

SYMPTOMS:
Convulsions, red face, hallucinations, coma.
WHAT TO DO:
- Dial 0 (operator) or 911 (emergency) for an ambulance or medical help. Then give first aid immediately.
- If patient is unconscious and not breathing, give mouth-to-mouth breathing. If there is no heartbeat, use cardiac massage and mouth-to-mouth breathing (CPR). Don't try to make patient vomit. If you can't get help quickly, take patient to nearest emergency facility.
- See emergency information on inside covers.

 POSSIBLE ADVERSE REACTIONS OR SIDE EFFECTS

SYMPTOMS	WHAT TO DO
Life-threatening: None expected.	
Common: Drowsiness; dizziness; nausea; dry mouth, nose, throat.	Continue. Tell doctor at next visit.
Infrequent:	
• Changes in vision.	Discontinue. Call doctor right away.
• Less tolerance for contact lenses, urination difficulty.	Continue. Call doctor when convenient.
• Appetite loss.	Continue. Tell doctor at next visit.
Rare: Nightmares, agitation, irritability, sore throat, fever, rapid heartbeat, unusual bleeding or bruising, fatigue, weakness.	Discontinue. Call doctor right away.

WARNINGS & PRECAUTIONS

Don't take if:
You are allergic to any antihistamine.

Before you start, consult your doctor:
- If you have glaucoma.
- If you have enlarged prostate.
- If you have asthma.
- If you have kidney disease.
- If you have peptic ulcer.
- If you will have surgery within 2 months, including dental surgery, requiring general or spinal anesthesia.

Over age 60:
Don't exceed recommended dose. Adverse reactions and side effects may be more frequent and severe than in younger persons, especially urination difficulty, diminished alertness and other brain and nervous-system symptoms.

Pregnancy:
No proven harm to unborn child. Avoid if possible.

Breast-feeding:
Drug passes into milk. Avoid drug or discontinue nursing until you finish medicine. Consult doctor for advice on maintaining milk supply.

Infants & children:
Not recommended for premature or newborn infants. Otherwise, no problems expected.

Prolonged use:
Avoid. May damage bone marrow and nerve cells.

Skin & sunlight:
May cause rash or intensify sunburn in areas exposed to sun or sunlamp.

Driving, piloting or hazardous work:
Don't drive or pilot aircraft until you learn how medicine affects you. Don't work around dangerous machinery. Don't climb ladders or work in high places. Danger increases if you drink alcohol or take medicine affecting alertness and reflexes, such as antihistamines, tranquilizers, sedatives, pain medicine, narcotics and mind-altering drugs.

Discontinuing:
No problems expected.

Others:
May mask symptoms of hearing damage from aspirin, other salicylates, cisplatin, paromomycin, vancomycin or anticonvulsants. Consult doctor if you use these.

POSSIBLE INTERACTION WITH OTHER DRUGS

GENERIC NAME OR DRUG CLASS	COMBINED EFFECT
Anticholinergics*	Increased anticholinergic effect.
Anticoagulants, oral*	Decreased carbinoxamine.
Antidepressants*	Increased carbinoxamine effect. Excess sedation. Avoid.
Antihistamines, other*	Excess sedation. Avoid.
Carteolol	Decreased antihistamine effect.
Dronabinol	Increased effects of both drugs. Avoid.
Hypnotics*	Excess sedation. Avoid.
MAO inhibitors*	Increased carbinoxamine effect.
Mind-altering drugs*	Excess sedation. Avoid.
Molindone	Increased antihistamine effect.
Nabilone	Greater depression of central nervous system.
Narcotics*	Excess sedation. Avoid.
Procarbazine	May increase sedation.
Sedatives*	Excess sedation. Avoid.
Sleep inducers*	Excess sedation. Avoid.
Sotalol	Increased antihistamine effect.
Tranquilizers*	Excess sedation. Avoid.

POSSIBLE INTERACTION WITH OTHER SUBSTANCES

INTERACTS WITH	COMBINED EFFECT
Alcohol:	Excess sedation. Avoid.
Beverages: Caffeine drinks.	Less carbinoxamine sedation.
Cocaine:	Decreased carbinoxamine effect. Avoid.
Foods:	None expected.
Marijuana:	Excess sedation. Avoid.
Tobacco:	None expected.

CARBOL-FUCHSIN (Topical)

BRAND NAMES

Castel Plus   Castilani Pain

BASIC INFORMATION

Habit forming? No
Prescription needed? Yes
Available as generic? Yes
Drug class: Antifungal; drying agent

 ## USES

Treats fungal infections of skin and nails including athlete's foot and ringworm. Also used as drying agent for ulcerations in skin.

 ## DOSAGE & USAGE INFORMATION

How to use:
* Bathe and dry area to be treated.
* Apply solution with cotton applicator or swab to affected areas.
* Protect from normal skin.
* Do not bandage or wrap fingers or toes.

When to use:
1 to 3 times a day according to instructions.

If you forget a dose:
Use as soon as you remember.

What drug does:
* Kills fungi on contact.
* Basic fuchsin (a dye) stimulates growth of new skin.
* Acts as mild anesthetic and kills some bacteria.

Time lapse before drug works:
May require daily treatment for several months or more.

Don't use with:
Other skin preparations without telling your doctor.

 ## OVERDOSE

SYMPTOMS:
None expected.
WHAT TO DO:
Not for internal use. If child accidentally swallows, call poison-control center.

 ## POSSIBLE ADVERSE REACTIONS OR SIDE EFFECTS

SYMPTOMS	WHAT TO DO
Life-threatening	None expected.
Common	None expected.

Infrequent
* After beginning this medicine, skin irritation appears.   Discontinue. Call doctor right away.
* Mild, temporary stinging.   Continue. Call doctor when convenient.

Rare
None expected.

CARBOL-FUCHSIN (Topical)

WARNINGS & PRECAUTIONS

Don't use if:
You are allergic to carbol-fuchsin.

Before you start, consult your doctor:
If you are allergic to anything.

Over age 60:
No problems expected, but check with doctor.

Pregnancy:
No problems expected, but check with doctor.

Breast-feeding:
No problems expected, but check with doctor.

Infants & children:
No problems expected, but check with doctor.

Prolonged use:
No problems expected, but check with doctor.

Skin & sunlight:
No problems expected, but check with doctor.

Driving, piloting or hazardous work:
No problems expected, but check with doctor.

Discontinuing:
No problems expected, but check with doctor.

Others:
- Stains clothing.
- May discolor hair slightly.
- Heat and moisture in bathroom medicine cabinet can cause breakdown of medicine. Store someplace else.
- Keep cool, but don't freeze.

POSSIBLE INTERACTION WITH OTHER DRUGS

GENERIC NAME OR DRUG CLASS	COMBINED EFFECT
None expected.	

POSSIBLE INTERACTION WITH OTHER SUBSTANCES

INTERACTS WITH	COMBINED EFFECT
Alcohol:	None expected.
Beverages:	None expected.
Cocaine:	None expected.
Foods:	None expected.
Marijuana:	None expected.
Tobacco:	None expected.

CARBONIC ANHYDRASE INHIBITORS

BRAND AND GENERIC NAMES

Acetazolam
ACETAZOLAMIDE
Ak-Zol
Apo-Acetazolamide
Cetazol
Daranide
Dazamide

Diamox
Diamox Sequels
DICHLORPHENAMIDE
METHAZOLAMIDE
Neptazane
Oratrol

BASIC INFORMATION

Habit forming? No
Prescription needed? Yes
Available as generic? Yes
Drug class: Carbonic anhydrase inhibitor*

USES

- Treatment of glaucoma.
- Treatment of epileptic seizures.
- Treatment of body-fluid retention.
- Treatment for shortness of breath, insomnia and fatigue in high altitudes.

DOSAGE & USAGE INFORMATION

How to take:
- Sustained-release tablets—Swallow whole with liquid or food to lessen stomach irritation.
- Extended-release capsules—Swallow whole with liquid.

When to take:
- 1 dose per day—At the same time each morning.
- More than 1 dose per day—Take last dose several hours before bedtime.

If you forget a dose:
Take as soon as you remember. Continue regular schedule.

Continued next column

OVERDOSE

SYMPTOMS:
Drowsiness, confusion, excitement, nausea, vomiting, numbness in hands and feet, coma.
WHAT TO DO:
- Call your doctor or poison-control center for advice if you suspect overdose, even if not sure. Symptoms may not appear until damage has occurred.
- See emergency information on inside covers.

What drug does:
- Inhibits action of carbonic anhydrase, an enzyme. This lowers the internal eye pressure by decreasing fluid formation in the eye.
- Forces sodium and water excretion, reducing body fluid.

Time lapse before drug works:
2 hours.

Don't take with:
- Non-prescription drugs without consulting doctor.
- See Interaction column and consult doctor.

POSSIBLE ADVERSE REACTIONS OR SIDE EFFECTS

SYMPTOMS	WHAT TO DO
Life-threatening: Convulsions.	Seek emergency treatment immediately.
Common: None expected.	
Infrequent: • Back pain, sedation.	Discontinue. Call doctor right away.
• Fatigue, weakness, tingling or burning in feet or hands.	Continue. Call doctor when convenient.
Rare: • Headache; mood changes; nervousness; clumsiness; trembling; confusion; hives, itch, rash; sores; ringing in ears; hoarseness; dry mouth; thirst; sore throat; fever; appetite change; nausea; vomiting; black, tarry stool; breathing difficulty; irregular or weak heartbeat; easy bleeding or bruising; muscle cramps; painful or frequent urination; blood in urine.	Discontinue. Call doctor right away.
• Depression.	Continue. Call doctor when convenient.

CARBONIC ANHYDRASE INHIBITORS

WARNINGS & PRECAUTIONS

Don't take if:
- You are allergic to any carbonic anhydrase inhibitor.
- You have liver or kidney disease.
- You have Addison's disease (adrenal gland failure).
- You have diabetes.

Before you start, consult your doctor:
- If you have gout or lupus.
- If you are allergic to any sulfa drug.
- If you will have surgery within 2 months, including dental surgery, requiring general or spinal anesthesia.

Over age 60:
- Don't exceed recommended dose.
- If you take a digitalis preparation, eat foods high in potassium content or take a potassium supplement.

Pregnancy:
No proven harm to unborn child. Avoid if possible, especially first 3 months.

Breast-feeding:
Avoid drug or don't nurse your infant.

Infants & children:
Not recommended for children younger than 12.

Prolonged use:
May cause kidney stones, vision change, loss of taste and smell, jaundice or weight loss.

Skin & sunlight:
No problems expected.

Driving, piloting or hazardous work:
Avoid if you feel drowsy or dizzy. Otherwise, no problems expected.

Discontinuing:
Don't discontinue without medical advice.

Others:
Medicine may increase sugar levels in blood and urine. Diabetics may need insulin adjustment.

POSSIBLE INTERACTION WITH OTHER DRUGS

GENERIC NAME OR DRUG CLASS	COMBINED EFFECT
Amphetamines *	Increased amphetamine effect.
Anticonvulsants *	Increased loss of bone minerals.
Antidepressants, tricyclic (TCA) *	Increased anti-depressant effect.
Antidiabetics, oral *	Increased potassium loss.
Aspirin	Decreased aspirin effect.
Ciprofloxacin	May cause kidney dysfunction.
Cortisone drugs *	Increased potassium loss.
Digitalis preparations *	Possible digitalis toxicity.
Diuretics *	Increased potassium loss.
Lithium	Decreased lithium effect.
Methenamine	Decreased methenamine effect.
Mexiletene	May slow elimination of mexiletene and cause need to adjust dosage.
Quinidine	Increased quinidine effect.
Salicylates *	Salicylate toxicity.
Sympathomimetics *	Increased sympatho-mimetic effect.

POSSIBLE INTERACTION WITH OTHER SUBSTANCES

INTERACTS WITH	COMBINED EFFECT
Alcohol:	None expected.
Beverages:	None expected.
Cocaine:	Avoid. Decreased carbonic anhydrase inhibitor effect.
Foods: Potassium-rich foods. *	Eat these to decrease potassium loss.
Marijuana:	Avoid. Increased carbonic anhydrase inhibitor effect.
Tobacco:	May decrease absorption of carbonic anhydrase inhibitors.

CARISOPRODOL

BRAND NAMES

Rela
Soma

Soma Compound
Soprodol

BASIC INFORMATION

Habit forming? Possibly
Prescription needed? Yes
Available as generic? Yes
Drug class: Muscle relaxant (skeletal)

USES

Adjunctive treatment to rest, analgesics, and physical therapy for muscle spasms.

DOSAGE & USAGE INFORMATION

How to take:
Tablet—Swallow with liquid.

When to take:
As needed, no more often than every 4 hours.

If you forget a dose:
Take as soon as you remember. Wait 4 hours for next dose.

What drug does:
Blocks body's pain messages to brain. Also causes sedation.

Time lapse before drug works:
60 minutes.

Don't take with:
See Interaction column and consult doctor.

OVERDOSE

SYMPTOMS:
Nausea, vomiting, diarrhea, headache. May progress to severe weakness, difficult breathing, sensation of paralysis, coma.
WHAT TO DO:
- Dial 0 (operator) or 911 (emergency) for an ambulance or medical help. Then give first aid immediately.
- See emergency information on inside covers.

POSSIBLE ADVERSE REACTIONS OR SIDE EFFECTS

SYMPTOMS	WHAT TO DO
Life-threatening: Hives, rash, intense itching, faintness soon after a dose (anaphylaxis); extreme weakness, transient paralysis, temporary vision loss.	Seek emergency treatment immediately.
Common: • Drowsiness, fainting, dizziness.	Continue. Call doctor when convenient.
• Orange or red-purple urine.	No action necessary.
Infrequent: Agitation, constipation or diarrhea, nausea, cramps, vomiting, wheezing, shortness of breath, headache, depression.	Discontinue. Call doctor right away.
Rare: • Black, tarry or bloody stool.	Discontinue. Seek emergency treatment.
• Rash, hives, or itch; sore throat; fever; jaundice; tiredness; weakness; hiccups.	Discontinue. Call doctor right away.

WARNINGS & PRECAUTIONS

Don't take if:
- You are allergic to any skeletal-muscle relaxant.
- You have porphyria.

Before you start, consult your doctor:
- If you have had liver or kidney disease.
- If you plan pregnancy within medication period.
- If you are allergic to tartrazine dye.

Over age 60:
Adverse reactions and side effects may be more frequent and severe than in younger persons.

Pregnancy:
Safety not proven. Avoid if possible.

Breast-feeding:
Drug passes into milk. Avoid drug or discontinue nursing until you finish medicine. Consult doctor for advice on maintaining milk supply.

Infants & children:
Not recommended.

Prolonged use:
Periodic liver-function tests recommended if you use this drug for a long time.

Skin & sunlight:
No problems expected.

Driving, piloting or hazardous work:
Don't drive or pilot aircraft until you learn how medicine affects you. Don't work around dangerous machinery. Don't climb ladders or work in high places. Danger increases if you drink alcohol or take medicine affecting alertness and reflexes, such as antihistamines, tranquilizers, sedatives, pain medicine, narcotics and mind-altering drugs.

Discontinuing:
Don't discontinue without doctor's advice until you complete prescribed dose, even though symptoms diminish or disappear.

Others:
No problems expected.

POSSIBLE INTERACTION WITH OTHER DRUGS

GENERIC NAME OR DRUG CLASS	COMBINED EFFECT
Antidepressants*	Increased sedation.
Antihistamines*	Increased sedation.
Dronabinol	Increased effect of dronabinol on central nervous system. Avoid combination.
Mind-altering drugs*	Increased sedation.
Muscle relaxants, others*	Increased sedation.
Narcotics*	Increased sedation.
Sedatives*	Increased sedation.
Sleep inducers*	Increased sedation.
Tranquilizers*	Increased sedation.

POSSIBLE INTERACTION WITH OTHER SUBSTANCES

INTERACTS WITH	COMBINED EFFECT
Alcohol:	Increased sedation.
Beverages:	None expected.
Cocaine:	Lack of coordination, increased sedation.
Foods:	None expected.
Marijuana:	Lack of coordination, drowsiness, fainting.
Tobacco:	None expected.

*See Glossary

CARTEOLOL

BRAND NAMES

Cartrol

BASIC INFORMATION

Habit forming? No
Prescription needed? Yes
Available as generic? Yes
Drug class: Beta-adrenergic blocker

USES

- Reduces angina attacks.
- Stabilizes irregular heartbeat.
- Lowers blood pressure.
- Reduces frequency of migraine headaches. (Does not relieve headache pain.)
- Other uses prescribed by your doctor.

DOSAGE & USAGE INFORMATION

How to take:
Tablet, liquid or extended-release capsule—Swallow with liquid. If you can't swallow whole, crumble tablet or open capsule and take with liquid or food. Don't crush capsule.

When to take:
As directed by your doctor.

If you forget a dose:
Take as soon as you remember. Return to regular schedule, but allow 3 hours between doses.

What drug does:
- Blocks certain actions of sympathetic nervous system.
- Lowers heart's oxygen requirements.
- Slows nerve impulses through heart.
- Reduces blood vessel contraction in heart, scalp and other body parts.

Time lapse before drug works:
1 to 4 hours.

Don't take with:
Non-prescription drugs or drugs in Interaction column without consulting doctor.

OVERDOSE

SYMPTOMS:
Weakness, slow or weak pulse, blood-pressure drop, fainting, difficulty breathing, convulsions, cold and sweaty skin.
WHAT TO DO:
- Dial 0 (operator) or 911 (emergency) for an ambulance or medical help. Then give first aid immediately.
- See emergency information on inside covers.

POSSIBLE ADVERSE REACTIONS OR SIDE EFFECTS

SYMPTOMS	WHAT TO DO
Life-threatening:	
Congestive heart failure.	Discontinue. Seek emergency treatment.
Common:	
• Pulse slower than 50 beats per minute.	Discontinue. Call doctor right away.
• Drowsiness, fatigue, numbness or tingling of fingers or toes, dizziness, diarrhea, nausea, weakness.	Continue. Call doctor when convenient.
• Cold hands or feet; dry mouth, eyes and skin.	Continue. Tell doctor at next visit.
Infrequent:	
• Hallucinations, nightmares, insomnia, headache, difficult breathing, joint pain, anxiety.	Discontinue. Call doctor right away.
• Confusion, reduced alertness, depression, impotence.	Continue. Call doctor when convenient.
• Constipation.	Continue. Tell doctor at next visit.
Rare:	
• Rash, sore throat, fever.	Discontinue. Call doctor right away.
• Unusual bleeding and bruising; dry, burning eyes; impotence.	Continue. Call doctor when convenient.

WARNINGS & PRECAUTIONS

Don't take if:
- You are allergic to any beta-adrenergic blocker.
- You have asthma.
- You have hay fever symptoms.
- You have taken MAO inhibitors in past 2 weeks.

Before you start, consult your doctor:
- If you have heart disease or poor circulation to the extremities.
- If you have hay fever, asthma, chronic bronchitis, emphysema.
- If you have overactive thyroid function.
- If you have impaired liver or kidney function.
- If you will have surgery within 2 months, including dental surgery, requiring general or spinal anesthesia.
- If you have diabetes or hypoglycemia.

Over age 60:
Adverse reactions and side effects may be more frequent and severe than in younger persons.

Pregnancy:
Risk to unborn child outweighs drug benefits. Don't use.

Breast-feeding:
Drug passes into milk. Avoid drug or discontinue nursing until you finish medicine. Consult doctor for advice on maintaining milk supply.

Infants & children:
Not recommended.

Prolonged use:
Weakens heart muscle contractions.

Skin & sunlight:
No problems expected.

Driving, piloting or hazardous work:
Don't drive or pilot aircraft until you learn how medicine affects you. Don't work around dangerous machinery. Don't climb ladders or work in high places. Danger increases if you drink alcohol or take medicine affecting alertness and reflexes.

Discontinuing:
Don't discontinue without consulting doctor. Dose may require gradual reduction if you have taken drug for a long time. Doses of other drugs may also require adjustment.

Others:
May mask hypoglycemia.

POSSIBLE INTERACTION WITH OTHER DRUGS

GENERIC NAME OR DRUG CLASS	COMBINED EFFECT
ACE inhibitors: captopril, enalapril, lisinopril*	Increased antihypertensive effects of both drugs. Dosages may require adjustment.
Antidiabetics*	Increased antidiabetic effect.
Antihistamines*	Decreased antihistamine effect.
Antihypertensives*	Increased antihypertensive effect.
Barbiturates*	Increased barbiturate effect. Dangerous sedation.
Beta-agonists*	Decreased beta-agonist effect.
Betaxolol eyedrops	Possible increased carteolol effect.
Diclofenac	Decreased antihypertensive effect of carteolol.
Digitalis preparations*	Can either increase or decrease heart rate. Improves irregular heartbeat.
Encainide	Increased effect of toxicity on heart muscle.
Indomethacin	Decreased effect of carteolol.

Continued on page 1081

POSSIBLE INTERACTION WITH OTHER SUBSTANCES

INTERACTS WITH	COMBINED EFFECT
Alcohol:	Excessive blood-pressure drop. Avoid.
Beverages:	None expected.
Cocaine:	Irregular heartbeat. Avoid.
Foods:	None expected.
Marijuana:	Daily use—Impaired circulation to hands and feet.
Tobacco:	Possible irregular heartbeat.

*See Glossary

CASCARA

BRAND NAMES

Aromatic Cascara
  Fluidextract
Cascara Sagrada
Cas-Evac

Milk of
  Magnesia-Cascara
Peri-Colace

BASIC INFORMATION

Habit forming? No
Prescription needed? No
Available as generic? Yes
Drug class: Laxative (stimulant)

 USES

Constipation relief.

 DOSAGE & USAGE INFORMATION

How to take:
- Tablet—Swallow with liquid. If you can't swallow whole, chew or crumble tablet and take with liquid or food.
- Liquid—Drink 6 to 8 glasses of water each day, in addition to one taken with each dose.

When to take:
Usually at bedtime with a snack, unless directed otherwise.

If you forget a dose:
Take as soon as you remember.

What drug does:
Acts on smooth muscles of intestine wall to cause vigorous bowel movement.

Time lapse before drug works:
6 to 10 hours.

Don't take with:
- See Interaction column and consult doctor.
- Don't take within 2 hours of taking another medicine. Laxative interferes with medicine absorption.

 OVERDOSE

SYMPTOMS:
Vomiting, electrolyte depletion.
WHAT TO DO:
Overdose unlikely to threaten life. If person takes much larger amount than prescribed, call doctor, poison-control center or hospital emergency room for instructions.

 POSSIBLE ADVERSE REACTIONS OR SIDE EFFECTS

SYMPTOMS	WHAT TO DO
Life-threatening: None expected.	
Common: Rectal irritation.	Continue. Call doctor when convenient.
Infrequent: • Dangerous potassium loss.	Discontinue. Call doctor right away.
• Belching, cramps, nausea.	Continue. Call doctor when convenient.
Rare: • Irritability, confusion, headache, rash, breathing difficulty, irregular heartbeat, muscle cramps, unusual tiredness or weakness.	Discontinue. Call doctor right away.
• Burning on urination.	Continue. Call doctor when convenient.
• Discoloration of urine.	No action necessary.

WARNINGS & PRECAUTIONS

Don't take if:
- You have symptoms of appendicitis, inflamed bowel or intestinal blockage.
- You are allergic to a stimulant laxative.
- You have missed a bowel movement for only 1 or 2 days.

Before you start, consult your doctor:
- If you have a colostomy or ileostomy.
- If you have congestive heart disease.
- If you have diabetes.
- If you have high blood pressure.
- If you have a laxative habit.
- If you have rectal bleeding.
- If you take other laxatives.

Over age 60:
Adverse reactions and side effects may be more frequent and severe than in younger persons.

Pregnancy:
Risk to mother and unborn child outweighs drug benefits. Don't use.

Breast-feeding:
Drug passes into milk. Avoid drug or discontinue nursing until you finish medicine. Consult doctor for advice on maintaining milk supply.

Infants & children:
Use only under medical supervision.

Prolonged use:
Don't take for more than 1 week unless under a doctor's supervision. May cause laxative dependence.

Skin & sunlight:
No problems expected.

Driving, piloting or hazardous work:
No problems expected.

Discontinuing:
May be unnecessary to finish medicine. Follow doctor's instructions.

Others:
Don't take to "flush out" your system or as a "tonic."

POSSIBLE INTERACTION WITH OTHER DRUGS

GENERIC NAME OR DRUG CLASS	COMBINED EFFECT
Antacids*	Irritation of stomach or small intestine.
Digoxin	Increased toxicity due to decreased potassium level.
Diuretics*	May cause dangerous low potassium level.
Ranitidine	Irritation of stomach or small intestine.

POSSIBLE INTERACTION WITH OTHER SUBSTANCES

INTERACTS WITH	COMBINED EFFECT
Alcohol:	None expected.
Beverages:	None expected.
Cocaine:	None expected.
Foods:	None expected.
Marijuana:	None expected.
Tobacco:	None expected.

CASTOR OIL

BRAND NAMES

Alphamul	Hydrisinol
Emulsoil	Kellogg's Castor Oil
Fleet Flavored	Neoloid
Castor Oil	Purge
Fleet Prep Kit	Stimuzyme Plus
Granulex	Unisoil

BASIC INFORMATION

Habit forming? No
Prescription needed? No
Available as generic? Yes
Drug class: Laxative (stimulant)

 ## USES

Constipation relief.

 ## DOSAGE & USAGE INFORMATION

How to take:
Liquid or capsules—Drink 6 to 8 glasses of water each day, in addition to one taken with each dose.

When to take:
Usually at bedtime with a snack, unless directed otherwise.

If you forget a dose:
Take as soon as you remember.

What drug does:
Acts on smooth muscles of intestine wall to cause vigorous bowel movement.

Time lapse before drug works:
2 to 6 hours.

Don't take with:
* See Interaction column and consult doctor.
* Don't take within 2 hours of taking another medicine. Laxative interferes with medicine absorption.

 ## OVERDOSE

SYMPTOMS:
Vomiting, electrolyte depletion.
WHAT TO DO:
Overdose unlikely to threaten life. If person takes much larger amount than prescribed, call doctor, poison-control center or hospital emergency room for instructions.

 ## POSSIBLE ADVERSE REACTIONS OR SIDE EFFECTS

SYMPTOMS	WHAT TO DO
Life-threatening:	
None expected.	
Common:	
Rectal irritation.	Continue. Call doctor when convenient.
Infrequent:	
• Dangerous potassium loss.	Discontinue. Call doctor right away.
• Belching, cramps, nausea.	Continue. Call doctor when convenient.
Rare:	
• Irritability, headache, confusion, rash, breathing difficulty, irregular heartbeat, muscle cramps, unusual tiredness or weakness.	Discontinue. Call doctor right away.
• Burning on urination.	Continue. Call doctor when convenient.

WARNINGS & PRECAUTIONS

Don't take if:
- You have symptoms of appendicitis, inflamed bowel or intestinal blockage.
- You are allergic to a stimulant laxative.
- You have missed a bowel movement for only 1 or 2 days.

Before you start, consult your doctor:
- If you have a colostomy or ileostomy.
- If you have congestive heart disease.
- If you have diabetes.
- If you have high blood pressure.
- If you have a laxative habit.
- If you have rectal bleeding.
- If you take other laxatives.

Over age 60:
Adverse reactions and side effects may be more frequent and severe than in younger persons.

Pregnancy:
Risk to mother and unborn child outweighs drug benefits. Don't use.

Breast-feeding:
Drug passes into milk. Avoid drug or discontinue nursing until you finish medicine. Consult doctor for advice on maintaining milk supply.

Infants & children:
Use only under medical supervision.

Prolonged use:
Don't take for more than 1 week unless under doctor's supervision. May cause laxative dependence.

Skin & sunlight:
No problems expected.

Driving, piloting or hazardous work:
No problems expected.

Discontinuing:
May be unnecessary to finish medicine. Follow doctor's instructions.

Others:
Don't take to "flush out" your system or as a "tonic."

POSSIBLE INTERACTION WITH OTHER DRUGS

GENERIC NAME OR DRUG CLASS	COMBINED EFFECT
Antihypertensives*	May cause dangerous low potassium level.
Diuretics*	May cause dangerous low potassium level.

POSSIBLE INTERACTION WITH OTHER SUBSTANCES

INTERACTS WITH	COMBINED EFFECT
Alcohol:	None expected.
Beverages:	None expected.
Cocaine:	None expected.
Foods:	None expected.
Marijuana:	None expected.
Tobacco:	None expected.

*See Glossary

CEFACLOR

BRAND NAMES

Ceclor

BASIC INFORMATION

Habit forming? No
Prescription needed? Yes
Available as generic? No
Drug class: Antibiotic (cephalosporin)

 ## USES

Treatment of bacterial infections. Will not cure viral infections such as cold and flu.

 ## DOSAGE & USAGE INFORMATION

How to take:
- Capsule—Swallow with liquid. If you can't swallow whole, open capsule and take with liquid or food.
- Liquid—Use measuring spoon.

When to take:
- At same times each day, 1 hour before or 2 hours after eating.
- Take until gone or as directed.

If you forget a dose:
Take as soon as you remember or double next dose. Return to regular schedule.

What drug does:
Kills susceptible bacteria.

Time lapse before drug works:
May require several days to affect infection.

Don't take with:
See Interaction column and consult doctor.

 ## OVERDOSE

SYMPTOMS:
Abdominal cramps, nausea, vomiting, severe diarrhea with mucus or blood in stool.
WHAT TO DO:
Overdose unlikely to threaten life. If person takes much larger amount than prescribed, call doctor, poison-control center or hospital emergency room for instructions.

 ## POSSIBLE ADVERSE REACTIONS OR SIDE EFFECTS

SYMPTOMS	WHAT TO DO
Life-threatening:	
Hives, rash, intense itching, faintness soon after a dose (anaphylaxis); difficulty breathing.	Seek emergency treatment immediately.
Common:	
Rash, redness, itching.	Discontinue. Call doctor right away.
Infrequent:	
Rectal itching, oral or vaginal candidiasis.	Continue. Call doctor when convenient.
Rare:	
Mild nausea, vomiting, cramps, severe diarrhea with mucus or blood in stool, unusual weakness, tiredness, weight loss, fever.	Discontinue. Call doctor right away.

WARNINGS & PRECAUTIONS

Don't take if:
You are allergic to any cephalosporin antibiotic.

Before you start, consult your doctor:
- If you are allergic to any penicillin antibiotic.
- If you have a kidney disorder.
- If you have colitis or enteritis.

Over age 60:
Adverse reactions and side effects may be more frequent and severe than in younger persons. More likely to itch around rectum and genitals.

Pregnancy:
No proven harm to unborn child. Avoid if possible.

Breast-feeding:
Drug passes into milk. Avoid drug or discontinue nursing until you finish medicine. Consult doctor for advice on maintaining milk supply.

Infants & children:
No special warnings.

Prolonged use:
Kills beneficial bacteria that protect body against other germs. Unchecked germs may cause secondary infections.

Skin & sunlight:
No problems expected.

Driving, piloting or hazardous work:
No problems expected.

Discontinuing:
Don't discontinue without doctor's advice until you complete prescribed dose, even though symptoms diminish or disappear.

Others:
No problems expected.

POSSIBLE INTERACTION WITH OTHER DRUGS

GENERIC NAME OR DRUG CLASS	COMBINED EFFECT
Anticoagulants*	Increased anticoagulant effect.
Erythromycin	Decreased antibiotic effect of cefaclor.
Chloramphenicol	Decreased antibiotic effect of cefaclor.
Clindamycin	Decreased antibiotic effect of cefaclor.
Probenecid	Increased cefaclor effect.
Tetracyclines*	Decreased antibiotic effect of cefaclor.

POSSIBLE INTERACTION WITH OTHER SUBSTANCES

INTERACTS WITH	COMBINED EFFECT
Alcohol:	Increased kidney toxicity.
Beverages:	None expected.
Cocaine:	None expected, but cocaine may slow body's recovery. Avoid.
Foods:	Slow absorption. Take with liquid 1 hour before or 2 hours after eating.
Marijuana:	None expected, but marijuana may slow body's recovery. Avoid.
Tobacco:	None expected.

CEFADROXIL

BRAND NAMES

Duricef   **Ultracef**

BASIC INFORMATION

Habit forming? No
Prescription needed? Yes
Available as generic? No
Drug class: Antibiotic (cephalosporin)

 ## USES

Treatment of bacterial infections. Will not cure viral infections such as cold and flu.

 ## DOSAGE & USAGE INFORMATION

How to take:
* Capsule—Swallow with liquid. If you can't swallow whole, open capsule and take with liquid or food.
* Liquid—Use measuring spoon.

When to take:
* At same times each day, 1 hour before or 2 hours after eating.
* Take until gone or as directed.

If you forget a dose:
Take as soon as you remember or double next dose. Return to regular schedule.

What drug does:
Kills susceptible bacteria.

Time lapse before drug works:
May require several days to affect infection.

Don't take with:
See Interaction column and consult doctor.

 ## OVERDOSE

SYMPTOMS:
Abdominal cramps, nausea, vomiting, severe diarrhea with mucus or blood in stool.
WHAT TO DO:
Overdose unlikely to threaten life. If person takes much larger amount than prescribed, call doctor, poison-control center or hospital emergency room for instructions.

 ## POSSIBLE ADVERSE REACTIONS OR SIDE EFFECTS

SYMPTOMS	WHAT TO DO
Life-threatening: Hives, rash, intense itching, faintness soon after a dose (anaphylaxis); difficulty breathing.	Seek emergency treatment immediately.
Common: Rash, redness, itching.	Discontinue. Call doctor right away.
Infrequent: Rectal itching.	Continue. Call doctor when convenient.
Rare: Mild nausea, vomiting, cramps, severe diarrhea with mucus or blood in stool, unusual weakness, tiredness, weight loss, fever, oral or vaginal candidiasis.	Discontinue. Call doctor right away.

WARNINGS & PRECAUTIONS

Don't take if:
You are allergic to any cephalosporin antibiotic.

Before you start, consult your doctor:
- If you are allergic to any penicillin antibiotic.
- If you have a kidney disorder.
- If you have colitis or enteritis.

Over age 60:
Adverse reactions and side effects may be more frequent and severe than in younger persons. More likely to itch around rectum and genitals.

Pregnancy:
No proven harm to unborn child. Avoid if possible.

Breast-feeding:
Drug passes into milk. Avoid drug or discontinue nursing until you finish medicine. Consult doctor for advice on maintaining milk supply.

Infants & children:
No special warnings.

Prolonged use:
Kills beneficial bacteria that protect body against other germs. Unchecked germs may cause secondary infections.

Skin & sunlight:
No problems expected.

Driving, piloting or hazardous work:
No problems expected.

Discontinuing:
Don't discontinue without doctor's advice until you complete prescribed dose, even though symptoms diminish or disappear.

Others:
No problems expected.

POSSIBLE INTERACTION WITH OTHER DRUGS

GENERIC NAME OR DRUG CLASS	COMBINED EFFECT
Anticoagulants*	Increased anticoagulant effect.
Erythromycin	Decreased antibiotic effect of cefadroxil.
Chloramphenicol	Decreased antibiotic effect of cefadroxil.
Clindamycin	Decreased antibiotic effect of cefadroxil.
Probenecid	Increased cefadroxil effect.
Tetracyclines*	Decreased antibiotic effect of cefadroxil.

POSSIBLE INTERACTION WITH OTHER SUBSTANCES

INTERACTS WITH	COMBINED EFFECT
Alcohol:	Increased kidney toxicity.
Beverages:	None expected.
Cocaine:	None expected, but cocaine may slow body's recovery. Avoid.
Foods:	Slow absorption. Take with liquid 1 hour before or 2 hours after eating.
Marijuana:	None expected, but marijuana may slow body's recovery. Avoid.
Tobacco:	None expected.

CEPHALEXIN

BRAND NAMES

Ceporex	Keflex
Keflet	Novolexin

BASIC INFORMATION

Habit forming? No
Prescription needed? Yes
Available as generic? Yes
Drug class: Antibiotic (cephalosporin)

USES

Treatment of bacterial infections. Will not cure viral infections such as cold and flu.

DOSAGE & USAGE INFORMATION

How to take:
- Capsule—Swallow with liquid. If you can't swallow whole, open capsule and take with liquid or food.
- Liquid—Use measuring spoon.

When to take:
- At same times each day, 1 hour before or 2 hours after eating.
- Take until gone or as directed.

If you forget a dose:
Take as soon as you remember or double next dose. Return to regular schedule.

What drug does:
Kills susceptible bacteria.

Time lapse before drug works:
May require several days to affect infection.

Don't take with:
See Interaction column and consult doctor.

OVERDOSE

SYMPTOMS:
Abdominal cramps, nausea, vomiting, severe diarrhea with mucus or blood in stool.
WHAT TO DO:
Overdose unlikely to threaten life. If person takes much larger amount than prescribed, call doctor, poison-control center or hospital emergency room for instructions.

POSSIBLE ADVERSE REACTIONS OR SIDE EFFECTS

SYMPTOMS	WHAT TO DO
Life-threatening:	
Hives, rash, intense itching, faintness soon after a dose (anaphylaxis); difficulty breathing.	Seek emergency treatment immediately.
Common:	
Rash, redness, itching.	Discontinue. Call doctor right away.
Infrequent:	
Rectal itching.	Continue. Call doctor when convenient.
Rare:	
Mild nausea, vomiting, cramps, severe diarrhea with mucus or blood in stool, unusual weakness, tiredness, weight loss, fever, oral or vaginal candidiasis.	Discontinue. Call doctor right away.

WARNINGS & PRECAUTIONS

Don't take if:
You are allergic to any cephalosporin antibiotic.

Before you start, consult your doctor:
• If you are allergic to any penicillin antibiotic.
• If you have a kidney disorder.
• If you have colitis or enteritis.

Over age 60:
Adverse reactions and side effects may be more frequent and severe than in younger persons. More likely to itch around rectum and genitals.

Pregnancy:
No proven harm to unborn child. Avoid if possible.

Breast-feeding:
Drug passes into milk. Avoid drug or discontinue nursing until you finish medicine. Consult doctor for advice on maintaining milk supply.

Infants & children:
No special warnings.

Prolonged use:
Kills beneficial bacteria that protect body against other germs. Unchecked germs may cause secondary infections.

Skin & sunlight:
No problems expected.

Driving, piloting or hazardous work:
No problems expected.

Discontinuing:
Don't discontinue without doctor's advice until you complete prescribed dose, even though symptoms diminish or disappear.

Others:
No problems expected.

POSSIBLE INTERACTION WITH OTHER DRUGS

GENERIC NAME OR DRUG CLASS	COMBINED EFFECT
Anticoagulants*	Increased anticoagulant effect.
Erythromycin	Decreased antibiotic effect of cephalexin.
Chloramphenicol	Decreased antibiotic effect of cephalexin.
Clindamycin	Decreased antibiotic effect of cephalexin.
Probenecid	Increased cephalexin effect.
Tetracyclines*	Decreased antibiotic effect of cephalexin.

POSSIBLE INTERACTION WITH OTHER SUBSTANCES

INTERACTS WITH	COMBINED EFFECT
Alcohol:	Increased kidney toxicity.
Beverages:	None expected.
Cocaine:	None expected, but cocaine may slow body's recovery. Avoid.
Foods:	Slow absorption. Take with liquid 1 hour before or 2 hours after eating.
Marijuana:	None expected, but marijuana may slow body's recovery. Avoid.
Tobacco:	None expected.

CEPHRADINE

BRAND NAMES

Anspor   Velosef

BASIC INFORMATION

Habit forming? No
Prescription needed? Yes
Available as generic? Yes
Drug class: Antibiotic (cephalosporin)

 USES

Treatment of bacterial infections. Will not cure
viral infections such as cold and flu.

 DOSAGE & USAGE INFORMATION

How to take:
• Capsule—Swallow with liquid. If you can't
  swallow whole, open capsule and take with
  liquid or food.
• Liquid—Use measuring spoon.

When to take:
• At same times each day, 1 hour before or 2
  hours after eating.
• Take until gone or as directed.

If you forget a dose:
Take as soon as you remember or double next
dose. Return to regular schedule.

What drug does:
Kills susceptible bacteria.

Time lapse before drug works:
May require several days to affect infection.

Don't take with:
See Interaction column and consult doctor.

 OVERDOSE

SYMPTOMS:
Abdominal cramps, nausea, vomiting,
severe diarrhea with mucus or blood in
stool.
WHAT TO DO:
Overdose unlikely to threaten life. If person
takes much larger amount than prescribed,
call doctor, poison-control center or hospital
emergency room for instructions.

 POSSIBLE ADVERSE REACTIONS OR SIDE EFFECTS

SYMPTOMS	WHAT TO DO
Life-threatening: Hives, rash, intense itching, faintness soon after a dose (anaphylaxis); difficulty breathing.	Seek emergency treatment immediately.
Common: Rash, redness, itching.	Discontinue. Call doctor right away.
Infrequent: Rectal itching.	Continue. Call doctor when convenient.
Rare: Mild nausea, vomiting, cramps, severe diarrhea with mucus or blood in stool, unusual weakness, tiredness, weight loss, fever, oral or vaginal candidiasis.	Discontinue. Call doctor right away.

WARNINGS & PRECAUTIONS

Don't take if:
You are allergic to any cephalosporin antibiotic.

Before you start, consult your doctor:
• If you are allergic to any penicillin antibiotic.
• If you have a kidney disorder.
• If you have colitis or enteritis.

Over age 60:
Adverse reactions and side effects may be more frequent and severe than in younger persons. More likely to itch around rectum and genitals.

Pregnancy:
No proven harm to unborn child. Avoid if possible.

Breast-feeding:
Drug passes into milk. Avoid drug or discontinue nursing until you finish medicine. Consult doctor for advice on maintaining milk supply.

Infants & children:
No special warnings.

Prolonged use:
Kills beneficial bacteria that protect body against other germs. Unchecked germs may cause secondary infections.

Skin & sunlight:
No problems expected.

Driving, piloting or hazardous work:
No problems expected.

Discontinuing:
Don't discontinue without doctor's advice until you complete prescribed dose, even though symptoms diminish or disappear.

Others:
No problems expected.

POSSIBLE INTERACTION WITH OTHER DRUGS

GENERIC NAME OR DRUG CLASS	COMBINED EFFECT
Anticoagulants*	Increased anticoagulant effect.
Erythromycin	Decreased antibiotic effect of cephradine.
Chloramphenicol	Decreased antibiotic effect of cephradine.
Clindamycin	Decreased antibiotic effect of cephradine.
Probenecid	Increased cephradine effect.
Tetracyclines*	Decreased antibiotic effect of cephradine.

POSSIBLE INTERACTION WITH OTHER SUBSTANCES

INTERACTS WITH	COMBINED EFFECT
Alcohol:	Increased kidney toxicity.
Beverages:	None expected.
Cocaine:	None expected, but cocaine may slow body's recovery. Avoid.
Foods:	Slow absorption. Take with liquid 1 hour before or 2 hours after eating.
Marijuana:	None expected, but marijuana may slow body's recovery. Avoid.
Tobacco:	None expected.

*See Glossary

CHARCOAL, ACTIVATED

BRAND NAMES

Acta-Char
Acta-Char Liquid
Actidose-Aqua
Aqueous Charcodote
Arm-a-Char
Charcoaid

Charcoalanti Dote
Charcocaps
Charcodote
Insta-Char
Liquid-Antidose

BASIC INFORMATION

Habit forming? No
Prescription needed? No
Available as generic? Yes
Drug class: Antidote (adsorbent)

 USES

- Treatment of poisonings from medication.
- Treatment (infrequent) for diarrhea or excessive gaseousness.

 DOSAGE & USAGE INFORMATION

How to take:
- Tablet or capsule—Swallow with liquid. If you can't swallow whole, crumble tablet or open capsule and take with liquid or food.
- Liquid—Take as directed on label.

When to take:
- For poisoning—Take immediately after poisoning. If your doctor or emergency poison control center has also recommended syrup of ipecac, don't take charcoal for 30 minutes or until vomiting from ipecac stops.
- For diarrhea or gas—Take at same times each day.
- Take one or more hours after taking other medicines.

If you forget a dose:
- For poisonings—Not applicable.
- For diarrhea or gas—Take as soon as you remember up to 2 hours late. If more than 2 hours, wait for next scheduled dose (don't double this dose).

Continued next column

 OVERDOSE

SYMPTOMS:
None expected.
WHAT TO DO:
Overdose unlikely to threaten life. If person takes much larger amount than prescribed, call doctor, poison-control center or hospital emergency room for instructions.

What drug does:
- Helps prevent poison from being absorbed from stomach and intestines.
- Helps absorb gas in intestinal tract.

Time lapse before drug works:
Begins immediately.

Don't take with:
Ice cream or sherbet.

 POSSIBLE ADVERSE REACTIONS OR SIDE EFFECTS

SYMPTOMS	WHAT TO DO
Life-threatening: None expected.	
Always: Black bowel movements.	No action necessary.
Infrequent: None expected.	
Rare: Unless taken with cathartic, can cause constipation when taken for overdose.	Take a laxative after crisis is over.

WARNINGS & PRECAUTIONS

Don't take if:
The poison was lye or other strong alkali, strong acids (such as sulfuric acid), cyanide, iron, ethyl alcohol or methyl alcohol. Charcoal will not prevent these poisons from causing ill effects.

Before you start, consult your doctor:
If you are taking it as an antidote for poison.

Over age 60:
No problems expected.

Pregnancy:
No problems expected.

Breast-feeding:
No problems expected.

Infants & children:
Don't give to children for more than 3 or 4 days for diarrhea. Continuing for longer periods can interfere with normal nutrition.

Prolonged use:
No problems expected.

Skin & sunlight:
No problems expected.

Driving, piloting or hazardous work:
No problems expected.

Discontinuing:
No problems expected.

Others:
No problems expected.

POSSIBLE INTERACTION WITH OTHER DRUGS

GENERIC NAME OR DRUG CLASS	COMBINED EFFECT
Any medicine taken at the same time	May decrease absorption of medicine.

POSSIBLE INTERACTION WITH OTHER SUBSTANCES

INTERACTS WITH	COMBINED EFFECT
Alcohol:	None expected.
Beverages:	None expected.
Cocaine:	None expected.
Foods: Ice cream or sherbet.	Decreased charcoal effect.
Marijuana:	None expected.
Tobacco:	None expected.

CHLOPHEDIANOL

BRAND NAMES

Ulo   Ulone

BASIC INFORMATION

Habit forming? No
Prescription needed? Yes
Available as generic? No
Drug class: Cough suppressant

 ## USES

Reduces non-productive cough due to bronchial irritation.

 ## DOSAGE & USAGE INFORMATION

How to take:
Take syrup without diluting. Don't drink fluids immediately after medicine.

When to take:
3 or 4 times a day when needed. No more often than every 3 hours.

If you forget a dose:
Take as soon as you remember up to 2 hours late. If more than 2 hours, wait for next scheduled dose (don't double this dose).

What drug does:
Reduces cough reflex by direct effect on cough center in brain, and by local anesthetic action.

Time lapse before drug works:
30 minutes to 1 hour.

Don't take with:
- Alcohol or brain depressant or stimulant drugs.
- See Interaction column and consult doctor.

 ## OVERDOSE

SYMPTOMS:
Blurred vision, hallucinations, coma.
WHAT TO DO:
- Dial 0 (operator) or 911 (emergency) for an ambulance or medical help. Then give first aid immediately.
- If patient is unconscious and not breathing, give mouth-to-mouth breathing. If there is no heartbeat, use cardiac massage and mouth-to-mouth breathing (CPR). Don't try to make patient vomit. If you can't get help quickly, take patient to nearest emergency facility.
- See emergency information on inside covers.

 ## POSSIBLE ADVERSE REACTIONS OR SIDE EFFECTS

SYMPTOMS	WHAT TO DO
Life-threatening None expected.	
Common: Difficult urination in older men with enlarged prostate.	Continue. Call doctor when convenient.
Infrequent: None expected.	
Rare:	
• Hallucinations, drowsiness, rash or hives, nausea, vomiting, irregular heartbeat.	Discontinue. Call doctor right away.
• Nightmares, excitement or irritability, blurred vision, dry mouth.	Continue. Call doctor when convenient.

WARNINGS & PRECAUTIONS

Don't take if:
You are allergic to chlophedianol.

Before you start, consult your doctor:
- If medicine is for hyperactive child who takes medicine for treatment.
- If your cough brings up sputum (phlegm).
- If you have heart disease.
- If you will have surgery within 2 months, including dental surgery, requiring general or spinal anesthesia.

Over age 60:
Adverse reactions and side effects may be more frequent and severe than in younger persons.

Pregnancy:
Risk to unborn child outweighs drug benefits. Don't use.

Breast-feeding:
Unknown whether medicine filters into milk. Consult doctor.

Infants & children:
Not recommended for children under age 2.

Prolonged use:
Not recommended. If cough persists despite medicine, consult doctor.

Skin & sunlight:
No problems expected.

Driving, piloting or hazardous work:
Don't drive or pilot aircraft until you learn how medicine affects you. Don't work around dangerous machinery. Don't climb ladders or work in high places. Danger increases if you drink alcohol or take medicine affecting alertness and reflexes, such as antihistamines, tranquilizers, sedatives, pain medicine, narcotics and mind-altering drugs.

Discontinuing:
May be unnecessary to finish medicine. Follow doctor's instructions.

Others:
Consult doctor if cough persists despite medication for 7 days or if fever, skin rash or headache accompany cough.

POSSIBLE INTERACTION WITH OTHER DRUGS

GENERIC NAME OR DRUG CLASS	COMBINED EFFECT
Anticonvulsants*	Interferes with actions of both.
Antidepressants, tricyclic (TCA)*	Excess sedation.
Appetite suppressants*	Excess stimulation.
Central nervous system depressants* (antidepressants,* antihistamines,* muscle relaxants,* narcotics,* pain pills, sedatives,* sleeping pills, tranquilizers*)	Excess sedation.
MAO inhibitors*	Excess sedation.
Sympathomimetics*	Excess stimulation.

POSSIBLE INTERACTION WITH OTHER SUBSTANCES

INTERACTS WITH	COMBINED EFFECT
Alcohol:	Excess sedation. Avoid.
Beverages: Coffee, tea, cocoa, cola.	Excess stimulation. Avoid.
Cocaine:	Increased chance of toxic stimulation. Avoid.
Foods:	None expected.
Marijuana:	Increased chance of toxic stimulation. Avoid.
Tobacco:	Decreased effect of chlophedianol.

*See Glossary

CHLORAL HYDRATE

BRAND NAMES

Aquachloral
Aquachloral
  Supprettes
Colidrate

Noctec
Novochlorhydrate
Oradrate
SK-Chloral Hydrate

BASIC INFORMATION

Habit forming? Yes
Prescription needed? Yes
Available as generic? Yes
Drug class: Hypnotic

USES

* Reduces anxiety.
* Relieves insomnia.

DOSAGE & USAGE INFORMATION

How to take:
* Syrup or capsule—Swallow with milk or food to lessen stomach irritation.
* Suppositories—Remove wrapper and moisten suppository with water. Gently insert larger end into rectum. Push well into rectum with finger.

When to take:
At the same time each day.

If you forget a dose:
Take as soon as you remember up to 2 hours late. If more than 2 hours, wait for next scheduled dose (don't double this dose).

Continued next column

OVERDOSE

SYMPTOMS:
Confusion, weakness, breathing difficulty, throat irritation, jaundice, stagger, slow or irregular heartbeat, unconsciousness, coma.
WHAT TO DO:
* Dial 0 (operator) or 911 (emergency) for an ambulance or medical help. Then give first aid immediately.
* If patient is unconscious and not breathing, give mouth-to-mouth breathing. If there is no heartbeat, use cardiac massage and mouth-to-mouth breathing (CPR). Don't try to make patient vomit. If you can't get help quickly, take patient to nearest emergency facility.
* See emergency information on inside covers.

What drug does:
Affects brain centers that control wakefulness and alertness.

Time lapse before drug works:
30 to 60 minutes.

Don't take with:
See Interaction column and consult doctor.

POSSIBLE ADVERSE REACTIONS OR SIDE EFFECTS

SYMPTOMS	WHAT TO DO
Life-threatening: None expected.	
Common: Nausea, stomach pain, vomiting.	Discontinue. Call doctor right away.
Infrequent: "Hangover" effect, clumsiness or unsteadiness, drowsiness, dizziness, lightheadedness.	Continue. Call doctor when convenient.
Rare: • Hallucinations, agitation, confusion. leukopenia (white blood cells causing sore throat and fever).	Discontinue. Call doctor right away.
• Hives, rash.	Continue. Call doctor when convenient.

WARNINGS & PRECAUTIONS

Don't take if:
You are allergic to chloral hydrate.

Before you start, consult your doctor:
- If you have had liver, kidney or heart trouble.
- If you are prone to stomach upsets (if medicine is in oral form).
- If you are allergic to tartrazine dye.
- If you have colitis or a rectal inflammation (if medicine is in suppository form).

Over age 60:
Adverse reactions and side effects may be more frequent and severe than in younger persons. More likely to have "hangover" effect.

Pregnancy:
Risk to unborn child outweighs drug benefits. Unborn child may become addicted to drug. Don't use.

Breast-feeding:
Drug filters into milk. May harm child. Avoid.

Infants & children:
Use only under medical supervision.

Prolonged use:
Addiction and possible kidney damage.

Skin & sunlight:
No problems expected.

Driving, piloting or hazardous work:
Don't drive or pilot aircraft until you learn how medicine affects you. Don't work around dangerous machinery. Don't climb ladders or work in high places. Danger increases if you drink alcohol or take medicine affecting alertness and reflexes, such as antihistamines, tranquilizers, sedatives, pain medicine, narcotics and mind-altering drugs.

Discontinuing:
Don't discontinue without consulting doctor. Dose may require gradual reduction if you have taken drug for a long time. Doses of other drugs may also require adjustment.

Others:
Frequent kidney-function tests recommended when drug is used for long time.

POSSIBLE INTERACTION WITH OTHER DRUGS

GENERIC NAME OR DRUG CLASS	COMBINED EFFECT
Anticoagulants, oral*	Possible hemorrhaging.
Antidepressants*	Increased chloral hydrate effect.
Antihistamines*	Increased chloral hydrate effect.
Ethinamate	Dangerous increased effects of ethinamate. Avoid combining.
Fluoxetine	Increased depressant effects of both drugs.
Guanfacine	May increase depressant effects of either drug.
Leucovorin	High alcohol content of leucovorin may cause adverse effects.
MAO inhibitors*	Increased chloral hydrate effect.
Methyprylon	Increased sedative effect, perhaps to dangerous level. Avoid.
Mind-altering drugs*	Increased chloral hydrate effect.
Molindone	Increased tranquilizer effect.
Nabilone	Greater depression of central nervous system.
Narcotics*	Increased chloral hydrate effect.
Pain relievers*	Increased chloral hydrate effect.
Phenothiazines*	Increased chloral hydrate effect.
Sedatives*	Increased chloral hydrate effect.
Sleep inducers*	Increased chloral hydrate effect.
Tranquilizers*	Increased chloral hydrate effect.

POSSIBLE INTERACTION WITH OTHER SUBSTANCES

INTERACTS WITH	COMBINED EFFECT
Alcohol:	Increased sedative effect of both. Avoid.
Beverages:	None expected.
Cocaine:	Decreased chloral hydrate effect. Avoid.
Foods:	None expected.
Marijuana:	May severely impair mental and physical functioning. Avoid.
Tobacco:	None expected.

*See Glossary

CHLORAMBUCIL

BRAND NAMES

Leukeran

BASIC INFORMATION

Habit forming? No
Prescription needed? Yes
Available as generic? No
Drug class: Antineoplastic,
  immunosuppressant

 USES

- Treatment for some kinds of cancer.
- Suppresses immune response after transplant and in immune disorders.

 DOSAGE & USAGE INFORMATION

How to take:
Tablet—Swallow with liquid after light meal. Don't drink fluids with meals. Drink extra fluids between meals. Avoid sweet or fatty foods.

When to take:
At the same time each day.

If you forget a dose:
Take as soon as you remember. Don't ever double dose.

What drug does:
Inhibits abnormal cell reproduction. May suppress immune system.

Time lapse before drug works:
Up to 6 weeks for full effect.

Don't take with:
See Interaction column and consult doctor.

 OVERDOSE

SYMPTOMS:
Bleeding, chills, fever, vomiting, abdominal pain, ataxia, collapse, stupor, seizure.
WHAT TO DO:
- Dial 0 (operator) or 911 (emergency) for an ambulance or medical help. Then give first aid immediately.
- If patient is unconscious and not breathing, give mouth-to-mouth breathing. If there is no heartbeat, use cardiac massage and mouth-to-mouth breathing (CPR). Don't try to make patient vomit. If you can't get help quickly, take patient to nearest emergency facility.
- See emergency information on inside covers.

 POSSIBLE ADVERSE REACTIONS OR SIDE EFFECTS

SYMPTOMS	WHAT TO DO
Life-threatening: None expected.	
Common:	
• Unusual bleeding or bruising, mouth sores with sore throat, chills and fever, black stools, mouth and lip sores, menstrual irregularities.	Discontinue. Call doctor right away.
• Hair loss, joint pain.	Continue. Call doctor when convenient.
• Nausea, vomiting, diarrhea (unavoidable), tiredness, weakness.	Continue. Tell doctor at next visit.
Infrequent:	
• Mental confusion, shortness of breath; may increase chance of developing leukemia.	Continue. Call doctor when convenient.
• Cough.	Continue. Tell doctor at next visit.
Rare:	
Jaundice.	Discontinue. Call doctor right away.

WARNINGS & PRECAUTIONS

Don't take if:
- You have had hypersensitivity to alkylating antineoplastic drugs.
- Your physician has not explained serious nature of your medical problem and risks of taking this medicine.

Before you start, consult your doctor:
- If you have gout.
- If you have had kidney stones.
- If you have active infection.
- If you have impaired kidney or liver function.
- If you have taken other antineoplastic drugs or had radiation treatment in last 3 weeks.

Over age 60:
Adverse reactions and side effects may be more frequent and severe than in younger persons.

Pregnancy:
Consult doctor. Risk to child is significant.

Breast-feeding:
Drug passes into milk. Don't nurse.

Infants & children:
Use only under care of medical supervisors who are experienced in anticancer drugs.

Prolonged use:
Adverse reactions more likely the longer drug is required.

Skin & sunlight:
No problems expected.

Driving, piloting or hazardous work:
No problems expected.

Discontinuing:
Don't discontinue without doctor's advice until you complete prescribed dose, even though symptoms diminish or disappear. Some side effects may follow discontinuing. Report to doctor blurred vision, convulsions, confusion, persistent headache.

Others:
May cause sterility.

POSSIBLE INTERACTION WITH OTHER DRUGS

GENERIC NAME OR DRUG CLASS	COMBINED EFFECT
Antigout drugs*	Decreased antigout effect.
Antineoplastic drugs, other*	Increased effect of all drugs (may be beneficial).
Chloramphenicol	Increased likelihood of toxic effects of both drugs.
Cyclosporine	May increase risk of infection.
Lovastatin	Increased heart and kidney damage.

POSSIBLE INTERACTION WITH OTHER SUBSTANCES

INTERACTS WITH	COMBINED EFFECT
Alcohol:	May increase chance of intestinal bleeding.
Beverages:	No problems expected.
Cocaine:	Increases chance of toxicity.
Foods:	Reduces irritation in stomach.
Marijuana:	No problems expected.
Tobacco:	Increases lung toxicity.

*See Glossary

CHLORAMPHENICOL

BRAND NAMES

Amphicol	Mychel
Antibiopto	Mychel-S
Chloromycetin	Nova-Phenicol
Chloroptic	Novochlorocap
Econochlor	Ophthochlor
Fenicol	Ophthocort
Isopto Fenicol	Pentamycetin
Minims	Sopamycetin

BASIC INFORMATION

Habit forming? No
Prescription needed? Yes
Available as generic? Yes
Drug class: Antibiotic

USES

Treatment of infections susceptible to chloramphenicol.

DOSAGE & USAGE INFORMATION

How to take:
- Suspension or capsule—Swallow with liquid.
- Eye or ear solution or cream—Follow label instructions.

When to take:
Capsule—1 hour before or 2 hours after eating.

If you forget a dose:
Take as soon as you remember up to 2 hours late. If more than 2 hours, wait for next scheduled dose (don't double this dose).

What drug does:
Prevents bacteria from growing and reproducing. Will not kill viruses.

Time lapse before drug works:
2 to 5 days, depending on type and severity of infection.

Don't take with:
See Interaction column and consult doctor.

OVERDOSE

SYMPTOMS:
Nausea, vomiting, diarrhea.
WHAT TO DO:
Overdose unlikely to threaten life. If person takes much larger amount than prescribed, call doctor, poison-control center or hospital emergency room for instructions.

POSSIBLE ADVERSE REACTIONS OR SIDE EFFECTS

SYMPTOMS	WHAT TO DO
Life-threatening: Hives, rash, intense itching, faintness soon after a dose (anaphylaxis).	Seek emergency treatment immediately.
Common: None expected.	
Infrequent: • Swollen face or extremities; diarrhea; nausea; vomiting; numbness, tingling, burning pain or weakness in hands and feet.	Discontinue. Call doctor right away.
• Headache, confusion.	Continue. Call doctor when convenient.
Rare: Pain, blurred vision, possible vision loss, sore throat, fever, jaundice, anemia.	Discontinue. Call doctor right away.

WARNINGS & PRECAUTIONS

Don't take if:
- You are allergic to chloramphenicol.
- It is prescribed for a minor disorder such as flu, cold or mild sore throat.

Before you start, consult your doctor:
- If you have had a blood disorder or bone-marrow disease.
- If you have had kidney or liver disease.
- If you have diabetes.

Over age 60:
Adverse reactions and side effects may be more frequent and severe than in younger persons, particularly skin irritation around rectum.

Pregnancy:
Risk to unborn child outweighs drug benefits. Don't use.

Breast-feeding:
Drug passes into milk. Avoid drug or discontinue nursing until you finish medicine. Consult doctor for advice on maintaining milk supply.

Infants & children:
Don't give to infants younger than 2.

Prolonged use:
You may become more susceptible to infections caused by germs not responsive to chloramphenicol.

Skin & sunlight:
No problems expected.

Driving, piloting or hazardous work:
Don't drive or pilot aircraft until you learn how medicine affects you. Don't work around dangerous machinery. Don't climb ladders or work in high places. Danger increases if you drink alcohol or take medicine affecting alertness and reflexes.

Discontinuing:
Don't discontinue without doctor's advice until you complete prescribed dose, even though symptoms diminish or disappear.

Others:
- Chloramphenicol can cause serious anemia. Frequent laboratory blood studies, liver and kidney tests recommended.
- Second medical opinion recommended before starting.

POSSIBLE INTERACTION WITH OTHER DRUGS

GENERIC NAME OR DRUG CLASS	COMBINED EFFECT
Anticoagulants*	Increased anticoagulant effect.
Antidiabetics, oral*	Increased antidiabetic effect.
Cephalosporins*	Decreased penicillin effect.
Cyclophosphamide	Increased cyclophosphamide effect.
Flecainide	Possible decreased blood-cell production in bone marrow.
Lisinopril	Possible blood disorders.
Penicillins*	Decreased penicillin effect.
Phenobarbital	Increased phenobarbital effect.
Phenytoin	Increased phenytoin effect.
Rifampin	Decreased chloramphenicol effect.
Tocainide	Possible decreased blood-cell production in bone marrow.

POSSIBLE INTERACTION WITH OTHER SUBSTANCES

INTERACTS WITH	COMBINED EFFECT
Alcohol:	Possible liver problems. May cause disulfiram reaction.*
Beverages:	None expected.
Cocaine:	No proven problems.
Foods:	None expected.
Marijuana:	None expected.
Tobacco:	None expected.

*See Glossary

CHLORDIAZEPOXIDE

BRAND AND GENERIC NAMES

Apo-Chlordiazepoxide	Murcil
CHLORDIAZEPOXIDE	Novopoxide
Libritabs	Reposans
Librium	Sereen
Lipoxide	SK-Lygen
Medilium	Solium

BASIC INFORMATION

Habit forming? Yes
Prescription needed? Yes
Available as generic? Yes
Drug class: Tranquilizer (benzodiazepine)

USES

- Treatment for nervousness or tension.
- Treatment for muscle spasm.
- Treatment for convulsive disorders.

DOSAGE & USAGE INFORMATION

How to take:
Tablet or capsule—Swallow with liquid. If you can't swallow whole, crumble tablet or open capsule and take with liquid or food.

When to take:
At the same time each day, according to instructions on prescription label.

If you forget a dose:
Take as soon as you remember up to 2 hours late. If more than 2 hours, wait for next scheduled dose (don't double this dose).

Continued next column

OVERDOSE

SYMPTOMS:
Drowsiness, weakness, tremor, stupor, coma.
WHAT TO DO:
- Dial 0 (operator) or 911 (emergency) for an ambulance or medical help. Then give first aid immediately.
- If patient is unconscious and not breathing, give mouth-to-mouth breathing. If there is no heartbeat, use cardiac massage and mouth-to-mouth breathing (CPR). Don't try to make patient vomit. If you can't get help quickly, take patient to nearest emergency facility.
- See emergency information on inside covers.

What drug does:
Affects limbic system of brain—part that controls emotions.

Time lapse before drug works:
2 hours. May take 6 weeks for full benefit.

Don't take with:
See Interaction column and consult doctor.

POSSIBLE ADVERSE REACTIONS OR SIDE EFFECTS

SYMPTOMS	WHAT TO DO
Life-threatening: None expected.	
Common: Clumsiness, drowsiness, dizziness.	Continue. Call doctor when convenient.
Infrequent: • Hallucinations, confusion, irritability, depression, rash, itch, vision changes.	Discontinue. Call doctor right away.
• Constipation or diarrhea, nausea, vomiting, difficult urination, vivid dreams.	Continue. Call doctor when convenient.
Rare: • Slow heartbeat, breathing difficulty.	Discontinue. Seek emergency treatment.
• Mouth, throat ulcers; jaundice.	Discontinue. Call doctor right away.
• Decreased libido.	Continue. Call doctor when convenient.

CHLORDIAZEPOXIDE

WARNINGS & PRECAUTIONS

Don't take if:
- You are allergic to any benzodiazepine.
- You have myasthenia gravis.
- You are active or recovering alcoholic.
- Patient is younger than 6 months.

Before you start, consult your doctor:
- If you have liver, kidney or lung disease.
- If you have diabetes, epilepsy or porphyria.

Over age 60:
Adverse reactions and side effects may be more frequent and severe than in younger persons. You need smaller doses for shorter periods of time. May develop agitation, rage or 'hangover' effect.

Pregnancy:
Risk to unborn child outweighs drug benefits. Don't use.

Breast-feeding:
Drug passes into milk. Avoid drug or discontinue nursing until you finish medicine. Consult doctor for advice on maintaining milk supply.

Infants & children:
Use only under medical supervision for children older than 6 months.

Prolonged use:
May impair liver function.

Skin & sunlight:
No problems expected.

Driving, piloting or hazardous work:
Don't drive or pilot aircraft until you learn how medicine affects you. Don't work around dangerous machinery. Don't climb ladders or work in high places. Danger increases if you drink alcohol or take medicine affecting alertness and reflexes.

Discontinuing:
Don't discontinue without consulting doctor. Dose may require gradual reduction if you have taken drug for a long time. Doses of other drugs may also require adjustment.

Others:
- Hot weather, heavy exercise and profuse sweat may reduce excretion and cause overdose.
- Blood sugar may rise in diabetics, requiring insulin adjustment.

POSSIBLE INTERACTION WITH OTHER DRUGS

GENERIC NAME OR DRUG CLASS	COMBINED EFFECT
Antidepressants*	Increased sedative effect of both drugs.
Antihistamines*	Increased sedative effect of both drugs.
Antihypertensives*	Excessively low blood pressure.
Contraceptives, oral*	Increased chlordiazepoxide effect.
Disulfiram	Increased chlordiazepoxide effect.
Dronabinol	Increased effects of both drugs. Avoid.
Erythromycin	Increased chlordiazepoxide effect.
Ketoconazole	Increased chlordiazepoxide effect.
Levodopa	Possible decreased levodopa effect.
MAO inhibitors*	Convulsions, deep sedation, rage.
Molindone	Increased tranquilizer effect.
Nabilone	Greater depression of the central nervous system.
Narcotics*	Increased sedative effect of both drugs.
Nizatidine	Increased effect and toxicity of chlordiazepoxide.
Probenecid	Increased chlordiazepoxide effect.
Sedatives*	Increased sedative effect of both drugs.
Sleep inducers*	Increased sedative effect of both drugs.
Tranquilizers*	Increased sedative effect of both drugs.

POSSIBLE INTERACTION WITH OTHER SUBSTANCES

INTERACTS WITH	COMBINED EFFECT
Alcohol:	Heavy sedation. Avoid.
Beverages:	None expected.
Cocaine:	Decreased chlordiazepoxide effect.
Foods:	None expected.
Marijuana:	Heavy sedation. Avoid.
Tobacco:	Decreased chlordiazepoxide effect.

*See Glossary

CHLORDIAZEPOXIDE & AMITRIPTYLINE

BRAND NAMES

Limbitrol   Limbitrol DS

BASIC INFORMATION

Habit forming? Yes
Prescription needed? Yes
Available as generic? No
Drug class: Antidepressant, tranquilizer
(benzodiazepine)

 USES

- Treatment for nervousness or tension.
- Gradually relieves, but doesn't cure, symptoms of depression.

 DOSAGE & USAGE INFORMATION

How to take:
Tablet—Swallow with liquid. If you can't swallow whole, crumble tablet and take with liquid or food.

When to take:
At the same time each day, according to instructions on prescription label.

If you forget a dose:
Bedtime dose—If you forget your once-a-day bedtime dose, don't take it more than 3 hours late. If more than 3 hours, wait for next scheduled dose (don't double this dose).

What drug does:
Affects limbic system of brain—part that controls emotions.

Continued next column

 OVERDOSE

SYMPTOMS:
Drowsiness, weakness, tremor, hallucinations, convulsions, stupor, coma.
WHAT TO DO:
- **Dial 0 (operator) or 911 (emergency) for an ambulance or medical help. Then give first aid immediately.**
- **If patient is unconscious and not breathing, give mouth-to-mouth breathing. If there is no heartbeat, use cardiac massage and mouth-to-mouth breathing (CPR). Don't try to make patient vomit. If you can't get help quickly, take patient to nearest emergency facility.**
- **See emergency information on inside covers.**

Time lapse before drug works:
Begins in 1 to 2 weeks. May require 4 to 6 weeks for maximum benefit.

Don't take with:
- Non-prescription drugs without consulting doctor.
- See Interaction column and consult doctor.

 POSSIBLE ADVERSE REACTIONS OR SIDE EFFECTS

SYMPTOMS	WHAT TO DO
Life-threatening:	
Slow heartbeat, irregular breathing.	Seek emergency treatment immediately.
Common:	
• Clumsiness, drowsiness, dizziness, headache, insomnia, dry mouth or unpleasant taste, constipation, fatigue, weakness.	Continue. Call doctor when convenient.
• "Sweet tooth."	Continue. Tell doctor at next visit.
Infrequent:	
• Hallucinations, confusion, irritability, depression, rash, itch, vision changes, blurred vision, eye pain, jaundice.	Discontinue. Call doctor right away.
• Constipation, difficult urination, diarrhea, nausea, vomiting, vivid dreams, indigestion.	Continue. Call doctor when convenient.
Rare:	
• Mouth or throat ulcers, fever.	Discontinue. Call doctor right away.
• Decreased libido.	Continue. Call doctor when convenient.

 WARNINGS & PRECAUTIONS

Don't take if:
- You are allergic to any benzodiazepine or tricyclic antidepressant.
- You have myasthenia gravis, glaucoma, taken MAO inhibitors within 2 weeks, had a heart attack within 6 weeks.
- You are active or recovering alcoholic.
- Patient is younger than 12.

Before you start, consult your doctor:
- If you have liver, kidney or lung disease, diabetes, epilepsy, porphyria, enlarged prostate, heart disease, high blood pressure, stomach or intestinal problems, overactive thyroid, asthma.

CHLORDIAZEPOXIDE & AMITRIPTYLINE

- If you will have surgery within 2 months, including dental surgery, requiring general or spinal anesthesia.

Over age 60:
More likely to develop urination difficulty and more side effects.

Pregnancy:
Risk to unborn child outweighs drug benefits. Don't use.

Breast-feeding:
Drug passes into milk. Avoid drug or discontinue nursing until you finish medicine. Consult doctor for advice on maintaining milk supply.

Infants & children:
Use only under medical supervision for children older than 6 months.

Prolonged use:
May impair liver function.

Skin & sunlight:
May cause rash or intensify sunburn in areas exposed to sun or sunlamp.

Driving, piloting or hazardous work:
Don't drive or pilot aircraft until you learn how medicine affects you. Don't work around dangerous machinery. Don't climb ladders or work in high places. Danger increases if you drink alcohol or take medicine affecting alertness and reflexes, such as antihistamines, tranquilizers, sedatives, pain medicine, narcotics and mind-altering drugs.

Discontinuing:
Don't discontinue without consulting doctor. Dose may require gradual reduction if you have taken drug for a long time. Doses of other drugs may also require adjustment.

Others:
- Hot weather, heavy exercise and profuse sweat may reduce excretion and cause overdose.
- Blood sugar may rise in diabetics, requiring insulin adjustment.

 POSSIBLE INTERACTION WITH OTHER DRUGS

GENERIC NAME OR DRUG CLASS	COMBINED EFFECT
Anticoagulants, oral*	Increased anticoagulant effect.
Anticonvulsants*	Change in seizure frequency or severity.
Anticholinergics*	Increased anticholinergic effect.
Antidepressants*	Increased sedative effect of both drugs.
Antihistamines*	Increased sedative effect of both drugs.
Antihypertensives*	Excessively low blood pressure.
Barbiturates*	Decreased antidepressant effect.
Cimetidine	Excess sedation.
Clonidine	Decreased clonidine effect.
Contraceptives, oral*	Increased chlordiazepoxide effect.
Disulfiram	Increased chlordiazepoxide effect.
Diuretics*	Increased antidepressant effect.
Dronabinol	Increased effect of both drugs.
Erythromycin	Increased chlordiazepoxide effect.
Ethchlorvynol	Delirium.
Guanethidine	Decreased guanethidine effect.
Ketoconazole	Increased chlordiazepoxide effect.
Levodopa	Possible decreased levodopa effect.
MAO inhibitors*	Convulsions, deep sedation, rage.
Methyldopa	Decreased methyldopa effect.
Nabilone	Greater depression of central nervous system.

Continued page 1081

 POSSIBLE INTERACTION WITH OTHER SUBSTANCES

INTERACTS WITH	COMBINED EFFECT
Alcohol: Beverages or medicines with alcohol.	Excessive intoxication. Avoid.
Beverages:	None expected.
Cocaine:	Excessive intoxication. Avoid.
Foods:	None expected.
Marijuana:	Excessive drowsiness. Avoid.
Tobacco:	Decreased chlordiazepoxide effect.

*See Glossary

CHLORDIAZEPOXIDE & CLIDINIUM

BRAND NAMES

Apo-Chlorax	Corium
Clindex	Librax
Clinoxide	Lidox
Clipoxide	

BASIC INFORMATION

Habit forming? Yes
Prescription needed? Yes
Available as generic? No
Drug class: Tranquilizer (benzodiazepine), antispasmodic, anticholinergic

USES

- Reduces spasms of digestive system, bladder and urethra.
- Treatment for nervousness or tension.
- Treatment for muscle spasm.

DOSAGE & USAGE INFORMATION

How to take:
Capsule—Swallow with liquid. If you can't swallow whole, open capsule and take with liquid or food.

When to take:
At the same time each day, according to instructions on prescription label.

If you forget a dose:
Take as soon as you remember up to 2 hours late. If more than 2 hours, wait for next scheduled dose (don't double this dose).

Continued next column

OVERDOSE

SYMPTOMS:
Dilated pupils, rapid pulse and breathing, dizziness, drowsiness, weakness, tremor, stupor, fever, hallucinations, confusion, slurred speech, agitation, flushed face, convulsions, coma.
WHAT TO DO:
- **Dial 0 (operator) or 911 (emergency) for an ambulance or medical help. Then give first aid immediately.**
- **If patient is unconscious and not breathing, give mouth-to-mouth breathing. If there is no heartbeat, use cardiac massage and mouth-to-mouth breathing (CPR). Don't try to make patient vomit. If you can't get help quickly, take patient to nearest emergency facility.**
- **See emergency information on inside covers.**

What drug does:
- Blocks nerve impulses at parasympathetic nerve endings, preventing muscle contractions and gland secretions of organs involved.
- Affects limbic system of brain—part that controls emotions.

Time lapse before drug works:
15 to 30 minutes.

Don't take with:
See Interaction column and consult doctor.

POSSIBLE ADVERSE REACTIONS OR SIDE EFFECTS

SYMPTOMS	WHAT TO DO
Life-threatening:	
Slow or rapid heartbeat, breathing difficulty.	Discontinue. Seek emergency treatment.
Common:	
• Clumsiness, drowsiness, dizziness, delirium.	Discontinue. Call doctor right away.
• Dry mouth, throat, nose.	Continue. Tell doctor at next visit.
Infrequent:	
• Hallucinations, confusion, irritability, depression, rash, itch, vision changes, vomiting.	Discontinue. Call doctor right away.
• Constipation, diarrhea, nausea, urination difficulty, vivid dreams, impotence.	Continue. Call doctor when convenient.
Rare:	
• Jaundice, rash or hives, eye pain, blurred vision.	Discontinue. Call doctor right away.
• Decreased libido.	Continue. Call doctor when convenient.

WARNINGS & PRECAUTIONS

Don't take if:
- You are allergic to any anticholinergic or any benzodiazepine.
- You have trouble with stomach bloating, difficulty emptying your bladder completely, narrow-angle glaucoma, severe ulcerative colitis, myasthenia gravis.
- You are active or recovering alcoholic.
- Patient is younger than 6 months.

Before you start, consult your doctor:
- If you have open-angle glaucoma, angina, chronic bronchitis or asthma, hiatal hernia, enlarged prostate, myasthenia gravis, peptic ulcer, liver, kidney or lung disease, diabetes, epilepsy or porphyria.

- If you will have surgery within 2 months, including dental surgery, requiring general or spinal anesthesia.

Over age 60:
Adverse reactions and side effects may be more frequent and severe than in younger persons.

Pregnancy:
Risk to unborn child outweighs drug benefits. Don't use.

Breast-feeding:
Drug passes into milk. Avoid drug or discontinue nursing until you finish medicine. Consult doctor for advice on maintaining milk supply.

Infants & children:
Use only under medical supervision.

Prolonged use:
- Chronic constipation, possible fecal impaction.
- May impair liver function.

Skin & sunlight:
No problems expected.

Driving, piloting or hazardous work:
Don't drive or pilot aircraft until you learn how medicine affects you. Don't work around dangerous machinery. Don't climb ladders or work in high places. Danger increases if you drink alcohol or take medicine affecting alertness and reflexes, such as antihistamines, tranquilizers, sedatives, pain medicine, narcotics and mind-altering drugs.

Discontinuing:
Don't discontinue without consulting doctor. Dose may require gradual reduction if you have taken drug for a long time. Doses of other drugs may also require adjustment.

Others:
- Hot weather, heavy exercise and profuse sweat may reduce excretion and cause overdose.
- Blood sugar may rise in diabetics, requiring insulin adjustment.

POSSIBLE INTERACTION WITH OTHER DRUGS

GENERIC NAME OR DRUG CLASS	COMBINED EFFECT
Amantadine	Increased clidinium effect.
Antacids*	Decreased clidinium effect.
Anticholinergics, other*	Increased clidinium effect.
Antidepressants*	Increased sedative effect of both drugs.
Antihistamines*	Increased sedative effect of both drugs.
Antihypertensives*	Excessively low blood pressure.
Contraceptives, oral*	Increased chlordiazepoxide effect.
Disulfiram	Increased chlordiazepoxide effect.
Dronabinol	Increased effects of both drugs. Avoid.
Erythromycin	Increased chlordiazepoxide effect.
Haloperidol	Increased internal-eye pressure.
Ketoconazole	Increased chlordiazepoxide effect.
Levodopa	Possible decreased levodopa effect.
MAO inhibitors*	Convulsions, deep sedation, rage.
Meperidine	Increased clidinium effect.
Methylphenidate	Increased clidinium effect.
Nabilone	Greater depression of central nervous system.
Narcotics*	Increased sedative effect of both drugs.
Nitrates*	Increased internal-eye pressure.
Nizatidine	Increased nizatidine effect.
Orphenadrine	Increased clidinium effect.

Continued page 1081

POSSIBLE INTERACTION WITH OTHER SUBSTANCES

INTERACTS WITH	COMBINED EFFECT
Alcohol:	Heavy sedation. Avoid.
Beverages:	None expected.
Cocaine:	Excessively rapid heartbeat. Avoid.
Foods:	None expected.
Marijuana:	Drowsiness and dry mouth, heavy sedation. Avoid.
Tobacco:	Decreased chlordiazepoxide effect.

*See Glossary

CHLOROQUINE

BRAND NAMES

Aralen

BASIC INFORMATION

Habit forming? No
Prescription needed? Yes
Available as generic? Yes
Drug class: Antiprotozoal, antirheumatic

USES

- Treatment for protozoal infections, such as malaria and amebiasis.
- Treatment for some forms of arthritis and lupus.

DOSAGE & USAGE INFORMATION

How to take:
Tablet—Swallow with food or milk to lessen stomach irritation.

When to take:
- Depends on condition. Is adjusted during treatment.
- Malaria prevention—Begin taking medicine 2 weeks before entering areas with malaria.

If you forget a dose:
- 1 or more doses a day—Take as soon as you remember up to 2 hours late. If more than 2 hours, wait for next scheduled dose (don't double this dose).
- 1 dose weekly—Take as soon as possible, then return to regular dosing schedule.

What drug does:
- Inhibits parasite multiplication.
- Decreases inflammatory response in diseased joint.

Time lapse before drug works:
1 to 2 hours.

Don't take with:
See Interaction column and consult doctor.

OVERDOSE

SYMPTOMS:
Severe breathing difficulty, drowsiness, faintness, headache, seizures.
WHAT TO DO:
- **Dial 0 (operator) or 911 (emergency) for an ambulance or medical help. Then give first aid immediately.**
- **See emergency information on inside covers.**

POSSIBLE ADVERSE REACTIONS OR SIDE EFFECTS

SYMPTOMS	WHAT TO DO
Life-threatening: None expected.	
Common: Headache.	Continue. Tell doctor at next visit.
Infrequent:	
• Blurred or changed vision.	Discontinue. Call doctor right away.
• Rash or itch, diarrhea, nausea, vomiting, decreased blood pressure.	Continue. Call doctor when convenient.
Rare:	
• Mood or mental changes, seizures, sore throat, fever, unusual bleeding or bruising, muscle weakness, convulsions.	Discontinue. Call doctor right away.
• Ringing or buzzing in ears, hearing loss, headache, decreased blood pressure.	Continue. Call doctor when convenient.

228

WARNINGS & PRECAUTIONS

Don't take if:
You are allergic to chloroquine or hydroxychloroquine.

Before you start, consult your doctor:
- If you plan to become pregnant within the medication period.
- If you have blood disease.
- If you have eye or vision problems.
- If you have a G6PD deficiency.
- If you have liver disease.
- If you have nerve or brain disease (including seizure disorders).
- If you have porphyria.
- If you have psoriasis.
- If you have stomach or intestinal disease.
- If you drink more than 3 oz. of alcohol daily.

Over age 60:
Adverse reactions and side effects may be more frequent and severe than in younger persons.

Pregnancy:
Risk to unborn child outweighs drug benefits. Don't use.

Breast-feeding:
Drug passes into milk. Avoid drug or discontinue nursing.

Infants & children:
Not recommended. Dangerous.

Prolonged use:
Permanent damage to the retina (back part of the eye) or nerve deafness.

Skin & sunlight:
May cause rash or intensify sunburn in areas exposed to sun or sunlamp.

Driving, piloting or hazardous work:
Don't drive or pilot aircraft until you learn how medicine affects you. Don't work around dangerous machinery. Don't climb ladders or work in high places. Danger increases if you drink alcohol or take medicine affecting alertness and reflexes.

Discontinuing:
Don't discontinue without doctor's advice until you complete prescribed dose, even though symptoms diminish or disappear.

Others:
- Periodic physical and blood examinations recommended.
- If you are in a malaria area for a long time, you may need to change to another preventive drug every 2 years.

POSSIBLE INTERACTION WITH OTHER DRUGS

GENERIC NAME OR DRUG CLASS	COMBINED EFFECT
Estrogens*	Possible liver toxicity.
Gold compounds*	Risk of severe rash and itch.
Kaolin	Decreased absorption of chloroquine.
Magnesium trisilicate	Decreased absorption of chloroquine.
Penicillamine	Possible blood or kidney toxicity.

POSSIBLE INTERACTION WITH OTHER SUBSTANCES

INTERACTS WITH	COMBINED EFFECT
Alcohol:	Possible liver toxicity. Avoid.
Beverages:	None expected.
Cocaine:	None expected.
Foods:	None expected.
Marijuana:	None expected.
Tobacco:	None expected.

*See Glossary

CHLOROTHIAZIDE

BRAND NAMES

Aldoclor
Chloroserpine
Diupres
Diuril
SK-Chlorothiazide

BASIC INFORMATION

Habit forming? No
Prescription needed? Yes
Available as generic? Yes
Drug class: Antihypertensive, diuretic
(thiazide)

USES

- Controls, but doesn't cure, high blood pressure.
- Reduces fluid retention (edema) caused by conditions such as heart disorders and liver disease.

DOSAGE & USAGE INFORMATION

How to take:
Tablet or liquid—Swallow with liquid. If you can't swallow whole, crumble tablet and take with liquid or food. Don't exceed dose.

When to take:
At the same time each day.

If you forget a dose:
Take as soon as you remember up to 2 hours late. If more than 2 hours, wait for next scheduled dose (don't double this dose).

What drug does:
- Forces sodium and water excretion, reducing body fluid.
- Relaxes muscle cells of small arteries.
- Reduced body fluid and relaxed arteries lower blood pressure.

Time lapse before drug works:
4 to 6 hours. May require several weeks to lower blood pressure.

Continued next column

OVERDOSE

SYMPTOMS:
Cramps, weakness, drowsiness, weak pulse, coma.
WHAT TO DO:
- Dial 0 (operator) or 911 (emergency) for an ambulance or medical help. Then give first aid immediately.
- See emergency information on inside covers.

Don't take with:
- See Interaction column and consult doctor.
- Non-prescription drugs without consulting doctor.

POSSIBLE ADVERSE REACTIONS OR SIDE EFFECTS

SYMPTOMS	WHAT TO DO
Life-threatening: None expected.	
Common: None expected.	
Infrequent:	
• Blurred vision, severe abdominal pain, nausea, vomiting, irregular heartbeat, weak pulse.	Discontinue. Call doctor right away.
• Dizziness, mood changes, headaches, weakness, tiredness, weight changes.	Continue. Call doctor when convenient.
• Dry mouth, thirst.	Continue. Tell doctor at next visit.
Rare:	
• Rash or hives.	Discontinue. Seek emergency treatment.
• Jaundice.	Discontinue. Call doctor right away.
• Sore throat, fever.	Continue. Tell doctor at next visit.

WARNINGS & PRECAUTIONS

Don't take if:
You are allergic to any thiazide diuretic drug.

Before you start, consult your doctor:
- If you are allergic to any sulfa drug.
- If you have gout.
- If you have liver, pancreas or kidney disorder.

Over age 60:
Adverse reactions and side effects may be more frequent and severe than in younger persons, especially dizziness and excessive potassium loss.

Pregnancy:
Risk to unborn child outweighs drug benefits. Don't use.

Breast-feeding:
Drug passes into milk. Avoid drug or discontinue nursing.

Infants & children:
No problems expected.

Prolonged use:
You may need medicine to treat high blood pressure for the rest of your life.

Skin & sunlight:
May cause rash or intensify sunburn in areas exposed to sun or sunlamp.

Driving, piloting or hazardous work:
Don't drive or pilot aircraft until you learn how medicine affects you. Don't work around dangerous machinery. Don't climb ladders or work in high places. Danger increases if you drink alcohol or take medicine affecting alertness and reflexes, such as antihistamines, tranquilizers, sedatives, pain medicine, narcotics and mind-altering drugs.

Discontinuing:
Don't discontinue without medical advice.

Others:
- Hot weather and fever may cause dehydration and drop in blood pressure. Dose may require temporary adjustment. Weigh daily and report any unexpected weight decreases to your doctor.
- May cause rise in uric acid, leading to gout.
- May cause blood-sugar rise in diabetics.

 ## POSSIBLE INTERACTION WITH OTHER DRUGS

GENERIC NAME OR DRUG CLASS	COMBINED EFFECT
ACE inhibitors: captopril, enalapril, lisinopril*	Decreased blood pressure.
Allopurinol	Decreased allopurinol effect.
Amiodarone	Increased risk of heartbeat irregularity due to low potassium.
Amphotericin B	Increased potassium.
Antidepressants, tricyclic (TCA)*	Dangerous drop in blood pressure. Avoid combination unless under medical supervision.
Antidiabetic agents, oral*	Increased blood sugar.
Antihypertensives*	Increased hypertensive effect.
Barbiturates*	Increased chlorothiazide effect.
Beta-adrenergic blockers*	Increased antihypertensive effect. Dosages of both drugs may require adjustments.

Calcium supplements*	Increased calcium in blood.
Carteolol	Increased antihypertensive effect.
Cholestyramine	Decreased chlorothiazide effect.
Colestipol	Decreased chlorothiazide effect.
Cortisone drugs*	Excessive potassium loss that causes dangerous heart rhythms.
Digitalis preparations*	Excessive potassium loss that causes dangerous heart rhythms.
Diuretics, thiazide*	Increased effect of other thiazide diuretics.
Indapamide	Increased diuretic effect.
Indomethacin	Decreased chlorothiazide effect.
Lithium	Increased effect of lithium.
MAO inhibitors*	Increased chlorothiazide effect.

Continued page 1081

 ## POSSIBLE INTERACTION WITH OTHER SUBSTANCES

INTERACTS WITH	COMBINED EFFECT
Alcohol:	Dangerous blood-pressure drop.
Beverages:	None expected.
Cocaine	Increased risk of heart block and high blood pressure.
Foods: Licorice.	Excessive potassium loss that causes dangerous heart rhythms.
Marijuana:	May increase blood pressure.
Tobacco:	None expected.

*See Glossary

231

CHLOROTRIANISENE

BRAND NAMES

TACE

BASIC INFORMATION

Habit forming? No
Prescription needed? Yes
Available as generic? No
Drug class: Female sex hormone (estrogen)

 ## USES

- Treatment for symptoms of menopause and menstrual-cycle irregularity.
- Replacement for female hormone deficiency.
- Treatment for cancer of prostate.

 ## DOSAGE & USAGE INFORMATION

How to take:
Capsule—Swallow with liquid. If you can't swallow whole, open capsule and take with liquid or food.

When to take:
At the same time each day.

If you forget a dose:
Take as soon as you remember up to 12 hours late. If more than 12 hours, wait for next scheduled dose (don't double this dose).

What drug does:
Restores normal estrogen level in tissues.

Time lapse before drug works:
10 to 20 days.

Don't take with:
See Interaction column and consult doctor.

 ## OVERDOSE

SYMPTOMS:
Nausea, vomiting, fluid retention, breast enlargement and discomfort, abnormal vaginal bleeding.
WHAT TO DO:
Overdose unlikely to threaten life. If person takes much larger amount than prescribed, call doctor, poison-control center or hospital emergency room for instructions.

 ## POSSIBLE ADVERSE REACTIONS OR SIDE EFFECTS

SYMPTOMS	WHAT TO DO
Life-threatening: None expected.	
Common: • Stomach cramps.	Discontinue. Call doctor right away.
• Appetite loss.	Continue. Call doctor when convenient.
• Swollen ankles or feet; swollen, tender breasts; nausea; diarrhea.	Continue. Tell doctor at next visit.
Infrequent: • Rash, stomach or side pain.	Discontinue. Call doctor right away.
• Depression, vomiting, dizziness, irritability, breast lumps.	Continue. Call doctor when convenient.
• Brown blotches on skin, hair loss, vaginal discharge or bleeding, changes in sex drive.	Continue. Tell doctor at next visit.
Rare: Jaundice.	Discontinue. Call doctor right away.

WARNINGS & PRECAUTIONS

Don't take if:
- You are allergic to any estrogen-containing drugs.
- You have impaired liver function.
- You have had blood clots, stroke or heart attack.
- You have unexplained vaginal bleeding.

Before you start, consult your doctor:
- If you have had cancer of breast or reproductive organs, fibrocystic breast disease, fibroid tumors of the uterus or endometriosis.
- If you have had migraine headaches, epilepsy or porphyria.
- If you have diabetes, high blood pressure, asthma, congestive heart failure, kidney disease or gallstones.
- If you plan to become pregnant within 3 months.

Over age 60:
Controversial. You and your doctor must decide if drug risks outweigh benefits.

Pregnancy:
Risk to unborn child outweighs drug benefits. Don't use.

Breast-feeding:
Drug filters into milk. May harm child. Avoid.

Infants & children:
Not recommended.

Prolonged use:
Increased growth of fibroid tumors of uterus. Possible association with cancer of uterus.

Skin & sunlight:
May cause rash or intensify sunburn in areas exposed to sun or sunlamp.

Driving, piloting or hazardous work:
No problems expected.

Discontinuing:
You may need to discontinue chlorotrianisene periodically. Consult your doctor.

Others:
In rare instances, may cause blood clot in lung, brain or leg. Symptoms are *sudden* severe headache, coordination loss, vision change, chest pain, breathing difficulty, slurred speech, pain in legs or groin. Seek emergency treatment immediately.

POSSIBLE INTERACTION WITH OTHER DRUGS

GENERIC NAME OR DRUG CLASS	COMBINED EFFECT
Anticoagulants, oral*	Decreased anti-coagulant effect.
Anticonvulsants, hydantoin*	Increased seizures.
Antidiabetics, oral*	Unpredictable increase or decrease in blood sugar.
Antifibrinolytic agents*	Increased possibility of blood clotting.
Carbamazepine	Increased seizures.
Clofibrate	Decreased clofibrate effect.
Meprobamate	Increased chloro-trianisene effect.
Phenobarbital	Decreased chloro-trianisene effect.
Phenytoin	Decreased chloro-trianisene effect.
Primidone	Decreased chloro-trianisene effect.
Rifampin	Decreased chloro-trianisene effect.
Thyroid hormones*	Decreased thyroid effect.
Terazosin	Decreases effectiveness of terazosin.
Ursodiol	Decreased effect of ursodiol.

POSSIBLE INTERACTION WITH OTHER SUBSTANCES

INTERACTS WITH	COMBINED EFFECT
Alcohol:	None expected.
Beverages:	None expected.
Cocaine:	No proven problems.
Foods:	None expected.
Marijuana:	Possible menstrual irregularities and bleeding between periods.
Tobacco:	Increased risk of blood clots leading to stroke or heart attack.

CHLORPHENESIN

BRAND NAMES

Maolate   Mycil

BASIC INFORMATION

Habit forming? Possibly
Prescription needed? Yes
Available as generic? No
Drug class: Muscle relaxant (skeletal)

 ## USES

Adjunctive treatment to rest, analgesics and physical therapy for muscle spasm.

 ## DOSAGE & USAGE INFORMATION

How to take:
Tablet—Swallow with liquid.

When to take:
As needed, no more often than every 4 hours.

If you forget a dose:
Take as soon as you remember. Wait 4 hours for next dose.

What drug does:
Blocks body's pain messages to brain. Also causes sedation.

Time lapse before drug works:
60 minutes.

Don't take with:
See Interaction column and consult doctor.

 ## OVERDOSE

SYMPTOMS:
Nausea, vomiting, sedation.
WHAT TO DO:
- Dial 0 (operator) or 911 (emergency) for an ambulance or medical help. Then give first aid immediately.
- See emergency information on inside covers.

 ## POSSIBLE ADVERSE REACTIONS OR SIDE EFFECTS

SYMPTOMS	WHAT TO DO
Life-threatening: Hives, rash, intense itching, faintness soon after a dose (anaphylaxis); extreme weakness, transient paralysis, temporary vision loss.	Seek emergency treatment immediately.
Common: • Drowsiness, fainting, dizziness, confusion.	Continue. Call doctor when convenient.
• Orange or red-purple urine.	No action necessary.
Infrequent: Agitation, constipation or diarrhea, nausea, cramps, vomiting, wheezing, shortness of breath, headache, depression.	Discontinue. Call doctor right away.
Rare: • Bloody or tarry, black stool.	Discontinue. Seek emergency treatment.
• Rash, hives or itch; sore throat, fever; jaundice; tiredness; weakness; hiccups.	Discontinue. Call doctor right away.

WARNINGS & PRECAUTIONS

Don't take if:
- You are allergic to any skeletal-muscle relaxant.
- You have porphyria.

Before you start, consult your doctor:
- If you have had liver or kidney disease.
- If you plan pregnancy within medication period.
- If you are allergic to tartrazine dye.
- If you will have surgery within 2 months, including dental surgery, requiring general or spinal anesthesia.

Over age 60:
Adverse reactions and side effects may be more frequent and severe than in younger persons.

Pregnancy:
Safety not proven.. Avoid if possible.

Breast-feeding:
Drug passes into milk. Avoid drug or discontinue nursing until you finish medicine. Consult doctor for advice on maintaining milk supply.

Infants & children:
Not recommended.

Prolonged use:
- Periodic liver-function tests recommended if you use this drug for a long time.
- Safety beyond 8 weeks of treatment not established.

Skin & sunlight:
No problems expected.

Driving, piloting or hazardous work:
Don't drive or pilot aircraft until you learn how medicine affects you. Don't work around dangerous machinery. Don't climb ladders or work in high places. Danger increases if you drink alcohol or take medicine affecting alertness and reflexes, such as antihistamines, tranquilizers, sedatives, pain medicine, narcotics and mind-altering drugs.

Discontinuing:
Don't discontinue without doctor's advice until you complete prescribed dose, even though symptoms diminish or disappear.

Others:
No problems expected.

POSSIBLE INTERACTION WITH OTHER DRUGS

GENERIC NAME OR DRUG CLASS	COMBINED EFFECT
Antidepressants*	Increased sedation.
Antihistamines*	Increased sedation.
Dronabinol	Increased effects of dronabinol on central nervous system. Avoid combination.
Mind-altering drugs*	Increased sedation.
Muscle relaxants, other*	Increased sedation.
Narcotics*	Increased sedation.
Sedatives*	Increased sedation.
Sleep inducers*	Increased sedation.
Tranquilizers*	Increased sedation.

POSSIBLE INTERACTION WITH OTHER SUBSTANCES

INTERACTS WITH	COMBINED EFFECT
Alcohol:	Increased sedation. Avoid.
Beverages:	None expected.
Cocaine:	Lack of coordination, increased sedation. Avoid.
Foods:	None expected.
Marijuana:	Lack of coordination, drowsiness, fainting. Avoid.
Tobacco:	None expected.

CHLORPHENIRAMINE

BRAND NAMES

See complete list of brand names in the *Brand Name Directory*, page 1060.

BASIC INFORMATION

Habit forming? No
Prescription needed? No
Available as generic? Yes
Drug class: Antihistamine

USES

- Reduces allergic symptoms such as hay fever, hives, rash or itching.
- Prevents motion sickness, nausea, vomiting.
- Induces sleep.

DOSAGE & USAGE INFORMATION

How to take:
- Tablet or syrup—Swallow with liquid or food to lessen stomach irritation.
- Extended-release tablets or capsules—Swallow each dose whole.
- Chewable tablets—Chew well before swallowing.

When to take:
Varies with form. Follow label directions.

If you forget a dose:
Take as soon as you remember up to 2 hours late. If more than 2 hours, wait for next scheduled dose (don't double this dose).

What drug does:
Blocks action of histamine after an allergic response triggers histamine release in sensitive cells.

Time lapse before drug works:
30 minutes.

Don't take with:
See Interaction column and consult doctor.

OVERDOSE

SYMPTOMS:
Convulsions, red face, hallucinations, coma.
WHAT TO DO:
- **Dial 0 (operator) or 911 (emergency) for an ambulance or medical help. Then give first aid immediately.**
- **See emergency information on inside covers.**

POSSIBLE ADVERSE REACTIONS OR SIDE EFFECTS

SYMPTOMS	WHAT TO DO
Life-threatening: None expected.	
Common: Drowsiness; dizziness; dry mouth, nose, throat; nausea.	Continue. Tell doctor at next visit.
Infrequent:	
• Vision changes.	Discontinue. Call doctor right away.
• Less tolerance for contact lenses, difficult urination.	Continue. Call doctor when convenient.
• Appetite loss.	Continue. Tell doctor at next visit.
Rare: Nightmares, agitation, irritability, sore throat, fever, rapid heartbeat, unusual bleeding or bruising, fatigue, weakness.	Discontinue. Call doctor right away.

WARNINGS & PRECAUTIONS

Don't take if:
You are allergic to any antihistamine.

Before you start, consult your doctor:
- If you have glaucoma.
- If you have enlarged prostate.
- If you have asthma.
- If you have kidney disease.
- If you have peptic ulcer.
- If you will have surgery within 2 months, including dental surgery, requiring general or spinal anesthesia.

Over age 60:
Don't exceed recommended dose. Adverse reactions and side effects may be more frequent and severe than in younger persons, especially urination difficulty, diminished alertness and other brain and nervous-system symptoms.

Pregnancy:
No proven harm to unborn child. Avoid if possible.

Breast-feeding:
Drug passes into milk. Avoid drug or discontinue nursing until you finish medicine. Consult doctor for advice on maintaining milk supply.

Infants & children:
Not recommended for premature or newborn infants. Otherwise, no problems expected.

Prolonged use:
Avoid. May damage bone marrow and nerve cells.

Skin & sunlight:
May cause rash or intensify sunburn in areas exposed to sun or sunlamp.

Driving, piloting or hazardous work:
Don't drive or pilot aircraft until you learn how medicine affects you. Don't work around dangerous machinery. Don't climb ladders or work in high places. Danger increases if you drink alcohol or take medicine affecting alertness and reflexes, such as antihistamines, tranquilizers, sedatives, pain medicine, narcotics and mind-altering drugs.

Discontinuing:
No problems expected.

Others:
May mask symptoms of hearing damage from aspirin, other salicylates, cisplatin, paromomycin, vancomycin or anticonvulsants. Consult doctor if you use these.

POSSIBLE INTERACTION WITH OTHER DRUGS

GENERIC NAME OR DRUG CLASS	COMBINED EFFECT
Anticoagulants, oral*	Decreased chlorpheniramine effect.
Anticholinergics*	Increased anticholinergic effect.
Antidepressants*	Excess sedation. Avoid.
Antihistamines, other*	Excess sedation. Avoid.
Carteolol	Decreased antihistamine effect.
Dronabinol	Increased effects of both drugs. Avoid.
Hypnotics*	Excess sedation. Avoid.
MAO inhibitors*	Increased chlorpheniramine effect.
Mind-altering drugs*	Excess sedation. Avoid.
Molindone	Increased antihistamine effect.
Nabilone	Greater depression of central nervous system.
Narcotics*	Excess sedation. Avoid.
Procarbazine	May increase sedation.
Sedatives*	Excess sedation. Avoid.
Sleep inducers*	Excess sedation. Avoid.
Sotalol	Increased antihistamine effect.
Tranquilizers*	Excess sedation. Avoid.

POSSIBLE INTERACTION WITH OTHER SUBSTANCES

INTERACTS WITH	COMBINED EFFECT
Alcohol:	Excess sedation. Avoid.
Beverages: Caffeine drinks.	Less chlorpheniramine sedation.
Cocaine:	Decreased chlorpheniramine effect. Avoid.
Foods:	None expected.
Marijuana:	Excess sedation. Avoid.
Tobacco:	None expected.

*See Glossary

CHLORPROMAZINE

BRAND NAMES

Apo-Chlorpromazine
Chloramead
Chlor-Promanyl
Chlorprom
Clorazine
Largactil
Novochlorpromazine
Ormazine
Promapar
Promaz
Promosol
Thorazine
Thor-Prom

BASIC INFORMATION

Habit forming? No
Prescription needed? Yes
Available as generic? Yes
**Drug class: Tranquilizer, antiemetic
(phenothiazine)**

 ## USES

- Stops nausea, vomiting, hiccups.
- Reduces anxiety, agitation.

 ## DOSAGE & USAGE INFORMATION

How to take:
- Tablet or extended-release capsule—Swallow with liquid or food to lessen stomach irritation.
- Suppositories—Remove wrapper and moisten suppository with water. Gently insert into rectum, large end first.
- Drops or liquid—Dilute dose in beverage.

When to take:
- Nervous and mental disorders—Take at the same times each day.
- Nausea and vomiting—Take as needed, no more often than every 4 hours.

If you forget a dose:
- Nervous and mental disorders—Take up to 2 hours late. If more than 2 hours, wait for next scheduled dose (don't double this dose).
- Nausea and vomiting—Take as soon as you remember. Wait 4 hours for next dose.

Continued next column

 ## OVERDOSE

SYMPTOMS:
Stupor, convulsions, coma.
WHAT TO DO:
- **Dial 0 (operator) or 911 (emergency) for an ambulance or medical help. Then give first aid immediately.**
- **See emergency information on inside covers.**

What drug does:
- Suppresses brain's vomiting center.
- Suppresses brain centers that control abnormal emotions and behavior.

Time lapse before drug works:
- Nausea and vomiting—1 hour or less.
- Nervous and mental disorders—4 to 6 weeks.

Don't take with:
- Antacid or medicine for diarrhea.
- Non-prescription drug for cough, cold or allergy.
- See Interaction column and consult doctor.

 ## POSSIBLE ADVERSE REACTIONS OR SIDE EFFECTS

SYMPTOMS	WHAT TO DO
Life-threatening:	
Uncontrolled muscle movements of tongue, face and other muscles (neuroleptic malignant syndrome, rare).	Discontinue. Seek emergency treatment.
Common:	
• Muscle spasms of face and neck, unsteady gait.	Discontinue. Seek emergency treatment.
• Restlessness, tremor, drowsiness.	Discontinue. Call doctor right away.
• Decreased sweating, dry mouth, stuffy nose, constipation.	Continue. Call doctor when convenient.
Infrequent:	
• Fainting.	Discontinue. Seek emergency treatment.
• Rash.	Discontinue. Call doctor right away.
• Difficult urination, diminished sex drive, swollen breasts, menstrual irregularities.	Continue. Call doctor when convenient.
Rare:	
Vision changes, sore throat, fever, jaundice, abdominal pain, constipation.	Discontinue. Call doctor right away.

WARNINGS & PRECAUTIONS

Don't take if:
- You are allergic to any phenothiazine.
- You have a blood or bone-marrow disease.

Before you start, consult your doctor:
- If you will have surgery within 2 months, including dental surgery, requiring general or spinal anesthesia.
- If you have asthma, emphysema or other lung disorder; glaucoma; or prostate trouble.
- If you take non-prescription ulcer medicine, asthma medicine or amphetamines.

Over age 60:
Adverse reactions and side effects may be more frequent and severe than in younger persons. More likely to develop involuntary movement of jaws, lips, tongue, chewing. Report this to your doctor immediately. Early treatment can help.

Pregnancy:
Risk to unborn child outweighs drug benefits. Don't use.

Breast-feeding:
Drug passes into milk. Avoid drug or discontinue nursing until you finish medicine. Consult doctor for advice on maintaining milk supply.

Infants & children:
Don't give to children younger than 2.

Prolonged use:
May lead to tardive dyskinesia (involuntary movement of jaws, lips, tongue, chewing).

Skin & sunlight:
May cause rash or intensify sunburn in areas exposed to sun or sunlamp. Skin may remain sensitive for 3 months after discontinuing.

Driving, piloting or hazardous work:
Don't drive or pilot aircraft until you learn how medicine affects you. Don't work around dangerous machinery. Don't climb ladders or work in high places. Danger increases if you drink alcohol or take medicine affecting alertness and reflexes.

Discontinuing:
- Nervous and mental disorders—Don't discontinue without doctor's advice until you complete prescribed dose, even though symptoms diminish or disappear.
- Nausea and vomiting—May be unnecessary to finish medicine. Follow doctor's instructions.

Others:
No problems expected.

POSSIBLE INTERACTION WITH OTHER DRUGS

GENERIC NAME OR DRUG CLASS	COMBINED EFFECT
Anticholinergics*	Increased anti-cholinergic effect.
Antidepressants, tricyclic (TCA)*	Increased chlorpromazine effect.
Antihistamines*	Increased antihistamine effect.
Appetite suppressants*	Decreased suppressant effect.
Calcium supplements*	Decreased chlorpromazine effect.
Dronabinol	Increased effects of both drugs. Avoid.
Guanethidine	Increased guanethidine effect.
Levodopa	Decreased levodopa effect.
Mind-altering drugs*	Increased effect of mind-altering drugs.
Molindone	Increased tranquilizer effect.
Nabilone	Greater depression of central nervous system.
Narcotics*	Increased narcotic effect.
Phenytoin	Increased phenytoin effect.
Procarbazine	Increased sedation.
Quinidine	Impaired heart function. Dangerous mixture.
Sedatives*	Increased sedation.
Tranquilizers* (other)	Increased tranquilizer effect.

POSSIBLE INTERACTION WITH OTHER SUBSTANCES

INTERACTS WITH	COMBINED EFFECT
Alcohol:	Dangerous oversedation.
Beverages:	None expected.
Cocaine:	Decreased chlorpromazine effect. Avoid.
Foods:	None expected.
Marijuana:	Drowsiness. May increase antinausea effect.
Tobacco:	None expected.

*See Glossary

CHLORPROPAMIDE

BRAND NAMES

Apo-Chlorpropamide
Chloromide
Chloronase
Diabinese

Glucamide
Novopropamide
Stabinol

BASIC INFORMATION

Habit forming? No
Prescription needed? Yes
Available as generic? Yes
Drug class: Antidiabetic (oral), sulfonurea

USES

Treatment for diabetes insipidus and diabetes in adults who can't control blood sugar by diet, weight loss and exercise.

DOSAGE & USAGE INFORMATION

How to take:
Tablet—Swallow with liquid or food to lessen stomach irritation. If you can't swallow whole, crumble tablet and take with liquid or food.

When to take:
At the same times each day.

If you forget a dose:
Take as soon as you remember up to 2 hours late. If more than 2 hours, wait for next scheduled dose (don't double this dose).

What drug does:
Stimulates pancreas to produce more insulin. Insulin in blood forces cells to use sugar in blood.

Time lapse before drug works:
3 to 4 hours. May require 2 weeks for maximum benefit.

Don't take with:
See Interaction column and consult doctor.

OVERDOSE

SYMPTOMS:
Excessive hunger, nausea, anxiety, cool skin, cold sweats, drowsiness, rapid heartbeat, weakness, unconsciousness, coma.
WHAT TO DO:
- Dial 0 (operator) or 911 (emergency) for an ambulance or medical help. Then give first aid immediately.
- See emergency information on inside covers.

POSSIBLE ADVERSE REACTIONS OR SIDE EFFECTS

SYMPTOMS	WHAT TO DO
Life-threatening: None expected.	
Common:	
• Dizziness.	Discontinue. Call doctor right away.
• Diarrhea, appetite loss, nausea, stomach pain, heartburn.	Continue. Call doctor when convenient.
Infrequent: Low blood sugar (hunger, anxiety, cold sweats, rapid pulse).	Discontinue. Seek emergency treatment.
Rare: Fatigue, itching or rash, sore throat, fever, ringing in ears, unusual bleeding or bruising, jaundice, edema, weakness, confusion.	Discontinue. Call doctor right away.

WARNINGS & PRECAUTIONS

Don't take if:
- You are allergic to any sulfonurea.
- You have impaired kidney or liver function.

Before you start, consult your doctor:
- If you have a severe infection.
- If you have thyroid disease.
- If you take insulin.
- If you have heart disease.

Over age 60:
Dose usually smaller than for younger adults. Avoid "low-blood-sugar" episodes because repeated ones can damage brain permanently.

Pregnancy:
No proven harm to unborn child. Avoid if possible.

Breast-feeding:
Drug filters into milk. May lower baby's blood sugar. Avoid.

Infants & children:
Don't give to infants or children.

Prolonged use:
None expected.

Skin & sunlight:
May cause rash or intensify sunburn in areas exposed to sun or sunlamp.

Driving, piloting or hazardous work:
No problems expected unless you develop hypoglycemia (low blood sugar). If so, avoid driving or hazardous activity.

Discontinuing:
Don't discontinue without consulting doctor. Dose may require gradual reduction if you have taken drug for a long time. Doses of other drugs may also require adjustment.

Others:
Don't exceed recommended dose. Hypoglycemia (low blood sugar) may occur, even with proper dose schedule. You must balance medicine, diet and exercise.

 ## POSSIBLE INTERACTION WITH OTHER DRUGS

GENERIC NAME OR DRUG CLASS	COMBINED EFFECT
Androgens*	Increased chlor-propamide effect.
Anticoagulants, oral*	Unpredictable prothrombin times.*
Anticonvulsants, hydantoin*	Decreased chlor-propamide effect.
Aspirin	Increased chlor-propamide effect.
Beta-adrenergic blockers*	Possible increased difficulty in regulating blood-sugar levels. Increased chlorpropa-mide effect.
Bismuth subsalicylate	Increased insulin effect. May require dosage adjustment.
Chloramphenicol	Increased chlorpropa-mide effect.
Cimetidine	Possible increased chlorpropamide effect.
Clofibrate	Increased chlorpropa-mide effect.
Contraceptives, oral*	Decreased chlor-propamide effect.
Cortisone drugs*	Decreased chlor-propamide effect.
Digoxin	Possible decreased digoxin effect.
Diuretics, thiazide and loop*	Decreased chlor-propamide effect.
Epinephrine	Decreased chlor-propamide effect.
Estrogens*	Decreased chlor-propamide effect.
Guanethidine	Increased chlor-propamide effect.
Insulin	Increased chlor-propamide effect.
Isoniazid	Decreased chlor-propamide effect.
Labetalol	Increased antidiabetic effect, may mask hypoglycemia.
MAO inhibitors*	Increased chlor-propamide effect.
Nicotinic acid	Decreased chlor-propamide effect.
Non-steroidal anti-inflammatory drugs (NSAIDs)*	Increased chlor-propamide effect.
Oxyphenbutazone	Increased chlor-propamide effect.
Phenothiazines*	Decreased chlor-propamide effect.
Phenylbutazone	Increased chlor-propamide effect.
Phenytoin	Decreased chlor-propamide effect.
Probenecid	Increased chlor-propamide effect.
Pyrazinamide	Decreased chlor-propamide effect.
Ranitidine	Possible increased chlorpropamide effect.
Rifampin	Decreased chlor-propamide effect.
Sulfa drugs*	Increased chlor-propamide effect.
Thyroid hormones*	Decreased chlor-propamide effect.

 ## POSSIBLE INTERACTION WITH OTHER SUBSTANCES

INTERACTS WITH	COMBINED EFFECT
Alcohol:	Disulfiram reaction.* Avoid.
Beverages:	None expected.
Cocaine:	No proven problems.
Foods:	None expected.
Marijuana:	Decreased chlorpro-pamide effect. Avoid.
Tobacco:	None expected.

CHLORPROTHIXENE

BRAND NAMES

Taractan   Tarasan

BASIC INFORMATION

Habit forming? No
Prescription needed? Yes
Available as generic? No
Drug class: Tranquilizer (thioxanthine), antiemetic

USES

- Reduces anxiety, agitation, psychosis.
- Stops vomiting, hiccups.

DOSAGE & USAGE INFORMATION

How to take:
- Tablet or sustained-release capsule—Swallow with liquid. If you can't swallow whole, crumble tablet and take with liquid or food.
- Syrup—Dilute dose in beverage before swallowing.

When to take:
At the same time each day.

If you forget a dose:
Take as soon as you remember up to 2 hours late. If more than 2 hours, wait for next scheduled dose (don't double this dose).

What drug does:
Corrects imbalance of nerve impulses.

Continued next column

OVERDOSE

SYMPTOMS:
Drowsiness, dizziness, weakness, muscle rigidity, twitching, tremors, confusion, dry mouth, blurred vision, rapid pulse, shallow breathing, low blood pressure, convulsions, coma.

WHAT TO DO:
- Dial 0 (operator) or 911 (emergency) for an ambulance or medical help. Then give first aid immediately.
- If patient is unconscious and not breathing, give mouth-to-mouth breathing. If there is no heartbeat, use cardiac massage and mouth-to-mouth breathing (CPR). Don't try to make patient vomit. If you can't get help quickly, take patient to nearest emergency facility.
- See emergency information on inside covers.

Time lapse before drug works:
3 weeks.

Don't take with:
See Interaction column and consult doctor.

POSSIBLE ADVERSE REACTIONS OR SIDE EFFECTS

SYMPTOMS	WHAT TO DO
Life-threatening:	
Uncontrollable movements of head, neck, arms, legs (rarely).	Discontinue. Seek emergency treatment.
Common:	
• Fainting; jerky, involuntary movements; restlessness; blurred vision; rapid heartbeat.	Discontinue. Call doctor right away.
• Dizziness, drowsiness, constipation, muscle spasms, shuffling walk, decreased sweating.	Continue. Call doctor when convenient.
• Dry mouth, stuffy nose.	Continue. Tell doctor at next visit.
Infrequent:	
• Rash.	Discontinue. Call doctor right away.
• Less sexual ability, difficult urination.	Continue. Call doctor when convenient.
• Menstrual irregularities, swollen breasts.	Continue. Tell doctor at next visit.
Rare:	
Sore throat, fever, jaundice, abdominal pain, constipation.	Discontinue. Call doctor right away.

WARNINGS & PRECAUTIONS

Don't take if:
- You are allergic to any thioxanthine or phenothiazine tranquilizer.
- You have serious blood disorder.
- You have Parkinson's disease.
- Patient is younger than 12.

Before you start, consult your doctor:
- If you have had liver or kidney disease.
- If you have epilepsy, glaucoma or prostate trouble.
- If you have high blood pressure or heart disease (especially angina).
- If you use alcohol daily.
- If you will have surgery within 2 months, including dental surgery, requiring general or spinal anesthesia.

Over age 60:
Adverse reactions and side effects may be more frequent and severe than in younger persons.

Pregnancy:
No proven harm to unborn child. Avoid if possible.

Breast-feeding:
Studies inconclusive. Consult your doctor.

Infants & children:
Not recommended.

Prolonged use:
- Pigment deposits in lens and retina of eye.
- Involuntary movements of jaws, lips, tongue (tardive dyskinesia).

Skin & sunlight:
May cause rash or intensify sunburn in areas exposed to sun or sunlamp.

Driving, piloting or hazardous work:
Don't drive or pilot aircraft until you learn how medicine affects you. Don't work around dangerous machinery. Don't climb ladders or work in high places. Danger increases if you drink alcohol or take medicine affecting alertness and reflexes.

Discontinuing:
Don't discontinue without consulting doctor. Dose may require gradual reduction if you have taken drug for a long time. Doses of other drugs may also require adjustment.

Others:
Hot temperatures increase chance of heat stroke.

POSSIBLE INTERACTION WITH OTHER DRUGS

GENERIC NAME OR DRUG CLASS	COMBINED EFFECT
Anticholinergics*	Increased anticholinergic effect.
Anticonvulsants*	Change in seizure pattern.
Antidepressants, tricyclic (TCA)*	Increased chlorprothixene effect. Excessive sedation.
Antihistamines*	Increased chlorprothixene effect. Excessive sedation.
Antihypertensives*	Excessively low blood pressure.
Barbiturates*	Increased chlorprothixene effect. Excessive sedation.
Bethanechol	Decreased bethanechol effect.
Dronabinol	Increased effects of both drugs. Avoid.
Guanethidine	Decreased guanethidine effect.
Levodopa	Decreased levodopa effect.
MAO inhibitors*	Excessive sedation.
Mind-altering drugs*	Increased chlorprothixene effect. Excessive sedation.
Narcotics*	Increased chlorprothixene effect. Excessive sedation.
Procarbazine	Increased sedation.
Sedatives*	Increased chlorprothixene effect. Excessive sedation.
Sleep inducers*	Increased chlorprothixene effect. Excessive sedation.
Tranquilizers*	Increased chlorprothixene effect. Excessive sedation.

POSSIBLE INTERACTION WITH OTHER SUBSTANCES

INTERACTS WITH	COMBINED EFFECT
Alcohol:	Excessive brain depression. Avoid.
Beverages:	None expected.
Cocaine:	Decreased chlorprothixene effect. Avoid.
Foods:	None expected.
Marijuana:	Daily use—Fainting likely, possible psychosis.
Tobacco:	None expected.

*See Glossary

CHLORTHALIDONE

BRAND NAMES

Apo-Chlorthalide	Novothalidone
Apo-Chlorthalidone	Regroton
Combipres	Tenoretic
Demi-Regroton	Thalitone
Hygroton	Uridon

BASIC INFORMATION

Habit forming? No
Prescription needed? Yes
Available as generic? Yes
Drug class: Antihypertensive, diuretic (thiazide)

USES

- Controls, but doesn't cure, high blood pressure.
- Reduces fluid retention (edema) caused by conditions such as heart disorders and liver disease.

DOSAGE & USAGE INFORMATION

How to take:
Tablet—Swallow with liquid. If you can't swallow whole, crumble tablet and take with liquid or food. Don't exceed dose.

When to take:
At the same time each day.

If you forget a dose:
Take as soon as you remember up to 2 hours late. If more than 2 hours, wait for next scheduled dose (don't double this dose).

What drug does:
- Forces sodium and water excretion, reducing body fluid.
- Relaxes muscle cells of small arteries.
- Reduced body fluid and relaxed arteries lower blood pressure.

Continued next column

OVERDOSE

SYMPTOMS:
Cramps, weakness, drowsiness, weak pulse, coma.
WHAT TO DO:
- Dial 0 (operator) or 911 (emergency) for an ambulance or medical help. Then give first aid immediately.
- See emergency information on inside covers.

Time lapse before drug works:
4 to 6 hours. May require several weeks to lower blood pressure.

Don't take with:
- See Interaction column and consult doctor.
- Non-prescription drugs without consulting doctor.

POSSIBLE ADVERSE REACTIONS OR SIDE EFFECTS

SYMPTOMS	WHAT TO DO
Life-threatening: None expected.	
Common: None expected.	
Infrequent:	
• Blurred vision, severe abdominal pain, nausea, vomiting, irregular heartbeat, weak pulse.	Discontinue. Call doctor right away.
• Dizziness, mood changes, headaches, weakness, tiredness, weight changes.	Continue. Call doctor when convenient.
• Dry mouth, thirst.	Continue. Tell doctor at next visit.
Rare:	
• Rash or hives.	Discontinue. Seek emergency treatment.
• Jaundice, sore throat, fever.	Discontinue. Call doctor right away.

WARNINGS & PRECAUTIONS

Don't take if:
You are allergic to any thiazide diuretic drug.

Before you start, consult your doctor:
- If you are allergic to any sulfa drug.
- If you have gout.
- If you have liver, pancreas or kidney disorder.

Over age 60:
Adverse reactions and side effects may be more frequent and severe than in younger persons, especially dizziness and excessive potassium loss.

Pregnancy:
Risk to unborn child outweighs drug benefits. Don't use.

Breast-feeding:
Drug passes into milk. Avoid this medicine or discontinue nursing.

Infants & children:
No problems expected.

Prolonged use:
You may need medicine to treat high blood pressure for the rest of your life.

Skin & sunlight:
May cause rash or intensify sunburn in areas exposed to sun or sunlamp.

Driving, piloting or hazardous work:
Don't drive or pilot aircraft until you learn how medicine affects you. Don't work around dangerous machinery. Don't climb ladders or work in high places. Danger increases if you drink alcohol or take medicine affecting alertness and reflexes, such as antihistamines, tranquilizers, sedatives, pain medicine, narcotics and mind-altering drugs.

Discontinuing:
Don't discontinue without medical advice.

Others:
- Hot weather and fever may cause dehydration and drop in blood pressure. Dose may require temporary adjustment. Weigh daily and report any unexpected weight decreases to your doctor.
- May cause rise in uric acid, leading to gout.
- May cause blood-sugar rise in diabetics.

 POSSIBLE INTERACTION WITH OTHER DRUGS

GENERIC NAME OR DRUG CLASS	COMBINED EFFECT
ACE inhibitors: captopril, enalapril, lisinopril*	Possible excessive potassium in blood.
Allopurinol	Decreased allopurinol effect.
Amiodarone	Increased risk of heartbeat irregularity due to low potassium.
Amphotericin B	Increased potassium.
Antidepressants, tricyclic (TCA)*	Dangerous drop in blood pressure. Avoid combination unless under medical supervision.
Antidiabetic agents*	Increased blood sugar.
Antihypertensives*	Decreased blood pressure.
Barbiturates*	Increased chlorthalidone effect.
Beta-adrenergic blockers*	Increased antihypertensive effect. Dosages of both drugs may require adjustments.
Calcium supplements*	Increased calcium in blood.
Carteolol	Increased antihypertensive effect.
Cholestyramine	Decreased chlorthalidone effect.
Colestipol	Decreased chlorthalidone effect.
Cortisone drugs*	Excessive potassium loss that causes dangerous heart rhythms.
Digitalis preparations*	Excessive potassium loss that causes dangerous heart rhythms.
Diuretics, thiazide*	Increased effect of other thiazide diuretics.
Indapamide	Increased diuretic effect.
Indomethacin	Decreased chlorthalidone effect.
Lithium	Increased effect of lithium.
MAO inhibitors*	Increased chlorthalidone effect.
Nicardipine	Blood-pressure drop. Dosages may require adjustment.
Nitrates*	Excessive blood-pressure drop.
Opiates*	Dizziness or weakness when standing up after sitting or lying down.
Pentoxifylline	Increased antihypertensive effect.
Potassium supplements*	Decreased potassium effect.

Continued page 1082

POSSIBLE INTERACTION WITH OTHER SUBSTANCES

INTERACTS WITH	COMBINED EFFECT
Alcohol:	Dangerous blood-pressure drop.
Beverages:	None expected.
Cocaine:	Increased risk of heart block and high blood pressure.
Foods: Licorice.	Excessive potassium loss that causes dangerous heart rhythms.
Marijuana:	May increase blood pressure.
Tobacco:	None expected.

*See Glossary

CHLORZOXAZONE

BRAND NAMES

Algisin	Paraflex
Chlorzone Forte	Parafon Forte DSC

BASIC INFORMATION

Habit forming? Possibly
Prescription needed? Yes
Available as generic? Yes
Drug class: Muscle relaxant (skeletal)

 USES

Adjunctive treatment to rest, analgesics and physical therapy for muscle spasm.

 DOSAGE & USAGE INFORMATION

How to take:
Tablet—Swallow with liquid.

When to take:
As needed, no more often than every 4 hours.

If you forget a dose:
Take as soon as you remember. Wait 4 hours for next dose.

What drug does:
Blocks body's pain messages to brain. Also causes sedation.

Time lapse before drug works:
60 minutes.

Don't take with:
See Interaction column and consult doctor.

 OVERDOSE

SYMPTOMS:
Nausea, vomiting, diarrhea, headache, severe weakness, breathing difficulty, sensation of paralysis.
WHAT TO DO:
Overdose unlikely to threaten life.
Depending on severity of symptoms and amount taken, call doctor, poison-control center or hospital emergency room for instructions.

 POSSIBLE ADVERSE REACTIONS OR SIDE EFFECTS

SYMPTOMS	WHAT TO DO
Life-threatening: Hives, rash, intense itching, faintness soon after a dose (anaphylaxis); extreme weakness, transient paralysis, temporary loss of vision.	Seek emergency treatment immediately.
Common: • Drowsiness, dizziness. • Orange or red-purple urine.	Continue. Call doctor when convenient. No action necessary.
Infrequent: Agitation, constipation or diarrhea, nausea, cramps, vomiting, headache, depression.	Discontinue. Call doctor right away.
Rare: • Bloody or tarry, black stool. • Rash or itch, sore throat, fever, jaundice, tiredness, weakness, bleeding in skin, hiccups.	Discontinue. Seek emergency treatment. Discontinue. Call doctor right away.

CHLORZOXAZONE

WARNINGS & PRECAUTIONS

Don't take if:
You are allergic to any skeletal-muscle relaxant.

Before you start, consult your doctor:
- If you have had liver disease.
- If you plan pregnancy within medication period.
- If you are allergic to tartrazine dye.

Over age 60:
Adverse reactions and side effects may be more frequent and severe than in younger persons.

Pregnancy:
Safety not proven. Avoid if possible.

Breast-feeding:
Drug passes into milk. Avoid drug or discontinue nursing until you finish medicine. Consult doctor for advice on maintaining milk supply.

Infants & children:
Not recommended.

Prolonged use:
No problems expected.

Skin & sunlight:
No problems expected.

Driving, piloting or hazardous work:
Don't drive or pilot aircraft until you learn how medicine affects you. Don't work around dangerous machinery. Don't climb ladders or work in high places. Danger increases if you drink alcohol or take medicine affecting alertness and reflexes, such as antihistamines, tranquilizers, sedatives, pain medicine, narcotics and mind-altering drugs.

Discontinuing:
Don't discontinue without doctor's advice until you complete prescribed dose, even though symptoms diminish or disappear.

Others:
Periodic liver-function tests recommended if you use this drug for a long time.

POSSIBLE INTERACTION WITH OTHER DRUGS

GENERIC NAME OR DRUG CLASS	COMBINED EFFECT
Antidepressants*	Increased sedation.
Antihistamines*	Increased sedation.
Dronabinol	Increased effect of dronabinol on central nervous system. Avoid combination.
Ethinamate	Dangerous increased effects of ethinamate. Avoid combining.
Fluoxetine	Increased depressant effects of both drugs.
Guanfacine	May increase depressant effects of either drug.
Leucovorin	High alcohol content of leucovorin may cause adverse effects.
MAO inhibitors*	Increased effect of both drugs.
Methyprylon	Increased sedative effect, perhaps to dangerous level. Avoid.
Mind-altering drugs*	Increased sedation.
Muscle relaxants, others*	Increased sedation.
Nabilone	Greater depression of central nervous system.
Narcotics*	Increased sedation.
Sedatives*	Increased sedation.
Sleep inducers*	Increased sedation
Tranquilizers*	Increased sedation.

POSSIBLE INTERACTION WITH OTHER SUBSTANCES

INTERACTS WITH	COMBINED EFFECT
Alcohol:	Increased sedation.
Beverages:	No problems expected.
Cocaine:	Lack of coordination.
Foods:	No problems expected.
Marijuana:	Lack of coordination, drowsiness, fainting.
Tobacco:	No problems expected.

*See Glossary

247

CHLORZOXAZONE & ACETAMINOPHEN

BRAND NAMES

Blanex
Chlorofon-F
Chlorzone Forte
Chlorzoxazone
  with APAP
Flexaphen
Flexin

Lobac
Mus-Lax
Paracet Forte
Parafon Forte
Polyflex
Zoxaphen

BASIC INFORMATION

Habit forming? Possibly
Prescription needed? Yes
Available as generic? Yes
**Drug class: Muscle relaxant (skeletal),
analgesic, fever-reducer**

USES

- Adjunctive treatment to rest, analgesics and physical therapy for muscle spasms.
- Treatment of mild to moderate pain and fever.

DOSAGE & USAGE INFORMATION

How to take:
Tablet—Swallow with liquid.

When to take:
As needed, no more often than every 3 hours.

If you forget a dose:
Take as soon as you remember. Wait 3 hours for next dose.

Continued next column

OVERDOSE

SYMPTOMS:
Nausea, vomiting, diarrhea, anorexia, headache, severe weakness, unusual increase in sweating, fainting, breathing difficulty, irritability, convulsions, sensation of paralysis, coma.
WHAT TO DO:
- **Overdose unlikely to threaten life. Depending on severity of symptoms and amount taken, call doctor, poison-control center or hospital emergency room for instructions.**
- **Dial 0 (operator) or 911 (emergency) for an ambulance or medical help. Then give first aid immediately.**
- **See emergency information on inside covers.**

What drug does:
- Blocks body's pain messages to brain. Also causes sedation.
- May affect hypothalamus, the part of the brain that helps regulate body heat and receives body's pain messages.

Time lapse before drug works:
15 to 30 minutes. May last 4 hours.

Don't take with:
- Other drugs with acetaminophen. Too much acetaminophen can damage liver and kidneys.
- See Interaction column and consult doctor.

POSSIBLE ADVERSE REACTIONS OR SIDE EFFECTS

SYMPTOMS	WHAT TO DO
Life-threatening: Hives, rash, intense itching, faintness soon after a dose (anaphylaxis); extreme weakness, transient paralysis, temporary loss of vision.	Seek emergency treatment immediately.
Common: Dizziness, lightheadedness, drowsiness.	Discontinue. Call doctor right away.
Infrequent: • Difficult or frequent urination.	Discontinue. Call doctor right away.
• Nervousness, restlessness, irritability, headache, indigestion, depression, agitation, constipation.	Continue. Call doctor when convenient.
Rare: • Sudden decrease in urine output; swelling of lips, face or tongue.	Discontinue. Seek emergency treatment.
• Bloody or black stools, jaundice, unusual bleeding or bruising, sore mouth or throat, fever, hiccups.	Discontinue. Call doctor right away.

CHLORZOXAZONE & ACETAMINOPHEN

WARNINGS & PRECAUTIONS

Don't take if:
- You are allergic to any skeletal-muscle relaxant or acetaminophen.
- Your symptoms don't improve after 2 days use. Call your doctor.

Before you start, consult your doctor:
- If you have had liver disease.
- If you have kidney disease or liver damage.
- If you plan pregnancy within medication period.
- If you are allergic to tartrazine dye.

Over age 60:
- Adverse reactions and side effects may be more frequent and severe than in younger persons.
- Don't exceed recommended dose. You can't eliminate drug as efficiently as younger persons.

Pregnancy:
Safety not proven. Avoid if possible.

Breast-feeding:
Drug passes into milk. Avoid drug or discontinue nursing until you finish medicine. Consult doctor for advice on maintaining milk supply.

Infants & children:
Not recommended.

Prolonged use:
May affect blood system and cause anemia. Limit use to 5 days for children 12 and under, and 10 days for adults.

Skin & sunlight:
No problems expected.

Driving, piloting or hazardous work:
Don't drive or pilot aircraft until you learn how medicine affects you. Don't work around dangerous machinery. Don't climb ladders or work in high places. Danger increases if you drink alcohol or take medicine affecting alertness and reflexes, such as antihistamines, tranquilizers, sedatives, pain medicine, narcotics and mind-altering drugs.

Discontinuing:
Don't discontinue without consulting your doctor. Dose may require gradual reduction if you have taken drug for a long time. Doses of other drugs may also require adjustment.

Others:
Periodic liver-function tests recommended if you use this drug for a long time.

POSSIBLE INTERACTION WITH OTHER DRUGS

GENERIC NAME OR DRUG CLASS	COMBINED EFFECT
Anticoagulants, oral*	May increase anticoagulant effect. If combined frequently, prothrombin time should be monitored.
Antidepressants*	Increased sedation.
Antihistamines*	Increased sedation.
Dronabinol	Increased effect of dronabinol on central nervous system. Avoid combination.
MAO inhibitors*	Increased effect (but safety not established) of both drugs.
Mind-altering drugs*	Increased sedation.
Muscle relaxants, others*	Increased sedation.
Narcotics*	Increased sedation.
Phenobarbital	Quicker elimination and decreased effects of acetaminophen.
Sedatives*	Increased sedation.
Sleep inducers*	Increased sedation.

Continued page 1082

POSSIBLE INTERACTION WITH OTHER SUBSTANCES

INTERACTS WITH	COMBINED EFFECT
Alcohol:	Drowsiness, increased sedation. Long-term use may cause toxic effect in liver.
Beverages:	No problems expected.
Cocaine:	Lack of coordination. May slow body's recovery. Avoid.
Foods:	No problems expected.
Marijuana:	Increased pain relief, lack of coordination, drowsiness, fainting. May slow body's recovery. Avoid.
Tobacco:	No problems expected.

CHOLESTYRAMINE

BRAND NAMES

Questran

BASIC INFORMATION

Habit forming? No
Prescription needed? Yes
Available as generic? No
Drug class: Antihyperlipidemic, antipruritic

 ## USES

- Removes excess bile acids that occur with some liver problems. Reduces persistent itch caused by bile acids.
- Lowers cholesterol level.
- Treatment of one form of colitis (rare).

 ## DOSAGE & USAGE INFORMATION

How to take:
Powder, granules—Sprinkle into 8 oz. liquid. Let stand for 2 minutes, then mix with liquid before swallowing. Or mix with cereal, soup or pulpy fruit. Don't swallow dry.

When to take:
- 3 or 4 times a day on an empty stomach, 1 hour before or 2 hours after eating.
- If taking other medicines, take 1 hour before or 4 to 6 hours after taking cholestyramine.

If you forget a dose:
Take as soon as you remember up to 2 hours late. If more than 2 hours, wait for next scheduled dose (don't double this dose).

What drug does:
Binds with bile acids to prevent their absorption.

Time lapse before drug works:
- Cholesterol reduction—1 day.
- Bile-acid reduction—3 to 4 weeks.

Don't take with:
- Any drug or vitamin simultaneously. Space doses 2 hours apart.
- See Interaction column and consult doctor.

 ## OVERDOSE

SYMPTOMS:
Increased side effects and adverse reactions.
WHAT TO DO:
Overdose unlikely to threaten life.
Depending on severity of symptoms and amount taken, call doctor, poison-control center or hospital emergency room for instructions.

 ## POSSIBLE ADVERSE REACTIONS OR SIDE EFFECTS

SYMPTOMS	WHAT TO DO
Life-threatening: None expected.	
Common: Constipation.	Continue. Call doctor when convenient.
Infrequent: Belching, bloating, diarrhea, mild nausea, vomiting, stomach pain.	Discontinue. Call doctor right away.
Rare:	
• Severe stomach pain; nausea; vomiting; black, tarry stool.	Discontinue. Seek emergency treatment.
• Rash, hives, dermatitis, hiccups.	Discontinue. Call doctor right away.
• Sore tongue.	Continue. Call doctor when convenient.

CHOLESTYRAMINE

WARNINGS & PRECAUTIONS

Don't take if:
You are allergic to cholestyramine.

Before you start, consult your doctor:
- If you plan to become pregnant within medication period.
- If you have angina, heart or blood-vessel disease.
- If you have stomach problems (including ulcer).
- If you have tartrazine sensitivity.
- If you have constipation or hemorrhoids.
- If you have kidney disease.

Over age 60:
Adverse reactions and side effects may be more frequent and severe than in younger persons.

Pregnancy:
No proven harm to unborn child. Avoid if possible.

Breast-feeding:
No problems expected, but consult doctor.

Infants & children:
Not recommended.

Prolonged use:
May decrease absorption of folic acid.

Skin & sunlight:
No problems expected.

Driving, piloting or hazardous work:
No problems expected.

Discontinuing:
Don't discontinue without doctor's advice until you complete prescribed dose, even though symptoms diminish or disappear.

Others:
No problems expected.

POSSIBLE INTERACTION WITH OTHER DRUGS

GENERIC NAME OR DRUG CLASS	COMBINED EFFECT
Anticoagulants, oral*	Increased anti-coagulant effect.
Digitalis preparations*	Decreased digitalis effect.
Indapamide	Decreased indapamide effect.
Thiazides*	Decreased absorption of cholestyramine.
Thyroid hormones*	Decreased thyroid effect.
Trimethoprim	Decreased absorption of cholestyramine.
Ursodiol	Decreased absorption of ursodiol.
Vitamins	Decreased absorption of fat-soluble vitamins (A,D,E,K).
All other medicines	Decreased absorption, so dosages or dosage intervals may require adjustment.

POSSIBLE INTERACTION WITH OTHER SUBSTANCES

INTERACTS WITH	COMBINED EFFECT
Alcohol:	None expected.
Beverages:	None expected.
Cocaine:	None expected.
Foods:	Absorption of vitamins in foods decreased. Take vitamin supplements, particularly A, D, E & K.
Marijuana:	None expected.
Tobacco:	None expected.

CIMETIDINE

BRAND NAMES

Apo-Cimetidine   Peptol
Novo-Cimetine   Tagamet

BASIC INFORMATION

Habit forming? No
Prescription needed? Yes
Available as generic? No
Drug class: Histamine H-2 antagonist

 ## USES

Treatment for duodenal ulcers and other conditions in which stomach produces excess hydrochloric acid.

 ## DOSAGE & USAGE INFORMATION

How to take:
Tablet or liquid—Swallow with liquid.

When to take:
- 1 dose per day—Take at bedtime.
- 2 or more doses per day—Take at the same times each day.

If you forget a dose:
Take as soon as you remember up to 2 hours late. If more than 2 hours, wait for next scheduled dose (don't double this dose).

What drug does:
Blocks histamine release so stomach secretes less acid.

Time lapse before drug works:
Begins in 30 minutes. May require several days to relieve pain.

Don't take with:
See Interaction column and consult doctor.

 ## OVERDOSE

SYMPTOMS:
Confusion, slurred speech, breathing difficulty, rapid heartbeat, delirium.
WHAT TO DO:
Overdose unlikely to threaten life. If person takes much larger amount than prescribed, call doctor, poison-control center or hospital emergency room for instructions.

 ## POSSIBLE ADVERSE REACTIONS OR SIDE EFFECTS

SYMPTOMS	WHAT TO DO
Life-threatening: None expected.	
Common: None expected.	
Infrequent:	
• Diarrhea, jaundice.	Discontinue. Call doctor right away.
• Dizziness or headache, diarrhea, decreased sperm production.	Continue. Call doctor when convenient.
• Diminished sex drive, breast swelling and soreness in males, unusual milk flow in females, hair loss.	Continue. Tell doctor at next visit.
Rare: Confusion; rash, hives; sore throat, fever; slow, fast or irregular heartbeat; unusual bleeding or bruising; muscle cramps or pain; fatigue; weakness; peripheral neuritis; chronic kidney disease.	Discontinue. Call doctor right away.

WARNINGS & PRECAUTIONS

Don't take if:
You are allergic to cimetidine or other histamine H-2 antagonist.

Before you start, consult your doctor:
- If you plan to become pregnant during medication period.
- If you take aspirin. Aspirin may irritate stomach.

Over age 60:
Adverse reactions and side effects may be more frequent and severe than in younger persons.

Pregnancy:
No proven harm to unborn child. Avoid if possible.

Breast-feeding:
No problems expected.

Infants & children:
Not recommended.

Prolonged use:
Possible liver damage.

Skin & sunlight:
No problems expected.

Driving, piloting or hazardous work:
Don't drive or pilot aircraft until you learn how medicine affects you. Don't work around dangerous machinery. Don't climb ladders or work in high places. Danger increases if you drink alcohol or take medicine affecting alertness and reflexes, such as antihistamines, tranquilizers, sedatives, pain medicine, narcotics and mind-altering drugs.

Discontinuing:
Don't discontinue without consulting doctor. Dose may require gradual reduction if you have taken drug for a long time. Doses of other drugs may also require adjustment.

Others:
Patients on kidney dialysis—Take at end of dialysis treatment.

POSSIBLE INTERACTION WITH OTHER DRUGS

GENERIC NAME OR DRUG CLASS	COMBINED EFFECT
Alprazolam	Increased effect and toxicity of alprazolam.
Antacids *	Decreased cimetidine absorption.
Anticoagulants, oral *	Increased anti-coagulant effect.
Anticholinergics *	Increased cimetidine effect.

Carbamazepine	Increased effect and toxicity of carbamazepine.
Carmustine (BCNU)	Severe impairment of red-blood-cell production; some interference with white-blood-cell formation.
Chlordiazepoxide	Increased effect and toxicity of chlordiazepoxide.
Diazepam	Increased effect and toxicity of diazepam.
Digitalis preparations *	Increased digitalis effect.
Encainide	Increased effect of cimetidine.
Flurazepam	Increased effect and toxicity of flurazepam.
Glipizide	Increased effect and toxicity of glipizide.

Continued page 1082

POSSIBLE INTERACTION WITH OTHER SUBSTANCES

INTERACTS WITH	COMBINED EFFECT
Alcohol:	No interactions expected, but alcohol may slow body's recovery. Avoid.
Beverages: Milk.	Enhanced effectiveness. Small amounts useful for taking medication.
Caffeine drinks.	May increase acid secretion and delay healing.
Cocaine:	Decreased cimetidine effect.
Foods:	Enhanced effectiveness. Protein-rich foods should be eaten in moderation to minimize secretion of stomach acid.
Marijuana:	Increased chance of low sperm count. Marijuana may slow body's recovery. Avoid.
Tobacco:	Reverses cimetidine effect. Tobacco may slow body's recovery. Avoid.

*See Glossary

CINOXACIN

BRAND NAMES

Azolinic Acid   Cinobactin
Cinobac

BASIC INFORMATION

Habit forming? No
Prescription needed? Yes
Available as generic? No
Drug class: Urinary anti-infective

USES

Treatment for urinary-tract infections.

DOSAGE & USAGE INFORMATION

How to take:
Capsules—Swallow with food or milk to lessen stomach irritation. If you can't swallow whole, open capsule and take with liquid or food.

When to take:
At the same times each day.

If you forget a dose:
Take as soon as you remember up to 2 hours late. If more than 2 hours, wait for next scheduled dose (don't double this dose).

What drug does:
Destroys bacteria susceptible to cinoxacin.

Time lapse before drug works:
1 to 2 weeks.

Don't take with:
See Interaction column and consult doctor.

OVERDOSE

SYMPTOMS:
Lethargy, stomach upset, behavioral changes, convulsions and stupor.
WHAT TO DO:
- Dial 0 (operator) or 911 (emergency) for an ambulance or medical help. Then give first aid immediately.
- If patient is unconscious and not breathing, give mouth-to-mouth breathing. If there is no heartbeat, use cardiac massage and mouth-to-mouth breathing (CPR). Don't try to make patient vomit. If you can't get help quickly, take patient to nearest emergency facility.
- See emergency information on inside covers.

POSSIBLE ADVERSE REACTIONS OR SIDE EFFECTS

SYMPTOMS	WHAT TO DO
Life-threatening: Hives, rash, intense itching, faintness soon after a dose (anaphylaxis).	Seek emergency treatment immediately.
Common: Rash, itch; decreased, blurred or double vision; halos around lights or excess brightness; changes in color vision; nausea, vomiting, diarrhea.	Discontinue. Call doctor right away.
Infrequent: Dizziness, drowsiness, headache, ringing in ears, insomnia.	Continue. Call doctor when convenient.
Rare: • Severe stomach pain, seizures, psychosis, joint pain, numbness or tingling in hands or feet (infants and children).	Discontinue. Call doctor right away.
• Headache, dizziness.	Continue. Call doctor when convenient.

WARNINGS & PRECAUTIONS

Don't take if:
- You are allergic to cinoxacin or nalidixic acid.
- You have a seizure disorder (epilepsy, convulsions).

Before you start, consult your doctor:
- If you plan to become pregnant during medication period.
- If you have or have had kidney or liver disease.
- If you have impaired circulation to the brain (hardened arteries).

Over age 60:
Adverse reactions and side effects may be more frequent and severe than in younger persons.

Pregnancy:
Risk to unborn child outweighs drug benefits. Don't use, especially during first 3 months.

Breast-feeding:
No problems expected, unless you have impaired kidney function. Consult doctor.

Infants & children:
Don't give to infants younger than 3 months.

Prolonged use:
No problems expected.

Skin & sunlight:
- May cause sunlight to hurt eyes.
- May cause rash or intensify sunburn in areas exposed to sun or sunlamp.

Driving, piloting or hazardous work:
Avoid if you feel drowsy, dizzy or have vision problems. Otherwise, no problems expected.

Discontinuing:
Don't discontinue without consulting doctor. Dose may require gradual reduction if you have taken drug for a long time. Doses of other drugs may also require adjustment.

Others:
Periodic blood counts, liver-function and kidney-function tests recommended.

POSSIBLE INTERACTION WITH OTHER DRUGS

GENERIC NAME OR DRUG CLASS	COMBINED EFFECT
Probenecid	Decreased elimination.

POSSIBLE INTERACTION WITH OTHER SUBSTANCES

INTERACTS WITH	COMBINED EFFECT
Alcohol:	Impaired alertness, judgment and coordination.
Beverages:	None expected.
Cocaine:	Impaired judgment and coordination.
Foods:	None expected.
Marijuana:	Impaired alertness, judgment and coordination.
Tobacco:	None expected.

CIPROFLOXACIN

BRAND NAMES

Cipro

BASIC INFORMATION

Habit forming? No
Prescription needed? Yes
Available as generic? No
Drug class: Antibacterial (antibiotic)

 ## USES

Treats a wide range of germs that may cause diarrhea, pneumonia, skin and soft tissue infections, urinary tract infections, bone infections.

 ## DOSAGE & USAGE INFORMATION

How to take:
Tablets—Take with full glass of water on empty stomach.

When to take:
As directed by your doctor.

If you forget a dose:
Take as soon as you remember up to 2 hours late. If more than 2 hours, wait for next scheduled dose (don't double this dose).

What drug does:
Destroys bacteria in the body, probably by promoting DNA breakage in germs.

Time lapse before drug works:
1 to 2 hours.

Don't take with:
• Food or antacids.
• See Interaction column and consult doctor.

 ## OVERDOSE

SYMPTOMS:
Convulsions.
WHAT TO DO:
• Dial 0 (operator) or 911 (emergency) for an ambulance or medical help. Then give first aid immediately.
• If patient is unconscious and not breathing, give mouth-to-mouth breathing. If there is no heartbeat, use cardiac massage and mouth-to-mouth breathing (CPR). Don't try to make patient vomit. If you can't get help quickly, take patient to nearest emergency facility.
• See emergency information on inside covers.

 ## POSSIBLE ADVERSE REACTIONS OR SIDE EFFECTS

SYMPTOMS	WHAT TO DO
Life-threatening:	
Hives, rash, intense itching, faintness soon after a dose (anaphylaxis).	Seek emergency treatment immediately.
Common:	
Abdominal discomfort, diarrhea, vomiting	Discontinue. Call doctor right away.
Infrequent:	
• Blood in urine, back pain.	Discontinue. Call doctor right away.
• Drowsiness, joint pain, skin rash, insomnia.	Continue. Call doctor when convenient.
Rare:	
Sun sensitivity.	Discontinue. Call doctor right away.

WARNINGS & PRECAUTIONS

Don't take if:
You are allergic to ciprofloxacin, nalidixic acid or norfloxacin.

Before you start, consult your doctor:
If you have any disorder of the central nervous system such as epilepsy or stroke.

Over age 60:
Adverse reactions and side effects may be more frequent and severe than in younger persons. You may need smaller doses for shorter periods of time.

Pregnancy:
Studies inconclusive on harm to unborn child. Not recommended for use during pregnancy.

Breast-feeding:
Not recommended.

Infants & children:
Not recommended.

Prolonged use:
No documented problems.

Skin & sunlight:
Rare adverse reaction to sunlight or sun lamp. Avoid over-exposure.

Driving, piloting or hazardous work:
Don't drive or pilot aircraft until you learn how medicine affects you. Don't work around dangerous machinery. Don't climb ladders or work in high places. Danger increases if you drink alcohol or take medicine affecting alertness and reflexes, such as antihistamines, tranquilizers, sedatives, pain medicine, narcotics and mind-altering drugs.

Discontinuing:
Don't discontinue without consulting doctor. Dose may require gradual reduction if you have taken drug for a long time. Doses of other drugs may also require adjustment.

Others:
May affect accuracy of laboratory test values for SGOT, serum bilirubin, serum creatinine and LDH.

POSSIBLE INTERACTION WITH OTHER DRUGS

GENERIC NAME OR DRUG CLASS	COMBINED EFFECT
Antacids*	May cause kidney dysfunction.
Carbonic anyhdrase inhibitors*	May cause kidney dysfunction.
Probenecid	May cause kidney dysfunction.
Theophylline	May increase possibility of central nervous system poisoning, such as nausea, vomiting, restlessness, palpitations.

POSSIBLE INTERACTION WITH OTHER SUBSTANCES

INTERACTS WITH	COMBINED EFFECT
Alcohol:	Increased possibility of central nervous system poisoning.
Beverages:	None expected.
Cocaine:	Increased possibility of central nervous system poisoning.
Foods:	None expected.
Marijuana:	Increased possibility of central nervous system poisoning.
Tobacco:	Increased possibility of central nervous system poisoning.

CITRATES

BRAND AND GENERIC NAMES

Albright's Solution
Bicitra
Citrolith
Modified Shohl's
   Solution
Oracit
Polycitra
Polycitra-K
Polycitra-LC-
   Sugar-free
POTASSIUM
   CITRATE

POTASSIUM
   CITRATE &
   CITRIC ACID
POTASSIUM
   CITRATE &
   SODIUM CITRATE
SODIUM CITRATE &
   CITRIC ACID
TRICITRATES
Urocit-K

BASIC INFORMATION

Habit forming? No
Prescription needed? Yes
Available as generic? No
Drug class: Urinary alkalizer, anti-urolithic
   (kidney stone)

 USES

- To make urine more alkaline (less acid).
- To treat or prevent recurrence of some types
  of kidney stones.

 DOSAGE & USAGE INFORMATION

How to take:
Liquid—Swallow with liquid.

When to take:
On full stomach, usually after meals or with food.

If you forget a dose:
Take as soon as you remember up to 2 hours
late. If more than 2 hours, wait for next
scheduled dose (don't double this dose).

Continued next column

 OVERDOSE

SYMPTOMS:
Convulsions, coma.
WHAT TO DO:
- Dial 0 (operator) or 911 (emergency) for
  an ambulance or medical help. Then give
  first aid immediately.
- See emergency information on inside
  covers.

What drug does:
Increases urinary alkalinity by excretion of
bicarbonate ions.

Time lapse before drug works:
1 hour.

Don't take with:
- Any medicine that will decrease mental
  alertness or reflexes, such as alcohol, other
  mind-altering drugs, cough/cold medicines,
  antihistamines, allergy medicine, sedatives,
  tranquilizers (sleeping pills or "downers"),
  barbiturates, seizure medicine, narcotics, other
  prescription medicine for pain, muscle
  relaxants, anesthetics.
- See Interaction column and consult doctor.

 POSSIBLE ADVERSE REACTIONS OR SIDE EFFECTS

SYMPTOMS	WHAT TO DO
Life-threatening:	
Black, tarry stools; vomiting blood; severe abdominal cramps; irregular heartbeat; shortness of breath.	Discontinue. Seek emergency treatment.
Common:	
Nausea or vomiting.	Continue. Call doctor when convenient.
Infrequent:	
Confusion, dizziness, swollen feet and ankles, irritability, depression, muscle pain, nervousness, numbness or tingling in hands or feet, unpleasant taste, weakness.	Discontinue. Call doctor right away.
Rare:	
Increases potassium.	Monitor potassium with frequent laboratory studies.

WARNINGS & PRECAUTIONS

Don't take if:
You are allergic to any citrate.

Before you start, consult your doctor:
- If you have any disease involving the adrenal glands, diabetes, chronic diarrhea, heart problems, hypertension, kidney disease, stomach ulcer or gastritis, urinary tract infection, toxemia of pregnancy.
- If you plan strenuous exercise.

Over age 60:
Adverse reactions and side effects may be more frequent and severe than in younger persons. Ask doctor about smaller doses.

Pregnancy:
Safety to unborn child unestablished. Avoid if possible.

Breast-feeding:
Safety during lactation not established. Consult doctor.

Infants & children:
Use only under close medical supervision.

Prolonged use:
Adverse reactions more likely.

Skin & sunlight:
No problems expected.

Driving, piloting or hazardous work:
Don't drive or pilot aircraft until you learn how medicine affects you. Don't work around dangerous machinery. Don't climb ladders or work in high places. Danger increases if you drink alcohol or take medicine affecting alertness and reflexes, such as antihistamines, tranquilizers, sedatives, pain medicine, narcotics and mind-altering drugs.

Discontinuing:
Don't discontinue without consulting doctor. Dose may require gradual reduction if you have taken drug for a long time. Doses of other drugs may also require adjustment.

Others:
- Drink at least 8 ounces of water or other liquid (except milk) every hour while awake.
- Liquid may be chilled (don't freeze) to improve taste.

 ## POSSIBLE INTERACTION WITH OTHER DRUGS

GENERIC NAME OR DRUG CLASS	COMBINED EFFECT
Amphetamines*	Increased amphetamine effect.
Antacids*	Toxic effect of citrates (alkalosis).
Calcium supplements*	Increases risk of kidney stones.
Methenamine	Decreases effects of methenamine.
Mexiletine	May slow elimination of mexiletine and cause need to adjust dosage.
Quinidine	Prolongs quinidine effect.

 ## POSSIBLE INTERACTION WITH OTHER SUBSTANCES

INTERACTS WITH	COMBINED EFFECT
Alcohol:	Will decrease mental alertness.
Beverages: Salt-free milk.	May cause potassium toxicity.
Cocaine:	No proven problems.
Foods: Milk, cheese, ice cream, yogurt, buttermilk, salty foods, salt, salt substitutes.	May increase likelihood of kidney stones.
Marijuana:	No proven problems.
Tobacco:	Increases likelihood of stomach irritation.

CLEMASTINE

BRAND NAMES

Tavist

BASIC INFORMATION

Habit forming? No
Prescription needed? No
Available as generic? No
Drug class: Antihistamine

 ## USES

Reduces allergic symptoms such as hay fever, hives, rash or itching.

 ## DOSAGE & USAGE INFORMATION

How to take:
Tablet or syrup—Swallow with liquid or food to lessen stomach irritation.

When to take:
Varies with form. Follow label directions.

If you forget a dose:
Take as soon as you remember up to 2 hours late. If more than 2 hours, wait for next scheduled dose (don't double this dose).

What drug does:
Blocks action of histamine after an allergic response triggers histamine release in sensitive cells.

Time lapse before drug works:
30 minutes.

Don't take with:
See Interaction column and consult doctor.

 ## OVERDOSE

SYMPTOMS:
Convulsions, red face, hallucinations, coma.
WHAT TO DO:
- **Dial 0 (operator) or 911 (emergency) for an ambulance or medical help. Then give first aid immediately.**
- **If patient is unconscious and not breathing, give mouth-to-mouth breathing. If there is no heartbeat, use cardiac massage and mouth-to-mouth breathing (CPR). Don't try to make patient vomit. If you can't get help quickly, take patient to nearest emergency facility.**
- **See emergency information on inside covers.**

 ## POSSIBLE ADVERSE REACTIONS OR SIDE EFFECTS

SYMPTOMS	WHAT TO DO
Life-threatening: None expected.	
Common: Drowsiness; dizziness; dry mouth, nose, throat; nausea.	Continue. Tell doctor at next visit.
Infrequent: • Vision changes.	Discontinue. Call doctor right away.
• Less tolerance for contact lenses; difficult urination.	Continue. Call doctor when convenient.
• Appetite loss.	Continue. Tell doctor at next visit.
Rare: Nightmares, agitation, irritability; sore throat, fever; rapid heartbeat; unusual bleeding or bruising; fatigue, weakness.	Discontinue. Call doctor right away.

WARNINGS & PRECAUTIONS

Don't take if:
You are allergic to any antihistamine.

Before you start, consult your doctor:
- If you have glaucoma.
- If you have enlarged prostate.
- If you have asthma.
- If you have kidney disease.
- If you have peptic ulcer.
- If you will have surgery within 2 months, including dental surgery, requiring general or spinal anesthesia.

Over age 60:
Don't exceed recommended dose. Adverse reactions and side effects may be more frequent and severe than in younger persons, especially urination difficulty, diminished alertness and other brain and nervous-system symptoms.

Pregnancy:
No proven harm to unborn child. Avoid if possible.

Breast-feeding:
Drug passes into milk. Avoid drug or discontinue nursing until you finish medicine. Consult doctor for advice on maintaining milk supply.

Infants & children:
Not recommended for premature or newborn infants. Otherwise, no problems expected.

Prolonged use:
Avoid. May damage bone marrow and nerve cells.

Skin & sunlight:
May cause rash or intensify sunburn in areas exposed to sun or sunlamp.

Driving, piloting or hazardous work:
Don't drive or pilot aircraft until you learn how medicine affects you. Don't work around dangerous machinery. Don't climb ladders or work in high places. Danger increases if you drink alcohol or take medicine affecting alertness and reflexes, such as antihistamines, tranquilizers, sedatives, pain medicine, narcotics and mind-altering drugs.

Discontinuing:
No problems expected.

Others:
May mask symptoms of hearing damage from aspirin, other salicylates, cisplatin, paromomycin, vancomycin or anticonvulsants. Consult doctor if you use these.

POSSIBLE INTERACTION WITH OTHER DRUGS

GENERIC NAME OR DRUG CLASS	COMBINED EFFECT
Anticholinergics*	Increased anti-cholinergic effect.
Antidepressants*	Excess sedation. Avoid.
Antihistamines, other*	Excess sedation. Avoid.
Carteolol	Decreased anti-histamine effect.
Dronabinol	Increased effects of both drugs. Avoid.
Hypnotics*	Excess sedation. Avoid.
MAO inhibitors*	Increased clemastine effect.
Mind-altering drugs*	Excess sedation. Avoid.
Molindone	Increased antihistamine effect.
Nabilone	Greater depression of central nervous system.
Narcotics*	Excess sedation. Avoid.
Sedatives*	Excess sedation. Avoid.
Sleep inducers*	Excess sedation. Avoid.
Sotalol	Increased antihistamine effect.
Tranquilizers*	Excess sedation. Avoid.

POSSIBLE INTERACTION WITH OTHER SUBSTANCES

INTERACTS WITH	COMBINED EFFECT
Alcohol:	Excess sedation. Avoid.
Beverages: Caffeine drinks.	Less clemastine sedation.
Cocaine:	Decreased clemastine effect. Avoid.
Foods:	None expected.
Marijuana:	Excess sedation. Avoid.
Tobacco:	None expected.

*See Glossary

CLIDINIUM

BRAND NAMES

Clipoxide   Quarzan
Librax

BASIC INFORMATION

Habit forming? No
Prescription needed?
  Low strength: No
  High strength: Yes
Available as generic? No
Drug class: Antispasmodic, anticholinergic

 ## USES

Reduces spasms of digestive system, bladder
and urethra.

 ## DOSAGE & USAGE INFORMATION

How to take:
Capsule—Swallow with liquid or food to lessen
stomach irritation.

When to take:
30 minutes before meals (unless directed
otherwise by doctor).

If you forget a dose:
Take as soon as you remember up to 2 hours
late. If more than 2 hours, wait for next
scheduled dose (don't double this dose).

What drug does:
Blocks nerve impulses at parasympathetic nerve
endings, preventing muscle contractions and
gland secretions of organs involved.

Time lapse before drug works:
15 to 30 minutes.

Don't take with:
See Interaction column and consult doctor.

 ## OVERDOSE

SYMPTOMS:
**Dilated pupils, rapid pulse and breathing,
dizziness, fever, hallucinations, confusion,
slurred speech, agitation, flushed face,
convulsions, coma.**
WHAT TO DO:
- **Dial 0 (operator) or 911 (emergency) for
  an ambulance or medical help. Then give
  first aid immediately.**
- **See emergency information on inside
  covers.**

 ## POSSIBLE ADVERSE REACTIONS OR SIDE EFFECTS

SYMPTOMS	WHAT TO DO
Life-threatening:	
None expected.	
Common:	
• Confusion, delirium, rapid heartbeat.	Discontinue. Call doctor right away.
• Nausea, vomiting, decreased sweating.	Continue. Call doctor when convenient.
• Constipation.	Continue. Tell doctor at next visit.
• Dryness in ears, nose, throat.	No action necessary.
Infrequent:	
• Nasal congestion, altered taste.	Discontinue. Call doctor right away.
• Difficult urination, headache, impotence.	Continue. Call doctor when convenient.
Rare:	
Rash or hives, pain, blurred vision.	Discontinue. Call doctor right away.

WARNINGS & PRECAUTIONS

Don't take if:
- You are allergic to any anticholinergic.
- You have trouble with stomach bloating.
- You have difficulty emptying your bladder completely.
- You have narrow-angle glaucoma.
- You have severe ulcerative colitis.

Before you start, consult your doctor:
- If you have open-angle glaucoma.
- If you have angina, chronic bronchitis or asthma, hiatal hernia, liver disease, enlarged prostate, myasthenia gravis, peptic ulcer.
- If you will have surgery within 2 months, including dental surgery, requiring general or spinal anesthesia.

Over age 60:
Adverse reactions and side effects may be more frequent and severe than in younger persons.

Pregnancy:
Studies inconclusive on harm to unborn child. Animal studies show fetal abnormalities. Decide with your doctor whether drug benefits justify risk to unborn child.

Breast-feeding:
Drug passes into milk and decreases milk flow. Avoid drug or discontinue nursing until you finish medicine. Consult doctor for advice on maintaining milk supply.

Infants & children:
Use only under medical supervision.

Prolonged use:
Chronic constipation, possible fecal impaction. Consult doctor immediately.

Skin & sunlight:
No problems expected.

Driving, piloting or hazardous work:
Don't drive or pilot aircraft until you learn how medicine affects you. Don't work around dangerous machinery. Don't climb ladders or work in high places. Danger increases if you drink alcohol or take medicine affecting alertness and reflexes, such as antihistamines, tranquilizers, sedatives, pain medicine, narcotics, or mind-altering drugs.

Discontinuing:
May be unnecessary to finish medicine. Follow doctor's instructions.

Others:
No problems expected.

POSSIBLE INTERACTION WITH OTHER DRUGS

GENERIC NAME OR DRUG CLASS	COMBINED EFFECT
Amantadine	Increased clidinium effect.
Antacids*	Decreased clidinium effect.
Anticholinergics, other*	Increased clidinium effect.
Antidepressants, tricyclic (TCA)*	Increased clidinium effect. Increased sedation.
Antihistamines*	Increased clidinium effect.
Haloperidol	Increased internal-eye pressure.
MAO inhibitors*	Increased clidinium effect.
Meperidine	Increased clidinium effect.
Methylphenidate	Increased clidinium effect.
Molindone	Increased anti-cholinergic effect.
Nitrates*	Increased internal-eye pressure.
Nizatidine	Increased nizatidine effect.
Orphenadrine	Increased clidinium effect.
Phenothiazines*	Increased clidinium effect.

Continued page 1082

POSSIBLE INTERACTION WITH OTHER SUBSTANCES

INTERACTS WITH	COMBINED EFFECT
Alcohol:	None expected.
Beverages:	None expected.
Cocaine:	Excessively rapid heartbeat. Avoid.
Foods:	None expected.
Marijuana:	Drowsiness and dry mouth.
Tobacco:	None expected.

CLINDAMYCIN

BRAND NAMES

Cleocin   Dalacin C
Cleocin-T

BASIC INFORMATION

Habit forming? No
Prescription needed? Yes
Available as generic? No
Drug class: Antibiotic (lincomycin)

 USES

- Treatment of bacterial infections that are susceptible to clindamycin.
- Topical treatment for acne. Follow instructions on package.

 DOSAGE & USAGE INFORMATION

How to take:
Capsule or liquid—Swallow with liquid 1 hour before or 2 hours after eating.

When to take:
At the same times each day.

If you forget a dose:
Take as soon as you remember up to 2 hours late. If more than 2 hours, wait for next scheduled dose (don't double this dose).

What drug does:
Destroys susceptible bacteria. Does not kill viruses.

Time lapse before drug works:
3 to 5 days.

Don't take with:
See Interaction column and consult doctor.

 OVERDOSE

SYMPTOMS:
Severe nausea, vomiting, diarrhea.
WHAT TO DO:
Overdose unlikely to threaten life. If person takes much larger amount than prescribed, call doctor, poison-control center or hospital emergency room for instructions.

 POSSIBLE ADVERSE REACTIONS OR SIDE EFFECTS

SYMPTOMS	WHAT TO DO
Life-threatening:	
Hives, wheezing, faintness (rarely) itching, coma.	Seek emergency treatment immediately.
Common:	
None expected.	
Infrequent:	
• Unusual thirst; vomiting; stomach cramps; severe and watery diarrhea with blood or mucus; weight loss, painful, swollen joints; fever; jaundice; tiredness; weakness.	Discontinue. Call doctor right away.
• White patches in mouth; rash, itch around groin, rectum or armpits; vaginal discharge, itching.	Continue. Call doctor when convenient.
Rare:	
Agranulocytosis, leukopenia (low white blood cells causing sore throat and fever).	Discontinue. Call doctor right away.

WARNINGS & PRECAUTIONS

Don't take if:
- You are allergic to lincomycins.
- You have had ulcerative colitis.
- Prescribed for infant under 1 month old.

Before you start, consult your doctor:
- If you have had yeast infections of mouth, skin or vagina.
- If you will have surgery within 2 months, including dental surgery, requiring general or spinal anesthesia.
- If you have kidney or liver disease.
- If you have allergies of any kind.

Over age 60:
Adverse reactions and side effects may be more frequent and severe than in younger persons.

Pregnancy:
Risk to unborn child outweighs drug benefits. Don't use.

Breast-feeding:
Drug passes into milk. Avoid drug or discontinue nursing until you finish medicine. Consult doctor for advice on maintaining milk supply.

Infants & children:
Don't give to infants younger than 1 month. Use for children only under medical supervision.

Prolonged use:
- Severe colitis with diarrhea and bleeding.
- You may become more susceptible to infections caused by germs not responsive to clindamycin.

Skin & sunlight:
No problems expected.

Driving, piloting or hazardous work:
No problems expected.

Discontinuing:
Don't discontinue without doctor's advice until you complete prescribed dose, even though symptoms diminish or disappear.

Others:
No problems expected.

 ## POSSIBLE INTERACTION WITH OTHER DRUGS

GENERIC NAME OR DRUG CLASS	COMBINED EFFECT
Antidiarrheal preparations*	Decreased clindamycin effect.
Chloramphenicol	Decreased clindamycin effect.
Diphenoxylate	May delay removal of toxins from colon in cases of diarrhea caused by side effects of clindamycin.
Erythromycin	Decreased clindamycin effect.
Loperamide	May delay removal of toxins from colon in cases of diarrhea caused by side effects of clindamycin.
Muscle blocking drugs*	Increased actions of muscle blockers.

 ## POSSIBLE INTERACTION WITH OTHER SUBSTANCES

INTERACTS WITH	COMBINED EFFECT
Alcohol:	None expected.
Beverages:	None expected.
Cocaine:	None expected.
Foods:	None expected.
Marijuana:	None expected.
Tobacco:	None expected.

*See Glossary

CLOFIBRATE

BRAND NAMES

Atromid-S	Liprinal
Claripex	Novofibrate

BASIC INFORMATION

Habit forming? No
Prescription needed? Yes
Available as generic? Yes
Drug class: Antihyperlipidemic

USES

Reduces fatty substances in the blood (triglycerides).

DOSAGE & USAGE INFORMATION

How to take:
Capsule—Swallow with liquid or food to lessen stomach irritation.

When to take:
At the same times each day.

If you forget a dose:
Take as soon as you remember up to 2 hours late. If more than 2 hours, wait for next scheduled dose (don't double this dose).

What drug does:
Inhibits formation of fatty substances.

Time lapse before drug works:
3 months or more.

Don't take with:
See Interaction column and consult doctor.

OVERDOSE

SYMPTOMS:
Diarrhea, headache, muscle pain.
WHAT TO DO:
Overdose unlikely to threaten life. If person takes much larger amount than prescribed, call doctor, poison-control center or hospital emergency room for instructions.

POSSIBLE ADVERSE REACTIONS OR SIDE EFFECTS

SYMPTOMS	WHAT TO DO
Life-threatening:	
None expected.	
Common:	
None expected.	
Infrequent:	
• Chest pain, shortness of breath, irregular heartbeat, gallstones, nausea, flu-like illness.	Discontinue. Call doctor right away.
• Vomiting, diarrhea, stomach pain.	Continue. Call doctor when convenient.
Rare:	
• Cardiac arrythmias, angina.	Discontinue. Seek emergency treatment.
• Rash, itch; mouth or lip sores; sore throat; swollen feet, legs; blood in urine; painful urination; fever; chills, anemia.	Discontinue. Call doctor right away.
• Dizziness, weakness, drowsiness, muscle cramps, headache, dryness, diminished sex drive, hair loss.	Continue. Call doctor when convenient.

WARNINGS & PRECAUTIONS

Don't take if:
- You are allergic to any clofibrate.
- You have had serious liver disease.

Before you start, consult your doctor:
- If you have had liver or kidney disease.
- If you have had peptic-ulcer disease.
- If you have diabetes.

Over age 60:
Adverse reactions and side effects may be more frequent and severe than in younger persons. May develop flu-like symptoms.

Pregnancy:
Risk to unborn child outweighs drug benefits. Don't use.

Breast-feeding:
May harm child. Avoid.

Infants & children:
Not recommended.

Prolonged use:
- May cause gall bladder infection.
- Possible cause of stomach cancer.

Skin & sunlight:
No problems expected.

Driving, piloting or hazardous work:
Avoid if you feel drowsy or dizzy. Otherwise, no problems expected.

Discontinuing:
Don't discontinue without doctor's advice until you complete prescribed dose, even though symptoms diminish or disappear.

Others:
- Periodic blood-cell counts and liver-function studies recommended if you take clofibrate for a long time.
- Some studies question effectiveness. Many studies warn against toxicity.

POSSIBLE INTERACTION WITH OTHER DRUGS

GENERIC NAME OR DRUG CLASS	COMBINED EFFECT
Anticoagulants, oral*	Increased anticoagulant effect. Dose reduction of anticoagulant necessary.
Antidiabetics, oral*	Increased antidiabetic effect.
Contraceptives, oral*	Decreased clofibrate effect.
Estrogens*	Decreased clofibrate effect.
Furosemide	Possible toxicity of both drugs.
Insulin	Increased insulin effect.
Probenecid	Increased effect and toxicity of clofibrate.
Thyroid hormones*	Increased clofibrate effect.
Ursodiol	Decreased effect of ursodiol.

POSSIBLE INTERACTION WITH OTHER SUBSTANCES

INTERACTS WITH	COMBINED EFFECT
Alcohol:	None expected.
Beverages:	None expected.
Cocaine:	None expected.
Foods: Fatty foods.	Decreased clofibrate effect.
Marijuana:	None expected.
Tobacco:	None expected.

CLOMIPHENE

BRAND NAMES

Clomid   Serophene

BASIC INFORMATION

Habit forming? No
Prescription needed? Yes
Available as generic? No
Drug class: Gonad stimulant

 USES

- Treatment for men with low sperm counts.
- Treatment for ovulatory failure in women who wish to become pregnant.

 DOSAGE & USAGE INFORMATION

How to take:
Tablet—Swallow with liquid.

When to take:
- Men—Take at the same time each day.
- Women—If you are to begin treatment on "Day 5," count your first menstrual day as "Day 1." Take a tablet each day for 5 days.

If you forget a dose:
Take as soon as you remember. If you forget a day, double next dose. If you miss 2 or more doses, consult doctor.

What drug does:
Antiestrogen effect stimulates ovulation and sperm production.

Time lapse before drug works:
Usually 3 to 6 months. Ovulation may occur 6 to 10 days after last day of treatment in any cycle.

Don't take with:
No restrictions.

 OVERDOSE

SYMPTOMS:
Increased severity of adverse reactions and side effects.
WHAT TO DO:
Overdose unlikely to threaten life. If person takes much larger amount than prescribed, call doctor, poison-control center or hospital emergency room for instructions.

 POSSIBLE ADVERSE REACTIONS OR SIDE EFFECTS

SYMPTOMS	WHAT TO DO
Life-threatening: None expected.	
Common:	
• Bloating, stomach pain, pelvic pain.	Discontinue. Call doctor right away.
• Hot flashes.	Continue. Tell doctor at next visit.
Infrequent:	
• Rash, itch, vomiting, jaundice.	Discontinue. Call doctor right away.
• Constipation, diarrhea, increased appetite, heavy menstrual flow, frequent urination, breast discomfort, weight change, hair loss, nausea.	Continue. Call doctor when convenient.
Rare:	
• Vision changes.	Discontinue. Call doctor right away.
• Dizziness, headache, tiredness, depression, nervousness.	Continue. Call doctor when convenient.

WARNINGS & PRECAUTIONS

Don't take if:
You are allergic to clomiphene.

Before you start, consult your doctor:
- If you have an ovarian cyst, fibroid uterine tumors or unusual vaginal bleeding.
- If you have inflamed veins caused by blood clots.
- If you have liver disease.
- If you are depressed.

Over age 60:
Not recommended.

Pregnancy:
Stop taking at first sign of pregnancy.

Breast-feeding:
Not used.

Infants & children:
Not used.

Prolonged use:
Not recommended.

Skin & sunlight:
No problems expected.

Driving, piloting or hazardous work:
- Avoid if you feel dizzy.
- May cause blurred vision.

Discontinuing:
May be unnecessary to finish medicine. Follow doctor's instructions.

Others:
- Have a complete pelvic examination before treatment.
- If you become pregnant, twins or triplets are possible.

POSSIBLE INTERACTION WITH OTHER DRUGS

GENERIC NAME OR DRUG CLASS	COMBINED EFFECT
Thyroglobulin	May increase serum thyroglobulin.
Thyroxine (T-4)	May increase serum thyroxine.

POSSIBLE INTERACTION WITH OTHER SUBSTANCES

INTERACTS WITH	COMBINED EFFECT
Alcohol:	None expected.
Beverages:	None expected.
Cocaine:	None expected.
Foods:	None expected.
Marijuana:	None expected.
Tobacco:	None expected.

CLONIDINE

BRAND NAMES

Catapres
Catapres-TTS

Combipres
Dixarit

BASIC INFORMATION

Habit forming? No
Prescription needed? Yes
Available as generic? Yes
Drug class: Antihypertensive

 ## USES

- Treatment of high blood pressure and congestive heart failure.
- Treatment of dysmenorrhea and menopausal "hot flashes."
- Treatment of narcotic withdrawal syndrome.
- Prevention of vascular headaches.

 ## DOSAGE & USAGE INFORMATION

How to take:
- Tablet—Swallow with liquid.
- Patches that attach to skin—Apply to clean, dry, hairless skin on arm or trunk.

When to take:
Daily dose at bedtime.

If you forget a dose:
Bedtime dose—If you forget your once-a-day dose, take it as soon as you remember. *Don't* double dose.

What drug does:
Relaxes and allows expansion of blood vessel walls.

Continued next column

 ## OVERDOSE

SYMPTOMS:
Vomiting, fainting, slow heartbeat, coma, diminished reflexes.
WHAT TO DO:
- **Dial 0 (operator) or 911 (emergency) for an ambulance or medical help. Then give first aid immediately.**
- **If patient is unconscious and not breathing, give mouth-to-mouth breathing. If there is no heartbeat, use cardiac massage and mouth-to-mouth breathing (CPR). Don't try to make patient vomit. If you can't get help quickly, take patient to nearest emergency facility.**
- **See emergency information on inside covers.**

Time lapse before drug works:
1 to 3 hours.

Don't take with:
- Non-prescription medicines containing alcohol.
- See Interaction column and consult doctor.

 ## POSSIBLE ADVERSE REACTIONS OR SIDE EFFECTS

SYMPTOMS	WHAT TO DO
Life-threatening: None expected.	
Common:	
• Dizziness, weight gain, drowsiness, lightheadedness upon rising from sitting or lying, swollen breasts.	Continue. Call doctor when convenient.
• Dry mouth.	Continue. Tell doctor at next visit.
Infrequent:	
• Abnormal heart rhythm.	Discontinue. Call doctor right away.
• Headache; painful glands in neck; nightmares; nausea; vomiting; cold fingers and toes; dry, burning eyes.	Continue. Call doctor when convenient.
• Insomnia, constipation, appetite loss, diminished sex drive.	Continue. Tell doctor at next visit.
Rare:	
• Rash, itch.	Discontinue. Call doctor right away.
• Depression.	Continue. Call doctor when convenient.

 ## WARNINGS & PRECAUTIONS

Don't take if:
- You are allergic to any alpha-adrenergic blocker.
- You are under age 12.

Before you start, consult your doctor:
- If you will have surgery within 2 months, including dental surgery, requiring general or spinal anesthesia.
- If you have heart disease or chronic kidney disease.
- If you have a peripheral circulation disorder (intermittent claudication, Buerger's disease).
- If you have history of depression.

Over age 60:
Adverse reactions and side effects may be more frequent and severe than in younger persons.

Pregnancy:
Studies inconclusive on harm to unborn child. Animal studies show fetal abnormalities. Decide with your doctor whether drug benefits justify risk to unborn child.

Breast-feeding:
Unknown whether safe or not. Consult doctor.

Infants & children:
Use only under careful medical supervision after age 12. Avoid before age 12.

Prolonged use:
- Don't discontinue without consulting doctor. Dose may require gradual reduction if you have taken drug for a long time. Doses of other drugs may also require adjustment.
- Continued use may cause fluid retention, requiring addition of diuretic to treatment program.
- Request yearly eye examinations.

Skin & sunlight:
No problems expected.

Driving, piloting or hazardous work:
Don't drive or pilot aircraft until you learn how medicine affects you. Don't work around dangerous machinery. Don't climb ladders or work in high places. Danger increases if you drink alcohol or take medicine affecting alertness and reflexes.

Discontinuing:
Don't discontinue abruptly. May cause rebound high blood pressure, anxiety, chest pain, insomnia, headache, nausea, irregular heartbeat, flushed face, sweating.

Others:
No problems expected.

POSSIBLE INTERACTION WITH OTHER DRUGS

GENERIC NAME OR DRUG CLASS	COMBINED EFFECT
ACE Inhibitors: captopril, enalapril, lisinopril*	Possible excessive potassium in blood.
Antidepressants, tricyclic (TCA)*	Decreased clonidine effect.
Antihypertensives, other*	Excessive blood-pressure drop.
Appetite suppressants*	Decreased clonidine effect.
Beta-adrenergic blockers*	Possible precipitous change in blood pressure.
Carteolol	Increased antihypertensive effect.
Diuretics*	Excessive blood-pressure drop.
Ethinamate	Dangerous increased effects of ethinamate. Avoid combining.
Fenfluramine	Possible increased clonidine effect.
Fluoxetine	Increased depressant effects of both drugs.
Guanfacine	Blood-pressure control impaired.
Leucovorin	High alcohol content of leucovorin may cause adverse effects.
Methyprylon	Increased sedative effect, perhaps to dangerous level. Avoid.
Nabilone	Greater depression of central nervous system.
Nicardipine	Blood-pressure drop. Dosages may require adjustment.
Nitrates*	Possible excessive blood-pressure drop.
Sotalol	Increased antihypertensive effect.
Terazosin	Decreases effectiveness of terazosin.

POSSIBLE INTERACTION WITH OTHER SUBSTANCES

INTERACTS WITH	COMBINED EFFECT
Alcohol:	Increased sensitivity to sedative effect of alcohol and very low blood pressure. Avoid.
Beverages: Caffeine-containing drinks.	Decreased clonidine effect.
Cocaine	Increased risk of heart block and high blood pressure.
Foods:	No problems expected.
Marijuana:	Weakness on standing.
Tobacco:	No problems expected.

CLONIDINE & CHLORTHALIDONE

BRAND NAMES

Combipres

BASIC INFORMATION

Habit forming? No
Prescription needed? Yes
Available as generic? No
Drug class: Antihypertensive

USES

- Treatment of high blood pressure.
- Reduces fluid retention (edema) caused by conditions such as heart disorders and liver disease.

DOSAGE & USAGE INFORMATION

How to take:
Tablet—Swallow with liquid. If you can't swallow whole, crumble tablet and take with liquid or food. Don't exceed dose.

When to take:
At the same time each day.

If you forget a dose:
Take as soon as you remember up to 2 hours late. If more than 2 hours, wait for next scheduled dose (don't double this dose).

What drug does:
- Relaxes and allows expansion of blood vessel walls.

Continued next column

OVERDOSE

SYMPTOMS:
Vomiting; fainting; rapid, irregular, slow heartbeat; diminished reflexes; cramps; weakness; drowsiness; weak pulse; coma.
WHAT TO DO:
- **Dial 0 (operator) or 911 (emergency) for an ambulance or medical help. Then give first aid immediately.**
- **If patient is unconscious and not breathing, give mouth-to-mouth breathing. If there is no heartbeat, use cardiac massage and mouth-to-mouth breathing (CPR). Don't try to make patient vomit. If you can't get help quickly, take patient to nearest emergency facility.**
- **See emergency information on inside covers.**

- Forces sodium and water excretion, reducing body fluid.
- Reduced body fluid and relaxed arteries lower blood pressure.

Time lapse before drug works:
4 to 6 hours. May require several weeks to lower blood pressure.

Don't take with:
Any medicine that will decrease mental alertness such as alcohol, antihistamines, cold/cough medicines, sedatives, tranquilizers, narcotics, prescription pain medicine, barbiturates, seizure medicine, anesthetics.

POSSIBLE ADVERSE REACTIONS OR SIDE EFFECTS

SYMPTOMS	WHAT TO DO
Life-threatening: Irregular heartbeat, weak pulse.	Discontinue. Seek emergency treatment.
Common: Dry mouth, increased thirst, muscle cramps, nausea or vomiting, mood changes, drowsiness.	Discontinue. Call doctor right away.
Infrequent: Vomiting, diminished sex desire and performance, insomnia, dizziness, diarrhea, constipaion, appetite loss.	Continue. Call doctor when convenient.
Rare: • Jaundice; easy bruising or bleeding; sore throat, fever, mouth ulcers; rash or hives; joint pain; flank pain; abdominal pain.	Discontinue. Call doctor right away.
• Cold fingers and toes, nightmares, vomiting.	Continue. Call doctor when convenient.

WARNINGS & PRECAUTIONS

Don't take if:
- You are allergic to any thiazide diuretic drug or alpha-adrenergic blocker.
- You are under age 12.

Before you start, consult your doctor:
- If you are allergic to any sulfa drug.
- If you have gout, liver, pancreas or kidney disorder, a peripheral circulation disorder (intermittent claudication, Buerger's disease), history of depression, heart disease.

- If you will have surgery within 2 months, including dental surgery, requiring general or spinal anesthesia.

Over age 60:
Adverse reactions and side effects may be more frequent and severe than in younger persons, especially dizziness and excessive potassium loss.

Pregnancy:
Risk to unborn child outweighs drug benefits. Don't use.

Breast-feeding:
Drug passes into milk. Avoid drug or discontinue nursing until you finish medicine. Consult doctor for advice on maintaining milk supply.

Infants & children:
Use only after careful medical supervision after age 12. Avoid before age 12.

Prolonged use:
- Don't discontinue without consulting doctor. Dose may require gradual reduction if you have taken drug for a long time. Doses of other drugs may also require adjustment.
- Continued use may cause fluid retention, requiring addition of diuretic to treatment program.
- Request yearly eye examinations.

Skin & sunlight:
May cause rash or intensify sunburn in areas exposed to sun or sunlamp.

Driving, piloting or hazardous work:
Don't drive or pilot aircraft until you learn how medicine affects you. Don't work around dangerous machinery. Don't climb ladders or work in high places. Danger increases if you drink alcohol or take medicine affecting alertness and reflexes, such as antihistamines, tranquilizers, sedatives, pain medicine, narcotics and mind-altering drugs.

Discontinuing:
Don't discontinue abruptly. May cause rebound high blood pressure, anxiety, chest pain, insomnia, headache, nausea, irregular heartbeat, flushed face, sweating.

Others:
- Hot weather and fever may cause dehydration and drop in blood pressure. Dose may require temporary adjustment. Weigh daily and report any unexpected weight decreases to your doctor.
- May cause rise in uric acid, leading to gout.
- May cause blood-sugar rise in diabetics.

 ## POSSIBLE INTERACTION WITH OTHER DRUGS

GENERIC NAME OR DRUG CLASS	COMBINED EFFECT
ACE inhibitors: captopril, enalapril, lisinopril*	Possible excessive potassium in blood.
Allopurinol	Decreased allopurinol effect.
Antidepressants, tricyclic (TCA)*	Dangerous drop in blood pressure. Avoid combination unless under medical supervision.
Antihypertensives, other*	Excessive blood pressure drop.
Appetite suppressants*	Decreased clonidine effect.
Barbiturates*	Increased chlorthalidone effect.
Beta-adrenergic blockers*	Possible precipitous change in blood pressure.
Carteolol	Increased antihypertensive effect.

Continued page 1083

 ## POSSIBLE INTERACTION WITH OTHER SUBSTANCES

INTERACTS WITH	COMBINED EFFECT
Alcohol:	Increased sensitivity to sedative effect of alcohol and very low blood pressure. Avoid.
Beverages: Caffeine-containing drinks.	Decreased clonidine effect.
Cocaine	Increased risk of heart block and high blood pressure.
Foods: Licorice.	Excessive potassium loss that causes dangerous heart rhythm.
Marijuana:	Weakness on standing. May increase blood pressure.
Tobacco:	None expected.

CLORAZEPATE

BRAND NAMES

Novoclopate
Tranxene

Tranxene-SD
Tranxene T-Tab

BASIC INFORMATION

Habit forming? Yes
Prescription needed? Yes
Available as generic? Yes
Drug class: Tranquilizer (benzodiazepine)

USES

- Treatment for nervousness or tension.
- Treatment for convulsive disorders.

DOSAGE & USAGE INFORMATION

How to take:
Tablet or capsule—Swallow with liquid. If you can't swallow whole, crumble tablet or open capsule and take with liquid or food.

When to take:
At the same time each day, according to instructions on prescription label.

If you forget a dose:
Take as soon as you remember up to 2 hours late. If more than 2 hours, wait for next scheduled dose (don't double this dose).

What drug does:
Affects limbic system of brain—part that controls emotions.

Time lapse before drug works:
2 hours. May take 6 weeks for full benefit.

Don't take with:
See Interaction column and consult doctor.

OVERDOSE

SYMPTOMS:
Drowsiness, weakness, tremor, stupor, coma.
WHAT TO DO:
- **Dial 0 (operator) or 911 (emergency) for an ambulance or medical help. Then give first aid immediately.**
- **If patient is unconscious and not breathing, give mouth-to-mouth breathing. If there is no heartbeat, use cardiac massage and mouth-to-mouth breathing (CPR). Don't try to make patient vomit. If you can't get help quickly, take patient to nearest emergency facility.**
- **See emergency information on inside covers.**

POSSIBLE ADVERSE REACTIONS OR SIDE EFFECTS

SYMPTOMS	WHAT TO DO
Life-threatening: None expected.	
Common: Clumsiness, drowsiness, dizziness.	Continue. Call doctor when convenient.
Infrequent:	
• Hallucinations, confusion, depression, irritability, rash, itch, vision changes.	Discontinue. Call doctor right away.
• Constipation or diarrhea, nausea, vomiting, difficult urination, vivid dreams.	Continue. Call doctor when convenient.
Rare:	
• Slow heartbeat, breathing difficulty.	Discontinue. Seek emergency treatment.
• Mouth, throat ulcers; jaundice, decreased libido.	Discontinue. Call doctor right away.

WARNINGS & PRECAUTIONS

Don't take if:
- You are allergic to any benzodiazepine.
- You have myasthenia gravis.
- You are active or recovering alcoholic.
- Patient is younger than 6 months.

Before you start, consult your doctor:
- If you have liver, kidney or lung disease.
- If you have diabetes, epilepsy or porphyria.

Over age 60:
Adverse reactions and side effects may be more frequent and severe than in younger persons. You need smaller doses for shorter periods of time. May develop agitation, rage or "hangover" effect.

Pregnancy:
Risk to unborn child outweighs drug benefits. Don't use.

Breast-feeding:
Drug passes into milk. Avoid drug or discontinue nursing until you finish medicine. Consult doctor for advice on maintaining milk supply.

Infants & children:
Use only under medical supervision for children older than 6 months.

Prolonged use:
May impair liver function.

Skin & sunlight:
No problems expected.

Driving, piloting or hazardous work:
Don't drive or pilot aircraft until you learn how medicine affects you. Don't work around dangerous machinery. Don't climb ladders or work in high places. Danger increases if you drink alcohol or take medicine affecting alertness and reflexes.

Discontinuing:
Don't discontinue without consulting doctor. Dose may require gradual reduction if you have taken drug for a long time. Doses of other drugs may also require adjustment.

Others:
- Hot weather, heavy exercise and profuse sweat may reduce excretion and cause overdose.
- Blood sugar may rise in diabetics, requiring insulin adjustment.

POSSIBLE INTERACTION WITH OTHER DRUGS

GENERIC NAME OR DRUG CLASS	COMBINED EFFECT
Antidepressants*	Increased sedative effect of both drugs.
Antihistamines*	Increased sedative effect of both drugs.
Antihypertensives*	Excessively low blood pressure.
Contraceptives, oral*	Increased clorazepate effect.
Disulfiram	Increased clorazepate effect.
Dronabinol	Increased effects of both drugs. Avoid.
Erythromycin	Increased clorazepate effect.
Ketoconazole	Increased clorazepate effect.
Levodopa	Possible decreased levodopa effect.
MAO inhibitors*	Convulsions, deep sedation, rage.
Molindone	Increased tranquilizer effect.
Nabilone	Greater depression of central nervous system.
Narcotics*	Increased sedative effect of both drugs.
Probenecid	Increased clorazepate effect.
Sedatives*	Increased sedative effect of both drugs.
Sleep inducers*	Increased sedative effect of both drugs.
Tranquilizers*	Increased sedative effect of both drugs.

POSSIBLE INTERACTION WITH OTHER SUBSTANCES

INTERACTS WITH	COMBINED EFFECT
Alcohol:	Heavy sedation. Avoid.
Beverages:	None expected.
Cocaine:	Decreased clorazepate effect.
Foods:	None expected.
Marijuana:	Heavy sedation. Avoid.
Tobacco:	Decreased clorazepate effect.

CLOTRIMAZOLE (Oral-Local)

BRAND NAMES

Mycelex

BASIC INFORMATION

Habit forming? No
Prescription needed? Yes
Available as generic? No
Drug class: Antifungal

 ## USES

- Treats thrush; white mouth (candidiasis).
- Used primarily in immunosuppressed patients to treat and prevent infection.

 ## DOSAGE & USAGE INFORMATION

How to take:
Lozenges—Dissolve slowly and completely in the mouth, 5 times a day. Swallow saliva during this time. Don't swallow lozenge whole, don't chew.

When to take:
14 days or longer.

If you forget a dose:
Take as soon as you remember up to 2 hours late. If more than 2 hours, wait for next scheduled dose (don't double this dose).

What drug does:
Kills fungus by interfering with cell wall membrane and its permeability.

Time lapse before drug works:
1 to 3 hours.

Don't take with:
See Interaction column and consult doctor.

 ## OVERDOSE

SYMPTOMS:
None expected, but if large dose has been taken, follow instructions below.
WHAT TO DO:
- Dial 0 (operator) or 911 (emergency) for an ambulance or medical help. Then give first aid immediately.
- See emergency information on inside covers.

 ## POSSIBLE ADVERSE REACTIONS OR SIDE EFFECTS

SYMPTOMS	WHAT TO DO
Life-threatening: None expected.	
Common: None expected.	
Infrequent: Abdominal pain, diarrhea, nausea, vomiting.	Discontinue. Call doctor right away.
Rare: None expected.	

WARNINGS & PRECAUTIONS

Don't take if:
You have severe liver disease.

Before you start, consult your doctor:
If you have had a recent organ transplant.

Over age 60:
Adverse reactions and side effects may be more frequent and severe than in younger persons. You may need smaller doses for shorter periods of time.

Pregnancy:
Risk to unborn child outweighs drug benefits. Don't use.

Breast-feeding:
Drug passes into milk. Avoid drug or discontinue nursing until you finish medicine. Consult doctor for advice on maintaining milk supply.

Infants & children:
Use only under medical supervision for children younger than 4 or 5 years.

Prolonged use:
No problems expected.

Skin & sunlight:
No problems expected.

Driving, piloting or hazardous work:
Don't drive or pilot aircraft until you learn how medicine affects you. Don't work around dangerous machinery. Don't climb ladders or work in high places. Danger increases if you drink alcohol or take medicine affecting alertness and reflexes.

Discontinuing:
Don't discontinue without consulting doctor. Dose may require gradual reduction if you have taken drug for a long time. Doses of other drugs may also require adjustment.

Others:
* Continue for full term of treatment. May require several months.
* Check with physician if not improved in 1 week.

POSSIBLE INTERACTION WITH OTHER DRUGS

GENERIC NAME OR DRUG CLASS	COMBINED EFFECT
None expected.	

POSSIBLE INTERACTION WITH OTHER SUBSTANCES

INTERACTS WITH	COMBINED EFFECT
Alcohol:	Decreased effects of clotrimazole.
Beverages:	None expected.
Cocaine:	Decreased effects of clotrimazole.
Foods:	None expected.
Marijuana:	Decreased effects of clotrimazole.
Tobacco:	Decreased effects of clotrimazole.

CLOXACILLIN

BRAND NAMES

Apo-Cloxi	Novocloxin
Bactopen	Orbenin
Cloxapen	Tegopen
Cloxilean	

BASIC INFORMATION

Habit forming? No
Prescription needed? Yes
Available as generic? Yes
Drug class: Antibiotic (penicillin)

USES

Treatment of bacterial infections that are susceptible to cloxacillin.

DOSAGE & USAGE INFORMATION

How to take:
- Capsules—Swallow with liquid on an empty stomach 1 hour before or 2 hours after eating.
- Liquid—Take with cold beverage. Liquid form is perishable and effective for only 7 days at room temperature. Effective for 14 days if stored in refrigerator. Don't freeze.

When to take:
Follow instructions on prescription label or side of package. Doses should be evenly spaced. For example, 4 times a day means every 6 hours.

If you forget a dose:
Take as soon as you remember. Continue regular schedule.

What drug does:
Destroys susceptible bacteria. Does not kill viruses.

Time lapse before drug works:
May be several days before medicine affects infection.

Don't take with:
See Interaction column and consult doctor.

OVERDOSE

SYMPTOMS:
Severe diarrhea, nausea or vomiting.
WHAT TO DO:
Overdose unlikely to threaten life. If person takes much larger amount than prescribed, call doctor, poison-control center or hospital emergency room for instructions.

POSSIBLE ADVERSE REACTIONS OR SIDE EFFECTS

SYMPTOMS	WHAT TO DO
Life-threatening: Hives, rash, intense itching, faintness soon after a dose (anaphylaxis).	Seek emergency treatment immediately.
Common: Dark or discolored tongue.	Continue. Tell doctor at next visit.
Infrequent: Mild nausea, vomiting, diarrhea.	Continue. Call doctor when convenient.
Rare: Unexplained bleeding.	Discontinue. Call doctor right away.

WARNINGS & PRECAUTIONS

Don't take if:
You are allergic to cloxacillin, cephalosporin antibiotics, other penicillins or penicillamine. Life-threatening reaction may occur.

Before you start, consult your doctor:
If you are allergic to any substance or drug.

Over age 60:
You may have skin reactions, particularly around genitals and anus.

Pregnancy:
Studies inconclusive on harm to unborn child. Animal studies show fetal abnormalities. Decide with your doctor whether drug benefits justify risk to unborn child.

Breast-feeding:
Drug passes into milk. Child may become sensitive to penicillins and have allergic reactions to penicillin drugs. Avoid cloxacillin or discontinue nursing until you finish medicine. Consult doctor for advice on maintaining milk supply.

Infants & children:
No problems expected.

Prolonged use:
You may become more susceptible to infections caused by germs not responsive to cloxacillin.

Skin & sunlight:
No problems expected.

Driving, piloting or hazardous work:
Usually not dangerous. Most hazardous reactions likely to occur a few minutes after taking cloxacillin.

Discontinuing:
Don't discontinue without doctor's advice until you complete prescribed dose, even though symptoms diminish or disappear.

Others:
No problems expected.

POSSIBLE INTERACTION WITH OTHER DRUGS

GENERIC NAME OR DRUG CLASS	COMBINED EFFECT
Beta-adrenergic blockers*	Increased chance of anaphylaxis (see emergency information on inside front cover).
Chloramphenicol	Decreased effect of both drugs.
Erythromycins*	Decreased effect of both drugs.
Loperamide	Decreased cloxacillin effect.
Paromomycin	Decreased effect of both drugs.
Tetracyclines*	Decreased effect of both drugs.
Troleandomycin	Decreased effect of both drugs.

POSSIBLE INTERACTION WITH OTHER SUBSTANCES

INTERACTS WITH	COMBINED EFFECT
Alcohol:	Occasional stomach irritation.
Beverages:	None expected.
Cocaine:	No proven problems.
Foods:	None expected.
Marijuana:	No proven problems.
Tobacco:	None expected.

*See Glossary

COCAINE

BRAND NAMES

Cocaine

BASIC INFORMATION

Habit forming? Yes
Prescription needed? Yes
Available as generic? Yes
Drug class: Anesthetic, local

USES

Provides local anesthesia to the nose, mouth or throat to allow some types of surgery or examinations without pain.

DOSAGE & USAGE INFORMATION

How to use:
Used only under doctor's supervision, it's applied by spray or cotton swab directly to the area being anesthetized.

When to use:
Immediately before special examinations or surgery.

If you forget a dose:
Not applicable.

What drug does:
- Blocks conduction of nerve impulses to brain.
- Reduces swelling, bleeding and congestion at operation site.

Time lapse before drug works:
Immediate.

Don't use with:
See Interaction column and consult doctor.

OVERDOSE

SYMPTOMS:
Abdominal pain, chills, confusion, lightheadedness, dizziness, severe nervousness or restlessness, fast or irregular heartbeat, severe headache, sweating, twitching, dilated pupils, bulging eyes.
WHAT TO DO:
- **Tell your doctor immediately if any of the above occurs after cocaine has been applied.**
- **Dial 0 (operator) or 911 (emergency) for an ambulance or medical help. Then give first aid immediately.**
- **See emergency information on inside covers.**

POSSIBLE ADVERSE REACTIONS OR SIDE EFFECTS

SYMPTOMS	WHAT TO DO
Life-threatening: Blue discoloration of skin, lips, nails; irregular, weak heartbeat; chest pain; seizure; loss of bowel and bladder control.	Seek emergency treatment immediately.
Common: Abdominal pain, dizziness, confusion, agitation, irritability, hallucinations, fast or irregular heartbeat, headache, euphoria, psychotic behavior, trembling, large pupils.	Discontinue. Seek medical help if symptoms don't quickly subside.
Infrequent: Taste or smell loss after application to nose or mouth.	Nothing. This is a normal effect.
Rare: None expected.	

WARNINGS & PRECAUTIONS

Don't take if:
You are allergic to cocaine.

Before you start, consult your doctor:
- If you are allergic to anything.
- If you are taking *any* other medicine.
- If you have any acute illness or history of cancer, convulsions, irregular heartbeat, heart disease, blood vessel disease, high blood pressure, liver disease, heart attack history, hyperthyroidism (overactive thyroid gland).
- If you have recently used an insecticide.
- If you have had glaucoma or are using eye drops for glaucoma (such as Betoptic, Betagan, Timoptic).
- If you have a throat infection.

Over age 60:
More sensitive to drug. May cause impaired thinking, hallucinations, nightmares. Consult doctor about any of these.

Pregnancy:
Risk to unborn child outweighs any possible drug benefits. Don't use.

Breast-feeding:
Risk outweighs any possible drug benefits. Don't use.

Infants & children:
Not recommended for children 6 and younger. Use for older children only under doctor's supervision.

Prolonged use:
Addiction.

Skin & sunlight:
No problems expected.

Driving, piloting or hazardous work:
Don't drive or pilot aircraft for 24 hours after cocaine has been used for local anesthesia. Don't work around dangerous machinery. Don't climb ladders or work in high places. Danger increases if you drink alcohol or take medicine affecting alertness and reflexes, such as antihistamines, tranquilizers, sedatives, pain medicine, narcotics and mind-altering drugs.

Discontinuing:
No problems expected.

Others:
- In some people, even small amounts of cocaine can cause serious adverse reactions.
- Cocaine is used only under the direct supervision of your doctor.

POSSIBLE INTERACTION WITH OTHER DRUGS

GENERIC NAME OR DRUG CLASS	COMBINED EFFECT
Anesthetics*	Increased risk of heartbeat irregularity.
Antidepressants, tricyclic (TCA)*	Increased risk of heartbeat irregularity.
Antihypertensives*	Increased risk of heart block and high blood pressure.
Central nervous system stimulants*	Convulsions or excessive nervousness.
Digitalis preparations*	Increased risk of heartbeat irregularity.
Insecticides	Increased risk of toxicity.
Levodopa	Increased risk of heartbeat irregularity.
MAO inhibitors*	Increased risk of toxicity.
Methyldopa	Increased risk of heartbeat irregularity.
Nitrates*	Reduced effectiveness of nitrates.
Sympathomimetics*	High risk of heartbeat irregularities and high blood pressure.

POSSIBLE INTERACTION WITH OTHER SUBSTANCES

INTERACTS WITH	COMBINED EFFECT
Alcohol:	Dangerous interaction. Don't use.
Beverages: Caffeine drinks.	Dangerous interaction. Don't use.
Cocaine: Orally.	Increased chance of adverse reactions.
Foods:	No proven problems.
Marijuana:	Dangerous interaction. Don't use.
Tobacco:	Increased likelihood of irregular or rapid heartbeat.

COLCHICINE

BRAND NAMES

ColBenemid   Novocolchine
Col-Probenecid

BASIC INFORMATION

Habit forming? No
Prescription needed? Yes
Available as generic? Yes
Drug class: Antigout

 USES

- Relieves joint pain, inflammation, swelling of gout.
- Also used for familial Mediterranean fever, dermatitis herpetiformis.

 DOSAGE & USAGE INFORMATION

How to take:
Tablet—Swallow with liquid or food to lessen stomach irritation.

When to take:
- As prescribed. Stop taking when pain stops or at first sign of digestive upset. Wait at least 3 days between treatments.
- Don't take more than 8 doses.

If you forget a dose:
Don't double next dose. Consult doctor.

What drug does:
Decreases acidity of joint tissues and prevents deposits of uric-acid crystals.

Time lapse before drug works:
12 to 48 hours.

Don't take with:
See Interaction column and consult doctor.

 OVERDOSE

SYMPTOMS:
Bloody urine, diarrhea, muscle weakness, fever, shortness of breath, stupor, convulsions, coma.
WHAT TO DO:
- **Dial 0 (operator) or 911 (emergency) for an ambulance or medical help. Then give first aid immediately.**
- **See emergency information on inside covers.**

 POSSIBLE ADVERSE REACTIONS OR SIDE EFFECTS

SYMPTOMS	WHAT TO DO
Life-threatening: None expected.	
Common: Diarrhea, nausea, vomiting, abdominal pain.	Discontinue. Call doctor right away.
Infrequent: • Rash, itch, unusual bruising, blood in urine.	Discontinue. Call doctor right away.
• Numbness, tingling, pain or weakness in hands or feet; unusual tiredness or weakness; fever; hair loss.	Continue. Call doctor when convenient.
Rare: Jaundice, aplastic anemia (low red blood cells), agranulocytosis (low white blood cells).	Discontinue. Call doctor right away.

WARNINGS & PRECAUTIONS

Don't take if:
You are allergic to colchicine.

Before you start, consult your doctor:
- If you have had peptic ulcers or ulcerative colitis.
- If you have heart, liver or kidney disease.
- If you will have surgery within 2 months, including dental surgery, requiring general or spinal anesthesia.

Over age 60:
Adverse reactions and side effects may be more frequent and severe than in younger persons. Colchicine has a narrow margin of safety for people in this age group.

Pregnancy:
Risk to unborn child outweighs drug benefits. Don't use.

Breast-feeding:
No problems expected, but consult doctor.

Infants & children:
Not recommended.

Prolonged use:
- Permanent hair loss.
- Anemia. Request blood counts.
- Numbness or tingling in hands and feet.

Skin & sunlight:
No problems expected.

Driving, piloting or hazardous work:
Don't drive or pilot aircraft until you learn how medicine affects you. Don't work around dangerous machinery. Don't climb ladders or work in high places. Danger increases if you drink alcohol or take medicine affecting alertness and reflexes, such as antihistamines, tranquilizers, sedatives, pain medicine, narcotics and mind-altering drugs.

Discontinuing:
- May be unnecessary to finish medicine. Follow doctor's instructions.
- Stop taking if digestive upsets occur before symptoms are relieved.

Others:
- Limit each course of treatment to 8 mg. Don't exceed 3 mg. per 24 hours.
- Possible sperm damage. May cause birth defects if child conceived while father taking colchicine.

POSSIBLE INTERACTION WITH OTHER DRUGS

GENERIC NAME OR DRUG CLASS	COMBINED EFFECT
Anticoagulants*	Increased anticoagulant effect.
Diuretics*	Decreased antigout effect of colchicine.
Phenylbutazone	Increased chance of ulcers in gastro-intestinal tract.
Vitamin B-12	Decreased absorption of vitamin B-12.

POSSIBLE INTERACTION WITH OTHER SUBSTANCES

INTERACTS WITH	COMBINED EFFECT
Alcohol:	Increased risk of gastrointestinal toxicity.
Beverages: Herbal teas.	Increased colchicine effect. Avoid.
Cocaine:	Overstimulation. Avoid.
Foods:	No proven problems.
Marijuana:	Decreased colchicine effect.
Tobacco:	No proven problems.

COLESTIPOL

BRAND NAMES

Colestid

BASIC INFORMATION

Habit forming? No
Prescription needed? Yes
Available as generic? No
Drug class: Antihyperlipidemic

 ## USES

- Reduces cholesterol level in blood in patients with type IIa hyperlipidemia.
- Treats overdose of digitalis.
- Reduces skin itching associated with some forms of liver disease.
- Treats diarrhea after some surgical operations.
- Treatment of one form of colitis (rare).

 ## DOSAGE & USAGE INFORMATION

How to take:
Mix well with 6 ounces or more or water or liquid, or in soups, pulpy fruits, with milk or in cereals. Will not dissolve.

When to take:
- Before meals.
- If taking other medicine, take it 1 hour before or 4 to 6 hours after taking colestipol.

If you forget a dose:
Take as soon as you remember up to 2 hours late. If more than 2 hours, wait for next scheduled dose (don't double this dose).

What drug does:
Binds with bile acids in intestines, preventing reabsorption.

Time lapse before drug works:
3 to 12 months.

Don't take with:
See Interaction column and consult doctor.

 ## OVERDOSE

SYMPTOMS:
Fecal impaction.
WHAT TO DO:
Overdose unlikely to threaten life. If person takes much larger amount than prescribed, call doctor, poison-control center or hospital emergency room for instructions.

 ## POSSIBLE ADVERSE REACTIONS OR SIDE EFFECTS

SYMPTOMS	WHAT TO DO
Life-threatening: None expected.	
Common: None expected.	
Infrequent:	
• Black, tarry stools from gastrointestinal bleeding.	Discontinue. Seek emergency treatment.
• Severe abdominal pain.	Discontinue. Call doctor right away.
• Constipation, belching, diarrhea, nausea, unexpected weight loss.	Continue. Call doctor when convenient.
Rare:	
Hives, dermatitis, hiccups.	Discontinue. Call doctor right away.

WARNINGS & PRECAUTIONS

Don't take if:
You are allergic to colestipol.

Before you start, consult your doctor:
- If you have liver disease such as cirrhosis.
- If you are jaundiced.
- If you will have surgery within 2 months, including dental surgery, requiring general or spinal anesthesia.
- If you are constipated.
- If you have peptic ulcer.
- If you have coronary artery disease.

Over age 60:
Constipation more likely. Other adverse effects more likely.

Pregnancy:
No proven harm to unborn child. Avoid if possible.

Breast-feeding:
No proven harm to child. Consult doctor.

Infants & children:
Only under expert medical supervision.

Prolonged use:
- Request lab studies to determine serum cholesterol and serum triglycerides.
- May decrease absorption of folic acid.

Skin & sunlight:
No problems expected.

Driving, piloting or hazardous work:
No problems expected.

Discontinuing:
Don't discontinue without consulting doctor. Dose may require gradual reduction if you have taken drug for a long time. Doses of other drugs may also require adjustment, particularly digitalis.

Others:
This medicine does not cure disorders, but helps to control them.

POSSIBLE INTERACTION WITH OTHER DRUGS

GENERIC NAME OR DRUG CLASS	COMBINED EFFECT
Anticoagulants, oral*	Decreased anticoagulant effect.
Digitalis preparations*	Decreased absorption.
Diuretics, thiazide*	Decreased absorption.
Penicillins*	Decreased absorption.
Tetracyclines*	Decreased absorption.
Thiazides*	Decreased absorption of colestipol.
Trimethoprim	Decreased absorption of colestipol.
Ursodiol	Decreased absorption of ursodiol.
Vitamins	Decreased absorption of fat-soluble vitamins (A,D,E,K)
Other medicines	May delay or reduce absorption.

POSSIBLE INTERACTION WITH OTHER SUBSTANCES

INTERACTS WITH	COMBINED EFFECT
Alcohol:	None expected.
Beverages:	None expected.
Cocaine:	None expected.
Foods:	Interferes with absorption of vitamins. Take supplements.
Marijuana:	None expected.
Tobacco:	None expected.

*See Glossary

CONJUGATED ESTROGENS

BRAND NAMES

C.E.S.   Premarin
C.S.D.   Progens
Conjugated
  Estrogens

BASIC INFORMATION

Habit forming? No
Prescription needed? Yes
Available as generic? Yes
Drug class: Female sex hormone (estrogen)

 ## USES

- Treatment for symptoms of menopause and menstrual-cycle irregularity.
- Replacement for female hormone deficiency.
- Treatment for estrogen-deficiency osteoporosis (bone softening from calcium loss).
- Treatment for cancer of prostate and breast.

 ## DOSAGE & USAGE INFORMATION

How to take:
- Tablet—Swallow with liquid. If you can't swallow whole, crumble tablet and take with liquid or food.
- Vaginal cream—Use as directed on label.

When to take:
At the same time each day.

If you forget a dose:
Take as soon as you remember up to 12 hours late. If more than 12 hours, wait for next scheduled dose (don't double this dose).

What drug does:
Restores normal estrogen level in tissues.

Time lapse before drug works:
10 to 20 days.

Don't take with:
See Interaction column and consult doctor.

 ## OVERDOSE

SYMPTOMS:
Nausea, vomiting, fluid retention, breast enlargement and discomfort, abnormal vaginal bleeding.
WHAT TO DO:
Overdose unlikely to threaten life. If person takes much larger amount than prescribed, call doctor, poison-control center or hospital emergency room for instructions.

 ## POSSIBLE ADVERSE REACTIONS OR SIDE EFFECTS

SYMPTOMS	WHAT TO DO
Life-threatening: None expected.	
Common:	
• Stomach cramps.	Discontinue. Call doctor right away.
• Appetite loss.	Continue. Call doctor when convenient.
• Nausea; diarrhea; swollen ankles or feet; swollen, tender breasts.	Continue. Tell doctor at next visit.
Infrequent:	
• Rash, stomach or side pain.	Discontinue. Call doctor right away.
• Depression, dizziness, headache, irritability, vomiting, breast lumps.	Continue. Call doctor when convenient.
• Brown blotches on skin, hair loss, vaginal discharge or bleeding, changes in sex drive.	Continue. Tell doctor at next visit.
Rare: Jaundice, hypercalcemia in breast cancer, intolerance of contact lenses.	Discontinue. Call doctor right away.

CONJUGATED ESTROGENS

WARNINGS & PRECAUTIONS

Don't take if:
- You are allergic to any estrogen-containing drugs.
- You have impaired liver function.
- You have had blood clots, stroke or heart attack.
- You have unexplained vaginal bleeding.

Before you start, consult your doctor:
- If you have had cancer of breast or reproductive organs, fibrocystic breast disease, fibroid tumors of the uterus or endometriosis.
- If you have had migraine headaches, epilepsy or porphyria.
- If you have diabetes, high blood pressure, asthma, congestive heart failure, kidney disease or gallstones.
- If you plan to become pregnant within 3 months.

Over age 60:
Controversial. You and your doctor must decide if drug risks outweigh benefits.

Pregnancy:
Risk to unborn child outweighs drug benefits. Don't use.

Breast-feeding:
Drug filters into milk. May harm child. Avoid.

Infants & children:
Not recommended.

Prolonged use:
Increased growth of fibroid tumors of uterus. Possible association with cancer of uterus.

Skin & sunlight:
May cause rash or intensify sunburn in areas exposed to sun or sunlamp.

Driving, piloting or hazardous work:
No problems expected.

Discontinuing:
You may need to discontinue estrogen periodically. Consult your doctor.

Others:
In rare instances, may cause blood clot in lung, brain or leg. Symptoms are *sudden* severe headache, coordination loss, vision change, chest pain, breathing difficulty, slurred speech, pain in legs or groin. Seek emergency treatment immediately.

POSSIBLE INTERACTION WITH OTHER DRUGS

GENERIC NAME OR DRUG CLASS	COMBINED EFFECT
Anticoagulants, oral*	Decreased anticoagulant effect.
Anticonvulsants, hydantoin*	Decreased estrogen effect.
Antidepressants, tricyclic (TCA)*	Increased toxicity of antidepressant.
Antidiabetics, oral*	Unpredictable increase or decrease in blood sugar.
Antifibrinolytic agents*	Increased possibility of blood clotting.
Carbamazepine	Decreased estrogen effect.
Clofibrate	Decreased clofibrate effect.
Insulin	Possible decreased insulin effect. May require dose adjustment.
Meprobamate	Increased effect of conjugated estrogens.
Phenobarbital	Decreased effect of conjugated estrogens.
Primidone	Decreased effect of conjugated estrogens.
Rifampin	Decreased effect of conjugated estrogens.
Vitamin C	Possible increased estrogen effect.
Terazosin	Decreases effectiveness of terazosin.
Thyroid hormones*	Decreased thyroid effect.
Ursodiol	Decreased effect of ursodiol.

POSSIBLE INTERACTION WITH OTHER SUBSTANCES

INTERACTS WITH	COMBINED EFFECT
Alcohol:	None expected.
Beverages:	None expected.
Cocaine:	No proven problems.
Foods:	None expected.
Marijuana:	Possible menstrual irregularities and bleeding between periods.
Tobacco:	Increased risk of blood clots leading to stroke or heart attack.

CONTRACEPTIVES (Oral)

BRAND NAMES

See complete list of brand names in the *Brand Name Directory*, page 1060.

BASIC INFORMATION

Habit forming? No
Prescription needed? Yes
Available as generic? No
Drug class: Female sex hormone, contraceptive

USES

- Prevents pregnancy.
- Regulates menstrual periods.

DOSAGE & USAGE INFORMATION

How to take:
Tablet—Swallow with liquid or food to lessen stomach irritation.

When to take:
At same time each day according to prescribed instructions, usually for 21 days of 28-day cycle.

If you forget a dose:
Call doctor's office for advice about additional protection against pregnancy.

What drug does:
- Alters mucus at cervix entrance to prevent sperm entry.
- Alters uterus lining to resist implantation of fertilized egg.
- Creates same chemical atmosphere in blood that exists during pregnancy, suppressing pituitary hormones which stimulate ovulation.

Time lapse before drug works:
10 days or more to provide contraception.

Don't take with:
- Tobacco
- See Interaction column and consult doctor.

OVERDOSE

SYMPTOMS:
Drowsiness
WHAT TO DO:
Overdose unlikely to threaten life. If person takes much larger amount than prescribed, call doctor, poison-control center or hospital emergency room for instructions.

POSSIBLE ADVERSE REACTIONS OR SIDE EFFECTS

SYMPTOMS	WHAT TO DO
Life-threatening: Stroke, chest pain.	Seek emergency treatment immediately.
Common: Brown blotches on skin; vaginal discharge, itch; fluid retention.	Continue. Call doctor when convenient.
Infrequent: • Headache; blood clots, pain, swelling in leg; muscle, joint pain, depression.	Discontinue. Call doctor right away.
• Blue tinge to objects, lights; appetite change; nausea; bloating; vomiting; pain; changed sex drive.	Continue. Call doctor when convenient.
Rare: • Clotting tendency.	Discontinue. Seek emergency treatment.
• Jaundice, rash, hives, itch, fever, hypercalcemia in breast cancer, intolerance of contact lenses, excess hair growth, voice change, enlarged clitoris in women.	Discontinue. Call doctor right away.
• Amenorrhea, insomnia, hair loss.	Continue. Call doctor when convenient.

WARNINGS & PRECAUTIONS

Don't take if:
- You are allergic to any female hormone.
- You have had heart disease, blood clots or stroke.
- You have liver disease.
- You have cancer of breast, uterus or ovaries.
- You have unexplained vaginal bleeding.

Before you start, consult your doctor:
- If you have fibrocystic disease of breast.
- If you have migraine headaches.
- If you have fibroid tumors of uterus.
- If you have epilepsy.
- If you have asthma.
- If you have high blood pressure.
- If you will have surgery within 2 months, including dental surgery, requiring general or spinal anesthesia.
- If you have endometriosis.
- If you have diabetes.
- If you have sickle-cell anemia.
- If you smoke cigarettes.

Over age 60:
Not used.

Pregnancy:
May harm child. Discontinue at first sign of pregnancy.

Breast-feeding:
Drug passes into milk. Avoid drug or discontinue nursing.

Infants & children:
Not recommended.

Prolonged use:
- Gallstones.
- Gradual blood-pressure rise.
- Possible difficulty becoming pregnant after discontinuing.

Skin & sunlight:
May cause rash or intensify sunburn in areas exposed to sun or sunlamp.

Driving, piloting or hazardous work:
No problems expected.

Discontinuing:
Don't become pregnant for 6 months after discontinuing.

Others:
Failure to take oral contraceptives for 1 day may cancel pregnancy protection. If you forget a dose, use other contraceptive measures and call doctor for instructions on re-starting oral contraceptive.

POSSIBLE INTERACTION WITH OTHER DRUGS

GENERIC NAME OR DRUG CLASS	COMBINED EFFECT
Ampicillin	Decreased contraceptive effect.
Anticoagulants*	Decreased anticoagulant effect.
Anticonvulsants, hydantoin*	Decreased contraceptive effect.
Antidepressants, tricyclic (TCA)*	Increased toxicity of antidepressants.
Antidiabetics*	Decreased antidiabetic effect.
Antifibronolytic agents*	Increased possibility of blood clotting.
Antihistamines*	Decreased contraceptive effect.
Barbiturates*	Decreased contraceptive effect.
Chloramphenicol	Decreased contraceptive effect.

Clofibrate	Decreased clofibrate effect.
Guanethidine	Decreased guanethidine effect.
Hypoglycemics, oral*	Decreased effect of hypoglycemics.
Insulin	Possibly decreased insulin effect.
Meperidine	Increased meperidine effect.
Meprobamate	Decreased contraceptive effect.
Mineral oil	Decreased contraceptive effect.
Non-steroidal anti-inflammatory drugs (NSAIDs)*	Decreased contraceptive effect.
Phenothiazines*	Increased phenothiazine effect.
Rifampin	Decreased contraceptive effect.
Terazosin	Decreases effectiveness of terazosin.
Tetracyclines*	Decreased contraceptive effect.
Ursodiol	Decreased effect of ursodiol.
Vitamin C	Possible increased contraceptive effect.

POSSIBLE INTERACTION WITH OTHER SUBSTANCES

INTERACTS WITH	COMBINED EFFECT
Alcohol:	No proven problems.
Beverages:	No proven problems.
Cocaine:	No proven problems.
Foods: Salt.	Increased edema (fluid retention).
Marijuana:	Increased bleeding between periods. Avoid.
Tobacco:	Possible heart attack, blood clots and stroke.

*See Glossary

CORTISONE

BRAND NAMES

Cortelan
Cortistab
Cortone Acetate

BASIC INFORMATION

Habit forming? No
Prescription needed? Yes
Available as generic? Yes
Drug class: Cortisone drug (adrenal corticosteroid)

 USES

- Reduces inflammation caused by many different medical problems.
- Treatment for some allergic diseases, blood disorders, kidney diseases, asthma and emphysema.
- Replaces corticosteroid deficiencies.

 DOSAGE & USAGE INFORMATION

How to take:
Tablet—Swallow with liquid or food to lessen stomach irritation. If you can't swallow whole, crumble tablet and take with liquid or food.

When to take:
At the same times each day. Take once-a-day or once-every-other-day doses in mornings.

If you forget a dose:
- Several-doses-per-day prescription—Take as soon as you remember up to 2 hours late. If more than 2 hours, wait for next scheduled dose (don't double this dose).
- Once-a-day dose or less—Wait for next dose. Double this dose.

What drug does:
Decreases inflammatory responses.

Time lapse before drug works:
2 to 4 days.

Don't take with:
See Interaction column and consult doctor.

 OVERDOSE

SYMPTOMS:
Headache, convulsions, heart failure.
WHAT TO DO:
- Dial 0 (operator) or 911 (emergency) for an ambulance or medical help. Then give first aid immediately.
- See emergency information on inside covers.

 POSSIBLE ADVERSE REACTIONS OR SIDE EFFECTS

SYMPTOMS	WHAT TO DO
Life-threatening:	
Hives, rash, intense itching, faintness soon after a dose (anaphylaxis).	Seek emergency treatment immediately.
Common:	
Acne, thirst, nausea, indigestion, vomiting, poor wound healing, decreased growth in children.	Continue. Call doctor when convenient.
Infrequent:	
• Bloody or black, tarry stool.	Discontinue. Seek emergency treatment.
• Blurred vision; halos around lights; sore throat, fever; muscle cramps; swollen legs, feet.	Discontinue. Call doctor right away.
• Mood changes, insomnia, fatigue, restlessness, frequent urination, weight gain, round face, weakness, TB recurrence, irregular menstrual periods.	Continue. Call doctor when convenient.
Rare:	
• Irregular heartbeat.	Discontinue. Seek emergency treatment.
• Rash, hallucinations, thrombophlebitis, pancreatitis, numbness or tingling in hands or feet, convulsions.	Discontinue. Call doctor right away.

 WARNINGS & PRECAUTIONS

Don't take if:
- You are allergic to any cortisone drug.
- You have tuberculosis or fungus infection.
- You have herpes infection of eyes, lips or genitals.

Before you start, consult your doctor:
- If you have had tuberculosis.
- If you have congestive heart failure.
- If you have diabetes, peptic ulcer, glaucoma, underactive thyroid, high blood pressure, myasthenia gravis, blood clots in legs or lungs.

Over age 60:
Adverse reactions and side effects may be more frequent and severe than in younger persons.

Likely to aggravate edema, diabetes or ulcers. Likely to cause cataracts and osteoporosis (softening of the bones).

Pregnancy:
Risk to unborn child outweighs drug benefits. Don't use.

Breast-feeding:
Drug passes into milk. Avoid drug or discontinue nursing until you finish medicine. Consult doctor for advice on maintaining milk supply.

Infants & children:
Use only under medical supervision.

Prolonged use:
- Retards growth in children.
- Possible glaucoma, cataracts, diabetes, fragile bones and thin skin.
- Functional dependence.

Skin & sunlight:
No problems expected.

Driving, piloting or hazardous work:
No problems expected.

Discontinuing:
- Don't discontinue without doctor's advice until you complete prescribed dose, even though symptoms diminish or disappear.
- Drug affects your response to surgery, illness, injury or stress for 2 years after discontinuing. Tell anyone who takes medical care of you within 2 years about drug.

Others:
Avoid immunizations if possible.

 POSSIBLE INTERACTION WITH OTHER DRUGS

GENERIC NAME OR DRUG CLASS	COMBINED EFFECT
Amphotericin B	Potassium depletion.
Anticholinergics*	Possible glaucoma.
Anticoagulants, oral*	Decreased anti-coagulant effect.
Anticonvulsants, hydantoin*	Decreased cortisone effect.
Antidiabetics, oral*	Decreased anti-diabetic effect.
Antihistamines*	Decreased cortisone effect.
Aspirin	Increased cortisone effect.
Attenuated virus vaccines*	Possible viral infection.
Barbiturates*	Decreased cortisone effect. Oversedation.

Chloral hydrate	Decreased cortisone effect.
Chlorthalidone	Potassium depletion.
Cholinergics*	Decreased cholinergic effect.
Cholestyramine	Decreased cortisone absorption effect.
Colestipol	Decreased cortisone absorption effect.
Contraceptives, oral*	Increased cortisone effect.
Cyclosporine	Increased risk of infection.
Diclofenac	Increased risk of stomach ulcer.
Digitalis preparations*	Dangerous potassium depletion. Possible digitalis toxicity.
Diuretics, thiazide*	Potassium depletion.
Ephedrine	Decreased cortisone effect.
Estrogens*	Increased cortisone effect.
Ethacrynic acid	Potassium depletion.
Furosemide	Potassium depletion.
Glutethimide	Decreased cortisone effect.
Indapamide	Possible excessive potassium loss, causing dangerous heartbeat irregularity.

Continued page 1083

 POSSIBLE INTERACTION WITH OTHER SUBSTANCES

INTERACTS WITH	COMBINED EFFECT
Alcohol:	Risk of stomach ulcers.
Beverages:	No proven problems.
Cocaine:	Overstimulation. Avoid.
Foods:	No proven problems.
Marijuana:	Decreased immunity.
Tobacco:	Increased cortisone effect. Possible toxicity.

*See Glossary

CROMOLYN

BRAND NAMES

Fivent
Intal
Nalcrom
Nasalcrom

Opticrom
Rynacrom
Sodium
Cromoblycate

BASIC INFORMATION

Habit forming? No
Prescription needed? Yes
Available as generic? No
Drug class: Antiasthmatic, anti-inflammatory

USES

- Prevents asthma attacks. Will not stop an active asthma attack.
- Treatment for inflammation of covering to eye and cornea.
- Reduces nasal allergic symptoms.

DOSAGE & USAGE INFORMATION

How to take:
- Inhaler—Follow instructions enclosed with inhaler. Don't swallow cartridges for inhaler. Gargle and rinse mouth after inhalations.
- Eye drops—Follow prescription instructions.
- Nasal solution—Follow prescription instructions.

When to take:
At the same times each day. If you also use a bronchodilator inhaler, use the bronchodilator before the cromolyn.

If you forget a dose:
Take as soon as you remember up to 2 hours late. If more than 2 hours, wait for next scheduled dose (don't double this dose).

What drug does:
Blocks histamine release from mast cells.

Time lapse before drug works:
- 4 weeks for prevention of asthma attacks.
- 1 to 2 weeks for nasal or eye symptoms.

Don't take with:
See Interaction column and consult doctor.

OVERDOSE

SYMPTOMS:
Increased side effects and adverse reactions listed.
WHAT TO DO:
Overdose unlikely to threaten life. If person inhales much larger amount than prescribed, call doctor, poison-control center or hospital emergency room for instructions.

POSSIBLE ADVERSE REACTIONS OR SIDE EFFECTS

SYMPTOMS	WHAT TO DO
Life-threatening: Hives, rash, intense itching, faintness soon after a dose (anaphylaxis).	Seek emergency treatment immediately.
Common: Hoarseness, cough, dry mouth.	Continue. Call doctor when convenient.
Infrequent: • Rash, hives, swallowing difficulty, nausea, vomiting, increased wheezing, joint pain or swelling, sneezing, nasal burning, weakness, muscle pain, difficult or painful urination.	Discontinue. Call doctor right away.
• Drowsiness, dizziness, headache, watery eyes, stuffy nose, throat irritation.	Continue. Call doctor when convenient.
Rare: Nosebleed.	Continue. Call doctor when convenient.

WARNINGS & PRECAUTIONS

Don't take if:
You are allergic to cromolyn, lactose, milk or milk products.

Before you start, consult your doctor:
• If you plan to become pregnant within medication period.
• If you have kidney or liver disease.

Over age 60:
Adverse reactions and side effects may be more frequent and severe than in younger persons.

Pregnancy:
Risk to unborn child outweighs drug benefits. Don't use.

Breast-feeding:
Drug passes into milk. Avoid drug or discontinue nursing.

Infants & children:
Use only under medical supervision.

Prolonged use:
No problems expected.

Skin & sunlight:
No problems expected.

Driving, piloting or hazardous work:
No problems expected.

Discontinuing:
No problems expected.

Others:
• Inhaler must be cleaned and work well for drug to be effective.
• This treatment does not stop an acute asthma attack. It may aggravate it.
• Eye drops:
Wash hands. Apply pressure to inside corner of eye with middle finger. Continue pressure for 1 minute after placing medicine in eye. Tilt head backward. Pull lower lid away from eye with index finger of the same hand. Drop eye drops into pouch and close eye. Don't blink. Keep eyes closed for 1 to 2 minutes. Don't touch applicator tip to any surface (including the eye). If you accidentally touch tip, clean with warm soap and water. Keep container tightly closed. Keep cool, but don't freeze. Wash hands immediately after using.

POSSIBLE INTERACTION WITH OTHER DRUGS

GENERIC NAME OR DRUG CLASS	COMBINED EFFECT
Beta-agonists*	Increased cromolyn effect.
Cortisone drugs*	Increased cortisone effect in treating asthma. Cortisone dose may be decreased.
Ipratroprium	Increased cromolyn effect.

POSSIBLE INTERACTION WITH OTHER SUBSTANCES

INTERACTS WITH	COMBINED EFFECT
Alcohol:	None expected.
Beverages:	None expected.
Cocaine:	None expected.
Foods:	None expected.
Marijuana:	None expected.
Tobacco:	None expected, but tobacco smoke aggravates asthma and eye irritation. Avoid.

CYCLACILLIN

BRAND NAMES

Cyclapen-W

BASIC INFORMATION

Habit forming? No
Prescription needed? Yes
Available as generic? No
Drug class: Antibiotic (penicillin)

USES

Treatment of bacterial infections that are susceptible to cyclacillin.

DOSAGE & USAGE INFORMATION

How to take:
- Tablet—Swallow with liquid on an empty stomach 1 hour before or 2 hours after eating.
- Liquid—Take with cold beverage. Liquid form is perishable and effective for only 7 days at room temperature. Effective for 14 days if stored in refrigerator. Don't freeze.

When to take:
Follow instructions on prescription label or side of package. Doses should be evenly spaced. For example, 4 times a day means every 6 hours.

If you forget a dose:
Take as soon as you remember. Continue regular schedule.

What drug does:
Destroys susceptible bacteria. Does not kill viruses.

Time lapse before drug works:
May be several days before medicine affects infection.

Don't take with:
See Interaction column and consult doctor.

OVERDOSE

SYMPTOMS:
Severe diarrhea, nausea or vomiting.
WHAT TO DO:
Overdose unlikely to threaten life. If person takes much larger amount than prescribed, call doctor, poison-control center or hospital emergency room for instructions.

POSSIBLE ADVERSE REACTIONS OR SIDE EFFECTS

SYMPTOMS	WHAT TO DO
Life-threatening: Hives, rash, intense itching, faintness soon after a dose (anaphylaxis).	Seek emergency treatment immediately.
Common: Dark or discolored tongue.	Continue. Tell doctor at next visit.
Infrequent: Mild nausea, vomiting, diarrhea.	Continue. Call doctor when convenient.
Rare: Unexplained bleeding.	Discontinue. Call doctor right away.

WARNINGS & PRECAUTIONS

Don't take if:
Your are allergic to cyclacillin, cephalosporin antibiotics, other penicillins or penicillamine. Life-threatening reaction may occur.

Before you start, consult your doctor:
If you are allergic to any substance or drug.

Over age 60:
You may have skin reactions, particularly around genitals and anus.

Pregnancy:
Studies inconclusive on harm to unborn child. Animal studies show fetal abnormalities. Decide with your doctor whether drug benefits justify risk to unborn child.

Breast-feeding:
Drug passes into milk. Child may become sensitive to penicillins and have allergic reactions to penicillin drugs. Avoid cyclacillin or discontinue nursing until you finish medicine. Consult doctor for advice on maintaining milk supply.

Infants & children:
No problems expected.

Prolonged use:
You may become more susceptible to infections caused by germs not responsive to cyclacillin.

Skin & sunlight:
No problems expected.

Driving, piloting or hazardous work:
Usually not dangerous. Most hazardous reactions likely to occur a few minutes after taking cyclacillin.

Discontinuing:
Don't discontinue without doctor's advice until you complete prescribed dose, even though symptoms diminish or disappear.

Others:
No problems expected.

POSSIBLE INTERACTION WITH OTHER DRUGS

GENERIC NAME OR DRUG CLASS	COMBINED EFFECT
Beta-adrenergic blockers*	Increased chance of anaphylaxis (see emergency information on inside front cover).
Chloramphenicol	Decreased effect of both drugs.
Erythromycins*	Decreased effect of both drugs.
Loperamide	Decreased cyclacillin effect.
Paromomycin	Decreased effect of both drugs.
Tetracyclines*	Decreased effect of both drugs.
Troleandomycin	Decreased effect of both drugs.

POSSIBLE INTERACTION WITH OTHER SUBSTANCES

INTERACTS WITH	COMBINED EFFECT
Alcohol:	Occasional stomach irritation.
Beverages:	None expected.
Cocaine:	No proven problems.
Foods:	Decreased effect of cyclacillin.
Marijuana:	No proven problems.
Tobacco:	None expected.

*See Glossary

295

CYCLANDELATE

BRAND NAMES

Cyclospasmol   Cyraso-400

BASIC INFORMATION

Habit forming? No
Prescription needed?
  U.S.: Yes
  Canada: No
Available as generic? Yes
Drug class: Vasodilator

 ## USES

Improves poor blood flow to extremities.

 ## DOSAGE & USAGE INFORMATION

How to take:
Tablet or capsule—Swallow with liquid. If you can't swallow whole, crumble tablet or open capsule and take with liquid or food.

When to take:
At the same time each day.

If you forget a dose:
Take as soon as you remember up to 2 hours late. If more than 2 hours, wait for next scheduled dose (don't double this dose).

What drug does:
Increases blood flow by relaxing and expanding blood-vessel walls.

Time lapse before drug works:
3 weeks.

Don't take with:
See Interaction column and consult doctor.

 ## OVERDOSE

SYMPTOMS:
Severe headache, dizziness; nausea, vomiting; flushed, hot face.
WHAT TO DO:
Overdose unlikely to threaten life. If person takes much larger amount than prescribed, call doctor, poison-control center or hospital emergency room for instructions.

 ## POSSIBLE ADVERSE REACTIONS OR SIDE EFFECTS

SYMPTOMS	WHAT TO DO
Life-threatening: None expected.	
Common: None expected.	
Infrequent:	
• Rapid heartbeat.	Discontinue. Call doctor right away.
• Dizziness; headache; weakness; flushed face; tingling in face, fingers or toes; unusual sweating.	Continue. Call doctor when convenient.
• Belching, heartburn, nausea or stomach pain.	Continue. Tell doctor at next visit.
Rare: None expected.	

WARNINGS & PRECAUTIONS

Don't take if:
You have had allergic reaction to cyclandelate.

Before you start, consult your doctor:
• If you have glaucoma.
• If you have had heart attack or stroke.

Over age 60:
Adverse reactions and side effects may be more frequent and severe than in younger persons.

Pregnancy:
No proven harm to unborn child. Avoid if possible.

Breast-feeding:
No proven problems. Consult doctor.

Infants & children:
Not recommended.

Prolonged use:
No problems expected.

Skin & sunlight:
No problems expected.

Driving, piloting or hazardous work:
Avoid if you feel dizzy or weak. Otherwise, no problems expected.

Discontinuing:
Don't discontinue without doctor's advice until you complete prescribed dose, even though symptoms diminish or disappear.

Others:
Response to drug varies. If your symptoms don't improve after 3 weeks of use, consult doctor.

POSSIBLE INTERACTION WITH OTHER DRUGS

GENERIC NAME OR DRUG CLASS	COMBINED EFFECT
None expected.	

POSSIBLE INTERACTION WITH OTHER SUBSTANCES

INTERACTS WITH	COMBINED EFFECT
Alcohol:	None expected.
Beverages:	None expected.
Cocaine:	Decreased cyclandelate effect. Avoid.
Foods:	None expected.
Marijuana:	None expected.
Tobacco:	May decrease cyclandelate effect.

CYCLIZINE

BRAND NAMES

Marezine   Marzine

BASIC INFORMATION

Habit forming? No
Prescription needed?
   U.S.: No
   Canada: Yes
Available as generic? No
Drug class: Antihistamine, antiemetic

 ## USES

Prevents motion sickness.

 ## DOSAGE & USAGE INFORMATION

How to take:
Tablet—Swallow with liquid or food to lessen
stomach irritation. If you can't swallow whole,
crumble tablet and chew or take with liquid or
food.

When to take:
30 minutes to 1 hour before traveling.

If you forget a dose:
Take as soon as you remember. Wait 4 hours for
next dose.

What drug does:
Reduces sensitivity of nerve endings in inner
ear, blocking messages to brain's vomiting
center.

Time lapse before drug works:
30 to 60 minutes.

Don't take with:
See Interaction column and consult doctor.

 ## OVERDOSE

SYMPTOMS:
Drowsiness, confusion, incoordination,
stupor, coma, weak pulse, shallow breathing
hallucinations.
WHAT TO DO:
● Dial 0 (operator) or 911 (emergency) for
  an ambulance or medical help. Then give
  first aid immediately.
● See emergency information on inside
  covers.

 ## POSSIBLE ADVERSE REACTIONS OR SIDE EFFECTS

SYMPTOMS	WHAT TO DO
Life-threatening: None expected.	
Common: Drowsiness.	Continue. Tell doctor at next visit.
Infrequent: ● Headache, diarrhea or constipation, nausea, fast heartbeat.	Continue. Call doctor when convenient.
● Dry mouth, nose, throat.	Continue. Tell doctor at next visit.
Rare: ● Rash or hives, jaundice.	Discontinue. Call doctor right away.
● Restlessness, excitement, insomnia, blurred vision, frequent or difficult urination, hallucinations.	Continue. Call doctor when convenient.
● Appetite loss, nausea.	Continue. Tell doctor at next visit.

 ## WARNINGS & PRECAUTIONS

Don't take if:
● You are allergic to meclizine, buclizine or
  cyclizine.
● You have taken MAO inhibitors in the past 2
  weeks.

Before you start, consult your doctor:
● If you have glaucoma.
● If you have prostate enlargement.
● If you have reacted badly to any antihistamine.

Over age 60:
Adverse reactions and side effects may be more
frequent and severe than in younger persons,
especially impaired urination from enlarged
prostate gland.

Pregnancy:
Studies inconclusive on harm to unborn child.
Animal studies show fetal abnormalities. Decide
with your doctor whether drug benefits justify
risk to unborn child.

Breast-feeding:
Drug passes into milk. Avoid drug or discontinue
nursing until you finish medicine. Consult doctor
for advice on maintaining milk supply.

Infants & children:
Safety not established. Avoid if under age 12.

Prolonged use:
No problems expected.

Skin & sunlight:
No problems expected.

Driving, piloting or hazardous work:
Don't fly aircraft. Don't drive until you learn how medicine affects you. Don't work around dangerous machinery. Don't climb ladders or work in high places. Danger increases if you drink alcohol or take medicine affecting alertness and reflexes, such as antihistamines, tranquilizers, sedatives, pain medicine, narcotics and mind-altering drugs.

Discontinuing:
No problems expected.

Others:
Some products contain tartrazine dye. Avoid if allergic (especially aspirin hypersensitivity).

POSSIBLE INTERACTION WITH OTHER DRUGS

GENERIC NAME OR DRUG CLASS	COMBINED EFFECT
Amphetamines*	May decrease drowsiness caused by cyclizine.
Anticholinergics*	Increased effect of both drugs.
Antidepressants, tricyclic (TCA)*	Increased effect of both drugs.
Carteolol	Decreased antihistamine effect.
Dronabinol	Increased cyclizine effect.
Ethinamate	Dangerous increased effects of ethinamate. Avoid combining.
Fluoxetine	Increased depressant effects of both drugs.
Guanfacine	May increase depressant effects of either drug.
Leucovorin	High alcohol content of leucovorin may cause adverse effects.
MAO inhibitors*	Increased cyclizine effect.
Methyprylon	Increased sedative effect, perhaps to dangerous level. Avoid.
Nabilone	Greater depression of central nervous system.
Narcotics*	Increased effect of both drugs.
Pain relievers*	Increased effect of both drugs.
Sedatives*	Increased effect of both drugs.
Sleep inducers*	Increased effect of both drugs.
Sotalol	Increased antihistamine effect.
Tranquilizers*	Increased effect of both drugs.

POSSIBLE INTERACTION WITH OTHER SUBSTANCES

INTERACTS WITH	COMBINED EFFECT
Alcohol:	Increased sedation. Avoid.
Beverages: Caffeine drinks.	May decrease drowsiness.
Cocaine:	None expected.
Foods:	None expected.
Marijuana:	Increased drowsiness, dry mouth.
Tobacco:	None expected.

CYCLOBENZAPRINE

BRAND NAMES

Flexeril

BASIC INFORMATION

Habit forming? No
Prescription needed? Yes
Available as generic? No
Drug class: Muscle relaxant (skeletal)

USES

Treatment for pain and limited motion caused by spasms in voluntary muscles.

DOSAGE & USAGE INFORMATION

How to take:
Tablet—Swallow with liquid.

When to take:
At the same time each day or according to label instructions.

If you forget a dose:
Take as soon as you remember. Wait 4 hours for next dose.

What drug does:
Blocks body's pain messages to brain. May also sedate.

Time lapse before drug works:
30 to 60 minutes.

Continued next column

OVERDOSE

SYMPTOMS:
Drowsiness, confusion, difficulty concentrating, visual problems, vomiting, blood-pressure drop, low body temperature, weak and rapid pulse, convulsions, coma.
WHAT TO DO:
- Dial 0 (operator) or 911 (emergency) for an ambulance or medical help. Then give first aid immediately.
- If patient is unconscious and not breathing, give mouth-to-mouth breathing. If there is no heartbeat, use cardiac massage and mouth-to-mouth breathing (CPR). Don't try to make patient vomit. If you can't get help quickly, take patient to nearest emergency facility.
- See emergency information on inside covers.

Don't take with:
- Non-prescription drugs without consulting doctor.
- See Interaction column and consult doctor.

POSSIBLE ADVERSE REACTIONS OR SIDE EFFECTS

SYMPTOMS	WHAT TO DO
Life-threatening: None expected.	
Common: Drowsiness, dizziness, dry mouth.	Continue. Call doctor when convenient.
Infrequent:	
• Blurred vision, fast heartbeat.	Discontinue. Call doctor right away.
• Insomnia, numbness in extremities, bad taste in mouth, fatigue, nausea, sweating.	Continue. Call doctor when convenient.
Rare:	
• Unsteadiness, confusion, depression, hallucinations, rash, itch, swelling, breathing difficulty.	Discontinue. Call doctor right away.
• Difficult urination. rash.	Continue. Call doctor when convenient.

WARNINGS & PRECAUTIONS

Don't take if:
- You are allergic to any skeletal-muscle relaxant.
- You have taken MAO inhibitors in last 2 weeks.
- You have had a heart attack within 6 weeks, or suffer from congestive heart failure.
- You have overactive thyroid.

Before you start, consult your doctor:
- If you have a heart problem.
- If you have reacted to tricyclic antidepressants.
- If you have glaucoma.
- If you have a prostate condition and urination difficulty.
- If you intend to pilot aircraft.

Over age 60:
Adverse reactions and side effects may be more frequent and severe than in younger persons. Avoid extremes of heat and cold.

Pregnancy:
Risk to unborn child outweighs drug benefits. Don't use.

Breast-feeding:
Drug passes into milk. Avoid drug or discontinue nursing until you finish medicine. Consult doctor for advice on maintaining milk supply.

Infants & children:
Don't use for children younger than 15.

Prolonged use:
Do not take for longer than 2 to 3 weeks.

Skin & sunlight:
May cause rash or intensify sunburn in areas exposed to sun or sunlamp.

Driving, piloting or hazardous work:
Don't drive or pilot aircraft until you learn how medicine affects you. Don't work around dangerous machinery. Don't climb ladders or work in high places. Danger increases if you drink alcohol or take medicine affecting alertness and reflexes.

Discontinuing:
May be unnecessary to finish medicine. Follow doctor's instructions.

Others:
No problems expected.

POSSIBLE INTERACTION WITH OTHER DRUGS

GENERIC NAME OR DRUG CLASS	COMBINED EFFECT
Anticholinergics*	Increased anti-cholinergic effect.
Antidepressants*	Increased sedation.
Antihistamines*	Increased anti-histamine effect.
Barbiturates*	Increased sedation.
Cimetidine	Possible increased cyclobenzaprine effect.
Clonidine	Decreased clonidine effect.
Dronabinol	Increased effect of dronabinol on central nervous system. Avoid combination.
Guanethidine	Decreased guanethidine effect.
MAO inhibitors*	High fever, convulsions, possible death.
Methyldopa	Decreased methyldopa effect.
Mind-altering drugs*	Increased mind-altering effect.

Narcotics*	Increased sedation.
Pain relievers*	Increased pain reliever effect.
Procainamide	Possible increased conduction disturbance.
Quinidine	Possible increased conduction disturbance.
Rauwolfia alkaloids*	Decreased effect of rauwolfia alkaloids.
Sedatives*	Increased sedative effect.
Sleep inducers*	Increased sedation.
Tranquilizers*	Increased tranquilizer effect.

POSSIBLE INTERACTION WITH OTHER SUBSTANCES

INTERACTS WITH	COMBINED EFFECT
Alcohol:	Depressed brain function. Avoid.
Beverages:	None expected.
Cocaine:	Decreased cyclobenzaprine effect.
Foods:	None expected.
Marijuana:	Occasional use—Drowsiness. Frequent use—Severe mental and physical impairment.
Tobacco:	None expected.

CYCLOPEGIC, MYDRIATIC (Ophthalmic)

BRAND AND GENERIC NAMES

AK Homatropine
Atropar Eye Drops
  & Ointment
ATROPINE
Atropine Care Eye
  Drops & Ointment
Atropisol
HOMATROPINE

Isopto
Isopto Atropine
Isopto Hyoscine
Minims
Minims Atropine
S.M.P. Atropine
SCOPOLAMINE

BASIC INFORMATION

Habit forming? No
Prescription needed? Yes
Available as generic? Yes, some
Drug class: Cyclopegic, mydriatic

USES

- Dilates pupil of the eye.
- Used before some eye examinations, before and after some eye surgical procedures and, rarely, to treat some eye problems such as glaucoma.

DOSAGE & USAGE INFORMATION

How to use:
Eye drops
- Wash hands.
- Apply pressure to inside corner of eye with middle finger.
- Continue pressure for 1 minute after placing medicine in eye.
- Tilt head backward. Pull lower lid away from eye with index finger of the same hand.
- Drop eye drops into pouch and close eye. Don't blink.
- Keep eyes closed for 1 to 2 minutes.

Continued next column

OVERDOSE

SYMPTOMS:
None expected.
WHAT TO DO:
Not intended for internal use. If child accidentally swallows, call poison-control center.

Eye ointment
- Wash hands.
- Pull lower lid down from eye to form a pouch.
- Squeeze tube to apply thin strip of ointment into pouch.
- Close eye for 1 to 2 minutes.
- Don't touch applicator tip to any surface (including the eye). If you accidentally touch tip, clean with warm soap and water.
- Keep container tightly closed.
- Keep cool, but don't freeze.
- Wash hands immediately after using.

When to use:
As directed on label.

If you forget a dose:
Use as soon as you remember.

What drug does:
Blocks normal response to sphincter muscle of the iris of the eye and the accommodative muscle of the ciliary body.

Time lapse before drug works:
Begins within 1 minute. Residual effects may last up to 14 days.

Don't use with:
Other eye medicines such as carbachol, demecarium, echothiopate, isoflurophate, physostigmine, pilocarpine.

POSSIBLE ADVERSE REACTIONS OR SIDE EFFECTS

SYMPTOMS	WHAT TO DO
Life-threatening: None expected.	
Common: • Increased sensitivity to light. • Burning eyes.	Continue. Call doctor when convenient. Continue. Tell doctor at next visit.
Infrequent: None expected.	
Rare (extremely): Symptoms of excess medicine absorbed by the body—Clumsiness, confusion, fever, flushed face, hallucinations, rash, slurred speech, swollen stomach (children), drowsiness, fast heartbeat.	Discontinue. Seek emergency treatment.

CYCLOPEGIC, MYDRIATIC (Ophthalmic)

WARNINGS & PRECAUTIONS

Don't use if:
You are allergic to cyclopentolate.

Before you start, consult your doctor:
- If medicine is for a brain-damaged child or child with Down's syndrome.
- If prescribed for a child with spastic paralysis.

Over age 60:
No problems expected.

Pregnancy:
Safety to unborn child unestablished. Avoid if possible.

Breast-feeding:
Safety unestablished. Avoid if possible.

Infants & children:
Use only under close medical supervision.

Prolonged use:
Avoid. May increase absorption into body.

Skin & sunlight:
Wear sunglasses to protect from sunlight and bright light.

Driving, piloting or hazardous work:
Don't drive or pilot aircraft until you learn how medicine affects you. Don't work around dangerous machinery. Don't climb ladders or work in high places. Danger increases if you drink alcohol or take medicine affecting alertness and reflexes, such as antihistamines, tranquilizers, sedatives, pain medicine, narcotics and mind-altering drugs.

Discontinuing:
Effects may last up to 14 days later.

Others:
Keep cool, but don't freeze.

POSSIBLE INTERACTION WITH OTHER DRUGS

GENERIC NAME OR DRUG CLASS	COMBINED EFFECT
Clinically significant interactions with oral or injected medicines unlikely.	

POSSIBLE INTERACTION WITH OTHER SUBSTANCES

INTERACTS WITH	COMBINED EFFECT
Alcohol:	None expected.
Beverages:	None expected.
Cocaine:	None expected.
Foods:	None expected.
Marijuana:	None expected.
Tobacco:	None expected.

CYCLOPENTOLATE (Ophthalmic)

BRAND NAMES

Ak-Pentolate
Cy clogyl

Minims
Cyclopentolate
Pentolair

BASIC INFORMATION

Habit forming? No
Prescription needed? Yes
Available as generic? Yes
Drug class: Cyclopegic (paralyzes eye accommodation to light), mydriatic (dilates pupil)

 ## USES

- Enlarges (dilates) pupil.
- Temporarily paralyzes the normal pupil accommodation to light before eye examinations and to treat some eye conditions.

 ## DOSAGE & USAGE INFORMATION

How to use:
Eye drops
- Wash hands.
- Apply pressure to inside corner of eye with middle finger.
- Continue pressure for 1 minute after placing medicine in eye.
- Tilt head backward. Pull lower lid away from eye with index finger of the same hand.
- Drop eye drops into pouch and close eye. Don't blink.
- Keep eyes closed for 1 to 2 minutes.
- Don't touch applicator tip to any surface (including the eye). If you accidentally touch tip, clean with warm soap and water.
- Keep container tightly closed.
- Keep cool, but don't freeze.
- Wash hands immediately after using.

When to use:
As directed on bottle.

Continued next column

 ## OVERDOSE

SYMPTOMS:
None expected.
WHAT TO DO:
Not intended for internal use. If child accidentally swallows, call poison-control center.

If you forget a dose:
Use as soon as you remember.

What drug does:
Blocks sphincter muscle of the iris and ciliary body.

Time lapse before drug works:
Within 30 to 60 minutes. Effects usually disappear in 24 hours.

Don't use with:
Other eye medicines such as carbachol, demecarium, echothiopate, isoflurophate, physostigmine, pilocarpine.

 ## POSSIBLE ADVERSE REACTIONS OR SIDE EFFECTS

SYMPTOMS	WHAT TO DO
Life-threatening: None expected.	
Common: • Increased sensitivity to light. • Burning eyes.	Continue. Call doctor when convenient. Continue. Tell doctor at next visit.
Infrequent: None expected.	
Rare (extremely): Symptoms of excess medicine absorbed by the body—Clumsiness, confusion, fever, flushed face, hallucinations, rash, slurred speech, swollen stomach (children), drowsiness, fast heartbeat.	Discontinue. Seek emergency treatment.

CYCLOPENTOLATE (Ophthalmic)

WARNINGS & PRECAUTIONS

Don't use if:
You are allergic to cyclopentolate.

Before you start, consult your doctor:
- If medicine is for a brain-damaged child or child with Down's syndrome.
- If prescribed for a child with spastic paralysis.

Over age 60:
No problems expected.

Pregnancy:
Safety to unborn child unestablished. Avoid if possible.

Breast-feeding:
Safety unestablished. Avoid if possible.

Infants & children:
Use only under close medical supervision.

Prolonged use:
Avoid. May increase absorption into body.

Skin & sunlight:
Wear sunglasses to protect from sunlight and bright light.

Driving, piloting or hazardous work:
Don't drive or pilot aircraft until you learn how medicine affects you. Don't work around dangerous machinery. Don't climb ladders or work in high places. Danger increases if you drink alcohol or take medicine affecting alertness and reflexes, such as antihistamines, tranquilizers, sedatives, pain medicine, narcotics and mind-altering drugs.

Discontinuing:
If effects last longer than 36 hours after last drops, consult doctor.

Others:
Keep cool, but don't freeze.

POSSIBLE INTERACTION WITH OTHER DRUGS

GENERIC NAME OR DRUG CLASS	COMBINED EFFECT
Clinically significant interactions with oral or injected medicines unlikely.	

POSSIBLE INTERACTION WITH OTHER SUBSTANCES

INTERACTS WITH	COMBINED EFFECT
Alcohol:	None expected.
Beverages:	None expected.
Cocaine:	None expected.
Foods:	None expected.
Marijuana:	None expected.
Tobacco:	None expected.

CYCLOPHOSPHAMIDE

BRAND NAMES

Cytoxan   Procytox
Neosar

BASIC INFORMATION

Habit forming? No
Available as generic? No
Prescription needed? No
Drug class: Immunosuppressant

USES

- Treatment for cancer.
- Treatment for severe rheumatoid arthritis.
- Treatment for blood-vessel disease.
- Treatment for skin disease.

DOSAGE & USAGE INFORMATION

How to take:
Tablet or liquid—Swallow with liquid. If you can't swallow whole, crumble tablet and take with liquid or food.

When to take:
Works best if taken first thing in morning. However, may take with food to lessen stomach irritation. Don't take at bedtime.

If you forget a dose:
Take as soon as you remember up to 12 hours late. If more than 12 hours, wait for next scheduled dose (don't double this dose).

What drug does:
- Kills cancer cells.
- Suppresses spread of cancer cells.
- Suppresses immune system.

Time lapse before drug works:
7 to 10 days continual use.

Don't take with:
See Interaction column and consult doctor.

OVERDOSE

SYMPTOMS:
Bloody urine, water retention, weight gain, severe infection.
WHAT TO DO:
Overdose unlikely to threaten life. If person takes much larger amount than prescribed, call doctor, poison-control center or hospital emergency room for instructions.

POSSIBLE ADVERSE REACTIONS OR SIDE EFFECTS

SYMPTOMS	WHAT TO DO
Life-threatening:	
Hives, rash, intense itching, faintness soon after a dose (anaphylaxis).	Seek emergency treatment immediately.
Common:	
• Sore throat, fever.	Discontinue. Call doctor right away.
• Dark skin, nails; nausea; appetite loss; vomiting; missed period.	Continue. Call doctor when convenient.
Infrequent:	
• Rash, hives, itch; shortness of breath; rapid heartbeat; cough; blood in urine, painful urination; pain in side; bleeding, bruising; increased sweating.	Discontinue. Call doctor right away.
• Confusion, agitation, headache, dizziness, flushed face, stomach pain, joint pain, fatigue, weakness.	Continue. Call doctor when convenient.
Rare:	
• Mouth, lip sores; black stool; unusual thirst.	Discontinue. Call doctor right away.
• Blurred vision, increased urination, hair loss.	Continue. Call doctor when convenient.

WARNINGS & PRECAUTIONS

Don't take if:
- You are allergic to any alkylating agent.
- You have an infection.
- You have bloody urine.
- You will have surgery within 2 months, including dental surgery, requiring general or spinal anesthesia.

Before you start, consult your doctor:
- If you have impaired liver or kidney function.
- If you have impaired bone-marrow or blood-cell production.
- If you have had chemotherapy or X-ray therapy.
- If you have taken cortisone drugs in the past year.

Over age 60:
Adverse reactions and side effects may be more frequent and severe than in younger persons. To reduce risk of chemical bladder inflammation, drink 8 to 10 glasses of water daily.

Pregnancy:
Risk to unborn child outweighs drug benefits. Don't use.

Breast-feeding:
Drug passes into milk. Avoid drug or discontinue nursing until you finish medicine. Consult doctor for advice on maintaining milk supply.

Infants & children:
Use only under medical supervision.

Prolonged use:
- Development of fibrous lung tissue.
- Possible jaundice.
- Swelling of feet, lower legs.
- Cancer.
- Infertility in men.

Skin & sunlight:
No problems expected.

Driving, piloting or hazardous work:
Avoid if you feel dizzy or have blurred vision. Otherwise, no problems expected.

Discontinuing:
Don't discontinue without consulting doctor. Dose may require gradual reduction if you have taken drug for a long time. Doses of other drugs may also require adjustment.

Others:
Frequently causes hair loss. After treatment ends, hair should grow back.

POSSIBLE INTERACTION WITH OTHER DRUGS

GENERIC NAME OR DRUG CLASS	COMBINED EFFECT
Allopurinol	Possible anemia.
Antidiabetics, oral*	Increased antidiabetic effect.
Cyclosporine	May increase risk of infection.
Digoxin	Possible decreased digoxin absorption.
Insulin	Increased insulin effect.
Lovastatin	Increased heart and kidney damage.
Phenobarbital	Increased cyclo-phosphamide effect.

POSSIBLE INTERACTION WITH OTHER SUBSTANCES

INTERACTS WITH	COMBINED EFFECT
Alcohol:	No problems expected.
Beverages:	No problems expected. Drink at least 2 quarts fluid every day.
Cocaine:	Increased danger of brain damage.
Foods:	None expected.
Marijuana:	Increased impairment of immunity.
Tobacco:	None expected.

*See Glossary

CYCLOSERINE

BRAND NAMES

Seromycin

BASIC INFORMATION

Habit forming? No
Prescription needed? Yes
Available as generic? No
Drug class: Antibacterial (antibiotic)

 USES

- Treats urinary tract infections.
- Treats tuberculosis.

 DOSAGE & USAGE INFORMATION

How to take:
Capsules—Swallow with liquid or food to lesson stomach irritation. If you can't swallow whole, open capsule and take with liquid or food.

When to take:
- Once or twice daily.
- At the same time each day after meals to prevent stomach irritation.

If you forget a dose:
Take as soon as you remember up to 2 hours late. If more than 2 hours, wait for next scheduled dose (don't double this dose).

What drug does:
Interferes with bacterial wall synthesis and keeps germs from multiplying.

Time lapse before drug works:
3 to 4 hours.

Don't take with:
See Interaction column and consult doctor.

 OVERDOSE

SYMPTOMS:
Seizures.
WHAT TO DO:
- Dial 0 (operator) or 911 (emergency) for an ambulance or medical help. Then give first aid immediately.
- See emergency information on inside covers.

 POSSIBLE ADVERSE REACTIONS OR SIDE EFFECTS

SYMPTOMS	WHAT TO DO
Life-threatening: Seizures, muscle twitching or trembling.	Seek emergency treatment immediately.
Common: Gum inflammation, pale skin, depression, confusion, dizziness, restlessness, anxiety, nightmares, severe headache.	Discontinue. Call doctor right away.
Infrequent: Visual changes; sun sensitivity; skin rash; numbness, tingling or burning in hands and feet; jaundice.	Continue. Call doctor when convenient.
Rare: Seizures, thoughts of suicide.	Discontinue. Seek emergency treatment.

WARNINGS & PRECAUTIONS

Don't take if:
- You are an alcoholic.
- You have a convulsive disorder.

Before you start, consult your doctor:
- If you are depressed.
- If you have kidney disease.
- If you have severe anxiety.

Over age 60:
Adverse reactions and side effects may be more frequent and severe than in younger persons. You may need smaller doses for shorter periods of time.

Pregnancy:
Safety not established. Consult your doctor.

Breast-feeding:
Drug passes into milk. Avoid drug or discontinue nursing until you finish medicine. Consult doctor for advice on maintaining milk supply.

Infants & children:
No information available.

Prolonged use:
- May cause liver or kidney damage.
- May cause anemia.

Skin & sunlight:
May cause hypersensitivity to sun exposure.

Driving, piloting or hazardous work:
Don't drive or pilot aircraft until you learn how medicine affects you. Don't work around dangerous machinery. Don't climb ladders or work in high places. Danger increases if you drink alcohol or take medicine affecting alertness and reflexes.

Discontinuing:
Don't discontinue without consulting doctor. Dose may require gradual reduction if you have taken drug for a long time. Doses of other drugs may also require adjustment.

Others:
- May have to take anticonvulsants, sedatives and/or pyridoxine to prevent or minimize toxic effects on the brain.
- If you must take more than 500 mg per day, toxicity is much more likely to occur.

POSSIBLE INTERACTION WITH OTHER DRUGS

GENERIC NAME OR DRUG CLASS	COMBINED EFFECT
Ethionamide	Increased risk of seizures.
Isoniazid	Increased risk of central nervous system effects.
Pyridoxine	Reduces effects of pyridoxine. Since pyridoxine is a vital vitamin, patients on cycloserine require pyridoxine supplements to prevent anemia or peripheral neuritis.

POSSIBLE INTERACTION WITH OTHER SUBSTANCES

INTERACTS WITH	COMBINED EFFECT
Alcohol:	Toxic. May increase risk of seizures. Avoid.
Beverages:	None expected. All beverages except those with alcohol.
Cocaine:	Toxic. Avoid.
Foods:	None expected.
Marijuana:	May increase risk of seizures.
Tobacco:	May decrease effect of cycloserine.

CYCLOSPORINE

BRAND NAMES

Sandimmune

BASIC INFORMATION

Habit forming? No
Prescription needed? Yes
Available as generic? No
Drug class: Immunosuppressant

 ## USES

Suppresses the immune response in patients who have transplants of the heart, lung, kidney, liver, pancreas. Cyclosporine treats rejection as well as helps prevent it.

 ## DOSAGE & USAGE INFORMATION

How to take:
- Oral solution—Take after meals with liquid to decrease stomach irritation. May mix with milk, chocolate milk or orange juice.
- Use special dropper for exact dosage.

When to take:
At the same time each day, according to instructions on prescription label.

If you forget a dose:
Take as soon as you remember up to 2 hours late. If more than 2 hours, wait for next scheduled dose (don't double this dose).

What drug does:
Exact mechanism is unknown, but believed to inhibit interluken II to affect T-lymphocytes.

Time lapse before drug works:
3 to 3-1/2 hours.

Don't take with:
See Interaction column and consult doctor.

 ## OVERDOSE

SYMPTOMS:
Irregular heartbeat, seizures, coma.
WHAT TO DO:
- Dial 0 (operator) or 911 (emergency) for an ambulance or medical help. Then give first aid immediately.
- See emergency information on inside covers.

 ## POSSIBLE ADVERSE REACTIONS OR SIDE EFFECTS

SYMPTOMS	WHAT TO DO
Life-threatening:	
Seizures, wheezing with shortness of breath.	Discontinue. Seek emergency treatment.
Common:	
• Gum inflammation, blood in urine, jaundice.	Continue. Call doctor when convenient.
• Increased hair growth.	Continue. Tell doctor at next visit.
Infrequent:	
• Fever, chills, sore throat, shortness of breath.	Discontinue. Call doctor right away.
• Frequent urination.	Continue. Call doctor when convenient.
Rare:	
• Confusion, irregular heartbeat, numbness of hands and feet, nervousness, face flushing, severe abdominal pain, weakness.	Discontinue. Call doctor right away.
• Acne, headache.	Continue. Call doctor when convenient.

WARNINGS & PRECAUTIONS

Don't take if:
- You have chicken pox.
- You have shingles (herpes zoster).

Before you start, consult your doctor:
- If you have liver problems.
- If you have an infection.
- If you have kidney disease.

Over age 60:
No special problems expected.

Pregnancy:
Safety not established. Consult your doctor.

Breast-feeding:
Drug passes into milk. Avoid drug or discontinue nursing until you finish medicine. Consult doctor for advice on maintaining milk supply.

Infants & children:
No problems expected.

Prolonged use:
Can cause reduced function of kidney.

Skin & sunlight:
No problems expected.

Driving, piloting or hazardous work:
Don't drive or pilot aircraft until you learn how medicine affects you. Don't work around dangerous machinery. Don't climb ladders or work in high places. Danger increases if you drink alcohol or take medicine affecting alertness and reflexes.

Discontinuing:
Don't discontinue without consulting doctor. You probably will require this medicine for the remainder of your life.

Others:
- Request regular laboratory studies to measure levels of potassium, cyclosporine in blood, and to evaluate liver and kidney function.
- Check blood pressure. Cyclosporine sometimes causes hypertension.
- Don't store solution in the refrigerator.
- Avoid any immunizations except those specifically recommended by your doctor.
- Maintain good dental hygiene. Cyclosporine can cause gum problems.

POSSIBLE INTERACTION WITH OTHER DRUGS

GENERIC NAME OR DRUG CLASS	COMBINED EFFECT
Anticonvulsants*	Decreased effect of cyclosporine.
Immuno-suppressants* (adrenocorticoids, azathioprine, chlorambucil, cyclophosphamide, mercaptopurine, muromonab-CD3)	May increase risk of infection.
Ketoconazole	Increased risk of toxicity to kidney.
Lovastatin	Increased heart and kidney damage.
Medicines that may be toxic to kidneys (gold, NSAIDs* sulfonamides)	Increased risk of toxicity to kidneys.
Rifampin	Decreased effect of cyclosporine.
Virus vaccines	Increased adverse reactions to vaccine.

POSSIBLE INTERACTION WITH OTHER SUBSTANCES

INTERACTS WITH	COMBINED EFFECT
Alcohol:	May increase possibility of toxic effects. Avoid.
Beverages:	None expected.
Cocaine:	May increase possibility of toxic effects. Avoid.
Foods:	None expected.
Marijuana:	May increase possibility of toxic effects. Avoid.
Tobacco:	May increase possibility of toxic effects. Avoid.

*See Glossary

CYCLOTHIAZIDE

BRAND NAMES

Anhydron   Fluidil

BASIC INFORMATION

Habit forming? No
Prescription needed? Yes
Available as generic? No
Drug class: Antihypertensive, diuretic
(thiazide)

USES

- Controls, but doesn't cure, high blood pressure.
- Reduces fluid retention (edema) caused by conditions such as heart disorders and liver disease.

DOSAGE & USAGE INFORMATION

How to take:
Tablet—Swallow with liquid. If you can't swallow whole, crumble tablet and take with liquid or food.

When to take:
At the same time each day.

If you forget a dose:
Take as soon as you remember up to 2 hours late. If more than 2 hours, wait for next scheduled dose (don't double this dose).

What drug does:
- Forces sodium and water excretion, reducing body fluid.
- Relaxes muscle cells of small arteries.
- Reduced body fluid and relaxed arteries lower blood pressure.

Time lapse before drug works:
4 to 6 hours. May require several weeks to lower blood pressure.

Continued next column

OVERDOSE

SYMPTOMS:
Cramps, weakness, confusion, drowsiness, weak pulse, coma.
WHAT TO DO:
- Dial 0 (operator) or 911 (emergency) for an ambulance or medical help. Then give first aid immediately.
- See emergency information on inside covers.

Don't take with:
- See Interaction column and consult doctor.
- Non-prescription drugs without consulting doctor.

POSSIBLE ADVERSE REACTIONS OR SIDE EFFECTS

SYMPTOMS	WHAT TO DO
Life-threatening: None expected.	
Common: None expected.	
Infrequent: • Blurred vision, severe abdominal pain, nausea, vomiting, irregular heartbeat, weak pulse.	Discontinue. Call doctor right away.
• Dizziness, mood changes, headaches, weakness, tiredness, weight changes.	Continue. Call doctor when convenient.
• Dry mouth, thirst.	Continue. Tell doctor at next visit.
Rare: • Rash or hives.	Discontinue. Seek emergency treatment.
• Sore throat, fever, jaundice.	Discontinue. Call doctor right away.

WARNINGS & PRECAUTIONS

Don't take if:
You are allergic to any thiazide diuretic drugs.

Before you start, consult your doctor:
- If you are allergic to any sulfa drug or tartrazine dye.
- If you have gout, diabetes or systemic lupus erythematosus.
- If you have liver, pancreas or kidney disorder.

Over age 60:
Adverse reactions and side effects may be more frequent and severe than in younger persons, especially dizziness and excessive potassium loss.

Pregnancy:
Risk to unborn child outweighs drug benefits. Don't use.

Breast-feeding:
Drug passes into milk. Avoid drug or discontinue nursing.

Infants & children:
No problems expected.

Prolonged use:
You may need medicine to treat high blood pressure for the rest of your life.

Skin & sunlight:
May cause rash or intensify sunburn in areas exposed to sun or sunlamp.

Driving, piloting or hazardous work:
Don't drive or pilot aircraft until you learn how medicine affects you. Don't work around dangerous machinery. Don't climb ladders or work in high places. Danger increases if you drink alcohol or take medicine affecting alertness and reflexes, such as antihistamines, tranquilizers, sedatives, pain medicine, narcotics and mind-altering drugs.

Discontinuing:
Don't discontinue without medical advice.

Others:
- Hot weather and fever may cause dehydration and drop in blood pressure. Dose may require temporary adjustment. Weigh daily and report any unexpected weight decreases to your doctor.
- May cause rise in uric acid, leading to gout.
- May cause blood-sugar rise in diabetics.

 ## POSSIBLE INTERACTION WITH OTHER DRUGS

GENERIC NAME OR DRUG CLASS	COMBINED EFFECT
ACE Inhibitors: captopril, enalapril, lisinopril*	Decreased blood pressure.
Amiodarone and other medicines to treat irregular heartbeat	Increased risk of heartbeat irregularity due to low potassium.
Amphotericin B	Increased potassium.
Antidepressants, tricyclic (TCA)*	Dangerous drop in blood pressure. Avoid combination unless under medical supervision.
Antidiabetic agents, oral*	Increased blood sugar.
Antihypertensives*	Increased chlorthiazide effect or decreased blood pressure.
Beta-adrenergic blockers*	Increased antihypertensive effect. Dosages of both drugs may require adjustments.
Bumetanide	Increased diuretic effect.
Calcium supplements*	May increase calcium in blood.

Carteolol	Increased antihypertensive effect.
Cholestyramine	Decreased cyclothiazide effect.
Colestipol	Decreased cyclothiazide effect.
Cortisone drugs*	Excessive potassium loss that causes dangerous heart rhythms.
Digitalis preparations*	Excessive potassium loss that causes dangerous heart rhythms.
Diuretics, thiazide*	Increased effect of other thiazide diuretics.
Ethacrynic acid	Increased diuretic effect.
Furosemide	Decreased diuretic effect.
Hypoglycemics, oral*	Decreased ability to lower blood glucose.
Indapamide	Increased diuretic effect.
Indomethacin	Decreased cyclothiazide effect.
Insulin	Decreased ability to lower blood glucose.
Lithium	Increased effect of lithium.
MAO inhibitors*	Increased cyclothiazide effect.
Metolazone	Increased diuretic effect.

Continued page 1083

 ## POSSIBLE INTERACTION WITH OTHER SUBSTANCES

INTERACTS WITH	COMBINED EFFECT
Alcohol:	Dangerous blood-pressure drop.
Beverages:	None expected.
Cocaine:	Increased risk of heart block and high blood pressure.
Foods: Licorice.	Excessive potassium loss that causes dangerous heart rhythms.
Marijuana:	May increase blood pressure.
Tobacco:	None expected.

*See Glossary

CYCRIMINE

BRAND NAMES

Pagitane

BASIC INFORMATION

Habit forming? No
Prescription needed? Yes
Available as generic? No
Drug class: Antidyskinetic, antiparkinsonism

 USES

- Treatment of Parkinson's disease.
- Treatment of adverse effects of phenothiazines.

 DOSAGE & USAGE INFORMATION

How to take:
Tablets or capsules—Take with food to lessen stomach irritation.

When to take:
At the same times each day.

If you forget a dose:
Take as soon as you remember up to 2 hours late. If more than 2 hours, wait for next scheduled dose (don't double this dose).

What drug does:
- Balances chemical reactions necessary to send nerve impulses within base of brain.
- Improves muscle control and reduces stiffness.

Time lapse before drug works:
1 to 2 hours.

Continued next column

 OVERDOSE

SYMPTOMS:
Agitation, dilated pupils, hallucinations, dry mouth, rapid heartbeat, sleepiness.
WHAT TO DO:
- **Dial 0 (operator) or 911 (emergency) for an ambulance or medical help. Then give first aid immediately.**
- **If patient is unconscious and not breathing, give mouth-to-mouth breathing. If there is no heartbeat, use cardiac massage and mouth-to-mouth breathing (CPR). Don't try to make patient vomit. If you can't get help quickly, take patient to nearest emergency facility.**
- **See emergency information on inside covers.**

Don't take with:
- Non-prescription drugs for colds, cough or allergy.
- See Interaction column and consult doctor.

 POSSIBLE ADVERSE REACTIONS OR SIDE EFFECTS

SYMPTOMS	WHAT TO DO
Life-threatening: None expected.	
Common:	
• Blurred vision, light sensitivity, constipation, nausea, vomiting.	Continue. Call doctor when convenient.
• Difficult or painful urination.	Continue. Tell doctor at next visit.
Infrequent: None expected.	
Rare:	
• Rash, eye pain.	Discontinue. Call doctor right away.
• Confusion; dizziness; sore mouth or tongue; muscle cramps; numbness, weakness in hands or feet.	Continue. Call doctor when convenient.

WARNINGS & PRECAUTIONS

Don't take if:
You are allergic to any antidyskinetic.

Before you start, consult your doctor:
- If you have had glaucoma.
- If you have had high blood pressure or heart disease.
- If you have had impaired liver function.
- If you have had kidney disease or urination difficulty.

Over age 60:
More sensitive to drug. Aggravates symptoms of enlarged prostate. Causes impaired thinking, hallucinations, nightmares. Consult doctor about any of these.

Pregnancy:
Studies inconclusive on harm to unborn child. Animal studies show fetal abnormalities. Decide with your doctor whether drug benefits justify risk to unborn child.

Breast-feeding:
No problems expected.

Infants & children:
Not recommended for children 3 and younger. Use for older children only under doctor's supervision.

Prolonged use:
Possible glaucoma.

Skin & sunlight:
No problems expected.

Driving, piloting or hazardous work:
Don't drive or pilot aircraft until you learn how medicine affects you. Don't work around dangerous machinery. Don't climb ladders or work in high places. Danger increases if you drink alcohol or take medicine affecting alertness and reflexes, such as antihistamines, tranquilizers, sedatives, pain medicine, narcotics and mind-altering drugs.

Discontinuing:
Don't discontinue without consulting doctor. Dose may require gradual reduction if you have taken drug for a long time. Doses of other drugs may also require adjustment.

Others:
- Internal eye pressure should be measured regularly.
- Avoid becoming overheated.

POSSIBLE INTERACTION WITH OTHER DRUGS

GENERIC NAME OR DRUG CLASS	COMBINED EFFECT
Amantadine	Increased amantadine effect.
Antidepressants, tricyclic (TCA)*	Increased cycrimine effect. May cause glaucoma.
Antihistamines*	Increased cycrimine effect.
Levodopa	Increased levodopa effect. Improved results in treating Parkinson's disease.
Meperidine	Increased cycrimine effect.
MAO inhibitors*	Increased cycrimine effect.
Nabilone	Greater depression of central nervous system.
Orphenadrine	Increased cycrimine effect.
Phenothiazines*	Behavior changes.
Primidone	Excessive sedation.
Procainamide	Increased procainamide effect.
Quinidine	Increased cycrimine effect.
Tranquilizers*	Excessive sedation.

POSSIBLE INTERACTION WITH OTHER SUBSTANCES

INTERACTS WITH	COMBINED EFFECT
Alcohol:	None expected.
Beverages:	None expected.
Cocaine:	Decreased cycrimine effect. Avoid.
Foods:	None expected.
Marijuana:	None expected.
Tobacco:	None expected.

CYPROHEPTADINE

BRAND NAMES

Cyprodine   Vimicon
Periactin

BASIC INFORMATION

Habit forming? No
Prescription needed? Yes
Available as generic? Yes
Drug class: Antihistamine

 USES

- Reduces allergic symptoms such as hay fever, hives, rash or itching.
- Reduces symptoms of cold urticaria.

 DOSAGE & USAGE INFORMATION

How to take:
Tablet or syrup—Swallow with liquid or food to lessen stomach irritation.

When to take:
Varies with form. Follow label directions.

If you forget a dose:
Take as soon as you remember up to 2 hours late. If more than 2 hours, wait for next scheduled dose (don't double this dose).

What drug does:
Blocks action of histamine after an allergic response triggers histamine release in sensitive cells.

Time lapse before drug works:
30 minutes.

Don't take with:
See Interaction column and consult doctor.

 OVERDOSE

SYMPTOMS:
Convulsions, red face, hallucinations, coma.
WHAT TO DO:
- **Dial 0 (operator) or 911 (emergency) for an ambulance or medical help. Then give first aid immediately.**
- **If patient is unconscious and not breathing, give mouth-to-mouth breathing. If there is no heartbeat, use cardiac massage and mouth-to-mouth breathing (CPR). Don't try to make patient vomit. If you can't get help quickly, take patient to nearest emergency facility.**
- **See emergency information on inside covers.**

 POSSIBLE ADVERSE REACTIONS OR SIDE EFFECTS

SYMPTOMS	WHAT TO DO
Life-threatening: None expected.	
Common: Drowsiness, dizziness, dry mouth, nose, throat, nausea.	Continue. Tell doctor at next visit.
Infrequent:	
• Vision changes.	Discontinue. Call doctor right away.
• Less tolerance for contact lenses, difficult urination.	Continue. Call doctor when convenient.
• Appetite loss.	Continue. Tell doctor at next visit.
Rare: Nightmares, agitation, irritability, sore throat, fever, rapid heartbeat, unusual bleeding or bruising, fatigue, weakness.	Discontinue. Call doctor right away.

WARNINGS & PRECAUTIONS

Don't take if:
You are allergic to any antihistamine.

Before you start, consult your doctor:
- If you have glaucoma.
- If you have enlarged prostate.
- If you have asthma.
- If you have kidney disease.
- If you have peptic ulcer.
- If you will have surgery within 2 months, including dental surgery, requiring general or spinal anesthesia.

Over age 60:
Don't exceed recommended dose. Adverse reactions and side effects may be more frequent and severe than in younger persons, especially urination difficulty, diminished alertness and other brain and nervous-system symptoms.

Pregnancy:
No proven harm to unborn child. Avoid if possible.

Breast-feeding:
Drug passes into milk. Avoid drug or discontinue nursing until you finish medicine. Consult doctor for advice on maintaining milk supply.

Infants & children:
Not recommended for premature or newborn infants. Otherwise, no problems expected.

Prolonged use:
Avoid. May damage bone marrow and nerve cells.

Skin & sunlight:
May cause rash or intensify sunburn in areas exposed to sun or sunlamp.

Driving, piloting or hazardous work:
Don't drive or pilot aircraft until you learn how medicine affects you. Don't work around dangerous machinery. Don't climb ladders or work in high places. Danger increases if you drink alcohol or take medicine affecting alertness and reflexes, such as antihistamines, tranquilizers, sedatives, pain medicine, narcotics and mind-altering drugs.

Discontinuing:
No problems expected.

Others:
May mask symptoms of hearing damage from aspirin, other salicylates, cisplatin, paromomycin, vancomycin or anticonvulsants. Consult doctor if you use these.

POSSIBLE INTERACTION WITH OTHER DRUGS

GENERIC NAME OR DRUG CLASS	COMBINED EFFECT
Anticholinergics*	Increased anticholinergic effect.
Anticoagulants, oral*	Decreased cyproheptadine effect.
Antidepressants*	Excess sedation. Avoid.
Antihistamines, other*	Excess sedation. Avoid.
Carteolol	Decreased antihistamine effect.
Dronabinol	Increased effects of both drugs. Avoid.
Hypnotics*	Excess sedation. Avoid.
MAO inhibitors*	Increased cyproheptadine effect.
Mind-altering drugs*	Excess sedation. Avoid.
Molindone	Increased antihistamine effect.
Nabilone	Greater depression of central nervous system.
Narcotics*	Excess sedation. Avoid.
Procarbazine	May increase sedation.
Sedatives*	Excess sedation. Avoid.
Sleep inducers*	Excess sedation. Avoid.
Sotalol	Increased antihistamine effect.
Tranquilizers*	Excess sedation. Avoid.

POSSIBLE INTERACTION WITH OTHER SUBSTANCES

INTERACTS WITH	COMBINED EFFECT
Alcohol:	Excess sedation. Avoid.
Beverages: Caffeine drinks.	Less cyproheptadine sedation.
Cocaine:	Decreased cyproheptadine effect. Avoid.
Foods:	None expected.
Marijuana:	Excess sedation. Avoid.
Tobacco:	None expected.

*See Glossary

DANAZOL

BRAND NAMES

Cyclomen   Danocrine

BASIC INFORMATION

Habit forming? No
Prescription needed? Yes
Available as generic? No
Drug class: Gonadotropin inhibitor

USES

Treatment of endometriosis, fibrocystic breast disease, angioneurotic edema except in pregnant women, gynecomastia, infertility, excessive menstruation, precocious puberty.

DOSAGE & USAGE INFORMATION

How to take:
Capsule—Swallow with liquid or food to lessen stomach irritation. If you can't swallow whole, open capsule and take with liquid or food.

When to take:
At the same times each day.

If you forget a dose:
Take as soon as you remember (don't double dose).

What drug does:
Partially prevents output of pituitary follicle-stimulating hormone and lutenizing hormone reducing estrogen production.

Time lapse before drug works:
- 2 to 3 months to treat endometriosis.
- 1 to 2 months to treat other disorders.

Don't take with:
- Birth control pills.
- See Interaction column and consult doctor.

OVERDOSE

SYMPTOMS:
None expected.
WHAT TO DO:
Overdose unlikely to threaten life. If person takes much larger amount than prescribed, call doctor, poison-control center or hospital emergency room for instructions.

POSSIBLE ADVERSE REACTIONS OR SIDE EFFECTS

SYMPTOMS	WHAT TO DO
Life-threatening: None expected.	
Common: Menstrual irregularities.	Continue. Call doctor when convenient.
Infrequent:	
• Unnatural hair growth in women, nosebleeds.	Discontinue. Call doctor right away.
• Dizziness; deepened voice; hoarseness; flushed or red skin; muscle cramps; enlarged clitoris; decreased testicle size; vaginal burning, itching; swollen feet; decreased breast size.	Continue. Call doctor when convenient.
• Headache, acne, weight gain.	Continue. Tell doctor at next visit.
Rare: Jaundice, flushing, sweating, vaginitis, rash, nausea, vomiting, constipation.	Discontinue. Call doctor right away.

WARNINGS & PRECAUTIONS

Don't take if:
• You become pregnant.
• You have breast cancer.

Before you start, consult your doctor:
• If you take birth control pills.
• If you have diabetes.
• If you have heart disease.
• If you have epilepsy.
• If you have kidney disease.
• If you have liver disease.
• If you have migraine headaches.

Over age 60:
Adverse reactions and side effects may be more frequent and severe than in younger persons.

Pregnancy:
Risk to unborn child outweighs drug benefits. Don't use. Stop if you get pregnant.

Breast-feeding:
Unknown whether medicine filters into milk. Consult doctor.

Infants & children:
Not recommended.

Prolonged use:
Required for full effect. Don't discontinue without consulting doctor.

Skin & sunlight:
No problems expected.

Driving, piloting or hazardous work:
No problems expected.

Discontinuing:
Don't discontinue without consulting doctor. Menstrual periods may be absent for 2 to 3 months after discontinuation.

Others:
May alter blood-sugar levels in diabetic persons.

POSSIBLE INTERACTION WITH OTHER DRUGS

GENERIC NAME OR DRUG CLASS	COMBINED EFFECT
Anticoagulants, oral*	Increased anti-coagulant effect.
Antidiabetic agents, oral*	Decreased anti-diabetic effect.
Insulin	Decreased insulin effect.

POSSIBLE INTERACTION WITH OTHER SUBSTANCES

INTERACTS WITH	COMBINED EFFECT
Alcohol:	Excessive nervous system depression. Avoid.
Beverages: Caffeine.	Rapid, irregular heartbeat. Avoid.
Cocaine:	May interfere with expected action of danazol. Avoid.
Foods:	No problems expected.
Marijuana:	May interfere with expected action of danazol. Avoid.
Tobacco:	Rapid, irregular heartbeat. Avoid. Increased leg cramps.

DANTHRON

BRAND NAMES

AKshun
Dorbane
Dorbantyl L
Doxidan

Modane
Roydan
Roydan Mild

BASIC INFORMATION

Habit forming? No
Prescription needed? No
Available as generic? No
Drug class: Laxative (stimulant)

 USES

Constipation relief.

 DOSAGE & USAGE INFORMATION

How to take:
- Tablet—Swallow with liquid or food.
- Liquid—Drink 6 to 8 glasses of water each day, in addition to one taken with each dose.

When to take:
Usually at bedtime with a snack, unless directed otherwise.

If you forget a dose:
Take as soon as you remember.

What drug does:
Acts on smooth muscles of intestine wall to cause vigorous bowel movement.

Time lapse before drug works:
6 to 10 hours.

Don't take with:
- Don't take within 2 hours of taking another medicine. Laxative interferes with medicine absorption.
- See Interaction column and consult doctor.

 OVERDOSE

SYMPTOMS:
Vomiting, electrolyte depletion.
WHAT TO DO:
Overdose unlikely to threaten life. If person takes much larger amount than prescribed, call doctor, poison-control center or hospital emergency room for instructions.

 POSSIBLE ADVERSE REACTIONS OR SIDE EFFECTS

SYMPTOMS	WHAT TO DO
Life-threatening: None expected.	
Common: Rectal irritation.	Continue. Call doctor when convenient.
Infrequent:	
• Dangerous potassium loss.	Discontinue. Call doctor right away.
• Belching, cramps, nausea.	Continue. Call doctor when convenient.
Rare:	
• Irritability, confusion, headache, rash, breathing difficulty, irregular heartbeat, muscle cramps, unusual tiredness, weakness.	Discontinue. Call doctor right away.
• Burning on urination.	Continue. Call doctor when convenient.

WARNINGS & PRECAUTIONS

Don't take if:
- You have symptoms of appendicitis, inflamed bowel or intestinal blockage.
- You are allergic to a stimulant laxative.
- You have missed a bowel movement for only 1 or 2 days.

Before you start, consult your doctor:
- If you have a colostomy or ileostomy.
- If you have congestive heart disease.
- If you have diabetes.
- If you have high blood pressure.
- If you have a laxative habit.
- If you have rectal bleeding.
- If you take other laxatives.

Over age 60:
Adverse reactions and side effects may be more frequent and severe than in younger persons.

Pregnancy:
Risk to mother and unborn child outweighs drug benefits. Don't use.

Breast-feeding:
Drug passes into milk. Avoid drug or discontinue nursing until you finish medicine. Consult doctor for advice on maintaining milk supply.

Infants & children:
Use only under medical supervision.

Prolonged use:
Don't take for more than 1 week unless under a doctor's supervision. May cause laxative dependence.

Skin & sunlight:
No problems expected.

Driving, piloting or hazardous work:
No problems expected.

Discontinuing:
May be unnecessary to finish medicine. Follow doctor's instructions.

Others:
Don't take to "flush out" your system or as a "tonic."

POSSIBLE INTERACTION WITH OTHER DRUGS

GENERIC NAME OR DRUG CLASS	COMBINED EFFECT
Antihypertensives*	May cause dangerous low potassium level.
Digoxin	Increased possibility of digitalis toxicity.
Diuretics*	May cause dangerous low potassium level.
Docusate calcium	Liver toxicity.
Docusate sodium	Liver toxicity.

POSSIBLE INTERACTION WITH OTHER SUBSTANCES

INTERACTS WITH	COMBINED EFFECT
Alcohol:	None expected.
Beverages:	None expected.
Cocaine:	None expected.
Foods:	None expected.
Marijuana:	None expected.
Tobacco:	None expected.

*See Glossary

DANTROLENE

BRAND NAMES

Dantrium

BASIC INFORMATION

Habit forming? No
Prescription needed? Yes
Available as generic? No
Drug class: Muscle relaxant, antispastic

 USES

- Relieves muscle spasticity caused by diseases such as multiple sclerosis, cerebral palsy, stroke.
- Relieves muscle spasticity caused by injury to spinal cord.
- Relieves or prevents excess body temperature brought on by some surgical procedures.

 DOSAGE & USAGE INFORMATION

How to take:
Capsules—Swallow with liquid.

When to take:
Once a day for muscle spasticity during first 6 days. Later, every 6 hours. For excess temperature, follow label instructions.

If you forget a dose:
Take as soon as you remember up to 2 hours late. If more than 2 hours, wait for next scheduled dose (don't double this dose).

Continued next column

 OVERDOSE

SYMPTOMS:
Shortness of breath, bloody urine, chest pain, convulsions.
WHAT TO DO:
- **Dial 0 (operator) or 911 (emergency) for an ambulance or medical help. Then give first aid immediately.**
- **If patient is unconscious and not breathing, give mouth-to-mouth breathing. If there is no heartbeat, use cardiac massage and mouth-to-mouth breathing (CPR). Don't try to make patient vomit. If you can't get help quickly, take patient to nearest emergency facility.**
- **See emergency information on inside covers.**

What drug does:
Acts directly on muscles to prevent excess contractions.

Time lapse before drug works:
1 or more weeks.

Don't take with:
See Interaction column and consult doctor.

 POSSIBLE ADVERSE REACTIONS OR SIDE EFFECTS

SYMPTOMS	WHAT TO DO
Life-threatening: Seizure.	Seek emergency treatment immediately.
Common: Drowsiness, dizziness, weakness.	Discontinue. Call doctor right away.
Infrequent: • Rash, hives; black or bloody stools; chest pain; fast heartbeat; backache; blood in urine; painful, swollen feet; chills; fever.	Discontinue. Call doctor right away.
• Depression, confusion, headache, slurred speech, insomnia, nervousness, diarrhea, blurred vision, difficult swallowing, appetite loss, difficult urination, decreased sexual function in males.	Continue. Call doctor when convenient.
Rare: • Jaundice, anorexia, abdominal cramps, double vision.	Discontinue. Call doctor right away.
• Constipation.	Continue. Call doctor when convenient.

WARNINGS & PRECAUTIONS

Don't take if:
You are allergic to dantrolene or any muscle relaxant or antispastic medication.

Before you start, consult your doctor:
• If you have liver disease.
• If you have heart disease.
• If you have lung disease (especially emphysema).
• If you are over age 35.
• If you will have surgery within 2 months, including dental surgery, requiring general or spinal anesthesia.

Over age 60:
Adverse reactions and side effects may be more frequent and severe than in younger persons.

Pregnancy:
No proven harm to unborn child. Avoid if possible.

Breast-feeding:
Avoid nursing or discontinue until you finish drug.

Infants & children:
Only under close medical supervision.

Prolonged use:
Blood counts, G6PD tests before treatment begins in Negroes and Caucasians of Mediterranean heritage, liver function studies—all recommended periodically during prolonged use.

Skin & sunlight:
May cause rash or intensify sunburn in areas exposed to sun or sunlamp.

Driving, piloting or hazardous work:
Don't drive or pilot aircraft until you learn how medicine affects you. Don't work around dangerous machinery. Don't climb ladders or work in high places. Danger increases if you drink alcohol or take medicine affecting alertness and reflexes, such as antihistamines, tranquilizers, sedatives, pain medicine, narcotics and mind-altering drugs.

Discontinuing:
Don't discontinue without consulting doctor. Dose may require gradual reduction if you have taken drug for a long time. Doses of other drugs may also require adjustment.

Others:
No problems expected.

 ## POSSIBLE INTERACTION WITH OTHER DRUGS

GENERIC NAME OR DRUG CLASS	COMBINED EFFECT
Central nervous system depressants* (antidepressants,* antihistamines,* narcotics,* other muscle relaxants,* sedatives,* sleeping pills,* tranquilizers*)	Increased sedation, low blood pressure. Avoid.
Dronabinol	Increased effect of dronabinol on central nervous system. Avoid.

 ## POSSIBLE INTERACTION WITH OTHER SUBSTANCES

INTERACTS WITH	COMBINED EFFECT
Alcohol:	Increased sedation, low blood pressure. Avoid.
Beverages:	No problems expected.
Cocaine:	Increased spasticity. Avoid.
Foods:	No problems expected.
Marijuana:	Increased spasticity. Avoid.
Tobacco:	May interfere with absorption of medicine.

DAPSONE

BRAND NAMES

Aviosulfon   DDS

BASIC INFORMATION

Habit forming? No
Prescription needed? Yes
Available as generic? Yes
Drug class: Antibacterial (Antileprosy),
   Sulfone

USES

- Treatment of dermatitis herpetiformis.
- Treatment of leprosy.

DOSAGE & USAGE INFORMATION

How to take:
Tablet—Swallow with liquid or food to lessen
stomach irritation.

When to take:
Once a day at same time.

If you forget a dose:
Take as soon as you remember up to 2 hours
late. If more than 2 hours, wait for next
scheduled dose (don't double this dose).

What drug does:
Inhibits enzymes. Kills leprosy germs.

Time lapse before drug works:
- 3 years for leprosy.
- 1 to 2 weeks for dermatitis herpetiformis.

Don't take with:
See Interaction column and consult doctor.

OVERDOSE

SYMPTOMS:
**Bleeding, vomiting, seizures, cyanosis,
coma.**
WHAT TO DO:
- **Dial 0 (operator) or 911 (emergency) for
an ambulance or medical help. Then give
first aid immediately.**
- **If patient is unconscious and not
breathing, give mouth-to-mouth
breathing. If there is no heartbeat, use
cardiac massage and mouth-to-mouth
breathing (CPR). Don't try to make patient
vomit. If you can't get help quickly, take
patient to nearest emergency facility.**
- **See emergency information on inside
covers.**

POSSIBLE ADVERSE REACTIONS OR SIDE EFFECTS

SYMPTOMS	WHAT TO DO
Life-threatening:	
Fever, malaise, hepatitis, hepatic necrosis.	Seek emergency treatment immediately.
Common:	
• Rash.	Discontinue. Call doctor right away.
• Abdominal pain, appetite loss.	Continue. Call doctor when convenient.
Infrequent:	
Pale.	Discontinue. Call doctor right away.
Rare:	
• Dizziness; mental changes; sore throat; fever; difficult breathing; bleeding; jaundice; numbness, tingling, pain or burning in hands or feet; swelling of feet, hands, eyelids; blurred vision; infectious mono-like syndrome, anemia.	Discontinue. Call doctor right away.
• Headache; itching; nausea; vomiting; blue fingernails, lips.	Continue. Call doctor when convenient.

WARNINGS & PRECAUTIONS

Don't take if:
- You have G6PD deficiency.
- You are allergic to furosemide, thiazide diuretics, sulfonureas, carbonic anhydrase inhibitors, sulfonamides.

Before you start, consult your doctor:
- If you are anemic.
- If you have liver or kidney disease.
- If you are Negro or Caucasian with Mediterranean heritage.
- If you will have surgery within 2 months, including dental surgery, requiring general or spinal anesthesia.

Over age 60:
Adverse reactions and side effects may be more frequent and severe than in younger persons.

Pregnancy:
No problems expected.

Breast-feeding:
Consult doctor.

Infants & children:
Under close medical supervision only.

Prolonged use:
Request blood counts, liver function studies.

Skin & sunlight:
Exposure may cause illness with swelling, spots on skin, fever.

Driving, piloting or hazardous work:
Don't drive or pilot aircraft until you learn how medicine affects you. Don't work around dangerous machinery. Don't climb ladders or work in high places. Danger increases if you drink alcohol or take medicine affecting alertness and reflexes, such as antihistamines, tranquilizers, sedatives, pain medicine, narcotics and mind-altering drugs.

Discontinuing:
Don't discontinue without consulting doctor. Dose may require gradual reduction if you have taken drug for a long time. Doses of other drugs may also require adjustment.

Others:
No problems expected.

POSSIBLE INTERACTION WITH OTHER DRUGS

GENERIC NAME OR DRUG CLASS	COMBINED EFFECT
Activated charcoal	Decreased absorption of dapsone.
Aminobenzoic acid (PABA)	Decreased dapsone effect. Avoid.
Methotrexate	May increase hematologic toxicity.
Probenecid	Increased toxicity of dapsone.
Pyrimethamine	May increase hematologic toxicity.
Rifampin	Decreased effect of dapsone.
Trimethoprim	May increase hematologic toxicity.

POSSIBLE INTERACTION WITH OTHER SUBSTANCES

INTERACTS WITH	COMBINED EFFECT
Alcohol:	Increased chance of toxicity to liver.
Beverages:	No problems expected.
Cocaine:	Increased chance of toxicity. Avoid.
Foods:	No problems expected.
Marijuana:	Increased chance of toxicity. Avoid.
Tobacco:	May interfere with absorption of medicine.

DECONGESTANTS (Ophthalmic)

BRAND AND GENERIC NAMES

Ak-Con
Albalon
Allerest
Clear Eyes
Degest 2
Murine

Muro's Opcon
Naphcon
Naphcon Forte
TETRAHYDROZILINE
VasoClear
Vasocon

BASIC INFORMATION

Habit forming? No
Prescription needed? Yes, for some
Available as generic? Yes
Drug class: Decongestant (ophthalmic)

 ## USES

Treats eye redness, itching, burning or other
irritation due to dust, colds, allergies, rubbing
eyes, wearing contact lenses, swimming or eye
strain from close work, watching TV, reading.

 ## DOSAGE & USAGE INFORMATION

How to use:
Eye drops
• Wash hands.
• Apply pressure to inside corner of eye with
  middle finger.
• Tilt head backward. Pull lower lid away from
  eye with index finger of the same hand.
• Drop eye drops into pouch and close eye.
  Don't blink.
• Keep eyes closed for 1 to 2 minutes.
• Continue pressure for 1 minute after placing
  medicine in eye.
• Don't touch applicator tip to any surface
  (including the eye). If you accidentally touch
  tip, clean with warm soap and water.
• Keep container tightly closed.
• Keep cool, but don't freeze.
• Wash hands immediately after using.

When to use:
As directed. Usually every 3 or 4 hours.

Continued next column

 ## OVERDOSE

SYMPTOMS:
None expected.
WHAT TO DO:
Not intended for internal use. If child
accidentally swallows, call poison-control
center.

If you forget a dose:
Use as soon as you remember.

What drug does:
Acts on small blood vessels to make them
constrict or become smaller.

Time lapse before drug works:
2 to 10 minutes.

Don't use with:
Other eye drops without consulting your doctor.

 ## POSSIBLE ADVERSE REACTIONS OR SIDE EFFECTS

SYMPTOMS	WHAT TO DO
Life-threatening: None expected.	
Common: Increased eye irritation.	Discontinue. Call doctor right away.
Infrequent: None expected.	
Rare: Blurred vision, large pupils, weakness, drowsiness, decreased body temperature, slow heartbeat, dizziness, headache, nervousness, nausea.	Discontinue. Call doctor right away.

DECONGESTANTS (Ophthalmic)

 **WARNINGS &
PRECAUTIONS**

Don't use if:
You are allergic to any decongestant eye drops.

Before you start, consult your doctor:
- If you take antidepressants or maprolitine.
- If you have eye disease, infection or injury.
- If you have heart disease, high blood pressure, thyroid disease.

Over age 60:
No problems expected.

Pregnancy:
No problems expected, but check with doctor.

Breast-feeding:
No problems expected, but check with doctor.

Infants & children:
Don't use.

Prolonged use:
Don't use for more than 3 or 4 days.

Skin & sunlight:
No problems expected.

Driving, piloting or hazardous work:
No problems expected.

Discontinuing:
May not need all the medicine in container. If symptoms disappear, stop using.

Others:
- Keep cool, but don't freeze.
- Check with your doctor if eye irritation continues or becomes worse.

 **POSSIBLE INTERACTION
WITH OTHER DRUGS**

GENERIC NAME OR DRUG CLASS	COMBINED EFFECT
Clinically significant interactions with oral or injected medicines unlikely.	

 **POSSIBLE INTERACTION
WITH OTHER SUBSTANCES**

INTERACTS WITH	COMBINED EFFECT
Alcohol:	None expected.
Beverages:	None expected.
Cocaine:	None expected.
Foods:	None expected.
Marijuana:	None expected.
Tobacco:	Smoke may increase eye irritation. Avoid.

DEHYDROCHOLIC ACID

BRAND NAMES

Bilax	G.B.S.
Cholan-DH	Hepahydrin
Cholan-HMB	Neocholan
Decholin	Neolax
Dycholium	Trilax

BASIC INFORMATION

Habit forming? No
Prescription needed? No
Available as generic? Yes
Drug class: Laxative (stimulant)

 ## USES

Constipation relief.

 ## DOSAGE & USAGE INFORMATION

How to take:
Tablet or capsule—Swallow with liquid.

When to take:
Usually at bedtime with a snack, unless directed otherwise.

If you forget a dose:
Take as soon as you remember.

What drug does:
Acts on smooth muscles of intestine wall to cause vigorous bowel movement.

Time lapse before drug works:
6 to 10 hours.

Don't take with:
- See Interaction column and consult doctor.
- Don't take within 2 hours of taking another medicine. Laxative interferes with medicine absorption.

 ## OVERDOSE

SYMPTOMS:
Vomiting, electrolyte depletion.
WHAT TO DO:
Overdose unlikely to threaten life. If person takes much larger amount than prescribed, call doctor, poison-control center or hospital emergency room for instructions.

 ## POSSIBLE ADVERSE REACTIONS OR SIDE EFFECTS

SYMPTOMS	WHAT TO DO
Life-threatening: None expected.	
Common: Rectal irritation.	Continue. Call doctor when convenient.
Infrequent: • Dangerous potassium loss.	Discontinue. Call doctor right away.
• Belching, cramps, nausea.	Continue. Call doctor when convenient.
Rare: • Irritability, confusion, headache, rash, breathing difficulty, irregular heartbeat, muscle cramps, unusual tiredness or weakness.	Discontinue. Call doctor right away.
• Burning on urination.	Continue. Call doctor when convenient.

DEHYDROCHOLIC ACID

WARNINGS & PRECAUTIONS

Don't take if:
- You have symptoms of appendicitis, inflamed bowel or intestinal blockage.
- You are allergic to a stimulant laxative.
- You have missed a bowel movement for only 1 or 2 days.
- You have liver disease.

Before you start, consult your doctor:
- If you have a colostomy or ileostomy.
- If you have congestive heart disease.
- If you have diabetes.
- If you have an enlarged prostate.
- If you have a laxative habit.
- If you have rectal bleeding.
- If you take other laxatives.

Over age 60:
Adverse reactions and side effects may be more frequent and severe than in younger persons.

Pregnancy:
Risk to mother and unborn child outweighs drug benefits. Don't use.

Breast-feeding:
Drug passes into milk. Avoid drug or discontinue nursing until you finish medicine. Consult doctor for advice on maintaining milk supply.

Infants & children:
Use only under medical supervision.

Prolonged use:
Don't take for more than 1 week unless under a doctor's supervision. May cause laxative dependence.

Skin & sunlight:
No problems expected.

Driving, piloting or hazardous work:
No problems expected.

Discontinuing:
May be unnecessary to finish medicine. Follow doctor's instructions.

Others:
Don't take to "flush out" your system or as a "tonic."

POSSIBLE INTERACTION WITH OTHER DRUGS

GENERIC NAME OR DRUG CLASS	COMBINED EFFECT
Antihypertensives*	May cause dangerous low potassium level.
Diuretics*	May cause dangerous low potassium level.

POSSIBLE INTERACTION WITH OTHER SUBSTANCES

INTERACTS WITH	COMBINED EFFECT
Alcohol:	None expected.
Beverages:	None expected.
Cocaine:	None expected.
Foods:	None expected.
Marijuana:	None expected.
Tobacco:	None expected.

DEXAMETHASONE

BRAND NAMES

See complete list of brand names in the *Brand Name Directory*, page 1061.

BASIC INFORMATION

Habit forming? No
Prescription needed? Yes
Available as generic? Yes
Drug class: Cortisone drug (adrenal corticosteroid)

 ## USES

- Reduces inflammation caused by many different medical problems.
- Treatment for some allergic diseases, blood disorders, kidney diseases, asthma and emphysema.
- Replaces corticosteroid deficiencies.

 ## DOSAGE & USAGE INFORMATION

How to take:

- Tablet or liquid—Swallow with liquid or food to lessen stomach irritation. If you can't swallow whole, crumble tablet and take with liquid or food.
- Inhaler—Follow label instructions.

When to take:
At the same times each day. Take once-a-day or once-every-other-day doses in mornings.

If you forget a dose:

- Several-doses-per-day prescription—Take as soon as you remember up to 2 hours late. If more than 2 hours, wait for next scheduled dose (don't double this dose).
- Once-a-day dose or less—Wait for next dose. Double this dose.

What drug does:
Decreases inflammatory responses.

Time lapse before drug works:
2 to 4 days.

Don't take with:
See Interaction column and consult doctor.

 ## OVERDOSE

SYMPTOMS:
Headache, convulsions, heart failure.
WHAT TO DO:

- **Dial 0 (operator) or 911 (emergency) for an ambulance or medical help. Then give first aid immediately.**
- **See emergency information on inside covers.**

 ## POSSIBLE ADVERSE REACTIONS OR SIDE EFFECTS

SYMPTOMS	WHAT TO DO
Life-threatening: Hives, rash, intense itching, faintness soon after a dose (anaphylaxis).	Seek emergency treatment immediately.
Common: Poor wound healing, acne, thirst, nausea, indigestion, vomiting, decreased growth in children.	Continue. Call doctor when convenient.
Infrequent: • Bloody or black, tarry stool.	Discontinue. Seek emergency treatment.
• Blurred vision; halos around lights; sore throat, fever; muscle cramps; swollen legs, feet.	Discontinue. Call doctor right away.
• Mood changes, insomnia, fatigue, restlessness, frequent urination, weight gain, round face, weakness, TB recurrence, irregular menstrual periods.	Continue. Call doctor when convenient.
Rare: • Irregular heartbeat.	Discontinue. Seek emergency treatment.
• Rash, pancreatitis, numbness or tingling in hands or feet, thrombophlebitis, hallucinations, hiccups, convulsions.	Discontinue. Call doctor right away.

 ## WARNINGS & PRECAUTIONS

Don't take if:

- You are allergic to any cortisone drug.
- You have tuberculosis or fungus infection.
- You have herpes infection of eyes, lips or genitals.

Before you start, consult your doctor:

- If you have had tuberculosis.
- If you have congestive heart failure, diabetes, peptic ulcer, glaucoma, underactive thyroid, high blood pressure, myasthenia gravis.
- If you have blood clots in legs or lungs.

Over age 60:
Adverse reactions and side effects may be more frequent and severe than in younger persons. Likely to aggravate edema, diabetes or ulcers. Likely to cause cataracts and osteoporosis (softening of the bones).

Pregnancy:
Risk to unborn child outweighs drug benefits. Don't use.

Breast-feeding:
Drug passes into milk. Avoid drug or discontinue nursing until you finish medicine. Consult doctor for advice on maintaining milk supply.

Infants & children:
Use only under medical supervision.

Prolonged use:
- Retards growth in children.
- Possible glaucoma, cataracts, diabetes, fragile bones and thin skin.
- Functional dependence.

Skin & sunlight:
No problems expected.

Driving, piloting or hazardous work:
No problems expected.

Discontinuing:
- Don't discontinue without doctor's advice until you complete prescribed dose, even though symptoms diminish or disappear.
- Drug affects your response to surgery, illness, injury or stress for 2 years after discontinuing. Tell anyone who takes medical care of you within 2 years about drug.

Others:
Avoid immunizations if possible.

 POSSIBLE INTERACTION WITH OTHER DRUGS

GENERIC NAME OR DRUG CLASS	COMBINED EFFECT
Amphotericin B	Potassium depletion.
Anticholinergics*	Possible glaucoma.
Anticoagulants, oral*	Decreased anticoagulant effect.
Anticonvulsants, hydantoin*	Decreased dexamethasone effect.
Antidiabetics, oral*	Decreased antidiabetic effect.
Antihistamines*	Decreased dexamethasone effect.
Aspirin	Increased dexamethasone effect.
Attenuated virus vaccines*	Possible viral infection.

Barbiturates*	Decreased dexamethasone effect. Oversedation.
Chloral hydrate	Decreased dexamethasone effect.
Chlorthalidone	Potassium depletion.
Cholestyramine	Decreased dexamethasone effect.
Cholinergics*	Decreased cholinergic effect.
Colestipol	Decreased dexamethasone absorption.
Contraceptives, oral*	Increased dexamethasone effect.
Digitalis preparations*	Dangerous potassium depletion. Possible digitalis toxicity.
Diuretics, thiazide*	Potassium depletion.
Ephedrine	Decreased dexamethasone effect.
Estrogens*	Increased dexamethasone effect.
Ethacrynic acid	Potassium depletion.
Furosemide	Potassium depletion.
Glutethimide	Decreased dexamethasone effect.
Indapamide	Possible excessive potassium loss, causing dangerous heartbeat irregularity.
Indomethacin	Increased dexamethasone effect.
Insulin	Decreased insulin effect.
Isoniazid	Decreased isoniazid effect.

Continued page 1084

 POSSIBLE INTERACTION WITH OTHER SUBSTANCES

INTERACTS WITH	COMBINED EFFECT
Alcohol:	Risk of stomach ulcers.
Beverages:	No proven problems.
Cocaine:	Overstimulation. Avoid.
Foods:	No proven problems.
Marijuana:	Decreased immunity.
Tobacco:	Increased dexamethasone effect. Possible toxicity.

*See Glossary

DEXCHLORPHENIRAMINE

BRAND NAMES

Dexchlor
Polaramine

Polaramine
Repetabs

BASIC INFORMATION

Habit forming? No
Prescription needed? Yes
Available as generic? No
Drug class: Antihistamine

 ## USES

- Reduces allergic symptoms such as hay fever, hives, rash or itching.
- Induces sleep.

 ## DOSAGE & USAGE INFORMATION

How to take:
- Tablet or syrup—Swallow with liquid or food to lessen stomach irritation.
- Extended-release tablets—Swallow each dose whole. If you take regular tablets, you may chew or crush them.

When to take:
Varies with form. Follow label directions.

If you forget a dose:
Take as soon as you remember up to 2 hours late. If more than 2 hours, wait for next scheduled dose (don't double this dose).

What drug does:
Blocks action of histamine after an allergic response triggers histamine release in sensitive cells.

Continued next column

 ## OVERDOSE

SYMPTOMS:
Convulsions, red face, hallucinations, coma.
WHAT TO DO:
- **Dial 0 (operator) or 911 (emergency) for an ambulance or medical help. Then give first aid immediately.**
- **If patient is unconscious and not breathing, give mouth-to-mouth breathing. If there is no heartbeat, use cardiac massage and mouth-to-mouth breathing (CPR). Don't try to make patient vomit. If you can't get help quickly, take patient to nearest emergency facility.**
- **See emergency information on inside covers.**

Time lapse before drug works:
30 minutes.

Don't take with:
See Interaction column and consult doctor.

 ## POSSIBLE ADVERSE REACTIONS OR SIDE EFFECTS

SYMPTOMS	WHAT TO DO
Life-threatening: None expected.	
Common: Drowsiness; dizziness; dry mouth, nose, throat; nausea.	Continue. Tell doctor at next visit.
Infrequent: • Vision changes.	Discontinue. Call doctor right away.
• Less tolerance for contact lenses, difficult urination.	Continue. Call doctor when convenient.
• Appetite loss.	Continue. Tell doctor at next visit.
Rare: Nightmares, agitation, irritability, sore throat, fever, rapid heartbeat, unusual bleeding or bruising, fatigue, weakness.	Discontinue. Call doctor right away.

WARNINGS & PRECAUTIONS

Don't take if:
You are allergic to any antihistamine.

Before you start, consult your doctor:
- If you have glaucoma.
- If you have enlarged prostate.
- If you have asthma.
- If you have kidney disease.
- If you have peptic ulcer.
- If you will have surgery within 2 months, including dental surgery, requiring general or spinal anesthesia.

Over age 60:
Don't exceed recommended dose. Adverse reactions and side effects may be more frequent and severe than in younger persons, especially urination difficulty, diminished alertness and other brain and nervous-system symptoms.

Pregnancy:
No proven harm to unborn child. Avoid if possible.

Breast-feeding:
Drug passes into milk. Avoid drug or discontinue nursing until you finish medicine. Consult doctor for advice on maintaining milk supply.

Infants & children:
Not recommended for premature or newborn infants. Otherwise, no problems expected.

Prolonged use:
Avoid. May damage bone marrow and nerve cells.

Skin & sunlight:
May cause rash or intensify sunburn in areas exposed to sun or sunlamp.

Driving, piloting or hazardous work:
Don't drive or pilot aircraft until you learn how medicine affects you. Don't work around dangerous machinery. Don't climb ladders or work in high places. Danger increases if you drink alcohol or take medicine affecting alertness and reflexes, such as antihistamines, tranquilizers, sedatives, pain medicine, narcotics and mind-altering drugs.

Discontinuing:
No problems expected.

Others:
May mask symptoms of hearing damage from aspirin, other salicylates, cisplatin, paromomycin, vancomycin or anticonvulsants. Consult doctor if you use these.

POSSIBLE INTERACTION WITH OTHER DRUGS

GENERIC NAME OR DRUG CLASS	COMBINED EFFECT
Anticholinergics*	Increased anticholinergic effect.
Anticoagulants, oral*	Decreased dexchlorpheniramine effect.
Antidepressants*	Excess sedation. Avoid.
Antihistamines, other*	Excess sedation. Avoid.
Carteolol	Decreased antihistamine effect.
Dronabinol	Increased effects of both drugs. Avoid.
Hypnotics*	Excess sedation. Avoid.
MAO inhibitors*	Increased dexchlorpheniramine effect.
Mind-altering drugs*	Excess sedation. Avoid.
Molindone	Increased antihistamine effect.
Nabilone	Greater depression of central nervous system.
Narcotics*	Excess sedation. Avoid.
Procarbazine	May increase sedation.
Sedatives*	Excess sedation. Avoid.
Sleep inducers*	Excess sedation. Avoid.
Sotalol	Increased antihistamine effect.
Tranquilizers*	Excess sedation. Avoid.

POSSIBLE INTERACTION WITH OTHER SUBSTANCES

INTERACTS WITH	COMBINED EFFECT
Alcohol:	Excess sedation. Avoid.
Beverages: Caffeine drinks.	Decreased dexchlorpheniramine effect.
Cocaine:	Decreased dexchlorpheniramine effect. Avoid.
Foods:	None expected.
Marijuana:	Excess sedation. Avoid.
Tobacco:	None expected.

DEXTROAMPHETAMINE

BRAND NAMES

Amphaplex
Biphetamine
Declobese
Dexampex
Dexedrine
Eskatrol

Ferndex
Obetrol
Obotan
Oxydess II
Spancap No. 1

BASIC INFORMATION

Habit forming? Yes
Prescription needed? Yes
Available as generic? Yes
Drug class: Central nervous system
  stimulant (amphetamine)

 USES

- Prevents narcolepsy (attacks of uncontrollable sleepiness).
- Controls hyperactivity in children.

 DOSAGE & USAGE INFORMATION

How to take:
- Tablet or extended-release capsule—Swallow with liquid. If you can't swallow whole, crumble tablet or open capsule and take with liquid or food.
- Syrups—Take as directed on label.

When to take:
- At the same times each day.
- Short-acting form—Don't take later than 6 hours before bedtime.
- Long-acting form—Take on awakening.

If you forget a dose:
- Short-acting form—Take up to 2 hours late. If more than 2 hours, wait for next dose (don't double this dose).
- Long-acting form—Take as soon as you remember. Wait 20 hours for next dose.

Continued next column

 OVERDOSE

SYMPTOMS:
Rapid heartbeat, hyperactivity, high fever, hallucinations, suicidal or homicidal feelings, convulsions, coma.
WHAT TO DO:
- **Dial 0 (operator) or 911 (emergency) for an ambulance or medical help. Then give first aid immediately.**
- **See emergency information on inside covers.**

What drug does:
- Narcolepsy—Apparently affects brain centers to decrease fatigue or sleepiness and increase alertness and motor activity.
- Hyperactive children—Calms children, opposite to effect on narcoleptic adults.

Time lapse before drug works:
15 to 30 minutes.

Don't take with:
See Interaction column and consult doctor.

 POSSIBLE ADVERSE REACTIONS OR SIDE EFFECTS

SYMPTOMS	WHAT TO DO
Life-threatening: None expected.	
Common:	
• Irritability, insomnia, nervousness.	Continue. Call doctor when convenient.
• Dry mouth.	Continue. Tell doctor at next visit.
Infrequent:	
• Dizziness; lack of alertness; blurred vision; fast, pounding heartbeat; unusual sweating.	Discontinue. Call doctor right away.
• Headache.	Continue. Call doctor when convenient.
• Diarrhea or constipation, appetite loss, stomach pain, nausea, vomiting, weight loss, diminished sex drive, impotence.	Continue. Tell doctor at next visit.
Rare:	
• Pancytopenia (reduced blood cells of all kinds, causing weakness, paleness, sore throat and fever).	Discontinue. Seek emergency treatment.
• Rash, hives; chest pain or irregular heartbeat; uncontrollable movements of head, neck, arms, legs.	Discontinue. Call doctor right away.
• Mood changes, enlarged breasts.	Continue. Call doctor when convenient.

WARNINGS & PRECAUTIONS

Don't take if:
- You are allergic to any amphetamine or central-nervous-system stimulant.
- You will have surgery within 2 months, including dental surgery, requiring general or spinal anesthesia.

Before you start, consult your doctor:
- If you plan to become pregnant within medication period.
- If you have glaucoma.
- If you have heart or blood-vessel disease, or high blood pressure.
- If you have overactive thyroid, anxiety or tension.
- If you have a severe mental illness (especially children).

Over age 60:
Adverse reactions and side effects may be more frequent and severe than in younger persons.

Pregnancy:
Risk to unborn child outweighs drug benefits. Don't use.

Breast-feeding:
Drug passes into milk. Avoid drug or discontinue nursing.

Infants & children:
Not recommended for children under 12.

Prolonged use:
Habit forming.

Skin & sunlight:
No problems expected.

Driving, piloting or hazardous work:
Don't drive or pilot aircraft until you learn how medicine affects you. Don't work around dangerous machinery. Don't climb ladders or work in high places. Danger increases if you drink alcohol or take medicine affecting alertness and reflexes.

Discontinuing:
May be unnecessary to finish medicine. Follow doctor's instructions.

Others:
- This is a dangerous drug and must be closely supervised. Don't use for appetite control or depression. Potential for damage and abuse.
- During withdrawal phase, may cause prolonged sleep of several days.

 ## POSSIBLE INTERACTION WITH OTHER DRUGS

GENERIC NAME OR DRUG CLASS	COMBINED EFFECT
Anesthesias, general*	Irregular heartbeat.
Antidepressants, tricyclic (TCA)*	Decreased dextro-amphetamine effect.
Antihypertensives*	Decreased antihyper-tensive effect.
Barbiturates*	Decreased amphetamine effect.
Carbonic anhydrase inhibitors*	Increased dextro-amphetamine effect.
Guanadrel	Decreased guanadrel effect. Insulin requirements may change.
Guanethidine	Decreased guanethidine effect. Insulin requirements may change.
Haloperidol	Decreased dextro-amphetamine effect.
MAO inhibitors*	May severely increase blood pressure.
Nabilone	Greater depression of central nervous system.
Phenothiazines*	Decreased dextro-amphetamine effect.
Sodium bicarbonate	Increased dextro-amphetamine effect.

 ## POSSIBLE INTERACTION WITH OTHER SUBSTANCES

INTERACTS WITH	COMBINED EFFECT
Alcohol:	Decreased dextro-amphetamine effect. Avoid.
Beverages: Caffeine drinks.	Overstimulation. Avoid.
Cocaine:	Dangerous stimulation of nervous system. Avoid.
Foods:	None expected.
Marijuana:	Frequent use— Severely impaired mental function.
Tobacco:	None expected.

*See Glossary

DEXTROMETHORPHAN

BRAND NAMES

See complete list of brand names in the *Brand Name Directory*, page 1061.

BASIC INFORMATION

Habit forming? No
Prescription needed? No
Available as generic? No
Drug class: Cough suppressant

 ## USES

Suppresses cough associated with allergies or infections such as colds, bronchitis, flu and lung disorders.

 ## DOSAGE & USAGE INFORMATION

How to take:
- Chewable tablet—Chew well before swallowing.
- Lozenges or syrups—Take as directed on label.

When to take:
As needed, no more often than every 3 hours.

If you forget a dose:
Take as soon as you remember. Wait 3 hours for next dose.

What drug does:
Reduces sensitivity of brain's cough-control center, suppressing urge to cough.

Time lapse before drug works:
15 to 30 minutes.

Don't take with:
See Interaction column and consult doctor.

 ## OVERDOSE

SYMPTOMS:
Euphoria, overactivity, sense of intoxication, visual and auditory hallucinations, lack of coordination, stagger, stupor, shallow breathing.
WHAT TO DO:
- **Dial 0 (operator) or 911 (emergency) for an ambulance or medical help. Then give first aid immediately.**
- **See emergency information on inside covers.**

 ## POSSIBLE ADVERSE REACTIONS OR SIDE EFFECTS

SYMPTOMS	WHAT TO DO
Life-threatening: None expected.	
Common: None expected.	
Infrequent: None expected.	
Rare: Dizziness, drowsiness, rash, diarrhea, nausea or vomiting, stomach pain.	Discontinue. Call doctor right away.

WARNINGS & PRECAUTIONS

Don't take if:
You are allergic to any cough syrup containing dextromethorphan.

Before you start, consult your doctor:
- If you have asthma attacks.
- If you have impaired liver function.

Over age 60:
May become constipated, excessively drowsy or unsteady. If drug is used for cough, other treatment may be necessary to liquefy thick mucus in bronchial tubes.

Pregnancy:
No proven harm to unborn child. Avoid if possible.

Breast-feeding:
No proven problems. Consult doctor.

Infants & children:
Use only as label directs.

Prolonged use:
No problems expected.

Skin & sunlight:
No problems expected.

Driving, piloting or hazardous work:
Don't drive or pilot aircraft until you learn how medicine affects you. Don't work around dangerous machinery. Don't climb ladders or work in high places. Danger increases if you drink alcohol or take medicine affecting alertness and reflexes, such as antihistamines, tranquilizers, sedatives, pain medicine, narcotics and mind-altering drugs.

Discontinuing:
May be unnecessary to finish medicine. Follow doctor's instructions.

Others:
- If cough persists or if you cough blood or brown-yellow, thick mucus, call your doctor.
- Excessive use may lead to functional dependence.

POSSIBLE INTERACTION WITH OTHER DRUGS

GENERIC NAME OR DRUG CLASS	COMBINED EFFECT
MAO inhibitors*	Disorientation, high fever, drop in blood pressure and loss of consciousness.

POSSIBLE INTERACTION WITH OTHER SUBSTANCES

INTERACTS WITH	COMBINED EFFECT
Alcohol:	None expected.
Beverages:	None expected.
Cocaine:	Decreased dextromethorphan effect. Avoid.
Foods:	None expected.
Marijuana:	None expected.
Tobacco:	None expected.

*See Glossary

DIAZEPAM

BRAND NAMES

Apo-Diazepam	Rival
D-Tran	Serenack
E-Pam	Stress-Pam
Meval	Valium
Neo-Calme	Valrelease
Novodipam	Vivol
Q-Pam	

BASIC INFORMATION

Habit forming? Yes
Prescription needed? Yes
Available as generic? Yes
Drug class: Tranquilizer (benzodiazepine)

 USES

- Treatment for nervousness or tension.
- Treatment for muscle spasm.
- Treatment for convulsive disorders.

 DOSAGE & USAGE INFORMATION

How to take:
Tablet, extended-release capsule or liquid—Swallow with liquid. If you can't swallow whole, crumble tablet or open capsule and take with liquid or food.

When to take:
At the same time each day, according to instructions on prescription label.

If you forget a dose:
Take as soon as you remember up to 2 hours late. If more than 2 hours, wait for next scheduled dose (don't double this dose).

Continued next column

 OVERDOSE

SYMPTOMS:
Drowsiness, weakness, tremor, stupor, coma.
WHAT TO DO:
- **Dial 0 (operator) or 911 (emergency) for an ambulance or medical help. Then give first aid immediately.**
- **If patient is unconscious and not breathing, give mouth-to-mouth breathing. If there is no heartbeat, use cardiac massage and mouth-to-mouth breathing (CPR). Don't try to make patient vomit. If you can't get help quickly, take patient to nearest emergency facility.**
- **See emergency information on inside covers.**

What drug does:
Affects limbic system of brain—part that controls emotions.

Time lapse before drug works:
2 hours. May take 6 weeks for full benefit.

Don't take with:
See Interaction column and consult doctor.

 POSSIBLE ADVERSE REACTIONS OR SIDE EFFECTS

SYMPTOMS	WHAT TO DO
Life-threatening: None expected.	
Common: Clumsiness, drowsiness, dizziness.	Continue. Call doctor when convenient.
Infrequent:	
• Hallucinations, confusion, depression, irritability, rash, itch, vision changes.	Discontinue. Call doctor right away.
• Constipation or diarrhea, nausea, vomiting, difficult urination, vivid dreams.	Continue. Call doctor when convenient.
Rare:	
• Slow heartbeat, breathing difficulty.	Discontinue. Seek emergency treatment.
• Mouth, throat ulcers; jaundice.	Discontinue. Call doctor right away.
• Decreased libido.	Continue. Call doctor when convenient.

 WARNINGS & PRECAUTIONS

Don't take if:
- You are allergic to any benzodiazepine.
- You have myasthenia gravis.
- You are active or recovering alcoholic.
- Patient is younger than 6 months.

Before you start, consult your doctor:
- If you have liver, kidney or lung disease.
- If you have diabetes, epilepsy or porphyria.

Over age 60:
Adverse reactions and side effects may be more frequent and severe than in younger persons. You need smaller doses for shorter periods of time. May develop agitation, rage or "hangover" effect.

Pregnancy:
Risk to unborn child outweighs drug benefits. Don't use.

Breast-feeding:
Drug passes into milk. Avoid drug or discontinue nursing until you finish medicine. Consult doctor for advice on maintaining milk supply.

Infants & children:
Use only under medical supervision for children older than 6 months.

Prolonged use:
May impair liver function.

Skin & sunlight:
No problems expected.

Driving, piloting or hazardous work:
Don't drive or pilot aircraft until you learn how medicine affects you. Don't work around dangerous machinery. Don't climb ladders or work in high places. Danger increases if you drink alcohol or take medicine affecting alertness and reflexes.

Discontinuing:
Don't discontinue without consulting doctor. Dose may require gradual reduction if you have taken drug for a long time. Doses of other drugs may also require adjustment.

Others:
- Hot weather, heavy exercise and profuse sweat may reduce excretion and cause overdose.
- Blood sugar may rise in diabetics, requiring insulin adjustment.

POSSIBLE INTERACTION WITH OTHER DRUGS

GENERIC NAME OR DRUG CLASS	COMBINED EFFECT
Anticonvulsants*	Change in seizure frequency or severity.
Antidepressants*	Increased sedative effect of both drugs.
Antihistamines*	Increased sedative effect of both drugs.
Antihypertensives*	Excessively low blood pressure.
Contraceptives, oral*	Increased diazepam effect.
Disulfiram	Increased diazepam effect.
Dronabinol	Increased effects of both drugs. Avoid.
Erythromycin	Increased diazepam effect.
Ketoconazole	Increased diazepam effect.
Levodopa	Possible decreased levodopa effect.
MAO inhibitors*	Convulsions, deep sedation, rage.
Molindone	Increased tranquilizer effect.
Nabilone	Greater depression of central nervous system.
Narcotics*	Increased sedative effect of both drugs.
Nizatidine	Increased effect and toxicity of diazepam.
Probenecid	Increased diazepam effect.
Sedatives*	Increased sedative effect of both drugs.
Sleep inducers*	Increased sedative effect of both drugs.
Tranquilizers*	Increased sedative effect of both drugs.

POSSIBLE INTERACTION WITH OTHER SUBSTANCES

INTERACTS WITH	COMBINED EFFECT
Alcohol:	Heavy sedation. Avoid.
Beverages:	None expected.
Cocaine:	Decreased diazepam effect.
Foods:	None expected.
Marijuana:	Heavy sedation. Avoid.
Tobacco:	Decreased diazepam effect.

*See Glossary

DICLOFENAC

BRAND NAMES

Voltaren
Voltarol
Voltarol Retard

BASIC INFORMATION

Habit forming? No
Prescription needed? Yes
Available as generic? No
Drug class: Anti-inflammatory (non-steroid)

 USES

- Treatment for joint pain, stiffness, inflammation and swelling of arthritis and gout.
- Pain reliever.
- Treatment for dysmenorrhea (painful or difficult menstruation).
- Treats juvenile rheumatoid arthritis.

 DOSAGE & USAGE INFORMATION

How to take:
Tablet or capsule—Swallow with liquid or food to lessen stomach irritation. If you can't swallow whole, crumble tablet and take with liquid or food.

When to take:
At the same times each day.

If you forget a dose:
Take as soon as you remember up to 2 hours late. If more than 2 hours, wait for next scheduled dose (don't double this dose).

Continued next column

 OVERDOSE

SYMPTOMS:
Confusion, agitation, incoherence, convulsions, possible hemorrhage from stomach or intestine, coma.
WHAT TO DO:

- Dial 0 (operator) or 911 (emergency) for an ambulance or medical help. Then give first aid immediately.
- See emergency information on inside covers.

What drug does:
Reduces tissue concentration of prostaglandins (hormones which produce inflammation and pain).

Time lapse before drug works:
Begins in 4 to 24 hours. May require 3 weeks regular use for maximum benefit.

Don't take with:
See Interaction column and consult doctor.

 POSSIBLE ADVERSE REACTIONS OR SIDE EFFECTS

SYMPTOMS	WHAT TO DO
Life-threatening: Hives, rash, intense itching, faintness soon after a dose (anaphylaxis in aspirin-sensitive persons).	Seek emergency treatment immediately.
Common: • Dizziness, nausea, pain.	Continue. Call doctor when convenient.
• Headache.	Continue. Tell doctor at next visit.
Infrequent: Depression; drowsiness; ringing in ears; swollen feet, legs; constipation or diarrhea; vomiting.	Continue. Call doctor when convenient.
Rare: • Convulsions; confusion; rash, hives or itch; blurred vision; black, bloody, tarry stool; difficult breathing; tightness in chest; rapid heartbeat; unusual bleeding or bruising; blood in urine; jaundice; psychosis; frequent, painful urination; severe abdominal pain.	Discontinue. Call doctor right away.
• Fatigue, weakness, impotence, menstrual irregularities, swollen breasts in males.	Continue. Call doctor when convenient.

WARNINGS & PRECAUTIONS

Don't take if:
- You are allergic to aspirin or any non-steroid, anti-inflammatory drug.
- You have gastritis, peptic ulcer, enteritis, ileitis, ulcerative colitis, asthma, heart failure, high blood pressure or bleeding problems.
- Patient is younger than 15.

Before you start, consult your doctor:
- If you have epilepsy.
- If you have Parkinson's disease.
- If you have been mentally ill.
- If you have had kidney disease or impaired kidney function.

Over age 60:
Adverse reactions and side effects may be more frequent and severe than in younger persons.

Pregnancy:
Studies inconclusive on harm to unborn child. Decide with your doctor whether drug benefits justify risk to unborn child.

Breast-feeding:
May harm child. Avoid.

Infants & children:
Not recommended for anyone younger than 15. Use only under medical supervision.

Prolonged use:
- Eye damage.
- Reduced hearing.
- Sore throat, fever.
- Weight gain.

Skin & sunlight:
Possible increased sensitivity to sunlight.

Driving, piloting or hazardous work:
Don't drive or pilot aircraft until you learn how medicine affects you. Don't work around dangerous machinery. Don't climb ladders or work in high places. Danger increases if you drink alcohol or take medicine affecting alertness and reflexes, such as antihistamines, tranquilizers, sedatives, pain medicine, narcotics and mind-altering drugs.

Discontinuing:
Don't discontinue without consulting doctor. Dose may require gradual reduction if you have taken drug for a long time. Doses of other drugs may also require adjustment.

Others:
No problems expected.

POSSIBLE INTERACTION WITH OTHER DRUGS

GENERIC NAME OR DRUG CLASS	COMBINED EFFECT
ACE inhibitors: captopril, enalapril, lisinopril*	May decrease ACE inhibitor effect.
Anticoagulants, oral*	Increased risk of bleeding.
Aspirin	Increased risk of stomach ulcer.
Beta-adrenergic blockers*	Decreased antihypertensive effect.
Carteolol	Decreased antihypertensive effect of carteolol.
Cortisone drugs*	Increased risk of stomach ulcer.
Diuretics*	May decrease diuretic effect.
Lithium	Possible increase in effect and toxicity.
Methotrexate	May increase toxicity.
Minoxidil	Decreased minoxidil effect.
Oxyphenbutazone	Possible stomach ulcer.
Phenylbutazone	Possible stomach ulcer.
Probenecid	Increased diclofenac effect.
Sotalol	Decreased antihypertensive effect of sotalol.
Terazosin	Decreases effectiveness of terazosin. Causes sodium and fluid retention.
Thyroid hormones*	Rapid heartbeat, blood-pressure rise.

POSSIBLE INTERACTION WITH OTHER SUBSTANCES

INTERACTS WITH	COMBINED EFFECT
Alcohol:	Possible stomach ulcer or bleeding.
Beverages:	None expected.
Cocaine:	None expected.
Foods:	None expected.
Marijuana:	Increased pain relief from diclofenac.
Tobacco:	None expected.

*See Glossary

DICLOXACILLIN

BRAND NAMES

Dycill   Pathocil
Dynapen

BASIC INFORMATION

Habit forming? No
Prescription needed? Yes
Available as generic? Yes
Drug class: Antibiotic (penicillin)

USES

Treatment of bacterial infections that are susceptible to dicloxacillin.

DOSAGE & USAGE INFORMATION

How to take:
* Capsules—Swallow with liquid on an empty stomach 1 hour before or 2 hours after eating.
* Liquid—Take with cold beverage. Liquid form is perishable and effective for only 7 days at room temperature. Effective for 14 days if stored in refrigerator. Don't freeze.

When to take:
Follow instructions on prescription label or side of package. Doses should be evenly spaced. For example, 4 times a day means every 6 hours.

If you forget a dose:
Take as soon as you remember. Continue regular schedule.

What drug does:
Destroys susceptible bacteria. Does not kill viruses.

Time lapse before drug works:
May be several days before medicine affects infection.

Don't take with:
See Interaction column and consult doctor.

OVERDOSE

SYMPTOMS:
Severe diarrhea, nausea or vomiting.
WHAT TO DO:
Overdose unlikely to threaten life. If person takes much larger amount than prescribed, call doctor, poison-control center or hospital emergency room for instructions.

POSSIBLE ADVERSE REACTIONS OR SIDE EFFECTS

SYMPTOMS	WHAT TO DO
Life-threatening: Hives, rash, intense itching, faintness soon after a dose (anaphylaxis).	Seek emergency treatment immediately.
Common: Dark or discolored tongue.	Continue. Tell doctor at next visit.
Infrequent: Mild nausea, vomiting, diarrhea.	Continue. Call doctor when convenient.
Rare: Unexplained bleeding.	Discontinue. Call doctor right away.

WARNINGS & PRECAUTIONS

Don't take if:
You are allergic to dicloxacillin, cephalosporin antibiotics, other penicillins or penicillamine. Life-threatening reaction may occur.

Before you start, consult your doctor:
If you are allergic to any substance or drug.

Over age 60:
You may have skin reactions, particularly around genitals and anus.

Pregnancy:
Studies inconclusive on harm to unborn child. Animal studies show fetal abnormalities. Decide with your doctor whether drug benefits justify risk to unborn child.

Breast-feeding:
Drug passes into milk. Child may become sensitive to penicillins and have allergic reactions to penicillin drugs. Avoid dicloxacillin or discontinue nursing until you finish medicine. Consult doctor for advice on maintaining milk supply.

Infants & children:
No problems expected.

Prolonged use:
You may become more susceptible to infections caused by germs not responsive to dicloxacillin.

Skin & sunlight:
No problems expected.

Driving, piloting or hazardous work:
Usually not dangerous. Most hazardous reactions likely to occur a few minutes after taking dicloxacillin.

Discontinuing:
Don't discontinue without doctor's advice until you complete prescribed dose, even though symptoms diminish or disappear.

Others:
No problems expected.

POSSIBLE INTERACTION WITH OTHER DRUGS

GENERIC NAME OR DRUG CLASS	COMBINED EFFECT
Beta-adrenergic blockers*	Increased chance of anaphylaxis (see emergency information on inside front cover).
Chloramphenicol	Decreased effect of both drugs.
Erythromycins*	Decreased effect of both drugs.
Loperamide	Decreased dicloxacillin effect.
Paromomycin	Decreased effect of both drugs.
Tetracyclines*	Decreased effect of both drugs.
Troleandomycin	Decreased effect of both drugs.

POSSIBLE INTERACTION WITH OTHER SUBSTANCES

INTERACTS WITH	COMBINED EFFECT
Alcohol:	Occasional stomach irritation.
Beverages:	None expected.
Cocaine:	No proven problems.
Foods:	None expected.
Marijuana:	No proven problems.
Tobacco:	None expected.

DICYCLOMINE

BRAND NAMES

See complete list of brand names in the *Brand Name Directory*, page 1061.

BASIC INFORMATION

Habit forming? No
Prescription needed?
  Low strength: No
  High strength: Yes
Available as generic? Yes
Drug class: Antispasmodic, anticholinergic

 ## USES

Reduces spasms of digestive system, bladder and urethra.

 ## DOSAGE & USAGE INFORMATION

How to take:
Tablet, syrup or capsule—Swallow with liquid or food to lessen stomach irritation.

When to take:
30 minutes before meals (unless directed otherwise by doctor).

If you forget a dose:
Take as soon as you remember up to 2 hours late. If more than 2 hours, wait for next scheduled dose (don't double this dose).

What drug does:
Blocks nerve impulses at parasympathetic nerve endings, preventing muscle contractions and gland secretions of organs involved.

Time lapse before drug works:
15 to 30 minutes.

Don't take with:
See Interaction column and consult doctor.

 ## OVERDOSE

SYMPTOMS:
Dilated pupils, blurred vision, rapid pulse and breathing, dizziness, fever, hallucinations, confusion, slurred speech, agitation, flushed face, convulsions, coma.
WHAT TO DO:
- **Dial 0 (operator) or 911 (emergency) for an ambulance or medical help. Then give first aid immediately.**
- **See emergency information on inside covers.**

 ## POSSIBLE ADVERSE REACTIONS OR SIDE EFFECTS

SYMPTOMS	WHAT TO DO
Life-threatening: Hives, rash, intense itching, faintness soon after a dose (anaphylaxis).	Seek emergency treatment immediately.
Common:	
• Confusion, delirium, rapid heartbeat.	Discontinue. Call doctor right away.
• Nausea, vomiting, decreased sweating.	Continue. Call doctor when convenient.
• Constipation, loss of taste.	Continue. Tell doctor at next visit.
• Dry ears, nose, throat.	No action necessary.
Infrequent: Headache, difficult urination.	Continue. Call doctor when convenient.
Rare: Rash or hives, pain, blurred vision.	Discontinue. Call doctor right away.

 ## WARNINGS & PRECAUTIONS

Don't take if:
- You are allergic to any anticholinergic.
- You have trouble with stomach bloating.
- You have difficulty emptying your bladder completely.
- You have narrow-angle glaucoma.
- You have severe ulcerative colitis.

Before you start, consult your doctor:
- If you have open-angle glaucoma.
- If you have angina, chronic bronchitis or asthma.
- If you have hiatal hernia, liver disease, enlarged prostate, myasthenia gravis, peptic ulcer.
- If you will have surgery within 2 months, including dental surgery, requiring general or spinal anesthesia.

Over age 60:
Adverse reactions and side effects may be more frequent and severe than in younger persons.

Pregnancy:
Studies inconclusive on harm to unborn child. Animal studies show fetal abnormalities. Decide with your doctor whether drug benefits justify risk to unborn child.

DICYCLOMINE

Breast-feeding:
Drug passes into milk and decreases milk flow. Avoid drug or discontinue nursing until you finish medicine. Consult doctor for advice on maintaining milk supply.

Infants & children:
Use only under medical supervision.

Prolonged use:
Chronic constipation, possible fecal impaction. Consult doctor immediately.

Skin & sunlight:
No problems expected.

Driving, piloting or hazardous work:
Use disqualifies you for piloting aircraft. Otherwise, no problems expected.

Discontinuing:
May be unnecessary to finish medicine. Follow doctor's instructions.

Others:
No problems expected.

 ## POSSIBLE INTERACTION WITH OTHER DRUGS

GENERIC NAME OR DRUG CLASS	COMBINED EFFECT
Amantadine	Increased dicyclomine effect.
Antacids*	Decreased dicyclomine absorption effect.
Anticholinergics, other*	Increased dicyclomine effect.
Antidepressants, tricyclic (TCA)*	Increased dicyclomine effect. Increased sedation.
Antihistamines*	Increased dicyclomine effect.
Buclizine	Increased dicyclomine effect.
Cortisone drugs*	Increased internal-eye pressure.
Digitalis	Possible decreased absorption of digitalis.
Haloperidol	Increased internal-eye pressure.
MAO inhibitors*	Increased dicyclomine effect.
Meperidine	Increased dicyclomine effect.
Methylphenidate	Increased dicyclomine effect.

Nitrates*	Increased internal-eye pressure.
Nizatidine	Increased nizatidine effect.
Orphenadrine	Increased dicyclomine effect.
Phenothiazines*	Increased dicyclomine effect.
Pilocarpine	Loss of pilocarpine effect in glaucoma treatment.
Potassium supplements*	Possible intestinal ulcers with oral potassium tablets.
Quinidine	Increased dicyclomine effect.
Vitamin C	Decreased dicyclomine effect. Avoid large doses of vitamin C.

 ## POSSIBLE INTERACTION WITH OTHER SUBSTANCES

INTERACTS WITH	COMBINED EFFECT
Alcohol:	None expected.
Beverages:	None expected.
Cocaine:	Excessively rapid heartbeat. Avoid.
Foods:	None expected.
Marijuana:	Drowsiness and dry mouth.
Tobacco:	None expected.

*See Glossary

DIETHYLSTILBESTROL

BRAND NAMES

DES
Honvol
Stilbestrol

Stilphostrol
Stilbilium

BASIC INFORMATION

Habit forming? No
Prescription needed? Yes
Available as generic? Yes
Drug class: Female sex hormone (estrogen)

 USES

- Treatment for symptoms of menopause and menstrual-cycle irregularity.
- Replacement for female hormone deficiency.
- Treatment for cancer of prostate and breast.
- Used as morning-after pill for contraception.

 DOSAGE & USAGE INFORMATION

How to take:
- Tablet—Swallow with liquid. If you can't swallow whole, crumble tablet and take with liquid or food.
- Vaginal suppositories—Use as directed on label.

When to take:
At the same time each day.

If you forget a dose:
Take as soon as you remember up to 12 hours late. If more than 12 hours, wait for next scheduled dose (don't double this dose).

What drug does:
Restores normal estrogen level in tissues.

Time lapse before drug works:
10 to 20 days.

Don't take with:
See Interaction column and consult doctor.

 OVERDOSE

SYMPTOMS:
Nausea, vomiting, fluid retention, breast enlargement and discomfort, abnormal vaginal bleeding.
WHAT TO DO:
Overdose unlikely to threaten life. If person takes much larger amount than prescribed, call doctor, poison-control center or hospital emergency room for instructions.

 POSSIBLE ADVERSE REACTIONS OR SIDE EFFECTS

SYMPTOMS	WHAT TO DO
Life-threatening: None expected.	
Common:	
• Stomach cramps.	Discontinue. Call doctor right away.
• Appetite loss.	Continue. Call doctor when convenient.
• Nausea; diarrhea; swollen ankles and feet; tender, swollen breasts.	Continue. Tell doctor at next visit.
Infrequent:	
• Rash, stomach or side pain.	Discontinue. Call doctor right away.
• Depression, dizziness, headache, irritability, vomiting, breast lumps.	Continue. Call doctor when convenient.
• Brown blotches, hair loss, vaginal discharge or bleeding, changes in sex drive.	Continue. Tell doctor at next visit.
Rare: Jaundice, hyper-calcemia in breast cancer, intolerance of contact lenses.	Discontinue. Call doctor right away.

 WARNINGS & PRECAUTIONS

Don't take if:
- You are allergic to any estrogen-containing drugs.
- You have impaired liver function.
- You have had blood clots, stroke or heart attack.
- You have unexplained vaginal bleeding.

Before you start, consult your doctor:
- If you have had cancer of breast or reproductive organs, fibrocystic breast disease, fibroid tumors of the uterus or endometriosis.
- If you have had migraine headaches, epilepsy or porphyria.
- If you have diabetes, high blood pressure, asthma, congestive heart failure, kidney disease or gallstones.
- If you plan to become pregnant within 3 months.

Over age 60:
Controversial. You and your doctor must decide if drug risks outweigh benefits.

Pregnancy:
Risk to unborn child outweighs drug benefits. Don't use.

Breast-feeding:
Drug filters into milk. May harm child. Avoid.

Infants & children:
Not recommended.

Prolonged use:
Increased growth of fibroid tumors of uterus. Possible association with cancer of uterus.

Skin & sunlight:
May cause rash or intensify sunburn in areas exposed to sun or sunlamp.

Driving, piloting or hazardous work:
No problems expected.

Discontinuing:
You may need to discontinue diethylstilbestrol periodically. Consult your doctor.

Others:
In rare instances, may cause blood clot in lung, brain or leg. Symptoms are *sudden* severe headache, coordination loss, vision change, chest pain, breathing difficulty, slurred speech, pain in legs or groin. Seek emergency treatment immediately.

POSSIBLE INTERACTION WITH OTHER DRUGS

GENERIC NAME OR DRUG CLASS	COMBINED EFFECT
Anticoagulants, oral*	Decreased anticoagulant effect.
Anticonvulsants, hydantoin*	Decreased estrogen effect.
Antidepressants, tricyclic (TCA)*	Increased toxicity of antidepressants.
Antidiabetics, oral*	Unpredictable increase or decrease in blood sugar.
Antifibrinolytic agents*	Increased possibility of blood clotting.
Carbamazepine	Decreased estrogen effect.

Clofibrate	Decreased clofibrate effect.
Insulin	Possible decreased insulin effect. May require dosage adjustment.
Meprobamate	Increased diethyl-stilbestrol effect.
Phenobarbital	Decreased diethyl-stilbestrol effect.
Primidone	Decreased diethyl-stilbestrol effect.
Rifampin	Decreased diethyl-stilbestrol effect.
Terazosin	Decreases effectiveness of terazosin.
Thyroid hormones*	Decreased thyroid effect.
Ursodiol	Decreased effect of ursodiol.
Vitamin C	Possible increased estrogen effect.

POSSIBLE INTERACTION WITH OTHER SUBSTANCES

INTERACTS WITH	COMBINED EFFECT
Alcohol:	None expected.
Beverages:	None expected.
Cocaine:	No proven problems.
Foods:	None expected.
Marijuana:	Possible menstrual irregularities and bleeding between periods.
Tobacco:	Increased risk of blood clots leading to stroke or heart attack.

*See Glossary

DIFENOXIN & ATROPINE

BRAND NAMES

Motofen

BASIC INFORMATION

Habit forming? No
Prescription needed? Yes
Available as generic? No
Drug class: Antidiarrheal

USES

- Reduces spasms of digestive system.
- Treats severe diarrhea.

DOSAGE & USAGE INFORMATION

How to take:
Tablet—Swallow with liquid or food to lessen stomach irritation.

When to take:
After each loose stool or every 3 to 4 hours. No more than 5 tablets in 12 hours.

If you forget a dose:
Take as soon as you remember. Don't double this dose.

What drug does:
- Blocks nerve impulses at parasympathetic nerve endings, preventing muscle contractions and gland secretions of organs involved.
- Acts on brain to decrease spasm of smooth muscle.

Time lapse before drug works:
40 to 60 minutes.

Continued next column

OVERDOSE

SYMPTOMS:
Dilated pupils, rapid pulse and breathing, dizziness, fever, hallucinations, confusion, slurred speech, agitation, flushed face, convulsions, coma.
WHAT TO DO:
- **Dial 0 (operator) or 911 (emergency) for an ambulance or medical help. Then give first aid immediately.**
- **See emergency information on inside covers.**

Don't take with:
- Any medicine that will decrease mental alertness or reflexes, such as alcohol, other mind-altering drugs, cough/cold medicines, antihistamines, allergy medicine, sedatives, tranquilizers (sleeping pills or "downers") barbiturates, seizure medicine, narcotics, other prescription medicine for pain, muscle relaxants, anesthetics.
- See Interaction column and consult doctor.

POSSIBLE ADVERSE REACTIONS OR SIDE EFFECTS

SYMPTOMS	WHAT TO DO
Life-threatening: Shortness of breath, agitation, nervousness.	Discontinue. Seek emergency treatment.
Common: Dizziness, drowsiness.	Continue. Call doctor when convenient.
Infrequent: • Bloating; constipation; appetite loss; abdominal pain; blurred vision; warm, flushed skin; fast heartbeat; dry mouth.	Discontinue. Call doctor right away.
• Frequent urination, lightheadedness, dry skin, headache, insomnia.	Continue. Call doctor when convenient.
Rare: Weakness, confusion, fever.	Continue. Call doctor when convenient.

WARNINGS & PRECAUTIONS

Don't take if:
- You are allergic to any anticholinergic.
- You have trouble with stomach bloating, difficulty emptying your bladder completely, narrow-angle glaucoma, severe ulcerative colitis.
- You are dehydrated.

Before you start, consult your doctor:
- If you have open-angle glaucoma, angina, chronic bronchitis, asthma, liver disease, hiatal hernia, enlarged prostate, myasthenia gravis, peptic ulcer.
- If you will have surgery within 2 months, including dental surgery, requiring general or spinal anesthesia.

Over age 60:
Adverse reactions and side effects may be more frequent and severe than in younger persons.

Pregnancy:
Studies inconclusive on harm to unborn child. Animal studies show fetal abnormalities. Decide with your doctor whether drug benefits justify risk to unborn child.

Breast-feeding:
Drug passes into milk. Avoid drug or discontinue nursing until you finish medicine. Consult doctor for advice on maintaining milk supply.

Infants & children:
Use only under medical supervision.

Prolonged use:
Chronic constipation, possible fecal impaction. Consult doctor immediately.

Skin & sunlight:
No problems expected.

Driving, piloting or hazardous work:
Use disqualifies you for piloting aircraft. Otherwise, no problems expected.

Discontinuing:
May be unnecessary to finish medicine. Follow doctor's instructions.

Others:
Atropine included at doses below therapeutic level to prevent abuse.

 POSSIBLE INTERACTION WITH OTHER DRUGS

GENERIC NAME OR DRUG CLASS	COMBINED EFFECT
Addictive substances (narcotics,* others)	Increased chance of abuse.
Amantadine	Increased atropine effect.
Anticholinergics, other*	Increased atropine effect.
Antidepressants, tricyclic (TCA)*	Increased atropine effect. Increased sedation.
Antihistamines*	Increased atropine effect.
Antihypertensives*	Increased sedation.
Cortisone drugs*	Increased internal-eye pressure.
Ethinamate	Dangerous increased effects of ethinamate. Avoid combining.
Fluoxetine	Increased depressant effects of both drugs.
Guanfacine	May increase depressant effects of either drug.
Haloperidol	Increased internal-eye pressure.
Leucovorin	High alcohol content of leucovorin may cause adverse effects.
MAO inhibitors*	Increased atropine effect.
Meperidine	Increased atropine effect.
Methylphenidate	Increased atropine effect.
Methyprylon	Increased sedative effect, perhaps to dangerous level. Avoid.
Nabilone	Greater depression of central nervous system.
Nitrates*	Increased internal-eye pressure.
Orphenadrine	Increased atropine effect,
Phenothiazines*	Increased atropine effect.
Pilocarpine	Loss of pilocarpine effect in glaucoma treatment.
Potassium supplements*	Possible intestinal ulcers with oral potassium tablets.
Procainamide	Increased atropine effect.
Vitamin C	Decreased atropine effect. Avoid large doses of vitamin C.

 POSSIBLE INTERACTION WITH OTHER SUBSTANCES

INTERACTS WITH	COMBINED EFFECT
Alcohol:	Increased sedation. Avoid.
Beverages:	None expected.
Cocaine:	Excessively rapid heartbeat. Avoid.
Foods:	None expected.
Marijuana:	Drowsiness and dry mouth.
Tobacco:	May increase diarrhea. Avoid.

*See Glossary

DIFLUNISAL

BRAND NAMES

Dolobid

BASIC INFORMATION

Habit forming? No
Prescription needed? Yes
Available as generic? No
Drug class: Anti-inflammatory (non-steroid)

 USES

- Treatment for joint pain, stiffness, inflammation and swelling of arthritis and gout.
- Pain reliever.

 DOSAGE & USAGE INFORMATION

How to take:
Tablet—Swallow with liquid or food to lessen stomach irritation. If you can't swallow whole, crumble tablet and take with liquid or food.

When to take:
At the same times each day.

If you forget a dose:
Take as soon as you remember up to 2 hours late. If more than 2 hours, wait for next scheduled dose (don't double this dose).

What drug does:
Reduces tissue concentration of prostaglandins (hormones which produce inflammation and pain).

Time lapse before drug works:
Begins in 4 to 24 hours. May require 3 weeks regular use for maximum benefit.

Don't take with:
See Interaction column and consult doctor.

 OVERDOSE

SYMPTOMS:
Confusion, agitation, incoherence, convulsions, possible hemorrhage from stomach or intestine, coma.
WHAT TO DO:
- Dial 0 (operator) or 911 (emergency) for an ambulance or medical help. Then give first aid immediately.
- See emergency information on inside covers.

 POSSIBLE ADVERSE REACTIONS OR SIDE EFFECTS

SYMPTOMS	WHAT TO DO
Life-threatening: None expected.	
Common:	
• Dizziness, nausea, pain.	Continue. Call doctor when convenient.
• Headache.	Continue. Tell doctor at next visit.
Infrequent: Depression; drowsiness; ringing in ears; constipation or diarrhea; vomiting; swollen feet, legs.	Continue. Call doctor when convenient.
Rare:	
• Convulsions; confusion; rash, hives, or itch; blurred vision; bloody or black, tarry stools; difficult breathing; tightness in chest; rapid heartbeat; unusual bleeding or bruising; blood in urine; jaundice.	Discontinue. Call doctor right away.
• Urgent, frequent, painful or difficult urination; fatigue; weakness.	Continue. Call doctor when convenient.

WARNINGS & PRECAUTIONS

Don't take if:
- You are allergic to aspirin or any non-steroidal, anti-inflammatory drug.
- You have gastritis, peptic ulcer, enteritis, ileitis, ulcerative colitis, asthma, heart failure, high blood pressure or bleeding problems.
- Patient is younger than 15.

Before you start, consult your doctor:
- If you have epilepsy.
- If you have Parkinson's disease.
- If you have been mentally ill.
- If you have had kidney disease or impaired kidney function.

Over age 60:
Adverse reactions and side effects may be more frequent and severe than in younger persons.

Pregnancy:
Studies inconclusive on harm to unborn child. Animal studies show fetal abnormalities. Decide with your doctor whether drug benefits justify risk to unborn child.

Breast-feeding:
May harm child. Avoid.

Infants & children:
Not recommended for anyone younger than 15. Use only under medical supervision.

Prolonged use:
- Eye damage.
- Reduced hearing.
- Sore throat, fever.
- Weight gain.

Skin & sunlight:
No problems expected.

Driving, piloting or hazardous work:
Don't drive or pilot aircraft until you learn how medicine affects you. Don't work around dangerous machinery. Don't climb ladders or work in high places. Danger increases if you drink alcohol or take medicine affecting alertness and reflexes, such as antihistamines, tranquilizers, sedatives, pain medicine, narcotics and mind-altering drugs.

Discontinuing:
Don't discontinue without consulting doctor. Dose may require gradual reduction if you have taken drug for a long time. Doses of other drugs may also require adjustment.

Others:
No problems expected.

POSSIBLE INTERACTION WITH OTHER DRUGS

GENERIC NAME OR DRUG CLASS	COMBINED EFFECT
Antacids*	Decreased diflunisal effect.
Anticoagulants, oral*	Increased effect of anticoagulant.
Aspirin, other NSAIDs*	Increased risk of stomach ulcer.
Beta-adrenergic blockers*	Possible decreased antihypertensive effect.
Bismuth subsalicylate	Increased risk of salicylate toxicity.
Carteolol	Decreased antihypertensive effect of carteolol.
Cortisone drugs*	Increased risk of stomach ulcer.
Indomethacin	Increased possibility of intestinal hemorrhage.
Lisinopril	Decreased lisinopril effect.
Oxyphenbutazone	Possible stomach ulcer.
Phenylbutazone	Possible stomach ulcer.
Sotalol	Decreased antihypertensive effect of sotalol.
Terazosin	Decreases effectiveness of terazosin. Causes sodium and fluid retention.

POSSIBLE INTERACTION WITH OTHER SUBSTANCES

INTERACTS WITH	COMBINED EFFECT
Alcohol:	Possible stomach ulcer or bleeding.
Beverages:	None expected.
Cocaine:	Increased cocaine toxicity. Avoid.
Foods:	None expected.
Marijuana:	Increased pain relief from diflunisal.
Tobacco:	Decreased absorption of diflunisal. Avoid.

*See Glossary

DIGITALIS PREPARATIONS

BRAND AND GENERIC NAMES

Crystodigin
Crystogin
Digifortis
Digiglusin
DIGITALIS
DIGITOXIN
DIGOXIN

Gitaligen
GITALIN
Lanoxicaps
Lanoxin
Natigozine
Novodigoxin
Purodigin

BASIC INFORMATION

Habit forming? No
Prescription needed? Yes
Available as generic? Yes
Drug class: Digitalis preparations

USES

- Strengthens weak heart-muscle contractions to prevent congestive heart failure.
- Corrects irregular heartbeat.

DOSAGE & USAGE INFORMATION

How to take:
- Tablet or capsule—Swallow with liquid. If you can't swallow whole, crumble tablet or open capsule and take with liquid or food.
- Liquid—Dilute dose in beverage before swallowing.

When to take:
At the same time each day.

If you forget a dose:
Take as soon as you remember up to 12 hours late. If more than 12 hours, wait for next scheduled dose (don't double this dose).

What drug does:
- Strengthens heart-muscle contraction.
- Delays nerve impulses to heart.

Continued next column

OVERDOSE

SYMPTOMS:
Nausea, vomiting, diarrhea, vision disturbances, halos around lights, fatigue, irregular heartbeat, confusion, hallucinations, convulsions.
WHAT TO DO:
- **Dial 0 (operator) or 911 (emergency) for an ambulance or medical help. Then give first aid immediately.**
- **See emergency information on inside covers.**

Time lapse before drug works:
May require regular use for a week or more.

Don't take with:
- Non-prescription drugs without consulting doctor.
- See Interaction column and consult doctor.

POSSIBLE ADVERSE REACTIONS OR SIDE EFFECTS

SYMPTOMS	WHAT TO DO
Life-threatening: None expected.	
Common: Appetite loss, diarrhea.	Continue. Call doctor when convenient.
Infrequent: Drowsiness, lethargy, disorientation.	Discontinue. Call doctor right away.
Rare: • Rash, hives, cardiac arrhythmias, depression, hallucinations, psychosis.	Discontinue. Call doctor right away.
• Double or yellow-green vision; enlarged, sensitive male breasts; tiredness; weakness.	Continue. Call doctor when convenient.

WARNINGS & PRECAUTIONS

Don't take if:
- You are allergic to any digitalis preparation.
- Your heartbeat is slower than 50 beats per minute.

Before you start, consult your doctor:
- If you have taken another digitalis preparation in past 2 weeks.
- If you have taken a diuretic within 2 weeks.
- If you have liver or kidney disease.
- If you have a thyroid disorder.
- If you will have surgery within 2 months, including dental surgery, requiring general or spinal anesthesia.

Over age 60:
Adverse reactions and side effects may be more frequent and severe than in younger persons.

Pregnancy:
Studies inconclusive on harm to unborn child. Consult your doctor.

Breast-feeding:
Drug filters into milk. May harm child. Avoid.

Infants & children:
Use only under medical supervision.

Prolonged use:
No problems expected.

Skin & sunlight:
No problems expected.

Driving, piloting or hazardous work:
Possible vision disturbances. Otherwise, no problems expected.

Discontinuing:
Don't stop without doctor's advice.

Others:
Some digitalis products contain tartrazine dye. Avoid, especially if you are allergic to aspirin.

POSSIBLE INTERACTION WITH OTHER DRUGS

GENERIC NAME OR DRUG CLASS	COMBINED EFFECT
Amiodarone	Increased digitalis effect.
Amphotericin B	Decreased potassium. Increased toxicity of amphotericin B.
Antacids*	Decreased digitalis effect.
Anticonvulsants, hydantoin*	Increased digitalis effect at first, then decreased.
Anticholinergics*	Possible increased digitalis effect.
Beta-adrenergic blockers*	Increased digitalis effect.
Beta-agonists*	Increased risk of heartbeat irregularity.
Calcium supplements*	Decreased digitalis effects.
Carteolol	Can either increase or decrease heart rate. Improves irregular heartbeat.
Cholestyramine	Decreased digitalis effect.
Colestipol	Decreased digitalis effect.
Cortisone drugs*	Digitalis toxicity.
Disopyramide	Possible decreased digitalis effect.
Diuretics*	Possible digitalis toxicity. Excessive potassium loss that may cause irregular heartbeat.

GENERIC NAME OR DRUG CLASS	COMBINED EFFECT
Ephedrine	Disturbed heart rhythm. Avoid.
Epinephrine	Disturbed heart rhythm. Avoid.
Erythromycin	May increase digitalis absorption.
Flecainide	May increase digitalis blood level.
Fluoxetine	May cause confusion, agitation, convulsions and high blood pressure. Avoid combining.
Hydroxychloroquine	Possible increased digitalis toxicity.
Laxatives*	Decreased digitalis effect.
Metoclopramide	Decreased digitalis absorption.
Nicardipine	Increased digitalis effect. May need to reduce dose.
Nizatidine	Increased digitalis effect.
Oxyphenbutazone	Decreased digitalis effect.
Phenobarbital	Decreased digitalis effect.
Phenylbutazone	Decreased digitalis effect.
Potassium supplements*	Overdosage of either drug may cause severe heartbeat irregularity.
PTU/Metronidazole	Decreased digitalis effect.

Continued page 1084

POSSIBLE INTERACTION WITH OTHER SUBSTANCES

INTERACTS WITH	COMBINED EFFECT
Alcohol:	None expected.
Beverages: Caffeine drinks.	Irregular heartbeat. Avoid.
Cocaine:	Irregular heartbeat. Avoid.
Foods:	None expected.
Marijuana:	Decreased digitalis effect.
Tobacco:	Irregular heartbeat. Avoid.

*See Glossary

DILTIAZEM

BRAND NAMES

Cardizem

BASIC INFORMATION

Habit forming? No
Prescription needed? Yes
Available as generic? No
Drug class: Calcium-channel blocker,
  antiarrhythmic, antianginal

USES

- Prevents angina attacks.
- Stabilizes irregular heartbeat.
- Used after heart attacks to prevent spasm of coronary arteries.
- Treats high blood pressure.

DOSAGE & USAGE INFORMATION

How to take:
Sustained-release tablet—Swallow with liquid.

When to take:
At the same times each day 1 hour before or 2 hours after eating.

If you forget a dose:
Take as soon as you remember up to 2 hours late. If more than 2 hours, wait for next scheduled dose (don't double this dose).

What drug does:
- Reduces work that heart must perform.
- Reduces normal artery pressure.
- Increases oxygen to heart muscle.

Time lapse before drug works:
1 to 2 hours.

Don't take with:
See Interaction column and consult doctor.

OVERDOSE

SYMPTOMS:
Unusually fast or unusually slow heartbeat, loss of consciousness, cardiac arrest.
WHAT TO DO:
- Dial 0 (operator) or 911 (emergency) for an ambulance or medical help. Then give first aid immediately.
- See emergency information on inside covers.

POSSIBLE ADVERSE REACTIONS OR SIDE EFFECTS

SYMPTOMS	WHAT TO DO
Life-threatening: None expected.	
Common: Tiredness.	Continue. Tell doctor at next visit.
Infrequent:	
• Unusually slow or fast heartbeat, wheezing, cough, shortness of breath.	Discontinue. Call doctor right away.
• Dizziness; numbness or tingling in hands or feet; swollen ankles, feet or legs; difficult urination.	Continue. Call doctor when convenient.
• Nausea, constipation or diarrhea, vomiting, indigestion.	Continue. Tell doctor at next visit.
Rare:	
• Fainting, rash, jaundice, insomnia, depression, psychosis.	Discontinue. Call doctor right away.
• Vivid dreams, hair loss.	Continue. Call doctor when convenient.
• Headache.	Continue. Tell doctor at next visit.

WARNINGS & PRECAUTIONS

Don't take if:
You are allergic to any calcium-channel blocker.

Before you start, consult your doctor:
- If you have kidney or liver disease.
- If you have high or low blood pressure.
- If you have heart disease other than coronary artery disease.

Over age 60:
Adverse reactions and side effects may be more frequent and severe than in younger persons.

Pregnancy:
No proven harm to unborn child. Avoid if possible.

Breast-feeding:
No problems expected.

Infants & children:
Not recommended.

Prolonged use:
No problems expected.

Skin & sunlight:
May cause rash or intensify sunburn in areas exposed to sun or sunlamp.

Driving, piloting or hazardous work:
Avoid if you feel dizzy. Otherwise, no problems expected.

Discontinuing:
Don't discontinue without consulting doctor.

Others:
Learn to check your own pulse rate. If it drops to 50 beats per minute or lower, don't take diltiazem until you consult your doctor.

POSSIBLE INTERACTION WITH OTHER DRUGS

GENERIC NAME OR DRUG CLASS	COMBINED EFFECT
ACE inhibitors: captopril, enalapril, lisinopril*	Possible excessive potassium in blood. Dosages may require adjustment.
Antiarrhythmics*	Possible increased effect and toxicity of both drugs.
Antihypertensives*	Blood-pressure drop. Dosages may require adjustment.
Beta-adrenergic blockers*	Decreased angina attacks. Possible irregular heartbeat and congestive heart failure.
Carbamazepine	May increase carbamazepine effect and toxicity.
Cimetidine	Possible increased diltiazem effect and toxicity.
Diuretics*	Dangerous blood-pressure drop. Dosages may require adjustment.
Disopyramide	May cause dangerously slow, fast or irregular heartbeat.
Flecainide	Possible irregular heartbeat.
Lithium	Possible decreased lithium effect.
Nicardipine	Possible increased effect and toxicity of each drug.
Nitrates*	Reduced angina attacks.
Phenytoin	Possible decreased diltiazem effect.
Quinidine	Increased quinidine effect.
Rifampin	Decreased diltiazem effect.
Theophylline	May increase theophylline effect and toxicity.
Tocainide	Increased likelihood of adverse reactions from either drug.

POSSIBLE INTERACTION WITH OTHER SUBSTANCES

INTERACTS WITH	COMBINED EFFECT
Alcohol:	Dangerously low blood pressure.
Beverages:	None expected.
Cocaine:	Possible irregular heartbeat. Avoid.
Foods:	None expected.
Marijuana:	Possible irregular heartbeat. Avoid.
Tobacco:	Possible rapid heartbeat. Avoid.

*See Glossary

DIMENHYDRINATE

BRAND NAMES

See complete list of brand names in the *Brand Name Directory*, page 1061.

BASIC INFORMATION

Habit forming? No
Prescription needed?
 High strength: Yes
 Low strength: No
Available as generic? Yes
Drug class: Antihistamine

USES

- Reduces allergic symptoms such as hay fever, hives, rash or itching.
- Prevents motion sickness, nausea, vomiting.
- Induces sleep.

DOSAGE & USAGE INFORMATION

How to take:
Tablet or liquid—Swallow with liquid or food to lessen stomach irritation.

When to take:
Varies with form. Follow label directions.

If you forget a dose:
Take as soon as you remember up to 2 hours late. If more than 2 hours, wait for next scheduled dose (don't double this dose).

What drug does:
Blocks action of histamine after an allergic response triggers histamine release in sensitive cells.

Continued next column

OVERDOSE

SYMPTOMS:
Convulsions, red face, hallucinations, coma.
WHAT TO DO:
- **Dial 0 (operator) or 911 (emergency) for an ambulance or medical help. Then give first aid immediately.**
- **If patient is unconscious and not breathing, give mouth-to-mouth breathing. If there is no heartbeat, use cardiac massage and mouth-to-mouth breathing (CPR). Don't try to make patient vomit. If you can't get help quickly, take patient to nearest emergency facility.**
- **See emergency information on inside covers.**

Time lapse before drug works:
30 minutes.

Don't take with:
See Interaction column and consult doctor.

POSSIBLE ADVERSE REACTIONS OR SIDE EFFECTS

SYMPTOMS	WHAT TO DO
Life-threatening: Hives, rash, intense itching, faintness soon after a dose (anaphylaxis).	Seek emergency treatment immediately.
Common: Drowsiness; dizziness; dry mouth, eyes and nose; nausea.	Continue. Tell doctor at next visit.
Infrequent: • Change in vision.	Discontinue. Call doctor right away.
• Less tolerance for contact lenses, frequent urination, nausea.	Continue. Call doctor when convenient.
• Appetite loss, headache.	Continue. Tell doctor at next visit.
Rare: • Itchy skin, hives, swollen lips.	Discontinue. Seek emergency treatment.
• Nightmares, agitation, irritability, sore throat, fever, rapid heartbeat, unusual bleeding or bruising, fatigue, weakness, constipation, restlessness, hallucinations.	Discontinue. Call doctor right away.

DIMENHYDRINATE

WARNINGS & PRECAUTIONS

Don't take if:
You are allergic to any antihistamine.

Before you start, consult your doctor:
- If you have glaucoma.
- If you have enlarged prostate.
- If you have asthma.
- If you have kidney disease.
- If you have peptic ulcer.
- If you will have surgery within 2 months, including dental surgery, requiring general or spinal anesthesia.

Over age 60:
Don't exceed recommended dose. Adverse reactions and side effects may be more frequent and severe than in younger persons, especially urination difficulty, diminished alertness and other brain and nervous-system symptoms.

Pregnancy:
No proven harm to unborn child. Avoid if possible.

Breast-feeding:
Drug passes into milk. Avoid drug or discontinue nursing until you finish medicine. Consult doctor for advice on maintaining milk supply.

Infants & children:
Safety not established. Avoid if under 12 years old.

Prolonged use:
Avoid. May damage bone marrow and nerve cells.

Skin & sunlight:
May cause rash or intensify sunburn in areas exposed to sun or sunlamp.

Driving, piloting or hazardous work:
Don't drive or pilot aircraft until you learn how medicine affects you. Don't work around dangerous machinery. Don't climb ladders or work in high places. Danger increases if you drink alcohol or take medicine affecting alertness and reflexes, such as antihistamines, tranquilizers, sedatives, pain medicine, narcotics and mind-altering drugs.

Discontinuing:
No problems expected.

Others:
- May mask symptoms of hearing damage from aspirin, other salicylates, cisplatin, paromomycin, vancomycin or anticonvulsants. Consult doctor if you use these.
- Some products contain tartrazine dye. Avoid, especially if you are allergic to aspirin.

POSSIBLE INTERACTION WITH OTHER DRUGS

GENERIC NAME OR DRUG CLASS	COMBINED EFFECT
Anticholinergics*	Increased anticholinergic effect.
Antidepressants*	Excess sedation. Avoid.
Antihistamines, other*	Excess sedation. Avoid.
Carteolol	Decreased antihistamine effect.
Dronabinol	Increased effects of both drugs. Avoid.
Hypnotics*	Excess sedation. Avoid.
MAO inhibitors*	Increased dimenhydrinate effect.
Mind-altering drugs*	Excess sedation. Avoid.
Molindone	Increased antihistamine effect.
Nabilone	Greater depression of central nervous system.
Narcotics*	Excess sedation. Avoid.
Sedatives*	Excess sedation. Avoid.
Sleep inducers*	Excess sedation. Avoid.
Sotalol	Increased antihistamine effect.
Tranquilizers*	Excess sedation. Avoid.

POSSIBLE INTERACTION WITH OTHER SUBSTANCES

INTERACTS WITH	COMBINED EFFECT
Alcohol:	Excess sedation. Avoid.
Beverages: Caffeine drinks.	Less dimenhydrinate sedation.
Cocaine:	Decreased dimenhydrinate effect. Avoid.
Foods:	None expected.
Marijuana:	Excess sedation. Avoid.
Tobacco:	None expected.

*See Glossary

357

DINOPROSTONE (Vaginal)

BRAND NAMES

Prostin Ez

BASIC INFORMATION

Habit forming? No
Prescription needed? Yes
Available as generic? No
Drug class: Abortifacient (a prostoglandin), uterine stimulant

USES

- To induce abortion from 12th through 20th week of pregnancy. Sometimes used with other substances such as urea, hypertonic saline, oxytocin.
- To empty uterus of a dead fetus, resulting from a missed abortion.
- Reduces blood loss after delivery (sometimes).

DOSAGE & USAGE INFORMATION

How to use:
- Allow suppository to warm to room temperature prior to use.
- Insert suppository into vagina and remain lying down for 10 minutes.
- Take prescribed medicines for vomiting and diarrhea prior to taking dinoprostone.
- Frequently used during hospitalization to allow close monitoring of pulse, blood pressure and temperature.

When to use:
As directed by your doctor.

What drug does:
Stimulates contractions of the uterus and softens the cervix.

Time lapse before drug works:
Varies from patient to patient.

Don't use with:
Oxytocin or other medications to induce abortions.

OVERDOSE

SYMPTOMS:
Drop in blood pressure, wheezing, tightness in chest.
WHAT TO DO:
This medication is used only under medical supervision, so the necessary steps to treat overdose or hypersensitivity will be recognized and used by your doctor.

POSSIBLE ADVERSE REACTIONS OR SIDE EFFECTS

SYMPTOMS	WHAT TO DO
Life-threatening	
Excessive bleeding.	Discontinue. Seek emergency treatment.
Common	
• Fever that doesn't return to normal by 6 hours after using (about 50%).	Discontinue. Call doctor right away.
• Diarrhea (about 40%).	Continue. Call doctor when convenient.
• Nausea and vomiting (about 67%).	Continue. Call doctor when convenient.
Infrequent	
Chills, headache.	Continue. Call doctor when convenient.
Rare	
None expected.	

DINOPROSTONE (Vaginal)

 ## WARNINGS & PRECAUTIONS

Don't use if:
- You have had allergic or unusual reaction previously to dinoprostone.
- Membranes have ruptured.
- You have heart, liver or kidney disease.

Before you start, consult your doctor:
If you have anemia, asthma, lung disease, active heart disease, high blood pressure, low blood pressure, cervical stenosis, past surgery on the uterus, infected cervix, diabetes, epilepsy, glaucoma, liver disease, history of jaundice, acute pelvic inflammatory disease, kidney disease.

Over age 60:
Not used.

Infants & children:
Not used.

Prolonged use:
Not used.

Skin & sunlight:
No problems expected.

Driving, piloting or hazardous work:
Don't drive or pilot aircraft until you learn how medicine affects you. Don't work around dangerous machinery. Don't climb ladders or work in high places. Danger increases if you drink alcohol or take medicine affecting alertness and reflexes, such as antihistamines, tranquilizers, sedatives, pain medicine, narcotics and mind-altering drugs.

Discontinuing:
Some symptoms may be experienced such as unusual bleeding, fever, chills, foul-smelling vaginal discharge, abdominal pain. If any occur, notify your doctor immediately.

Others:
Make sure in your own mind that you are using this medication of your own free will, not the will of others imposed on you.

 ## POSSIBLE INTERACTION WITH OTHER DRUGS

GENERIC NAME OR DRUG CLASS	COMBINED EFFECT
Clinically significant interactions with oral or injected medicines unlikely.	

 ## POSSIBLE INTERACTION WITH OTHER SUBSTANCES

INTERACTS WITH	COMBINED EFFECT
Alcohol:	None expected.
Beverages:	None expected.
Cocaine:	None expected.
Foods:	None expected.
Marijuana:	None expected.
Tobacco:	None expected.

DIPHENYDRAMINE

BRAND NAMES

See complete list of brand names in the
Brand Name Directory, page 1061.

BASIC INFORMATION

Habit forming? No
Prescription needed?
   High strength: Yes
   Low strength: No
Available as generic? Yes
Drug class: Antihistamine

 USES

- Reduces allergic symptoms such as hay fever, hives, rash or itching.
- Prevents motion sickness, nausea, vomiting.
- Induces sleep.
- Reduces stiffness and tremors of Parkinson's disease.

 DOSAGE & USAGE INFORMATION

How to take:
- Tablet or capsule—Swallow with liquid or food to lessen stomach irritation.
- Syrup or elixir—Swallow with liquid to lesson stomach irritation.

When to take:
Varies with form. Follow label directions.

If you forget a dose:
Take as soon as you remember up to 2 hours late. If more than 2 hours, wait for next scheduled dose (don't double this dose).

What drug does:
Blocks action of histamine after an allergic response triggers histamine release in sensitive cells.

Continued next column

 OVERDOSE

SYMPTOMS:
Convulsions, red face, hallucinations, coma.
WHAT TO DO:
- **Dial 0 (operator) or 911 (emergency) for an ambulance or medical help. Then give first aid immediately.**
- **See emergency information on inside covers.**

Time lapse before drug works:
30 minutes.

Don't take with:
See Interaction column and consult doctor.

 POSSIBLE ADVERSE REACTIONS OR SIDE EFFECTS

SYMPTOMS	WHAT TO DO
Life-threatening: None expected.	
Common: Drowsiness; dizziness; dry mouth, nose, throat; nausea.	Continue. Tell doctor at next visit.
Infrequent:	
• Change in vision.	Discontinue. Call doctor right away.
• Less tolerance for contact lenses, painful or difficult urination.	Continue. Call doctor when convenient.
• Appetite loss.	Continue. Tell doctor at next visit.
Rare: Nightmares, agitation, irritability, sore throat, fever, rapid heartbeat, unusual bleeding or bruising, fatigue, weakness.	Discontinue. Call doctor right away.

DIPHENHYDRAMINE

WARNINGS & PRECAUTIONS

Don't take if:
You are allergic to any antihistamine.

Before you start, consult your doctor:
- If you have glaucoma.
- If you have enlarged prostate.
- If you have asthma.
- If you have kidney disease.
- If you have peptic ulcer.
- If you will have surgery within 2 months, including dental surgery, requiring general or spinal anesthesia.

Over age 60:
Don't exceed recommended dose. Adverse reactions and side effects may be more frequent and severe than in younger persons, especially urination difficulty, diminished alertness and other brain and nervous-system symptoms.

Pregnancy:
No proven harm to unborn child. Avoid if possible.

Breast-feeding:
Drug passes into milk. Avoid drug or discontinue nursing until you finish medicine. Consult doctor for advice on maintaining milk supply.

Infants & children:
Not recommended for premature or newborn infants. Otherwise, no problems expected.

Prolonged use:
Avoid. May damage bone marrow and nerve cells.

Skin & sunlight:
May cause rash or intensify sunburn in areas exposed to sun or sunlamp.

Driving, piloting or hazardous work:
Don't drive or pilot aircraft until you learn how medicine affects you. Don't work around dangerous machinery. Don't climb ladders or work in high places. Danger increases if you drink alcohol or take medicine affecting alertness and reflexes, such as antihistamines, tranquilizers, sedatives, pain medicine, narcotics and mind-altering drugs.

Discontinuing:
No problems expected.

Others:
May mask symptoms of hearing damage from aspirin, other salicylates, cisplatin, paromomycin, vancomycin or anticonvulsants. Consult doctor if you use these.

POSSIBLE INTERACTION WITH OTHER DRUGS

GENERIC NAME OR DRUG CLASS	COMBINED EFFECT
Anticholinergics*	Increased anticholinergic effect.
Anticoagulants, oral*	Decreased diphenhydramine effect.
Antidepressants*	Excess sedation. Avoid.
Antihistamines, other*	Excess sedation. Avoid.
Carteolol	Decreased antihistamine effect.
Dronabinol	Increased effects of both drugs. Avoid.
Hypnotics*	Excess sedation. Avoid.
MAO inhibitors*	Increased diphenhydramine effect.
Mind-altering drugs*	Excess sedation. Avoid.
Molindone	Increased sedative and antihistamine effect.
Nabilone	Greater depression of central nervous system.
Narcotics*	Excess sedation. Avoid.
Procarbazine	May increase sedation.
Sedatives*	Excess sedation. Avoid.
Sleep inducers*	Excess sedation. Avoid.
Sotalol	Increased antihistamine effect.
Tranquilizers*	Excess sedation. Avoid.

POSSIBLE INTERACTION WITH OTHER SUBSTANCES

INTERACTS WITH	COMBINED EFFECT
Alcohol:	Excess sedation. Avoid.
Beverages: Caffeine drinks.	Less diphenhydramine sedation.
Cocaine:	Decreased diphenhydramine effect. Avoid.
Foods:	None expected.
Marijuana:	Excess sedation. Avoid.
Tobacco:	None expected.

*See Glossary

DIPHENIDOL

BRAND NAMES

Vontrol

BASIC INFORMATION

Habit forming? No
Prescription needed? Yes
Available as generic? No
Drug class: Antiemetic, antivertigo

 USES

- Prevents motion sickness.
- Controls nausea and vomiting (do not use during pregnancy).

 DOSAGE & USAGE INFORMATION

How to take:
Tablet—Swallow with liquid or food to lessen stomach irritation. If you can't swallow whole, crumble tablet and chew or take with liquid or food.

When to take:
30 to 60 minutes before traveling.

If you forget a dose:
Take as soon as you remember. Wait 4 hours for next dose.

What drug does:
Reduces sensitivity of nerve endings in inner ear, blocking messages to brain's vomiting center.

Time lapse before drug works:
30 to 60 minutes.

Don't take with:
See Interaction column and consult doctor.

 OVERDOSE

SYMPTOMS:
Drowsiness, confusion, incoordination, weak pulse, shallow breathing, stupor, coma.
WHAT TO DO:
- Dial 0 (operator) or 911 (emergency) for an ambulance or medical help. Then give first aid immediately.
- See emergency information on inside covers.

 POSSIBLE ADVERSE REACTIONS OR SIDE EFFECTS

SYMPTOMS	WHAT TO DO
Life-threatening: None expected.	
Common: Drowsiness.	Continue. Tell doctor at next visit.
Infrequent: • Headache, diarrhea or constipation, fast heartbeat.	Continue. Call doctor when convenient.
• Dry mouth, nose, throat.	Continue. Tell doctor at next visit.
Rare: • Hallucinations, confusion.	Discontinue. Seek emergency treatment.
• Rash or hives, depression, jaundice.	Discontinue. Call doctor right away.
• Restlessness; excitement; insomnia; blurred vision; urgent, painful or difficult urination.	Continue. Call doctor when convenient.
• Appetite loss, nausea.	Continue. Tell doctor at next visit.

WARNINGS & PRECAUTIONS

Don't take if:
- You have severe kidney disease.
- You are allergic to diphenidol or meclizine.

Before you start, consult your doctor:
- If you have prostate enlargement.
- If you have glaucoma.
- If you have heart disease.
- If you have intestinal obstruction or ulcers in the gastrointestinal tract.
- If you have kidney disease.
- If you have low blood pressure.
- If you will have surgery within 2 months, including dental surgery, requiring general or spinal anesthesia.

Over age 60:
Adverse reactions and side effects may be more frequent and severe than in younger persons.

Pregnancy:
Animal studies show fetal abnormalities. Decide with your doctor whether drug benefits justify risk to unborn child.

Breast-feeding:
Drug passes into milk. Avoid drug or discontinue nursing until you finish medicine. Consult doctor for advice on maintaining milk supply.

Infants & children:
No problems expected.

Prolonged use:
No problems expected.

Skin & sunlight:
No problems expected.

Driving, piloting or hazardous work:
Don't fly aircraft. Don't drive until you learn how medicine affects you. Don't work around dangerous machinery. Don't climb ladders or work in high places. Danger increases if you drink alcohol or take medicine affecting alertness and reflexes, such as antihistamines, tranquilizers, sedatives, pain medicine, narcotics and mind-altering drugs.

Discontinuing:
No problems expected.

Others:
No problems expected.

POSSIBLE INTERACTION WITH OTHER DRUGS

GENERIC NAME OR DRUG CLASS	COMBINED EFFECT
Anticonvulsants*	Increased effect of both drugs.
Antidepressants, tricyclic (TCA)*	Increased sedative effect of both drugs.
Antihistamines*	Increased sedative effect of both drugs.
Atropine	Increased chance of toxic effect of atropine and atropine-like medicines.
Narcotics*	Increased sedative effect of both drugs.
Sedatives*	Increased sedative effect of both drugs.
Tranquilizers*	Increased sedative effect of both drugs.

POSSIBLE INTERACTION WITH OTHER SUBSTANCES

INTERACTS WITH	COMBINED EFFECT
Alcohol:	Increased sedation. Avoid.
Beverages: Caffeine.	May decrease drowsiness.
Cocaine:	Increased chance of toxic effects of cocaine. Avoid.
Foods:	None expected.
Marijuana:	Increased drowsiness, dry mouth.
Tobacco:	None expected.

DIPHENOXYLATE & ATROPINE

BRAND NAMES

Colonil	Lomotil
Diphenatol	Lonox
Enoxa	Lo-Trol
Latropine	Low-Quel
Lofene	Nor-Mil
Lomanate	SK-Diphenoxylate

BASIC INFORMATION

Habit forming? Yes
Prescription needed? Yes
Available as generic? Yes
Drug class: Antidiarrheal

 USES

Relieves diarrhea and intestinal cramps.

 DOSAGE & USAGE INFORMATION

How to take:
- Tablet—Swallow with liquid or food to lessen stomach irritation.
- Drops or liquid—Follow label instructions and use marked dropper.

When to take:
No more often than directed on label.

If you forget a dose:
Take as soon as you remember up to 2 hours late. If more than 2 hours, wait for next scheduled dose (don't double this dose).

What drug does:
Blocks digestive tract's nerve supply, which reduces propelling movements.

Continued next column

 OVERDOSE

SYMPTOMS:
Excitement, constricted pupils, shallow breathing, coma.
WHAT TO DO:
- Dial 0 (operator) or 911 (emergency) for an ambulance or medical help. Then give first aid immediately.
- If patient is unconscious and not breathing, give mouth-to-mouth breathing. If there is no heartbeat, use cardiac massage and mouth-to-mouth breathing (CPR). Don't try to make patient vomit. If you can't get help quickly, take patient to nearest emergency facility.
- See emergency information on inside covers.

Time lapse before drug works:
May require 12 to 24 hours of regular doses to control diarrhea.

Don't take with:
See Interaction column and consult doctor.

 POSSIBLE ADVERSE REACTIONS OR SIDE EFFECTS

SYMPTOMS	WHAT TO DO
Life-threatening:	
Hives, rash, intense itching, faintness soon after a dose (anaphylaxis).	Seek emergency treatment immediately.
Common:	
None expected.	
Infrequent:	
• Dry mouth, swollen gums, rapid heartbeat.	Discontinue. Call doctor right away.
• Dizziness, depression, drowsiness, rash or itch, blurred vision, decreased urination.	Continue. Call doctor when convenient.
Rare:	
Restlessness, flush, fever, headache, stomach pain, nausea, vomiting, bloating, constipation, numbness of hands or feet.	Discontinue. Call doctor right away.

DIPHENOXYLATE & ATROPINE

WARNINGS & PRECAUTIONS

Don't take if:
- You are allergic to diphenoxylate and atropine or any narcotic or anticholinergic.
- You have jaundice.
- You have infectious diarrhea or antibiotic-associated diarrhea.
- Patient is younger than 2.

Before you start, consult your doctor:
- If you have had liver problems.
- If you have ulcerative colitis.
- If you plan to become pregnant within medication period.
- If you have any medical disorder.
- If you take any medication, including non-prescription drugs.

Over age 60:
Adverse reactions and side effects may be more frequent and severe than in younger persons.

Pregnancy:
No proven harm to unborn child. Avoid because of many side effects.

Breast-feeding:
Drug passes into milk. Avoid drug or discontinue nursing until you finish medicine. Consult doctor for advice on maintaining milk supply.

Infants & children:
Don't give to infants or toddlers. Use only under doctor's supervision for children older than 2.

Prolonged use:
Habit forming.

Skin & sunlight:
No problems expected.

Driving, piloting or hazardous work:
Don't drive or pilot aircraft until you learn how medicine affects you. Don't work around dangerous machinery. Don't climb ladders or work in high places. Danger increases if you drink alcohol or take medicine affecting alertness and reflexes.

Discontinuing:
- May be unnecessary to finish medicine. Follow doctor's instructions.
- After discontinuing, consult doctor if you experience muscle cramps, nausea, vomiting, trembling, stomach cramps or unusual sweating.

Others:
If diarrhea lasts longer than 4 days, discontinue and call doctor.

POSSIBLE INTERACTION WITH OTHER DRUGS

GENERIC NAME OR DRUG CLASS	COMBINED EFFECT
Barbiturates*	Increased effect of both drugs.
Ethinamate	Dangerous increased effects of ethinamate. Avoid combining.
Fluoxetine	Increased depressant effects of both drugs.
Guanfacine	May increase depressant effects of either drug.
Leucovorin	High alcohol content of leucovorin may cause adverse effects.
MAO inhibitors*	May increase blood pressure excessively.
Methyprylon	Increased sedative effect, perhaps to dangerous level. Avoid.
Sedatives*	Increased effect of both drugs.
Tranquilizers*	Increased effect of both drugs.

POSSIBLE INTERACTION WITH OTHER SUBSTANCES

INTERACTS WITH	COMBINED EFFECT
Alcohol:	Depressed brain function. Avoid.
Beverages:	None expected.
Cocaine:	Decreased effect of diphenoxylate and atropine.
Foods:	None expected.
Marijuana:	None expected.
Tobacco:	None expected.

*See Glossary

DIPHENYLPYRALINE

BRAND NAMES

Diafen   Hispril

BASIC INFORMATION

Habit forming? No
Prescription needed?
  High strength: Yes
  Low strength: No
Available as generic? No
Drug class: Antihistamine

USES

- Reduces allergic symptoms such as hay fever, hives, rash or itching.
- Induces sleep.

DOSAGE & USAGE INFORMATION

How to take:
Extended-release capsules—Swallow each dose whole with liquid.

When to take:
Varies with form. Follow label directions.

If you forget a dose:
Take as soon as you remember up to 2 hours late. If more than 2 hours, wait for next scheduled dose (don't double this dose).

What drug does:
Blocks action of histamine after an allergic response triggers histamine release in sensitive cells.

Time lapse before drug works:
30 minutes.

Don't take with:
See Interaction column and consult doctor.

OVERDOSE

SYMPTOMS:
Convulsions, red face, hallucinations, coma.
WHAT TO DO:
- Dial 0 (operator) or 911 (emergency) for an ambulance or medical help. Then give first aid immediately.
- If patient is unconscious and not breathing, give mouth-to-mouth breathing. If there is no heartbeat, use cardiac massage and mouth-to-mouth breathing (CPR). Don't try to make patient vomit. If you can't get help quickly, take patient to nearest emergency facility.
- See emergency information on inside covers.

POSSIBLE ADVERSE REACTIONS OR SIDE EFFECTS

SYMPTOMS	WHAT TO DO
Life-threatening: None expected.	
Common: Drowsiness; dizziness; dry mouth, nose, throat; nausea.	Continue. Tell doctor at next visit.
Infrequent:	
• Change in vision.	Discontinue. Call doctor right away.
• Less tolerance for contact lenses, painful or difficult urination.	Continue. Call doctor when convenient.
• Appetite loss.	Continue. Tell doctor at next visit.
Rare: Nightmares, agitation, irritability, sore throat, fever, rapid heartbeat, unusual bleeding or bruising, fatigue, weakness.	Discontinue. Call doctor right away.

DIPHENYLPYRALINE

WARNINGS & PRECAUTIONS

Don't take if:
You are allergic to any antihistamine.

Before you start, consult your doctor:
• If you have glaucoma.
• If you have enlarged prostate.
• If you have asthma.
• If you have kidney disease.
• If you have peptic ulcer.
• If you will have surgery within 2 months, including dental surgery, requiring general or spinal anesthesia.

Over age 60:
Don't exceed recommended dose. Adverse reactions and side effects may be more frequent and severe than in younger persons, especially urination difficulty, diminished alertness and other brain and nervous-system symptoms.

Pregnancy:
No proven harm to unborn child. Avoid if possible.

Breast-feeding:
Drug passes into milk. Avoid drug or discontinue nursing until you finish medicine. Consult doctor for advice on maintaining milk supply.

Infants & children:
Not recommended for premature or newborn infants. Otherwise, no problems expected.

Prolonged use:
Avoid. May damage bone marrow and nerve cells.

Skin & sunlight:
May cause rash or intensify sunburn in areas exposed to sun or sunlamp.

Driving, piloting or hazardous work:
Don't drive or pilot aircraft until you learn how medicine affects you. Don't work around dangerous machinery. Don't climb ladders or work in high places. Danger increases if you drink alcohol or take medicine affecting alertness and reflexes, such as antihistamines, tranquilizers, sedatives, pain medicine, narcotics and mind-altering drugs.

Discontinuing:
No problems expected.

Others:
May mask symptoms of hearing damage from aspirin, other salicylates, cisplatin, paromomycin, vancomycin or anticonvulsants. Consult doctor if you use these.

POSSIBLE INTERACTION WITH OTHER DRUGS

GENERIC NAME OR DRUG CLASS	COMBINED EFFECT
Anticholinergics*	Increased anticholinergic effect.
Anticoagulants, oral*	Decreased diphenylpyraline effect.
Antidepressants*	Excess sedation. Avoid.
Antihistamines, other*	Excess sedation. Avoid.
Carteolol	Decreased antihistamine effect.
Dronabinol	Increased effects of both drugs. Avoid.
Hypnotics*	Excess sedation. Avoid.
MAO inhibitors*	Increased diphenylpyraline effect.
Mind-altering drugs*	Excess sedation. Avoid.
Molindone	Increased antihistamine effect.
Nabilone	Greater depression of central nervous system.
Narcotics*	Excess sedation. Avoid.
Procarbazine	May increase sedation.
Sedatives*	Excess sedation. Avoid.
Sleep inducers*	Excess sedation. Avoid.
Sotalol	Increased antihistamine effect.
Tranquilizers*	Excess sedation. Avoid.

POSSIBLE INTERACTION WITH OTHER SUBSTANCES

INTERACTS WITH	COMBINED EFFECT
Alcohol:	Excess sedation. Avoid.
Beverages: Caffeine drinks.	Less diphenylpyraline sedation.
Cocaine:	Decreased diphenylpyraline effect. Avoid.
Foods:	None expected.
Marijuana:	Excess sedation. Avoid.
Tobacco:	None expected.

DIPYRIDAMOLE

BRAND NAMES

Apo-Dipyridamole	Pyridamole
Persantine	SK-Dipyridamole

BASIC INFORMATION

Habit forming? No
Prescription needed?
  U.S.: Yes
  Canada: No
Available as generic? Yes
Drug class: Coronary vasodilator

USES

- May reduce frequency and intensity of angina attacks.
- Prevents blood clots after heart surgery.

DOSAGE & USAGE INFORMATION

How to take:
Tablet—Swallow with liquid. If you can't swallow whole, crumble tablet and take with liquid.

When to take:
1 hour before meals.

If you forget a dose:
Take as soon as you remember up to 2 hours late. If more than 2 hours, wait for next scheduled dose (don't double this dose).

What drug does:
- Probably dilates blood vessels to increase oxygen to heart.
- Prevents platelet clumping, which causes blood clots.

Continued next column

OVERDOSE

SYMPTOMS:
Decreased blood pressure; weak, rapid pulse; cold, clammy skin; collapse.
WHAT TO DO:
- Dial 0 (operator) or 911 (emergency) for an ambulance or medical help. Then give first aid immediately.
- If patient is unconscious and not breathing, give mouth-to-mouth breathing. If there is no heartbeat, use cardiac massage and mouth-to-mouth breathing (CPR). Don't try to make patient vomit. If you can't get help quickly, take patient to nearest emergency facility.
- See emergency information on inside covers.

Time lapse before drug works:
3 months of continual use.

Don't take with:
See Interaction column and consult doctor.

POSSIBLE ADVERSE REACTIONS OR SIDE EFFECTS

SYMPTOMS	WHAT TO DO
Life-threatening:	
None expected.	
Common:	
None expected.	
Infrequent:	
• Dizziness, fainting, headache.	Discontinue. Call doctor right away.
• Red flush, rash, nausea, vomiting, cramps, weakness.	Continue. Call doctor when convenient.
Rare:	
None expected.	

WARNINGS & PRECAUTIONS

Don't take if:
- You are allergic to dipyridamole.
- You are recovering from a heart attack.

Before you start, consult your doctor:
- If you have low blood pressure.
- If you have liver disease.

Over age 60:
Begin treatment with small doses.

Pregnancy:
No proven harm to unborn child. Avoid if possible.

Breast-feeding:
No proven problems. Consult doctor.

Infants & children:
Not recommended.

Prolonged use:
No problems expected.

Skin & sunlight:
No problems expected.

Driving, piloting or hazardous work:
Avoid if you feel dizzy. Otherwise, no problems expected.

Discontinuing:
Don't discontinue without doctor's advice until you complete prescribed dose, even though symptoms diminish or disappear.

Others:
Drug increases your ability to be active without angina pain. Avoid excessive physical exertion that might injure heart.

POSSIBLE INTERACTION WITH OTHER DRUGS

GENERIC NAME OR DRUG CLASS	COMBINED EFFECT
Anticoagulants, oral*	Increased anti-coagulant effect. Bleeding tendency.
Aspirin and combination drugs containing aspirin	Increased dipyridamole effect. Dose may need adjustment.

POSSIBLE INTERACTION WITH OTHER SUBSTANCES

INTERACTS WITH	COMBINED EFFECT
Alcohol:	May lower blood pressure excessively.
Beverages:	None expected.
Cocaine:	No proven problems.
Foods:	Decreased dipyridamole absorption unless taken 1 hour before eating.
Marijuana:	Daily use— Decreased dipyridamole effect.
Tobacco: Nicotine.	May decrease dipyridamole effect.

DISOPYRAMIDE

BRAND NAMES

Norpace
Norpace CR

Rythmodan
Rythmodan-LA

BASIC INFORMATION

Habit forming? No
Prescription needed? Yes
Available as generic? Yes
Drug class: Antiarrhythmic

 USES

Corrects heart rhythm disorders.

 DOSAGE & USAGE
INFORMATION

How to take:
Extended-release tablet or capsule—Swallow
with liquid. If you can't swallow whole, crumble
tablet or open capsule and take with liquid or
food.

When to take:
At the same times each day.

If you forget a dose:
Take as soon as you remember up to 2 hours
late. If more than 2 hours, wait for next
scheduled dose (don't double this dose).

What drug does:
Delays nerve impulses to heart to regulate
heartbeat.

Time lapse before drug works:
Begins in 30 to 60 minutes. Must use for 5 to 7
days to determine effectiveness.

Don't take with:
See Interaction column and consult doctor.

 OVERDOSE

SYMPTOMS:
Blood-pressure drop, irregular heartbeat,
apnea, loss of consciousness.
WHAT TO DO:
* Dial 0 (operator) or 911 (emergency) for
  an ambulance or medical help. Then give
  first aid immediately.
* If patient is unconscious and not
  breathing, give mouth-to-mouth
  breathing. If there is no heartbeat, use
  cardiac massage and mouth-to-mouth
  breathing (CPR). Don't try to make patient
  vomit. If you can't get help quickly, take
  patient to nearest emergency facility.
* See emergency information on inside
  covers.

 POSSIBLE
ADVERSE REACTIONS
OR SIDE EFFECTS

SYMPTOMS	WHAT TO DO
Life-threatening:	
Hives, rash, intense itching, faintness soon after a dose (anaphylaxis).	Seek emergency treatment immediately.
Common:	
• Hypoglycemia.	Discontinue. Call doctor right away.
• Dry mouth, constipation, painful or difficult urination, rapid weight gain, blurred vision.	Continue. Call doctor when convenient.
Infrequent:	
• Dizziness, fainting, confusion, chest pain, nervousness, depression, slow or fast heartbeat.	Discontinue. Call doctor right away.
• Swollen feet.	Continue. Call doctor when convenient.
Rare:	
• Shortness of breath, psychosis.	Discontinue. Seek emergency treatment.
• Rash, sore throat, fever, headache, jaundice, muscle weakness.	Discontinue. Call doctor right away.
• Eye pain, diminished sex drive, swollen breasts in men, numbness or tingling of hands and feet, bleeding tendency.	Continue. Call doctor when convenient.

DISOPYRAMIDE

 ## WARNINGS & PRECAUTIONS

Don't take if:
- You are allergic to disopyramide or any antiarrhythmic.
- You have second- or third-degree heart block.
- You have heart failure.

Before you start, consult your doctor:
- If you react unfavorably to other antiarrhythmic drugs.
- If you have had heart disease.
- If you have low blood pressure.
- If you have liver disease.
- If you have glaucoma.
- If you have enlarged prostate.
- If you have myasthenia gravis.
- If you take digitalis preparations or diuretics.

Over age 60:
- May require reduced dose.
- More likely to have difficulty urinating or be constipated.
- More likely to have blood-pressure drop.

Pregnancy:
No proven harm to unborn child. Avoid if possible.

Breast-feeding:
Drug passes into milk. Avoid drug or discontinue nursing until you finish medicine. Consult doctor for advice on maintaining milk supply.

Infants & children:
Safety not established. Don't use.

Prolonged use:
No problems expected.

Skin & sunlight:
No problems expected.

Driving, piloting or hazardous work:
Don't drive or pilot aircraft until you learn how medicine affects you. Don't work around dangerous machinery. Don't climb ladders or work in high places. Danger increases if you drink alcohol or take medicine affecting alertness and reflexes, such as antihistamines, tranquilizers, sedatives, pain medicine, narcotics, or mind-altering drugs.

Discontinuing:
Don't discontinue without doctor's advice until you complete prescribed dose, even though symptoms diminish or disappear.

Others:
If new illness, injury or surgery occurs, tell doctors of disopyramide use.

 ## POSSIBLE INTERACTION WITH OTHER DRUGS

GENERIC NAME OR DRUG CLASS	COMBINED EFFECT
Antiarrhythmics*	May increase effect and toxicity of each drug.
Anticholinergics*	Increased anticholinergic effect.
Anticoagulants, oral*	Possible increased anticoagulant effect.
Antihypertensives*	Increased antihypertensive effect.
Encainide	Increased effect of toxicity on the heart muscle.
Flecainide	Possible irregular heartbeat.
Nicardipine	May cause dangerously slow, fast or irregular heartbeat.
Phenobarbital	Increased metabolism, decreased disopyramide effect.
Phenytoin	Increased metabolism, decreased disopyramide effect.
Rifampin	Increased metabolism, decreased disopyramide effect.
Tocainide	Increased likelihood of adverse reactions with either drug.

 ## POSSIBLE INTERACTION WITH OTHER SUBSTANCES

INTERACTS WITH	COMBINED EFFECT
Alcohol:	Decreased blood pressure and blood sugar. Use caution.
Beverages:	None expected.
Cocaine:	Irregular heartbeat.
Foods:	None expected.
Marijuana:	Unpredictable. May decrease disopyramide effect.
Tobacco:	May decrease disopyramide effect.

*See Glossary

DISULFIRAM

BRAND NAMES

Antabuse

BASIC INFORMATION

Habit forming? No
Prescription needed? Yes
Available as generic? Yes
Drug class: None

 USES

Treatment for alcoholism. Will not cure alcoholism, but is a powerful deterrent to drinking.

 DOSAGE & USAGE INFORMATION

How to take:
Tablet—Swallow with liquid.

When to take:
Morning or bedtime. Avoid if you have used *any* alcohol, tonics, cough syrups, fermented vinegar, after-shave lotion or backrub solutions within 12 hours.

If you forget a dose:
Take as soon as you remember up to 12 hours late. If more than 12 hours, wait for next scheduled dose (don't double this dose).

What drug does:
In combination with alcohol, produces a metabolic change that causes severe, temporary toxicity.

Time lapse before drug works:
3 to 12 hours.

Don't take with:
- See Interaction column and consult doctor.
- Non-prescription drugs that contain *any* alcohol.

 OVERDOSE

SYMPTOMS:
Memory loss, behavior disturbances, lethargy, confusion and headaches; nausea, vomiting, stomach pain and diarrhea; weakness and unsteady walk; temporary paralysis.
WHAT TO DO:
- **Dial 0 (operator) or 911 (emergency) for an ambulance or medical help. Then give first aid immediately.**
- **See emergency information on inside covers.**

 POSSIBLE ADVERSE REACTIONS OR SIDE EFFECTS

SYMPTOMS	WHAT TO DO
Life-threatening: None expected.	
Common: Drowsiness.	Continue. Tell doctor at next visit.
Infrequent:	
• Eye pain, vision changes, stomach discomfort, throbbing headache, numbness in hands and feet.	Continue. Call doctor when convenient.
• Mood change, decreased sexual ability in men, tiredness.	Continue. Tell doctor at next visit.
• Bad taste in mouth (metal or garlic).	No action necessary.
Rare: Rash, jaundice.	Discontinue. Call doctor right away.

 WARNINGS & PRECAUTIONS

Don't take if:
- You are allergic to disulfiram (alcohol-disulfiram combination is not an allergic reaction).
- You have used alcohol in any form or amount within 12 hours.
- You have taken paraldehyde within 1 week.
- You have heart disease.

Before you start, consult your doctor:
- If you have allergies.
- If you plan to become pregnant within medication period.
- If no one has explained to you how disulfiram reacts.
- If you think you cannot avoid drinking.
- If you have diabetes, epilepsy, liver or kidney disease.
- If you take other drugs.

Over age 60:
Adverse reactions and side effects may be more frequent and severe than in younger persons.

Pregnancy:
Risk to unborn child outweighs drug benefits. Don't use.

Breast-feeding:
Studies inconclusive. Consult your doctor.

Infants & children:
Not recommended.

Prolonged use:
Periodic blood-cell counts and liver-function tests recommended if you take this drug a long time.

Skin & sunlight:
No problems expected.

Driving, piloting or hazardous work:
Avoid if you feel drowsy or have vision side effects. Otherwise, no restrictions.

Discontinuing:
Don't discontinue without consulting doctor. Dose may require gradual reduction if you have taken drug for a long time. Doses of other drugs may also require adjustment. Avoid alcohol at least 14 days following last dose.

Others:
No problems expected.

POSSIBLE INTERACTION WITH OTHER DRUGS

GENERIC NAME OR DRUG CLASS	COMBINED EFFECT
Anticoagulants*	Possible unexplained bleeding.
Anticonvulsants*	Excessive sedation.
Barbiturates*	Excessive sedation.
Cephalosporins*	Disulfiram reaction.*
Ethinamate	Dangerous increased effects of ethinamate. Avoid combining.
Fluoxetine	Increased depressant effects of both drugs.
Guanfacine	May increase depressant effects of either drug.
Isoniazid	Unsteady walk and disturbed behavior.
Leucovorin	High alcohol content of leucovorin may cause adverse effects.

Methyprylon	Increased sedative effect, perhaps to dangerous level. Avoid.
Metronidazole	Disulfiram reaction.*
Nabilone	Greater depression of central nervous system.
Sedatives*	Excessive sedation.

POSSIBLE INTERACTION WITH OTHER SUBSTANCES

INTERACTS WITH	COMBINED EFFECT
Alcohol: *Any* form or amount.	Possible life-threatening toxicity. See disulfiram reaction.*
Beverages: Punch or fruit drink that may contain alcohol.	Disulfiram reaction.*
Cocaine:	Increased disulfiram effect.
Foods: Sauces, fermented vinegar, marinades, desserts or other foods prepared with *any* alcohol.	Disulfiram reaction.*
Marijuana:	None expected.
Tobacco:	None expected.

DIVALPOREX

BRAND NAMES

Depakote   Epival

BASIC INFORMATION

Habit forming? No
Prescription needed? Yes
Available as generic? No
Drug class: Anticonvulsant

 USES

Controls petit mal (absence) seizures in
treatment of epilepsy.

 DOSAGE & USAGE INFORMATION

How to take:
Tablet—Swallow with liquid or food to lessen
stomach irritation.

When to take:
Once a day.

If you forget a dose:
Take as soon as you remember. Don't ever
double dose.

What drug does:
Increases concentration of gamma aminobutyric
acid, which inhibits nerve transmission in parts
of brain.

Time lapse before drug works:
1 to 4 hours.

Don't take with:
See Interaction column and consult doctor.

 OVERDOSE

SYMPTOMS:
Coma.
WHAT TO DO:
- Dial 0 (operator) or 911 (emergency) for
  an ambulance or medical help. Then give
  first aid immediately.
- If patient is unconscious and not
  breathing, give mouth-to-mouth
  breathing. If there is no heartbeat, use
  cardiac massage and mouth-to-mouth
  breathing (CPR). Don't try to make patient
  vomit. If you can't get help quickly, take
  patient to nearest emergency facility.
- See emergency information on inside
  covers.

 POSSIBLE ADVERSE REACTIONS OR SIDE EFFECTS

SYMPTOMS	WHAT TO DO
Life-threatening: None expected.	
Common: Menstrual irregularities, nausea, vomiting, abdominal cramps.	Continue. Call doctor when convenient.
Infrequent: • Rash, bloody spots under skin, hair loss, bleeding, easy bruising.	Discontinue. Call doctor right away.
• Drowsiness, weakness, easily upset emotionally, depression, psychic changes, headache, incoordination, nausea, vomiting, abdominal cramps, appetite change.	Continue. Call doctor when convenient.
Rare: • Double vision, unusual movements of eyes (nystagmus), jaundice, increased bleeding tendency, severe abdominal pain, edema (swelling of feet and legs).	Discontinue. Call doctor right away.
• Anemia.	Continue. Call doctor when convenient.

WARNINGS & PRECAUTIONS

Don't take if:
You are allergic to divalporex.

Before you start, consult your doctor:
- If you have blood, kidney or liver disease.
- If you will have surgery within 2 months, including dental surgery, requiring general or spinal anesthesia.

Over age 60:
Adverse reactions and side effects may be more frequent and severe than in younger persons.

Pregnancy:
No proven harm to unborn child. Avoid if possible.

Breast-feeding:
Unknown effect.

Infants & children:
Under close medical supervision only.

Prolonged use:
Request periodic blood tests, liver and kidney function tests.

Skin & sunlight:
No problems expected.

Driving, piloting or hazardous work:
Don't drive or pilot aircraft until you learn how medicine affects you. Don't work around dangerous machinery. Don't climb ladders or work in high places. Danger increases if you drink alcohol or take medicine affecting alertness and reflexes, such as antihistamines, tranquilizers, sedatives, pain medicine, narcotics and mind-altering drugs.

Discontinuing:
Don't discontinue without consulting doctor. Dose may require gradual reduction if you have taken drug for a long time. Doses of other drugs may also require adjustment.

Others:
No problems expected.

POSSIBLE INTERACTION WITH OTHER DRUGS

GENERIC NAME OR DRUG CLASS	COMBINED EFFECT
Anticoagulants*	Increases chance of bleeding.
Aspirin	Increases chance of bleeding.
Central nervous system depressants* (antidepressants,* antihistamines,* muscle relaxants,* narcotics,* sedatives,* sleeping pills,* tranquilizers*)	Increases sedative effect.
Clonazepam	May prolong seizure.
Dypiradamole	Increases chance of bleeding.
MAO inhibitors*	Increases sedative effect.
Nabilone	Greater depression of central nervous system.
Phenobarbital	Increases chance of toxicity.
Phenytoin	Unpredictable. May require increased or decreased dosage.
Primidone	Increases chance of toxicity.
Sulfinpyrazone	Increases chance of bleeding.

POSSIBLE INTERACTION WITH OTHER SUBSTANCES

INTERACTS WITH	COMBINED EFFECT
Alcohol:	Deep sedation. Avoid.
Beverages:	No problems expected.
Cocaine:	Increased brain sensitivity. Avoid.
Foods:	No problems expected.
Marijuana:	Increased brain sensitivity. Avoid.
Tobacco:	Increased brain sensitivity. Avoid.

*See Glossary

DOCUSATE CALCIUM

BRAND NAMES

Dioctocal
Doxidan
D-C-S

Pro-Cal-Sof
Surfak

BASIC INFORMATION

Habit forming? No
Prescription needed? No
Available as generic? Yes
Drug class: Laxative (emollient)

 ## USES

Constipation relief.

 ## DOSAGE & USAGE INFORMATION

How to take:
Capsule—Swallow with liquid. Don't open capsules.

When to take:
At the same time each day, preferably bedtime.

If you forget a dose:
Take as soon as you remember. Wait 12 hours for next dose. Return to regular schedule.

What drug does:
Makes stool hold fluid so it is easier to pass.

Time lapse before drug works:
2 to 3 days of continual use.

Don't take with:
- Other medicines at same time. Wait 2 hours.
- See Interaction column and consult doctor.

 ## OVERDOSE

SYMPTOMS:
Appetite loss, nausea, vomiting, diarrhea.
WHAT TO DO:
Overdose unlikely to threaten life. If person takes much larger amount than prescribed, call doctor, poison-control center or hospital emergency room for instructions.

 ## POSSIBLE ADVERSE REACTIONS OR SIDE EFFECTS

SYMPTOMS	WHAT TO DO
Life-threatening: None expected.	
Common: None expected.	
Infrequent: Throat irritation (liquid only), intestinal and stomach cramps.	Continue. Call doctor when convenient.
Rare: Rash.	Discontinue. Call doctor right away.

DOCUSATE CALCIUM

WARNINGS & PRECAUTIONS

Don't take if:
- You are allergic to any emollient laxative.
- You have abdominal pain and fever that might be appendicitis.

Before you start, consult your doctor:
- If you are taking other laxatives.
- To be sure constipation isn't a sign of a serious disorder.

Over age 60:
You must drink 6 to 8 glasses of fluid every 24 hours for drug to work.

Pregnancy:
No problems expected. Consult doctor.

Breast-feeding:
No problems expected.

Infants & children:
No problems expected.

Prolonged use:
Avoid. Overuse of laxatives may damage intestine lining.

Skin & sunlight:
No problems expected.

Driving, piloting or hazardous work:
No problems expected.

Discontinuing:
May be unnecessary to finish medicine. Follow doctor's instructions.

Others:
No problems expected.

POSSIBLE INTERACTION WITH OTHER DRUGS

GENERIC NAME OR DRUG CLASS	COMBINED EFFECT
Danthron	Possible liver damage.
Digitalis preparations*	Toxic absorption of digitalis.
Mineral oil	Increased mineral oil absorption into bloodstream. Avoid.
Phenolphthalein	Increased phenolphthalein absorption. Possible toxicity.

POSSIBLE INTERACTION WITH OTHER SUBSTANCES

INTERACTS WITH	COMBINED EFFECT
Alcohol:	None expected.
Beverages:	None expected.
Cocaine:	None expected.
Foods:	None expected.
Marijuana:	None expected.
Tobacco:	None expected.

*See Glossary

DOCUSATE POTASSIUM

BRAND NAMES

Dialose
Diocto-K

Kasof
Pro-Cal-Sof

BASIC INFORMATION

Habit forming? No
Prescription needed? No
Available as generic? Yes
Drug class: Laxative (emollient)

 ## USES

Constipation relief.

 ## DOSAGE & USAGE INFORMATION

How to take:
Capsule—Swallow with liquid. Don't open capsules.

When to take:
At the same time each day, preferably bedtime.

If you forget a dose:
Take as soon as you remember. Wait 12 hours for next dose. Return to regular schedule.

What drug does:
Makes stool hold fluid so it is easier to pass.

Time lapse before drug works:
2 to 3 days of continual use.

Don't take with:
- Other medicines at same time. Wait 2 hours.
- See Interaction column and consult doctor.

 ## OVERDOSE

SYMPTOMS:
Appetite loss, nausea, vomiting, diarrhea.
WHAT TO DO:
Overdose unlikely to threaten life. If person takes much larger amount than prescribed, call doctor, poison-control center or hospital emergency room for instructions.

 ## POSSIBLE ADVERSE REACTIONS OR SIDE EFFECTS

SYMPTOMS	WHAT TO DO
Life-threatening: None expected.	
Common: None expected.	
Infrequent: Throat irritation (liquid only), intestinal and stomach cramps.	Continue. Call doctor when convenient.
Rare: Rash.	Discontinue. Call doctor right away.

WARNINGS & PRECAUTIONS

Don't take if:
- You are allergic to any emollient laxative.
- You have abdominal pain and fever that might be appendicitis.

Before you start, consult your doctor:
- If you are taking other laxatives.
- To be sure constipation isn't a sign of a serious disorder.

Over age 60:
You must drink 6 to 8 glasses of fluid every 24 hours for drug to work.

Pregnancy:
No problems expected. Consult doctor.

Breast-feeding:
No problems expected.

Infants & children:
No problems expected.

Prolonged use:
Avoid. Overuse of laxatives may damage intestine lining.

Skin & sunlight:
No problems expected.

Driving, piloting or hazardous work:
No problems expected.

Discontinuing:
May be unnecessary to finish medicine. Follow doctor's instructions.

Others:
No problems expected.

POSSIBLE INTERACTION WITH OTHER DRUGS

GENERIC NAME OR DRUG CLASS	COMBINED EFFECT
Danthron	Possible liver damage.
Digitalis preparations*	Toxic absorption of digitalis.
Mineral oil	Increased mineral oil absorption into bloodstream. Avoid.
Phenolphthalein	Increased phenolphthalein absorption. Possible toxicity.

POSSIBLE INTERACTION WITH OTHER SUBSTANCES

INTERACTS WITH	COMBINED EFFECT
Alcohol:	None expected.
Beverages:	None expected.
Cocaine:	None expected.
Foods:	None expected.
Marijuana:	None expected.
Tobacco:	None expected.

*See Glossary

DOCUSATE SODIUM

BRAND NAMES

See complete list of brand names in the *Brand Name Directory*, page 1062.

BASIC INFORMATION

Habit forming? No
Prescription needed? No
Available as generic? Yes
Drug class: Laxative (emollient)

 ## USES

Constipation relief.

 ## DOSAGE & USAGE INFORMATION

How to take:
* Tablet or capsule—Swallow with liquid. Don't open capsules.
* Syrup—Take as directed on bottle.

When to take:
At the same time each day, preferably bedtime.

If you forget a dose:
Take as soon as you remember. Wait 12 hours for next dose. Return to regular schedule.

What drug does:
Makes stool hold fluid so it is easier to pass.

Time lapse before drug works:
2 to 3 days of continual use.

Don't take with:
* Other medicines at same time. Wait 2 hours.
* See Interaction column and consult doctor.

 ## OVERDOSE

SYMPTOMS:
Appetite loss, nausea, vomiting, diarrhea.
WHAT TO DO:
Overdose unlikely to threaten life. If person takes much larger amount than prescribed, call doctor, poison-control center or hospital emergency room for instructions.

 ## POSSIBLE ADVERSE REACTIONS OR SIDE EFFECTS

SYMPTOMS	WHAT TO DO
Life-threatening: None expected.	
Common: None expected.	
Infrequent: Throat irritation (liquid only), intestinal and stomach cramps.	Continue. Call doctor when convenient.
Rare: Rash.	Discontinue. Call doctor right away.

WARNINGS & PRECAUTIONS

Don't take if:
- You are allergic to any emollient laxative.
- You have abdominal pain and fever that might be appendicitis.

Before you start, consult your doctor:
- If you are taking other laxatives.
- To be sure constipation isn't a sign of a serious disorder.

Over age 60:
You must drink 6 to 8 glasses of fluid every 24 hours for drug to work.

Pregnancy:
No problems expected. Consult doctor.

Breast-feeding:
No problems expected.

Infants & children:
No problems expected.

Prolonged use:
Avoid. Overuse of laxatives may damage intestine lining.

Skin & sunlight:
No problems expected.

Driving, piloting or hazardous work:
No problems expected.

Discontinuing:
May be unnecessary to finish medicine. Follow doctor's instructions.

Others:
No problems expected.

POSSIBLE INTERACTION WITH OTHER DRUGS

GENERIC NAME OR DRUG CLASS	COMBINED EFFECT
Danthron	Possible liver damage.
Digitalis preparations*	Toxic absorption of digitalis.
Mineral oil	Increased mineral oil absorption into bloodstream. Avoid.
Phenolphthalein	Increased phenolphthalein absorption. Possible toxicity.

POSSIBLE INTERACTION WITH OTHER SUBSTANCES

INTERACTS WITH	COMBINED EFFECT
Alcohol:	None expected.
Beverages:	None expected.
Cocaine:	None expected.
Foods:	None expected.
Marijuana:	None expected.
Tobacco:	None expected.

*See Glossary

DOXYLAMINE

BRAND NAMES

Bendectin
Cremacoat 4
Decapryn

Unisom Nighttime
Sleep Aid

BASIC INFORMATION

Habit forming? No
Prescription needed? Yes
Available as generic? No
Drug class: Antihistamine

USES

* Reduces allergic symptoms such as hay fever, hives, rash or itching.
* Prevents motion sickness, nausea, vomiting.
* Induces sleep.

DOSAGE & USAGE INFORMATION

How to take:
Tablet—Swallow with liquid or food to lessen stomach irritation.

When to take:
Varies with form. Follow label directions.

If you forget a dose:
Take as soon as you remember up to 2 hours late. If more than 2 hours, wait for next scheduled dose (don't double this dose).

What drug does:
Blocks action of histamine after an allergic response triggers histamine release in sensitive cells.

Continued next column

OVERDOSE

SYMPTOMS:
Convulsions, red face, hallucinations, coma.
WHAT TO DO:
* Dial 0 (operator) or 911 (emergency) for an ambulance or medical help. Then give first aid immediately.
* If patient is unconscious and not breathing, give mouth-to-mouth breathing. If there is no heartbeat, use cardiac massage and mouth-to-mouth breathing (CPR). Don't try to make patient vomit. If you can't get help quickly, take patient to nearest emergency facility.
* See emergency information on inside covers.

Time lapse before drug works:
30 minutes.

Don't take with:
See Interaction column and consult doctor.

POSSIBLE ADVERSE REACTIONS OR SIDE EFFECTS

SYMPTOMS	WHAT TO DO
Life-threatening: None expected.	
Common: Drowsiness; dizziness; nausea; dry mouth, nose, throat.	Continue. Tell doctor at next visit.
Infrequent: • Change in vision.	Discontinue. Call doctor right away.
• Less tolerance for contact lenses, difficult urination.	Continue. Call doctor when convenient.
• Appetite loss.	Continue. Tell doctor at next visit.
Rare: Nightmares, agitation, irritability, sore throat, fever, rapid heartbeat, unusual bleeding or bruising, fatigue, weakness.	Discontinue. Call doctor right away.

WARNINGS & PRECAUTIONS

Don't take if:
You are allergic to any antihistamine.

Before you start, consult your doctor:
- If you have glaucoma.
- If you have enlarged prostate.
- If you have asthma.
- If you have kidney disease.
- If you have peptic ulcer.
- If you will have surgery within 2 months, including dental surgery, requiring general or spinal anesthesia.

Over age 60:
Don't exceed recommended dose. Adverse reactions and side effects may be more frequent and severe than in younger persons, especially urination difficulty, diminished alertness and other brain and nervous-system symptoms.

Pregnancy:
No proven harm to unborn child. Avoid if possible.

Breast-feeding:
Drug passes into milk. Avoid drug or discontinue nursing until you finish medicine. Consult doctor for advice on maintaining milk supply.

Infants & children:
Not recommended for premature or newborn infants. Otherwise, no problems expected.

Prolonged use:
Avoid. May damage bone marrow and nerve cells.

Skin & sunlight:
May cause rash or intensify sunburn in areas exposed to sun or sunlamp.

Driving, piloting or hazardous work:
Don't drive or pilot aircraft until you learn how medicine affects you. Don't work around dangerous machinery. Don't climb ladders or work in high places. Danger increases if you drink alcohol or take medicine affecting alertness and reflexes, such as antihistamines, tranquilizers, sedatives, pain medicine, narcotics and mind-altering drugs.

Discontinuing:
No problems expected.

Others:
May mask symptoms of hearing damage from aspirin, other salicylates, cisplatin, paromomycin, vancomycin or anticonvulsants. Consult doctor if you use these.

POSSIBLE INTERACTION WITH OTHER DRUGS

GENERIC NAME OR DRUG CLASS	COMBINED EFFECT
Anticholinergics*	Increased anticholinergic effect.
Anticoagulants, oral*	Decreased doxylamine effect.
Antidepressants*	Excess sedation. Avoid.
Antihistamines, other*	Excess sedation. Avoid.
Carteolol	Decreased antihistamine effect.
Dronabinol	Increased effects of both drugs. Avoid.
Hypnotics*	Excess sedation. Avoid.
MAO inhibitors*	Increased doxylamine effect.
Mind-altering drugs*	Excess sedation. Avoid.
Molindone	Increased sedative and antihistamine effect.
Nabilone	Greater depression of central nervous system.
Narcotics*	Excess sedation. Avoid.
Procarbazine	May increase sedation.
Sedatives*	Excess sedation. Avoid.
Sleep inducers*	Excess sedation. Avoid.
Sotalol	Increased antihistamine effect.
Tranquilizers*	Excess sedation. Avoid.

POSSIBLE INTERACTION WITH OTHER SUBSTANCES

INTERACTS WITH	COMBINED EFFECT
Alcohol:	Excess sedation. Avoid.
Beverages: Caffeine drinks.	Less doxylamine sedation.
Cocaine:	Decreased doxylamine effect. Avoid.
Foods:	None expected.
Marijuana:	Excess sedation. Avoid.
Tobacco:	None expected.

DRONABINOL

BRAND NAMES

Marinol

BASIC INFORMATION

Habit forming? Yes
Prescription needed? Yes
Available as generic? No
Drug class: Antiemetic

 ## USES

Prevents nausea and vomiting that may accompany taking anticancer medication (cancer chemotherapy). Should not be used unless other antinausea medicines fail.

 ## DOSAGE & USAGE INFORMATION

How to take:
Capsule—Swallow with liquid.

When to take:
Under supervision, a total of no more than 4 to 6 doses per day, every 2 to 4 hours after cancer chemotherapy for prescribed number of days.

If you forget a dose:
Take as soon as you remember up to 2 hours late. If more than 2 hours, wait for next scheduled dose (don't double this dose).

What drug does:
Affects nausea and vomiting center in brain to make it less irritable following cancer chemotherapy. Exact mechanism is unknown.

Time lapse before drug works:
2 to 4 hours.

Don't take with:
- Non-prescription drugs without consulting doctor.
- Drugs in interaction column without consulting doctor.

 ## OVERDOSE

SYMPTOMS:
Pounding, rapid heart rate; high or low blood pressure; confusion; hallucinations; drastic mood changes; nervousness or anxiety.
WHAT TO DO:
Overdose unlikely to threaten life. If person takes much larger amount than prescribed, call doctor, poison-control center or hospital emergency room for instructions.

 ## POSSIBLE ADVERSE REACTIONS OR SIDE EFFECTS

SYMPTOMS	WHAT TO DO
Life-threatening: None expected.	
Common:	
• Rapid, pounding heartbeat.	Discontinue. Call doctor right away.
• Dizziness, irritability, drowsiness, euphoria, decreased coordination.	Continue. Call doctor when convenient.
• Red eyes, dry mouth.	No action necessary.
Infrequent:	
• Depression, anxiety, nervousness, headache, hallucinations, dramatic mood changes.	Discontinue. Call doctor right away.
• Blurred or changed vision.	Continue. Call doctor when convenient.
Rare:	
• Rapid heartbeat, fainting, frequent or difficult urination, convulsions, shortness of breath.	Discontinue. Call doctor right away.
• Paranoia, nausea, loss of appetite, dizziness when standing after sitting or lying down, diarrhea.	Continue. Call doctor when convenient.

WARNINGS & PRECAUTIONS

Don't take if:
- Your nausea and vomiting is caused by anything other than cancer chemotherapy.
- You are sensitive or allergic to any form of marijuana or sesame oil.
- Your cycle of chemotherapy is longer than 7 consecutive days. Harmful side effects may occur.

Before you start, consult your doctor:
- If you have heart disease or high blood pressure.
- If you are an alcoholic or drug addict.
- If you are pregnant or intend to become pregnant.
- If you are nursing an infant.
- If you have schizophrenia or a manic-depressive disorder.

Over age 60:
Adverse reactions and side effects may be more frequent and severe than in younger persons.

Pregnancy:
No studies in humans. Avoid if possible.

Breast-feeding:
No studies in humans. Avoid if possible.

Infants & children:
Not recommended.

Prolonged use:
Avoid. Habit forming.

Skin & sunlight:
No problems expected.

Driving, piloting or hazardous work:
Don't drive or pilot aircraft until you learn how medicine affects you. Don't work around dangerous machinery. Don't climb ladders or work in high places. Danger increases if you drink alcohol or take medicine affecting alertness and reflexes, such as antihistamines, tranquilizers, sedatives, pain medicine, narcotics and mind-altering drugs.

Discontinuing:
Withdrawal effects such as irritability, insomnia, restlessness, sweating, diarrhea, hiccups, loss of appetite and hot flashes may follow abrupt withdrawal within 12 hours. Should they occur, these symptoms will probably subside within 96 hours.

Others:
Store in refrigerator.

POSSIBLE INTERACTION WITH OTHER DRUGS

GENERIC NAME OR DRUG CLASS	COMBINED EFFECT
Anesthetics*	Oversedation.
Anticonvulsants*	Oversedation.
Antidepressants, tricyclics (TCA)*	Oversedation.
Antihistamines*	Oversedation.
Barbiturates*	Oversedation.
Ethinamate	Dangerous increased effects of ethinamate. Avoid combining.
Fluoxetine	Increased depressant effects of both drugs.
Guanfacine	May increase depressant effects of either drug.
Leucovorin	High alcohol content of leucovorin may cause adverse effects.
Methyprylon	Increased sedative effect, perhaps to dangerous level. Avoid.
Molindone	Increased effects of both drugs. Avoid.
Muscle relaxants*	Oversedation.
Nabilone	Greater depression of central nervous system.
Narcotics*	Oversedation.
Sedatives*	Oversedation.
Tranquilizers*	Oversedation.

POSSIBLE INTERACTION WITH OTHER SUBSTANCES

INTERACTS WITH	COMBINED EFFECT
Alcohol:	Oversedation.
Beverages:	No problems expected.
Cocaine:	No problems expected.
Foods:	No problems expected.
Marijuana:	Oversedation.
Tobacco:	No problems expected.

*See Glossary

ENALAPRIL

BRAND NAMES

Vasotec

BASIC INFORMATION

Habit forming? No
Prescription needed? Yes
Available as generic? No
Drug class: Antihypertensive, ACE inhibitor*

USES

Treatment for high blood pressure and congestive heart failure.

DOSAGE & USAGE INFORMATION

How to take:
Tablet—Swallow with liquid. These are long-acting tablets. Food does not alter normal absorption from the gastrointestinal tract.

When to take:
Usually once a day, sometimes twice a day. Follow doctor's instructions.

If you forget a dose:
Take as soon as you remember up to 8 hours late. If more than 8 hours, wait for next scheduled dose (don't double this dose).

What drug does:
• Reduces resistance in arteries.
• Strengthens heartbeat.

Time lapse before drug works:
60 to 90 minutes.

Don't take with:
See Interaction column and consult doctor.

OVERDOSE

SYMPTOMS:
Fever, chills, sore throat, fainting, convulsions, coma.
WHAT TO DO:
• Dial 0 (operator) or 911 (emergency) for an ambulance or medical help. Then give first aid immediately.
• See emergency information on inside covers.

POSSIBLE ADVERSE REACTIONS OR SIDE EFFECTS

SYMPTOMS	WHAT TO DO
Life-threatening: None expected.	
Common: Rash, loss of taste.	Discontinue. Call doctor right away.
Infrequent: • Swelling of face, hands, mouth or feet.	Discontinue. Seek emergency treatment.
• Dizziness, fainting, chest pain, fast or irregular heartbeat.	Discontinue. Call doctor right away.
Rare: • Sore throat, cloudy urine, fever, chills.	Discontinue. Call doctor right away.
• Nausea, vomiting, indigestion, abdominal pain.	Continue. Call doctor when convenient.

WARNINGS & PRECAUTIONS

Don't take if:
• If you are allergic to enalapril or captopril.
• You have any autoimmune disease, including AIDS or lupus.
• You are receiving blood from a blood bank.
• You take drugs for cancer.
• You will have surgery within 2 months, including dental surgery, requiring general or spinal anesthesia.

Before you start, consult your doctor:
• If you have had a stroke.
• If you have angina, heart or blood-vessel disease, a high level of potassium in blood, kidney disease, lupus.
• If you are on a severe salt-restricted diet.

Over age 60:
Adverse reactions and side effects may be more frequent and severe than in younger persons.

Pregnancy:
Risk to unborn child outweighs drug benefits. Don't use.

Breast-feeding:
Drug passes into milk. Avoid drug or discontinue nursing until you finish medicine. Consult doctor for advice on maintaining milk supply.

Infants & children:
Not recommended.

Prolonged use:
May decrease white cells in blood or cause protein loss in urine. Request periodic laboratory blood counts and urine tests.

Skin & sunlight:
No problems expected.

Driving, piloting or hazardous work:
Avoid if you become dizzy or faint. Otherwise, no problems expected.

Discontinuing:
Don't discontinue without consulting doctor. Dose may require gradual reduction if you have taken drug for a long time. Doses of other drugs may also require adjustment.

Others:
- Stop taking diuretics or increase salt intake 1 week before starting enalapril.
- Avoid exercising in hot weather.

POSSIBLE INTERACTION WITH OTHER DRUGS

GENERIC NAME OR DRUG CLASS	COMBINED EFFECT
Amiloride	Possible excessive potassium in blood.
Antihypertensives, other*	Increased antihypertensive effect. Dosage of each may require adjustment.
Beta-adrenergic blockers*	Increased antihypertensive effect. Dosage of each may require adjustment.
Carteolol	Increased antihypertensive effects of both drugs. Dosages may require adjustments.
Chloramphenicol	Possible blood disorders.

Diuretics*	Possible severe blood-pressure drop with first dose.
Guanfacine	Increased effects of both drugs.
Lisinopril	Increased antihypertensive effect. Dosage of each may require adjustment.
Nicardipine	Possible excessive potassium in blood. Dosages may require adjustment.
Nitrates	Possible excessive blood-pressure drop.
Non-steroidal anti-inflammatory drugs (NSAIDs)*	Decreased enalapril effect.
Potassium supplements*	Possible increased potassium in blood.

Continued page 1084

POSSIBLE INTERACTION WITH OTHER SUBSTANCES

INTERACTS WITH	COMBINED EFFECT
Alcohol:	Possible excessive blood-pressure drop.
Beverages: Low-salt milk.	Possible excessive potassium in blood.
Cocaine:	Increased risk of heart block and high blood pressure.
Foods: Salt substitutes.	Possible excessive potassium.
Marijuana:	Increased dizziness.
Tobacco:	May decrease enalapril effect.

ENALAPRIL & HYDROCHLOROTHIAZIDE

BRAND NAMES

Vaseretic

BASIC INFORMATION

Habit forming? No
Prescription needed? Yes
Available as generic? No
Drug class: Antihypertensive, diuretic, ACE inhibitor*

USES

- Treatment for high blood pressure and congestive heart failure.
- Reduces fluid retention.

DOSAGE & USAGE INFORMATION

How to take:
Tablet—Swallow with liquid. These tablets are long-acting. Food does not alter normal absorption from the gastrointestinal tract.

When to take:
Usually once a day.

If you forget a dose:
Take as soon as you remember up to 18 hours late. If more than 18 hours, wait for next scheduled dose (don't double this dose).

What drug does:
- Forces sodium and water excretion, reducing body fluid.
- Relaxes muscle cells of small arteries.
- Reduced body fluid and relaxed arteries lower blood pressure.
- Reduces resistance in arteries.
- Strengthens heartbeat.

Time lapse before drug works:
4 to 6 hours. May require several weeks to lower blood pressure.

Continued next column

OVERDOSE

SYMPTOMS:
Cramps, weakness, drowsiness, weak pulse, fever, chills, sore throat, fainting, convulsions, coma.
WHAT TO DO:
- Dial 0 (operator) or 911 (emergency) for an ambulance or medical help. Then give first aid immediately.
- See emergency information on inside covers.

Don't take with:
- Non-prescription drugs without consulting doctor.
- See Interaction column and consult doctor.

POSSIBLE ADVERSE REACTIONS OR SIDE EFFECTS

SYMPTOMS	WHAT TO DO
Life-threatening:	
Irregular heartbeat (fast or uneven); difficulty breathing; hives, rash, intense itching, faintness soon after a dose (anaphylaxis).	Discontinue. Seek emergency treatment.
Common:	
• Dry mouth, thirst, tiredness, weakness, muscle cramps, vomiting, chest pain, skin rash, coughing.	Discontinue. Call doctor right away.
• Taste loss, dizziness.	Continue. Call doctor when convenient.
Infrequent:	
• Face, mouth, hands swelling.	Discontinue. Call doctor right away.
• Nausea, diarrhea.	Continue. Call doctor when convenient.
Rare:	
None expected.	

WARNINGS & PRECAUTIONS

Don't take if:
- You are allergic to enalapril, captopril, or any thiazide diuretic drug.
- You have any autoimmune disease, including AIDS or lupus.
- You are receiving blood from a blood bank.
- You take drugs for cancer.
- If you will have surgery within 2 months, including dental surgery, requiring general or spinal anesthesia.

Before you start, consult your doctor:
- If you have had a stroke.
- If you have angina, heart or blood-vessel disease, a high level of potassium in blood, lupus, gout, liver, pancreas or kidney disorder.
- If you are on a severe salt-restricted diet.
- If you are allergic to any sulfa drug.

Over age 60:
Adverse reactions and side effects may be more frequent and severe than in younger persons, especially dizziness and excessive potassium loss.

ENALAPRIL & HYDROCHLOROTHIAZIDE

Pregnancy:
Risk to unborn child outweighs drug benefits. Don't use.

Breast-feeding:
Drug passes into milk. Avoid drug or discontinue nursing until you finish medicine. Consult doctor for advice on maintaining milk supply.

Infants & children:
Not recommended.

Prolonged use:
May decrease white cells in blood or cause protein loss in urine. Request periodic laboratory blood counts and urine tests.

Skin & sunlight:
May cause rash or intensify sunburn in areas exposed to sun or sunlamp.

Driving, piloting or hazardous work:
Don't drive or pilot aircraft until you learn how medicine affects you. Don't work around dangerous machinery. Don't climb ladders or work in high places. Danger increases if you drink alcohol or take medicine affecting alertness and reflexes, such as antihistamines, tranquilizers, sedatives, pain medicine, narcotics and mind-altering drugs.

Discontinuing:
Don't discontinue without consulting doctor. Dose may require gradual reduction if you have taken drug for a long time. Doses of other drugs may also require adjustment.

Others:
- Hot weather and fever may cause dehydration and drop in blood pressure. Dose may require temporary adjustment. Weigh daily and report any unexpected weight decreases to your doctor.
- May cause rise in uric acid, leading to gout.
- May cause blood-sugar rise in diabetics.

POSSIBLE INTERACTION WITH OTHER DRUGS

GENERIC NAME OR DRUG CLASS	COMBINED EFFECT
Allopurinol	Decreased allopurinol effect.
Amiloride	Possible excessive potassium in blood.
Antidepressants, tricyclic (TCA)*	Dangerous drop in blood pressure. Avoid combination unless under medical supervision.
Antihypertensives, other*	Increased antihypertensive effect. Dosage of each may require adjustment.

Barbiturates*	Increased hydrochlorothiazide effect.
Beta-adrenergic blockers*	Increased antihypertensive effect. Dosages of both drugs may require adjustments.
Carteolol	Increased antihypertensive effect.
Chloramphenicol	Possible blood disorders.
Cholestyramine	Decreased hydrochlorothiazide effect.
Cortisone drugs*	Excessive potassium loss that causes dangerous heart rhythms.
Digitalis preparations*	Excessive potassium loss that causes dangerous heart rhythms.
Diuretics, thiazide*	Increased effect of other thiazide diuretics.
Indapamide	Increased diuretic effect.
Lisinopril	Increased antihypertensive effect. Dosage of each may require adjustment.
Lithium	Increased effect of lithium.

Continued page 1084

POSSIBLE INTERACTION WITH OTHER SUBSTANCES

INTERACTS WITH	COMBINED EFFECT
Alcohol:	Dangerous blood-pressure drop. Avoid.
Beverages: Low-salt milk.	Possible excessive potassium in blood.
Cocaine:	Increased risk of heart block and high blood pressure.
Foods: Salt substitutes.	Possible excessive potassium.
Marijuana:	Increased dizziness, may increase blood pressure.
Tobacco:	May decrease enalapril effect.

*See Glossary

ENCAINIDE

BRAND NAMES

Enkaid

BASIC INFORMATION

Habit forming? No
Prescription needed? Yes
Available as generic? No
Drug class: Antiarrhythmic

 USES

Stabilizes irregular heartbeat.

 DOSAGE & USAGE INFORMATION

How to take:
Capsules—Swallow with liquid or food to lessen stomach irritation. If you can't swallow whole, open capsule and take with liquid or food.

When to take:
At the same time each day, according to instructions on prescription label.

If you forget a dose:
Take as soon as you remember up to 2 hours late. If more than 2 hours, wait for next scheduled dose (don't double this dose).

What drug does:
- Increases refractory between muscle fiber contractions in the heart.
- Decreases excitability throughout the conducting system of the heart.

Time lapse before drug works:
1 to 3 hours. Peak effect in 30 to 90 minutes.

Don't take with:
See Interaction column and consult doctor.

 OVERDOSE

SYMPTOMS:
Very slow heartbeat, extreme weakness, seizures, loss of consciousness, cardiac arrest.
WHAT TO DO:
- Dial 0 (operator) or 911 (emergency) for an ambulance or medical help. Then give first aid immediately.
- See emergency information on inside covers.

 POSSIBLE ADVERSE REACTIONS OR SIDE EFFECTS

SYMPTOMS	WHAT TO DO
Life-threatening: Very fast or irregular heartbeat.	Seek emergency treatment immediately.
Common: None expected.	
Infrequent:	
• Chest pain, blurred or double vision, skin rash.	Discontinue. Call doctor right away.
• Dizziness, headache, tiredness or weakness, nausea.	Continue. Call doctor when convenient.
Rare:	
• Shortness of breath.	Discontinue. Call doctor right away.
• Swelling of lower legs and feet, trembling or shaking.	Continue. Call doctor when convenient.

WARNINGS & PRECAUTIONS

Don't take if:
- You have atrioventricular block and you do not have a pacemaker.
- You have right bundle branch block (by EKG).

Before you start, consult your doctor:
- If you have cardiomyopathy or congestive heart failure.
- If you have had a recent heart attack.
- If you have liver or kidney disease.
- If you have sick sinus syndrome. *
- If you have an alteration in potassium levels.

Over age 60:
No special problems expected.

Pregnancy:
No proven harm to unborn child, but avoid if possible.

Breast-feeding:
Drug passes into milk. Avoid drug or discontinue nursing until you finish medicine. Consult doctor for advice on maintaining milk supply.

Infants & children:
Effect not documented. Consult your pediatrician.

Prolonged use:
No problems expected.

Skin & sunlight:
No problems expected.

Driving, piloting or hazardous work:
Don't drive or pilot aircraft until you learn how medicine affects you. Don't work around dangerous machinery. Don't climb ladders or work in high places. Danger increases if you drink alcohol or take medicine affecting alertness and reflexes.

Discontinuing:
Don't discontinue without consulting doctor. Dose may require gradual reduction if you have taken drug for a long time. Doses of other drugs may also require adjustment.

Others:
Adverse effects may be dose related.

POSSIBLE INTERACTION WITH OTHER DRUGS

GENERIC NAME OR DRUG CLASS	COMBINED EFFECT
Antiarrhythmics*	Increased effect or toxicity on heart muscle.
Carteolol	Increased effect of toxicity on heart muscle.
Cimetidine	Increased effect of cimetidine.
Guanfacine	Increased effect of both drugs.
Nicardipine	Increased effect of toxicity on heart muscle.
Nizatidine	Increased effect of nizatidine.
Sotalol	Increased effect of toxicity on heart muscle.

POSSIBLE INTERACTION WITH OTHER SUBSTANCES

INTERACTS WITH	COMBINED EFFECT
Alcohol:	Heartbeat irregularities may increase.
Beverages:	None expected.
Cocaine:	Heartbeat irregularities may increase.
Foods:	No special problems expected.
Marijuana:	Heartbeat irregularities may increase.
Tobacco:	Heartbeat irregularities may increase.

*See Glossary

EPHEDRINE

BRAND NAMES

See complete list of brand names in the *Brand Name Directory*, page 1062.

BASIC INFORMATION

Habit forming? No
Prescription needed?
  Low strength: No
  High strength: Yes
Available as generic? Yes
Drug class: Sympathomimetic

USES

- Relieves bronchial asthma.
- Decreases congestion of breathing passages.
- Suppresses allergic reactions.

DOSAGE & USAGE INFORMATION

How to take:
- Tablet or capsule—Swallow with liquid. You may chew or crush tablet.
- Extended-release tablets or capsules— Swallow each dose whole.
- Syrup—Take as directed on bottle.
- Drops—Dilute dose in beverage.

When to take:
As needed, no more often than every 4 hours.

If you forget a dose:
Take up to 2 hours late. If more than 2 hours, wait for next dose (don't double this dose).

What drug does:
- Prevents cells from releasing allergy-causing chemicals (histamines).
- Relaxes muscles of bronchial tubes.
- Decreases blood-vessel size and blood flow, thus causing decongestion.

Time lapse before drug works:
30 to 60 minutes.

Continued next column

OVERDOSE

SYMPTOMS:
Severe anxiety, confusion, delirium, muscle tremors, rapid and irregular pulse.
WHAT TO DO:
- Dial 0 (operator) or 911 (emergency) for an ambulance or medical help. Then give first aid immediately.
- See emergency information on inside covers.

Don't take with:
- Non-prescription drugs with ephedrine, pseudoephedrine or epinephrine.
- Non-prescription drugs for cough, cold, allergy or asthma without consulting doctor.
- See Interaction column and consult doctor.

POSSIBLE ADVERSE REACTIONS OR SIDE EFFECTS

SYMPTOMS	WHAT TO DO
Life-threatening: None expected.	
Common:	
Nervousness, headache, paleness, rapid heartbeat.	Continue. Call doctor when convenient.
Insomnia.	Continue. Tell doctor at next visit.
Infrequent:	
Irregular heartbeat.	Discontinue. Call doctor right away.
Dizziness, appetite loss, nausea, vomiting, painful or difficult urination.	Continue. Call doctor when convenient.
Rare: None expected.	

WARNINGS & PRECAUTIONS

Don't take if:
You are allergic to ephedrine or any sympathomimetic drug.

Before you start, consult your doctor:
- If you have high blood pressure.
- If you have diabetes.
- If you have overactive thyroid gland.
- If you have difficulty urinating.
- If you have taken any MAO inhibitor in past 2 weeks.
- If you have taken digitalis preparations in the last 7 days.
- If you will have surgery within 2 months, including dental surgery, requiring general or spinal anesthesia.

Over age 60:
More likely to develop high blood pressure, heart-rhythm disturbances, angina and to feel drug's stimulant effects.

Pregnancy:
No proven harm to unborn child. Avoid if possible.

Breast-feeding:
Drug passes into milk. Avoid drug or discontinue nursing until you finish medicine. Consult doctor for advice on maintaining milk supply.

Infants & children:
No problems expected.

Prolonged use:
- Excessive doses—Rare toxic psychosis.
- Men with enlarged prostate gland may have more urination difficulty.

Skin & sunlight:
No problems expected.

Driving, piloting or hazardous work:
Avoid if you feel dizzy. Otherwise, no problems expected.

Discontinuing:
May be unnecessary to finish medicine. Follow doctor's instructions.

Others:
No problems expected.

POSSIBLE INTERACTION WITH OTHER DRUGS

GENERIC NAME OR DRUG CLASS	COMBINED EFFECT
Antidepressants, tricyclic (TCA)*	Increased effect of ephedrine. Excessive stimulation of heart and blood pressure.
Antihypertensives*	Decreased antihypertensive effect.
Beta-adrenergic blockers*	Decreased effects of both drugs.
Digitalis preparations*	Serious heart-rhythm disturbances.
Epinephrine	Increased epinephrine effect.
Ergot preparations*	Serious blood-pressure rise.
Guanadrel	Decreased effect of both drugs.
Guanethidine	Decreased effect of both drugs.
MAO inhibitors*	Increased ephedrine effect. Dangerous blood-pressure rise.
Methyldopa	Possible increased blood pressure.
Nitrates*	Possible decreased effects of both drugs.
Phenothiazines*	Possible increased ephedrine toxicity. Possible decreased ephedrine effect.
Pseudoephedrine	Increased pseudo-ephedrine effect.
Rauwolfia	Decreased rauwolfia effect.
Sympathomimetics*	Increased ephedrine effect.
Terazosin	Decreases effectiveness of terazosin.
Theophylline	Increased gastro-intestinal intolerance.

POSSIBLE INTERACTION WITH OTHER SUBSTANCES

INTERACTS WITH	COMBINED EFFECT
Alcohol:	None expected.
Beverages: Caffeine drinks.	Nervousness or insomnia.
Cocaine:	High risk of heartbeat irregularities and high blood pressure.
Foods:	None expected.
Marijuana:	Rapid heartbeat, possible heart-rhythm disturbance.
Tobacco:	None expected.

*See Glossary

EPINEPHRINE

BRAND NAMES

See complete list of brand names in the
Brand Name Directory, page 1062.

BASIC INFORMATION

Habit forming? No
Prescription needed? Yes
Available as generic?
  Nose drops, aerosol inhaler—Yes
  Eye drops, injection—Yes
Drug class: Sympathomimetic, antiglaucoma

USES

- Relieves allergic symptoms of anaphylaxis.
- Eases symptoms of acute bronchial spasms.
- Relieves congestion of nose, sinuses and throat.
- Reduces internal eye pressure.

DOSAGE & USAGE INFORMATION

How to take:
Eyedrops, nose drops, aerosol inhaler, injection—Use as directed on labels.

When to take:
As needed, no more often than label directs.

If you forget a dose:
If needed, take when you remember. Wait 3 hours for next dose.

What drug does:
- Contracts blood-vessel walls and raises blood pressure.
- Inhibits release of histamine.
- Dilates constricted bronchial tubes and decreases volume of blood in nasal tissue.
- Reduces fluid formation within the eye.

Time lapse before drug works:
1 to 2 minutes.

Continued next column

OVERDOSE

SYMPTOMS:
Tremor, rapid breathing, palpitations, extreme rise in blood pressure, irregular heartbeat, breathing difficulty, convulsions, coma.
WHAT TO DO:
- Dial 0 (operator) or 911 (emergency) for an ambulance or medical help. Then give first aid immediately.
- See emergency information on inside covers.

Don't take with:
- Non-prescription drugs without consulting doctor.
- See Interaction column and consult doctor.

POSSIBLE ADVERSE REACTIONS OR SIDE EFFECTS

SYMPTOMS	WHAT TO DO
Life-threatening: None expected.	
Common:	
• Headache, agitation, dizziness, insomnia, fast or pounding heartbeat.	Continue. Call doctor when convenient.
• Dry mouth and throat (inhaler only).	Continue. Tell doctor at next visit.
Infrequent:	
• Difficult breathing.	Discontinue. Call doctor right away.
• Shakiness, nausea, vomiting, cough or bronchial irritation (inhaler only), weakness, flushed face or redness.	Continue. Call doctor when convenient.
Rare:	
Chest pain, irregular heartbeat, sweating.	Discontinue. Call doctor right away.

WARNINGS & PRECAUTIONS

Don't take if:
- You are allergic to any sympathomimetic.
- You have narrow-angle glaucoma.
- You have had a stroke or heart attack within 3 weeks.
- You have heart-rhythm disturbance.

Before you start, consult your doctor:
- If you have high blood pressure, heart disease or have had a stroke.
- If you have diabetes.
- If you have overactive thyroid.

Over age 60:
- Use with caution if you have hardening of the arteries.
- If you have enlarged prostate, drug may increase urination difficulty.
- If you have Parkinson's disease, drug may temporarily increase rigidity and tremor.
- If you see "floaters" in field of vision, tell your doctor.

Pregnancy:
No proven harm to unborn child. Avoid if possible.

Breast-feeding:
Drug passes into milk. Avoid drug or discontinue nursing until you finish medicine. Consult doctor for advice on maintaining milk supply.

Infants & children:
Use only under medical supervision.

Prolonged use:
- You may stop responding to drug.
- Drug may reduce blood volume.
- Drug may damage eye retina and impair vision.

Skin & sunlight:
No problems expected.

Driving, piloting or hazardous work:
No problems expected. Use caution if you feel dizzy or nervous.

Discontinuing:
- May be unnecessary to finish medicine. Follow doctor's instructions.
- If drug fails to provide relief after several doses, discontinue. Don't increase dose or frequency.

Others:
- May temporarily raise blood sugar in diabetics.
- Excessive use can cause sudden death.
- Discard medicine if cloudy or discolored.

POSSIBLE INTERACTION WITH OTHER DRUGS

GENERIC NAME OR DRUG CLASS	COMBINED EFFECT
Albuterol	Increased effect of both drugs, especially harmful side effects.
Antidepressants, tricyclic (TCA)*	Increased epinephrine effect.
Antidiabetics, oral*	Decreased antidiabetic effect.
Antihistamines*	Increased epinephrine effect.
Beta-adrenergic blockers*	Decreased epinephrine effect.
Carbonic anhydrase inhibitors*	Increased epinephrine effect.
Digitalis preparations*	Possible irregular heartbeat.
Ephedrine	Increased ephedrine effect.
Guanadrel	Decreased guanadrel effect.
Guanethidine	Decreased guanethidine effect.
Insulin	Decreased insulin effect.
Isoproterenol	Dangerous to heart.
Loxapine	Rapid heart rate and severe drop in blood pressure.
MAO inhibitors*	Dangerous to heart.
Metaproterenol	Increased effect of both drugs, especially harmful side effects.
Methyldopa	Possible increased blood pressure.
Minoxidil	Decreased minoxidil effect.
Nitrates*	Possible decreased effects of both drugs.
Oxprenolol	Decreased effects of both drugs.
Phenothiazines*	Possible increased epinephrine toxicity. Possible decreased epinephrine effect.
Pilocarpine	Increased pilocarpine effect.
Rauwolfia alkaloids*	Increased epinephrine effect. Decreased rauwolfia effect.
Sympathomimetics*	Increased epinephrine effect.
Terazosin	Decreases effectiveness of terazosin.
Thyroid preparations*	Increased epinephrine effect.

POSSIBLE INTERACTION WITH OTHER SUBSTANCES

INTERACTS WITH	COMBINED EFFECT
Alcohol:	May increase urinary excretion of drug and reduce effectiveness.
Beverages:	None expected.
Cocaine:	High risk of heartbeat irregularities and high blood pressure.
Foods:	None expected.
Marijuana:	Increase in epinephrine's antiasthmatic effect.
Tobacco:	None expected.

*See Glossary

ERGOLOID MESYLATES

BRAND NAMES

Circanol
Deapril-ST
Dihydrogenated
  Ergot Alkaloids

Hydergine
Hydergine LC
Trigot

BASIC INFORMATION

Habit forming? No
Prescription needed? Yes
Available as generic? Yes
Drug class: Ergot preparation

USES

Treatment for reduced alertness, poor memory, confusion, depression or lack of motivation in the elderly.

DOSAGE & USAGE INFORMATION

How to take:
- Tablet—Swallow with liquid. If you can't swallow whole, crumble tablet and take with liquid or food.
- Liquid—Take as directed on label.
- Sublingual tablets—Dissolve tablet under tongue.

When to take:
At the same times each day.

If you forget a dose:
Take as soon as you remember up to 2 hours late. If more than 2 hours, wait for next scheduled dose (don't double this dose).

What drug does:
Stimulates brain-cell metabolism to increase use of oxygen and nutrients.

Time lapse before drug works:
Gradual improvements over 3 to 4 months.

Continued next column

OVERDOSE

SYMPTOMS:
Headache, flushed face, nasal congestion, nausea, vomiting, blood-pressure drop, weakness, collapse, coma.
WHAT TO DO:
- Dial 0 (operator) or 911 (emergency) for an ambulance or medical help. Then give first aid immediately.
- See emergency information on inside covers.

Don't take with:
- Non-prescription drugs containing alcohol without consulting doctor.
- See Interaction column and consult doctor.

POSSIBLE ADVERSE REACTIONS OR SIDE EFFECTS

SYMPTOMS	WHAT TO DO
Life-threatening: None expected.	
Common: Runny nose.	Continue. Tell doctor at next visit.
Infrequent:	
• Slow heartbeat, tingling fingers.	Discontinue. Call doctor right away.
• Nervousness, hostility, confusion, depression, blurred vision.	Continue. Call doctor when convenient.
Rare:	
• Fainting.	Discontinue. Seek emergency treatment.
• Rash, nausea, vomiting, stomach cramps.	Discontinue. Call doctor right away.
• Dizziness when getting up, fever, drowsiness, soreness under tongue, appetite loss.	Continue. Call doctor when convenient.

WARNINGS & PRECAUTIONS

Don't use if:
- If you are allergic to any ergot preparation.
- Your heartbeat is less than 60 beats per minute.
- Your systolic blood pressure is consistently below 100.

Before you start, consult your doctor:
If you have had low blood pressure.

Over age 60:
Primarily used in persons older than 60. Results unpredictable, but many patients show improved brain function.

Pregnancy:
Not recommended.

Breast-feeding:
Risk to nursing child outweighs drug benefits. Don't use.

Infants & children:
Not recommended.

Prolonged use:
No problems expected.

Skin & sunlight:
No problems expected.

Driving, piloting or hazardous work:
Avoid if you feel dizzy, faint or have blurred vision. Otherwise, no problems expected.

Discontinuing:
No problems expected.

Others:
No problems expected.

POSSIBLE INTERACTION WITH OTHER DRUGS

GENERIC NAME OR DRUG CLASS	COMBINED EFFECT
Antihypertensives*	Increased antihypertensive effect.
Beta-adrenergic blockers*	Excessive decrease in heartbeat and/or blood pressure.
Digitalis preparations*	Excessively slow heartbeat.

POSSIBLE INTERACTION WITH OTHER SUBSTANCES

INTERACTS WITH	COMBINED EFFECT
Alcohol:	Use caution. May drop blood pressure excessively.
Beverages:	None expected.
Cocaine:	Overstimulation. Avoid.
Foods:	None expected.
Marijuana:	Decreased effect of ergot alkaloids.
Tobacco:	None expected.

ERGONOVINE

BRAND NAMES

Ergometrine   Ergotrate

BASIC INFORMATION

Habit forming? No
Prescription needed? Yes
Available as generic? Yes
Drug class: Ergot preparation (uterine stimulant)

USES

Retards excessive post-delivery bleeding.

DOSAGE & USAGE INFORMATION

How to take:
Tablet—Swallow with liquid or food to lessen stomach irritation.

When to take:
At the same times each day.

If you forget a dose:
Don't take missed dose and don't double next one. Wait for next scheduled dose.

What drug does:
Causes smooth-muscle cells of uterine wall to contract and surround bleeding blood vessels of relaxed uterus.

Time lapse before drug works:
Tablets—20 to 30 minutes.

Don't take with:
See Interaction column and consult doctor.

OVERDOSE

SYMPTOMS:
Vomiting, diarrhea, weak pulse, low blood pressure, difficult breathing, angina, convulsions.
WHAT TO DO:
- Dial 0 (operator) or 911 (emergency) for an ambulance or medical help. Then give first aid immediately.
- If patient is unconscious and not breathing, give mouth-to-mouth breathing. If there is no heartbeat, use cardiac massage and mouth-to-mouth breathing (CPR). Don't try to make patient vomit. If you can't get help quickly, take patient to nearest emergency facility.
- See emergency information on inside covers.

POSSIBLE ADVERSE REACTIONS OR SIDE EFFECTS

SYMPTOMS	WHAT TO DO
Life-threatening: None expected.	
Common: Nausea, vomiting.	Discontinue. Call doctor right away.
Infrequent: • Confusion, ringing in ears, diarrhea, muscle cramps.	Discontinue. Call doctor right away.
• Unusual sweating.	Continue. Call doctor when convenient.
Rare: Sudden, severe headache; shortness of breath; chest pain; numb, cold hands and feet.	Discontinue. Seek emergency treatment.

WARNINGS & PRECAUTIONS

Don't take if:
You are allergic to any ergot preparation.

Before you start, consult your doctor:
- If you have coronary-artery or blood-vessel disease.
- If you have liver or kidney disease.
- If you have high blood pressure.
- If you have postpartum infection.

Over age 60:
Not recommended.

Pregnancy:
Risk to unborn child outweighs drug benefits. Don't use.

Breast-feeding:
Drug passes into milk. Avoid drug or discontinue nursing until you finish medicine. Consult doctor for advice on maintaining milk supply.

Infants & children:
Not recommended.

Prolonged use:
Not recommended.

Skin & sunlight:
No problems expected.

Driving, piloting or hazardous work:
No problems expected.

Discontinuing:
May be unnecessary to finish medicine. Follow doctor's instructions.

Others:
Drug should be used for short time only following childbirth or miscarriage.

POSSIBLE INTERACTION WITH OTHER DRUGS

GENERIC NAME OR DRUG CLASS	COMBINED EFFECT
Beta-adrenergic blockers*	Possible vasospasm (peripheral and cardiac).
Ergot preparations, other*	Increased ergonovine effect.

POSSIBLE INTERACTION WITH OTHER SUBSTANCES

INTERACTS WITH	COMBINED EFFECT
Alcohol:	None expected.
Beverages:	None expected.
Cocaine:	None expected.
Foods:	None expected.
Marijuana:	None expected.
Tobacco:	None expected.

*See Glossary

ERGOTAMINE

BRAND NAMES

Cafetrate-PB
Ergomar
Ergostat
Gynergen
Medihaler-
  Ergotamine

Migraine
Migral
Migrastat
Wigraine
Wigraine-PB
Wigrettes

BASIC INFORMATION

Habit forming? No
Prescription needed? Yes
Available as generic? No
Drug class: Vasoconstrictor, ergot
  preparation

 ## USES

Relieves pain of migraines and other headaches
caused by dilated blood vessels. Will not prevent
headaches.

 ## DOSAGE & USAGE INFORMATION

How to take:
- Tablet or sublingual tablet—Swallow with
  liquid, or let dissolve under tongue. If you
  can't swallow whole, crumble tablet and take
  with liquid or food.
- Suppositories—Remove wrapper and moisten
  suppository with water. Gently insert larger
  end into rectum. Push well into rectum with
  finger.
- Aerosol inhaler—Use only as directed on
  prescription label.
- Lie down in quiet, dark room after taking.

When to take:
At first sign of vascular or migraine headache.

Continued next column

 ## OVERDOSE

SYMPTOMS:
Tingling, cold extremities and muscle pain.
Progresses to nausea, vomiting, diarrhea,
cold skin, rapid and weak pulse, severe
numbness of extremities, confusion,
convulsions, coma.
WHAT TO DO:
- Dial 0 (operator) or 911 (emergency) for
  an ambulance or medical help. Then give
  first aid immediately.
- See emergency information on inside
  covers.

If you forget a dose:
Take as soon as you remember. Wait 4 hours for
next dose.

What drug does:
Constricts blood vessels in the head.

Time lapse before drug works:
30 to 60 minutes.

Don't take with:
See Interaction column and consult doctor.

 ## POSSIBLE ADVERSE REACTIONS OR SIDE EFFECTS

SYMPTOMS	WHAT TO DO
Life-threatening: None expected.	
Common: Dizziness, nausea, diarrhea, vomiting.	Continue. Call doctor when convenient.
Infrequent: Itchy or swollen skin; cold, pale hands or feet; pain or weakness in arms, legs, back.	Discontinue. Call doctor right away.
Rare: Anxiety or confusion; red or purple blisters, especially on hands, feet; change in vision; extreme thirst; stomach pain or bloating; unusually fast or slow heartbeat; possible chest pain; numbness or tingling in face, fingers, toes.	Discontinue. Call doctor right away.

WARNINGS & PRECAUTIONS

Don't take if:
You are allergic to any ergot preparation.

Before you start, consult your doctor:
- If you plan to become pregnant within medication period.
- If you have an infection.
- If you have angina, heart problems, high blood pressure, hardening of the arteries or vein problems.
- If you have kidney or liver disease.
- If you are allergic to other spray inhalants.

Over age 60:
Adverse reactions and side effects may be more frequent and severe than in younger persons.

Pregnancy:
Risk to unborn child outweighs drug benefits. Don't use.

Breast-feeding:
Drug filters into milk. May harm child. Avoid.

Infants & children:
Studies inconclusive on harm to children. Consult your doctor.

Prolonged use:
Cold skin, muscle pain, gangrene of hands and feet. This medicine not intended for uninterrupted use.

Skin & sunlight:
No problems expected.

Driving, piloting or hazardous work:
Don't drive or pilot aircraft until you learn how medicine affects you. Don't work around dangerous machinery. Don't climb ladders or work in high places. Danger increases if you drink alcohol or take medicine affecting alertness and reflexes, such as antihistamines, tranquilizers, sedatives, pain medicine, narcotics and mind-altering drugs.

Discontinuing:
May be unnecessary to finish medicine. Follow doctor's instructions.

Others:
Impaired blood circulation can lead to gangrene in intestines or extremities. Never exceed recommended dose.

POSSIBLE INTERACTION WITH OTHER DRUGS

GENERIC NAME OR DRUG CLASS	COMBINED EFFECT
Amphetamines*	Dangerous blood-pressure rise.
Beta-adrenergic blockers*	Narrowed arteries in heart if ergotamine is taken in high doses.
Ephedrine	Dangerous blood-pressure rise.
Epinephrine	Dangerous blood-pressure rise.
Pseudoephedrine	Dangerous blood-pressure rise.
Troleandomycin	Increased adverse reactions of ergotamine.

POSSIBLE INTERACTION WITH OTHER SUBSTANCES

INTERACTS WITH	COMBINED EFFECT
Alcohol:	Dilates blood vessels. Makes headache worse.
Beverages: Caffeine drinks.	May help relieve headache.
Cocaine:	Decreased ergotamine effect.
Foods: Any to which you are allergic.	May make headache worse. Avoid.
Marijuana:	Occasional use—Cool extremities. Regular use—Persistent chill.
Tobacco:	Decreased effect of ergotamine. Makes headache worse.

ERGOTAMINE, BELLADONNA & PHENOBARBITAL

BRAND NAMES

Bellergal
Bellergal-S

Bellergal Spacetabs

BASIC INFORMATION

Habit forming? Yes
Prescription needed? Yes
Available as generic? No
Drug class: Analgesic, antispasmodic, vasoconstrictor

USES

Reduces anxiety or nervous tension (low dose).

DOSAGE & USAGE INFORMATION

How to take:
- Tablet or extended-release tablet—Swallow with liquid, or let dissolve under tongue. If you can't swallow whole, crumble tablet or open capsule and take with liquid or food.
- Lie down in quiet, dark room after taking.

When to take:
At first sign of vascular or migraine headache.

If you forget a dose:
Take as soon as you remember. Wait 4 hours for next dose.

What drug does:
- Constricts blood vessels in the head.
- Blocks nerve impulses at parasympathetic nerve endings, preventing muscle contractions and gland secretions of organs involved.

Continued next column

OVERDOSE

SYMPTOMS:
Tingling, cold extremities; muscle pain; nausea; vomiting; diarrhea; cold skin; rapid and weak pulse; severe numbness of extremities; confusion; dilated pupils; rapid pulse and breathing; dizziness; fever; hallucinations; slurred speech; agitation; flushed face; convulsions; coma.
WHAT TO DO:
- **Dial 0 (operator) or 911 (emergency) for an ambulance or medical help. Then give first aid immediately.**
- **See emergency information on inside covers.**

Time lapse before drug works:
15 to 30 minutes.

Don't take with:
Non-prescription drugs without consulting doctor.

POSSIBLE ADVERSE REACTIONS OR SIDE EFFECTS

SYMPTOMS	WHAT TO DO
Life-threatening: Fast heartbeat, chest pain.	Discontinue. Seek emergency treatment.
Common: • Flushed skin, fever, drowsiness, bloating, depression, frequent urination.	Discontinue. Call doctor right away.
• Constipation, dizziness, drowsiness, "hangover" effect.	Continue. Call doctor when convenient.
Infrequent: Swollen feet and ankles, numbness or tingling in hands or feet, cold hands and feet, rash.	Discontinue. Call doctor right away.
Rare: Jaundice, weak legs, swallowing difficulty, dry mouth, increased sensitivity to sunlight, nausea, vomiting, decreased sweating.	Discontinue. Call doctor right away.

WARNINGS & PRECAUTIONS

Don't take if:
- You are allergic to any barbiturate, tartrazine dye, anticholinergic or ergot preparation.
- You have porphyria, trouble with stomach bloating, difficulty emptying your bladder completely, narrow-angle glaucoma, severe ulcerative colitis.

Before you start, consult your doctor:
- If you have epilepsy, kidney or liver damage, anemia, chronic pain, open-angle glaucoma, angina, fast heartbeat, heart problems, high blood pressure, hardening of the arteries, vein problems, chronic bronchitis, asthma, hiatal hernia, enlarged prostate, myasthenia gravis, peptic ulcer, an infection.

ERGOTAMINE, BELLADONNA & PHENOBARBITAL

- If you plan to become pregnant within medication period.
- If you will have surgery within 2 months, including dental surgery, requiring general or spinal anesthesia.

Over age 60:
Adverse reactions and side effects may be more frequent and severe than in younger persons.

Pregnancy:
Risk to unborn child outweighs drug benefits. Don't use.

Breast-feeding:
Drug passes into milk. Avoid drug or discontinue nursing until you finish medicine. Consult doctor for advice on maintaining milk supply.

Infants & children:
Not recommended.

Prolonged use:
- May cause addiction, anemia, chronic intoxication.
- May lower body temperature, making exposure to cold temperatures hazardous.
- Chronic constipation, possible fecal impaction.
- Cold skin, muscle pain, gangrene of hands and feet. This medicine not intended for uninterrupted use.

Skin & sunlight:
May cause rash or intensify sunburn in areas exposed to sun or sunlamp.

Driving, piloting or hazardous work:
Don't drive or pilot aircraft until you learn how medicine affects you. Don't work around dangerous machinery. Don't climb ladders or work in high places. Danger increases if you drink alcohol or take medicine affecting alertness and reflexes, such as antihistamines, tranquilizers, sedatives, pain medicine, narcotics and mind-altering drugs.

Discontinuing:
May be unnecessary to finish medicine. Follow doctor's instructions. If you develop withdrawal symptoms of hallucinations, agitation or sleeplessness after discontinuing, call doctor right away.

Others:
Impaired blood circulation can lead to gangrene in intestines or extremities. Never exceed recommended dose.

POSSIBLE INTERACTION WITH OTHER DRUGS

GENERIC NAME OR DRUG CLASS	COMBINED EFFECT
Amantadine	Increased belladonna effect.
Amphetamines*	Dangerous blood-pressure rise.
Anticholinergics, other*	Increased belladonna effect.
Anticoagulants, oral*	Decreased anti-coagulant effect.
Anticonvulsants*	Changed seizure patterns.
Antidepressants, tricyclics (TCA)*	Decreased anti-depressant effect. Possible dangerous oversedation.
Antidiabetics, oral*	Increased pheno-barbital effect.
Antihistamines*	Dangerous sedation. Avoid.
Aspirin	Decreased aspirin effect.
Beta-adrenergic blockers*	Narrowed arteries in heart if taken in large doses.
Contraceptives, oral*	Decreased contra-ceptive effect.
Cortisone drugs*	Decreased cortisone effect. Increased internal-eye pressure.

Continued page 1085

POSSIBLE INTERACTION WITH OTHER SUBSTANCES

INTERACTS WITH	COMBINED EFFECT
Alcohol:	Possible fatal oversedation. Avoid.
Beverages:	None expected.
Cocaine:	Excessively rapid heartbeat. Avoid.
Foods:	None expected.
Marijuana:	Drowsiness and dry mouth, excessive sedation. Avoid.
Tobacco:	None expected.

*See Glossary

ERGOTAMINE & CAFFEINE

BRAND NAMES

Cafatine	Ercaf
Cafergot	Ercatabs
Cafertabs	Ergo-Caff
Cafetrate	Wigraine

BASIC INFORMATION

Habit forming? No
Prescription needed? Yes
Available as generic? No
Drug class: Analgesic, stimulant (xanthine) vasoconstrictor

USES

Relieves pain of migraines and other headaches caused by dilated blood vessels. Will not prevent headaches.

DOSAGE & USAGE INFORMATION

How to take:
- Tablet—Swallow with liquid, or let dissolve under tongue. If you can't swallow whole, crumble tablet and take with liquid or food.
- Suppositories—Remove wrapper and moisten suppository with water. Gently insert larger end into rectum. Push well into rectum with finger.
- Lie down in quiet, dark room after taking.

When to take:
At first sign of vascular or migraine headache.

If you forget a dose:
Take as soon as you remember up to 2 hours late. If more than 2 hours, wait for next scheduled dose (don't double this dose).

What drug does:
- Constricts blood vessels in the head.
- Constricts blood-vessel walls.
- Stimulates central nervous system.

Continued next column

OVERDOSE

SYMPTOMS:
Tingling, cold extremities; muscle pain; nausea; vomiting; diarrhea; cold skin; severe numbness of extremities; confusion; excitement; rapid heartbeat; insomnia, hallucinations; convulsions; coma.
WHAT TO DO:
- Dial 0 (operator) or 911 (emergency) for an ambulance or medical help. Then give first aid immediately.
- See emergency information on inside covers.

Time lapse before drug works:
30 to 60 minutes.

Don't take with:
- Non-prescription drugs containing alcohol without consulting doctor.
- See Interaction column and consult doctor.

POSSIBLE ADVERSE REACTIONS OR SIDE EFFECTS

SYMPTOMS	WHAT TO DO
Life-threatening: Slow or fast heartbeat.	Discontinue. Seek emergency treatment.
Common: • Fast heartbeat.	Discontinue. Call doctor right away.
• Dizziness, nausea, diarrhea, vomiting, nervousness.	Continue. Call doctor when convenient.
Infrequent: Itchy skin; abdominal pain; cold hands and feet; weakness in arms, legs, back; confusion; irritability; indigestion; low blood sugar with weakness and trembling.	Discontinue. Call doctor right away.
Rare: Anxiety; red or purple blisters, especially on on hands and feet; change in vision; extreme thirst; numbness or tingling in hands or feet.	Discontinue. Call doctor right away.

WARNINGS & PRECAUTIONS

Don't take if:
- You are allergic to any stimulant or any ergot preparation.
- You have heart disease.
- You have active peptic ulcer of stomach or duodenum.

Before you start, consult your doctor:
- If you have irregular heartbeat, angina, heart problems, high blood pressure, hardening of the arteries or vein problems.
- If you have hypoglycemia (low blood sugar), epilepsy, an infection, kidney or liver disease.
- If you are allergic to spray inhalants.
- If you plan to become pregnant within medication period.

Over age 60:
Adverse reactions and side effects may be more frequent and severe than in younger persons, especially dizziness and excessive potassium loss.

Pregnancy:
Risk to unborn child outweighs drug benefits. Don't use.

Breast-feeding:
Drug passes into milk. Avoid drug or discontinue nursing until you finish medicine. Consult doctor for advice on maintaining milk supply.

Infants & children:
Not recommended.

Prolonged use:
Cold skin, muscle pain, stomach ulcers, gangrene of hands and feet. This medicine not intended for uninterrupted use.

Skin & sunlight:
No problems expected.

Driving, piloting or hazardous work:
Don't drive or pilot aircraft until you learn how medicine affects you. Don't work around dangerous machinery. Don't climb ladders or work in high places. Danger increases if you drink alcohol or take medicine affecting alertness and reflexes, such as antihistamines, tranquilizers, sedatives, pain medicine, narcotics and mind-altering drugs.

Discontinuing:
Will cause withdrawal symptoms of headache, irritability, drowsiness. Discontinue gradually if you use caffeine for a month or more.

Others:
- May produce or aggravate fibrocystic breast disease in women.
- Impaired blood circulation can lead to gangrene in intestines or extremities. Never exceed recommended dose.

POSSIBLE INTERACTION WITH OTHER DRUGS

GENERIC NAME OR DRUG CLASS	COMBINED EFFECT
Amphetamines*	Dangerous blood-pressure rise.
Beta-adrenergic blockers*	Narrowed arteries in heart if taken in large doses.
Cimetidine	Increased caffeine effect.
Contraceptives, oral*	Increased caffeine effect.
Ephedrine	Dangerous blood-pressure rise.
Epinephrine	Dangerous blood-pressure rise.
Isoniazid	Increased caffeine effect.
MAO inhibitors*	Dangerous blood-pressure rise.
Pseudoephedrine	Dangerous blood-pressure rise.
Sedatives*	Decreased sedative effect.
Sleep inducers*	Decreased sedative effect.
Sympathomimetics*	Overstimulation.
Thyroid hormones*	Increased thyroid effect.
Tranquilizers*	Decreased tranquilizer effect.
Troleandomycin	Increased adverse reactions of ergotamine.

POSSIBLE INTERACTION WITH OTHER SUBSTANCES

INTERACTS WITH	COMBINED EFFECT
Alcohol:	Dilates blood vessels. Makes headache worse.
Beverages: Caffeine drinks.	May help relieve headache.
Cocaine:	Overstimulation. Avoid.
Foods: Any to which you are allergic.	May make headache worse. Avoid.
Marijuana:	Occasional use—Cool extremities. Regular use—Persistent chill. Increased effect of both drugs. May lead to dangerous, rapid heartbeat. Avoid.
Tobacco:	Decreased effect of ergotamine and caffeine. Makes headache worse. Avoid.

*See Glossary

ERGOTAMINE, CAFFEINE, BELLADONNA & PENTOBARBITAL

BRAND NAMES

Cafatine PB
Cafergot-PB
Cafermine PB

Cafetrate PB
Migergot-PB

BASIC INFORMATION

Habit forming? Yes
Prescription needed? Yes
Available as generic? No
Drug class: Vasoconstrictor, stimulant (xanthine), sedative, antispasmodic

USES

- Relieves pain of migraines and other headaches caused by dilated blood vessels. Will not prevent headaches.
- Reduces anxiety or nervous tension (low dose).

DOSAGE & USAGE INFORMATION

How to take:
- Tablet—Swallow with liquid, or let dissolve under tongue. If you can't swallow whole, crumble tablet and take with liquid or food.
- Suppositories—Remove wrapper and moisten suppository with water. Gently insert larger end into rectum. Push well into rectum with finger.
- Lie down in quiet, dark room after taking.

When to take:
At first sign of vascular or migraine headache.

Continued next column

OVERDOSE

SYMPTOMS:
Tingling, cold extremities and muscle pain. Progresses to nausea, vomiting, diarrhea, insomnia, cold skin, rapid and weak pulse, severe numbness of extremities, confusion, convulsions, coma.
WHAT TO DO:
- **Dial 0 (operator) or 911 (emergency) for an ambulance or medical help. Then give first aid immediately.**
- **See emergency information on inside covers.**

If you forget a dose:
Take as soon as you remember up to 2 hours late. If more than 2 hours, wait for next scheduled dose (don't double this dose).

What drug does:
- Blocks nerve impulses at parasympathetic nerve endings, preventing muscle contractions and gland secretions of organs involved.
- May partially block nerve impulses at nerve-cell connections.
- Constricts blood-vessel walls.
- Stimulates central nervous system.

Time lapse before drug works:
15 to 30 minutes.

Don't take with:
- Non-prescription drugs without consulting doctor.
- See Interaction column and consult doctor.

POSSIBLE ADVERSE REACTIONS OR SIDE EFFECTS

SYMPTOMS	WHAT TO DO
Life-threatening:	
Extremely slow or fast heartbeat.	Discontinue. Seek emergency treatment.
Common:	
• Moderately fast heartbeat.	Discontinue. Call doctor right away.
• Dizziness, nausea, diarrhea, vomiting, nervousness, "hangover" effect.	Continue. Call doctor when convenient.
Infrequent:	
Itchy skin; rash; abdominal pain; cold hands and feet; weakness in arms, back, legs; confusion; irritability; indigestion; low blood sugar with weakness and trembling.	Discontinue. Call doctor right away.
Rare:	
Anxiety; red or purple blisters, especially in hands and feet; change in vision; extreme thirst; numbness or tingling in hands or feet; jaundice.	Discontinue. Call doctor right away.

ERGOTAMINE, CAFFEINE, BELLADONNA & PENTOBARBITAL

WARNINGS & PRECAUTIONS

Don't take if:
- You are allergic to any stimulant, ergot preparation, barbiturate or anticholinergic.
- You have heart disease, peptic ulcer of stomach or duodenum, porphyria, trouble with stomach bloating, difficulty emptying your bladder completely, narrow-angle glaucoma, severe ulcerative colitis.

Before you start, consult your doctor:
- If you have hypoglycemia (low blood sugar), an infection, angina, heart problems, high blood pressure, hardening of the arteries, vein problems, kidney or liver disease, epilepsy, asthma, anemia, chronic pain, open-angle glaucoma, chronic bronchitis, hiatal hernia, enlarged prostate, myasthenia gravis, peptic ulcer.
- If you plan to become pregnant within medication period.
- If you will have surgery within 2 months, including dental surgery, requiring general or spinal anesthesia.

Over age 60:
Adverse reactions and side effects may be more frequent and severe than in younger persons, especially dizziness and excessive potassium loss.

Pregnancy:
Risk to unborn child outweighs drug benefits. Don't use.

Breast-feeding:
Drug filters into milk. May harm child. Avoid.

Infants & children:
Not recommended.

Prolonged use:
- Stomach ulcers.
- Cold skin, muscle pain, gangrene of hands and feet. This medicine not intended for uninterrupted use.
- May cause addiction, anemia, chronic intoxication.
- May lower body temperature, making exposure to cold temperatures hazardous.
- Chronic constipation, possible fecal impaction.

Skin & sunlight:
May cause rash or intensify sunburn in areas exposed to sun or sunlamp.

Driving, piloting or hazardous work:
Don't drive or pilot aircraft until you learn how medicine affects you. Don't work around dangerous machinery. Don't climb ladders or work in high places. Danger increases if you drink alcohol or take medicine affecting alertness and reflexes, such as antihistamines, tranquilizers, sedatives, pain medicine, narcotics and mind-altering drugs.

Discontinuing:
May be unnecessary to finish medicine. Follow doctor's instructions. If you develop withdrawal symptoms of hallucinations, headache, agitation or sleeplessness after discontinuing, call doctor right away.

Others:
- Great potential for abuse.
- May produce or aggravate fibrocystic breast disease in women.
- Impaired blood circulation can lead to gangrene in intestines or extremities. Never exceed recommended dose.

POSSIBLE INTERACTION WITH OTHER DRUGS

GENERIC NAME OR DRUG CLASS	COMBINED EFFECT
Amantadine	Increased belladonna effect.
Amphetamines*	Dangerous blood-pressure rise.
Anticoagulants, oral*	Decreased anti-coagulant effect.

Continued page 1085

POSSIBLE INTERACTION WITH OTHER SUBSTANCES

INTERACTS WITH	COMBINED EFFECT
Alcohol:	Dilates blood vessels. Makes headache worse. Possible fatal oversedation. Avoid.
Beverages: Caffeine drinks.	May help relieve headache.
Cocaine:	Excessively rapid heartbeat. Avoid.
Foods: Any to which you are allergic.	May make headache worse. Avoid.
Marijuana:	Drowsiness and dry mouth, excessive sedation. Avoid. Occasional use—Cool extremities. Regular use—Persistent chill.
Tobacco:	Decreased effect of ergotamine. Makes headache worse.

*See Glossary

ERYTHROMYCINS

BRAND AND GENERIC NAMES

See complete list of brand names in the *Brand Name Directory*, page 1062.

BASIC INFORMATION

Habit forming? No
Prescription needed? Yes
Available as generic? Yes
Drug class: Antibiotic (erythromycin)

 ## USES

Treatment of infections responsive to erythromycin.

 ## DOSAGE & USAGE INFORMATION

How to take:
- Tablet or capsule—Swallow with liquid.
- Extended-release tablets or capsules—Swallow each dose whole. If you take regular tablets, you may chew or crush them.
- Liquid, drops, granules, skin ointment, eye ointment, skin solution—Follow prescription label directions.

When to take:
At the same times each day, 1 hour before or 2 hours after eating.

If you forget a dose:
- If you take 3 or more doses daily—Take as soon as you remember. Return to regular schedule.
- If you take 2 doses daily—Take as soon as you remember. Wait 5 to 6 hours for next dose. Return to regular schedule.

What drug does:
Prevents growth and reproduction of susceptible bacteria.

Time lapse before drug works:
2 to 5 days.

Don't take with:
See Interaction column and consult doctor.

 ## OVERDOSE

SYMPTOMS:
Nausea, vomiting, abdominal discomfort, diarrhea.
WHAT TO DO:
Overdose unlikely to threaten life. If person takes much larger amount than prescribed, call doctor, poison-control center or hospital emergency room for instructions.

 ## POSSIBLE ADVERSE REACTIONS OR SIDE EFFECTS

SYMPTOMS	WHAT TO DO
Life-threatening: None expected.	
Common: Gastrointestinal upset.	Discontinue. Call doctor right away.
Infrequent:	
• Diarrhea, nausea, stomach cramps, discomfort, vomiting.	Discontinue. Call doctor right away.
• Skin dryness, irritation, itch, stinging with use of skin solution, sore mouth or tongue.	Continue. Call doctor when convenient.
Rare:	
• Jaundice in adults, hearing loss.	Discontinue. Call doctor right away.
• Unusual tiredness or weakness.	Continue. Call doctor when convenient.

WARNINGS & PRECAUTIONS

Don't take if:
- You are allergic to any erythromycin.
- You have had liver disease or impaired liver function.

Before you start, consult your doctor:
If you have taken erythromycin estolate in the past.

Over age 60:
Adverse reactions and side effects may be more frequent and severe than in younger persons, especially skin reactions around genitals and anus.

Pregnancy:
No proven harm to unborn child. Avoid if possible.

Breast-feeding:
Drug passes into milk. Avoid drug or discontinue nursing until you finish medicine. Consult doctor for advice on maintaining milk supply.

Infants & children:
Use only under medical supervision.

Prolonged use:
You may become more susceptible to infections caused by germs not responsive to erythromycin.

Skin & sunlight:
No problems expected.

Driving, piloting or hazardous work:
No problems expected.

Discontinuing:
You must take full dose at least 10 consecutive days for streptococcal or staphylococcal infections.

Others:
No problems expected.

POSSIBLE INTERACTION WITH OTHER DRUGS

GENERIC NAME OR DRUG CLASS	COMBINED EFFECT
Aminophylline	Increased effect of aminophylline in blood.
Lincomycins*	Decreased lincomycin effect.
Oxtriphylline	Increased level of oxtriphylline in blood.
Penicillins*	Decreased penicillin effect.
Theophylline	Increased level of theophylline in blood.

POSSIBLE INTERACTION WITH OTHER SUBSTANCES

INTERACTS WITH	COMBINED EFFECT
Alcohol:	Possible liver damage.
Beverages:	None expected.
Cocaine:	None expected.
Foods:	None expected.
Marijuana:	None expected.
Tobacco:	None expected.

*See Glossary

ERYTHROMYCIN & SULFISOXAZOLE

BRAND NAMES

Pediazole

BASIC INFORMATION

Habit forming? No
Prescription needed? Yes
Available as generic? No
Drug class: Antibiotic (erythromycin), sulfa (sulfonamide)

 ## USES

Treatment of infections responsive to erythromycin and sulfa.

 ## DOSAGE & USAGE INFORMATION

How to take:
Suspension—Swallow with liquid. Instructions to take on empty stomach mean 1 hour before or 2 hours after eating. Shake carefully before measuring.

When to take:
At the same times each day, 1 hour before or 2 hours after eating.

If you forget a dose:
Take as soon as you remember up to 2 hours late. If more than 2 hours, wait for next scheduled dose (don't double this dose).

What drug does:
Prevents growth and reproduction of susceptible bacteria.

Time lapse before drug works:
2 to 5 days to affect infection.

Don't take with:
See Interaction column and consult doctor.

 ## OVERDOSE

SYMPTOMS:
Less urine, bloody urine, nausea, vomiting, abdominal discomfort, diarrhea, coma.
WHAT TO DO:
- Dial 0 (operator) or 911 (emergency) for an ambulance or medical help. Then give first aid immediately.
- See emergency information on inside covers.

 ## POSSIBLE ADVERSE REACTIONS OR SIDE EFFECTS

SYMPTOMS	WHAT TO DO
Life-threatening: None expected.	
Common: Headache, dizziness, itchy skin, rash, appetite loss, vomiting.	Discontinue. Call doctor right away.
Infrequent: Dryness, irritation, stinging with use of skin solution, mouth or tongue sore, diarrhea, nausea, abdominal cramps, vomiting, swallowing difficulty.	Continue. Call doctor when convenient.
Rare: • Jaundice, painful or difficult urination.	Discontinue. Call doctor right away.
• Weakness and unusual tiredness.	Continue. Call doctor when convenient.

 ## WARNINGS & PRECAUTIONS

Don't take if:
- You are allergic to any sulfa drug or any erythromycin.
- You have had liver disease or impaired liver function.

Before you start, consult your doctor:
- If you are allergic to carbonic anhydrase inhibitors, oral antidiabetics or thiazide diuretics.
- If you are allergic by nature.
- If you have liver or kidney disease, porphyria, developed anemia from use of any drug, taken erythromycin estolate in the past.

Over age 60:
Adverse reactions and side effects may be more frequent and severe than in younger persons, especially skin reactions around genitals and anus.

Pregnancy:
Risk to unborn child outweighs drug benefits. Don't use.

Breast-feeding:
Drug passes into milk. Avoid drug or discontinue nursing until you finish medicine. Consult doctor for advice on maintaining milk supply.

Infants & children:
Don't give to infants younger than 1 month.

Prolonged use:
- May enlarge thyroid gland.
- Request frequent blood counts, liver- and kidney-function studies.
- You may become more susceptible to infections caused by germs not responsive to erythromycin or sulfa.

Skin & sunlight:
May cause rash or intensify sunburn in areas exposed to sun or sunlamp.

Driving, piloting or hazardous work:
Avoid if you feel dizzy. Otherwise, no problems expected.

Discontinuing:
Don't discontinue without doctor's advice until you complete prescribed dose, even though symptoms diminish or disappear.

Others:
- Drink extra liquid each day to prevent adverse reactions.
- If you require surgery, tell anesthetist you take sulfa.

POSSIBLE INTERACTION WITH OTHER DRUGS

GENERIC NAME OR DRUG CLASS	COMBINED EFFECT
Aminobenzoate potassium	Possible decreased sulfisoxazole effect.
Aminophylline	Increased effect of aminophylline in blood.
Anticoagulants, oral*	Increased anti-coagulant effect.
Anticonvulsants, hydantoin*	Toxic effect on brain.
Aspirin	Increased sulfa effect.
Flecainide	Possible decreased blood-cell production in bone marrow.
Isoniazid	Possible anemia.
Lincomycins*	Decreased lincomycin effect.
Methenamine	Possible kidney blockage.
Methotrexate	Increased possibility of toxic side effects from methotrexate.
Oxtriphylline	Increased level of oxtriphylline in blood.

Oxyphenbutazone	Increased sulfa effect.
Para-aminosalicylic acid (PAS)	Decreased sulfa effect.
Penicillins*	Decreased penicillin effect.
Phenylbutazone	Increased sulfa effect.
Probenecid	Increased sulfa effect.
Sulfinpyrazone	Increased sulfa effect.
Theophylline	Increased level of theophylline in blood.
Tocainide	Possible decreased blood-cell production in bone marrow.
Trimethoprim	Increased sulfa effect.

POSSIBLE INTERACTION WITH OTHER SUBSTANCES

INTERACTS WITH	COMBINED EFFECT
Alcohol:	Increased alcohol effect. Possible liver damage.
Beverages: Less than 2 quarts of fluid daily.	Kidney damage.
Cocaine:	None expected.
Foods:	None expected.
Marijuana:	None expected.
Tobacco:	None expected.

ESTERIFIED ESTROGENS

BRAND NAMES

Amnestrogen	Estromed
Climestrone	Evex
Estratab	Menest
Estratest	Neo-Estrone

BASIC INFORMATION

Habit forming? No
Prescription needed? Yes
Available as generic? No
Drug class: Female sex hormone (estrogen)

 USES

- Treatment for symptoms of menopause and menstrual-cycle irregularity.
- Replacement for female hormone deficiency.
- Treatment for cancer of prostate and breast.

 DOSAGE & USAGE INFORMATION

How to take:
Tablet—Swallow with liquid. If you can't swallow whole, crumble tablet and take with liquid or food.

When to take:
At the same time each day.

If you forget a dose:
Take as soon as you remember up to 12 hours late. If more than 12 hours, wait for next scheduled dose (don't double this dose).

What drug does:
Restores normal estrogen level in tissues.

Time lapse before drug works:
10 to 20 days.

Don't take with:
See Interaction column and consult doctor.

 OVERDOSE

SYMPTOMS:
Nausea, vomiting, fluid retention, breast enlargement and discomfort, abnormal vaginal bleeding.
WHAT TO DO:
Overdose unlikely to threaten life. If person takes much larger amount than prescribed, call doctor, poison-control center or hospital emergency room for instructions.

 POSSIBLE ADVERSE REACTIONS OR SIDE EFFECTS

SYMPTOMS	WHAT TO DO
Life-threatening: None expected.	
Common:	
• Stomach cramps.	Discontinue. Call doctor right away.
• Appetite loss.	Continue. Call doctor when convenient.
• Nausea; diarrhea; swollen feet and ankles; tender, swollen breasts.	Continue. Tell doctor at next visit.
Infrequent:	
• Rash, stomach or side pain.	Discontinue. Call doctor right away.
• Depression, dizziness, headache, irritability, vomiting, breast lumps.	Continue. Call doctor when convenient.
• Brown blotches, hair loss, vaginal discharge or bleeding, changes in sex drive.	Continue. Tell doctor at next visit.
Rare:	
Jaundice, intolerance of contact lenses, hypercalcemia in breast cancer.	Discontinue. Call doctor right away.

 WARNINGS & PRECAUTIONS

Don't take if:
- You are allergic to any estrogen-containing drugs.
- You have impaired liver function.
- You have had blood clots, stroke or heart attack.
- You have unexplained vaginal bleeding.

Before you start, consult your doctor:
- If you have had cancer of breast or reproductive organs, fibrocystic breast disease, fibroid tumors of the uterus or endometriosis.
- If you have had migraine headaches, epilepsy or porphyria.
- If you have diabetes, high blood pressure, asthma, congestive heart failure, kidney disease or gallstones.
- If you plan to become pregnant within 3 months.

Over age 60:
Controversial. You and your doctor must decide if drug risks outweigh benefits.

Pregnancy:
Risk to unborn child outweighs drug benefits. Don't use.

Breast-feeding:
Drug filters into milk. May harm child. Avoid.

Infants & children:
Not recommended.

Prolonged use:
Increased growth of fibroid tumors of uterus. Possible association with cancer of uterus.

Skin & sunlight:
May cause rash or intensify sunburn in areas exposed to sun or sunlamp.

Driving, piloting or hazardous work:
No problems expected.

Discontinuing:
You may need to discontinue estrogen periodically. Consult your doctor.

Others:
In rare instances, may cause blood clot in lung, brain or leg. Symptoms are *sudden* severe headache, coordination loss, vision change, chest pain, breathing difficulty, slurred speech, pain in legs or groin. Seek emergency treatment immediately.

POSSIBLE INTERACTION WITH OTHER DRUGS

GENERIC NAME OR DRUG CLASS	COMBINED EFFECT
Anticoagulants, oral*	Decreased anticoagulant effect.
Anticonvulsants, hydantoin*	Decreased effect of esterified estrogens.
Antidepressants, tricyclic (TCA)*	Increased toxicity of antidepressant.
Antidiabetics, oral*	Unpredictable increase or decrease in blood sugar.
Antifibrinolytic agents*	Increased possibility of blood clotting.
Carbamazepine	Decreased effect of esterified estrogens.
Clofibrate	Decreased clofibrate effect.

Insulin	Possible decreased insulin effect. May require dosage adjustment.
Meprobamate	Increased effect of esterified estrogens.
Phenobarbital	Decreased effect of esterified estrogens.
Primidone	Decreased effect of esterified estrogens.
Rifampin	Decreased effect of esterified estrogens.
Terazosin	Decreases effectiveness of terazosin.
Thyroid hormones*	Decreased thyroid effect.
Ursodiol	Decreased effect of ursodiol.
Vitamin C	Possible increased effect of esterified estrogens.

POSSIBLE INTERACTION WITH OTHER SUBSTANCES

INTERACTS WITH	COMBINED EFFECT
Alcohol:	None expected.
Beverages:	None expected.
Cocaine:	No proven problems.
Foods:	None expected.
Marijuana:	Possible menstrual irregularities and bleeding between periods.
Tobacco:	Increased risk of blood clots leading to stroke or heart attack.

ESTRADIOL

BRAND NAMES

Delestrogen   Estrace

BASIC INFORMATION

Habit forming? No
Prescription needed? Yes
Available as generic? Yes
Drug class: Female sex hormone (estrogen)

 USES

- Treatment for symptoms of menopause and menstrual-cycle irregularity.
- Replacement for female hormone deficiency.
- Treatment for cancer of prostate and breast.

 DOSAGE & USAGE INFORMATION

How to take:
- Tablet—Swallow with liquid. If you can't swallow whole, crumble tablet and take with liquid or food.
- Transdermal patches—Follow package instructions.
- Vaginal cream—Use as directed on label.

When to take:
At the same time each day.

If you forget a dose:
Take as soon as you remember up to 12 hours late. If more than 12 hours, wait for next scheduled dose (don't double this dose).

What drug does:
Restores normal estrogen level in tissues.

Time lapse before drug works:
10 to 20 days.

Don't take with:
See Interaction column and consult doctor.

 OVERDOSE

SYMPTOMS:
Nausea, vomiting, fluid retention, breast enlargement and discomfort, abnormal vaginal bleeding.
WHAT TO DO:
Overdose unlikely to threaten life. If person takes much larger amount than prescribed, call doctor, poison-control center or hospital emergency room for instructions.

 POSSIBLE ADVERSE REACTIONS OR SIDE EFFECTS

SYMPTOMS	WHAT TO DO
Life-threatening: None expected.	
Common:	
• Stomach cramps.	Discontinue. Call doctor right away.
• Appetite loss.	Continue. Call doctor when convenient.
• Nausea; diarrhea; swollen feet and ankles; tender, swollen breasts.	Continue. Tell doctor at next visit.
Infrequent:	
• Rash, stomach or side pain.	Discontinue. Call doctor right away.
• Depression, dizziness, headache, irritability, vomiting, breast lumps.	Continue. Call doctor when convenient.
• Brown blotches, hair loss, vaginal discharge or bleeding, changes in sex drive.	Continue. Tell doctor at next visit.
Rare: Jaundice, intolerance of contact lenses, hypercalcemia in breast cancer.	Discontinue. Call doctor right away.

 WARNINGS & PRECAUTIONS

Don't take if:
- You are allergic to any estrogen-containing drugs.
- You have impaired liver function.
- You have had blood clots, stroke or heart attack.
- You have unexplained vaginal bleeding.

Before you start, consult your doctor:
- If you have had cancer of breast or reproductive organs, fibrocystic breast disease, fibroid tumors of the uterus or endometriosis.
- If you have had migraine headaches, epilepsy or porphyria.
- If you have diabetes, high blood pressure, asthma, congestive heart failure, kidney disease or gallstones.
- If you plan to become pregnant within 3 months.

Over age 60:
Controversial. You and your doctor must decide if drug risks outweigh benefits.

Pregnancy:
Risk to unborn child outweighs drug benefits. Don't use.

Breast-feeding:
Drug filters into milk. May harm child. Avoid.

Infants & children:
Not recommended.

Prolonged use:
Increased growth of fibroid tumors of uterus. Possible association with cancer of uterus.

Skin & sunlight:
May cause rash or intensify sunburn in areas exposed to sun or sunlamp.

Driving, piloting or hazardous work:
No problems expected.

Discontinuing:
You may need to discontinue estradiol periodically. Consult your doctor.

Others:
In rare instances, may cause blood clot in lung, brain or leg. Symptoms are *sudden* severe headache, coordination loss, vision change, chest pain, breathing difficulty, slurred speech, pain in legs or groin. Seek emergency treatment immediately.

POSSIBLE INTERACTION WITH OTHER DRUGS

GENERIC NAME OR DRUG CLASS	COMBINED EFFECT
Anticoagulants, oral*	Decreased anticoagulant effect.
Anticonvulsants, hydantoin*	Decreased estradiol effect.
Antidepressants, tricyclic (TCA)*	Increased toxicity of antidepressants.
Antidiabetics, oral*	Unpredictable increase or decrease in blood sugar.
Antifibrinolytic agents*	Increased possibility of blood clotting.
Carbamazepine	Decreased estradiol effect.
Clofibrate	Decreased clofibrate effect.

Insulin	Possible decreased insulin effect. May require dosage adjustment.
Meprobamate	Increased estradiol effect.
Phenobarbital	Decreased estradiol effect.
Primidone	Decreased estradiol effect.
Rifampin	Decreased estradiol effect.
Terazosin	Decreases effectiveness of terazosin.
Thyroid hormones*	Decreased thyroid effect.
Ursodiol	Decreased effect of ursodiol.
Vitamin C	Possible increased estradiol effect.

POSSIBLE INTERACTION WITH OTHER SUBSTANCES

INTERACTS WITH	COMBINED EFFECT
Alcohol:	None expected.
Beverages:	None expected.
Cocaine:	No proven problems.
Foods:	None expected.
Marijuana:	Possible menstrual irregularities and bleeding between periods.
Tobacco:	Increased risk of blood clots leading to stroke or heart attack.

ESTROGEN

BRAND NAMES

See complete list of brand names in the *Brand Name Directory*, page 1062.

BASIC INFORMATION

Habit forming? No
Prescription needed? Yes
Available as generic? Yes
Drug class: Female sex hormone (estrogen)

 ## USES

- Treatment for symptoms of menopause and menstrual-cycle irregularity.
- Treatment for estrogen-deficiency osteoporosis (bone softening from calcium loss).
- Treatment for DES-induced cancer.
- Treatment for atrophic vaginitis.

 ## DOSAGE & USAGE INFORMATION

How to take:
- Tablet or capsule—Swallow with liquid. If you can't swallow whole, crumble tablet or open capsule and take with liquid or food.
- Vaginal cream or suppositories—Use as directed on label.

When to take:
At the same time each day.

If you forget a dose:
Take as soon as you remember up to 12 hours late. If more than 12 hours, wait for next scheduled dose (don't double this dose).

What drug does:
Restores normal estrogen level in tissues.

Time lapse before drug works:
10 to 20 days.

Don't take with:
See Interaction column and consult doctor.

 ## OVERDOSE

SYMPTOMS:
Nausea, vomiting, fluid retention, breast enlargement and discomfort, abnormal vaginal bleeding.
WHAT TO DO:
Overdose unlikely to threaten life. If person takes much larger amount than prescribed, call doctor, poison-control center or hospital emergency room for instructions.

 ## POSSIBLE ADVERSE REACTIONS OR SIDE EFFECTS

SYMPTOMS	WHAT TO DO
Life-threatening:	
None expected.	
Common:	
• Stomach cramps.	Discontinue. Call doctor right away.
• Appetite loss.	Continue. Call doctor when convenient.
• Nausea; diarrhea; swollen feet and ankles; tender, swollen breasts.	Continue. Tell doctor at next visit.
Infrequent:	
• Rash, stomach or side pain.	Discontinue. Call doctor right away.
• Depression, dizziness, headache, irritability, vomiting, breast lumps.	Continue. Call doctor when convenient.
• Brown blotches, hair loss, vaginal discharge or bleeding, changes in sex drive.	Continue. Tell doctor at next visit.
Rare:	
Jaundice, intolerance of contact lenses, hypercalcemia in breast cancer.	Discontinue. Call doctor right away.

 ## WARNINGS & PRECAUTIONS

Don't take if:
- You are allergic to any estrogen-containing drugs.
- You have impaired liver function.
- You have had blood clots, stroke or heart attack.
- You have unexplained vaginal bleeding.

Before you start, consult your doctor:
- If you have had cancer of breast or reproductive organs, fibrocystic breast disease, fibroid tumors of the uterus or endometriosis.
- If you have had migraine headaches, epilepsy or porphyria.
- If you have diabetes, high blood pressure, asthma, congestive heart failure, kidney disease or gallstones.
- If you plan to become pregnant within 3 months.

Over age 60:
Controversial. You and your doctor must decide if drug risks outweigh benefits.

Pregnancy:
Risk to unborn child outweighs drug benefits. Don't use.

Breast-feeding:
Drug filters into milk. May harm child. Avoid.

Infants & children:
Not recommended.

Prolonged use:
Increased growth of fibroid tumors of uterus. Possible association with cancer of uterus.

Skin & sunlight:
May cause rash or intensify sunburn in areas exposed to sun or sunlamp.

Driving, piloting or hazardous work:
No problems expected.

Discontinuing:
You may need to discontinue estrogens periodically. Consult your doctor.

Others:
- In rare instances, may cause blood clot in lung, brain or leg. Symptoms are *sudden* severe headache, coordination loss, vision change, chest pain, breathing difficulty, slurred speech, pain in legs or groin. Seek emergency treatment immediately.
- Carefully read the paper called "Information for the Patient" that was given to you with your prescription. If you lose it, ask your pharmacist for a copy.

 POSSIBLE INTERACTION WITH OTHER DRUGS

GENERIC NAME OR DRUG CLASS	COMBINED EFFECT
Anticoagulants, oral*	Decreased anticoagulant effect.
Anticonvulsants, hydantoin*	Decreased estrogen effect.
Antidepressants, tricyclic (TCA)*	Increased toxicity of antidepressants.
Antidiabetics, oral*	Unpredictable increase or decrease in blood sugar.
Antifibrinolytic agents*	Increased possibility of blood clotting.
Carbamazepine	Decreased estrogen effect.
Clofibrate	Decreased clofibrate effect.
Guanfacine	May decrease antihypertensive effects of guanfacine.
Insulin	Possible decreased insulin effect. May require dosage adjustment.
Meprobamate	Increased estrogen effect.
Phenobarbital	Decreased estrogen effect.
Primidone	Decreased estrogen effect.
Rifampin	Decreased estrogen effect.
Terazosin	Decreases effectiveness of terazosin.
Thyroid hormones*	Decreased thyroid effect.
Ursodiol	Decreased effect of ursodiol.
Vitamin C	Possible increased estrogen effect.

 POSSIBLE INTERACTION WITH OTHER SUBSTANCES

INTERACTS WITH	COMBINED EFFECT
Alcohol:	None expected.
Beverages:	None expected.
Cocaine:	No proven problems.
Foods:	None expected.
Marijuana:	Possible menstrual irregularities and bleeding between periods.
Tobacco:	Increased risk of blood clots leading to stroke or heart attack.

ESTRONE

BRAND NAMES

Besterone	Kestrin Aqueous
Estaqua	Kestrone
Estrofol	Natural Estrogenic
Estroject	Substance
Estrone-A	Ogen
Estronol	Theelin
Femogen	Theelin Aqueous
Foygen Aqueous	Theogen
Gynogen	Unigen
Hormogen-A	Wehgen
Kestrin	

BASIC INFORMATION

Habit forming? No
Prescription needed? Yes
Available as generic? Yes
Drug class: Female sex hormone (estrogen)

USES

- Treatment for symptoms of menopause and menstrual-cycle irregularity.
- Replacement for female hormone deficiency.
- Treatment for prostate cancer.

DOSAGE & USAGE INFORMATION

How to take:
By injection under medical supervision.

When to take:
Varies according to doctor's instructions.

If you forget an injection:
Consult doctor.

What drug does:
Restores normal estrogen level in tissues.

Time lapse before drug works:
10 to 20 days.

Don't take with:
See Interaction column and consult doctor.

OVERDOSE

SYMPTOMS:
Nausea, vomiting, fluid retention, breast enlargement and discomfort, abnormal vaginal bleeding.
WHAT TO DO:
Overdose unlikely to threaten life. If person takes much larger amount than prescribed, call doctor, poison-control center or hospital emergency room for instructions.

POSSIBLE ADVERSE REACTIONS OR SIDE EFFECTS

SYMPTOMS	WHAT TO DO
Life-threatening: None expected.	
Common:	
• Stomach cramps.	Discontinue. Call doctor right away.
• Appetite loss.	Continue. Call doctor when convenient.
• Nausea; diarrhea; swollen feet and ankles; tender, swollen breasts.	Continue. Tell doctor at next visit.
Infrequent:	
• Rash, stomach or side pain.	Discontinue. Call doctor right away.
• Depression, dizziness, headache, irritability, vomiting, breast lumps.	Continue. Call doctor when convenient.
• Brown blotches, hair loss, vaginal discharge or bleeding, changes in sex drive.	Continue. Tell doctor at next visit.
Rare:	
Jaundice, intolerance of contact lenses, hypercalcemia in breast cancer.	Discontinue. Call doctor right away.

WARNINGS & PRECAUTIONS

Don't take if:
- You are allergic to any estrogen-containing drugs.
- You have impaired liver function.
- You have had blood clots, stroke or heart attack.
- You have unexplained vaginal bleeding.

Before you start, consult your doctor:
- If you have had cancer of breast or reproductive organs, fibrocystic breast disease, fibroid tumors of the uterus or endometriosis.
- If you have had migraine headaches, epilepsy or porphyria.
- If you have diabetes, high blood pressure, asthma, congestive heart failure, kidney disease or gallstones.
- If you plan to become pregnant within 3 months.

Over age 60:
Controversial. You and your doctor must decide if drug risks outweigh benefits.

Pregnancy:
Risk to unborn child outweighs drug benefits. Don't use.

Breast-feeding:
Drug filters into milk. May harm child. Avoid.

Infants & children:
Not recommended.

Prolonged use:
Increased growth of fibroid tumors of uterus. Possible association with cancer of uterus.

Skin & sunlight:
May cause rash or intensify sunburn in areas exposed to sun or sunlamp.

Driving, piloting or hazardous work:
No problems expected.

Discontinuing:
You may need to discontinue estrone periodically. Consult your doctor.

Others:
In rare instances, may cause blood clot in lung, brain or leg. Symptoms are *sudden* severe headache, coordination loss, vision change, chest pain, breathing difficulty, slurred speech, pain in legs or groin. Seek emergency treatment immediately.

POSSIBLE INTERACTION WITH OTHER DRUGS

GENERIC NAME OR DRUG CLASS	COMBINED EFFECT
Anticoagulants, oral*	Decreased anti-coagulant effect.
Anticonvulsants, hydantoin*	Decreased estrone effect.
Antidepressants, tricyclic (TCA)*	Increased toxicity of antidepressants.
Antidiabetics, oral*	Unpredictable increase or decrease in blood sugar.
Antifibrinolytic agents*	Increased possibility of blood clotting.
Carbamazepine	Decreased estrone effect.
Clofibrate	Decreased clofibrate effect.

Insulin	Possible decreased insulin effect. May require dosage adjustment.
Meprobamate	Increased estrone effect.
Phenobarbital	Decreased estrone effect.
Primidone	Decreased estrone effect.
Rifampin	Decreased estrone effect.
Terazosin	Decreases effectiveness of terazosin.
Thyroid hormones*	Decreased thyroid effect.
Ursodiol	Decreased effect of ursodiol.
Vitamin C	Possible increased estrogen effect.

POSSIBLE INTERACTION WITH OTHER SUBSTANCES

INTERACTS WITH	COMBINED EFFECT
Alcohol:	None expected.
Beverages:	None expected.
Cocaine:	No proven problems.
Foods:	None expected.
Marijuana:	Possible menstrual irregularities and bleeding between periods.
Tobacco:	Increased risk of blood clots leading to stroke or heart attack.

ESTROPIPATE

BRAND NAMES

Ogen

Piperazine Estrone
Sulfate

BASIC INFORMATION

Habit forming? No
Prescription needed? Yes
Available as generic? No
Drug class: Female sex hormone (estrogen)

 ## USES

- Treatment for symptoms of menopause and menstrual-cycle irregularity.
- Replacement for female hormone deficiency.

 ## DOSAGE & USAGE INFORMATION

How to take:
- Tablet—Swallow with liquid. if you can't swallow whole, crumble tablet and take with liquid or food.
- Vaginal cream—Use as directed on label.

When to take:
At the same time each day.

If you forget a dose:
Take as soon as you remember up to 12 hours late. If more than 12 hours, wait for next scheduled dose (don't double this dose).

What drug does:
Restores normal estrogen level in tissues.

Time lapse before drug works:
10 to 20 days.

Don't take with:
See Interaction column and consult doctor.

 ## OVERDOSE

SYMPTOMS:
Nausea, vomiting, fluid retention, breast enlargement and discomfort, abnormal vaginal bleeding.
WHAT TO DO:
Overdose unlikely to threaten life. If person takes much larger amount than prescribed, call doctor, poison-control center or hospital emergency room for instructions.

 ## POSSIBLE ADVERSE REACTIONS OR SIDE EFFECTS

SYMPTOMS	WHAT TO DO
Life-threatening: None expected.	
Common:	
• Stomach cramps.	Discontinue. Call doctor right away.
• Appetite loss.	Continue. Call doctor when convenient.
• Nausea; diarrhea; swollen feet and ankles; tender, swollen breasts.	Continue. Tell doctor at next visit.
Infrequent:	
• Rash, stomach or side pain.	Discontinue. Call doctor right away.
• Depression, dizziness, headache, irritability, vomiting, breast lumps.	Continue. Call doctor when convenient.
• Brown blotches, hair loss, vaginal discharge or bleeding, changes in sex drive.	Continue. Tell doctor at next visit.
Rare: Jaundice, intolerance of contact lenses, hypercalcemia in breast cancer.	Discontinue. Call doctor right away.

 ## WARNINGS & PRECAUTIONS

Don't take if:
- You are allergic to any estrogen-containing drugs.
- You have impaired liver function.
- You have had blood clots, stroke or heart attack.
- You have unexplained vaginal bleeding.

Before you start, consult your doctor:
- If you have had cancer of breast or reproductive organs, fibrocystic breast disease, fibroid tumors of the uterus or endometriosis.
- If you have had migraine headaches, epilepsy or porphyria.
- If you have diabetes, high blood pressure, asthma, congestive heart failure, kidney disease or gallstones.
- If you plan to become pregnant within 3 months.

Over age 60:
Controversial. You and your doctor must decide if drug risks outweigh benefits.

Pregnancy:
Risk to unborn child outweighs drug benefits. Don't use.

Breast-feeding:
Drug filters into milk. May harm child. Avoid.

Infants & children:
Not recommended.

Prolonged use:
Increased growth of fibroid tumors of uterus. Possible association with cancer of uterus.

Skin & sunlight:
May cause rash or intensify sunburn in areas exposed to sun or sunlamp.

Driving, piloting or hazardous work:
No problems expected.

Discontinuing:
You may need to discontinue estropipate periodically. Consult your doctor.

Others:
In rare instances, may cause blood clot in lung, brain or leg. Symptoms are *sudden* severe headache, coordination loss, vision change, chest pain, breathing difficulty, slurred speech, pain in legs or groin. Seek emergency treatment immediately.

POSSIBLE INTERACTION WITH OTHER DRUGS

GENERIC NAME OR DRUG CLASS	COMBINED EFFECT
Anticoagulants, oral*	Decreased anticoagulant effect.
Anticonvulsants, hydantoin*	Decreased estropipate effect.
Antidepressants, tricyclic (TCA)*	Increased toxicity of antidepressants.
Antidiabetics, oral*	Unpredictable increase or decrease in blood sugar.
Antifibrinolytic agents*	Increased possibility of blood clotting.
Carbamazepine	Decreased estropipate effect.
Clofibrate	Decreased clofibrate effect.
Insulin	Possible decreased insulin effect. May require dosage adjustment.
Meprobamate	Increased estropipate effect.
Phenobarbital	Decreased estropipate effect.
Primidone	Decreased estropipate effect.
Rifampin	Decreased estropipate effect.
Terazosin	Decreases effectiveness of terazosin.
Thyroid hormones*	Decreased thyroid effect.
Ursodiol	Decreased effect of ursodiol.
Vitamin C	Possible increased estrogen effect.

POSSIBLE INTERACTION WITH OTHER SUBSTANCES

INTERACTS WITH	COMBINED EFFECT
Alcohol:	None expected.
Beverages:	None expected.
Cocaine:	No proven problems.
Foods:	None expected.
Marijuana:	Possible menstrual irregularities and bleeding between periods.
Tobacco:	Increased risk of blood clots leading to stroke or heart attack.

*See Glossary

ETHACRYNIC ACID

BRAND NAMES

Edecrin

BASIC INFORMATION

Habit forming? No
Prescription needed? Yes
Available as generic? No
Drug class: Diuretic (loop diuretic);
antihypertensive

 USES

- Lowers blood pressure.
- Decreases fluid retention.

 DOSAGE & USAGE INFORMATION

How to take:
Tablet—Swallow with liquid or food to lessen stomach irritation. If you can't swallow whole, crumble tablet and take with liquid or food.

When to take:
- 1 dose a day—Take after breakfast.
- More than 1 dose a day—Take last dose no later than 6 p.m. unless otherwise directed.

If you forget a dose:
- 1 dose a day—Take as soon as you remember up to 12 hours late. If more than 12 hours, wait for next scheduled dose (don't double this dose).
- More than 1 dose a day—Take as soon as you remember up to 2 hours late. If more than 2 hours, wait for next scheduled dose (don't double this dose).

What drug does:
Increases elimination of sodium and water from body. Decreased body fluid reduces blood pressure.

Continued next column

 OVERDOSE

SYMPTOMS:
Weakness, lethargy, dizziness, confusion, nausea, vomiting, leg-muscle cramps, thirst, stupor, deep sleep, weak and rapid pulse, cardiac arrest.
WHAT TO DO:
- **Dial 0 (operator) or 911 (emergency) for an ambulance or medical help. Then give first aid immediately.**
- **See emergency information on inside covers.**

Time lapse before drug works:
1 hour to increase water loss. Requires 2 to 3 weeks to lower blood pressure.

Don't take with:
- Non-prescription drugs with aspirin.
- See Interaction column and consult doctor.

 POSSIBLE ADVERSE REACTIONS OR SIDE EFFECTS

SYMPTOMS	WHAT TO DO
Life-threatening: None expected.	
Common: Dizziness.	Continue. Call doctor when convenient.
Infrequent: Mood change, appetite loss, watery diarrhea, irregular heartbeat, muscle cramps, fatigue, weakness.	Discontinue. Call doctor right away.
Rare: Rash or hives, yellow vision, ringing in ears, hearing loss, sore throat, fever, dry mouth, thirst, side or stomach pain, nausea, vomiting, unusual bleeding or bruising, joint pain, numbness or tingling in hands or feet, jaundice.	Discontinue. Call doctor right away.

 WARNINGS & PRECAUTIONS

Don't take if:
You are allergic to ethacrynic acid.

Before you start, consult your doctor:
- If you are allergic to any sulfa drug.
- If you have liver or kidney disease.
- If you have gout.
- If you have diabetes.
- If you have impaired hearing.
- If you will have surgery within 2 months, including dental surgery, requiring general or spinal anesthesia.

Over age 60:
Adverse reactions and side effects may be more frequent and severe than in younger persons. Hot weather may cause need to reduce dosage.

Pregnancy:
Risk to unborn child outweighs drug benefits. Don't use.

Breast-feeding:
Drug filters into milk. May harm child. Avoid.

Infants & children:
Use only under medical supervision.

Prolonged use:
- Impaired balance of water, salt and potassium in blood and body tissues.
- Possible diabetes.

Skin & sunlight:
May cause rash or intensify sunburn in areas exposed to sun or sunlamp.

Driving, piloting or hazardous work:
No problems expected.

Discontinuing:
Don't discontinue without doctor's advice until you complete prescribed dose, even though symptoms diminish or disappear.

Others:
Frequent laboratory studies to monitor potassium level in blood recommended. Eat foods rich in potassium or take potassium supplements. Consult doctor.

POSSIBLE INTERACTION WITH OTHER DRUGS

GENERIC NAME OR DRUG CLASS	COMBINED EFFECT
Allopurinol	Decreased allopurinol effect.
Amiodarone	Increased risk of heartbeat irregularity due to low potassium.
Anticoagulants*	Abnormal clotting.
Antidepressants, tricyclic (TCA)*	Excessive blood-pressure drop.
Antidiabetics, oral*	Decreased anti-diabetic effect.
Antihypertensives*	Increased antihypertensive effect. Dosages may require adjustment.
Barbiturates*	Low blood pressure.
Calcium supplements*	Decreased calcium in blood.
Carteolol	Increased antihypertensive effect.
Cortisone drugs*	Excessive potassium loss.
Digitalis preparations*	Excessive potassium loss could lead to serious heart-rhythm disorders.

Diuretics*	Increased diuretic effect.
Insulin	Decreased insulin effect.
Lisinopril	Increased antihypertensive effect. Dosage of each may require adjustment.
Lithium	Increased lithium toxicity.
Narcotics*	Dangerous low blood pressure. Avoid.
Nicardipine	Blood-pressure drop. Dosages may require adjustment.
Nitrates*	Excessive blood-pressure drop.
Non-steroidal anti-inflammatory drugs (NSAIDs)*	Decreased ethacrynic acid effect.
Phenytoin	Decreased ethacrynic acid effect.
Potassium supplements*	Decreased potassium effect.
Probenecid	Decreased probenecid effect.
Salicylates* (including aspirin)	Dangerous salicylate retention.
Sedatives*	Increased ethacrynic acid effect.
Sotalol	Increased antihypertensive effect.
Terazosin	Decreases effectiveness of terazosin.

POSSIBLE INTERACTION WITH OTHER SUBSTANCES

INTERACTS WITH	COMBINED EFFECT
Alcohol:	Blood-pressure drop. Avoid.
Beverages:	None expected.
Cocaine:	Dangerous blood-pressure drop. Avoid.
Foods:	None expected.
Marijuana:	Increased thirst and urinary frequency, fainting.
Tobacco:	Decreased ethacrynic acid effect.

*See Glossary

ETHCHLORVYNOL

BRAND NAMES

Placidyl

BASIC INFORMATION

Habit forming? Yes
Prescription needed? Yes
Available as generic? No
Drug class: Sleep inducer (hypnotic)

 ## USES

Treatment of insomnia.

 ## DOSAGE & USAGE INFORMATION

How to take:
Capsules—Take with food or milk to lessen side effects.

When to take:
At or near bedtime.

If you forget a dose:
Bedtime dose—If you forget your once-a-day bedtime dose, don't take it more than 3 hours late.

What drug does:
Affects brain centers that control waking and sleeping.

Time lapse before drug works:
30 to 60 minutes.

Don't take with:
See Interaction column and consult doctor.

 ## OVERDOSE

SYMPTOMS:
Excitement, delirium, incoordination, excessive drowsiness, deep coma.
WHAT TO DO:
- **Dial 0 (operator) or 911 (emergency) for an ambulance or medical help. Then give first aid immediately.**
- **If patient is unconscious and not breathing, give mouth-to-mouth breathing. If there is no heartbeat, use cardiac massage and mouth-to-mouth breathing (CPR). Don't try to make patient vomit. If you can't get help quickly, take patient to nearest emergency facility.**
- **See emergency information on inside covers.**

 ## POSSIBLE ADVERSE REACTIONS OR SIDE EFFECTS

SYMPTOMS	WHAT TO DO
Life-threatening: None expected.	
Common:	
• Indigestion, nausea, vomiting, stomach pain.	Discontinue. Call doctor right away.
• Blurred vision, dizziness.	Continue. Call doctor when convenient.
• Unpleasant taste in mouth, fatigue, weakness.	Continue. Tell doctor at next visit.
Infrequent: Jitters, clumsiness, unsteadiness, drowsiness, confusion, rash, hives, unusual bleeding or bruising, facial numbness.	Discontinue. Call doctor right away.
Rare: Slow heartbeat, difficult breathing, fainting, jaundice.	Discontinue. Call doctor right away.

WARNINGS & PRECAUTIONS

Don't take if:
- You are allergic to any hypnotic.
- You have porphyria.
- Patient is younger than 12.

Before you start, consult your doctor:
- If you plan to become pregnant within medication period.
- If you have kidney or liver disease.

Over age 60:
Adverse reactions and side effects, especially a "hangover" effect, may be more frequent and severe than in younger persons.

Pregnancy:
Risk to unborn child outweighs drug benefits. Don't use.

Breast-feeding:
No problems expected, but observe child and ask doctor for guidance.

Infants & children:
Not recommended.

Prolonged use:
Impaired vision.

Skin & sunlight:
No problems expected.

Driving, piloting or hazardous work:
Don't drive or pilot aircraft until you learn how medicine affects you. Don't work around dangerous machinery. Don't climb ladders or work in high places. Danger increases if you drink alcohol or take medicine affecting alertness and reflexes.

Discontinuing:
- Don't discontinue without consulting doctor. Dose may require gradual reduction if you have taken drug for a long time. Doses of other drugs may also require adjustment.
- Many side effects may occur when you stop taking this drug, including irritability, muscle twitching, hallucinations or seizures. Consult your doctor.

Others:
No problems expected.

POSSIBLE INTERACTION WITH OTHER DRUGS

GENERIC NAME OR DRUG CLASS	COMBINED EFFECT
Anticoagulants, oral*	Decreased anticoagulant effect.
Antidepressants, tricyclic (TCA)*	Delirium and deep sedation.
Antihistamines*	Increased antihistamine effect.
Ethinamate	Dangerous increased effects of ethinamate. Avoid combining.
Fluoxetine	Increased depressant effects of both drugs.
Guanfacine	May increase depressant effects of either drug.
Leucovorin	High alcohol content of leucovorin may cause adverse effects.
MAO inhibitors*	Increased sedation.
Methyprylon	Increased sedative effect, perhaps to dangerous level. Avoid.
Molindone	Increased sedative effect.
Nabilone	Greater depression of central nervous system.
Narcotics*	Increased narcotic effect.
Pain relievers*	Increased effect of pain reliever.
Sedatives*	Increased sedative effect.
Tranquilizers*	Increased tranquilizer effect.

POSSIBLE INTERACTION WITH OTHER SUBSTANCES

INTERACTS WITH	COMBINED EFFECT
Alcohol:	Excessive depressant and sedative effect. Avoid.
Beverages:	None expected.
Cocaine:	Decreased ethchlorvynol effect.
Foods:	None expected.
Marijuana:	Occasional use—Drowsiness, unsteadiness, depressed function. Frequent use—Severe drowsiness, impaired physical and mental function.
Tobacco:	None expected.

*See Glossary

ETHINAMATE

BRAND NAMES

Valmid

BASIC INFORMATION

Habit forming? Yes
Prescription needed? Yes
Available as generic? No
Drug class: Sedative-hypnotic

 ## USES

Treats insomnia for short periods. Prolonged use is not recommended.

 ## DOSAGE & USAGE INFORMATION

How to take:
Capsules—Swallow with liquid or food to lessen stomach irritation. If you can't swallow whole, open capsule and take with liquid or food.

When to take:
At bedtime.

If you forget a dose:
Skip dose. Never double-dose.

What drug does:
Helps sleeplessness by an unknown mechanism of action.

Time lapse before drug works:
30 to 40 minutes.

Don't take with:
See Interaction column and consult doctor.

 ## OVERDOSE

SYMPTOMS:
Oversedation, coma.
WHAT TO DO:
- **Dial 0 (operator) or 911 (emergency) for an ambulance or medical help. Then give first aid immediately.**
- **See emergency information on inside covers.**

 ## POSSIBLE ADVERSE REACTIONS OR SIDE EFFECTS

SYMPTOMS	WHAT TO DO
Life-threatening:	
Coma, shortness of breath, slow heartbeat.	Seek emergency treatment immediately.
Common:	
None expected.	
Infrequent:	
• Unusual excitement (especially in children).	Discontinue. Seek emergency treatment.
• Allergic skin rash, upper abdominal discomfort, vomiting.	Discontinue. Call doctor right away.
Rare:	
• Excessive bleeding.	Discontinue. Call doctor right away.
• Daytime drowsiness.	Continue. Call doctor when convenient.

ETHINAMATE

WARNINGS & PRECAUTIONS

Don't take if:
- You are an alcoholic.
- You have a history of drug abuse of any sort.

Before you start, consult your doctor:
- If you have ever had significant depression.
- If you have uncontrolled pain.

Over age 60:
Adverse reactions and side effects may be more frequent and severe than in younger persons. You may need smaller doses for shorter periods of time.

Pregnancy:
Risk to unborn child outweighs drug benefits. Don't use.

Breast-feeding:
Unknown effects. Avoid.

Infants & children:
Not recommended.

Prolonged use:
May lead to habituation.

Skin & sunlight:
No problems expected.

Driving, piloting or hazardous work:
Don't drive or pilot aircraft until you learn how medicine affects you. Don't work around dangerous machinery. Don't climb ladders or work in high places. Danger increases if you drink alcohol or take medicine affecting alertness and reflexes.

Discontinuing:
Discontinue after maximum of 7 days. Don't resume without your doctor's recommendation.

Others:
Has not been shown to be effective after 1 week. If treatment must be repeated, allow 1 or more weeks between treatment periods.

POSSIBLE INTERACTION WITH OTHER DRUGS

GENERIC NAME OR DRUG CLASS	COMBINED EFFECT
Central nervous system (CNS) depressants*	Will dangerously increase the effects of ethinamate and any of the CNS drugs. Avoid combining.
Fluoxetine	Increased depressant effects of both drugs.
Guanfacine	May increase depressant effects of either drug.
Leucovorin	High alcohol content of leucovorin may cause adverse effects.
Methyprylon	Increased sedative effect, perhaps to dangerous level. Avoid.
Nabilone	Greater depression of central nervous system.

POSSIBLE INTERACTION WITH OTHER SUBSTANCES

INTERACTS WITH	COMBINED EFFECT
Alcohol:	Dangerous oversedation. Avoid.
Beverages: Any containing caffeine, such as coffee, tea or cocoa.	Decreases effects of ethinamate.
Cocaine:	Decreases effects of ethinamate and increases chance of toxicity. Avoid.
Foods:	No special problems expected.
Marijuana:	Decreases effects of ethinamate.
Tobacco:	No special problems expected.

ETHINYL ESTRADIOL

BRAND NAMES

Brevicon	Norette
Demulen	Norinyl
Estinyl	Norlestrin
Feminone	Ortho-Novum
Loestrin	Ovcon
Lo-Ovral	Ovral
Modicon	Tri-Norinyl

BASIC INFORMATION

Habit forming? No
Prescription needed? Yes
Available as generic? No
Drug class: Female sex hormone (estrogen)

 ## USES

- Treatment for symptoms of menopause and menstrual-cycle irregularity.
- Replacement for female hormone deficiency.
- Prevention of pregnancy.
- Treatment for cancer of breast and prostate.

 ## DOSAGE & USAGE INFORMATION

How to take:
Tablet—Swallow with liquid. If you can't swallow whole, crumble tablet and take with liquid or food.

When to take:
At the same time each day.

If you forget a dose:
Take as soon as you remember up to 12 hours late. If more than 12 hours, wait for next scheduled dose (don't double this dose).

What drug does:
- Restores normal estrogen level in tissues.
- Prevents pituitary gland from secreting hormone that causes ovary to ripen and release egg.

Continued next column

 ## OVERDOSE

SYMPTOMS:
Nausea, vomiting, fluid retention, breast enlargement and discomfort, abnormal vaginal bleeding.
WHAT TO DO:
Overdose unlikely to threaten life. If person takes much larger amount than prescribed, call doctor, poison-control center or hospital emergency room for instructions.

Time lapse before drug works:
10 to 20 days.

Don't take with:
See Interaction column and consult doctor.

 ## POSSIBLE ADVERSE REACTIONS OR SIDE EFFECTS

SYMPTOMS	WHAT TO DO
Life-threatening:	
None expected.	
Common:	
• Stomach cramps.	Discontinue. Call doctor right away.
• Appetite loss.	Continue. Call doctor when convenient.
• Nausea; diarrhea; swollen feet and ankles; tender, swollen breasts.	Continue. Tell doctor at next visit.
Infrequent:	
• Rash, stomach or side pain.	Discontinue. Call doctor right away.
• Depression, dizziness, headache, irritability, vomiting, breast lumps.	Continue. Call doctor when convenient.
• Brown blotches, hair loss, vaginal discharge or bleeding, changes in sex drive.	Continue. Tell doctor at next visit.
Rare:	
Jaundice, intolerance of contact lenses, hypercalcemia in breast cancer.	Discontinue. Call doctor right away.

 ## WARNINGS & PRECAUTIONS

Don't take if:
- You are allergic to any estrogen-containing drugs.
- You have impaired liver function.
- You have had blood clots, stroke or heart attack.
- You have unexplained vaginal bleeding.

Before you start, consult your doctor:
- If you have had cancer of breast or reproductive organs, fibrocystic breast disease, fibroid tumors of the uterus or endometriosis.
- If you have had migraine headaches, epilepsy or porphyria.
- If you have diabetes, high blood pressure, asthma, congestive heart failure, kidney disease or gallstones.
- If you plan to become pregnant within 3 months.

Over age 60:
Controversial. You and your doctor must decide if drug risks outweigh benefits.

Pregnancy:
Risk to unborn child outweighs drug benefits. Don't use.

Breast-feeding:
Drug filters into milk. May harm child. Avoid.

Infants & children:
Not recommended.

Prolonged use:
Increased growth of fibroid tumors of uterus. Possible association with cancer of uterus.

Skin & sunlight:
May cause rash or intensify sunburn in areas exposed to sun or sunlamp.

Driving, piloting or hazardous work:
No problems expected.

Discontinuing:
You may need to discontinue ethinyl estradiol periodically. Consult your doctor.

Others:
In rare instances, may cause blood clot in lung, brain or leg. Symptoms are *sudden* severe headache, coordination loss, vision change, chest pain, breathing difficulty, slurred speech, pain in legs or groin. Seek emergency treatment immediately.

POSSIBLE INTERACTION WITH OTHER DRUGS

GENERIC NAME OR DRUG CLASS	COMBINED EFFECT
Anticoagulants, oral*	Decreased anti-coagulant effect.
Anticonvulsants, hydantoin*	Decreased effect of ethinyl estradiol.
Antidepressants, tricyclic (TCA)*	Increased toxicity of antidepressants.
Antidiabetics, oral*	Unpredictable increase or decrease in blood sugar.
Antifibrinolytic agents*	Increased possibility of blood clotting.
Carbamazepine	Decreased effect of ethinyl estradiol.
Clofibrate	Decreased clofibrate effect.
Insulin	Possible decreased insulin effect. May require dosage adjustment.
Meprobamate	Increased effect of ethinyl estradiol.
Phenobarbital	Decreased effect of ethinyl estradiol.
Primidone	Decreased effect of ethinyl estradiol.
Rifampin	Decreased effect of ethinyl estradiol.
Terazosin	Decreases effectiveness of terazosin.
Thyroid hormones*	Decreased thyroid effect.
Ursodiol	Decreased effect of ursodiol.
Vitamin C	Possible increased estrogen effect.

POSSIBLE INTERACTION WITH OTHER SUBSTANCES

INTERACTS WITH	COMBINED EFFECT
Alcohol:	None expected.
Beverages:	None expected.
Cocaine:	No proven problems.
Foods:	None expected.
Marijuana:	Possible menstrual irregularities and bleeding between periods.
Tobacco:	Increased risk of blood clots leading to stroke or heart attack.

*See Glossary

ETHOPROPAZINE

BRAND NAMES

Parsidol   Parsitan

BASIC INFORMATION

Habit forming? No
Prescription needed? Yes
Available as generic? No
Drug class: Antidyskinetic, antiparkinsonism

USES

Treatment of Parkinson's disease.

DOSAGE & USAGE INFORMATION

How to take:
Tablets, elixir or sustained-release capsules—
Take with food to lessen stomach irritation.

When to take:
At the same times each day.

If you forget a dose:
Take as soon as you remember up to 2 hours
late. If more than 2 hours, wait for next
scheduled dose (don't double this dose).

What drug does:
- Balances chemical reactions necessary to
  send nerve impulses within base of brain.
- Improves muscle control and reduces
  stiffness.

Time lapse before drug works:
1 to 2 hours.

Continued next column

OVERDOSE

SYMPTOMS:
Agitation, dilated pupils, hallucinations, dry
mouth, rapid heartbeat, sleepiness.
WHAT TO DO:
- Dial 0 (operator) or 911 (emergency) for
  an ambulance or medical help. Then give
  first aid immediately.
- If patient is unconscious and not
  breathing, give mouth-to-mouth
  breathing. If there is no heartbeat, use
  cardiac massage and mouth-to-mouth
  breathing (CPR). Don't try to make patient
  vomit. If you can't get help quickly, take
  patient to nearest emergency facility.
- See emergency information on inside
  covers.

Don't take with:
- Non-prescription drugs for colds, cough or
  allergy.
- See Interaction column and consult doctor.

POSSIBLE ADVERSE REACTIONS OR SIDE EFFECTS

SYMPTOMS	WHAT TO DO
Life-threatening: None expected.	
Common:	
• Blurred vision, light sensitivity, constipation, nausea, vomiting.	Continue. Call doctor when convenient.
• Painful or difficult urination, dry mouth.	Continue. Tell doctor at next visit.
Infrequent: None expected.	
Rare:	
• Seizures.	Discontinue. Seek emergency treatment.
• Rash, eye pain, hallucinations, hives, jaundice, delusions, amnesia, paranoia, fever, swollen glands in neck.	Discontinue. Call doctor right away.
• Confusion; dizziness; sore mouth or tongue; muscle cramps; numbness, weakness in hands or feet.	Continue. Call doctor when convenient.

ETHOPROPAZINE

WARNINGS & PRECAUTIONS

Don't take if:
You are allergic to any antidyskinetic.

Before you start, consult your doctor:
- If you have had glaucoma.
- If you have had high blood pressure or heart disease.
- If you have had impaired liver function.
- If you have had kidney disease or urination difficulty.

Over age 60:
More sensitive to drug. Aggravates symptoms of enlarged prostate. Causes impaired thinking, hallucinations, nightmares. Consult doctor about any of these.

Pregnancy:
Studies inconclusive on harm to unborn child. Animal studies show fetal abnormalities. Decide with your doctor whether drug benefits justify risk to unborn child.

Breast-feeding:
No problems expected.

Infants & children:
Not recommended for children 3 and younger. Use for older children only under doctor's supervision.

Prolonged use:
Possible glaucoma.

Skin & sunlight:
No problems expected.

Driving, piloting or hazardous work:
Don't drive or pilot aircraft until you learn how medicine affects you. Don't work around dangerous machinery. Don't climb ladders or work in high places. Danger increases if you drink alcohol or take medicine affecting alertness and reflexes, such as antihistamines, tranquilizers, sedatives, pain medicine, narcotics and mind-altering drugs.

Discontinuing:
Don't discontinue without consulting doctor. Dose may require gradual reduction if you have taken drug for a long time. Doses of other drugs may also require adjustment.

Others:
- Internal eye pressure should be measured regularly.
- Avoid becoming overheated.

POSSIBLE INTERACTION WITH OTHER DRUGS

GENERIC NAME OR DRUG CLASS	COMBINED EFFECT
Amantadine	Increased amantadine effect.
Antacids*	Possible decreased absorption.
Anticholinergics, other*	Increased anticholinergic effect.
Antidepressants, tricyclic (TCA)*	Increased ethopropazine effect. May cause glaucoma.
Antihistamines*	Increased ethopropazine effect.
Digoxin	Increased toxicity of digoxin.
Disopyramide	Increased anticholinergic effect.
Haloperidol	Possible behavior changes.
Levodopa	Possible increased levodopa effect.
MAO inhibitors*	Increased ethopropazine effect.
Meperidine	Increased ethopropazine effect.
Nabilone	Greater depression of central nervous system.
Phenothiazines*	Behavior changes.
Primidone	Excessive sedation.
Quinidine	Increased ethopropazine effect.
Slow-k (extended-release potassium)	Increased risk of gastric irritation.
Tranquilizers*	Excessive sedation.

POSSIBLE INTERACTION WITH OTHER SUBSTANCES

INTERACTS WITH	COMBINED EFFECT
Alcohol:	None expected.
Beverages:	None expected.
Cocaine:	Decreased ethopropazine effect. Avoid.
Foods:	None expected.
Marijuana:	None expected.
Tobacco:	None expected.

ETHOSUXIMIDE

BRAND NAMES

Zarontin

BASIC INFORMATION

Habit forming? No
Prescription needed? Yes
Available as generic? No
Drug class: Anticonvulsant (succinimide)

USES

Controls seizures in treatment of epilepsy.

DOSAGE & USAGE INFORMATION

How to take:
Capsule or syrup—Swallow with liquid or food to lessen stomach irritation.

When to take:
Every day in regularly-spaced doses, according to prescription.

If you forget a dose:
Take as soon as you remember up to 2 hours late. If more than 2 hours, wait for next scheduled dose (don't double this dose).

What drug does:
Depresses nerve transmissions in part of brain that controls muscles.

Time lapse before drug works:
3 hours.

Don't take with:
See Interaction column and consult doctor.

OVERDOSE

SYMPTOMS:
Coma
WHAT TO DO:
- Dial 0 (operator) or 911 (emergency) for an ambulance or medical help. Then give first aid immediately.
- If patient is unconscious and not breathing, give mouth-to-mouth breathing. If there is no heartbeat, use cardiac massage and mouth-to-mouth breathing (CPR). Don't try to make patient vomit. If you can't get help quickly, take patient to nearest emergency facility.
- See emergency information on inside covers.

POSSIBLE ADVERSE REACTIONS OR SIDE EFFECTS

SYMPTOMS	WHAT TO DO
Life-threatening: None expected.	
Common: Nausea, vomiting, stomach cramps, appetite loss, dizziness, drowsiness.	Continue. Call doctor when convenient.
Infrequent: Headache, irritability, blurred vision, mood change.	Continue. Call doctor when convenient.
Rare: • Sore throat, fever, rash, unusual bleeding or bruising, eye or gum swelling, blood in urine, vaginal bleeding, depression, confusion.	Discontinue. Call doctor right away.
• Swollen lymph glands.	Continue. Call doctor when convenient.

WARNINGS & PRECAUTIONS

Don't take if:
You are allergic to any succinimide anticonvulsant.

Before you start, consult your doctor:
- If you plan to become pregnant within medication period.
- If you take other anticonvulsants.
- If you have blood disease.
- If you have kidney or liver disease.

Over age 60:
Adverse reactions and side effects may be more frequent and severe than in younger persons.

Pregnancy:
Risk to unborn child outweighs drug benefits. Don't use.

Breast-feeding:
Drug passes into milk. Avoid drug or discontinue nursing.

Infants & children:
Use only under medical supervision.

Prolonged use:
No problems expected.

Skin & sunlight:
No problems expected.

Driving, piloting or hazardous work:
Don't drive or pilot aircraft until you learn how medicine affects you. Don't work around dangerous machinery. Don't climb ladders or work in high places. Danger increases if you drink alcohol or take medicine affecting alertness and reflexes, such as antihistamines, tranquilizers, sedatives, pain medicine, narcotics and mind-altering drugs.

Discontinuing:
Don't discontinue without doctor's advice until you complete prescribed dose, even though symptoms diminish or disappear.

Others:
- Your response to medicine should be checked regularly by your doctor. Dose and schedule may have to be altered frequently to fit individual needs.
- Periodic blood-cell counts, kidney- and liver-function studies recommended.
- May discolor urine pink to red-brown. No action necessary.

POSSIBLE INTERACTION WITH OTHER DRUGS

GENERIC NAME OR DRUG CLASS	COMBINED EFFECT
Anticonvulsants, other*	Increased effect of both drugs.
Antidepressants, tricyclic (TCA)*	May provoke seizures.
Antipsychotics*	May provoke seizures.

POSSIBLE INTERACTION WITH OTHER SUBSTANCES

INTERACTS WITH	COMBINED EFFECT
Alcohol:	May provoke seizures.
Beverages:	None expected.
Cocaine:	May provoke seizures.
Foods:	None expected.
Marijuana:	May provoke seizures.
Tobacco:	None expected.

*See Glossary

ETHOTOIN

BRAND NAMES

Peganone

BASIC INFORMATION

Habit forming? No
Prescription needed? Yes
Available as generic? No
Drug class: Anticonvulsant (hydantoin)

 USES

- Prevents epileptic seizures.
- Stabilizes irregular heartbeat.

 DOSAGE & USAGE INFORMATION

How to take:
- Tablet—Swallow with liquid.
- Chewable tablets—Chew well before swallowing.
- Suspension—Shake well before taking with liquid.

When to take:
At the same time each day.

If you forget a dose:
- If drug taken 1 time per day—Take as soon as you remember up to 12 hours late. If more than 12 hours, wait for next scheduled dose (don't double this dose).
- If taken several times per day—Take as soon as possible, then return to regular schedule.

What drug does:
Promotes sodium loss from nerve fibers. This lessens excitability and inhibits spread of nerve impulses.

Time lapse before drug works:
7 to 10 days continual use.

Don't take with:
See Interaction column and consult doctor.

 OVERDOSE

SYMPTOMS:
Jerky eye movements; stagger; slurred speech; imbalance; drowsiness; blood-pressure drop; slow, shallow breathing; coma.
WHAT TO DO:
- **Dial 0 (operator) or 911 (emergency) for an ambulance or medical help. Then give first aid immediately.**
- **See emergency information on inside covers.**

 POSSIBLE ADVERSE REACTIONS OR SIDE EFFECTS

SYMPTOMS	WHAT TO DO
Life-threatening: None expected.	
Common: Mild dizziness, drowsiness, nausea, vomiting, constipation.	Continue. Call doctor when convenient.
Infrequent: • Hallucinations, confusion, slurred speech, stagger, rash, change in vision.	Discontinue. Call doctor right away.
• Headache, diarrhea, sleeplessness, muscle twitching.	Continue. Call doctor when convenient.
• Increased body and facial hair.	Continue. Tell doctor at next visit.
Rare: Sore throat, fever, unusual bleeding or bruising, stomach pain, jaundice, swollen lymph glands.	Discontinue. Call doctor right away.

 WARNINGS & PRECAUTIONS

Don't take if:
You are allergic to any hydantoin anticonvulsant.

Before you start, consult your doctor:
- If you have had impaired liver function or disease.
- If you will have surgery within 2 months, including dental surgery, requiring general or spinal anesthesia.

Over age 60:
Adverse reactions and side effects may be more frequent and severe than in younger persons.

Pregnancy:
Risk to unborn child outweighs drug benefits. Don't use.

Breast-feeding:
Drug passes into milk. Avoid drug or discontinue nursing until you finish medicine. Consult doctor for advice on maintaining milk supply.

Infants & children:
Use only under medical supervision.

Prolonged use:
- Weakened bones.
- Lymph gland enlargement.
- Possible liver damage.
- Numbness and tingling of hands and feet.

- Continual back-and-forth eye movements.
- Bleeding, swollen or tender gums.

Skin & sunlight:
May cause rash or intensify sunburn in areas exposed to sun or sunlamp.

Driving, piloting or hazardous work:
Don't drive or pilot aircraft until you learn how medicine affects you. Don't work around dangerous machinery. Don't climb ladders or work in high places. Danger increases if you drink alcohol or take medicine affecting alertness and reflexes.

Discontinuing:
Don't discontinue without consulting doctor. Dose may require gradual reduction if you have taken drug for a long time. Doses of other drugs may also require adjustment.

Others:
No problems expected.

POSSIBLE INTERACTION WITH OTHER DRUGS

GENERIC NAME OR DRUG CLASS	COMBINED EFFECT
Anticoagulants*	Increased effect of both drugs.
Antidepressants, tricyclic (TCA)*	Need to adjust ethotoin dose.
Barbiturates*	Changed seizure pattern.
Carbamazepine	Possible increased ethotoin metabolism.
Carbonic anhydrase inhibitors*	Increased chance of bone disease.
Chloramphenicol	Increased ethotoin effect.
Cimetidine	Increased ethotoin toxicity.
Contraceptives, oral*	Increased seizures.
Cortisone drugs*	Decreased cortisone effect.
Cyclosporine	May decrease cyclosporine effect.
Digitalis preparations*	Decreased digitalis effect.
Disopyramide	Decreased disopyramide effect.
Disulfiram	Increased ethotoin effect.
Estrogens*	Increased estrogen effect.

Furosemide	Decreased furosemide effect.
Glutethimide	Decreased ethotoin effect.
Griseofulvin	Increased griseofulvin effect.
Hypoglycemics, other*	Possible decreased hypoglycemic effect.
Isoniazid	Increased ethotoin effect.
Methadone	Decreased methadone effect.
Methotrexate	Increased methotrexate effect.
Methylphenidate	Increased ethotoin effect.
Nicardipine	Increased anti-convulsant effect.
Oxyphenbutazone	Increased ethotoin effect.
Para-aminosalicylic acid (PAS)	Increased ethotoin effect.
Phenothiazines*	Increased ethotoin effect.
Phenylbutazone	Increased ethotoin effect.
Propranolol	Increased propranolol effect.
Quinidine	Increased quinidine effect.
Sedatives*	Increased sedative effect.
Sulfa drugs*	Increased ethotoin effect.
Theophylline	Reduced anticonvulsant effect.

POSSIBLE INTERACTION WITH OTHER SUBSTANCES

INTERACTS WITH	COMBINED EFFECT
Alcohol:	Possible decreased anticonvulsant effect. Use with caution.
Beverages:	None expected.
Cocaine:	Possible seizures.
Foods:	None expected.
Marijuana:	Drowsiness, unsteadiness, decreased anticonvulsant effect.
Tobacco:	None expected.

*See Glossary

ETRETINATE

BRAND NAMES

Teglson

BASIC INFORMATION

Habit forming? No
Prescription needed? Yes
Available as generic? No
Drug class: Antipsoriatic

 USES

- Treats psoriasis in patients who don't respond well to standard or usual treatment.
- Treats arthritic symptoms sometimes associated with psoriasis.
- Treats ichthyosis.

 DOSAGE & USAGE INFORMATION

How to take:
Capsules—Swallow with liquid or food to lessen stomach irritation. If you can't swallow whole, open capsule and take with liquid or food.

When to take:
At the same time each day, according to instructions on prescription label.

If you forget a dose:
Take as soon as you remember up to 2 hours late. If more than 2 hours, wait for next scheduled dose (don't double this dose).

What drug does:
- Mechanism of action on skin is unknown, but positive effects on the disease have been documented. It probably reduces the production of protein in the outer layers of skin. It is chemically related to Retin-A.
- Also functions as an anti-inflammatory agent.

Continued next column

 OVERDOSE

SYMPTOMS:
None documented. If overdose is suspected, follow instructions below.
WHAT TO DO:
- Dial 0 (operator) or 911 (emergency) for an ambulance or medical help. Then give first aid immediately.
- See emergency information on inside covers.

Time lapse before drug works:
- 2 to 6 hours for effects to begin.
- Prolonged treatment, up to 2 to 4 weeks (sometimes with psoralens, ultraviolet light may be necessary to develop maximum benefit).

Don't take with:
See Interaction column and consult doctor.

 POSSIBLE ADVERSE REACTIONS OR SIDE EFFECTS

SYMPTOMS	WHAT TO DO
Life-threatening: None expected.	
Common:	
• Bone and joint pain, eye irritation.	Discontinue. Call doctor right away.
• Dry skin and eyes, nosebleeds, hair loss.	Continue. Call doctor when convenient.
Infrequent: Muscle cramps, blurred vision, hearing loss, dark-colored urine, jaundice, unusual bleeding or bruising.	Discontinue. Call doctor right away.
Rare:	
• Itching, peeling skin; inflamed nails; nausea; vomiting; headache.	Discontinue. Call doctor right away.
• Confusion, depression.	Continue. Call doctor when convenient.

WARNINGS & PRECAUTIONS

Don't take if:
If you are pregnant or expect to get pregnant soon.

Before you start, consult your doctor:
- If you have heart or blood vessel disease.
- If you have immediate family members with heart or blood vessel disease.
- If you have high plasma triglycerides.
- If you are an alcoholic.
- If you have diabetes mellitus.
- If you have liver disease.

Over age 60:
Adverse reactions and side effects may be more frequent and severe than in younger persons. You may need smaller doses for shorter periods of time.

Pregnancy:
Risk to unborn child outweighs drug benefits. Don't use.

Breast-feeding:
Drug passes into milk. Avoid drug or discontinue nursing until you finish medicine. Consult doctor for advice on maintaining milk supply.

Infants & children:
Don't use.

Prolonged use:
No problems expected, if used for no more than 4 months per treatment session.

Skin & sunlight:
May cause increased sensitivity to sunlight. Avoid when possible.

Driving, piloting or hazardous work:
Don't drive or pilot aircraft until you learn how medicine affects you. Don't work around dangerous machinery. Don't climb ladders or work in high places. Danger increases if you drink alcohol or take medicine affecting alertness and reflexes.

Discontinuing:
Don't discontinue without consulting doctor. Dose may require gradual reduction if you have taken drug for a long time. Doses of other drugs may also require adjustment.

Others:
- Courses of treatment are usually limited to 4 months, and repeating, if necessary, after a 4-month rest period.
- Don't donate blood during treatment or for several years thereafter.
- Likelihood of producing cancer is very low.
- During early treatment, psoriasis may appear to worsen.

POSSIBLE INTERACTION WITH OTHER DRUGS

GENERIC NAME OR DRUG CLASS	COMBINED EFFECT
Abrasive soaps or cleaners	Excessive drying effect on skin.
Acne preparations*	Excessive drying effect on skin.
Any topical preparation containing alcohol, such as after-shave lotions	Excessive drying effect on skin.
Isoretinoin	Increased toxicity.
Medicated cosmetics	Excessive drying effect on skin.
Methotrexate	Increased toxicity to liver.
Tetracyclines*	Increased adverse reactions of etretinate.
Tretinoin	Increased toxicity.
Vitamin A	Increased toxicity.

POSSIBLE INTERACTION WITH OTHER SUBSTANCES

INTERACTS WITH	COMBINED EFFECT
Alcohol:	May cause hypertriglyceridemia.
Beverages: Milk	Aids absorption of etretinate.
Cocaine:	None expected.
Foods: High-fat diet or milk products.	Aids absorption of etretinate.
Marijuana:	None expected.
Tobacco:	None expected.

*See Glossary

FAMOTIDINE

BRAND NAMES

Pepcid

BASIC INFORMATION

Habit forming? No
Prescription needed? Yes
Available as generic? No
Drug class: Antiulcer; stomach acid inhibitor

 USES

Treats duodenal ulcers, excess stomach acid secretion, Zollinger-Ellison syndrome, stomach ulcer, gastroesophageal reflux.

 DOSAGE & USAGE INFORMATION

How to take:
- Oral solution—Take after meals with liquid to decrease stomach irritation.
- Tablets—Swallow with liquid or food to lessen stomach irritation. If you can't swallow whole, crumble tablet and take with liquid or food.

When to take:
At the same time each day, according to instructions on prescription label.

If you forget a dose:
Take as soon as you remember up to 2 hours late. If more than 2 hours, wait for next scheduled dose (don't double this dose).

What drug does:
Decreases stomach acid production by interfering with action of histamine at H2-receptor sites.

Time lapse before drug works:
1 hour.

Don't take with:
See Interaction column and consult doctor.

 OVERDOSE

SYMPTOMS:
Fast, pounding heartbeat; seizures; coma.
WHAT TO DO:
- Dial 0 (operator) or 911 (emergency) for an ambulance or medical help. Then give first aid immediately.
- See emergency information on inside covers.

 POSSIBLE ADVERSE REACTIONS OR SIDE EFFECTS

SYMPTOMS	WHAT TO DO
Life-threatening:	
Quick swelling of eyelids (allergic reaction), tightness in chest.	Discontinue. Seek emergency treatment.
Common:	
None expected.	
Infrequent:	
• Upper abdominal pain.	Discontinue. Call doctor right away.
• Constipation, diarrhea, decreased sex drive, anxiety, depression.	Continue. Call doctor when convenient.
Rare:	
• Fast heartbeat, unusual bleeding or bruising, itching, skin rash.	Discontinue. Call doctor right away.
• Unusual taste in mouth, hair loss.	Continue. Call doctor when convenient.

WARNINGS & PRECAUTIONS

Don't take if:
You have severe kidney disease.

Before you start, consult your doctor:
If you have liver disease.

Over age 60:
Adverse reactions and side effects may be more frequent and severe than in younger persons. You may need smaller doses for shorter periods of time.

Pregnancy:
Risk to unborn child outweighs drug benefits. Don't use.

Breast-feeding:
Drug passes into milk. Avoid drug or discontinue nursing until you finish medicine. Consult doctor for advice on maintaining milk supply.

Infants & children:
Not recommended.

Prolonged use:
Not recommended.

Skin & sunlight:
No problems expected.

Driving, piloting or hazardous work:
Don't drive or pilot aircraft until you learn how medicine affects you. Don't work around dangerous machinery. Don't climb ladders or work in high places. Danger increases if you drink alcohol or take medicine affecting alertness and reflexes.

Discontinuing:
Don't discontinue without consulting doctor. Dose may require gradual reduction if you have taken drug for a long time. Doses of other drugs may also require adjustment.

Others:
May interfere with accurate results of skin testing for allergies.

POSSIBLE INTERACTION WITH OTHER DRUGS

GENERIC NAME OR DRUG CLASS	COMBINED EFFECT
Ketoconazole	Reduced absorption of ketoconazole. Take famotidine at least 2 hours after any dose of ketoconazole.

POSSIBLE INTERACTION WITH OTHER SUBSTANCES

INTERACTS WITH	COMBINED EFFECT
Alcohol:	Decreased effect of famotidine.
Beverages: Any containing caffeine, such as coffee, tea or cocoa.	Decreased effect of famotidine.
Cocaine:	Decreased effect of famotidine.
Foods:	None expected.
Marijuana:	Decreased effect of famotidine.
Tobacco:	Decreased effect of famotidine.

FENOPROFEN

BRAND NAMES

Fenopron   Progesic
Nalfon

BASIC INFORMATION

Habit forming? No
Available as generic? No
Prescription needed? Yes
Drug class: Anti-inflammatory (non-steroid)

USES

- Treatment for joint pain, stiffness, inflammation and swelling of arthritis and gout.
- Pain reliever.
- Treatment for dysmenorrhea (painful or difficult menstruation).
- Treats juvenile rheumatoid arthritis.

DOSAGE & USAGE INFORMATION

How to take:
Tablet or capsule—Swallow with liquid or food to lessen stomach irritation. If you can't swallow whole, crumble tablet or open capsule and take with liquid or food.

When to take:
At the same times each day.

If you forget a dose:
Take as soon as you remember up to 2 hours late. If more than 2 hours, wait for next scheduled dose (don't double this dose).

What drug does:
Reduces tissue concentration of prostaglandins (hormones which produce inflammation and pain).

Time lapse before drug works:
Begins in 4 to 24 hours. May require 3 weeks regular use for maximum benefit.

Don't take with:
See Interaction column and consult doctor.

OVERDOSE

SYMPTOMS:
Confusion, agitation, incoherence, convulsions, possible hemorrhage from stomach or intestine, coma.
WHAT TO DO:
- Dial 0 (operator) or 911 (emergency) for an ambulance or medical help. Then give first aid immediately.
- See emergency information on inside covers.

POSSIBLE ADVERSE REACTIONS OR SIDE EFFECTS

SYMPTOMS	WHAT TO DO
Life-threatening: Hives, rash, intense itching, faintness soon after a dose (anaphylaxis in aspirin-sensitive persons).	Seek emergency treatment immediately.
Common: • Dizziness, nausea, pain.	Continue. Call doctor when convenient.
• Headache.	Continue. Tell doctor at next visit.
Infrequent: Depression; drowsiness; ringing in ears; swollen feet, legs; constipation or diarrhea; vomiting.	Continue. Call doctor when convenient.
Rare: • Convulsions; confusion, rash, hives or itch; black or bloody, tarry stools; difficult breathing; tightness in chest; blurred vision; rapid heartbeat; unusual bleeding or bruising; blood in urine; jaundice; severe abdominal pain; psychosis.	Discontinue. Call doctor right away.
• Urgent, frequent or painful urination; fatigue; weakness; swollen breasts in males; impotence; menstrual irregularities.	Continue. Call doctor when convenient.

WARNINGS & PRECAUTIONS

Don't take if:
- You are allergic to aspirin or any non-steroid, anti-inflammatory drug.
- You have gastritis, peptic ulcer, enteritis, ileitis, ulcerative colitis, asthma, heart failure, high blood pressure or bleeding problems.
- Patient is younger than 15.

Before you start, consult your doctor:
- If you have epilepsy.
- If you have Parkinson's disease.
- If you have been mentally ill.
- If you have had kidney disease or impaired kidney function.

Over age 60:
Adverse reactions and side effects may be more frequent and severe than in younger persons.

Pregnancy:
Studies inconclusive on harm to unborn child. Decide with your doctor whether drug benefits justify risk to unborn child.

Breast-feeding:
May harm child. Avoid.

Infants & children:
Not recommended for anyone younger than 15. Use only under medical supervision.

Prolonged use:
- Eye damage.
- Reduced hearing.
- Sore throat, fever.
- Weight gain.

Skin & sunlight:
Increased sensitivity to sunlight.

Driving, piloting or hazardous work:
Don't drive or pilot aircraft until you learn how medicine affects you. Don't work around dangerous machinery. Don't climb ladders or work in high places. Danger increases if you drink alcohol or take medicine affecting alertness and reflexes, such as antihistamines, tranquilizers, sedatives, pain medicine, narcotics and mind-altering drugs.

Discontinuing:
Don't discontinue without consulting doctor. Dose may require gradual reduction if you have taken drug for a long time. Doses of other drugs may also require adjustment.

Others:
No problems expected.

POSSIBLE INTERACTION WITH OTHER DRUGS

GENERIC NAME OR DRUG CLASS	COMBINED EFFECT
ACE inhibitors: captopril, enalapril, lisinopril*	May decrease ACE inhibitor effect.
Anticoagulants, oral*	Increased risk of bleeding.
Aspirin	Increased risk of stomach ulcer.
Beta-adrenergic blockers*	Decreased antihypertensive effect.
Carteolol	Decreased antihypertensive effect of carteolol.
Cortisone drugs*	Increased risk of stomach ulcer.
Diuretics*	May decrease diuretic effect.
Lithium	Possible increased lithium effect and toxicity.
Methotrexate	May increase toxicity.
Oxyphenbutazone	Possible stomach ulcer.
Phenobarbital	Possible decreased fenoprofen effect.
Phenylbutazone	Possible stomach ulcer.
Probenecid	Increased fenoprofen effect.
Sotalol	Decreased antihypertensive effect of sotalol.
Terazosin	Decreased terazosin effect. Causes sodium and fluid retention.
Thyroid hormones*	Rapid heartbeat, blood-pressure rise.

POSSIBLE INTERACTION WITH OTHER SUBSTANCES

INTERACTS WITH	COMBINED EFFECT
Alcohol:	Possible stomach ulcer or bleeding.
Beverages:	None expected.
Cocaine:	None expected.
Foods:	None expected.
Marijuana:	Increased pain relief from fenoprofen.
Tobacco:	None expected.

*See Glossary

FERROUS FUMARATE

BRAND NAMES

See complete list of brand names in the *Brand Name Directory*, page 1063.

BASIC INFORMATION

Habit forming? No
Prescription needed?
  With folic acid: Yes
  Without folic acid: No
Available as generic? Yes
Drug class: Mineral supplement (iron)

USES

Treatment for dietary iron deficiency or iron-deficiency anemia from other causes.

DOSAGE & USAGE INFORMATION

How to take:
- Tablet, chewable tablet, extended-release capsule or liquid—Swallow with liquid or food to lessen stomach irritation. If you can't swallow whole, crumble tablet or open capsule and take with liquid or food. Place medicine far back on tongue to avoid staining teeth.
- Drops—Dilute dose in beverage before swallowing and drink through a straw.

When to take:
1 hour before or 2 hours after meals.

If you forget a dose:
Take up to 2 hours late. If more than 2 hours, wait for next dose (don't double this dose).

What drug does:
Stimulates bone-marrow production of hemoglobin (red-blood-cell pigment that carries oxygen to body cells).

Continued next column

OVERDOSE

SYMPTOMS:
Weakness, collapse; pallor, blue lips, hands and fingernails; weak, rapid heartbeat; shallow breathing; convulsions; coma.
WHAT TO DO:
- **Dial 0 (operator) or 911 (emergency) for an ambulance or medical help. Then give first aid immediately.**
- **See emergency information on inside covers.**

Time lapse before drug works:
3 to 7 days. May require 3 weeks for maximum benefit.

Don't take with:
- Multiple vitamin and mineral supplements.
- See Interaction column and consult doctor.

POSSIBLE ADVERSE REACTIONS OR SIDE EFFECTS

SYMPTOMS	WHAT TO DO
Life-threatening: Weak, rapid heartbeat.	Seek emergency treatment immediately.
Always: Gray or black stool.	No action necessary.
Common: Stained teeth with liquid iron.	No action necessary.
Infrequent:	
• Constipation or diarrhea, heartburn, nausea, vomiting.	Discontinue. Call doctor right away.
• Fatigue, weakness.	Continue. Call doctor when convenient.
• Dark urine.	Continue. Tell doctor at next visit.
Rare:	
• Throat or chest pain on swallowing, pain, cramps, blood in stool.	Discontinue. Call doctor right away.
• Drowsiness.	Continue. Call doctor when convenient.

WARNINGS & PRECAUTIONS

Don't take if:
- You are allergic to any iron supplement or tartrazine dye.
- You take iron injections.
- Your daily iron intake is high.
- You plan to take this supplement for a long time.
- You have acute hepatitis.
- You have hemosiderosis or hemochromatosis (conditions involving excess iron in body).
- You have hemolytic anemia.

Before you start, consult your doctor:
- If you plan to become pregnant within medication period.
- If you have had stomach surgery.
- If you have had peptic ulcer disease, enteritis or colitis.
- If you have had pancreatitis or hepatitis.

Over age 60:
May cause hemochromatosis (iron storage disease) with bronze skin, liver damage, diabetes, heart problems and impotence.

Pregnancy:
No proven harm to unborn child. Avoid if possible. Take only if your doctor prescribes supplement during last half of pregnancy.

Breast-feeding:
No problems expected. Take only if your doctor confirms you have a dietary deficiency or an iron-deficiency anemia.

Infants & children:
Use only under medical supervision. Overdose common and dangerous. Keep out of children's reach.

Prolonged use:
May cause hemochromatosis (iron storage disease) with bronze skin, liver damage, diabetes, heart problems and impotence.

Skin & sunlight:
No problems expected.

Driving, piloting or hazardous work:
No problems expected.

Discontinuing:
May be unnecessary to finish medicine. Follow doctor's instructions.

Others:
- Liquid form stains teeth. Mix with water or juice to lessen the effect. Brush with baking soda or hydrogen peroxide to help remove stain.
- Some products contain tartrazine dye. Avoid, especially if you are allergic to aspirin.

POSSIBLE INTERACTION WITH OTHER DRUGS

GENERIC NAME OR DRUG CLASS	COMBINED EFFECT
Acetohydroxamic acid	Decreased effects of both drugs.
Allopurinol	Possible excess iron storage in liver.
Antacids*	Poor iron absorption.
Chloramphenicol	Decreased effect of iron. Interferes with red-blood-cell and hemoglobin formation.
Cholestyramine	Decreased iron effect.
Iron supplements, other*	Possible excess iron storage in liver.
Penicillamine	Decreased penicillamine effect.
Tetracyclines*	Decreased tetracycline effect. Take iron 3 hours before or 2 hours after taking tetracycline.
Vitamin C	Increased iron effect.

POSSIBLE INTERACTION WITH OTHER SUBSTANCES

INTERACTS WITH	COMBINED EFFECT
Alcohol:	Increased iron absorption. May cause organ damage. Avoid or use in moderation.
Beverages: Milk, tea.	Decreased iron effect.
Cocaine:	None expected.
Foods: Dairy foods, eggs, whole-grain bread and cereal.	Decreased iron effect.
Marijuana:	None expected.
Tobacco:	None expected.

FERROUS GLUCONATE

BRAND NAMES

Apo-Ferrous
  Gluconate
Fergon
Ferralet
Ferralet Plus
Ferrous-G
Fertinic
Fosfree

Glytinic
I.L.X. B-12
Iromin-G
Megadose
Mission
Novoferrogluc
Simron

BASIC INFORMATION

Habit forming? No
Prescription needed?
  With folic acid: Yes
  Without folic acid: No
Available as generic? Yes
Drug class: Mineral supplement (iron)

USES

Treatment for dietary iron deficiency or iron-deficiency anemia from other causes.

DOSAGE & USAGE INFORMATION

How to take:
- Tablet, capsule or syrup—Swallow with liquid or food to lessen stomach irritation. If you can't swallow whole, crumble tablet or open capsule and take with liquid or food. Place medicine far back on tongue to avoid staining teeth.
- Elixir—Dilute dose in beverage before swallowing and drink through a straw.

When to take:
1 hour before or 2 hours after eating.

If you forget a dose:
Take up to 2 hours late. If more than 2 hours, wait for next dose (don't double this dose).

Continued next column

OVERDOSE

SYMPTOMS:
- **Moderate overdose—Stomach pain, vomiting, diarrhea, black stools, lethargy.**
- **Serious overdose—Weakness and collapse; pallor, weak and rapid heartbeat; shallow breathing; convulsions and coma.**

WHAT TO DO:
- **Dial 0 (operator) or 911 (emergency) for an ambulance or medical help. Then give first aid immediately.**
- **See emergency information on inside covers.**

What drug does:
Stimulates bone-marrow production of hemoglobin (red-blood-cell pigment that carries oxygen to body cells).

Time lapse before drug works:
3 to 7 days. May require 3 weeks for maximum benefit.

Don't take with:
- Multiple vitamin and mineral supplements.
- See Interaction column and consult doctor.

POSSIBLE ADVERSE REACTIONS OR SIDE EFFECTS

SYMPTOMS	WHAT TO DO
Life-threatening: Weak, rapid heartbeat.	Seek emergency treatment immediately.
Always: Gray or black stool.	No action necessary.
Common: Stained teeth with liquid iron.	No action necessary.
Infrequent:	
• Constipation or diarrhea, heartburn, nausea, vomiting.	Discontinue. Call doctor right away.
• Fatigue, weakness.	Continue. Call doctor when convenient.
Rare:	
• Blue lips, fingernails, palms of hands; pale, clammy skin.	Discontinue. Seek emergency treatment.
• Throat pain on swallowing, pain, cramps, blood in stool.	Discontinue. Call doctor right away.
• Drowsiness.	Continue. Call doctor when convenient.

WARNINGS & PRECAUTIONS

Don't take if:
- You are allergic to any iron supplement or tartrazine dye.
- You take iron injections.
- You have acute hepatitis, hemosiderosis or hemochromatosis (conditions involving excess iron in body).
- You have hemolytic anemia.

Before you start, consult your doctor:
- If you plan to become pregnant within medication period.
- If you have had stomach surgery.
- If you have had peptic ulcer, enteritis or colitis.

Over age 60:
May cause hemochromatosis (iron storage disease) with bronze skin, liver damage, diabetes, heart problems and impotence.

Pregnancy:
No proven harm to unborn child. Avoid if possible. Take only if your doctor advises supplement during last half of pregnancy.

Breast-feeding:
No problems expected. Take only if your doctor confirms you have a dietary deficiency or an iron-deficiency anemia.

Infants & children:
Use only under medical supervision. Overdose common and dangerous. Keep out of children's reach.

Prolonged use:
May cause hemochromatosis (iron storage disease) with bronze skin, liver damage, diabetes, heart problems and impotence.

Skin & sunlight:
No problems expected.

Driving, piloting or hazardous work:
No problems expected.

Discontinuing:
May be unnecessary to finish medicine. Follow doctor's instructions.

Others:
- Liquid form stains teeth. Mix with water or juice to lessen the effect. Brush with baking soda or hydrogen peroxide to help remove stain.
- Some products contain tartrazine dye. Avoid, especially if you are allergic to aspirin.

POSSIBLE INTERACTION WITH OTHER DRUGS

GENERIC NAME OR DRUG CLASS	COMBINED EFFECT
Acetohydroxamic acid	Decreased effects of both drugs.
Allopurinol	Possible excess iron storage in liver.
Antacids*	Poor iron absorption.
Chloramphenicol	Decreased effect of iron. Interferes with red-blood-cell and hemoglobin formation.
Cholestyramine	Decreased iron effect.
Iron supplements, other*	Possible excess iron storage in liver.
Tetracyclines*	Decreased tetracycline effect. Take iron 3 hours before or 2 hours after taking tetracycline.
Vitamin C	Increased iron effect.

POSSIBLE INTERACTION WITH OTHER SUBSTANCES

INTERACTS WITH	COMBINED EFFECT
Alcohol:	Increased iron absorption. May cause organ damage. Avoid or use in moderation.
Beverages: Milk, tea.	Decreased iron effect.
Cocaine:	None expected.
Foods: Dairy foods, eggs, whole-grain bread and cereal.	Decreased iron effect.
Marijuana:	None expected.
Tobacco:	None expected.

FERROUS SULFATE

BRAND NAMES

See complete list of brand names in the *Brand Name Directory*, page 1063.

BASIC INFORMATION

Habit forming? No
Prescription needed?
  With folic acid: Yes
  Without folic acid: No
Available as generic? Yes
Drug class: Mineral supplement (iron)

 ## USES

Treatment for dietary iron deficiency or iron-deficiency anemia from other causes.

 ## DOSAGE & USAGE INFORMATION

How to take:
- Tablet, capsule, or liquid—Swallow with liquid or food to lessen stomach irritation. Place medicine far back on tongue to avoid staining teeth.
- Drops—Dilute dose in beverage before swallowing and drink through a straw.
- Extended-release tablet or capsule—Swallow whole with liquid.

When to take:
1 hour before or 2 hours after meals.

If you forget a dose:
Take up to 2 hours late. If more than 2 hours, wait for next dose (don't double this dose).

What drug does:
Stimulates bone-marrow production of hemoglobin (red-blood-cell pigment that carries oxygen to body cells).

Time lapse before drug works:
3 to 7 days. May require 3 weeks for maximum benefit.

Continued next column

 ## OVERDOSE

SYMPTOMS:
Weakness, collapse; pallor, blue lips, hands and fingernails; weak, rapid heartbeat; shallow breathing; convulsions; coma.
WHAT TO DO:
- **Dial 0 (operator) or 911 (emergency) for an ambulance or medical help. Then give first aid immediately.**
- **See emergency information on inside covers.**

Don't take with:
- Multiple vitamin and mineral supplements.
- See Interaction column and consult doctor.

 ## POSSIBLE ADVERSE REACTIONS OR SIDE EFFECTS

SYMPTOMS	WHAT TO DO
Life-threatening: Weak, rapid heartbeat.	Seek emergency treatment immediately.
Always: Gray or black stool.	No action necessary.
Common: Stained teeth with liquid iron.	No action necessary.
Infrequent: • Constipation or diarrhea, heartburn, nausea, vomiting.	Discontinue. Call doctor right away.
• Fatigue, weakness.	Continue. Call doctor when convenient.
• Dark urine.	Continue. Tell doctor at next visit.
Rare: • Throat or chest pain on swallowing, pain, cramps, blood in stool.	Discontinue. Call doctor right away.
• Drowsiness.	Continue. Call doctor when convenient.

WARNINGS & PRECAUTIONS

Don't take if:
- You are allergic to any iron supplement or tartrazine dye.
- You take iron injections.
- Your daily iron intake is high.
- You plan to take this supplement for a long time.
- You have acute hepatitis.
- You have hemosiderosis or hemochromatosis (conditions involving excess iron in body).
- You have hemolytic anemia.

Before you start, consult your doctor:
- If you plan to become pregnant within medication period.
- If you have had stomach surgery.
- If you have had peptic ulcer disease, enteritis or colitis.
- If you have had pancreatitis or hepatitis.

Over age 60:
May cause hemochromatosis (iron storage disease) with bronze skin, liver damage, diabetes, heart problems and impotence.

Pregnancy:
No proven harm to unborn child. Avoid if possible. Take only if your doctor prescribes supplement during last half of pregnancy.

Breast-feeding:
No problems expected. Take only if your doctor confirms you have a dietary deficiency or an iron-deficiency anemia.

Infants & children:
Use only under medical supervision. Overdose common and dangerous. Keep out of children's reach.

Prolonged use:
May cause hemochromatosis (iron storage disease) with bronze skin, liver damage, diabetes, heart problems and impotence.

Skin & sunlight:
No problems expected.

Driving, piloting or hazardous work:
No problems expected.

Discontinuing:
May be unnecessary to finish medicine. Follow doctor's instructions.

Others:
- Liquid form stains teeth. Mix with water or juice to lessen the effect. Brush with baking soda or hydrogen peroxide to help remove stain.
- Some products contain tartrazine dye. Avoid, especially if you are allergic to aspirin.

POSSIBLE INTERACTION WITH OTHER DRUGS

GENERIC NAME OR DRUG CLASS	COMBINED EFFECT
Acetohydroxamic acid	Decreased effects of both drugs.
Allopurinol	Possible excess iron storage in liver.
Antacids*	Poor iron absorption.
Chloramphenicol	Decreased effect of iron. Interferes with red-blood-cell and hemoglobin formation.
Cholestyramine	Decreased iron effect.
Iron supplements, other*	Possible excess iron storage in liver.
Penicillamine	Decreased penicillamine effect.
Tetracyclines*	Decreased tetracycline effect. Take iron 3 hours before or 2 hours after taking tetracycline.
Vitamin C	Increased iron effect.

POSSIBLE INTERACTION WITH OTHER SUBSTANCES

INTERACTS WITH	COMBINED EFFECT
Alcohol:	Increased iron absorption. May cause organ damage. Avoid or use in moderation.
Beverages: Milk, tea.	Decreased iron effect.
Cocaine:	None expected.
Foods: Dairy foods, eggs, whole-grain bread and cereal.	Decreased iron effect.
Marijuana:	None expected.
Tobacco:	None expected.

FLAVOXATE

BRAND NAMES

Urispas

BASIC INFORMATION

Habit forming? No
Prescription needed? Yes
Available as generic? No
Drug class: Smooth-muscle relaxant, anticholinergic

 ## USES

Relieves urinary pain, urgency, nighttime urination, unusual frequency of urination associated with urinary system disorders.

 ## DOSAGE & USAGE INFORMATION

How to take:
Tablet—Swallow with liquid or food to lessen stomach irritation.

When to take:
30 minutes before meals (unless directed otherwise by doctor).

If you forget a dose:
Take as soon as you remember up to 2 hours late. If more than 2 hours, wait for next scheduled dose (don't double this dose).

What drug does:
Blocks nerve impulses at smooth muscle nerve endings, preventing muscle contractions and gland secretions of organs involved.

Time lapse before drug works:
15 to 30 minutes.

Don't take with:
See Interaction column and consult doctor.

 ## OVERDOSE

SYMPTOMS:
Dilated pupils, rapid pulse and breathing, dizziness, fever, hallucinations, confusion, slurred speech, agitation, flushed face, convulsions, coma.
WHAT TO DO:
- **Dial 0 (operator) or 911 (emergency) for an ambulance or medical help. Then give first aid immediately.**
- **See emergency information on inside covers.**

 ## POSSIBLE ADVERSE REACTIONS OR SIDE EFFECTS

SYMPTOMS	WHAT TO DO
Life-threatening: None expected.	
Common:	
• Confusion, delirium, rapid heartbeat.	Discontinue. Call doctor right away.
• Nausea, vomiting, less perspiration.	Continue. Call doctor when convenient.
• Constipation.	Continue. Tell doctor at next visit.
• Dry ears, nose, throat.	No action necessary.
Infrequent:	
• Unusual excitement, irritability, restlessness.	Discontinue. Call doctor right away.
• Headache, increased sensitivity to light, painful or difficult urination.	Continue. Call doctor when convenient.
Rare:	
• Shortness of breath.	Discontinue. Seek emergency treatment.
• Rash or hives; pain; blurred vision; sore throat, fever, mouth sores.	Discontinue. Call doctor right away.
• Dizziness.	Continue. Call doctor when convenient.

WARNINGS & PRECAUTIONS

Don't take if:
- You are allergic to any anticholinergic.
- You have trouble with stomach bloating.
- You have difficulty emptying your bladder completely.
- You have narrow-angle glaucoma.
- You have severe ulcerative colitis.

Before you start, consult your doctor:
- If you have open-angle glaucoma.
- If you have angina.
- If you have chronic bronchitis or asthma.
- If you have liver disease.
- If you have hiatal hernia.
- If you have enlarged prostate.
- If you have myasthenia gravis.
- If you have peptic ulcer.
- If you will have surgery within 2 months, including dental surgery, requiring general or spinal anesthesia.

Over age 60:
Adverse reactions and side effects, particularly mental confusion, may be more frequent and severe than in younger persons.

Pregnancy:
Studies inconclusive on harm to unborn child. Animal studies show fetal abnormalities. Decide with your doctor whether drug benefits justify risk to unborn child.

Breast-feeding:
Drug passes into milk. Avoid drug or discontinue nursing until you finish medicine. Consult doctor for advice on maintaining milk supply.

Infants & children:
Use only under medical supervision.

Prolonged use:
Chronic constipation, possible fecal impaction. Consult doctor immediately.

Skin & sunlight:
No problems expected.

Driving, piloting or hazardous work:
Use disqualifies you for piloting aircraft. Otherwise, no problems expected.

Discontinuing:
May be unnecessary to finish medicine. Follow doctor's instructions.

Others:
No problems expected.

POSSIBLE INTERACTION WITH OTHER DRUGS

GENERIC NAME OR DRUG CLASS	COMBINED EFFECT
Antimuscarinics*	Increased effect of flavoxate.
Central nervous system (CNS) depressants, other*	Increased effect of both drugs.
Ethinamate	Dangerous increased effects of ethinamate. Avoid combining.
Fluoxetine	Increased depressant effects of both drugs.
Guanfacine	May increase depressant effects of either drug.
Leucovorin	High alcohol content of leucovorin may cause adverse effects.
Methyprylon	Increased sedative effect, perhaps to dangerous level. Avoid.
Nabilone	Greater depression of central nervous system.
Nizatidine	Increased nizatidine effect.

POSSIBLE INTERACTION WITH OTHER SUBSTANCES

INTERACTS WITH	COMBINED EFFECT
Alcohol:	None expected.
Beverages:	None expected.
Cocaine:	Excessively rapid heartbeat. Avoid.
Foods:	None expected.
Marijuana:	Drowsiness, dry mouth.
Tobacco:	None expected.

FLECAINIDE ACETATE

BRAND NAMES

Tambocor

BASIC INFORMATION

Habit forming? No
Prescription needed? Yes
Available as generic? No
Drug class: Antiarrhythmic

 ## USES

Stabilizes irregular heartbeat.

 ## DOSAGE & USAGE INFORMATION

How to take:
Tablet—Swallow with liquid. If you can't swallow whole, crumble tablet and take with liquid or food.

When to take:
At the same time each day, according to instructions on prescription label. Take tablets approximately 12 hours apart.

If you forget a dose:
Take as soon as you remember up to 4 hours late. If more than 4 hours, wait for next scheduled dose (don't double this dose).

What drug does:
Decreases conduction of abnormal electrical activity in the heart muscle or its regulating systems.

Time lapse before drug works:
1 to 6 hours. May need doses daily for 2 to 3 days for maximum effect.

Continued next column

 ## OVERDOSE

SYMPTOMS:
Low blood pressure or unconsciousness, irregular or rapid heartbeat, sleepiness, tremor, sweating.
WHAT TO DO:
- Dial 0 (operator) or 911 (emergency) for an ambulance or medical help. Then give first aid immediately.
- If patient is unconscious and not breathing, give mouth-to-mouth breathing. If there is no heartbeat, use cardiac massage and mouth-to-mouth breathing (CPR). Don't try to make patient vomit. If you can't get help quickly, take patient to nearest emergency facility.
- See emergency information on inside covers.

Don't take with:
See Interaction column and consult doctor.

 ## POSSIBLE ADVERSE REACTIONS OR SIDE EFFECTS

SYMPTOMS	WHAT TO DO
Life-threatening: None expected.	
Common: Blurred vision, dizziness.	Continue. Call doctor when convenient.
Infrequent:	
• Chest pain, irregular heartbeat.	Discontinue. Seek emergency treatment.
• Shakiness, rash, nausea, vomiting.	Discontinue. Call doctor right away.
• Anxiety; depression; weakness; headache; appetite loss; weakness in muscles, bones, joints; swollen feet, ankles or legs; loss of taste; numbness or tingling in hands or feet.	Continue. Call doctor when convenient.
• Constipation.	Continue. Tell doctor at next visit.
Rare:	
• Shortness of breath.	Discontinue. Seek emergency treatment.
• Unusual bleeding or bruising; sore throat; jaundice; fever; chills; swelling of lips, mouth, tongue; rash; frequent urination; urinary retention; muscle ache.	Discontinue. Call doctor right away.
• Impotence.	Continue. Call doctor when convenient.

WARNINGS & PRECAUTIONS

Don't take if:
You are allergic to flecainide or a local anesthetic such as novocaine, xylocaine or other drug whose generic name ends with "caine."

Before you start, consult your doctor:
- If you have kidney disease.
- If you have liver disease.
- If you have had a heart attack in past 3 weeks.
- If you have a pacemaker.

Over age 60:
Adverse reactions and side effects may be more frequent and severe than in younger persons.

Pregnancy:
Studies inconclusive on harm to unborn child. Animal studies show fetal abnormalities. Decide with your doctor whether drug benefits justify risk to unborn child.

Breast-feeding:
No proven problems.

Infants & children:
Not recommended. Safety and dosage have not been established.

Prolonged use:
No proven problems.

Skin & sunlight:
No problems expected.

Driving, piloting or hazardous work:
Don't drive or pilot aircraft until you learn how medicine affects you. Don't work around dangerous machinery. Don't climb ladders or work in high places. Danger increases if you drink alcohol or take medicine affecting alertness and reflexes, such as antihistamines, tranquilizers, sedatives, pain medicine, narcotics and mind-altering drugs.

Discontinuing:
Don't discontinue without consulting doctor. Dose may require gradual reduction if you have taken drug for a long time. Doses of other drugs may also require adjustment.

Others:
Wear identification bracelet or carry an identification card with inscription of medicine you take.

POSSIBLE INTERACTION WITH OTHER DRUGS

GENERIC NAME OR DRUG CLASS	COMBINED EFFECT
Antacids* (high dose)	Possible increased flecainide acetate effect.
Antiarrhythmics, other*	Possible irregular heartbeat.
Beta-adrenergic blockers*	Possible decreased efficiency of heart-muscle contraction, leading to congestive heart failure.
Bone marrow depressants*	Possible decreased production of blood cells in bone marrow.
Carbonic anhydrase inhibitors*	Possible increased flecainide acetate effect.
Cimetidine	Increased effect of cimetidine.
Digitalis preparations*	Possible increased digitalis effect. Possible irregular heartbeat.
Disopyramide	Possible decreased efficiency of heart-muscle contraction, leading to congestive heart failure.
Encainide	Increased effect of toxicity on the heart muscle.
Nicardipine	Possible increased effect and toxicity of each drug.

Continued page 1086

POSSIBLE INTERACTION WITH OTHER SUBSTANCES

INTERACTS WITH	COMBINED EFFECT
Alcohol:	May further depress normal heart function.
Beverages: Caffeine-containing beverages.	Possible decreased flecainide effect.
Cocaine:	Possible decreased flecainide effect.
Foods:	None expected.
Marijuana:	Possible decreased flecainide effect.
Tobacco:	Possible decreased flecainide effect.

*See Glossary

FLUOROURACIL (Topical)

BRAND NAMES

Efudex   Fluoroplex

BASIC INFORMATION

Habit forming? No
Prescription needed? Yes
Available as generic? No
Drug class: Antineoplastic, topical

 ## USES

- Treats precancerous actinic keratoses on skin.
- Treats superficial basal cell carcinomas (skin cancers that don't spread to distant organs and, therefore, do not threaten life).

 ## DOSAGE & USAGE INFORMATION

How to use:
- Apply with cotton-tipped applicator.
- Cream, lotion, ointment—Bathe and dry area before use. Apply small amount and rub gently.
- Wash hands (if fingertips are used to apply) after applying medicine to other parts of body.

When to use:
Once or twice a day or as directed by doctor.

If you forget a dose:
Apply as soon as you remember. Resume basic schedule.

What drug does:
Selectively destroys actively proliferating cells.

Time lapse before drug works:
2 to 3 days.

Don't use with:
Other topical medications unless prescribed by your doctor.

 ## OVERDOSE

SYMPTOMS:
None expected.
WHAT TO DO:
Not for internal use. If child accidentally swallows, call poison-control center.

 ## POSSIBLE ADVERSE REACTIONS OR SIDE EFFECTS

SYMPTOMS	WHAT TO DO
Life-threatening	
None expected.	
Common	
• Skin redness or swelling.	Discontinue. Call doctor right away.
• After 1 or 2 weeks of use—Skin itching or oozing; rash, tenderness, soreness.	Continue. Call doctor when convenient.
Infrequent	
Skin darkening or scaling.	Continue. Call doctor when convenient.
Rare	
Watery eyes.	Discontinue. Call doctor right away.

WARNINGS & PRECAUTIONS

Don't use if:
You are allergic to fluorouracil.

Before you start, consult your doctor:
- If you have cloasma or acne rosacea.
- If you have any other skin problems.

Over age 60:
No problems expected.

Pregnancy:
No problems expected, but check with doctor.

Breast-feeding:
No problems expected, but check with doctor.

Infants & children:
No problems expected, but check with doctor.

Prolonged use:
No problems expected, but check with doctor.

Skin & sunlight:
Increased sensitivity to sunlight during treatment and for 1 to 2 months following. Avoid exposure if possible.

Driving, piloting or hazardous work:
No problems expected, but check with doctor.

Discontinuing:
Pink, smooth area remains after treatment (usually fades in 1 to 2 months).

Others:
- Skin lesions may need biopsy before treatment.
- Keep medicine out of eyes or mouth.
- Heat and moisture in bathroom medicine cabinet can cause breakdown of medicine. Store someplace else.

POSSIBLE INTERACTION WITH OTHER DRUGS

GENERIC NAME OR DRUG CLASS	COMBINED EFFECT
None expected.	

POSSIBLE INTERACTION WITH OTHER SUBSTANCES

INTERACTS WITH	COMBINED EFFECT
Alcohol:	None expected.
Beverages:	None expected.
Cocaine:	None expected.
Foods:	None expected.
Marijuana:	None expected.
Tobacco:	None expected.

FLUOXETINE

BRAND NAMES

Prozac

BASIC INFORMATION

Habit forming? No
Prescription needed? Yes
Available as generic? No
Drug class: Antidepressant

 USES

Treats mental depression, particularly in people who do not tolerate tricyclic antidepressants.

 DOSAGE & USAGE INFORMATION

How to take:
Capsules—Swallow with liquid or food to lessen stomach irritation. If you can't swallow whole, open capsule and take with liquid or food.

When to take:
In the morning at the same time each day.

If you forget a dose:
Take as soon as you remember up to 2 hours late. If more than 2 hours, wait for next scheduled dose (don't double this dose).

What drug does:
- Inhibits serotonin uptake in the central nervous system.
- Causes loss of appetite.

Time lapse before drug works:
1 to 3 weeks.

Don't take with:
- Any medicine that will change your level of consciousness or reflexes.
- See Interaction column and consult doctor.

 OVERDOSE

SYMPTOMS:
Seizures.
WHAT TO DO:
- Dial 0 (operator) or 911 (emergency) for an ambulance or medical help. Then give first aid immediately.
- See emergency information on inside covers.

 POSSIBLE ADVERSE REACTIONS OR SIDE EFFECTS

SYMPTOMS	WHAT TO DO
Life-threatening:	
Rash, itchy skin, breathing difficulty (allergic reaction), chest pain.	Seek emergency treatment immediately.
Common:	
Diarrhea, nervousness, drowsiness, headache, increased sweating.	Continue. Call doctor when convenient.
Infrequent:	
Chills, fever, joint or muscle pain, enlarged lymph glands, unusual excitability, blurred vision.	Discontinue. Call doctor right away.
Rare:	
• Convulsions.	Discontinue. Seek emergency treatment.
• Fast heartbeat, abdominal pain.	Discontinue. Call doctor right away.
• Nausea, vomiting, constipation, cough, decreased appetite.	Continue. Call doctor when convenient.

WARNINGS & PRECAUTIONS

Don't take if:
You have severe liver or kidney disease.

Before you start, consult your doctor:
If you have history of seizure disorders.

Over age 60:
Adverse reactions and side effects may be more frequent and severe than in younger persons. You may need smaller doses for shorter periods of time.

Pregnancy:
No proven effects. Don't take unless essential.

Breast-feeding:
Unknown effects.

Infants & children:
Not recommended.

Prolonged use:
No problems expected.

Skin & sunlight:
No problems expected.

Driving, piloting or hazardous work:
Don't drive or pilot aircraft until you learn how medicine affects you. Don't work around dangerous machinery. Don't climb ladders or work in high places. Danger increases if you drink alcohol or take medicine affecting alertness and reflexes.

Discontinuing:
Don't discontinue without consulting doctor. Dose may require gradual reduction if you have taken drug for a long time. Doses of other drugs may also require adjustment.

Others:
No problems expected.

POSSIBLE INTERACTION WITH OTHER DRUGS

GENERIC NAME OR DRUG CLASS	COMBINED EFFECT
Anticoagulants*	May cause confusion, agitation, convulsions, high blood pressure.
Central nervous system (CNS) depressants*	Increases depressant effect of both drugs.
Digitalis preparations*	May cause confusion, agitation, convulsions, high blood pressure.
MAO inhibitors*	May cause confusion, agitation, convulsions, high blood pressure.
Tryptophan	Increased chance of agitation, restlessness, stomach upsets.

POSSIBLE INTERACTION WITH OTHER SUBSTANCES

INTERACTS WITH	COMBINED EFFECT
Alcohol:	Possible toxicity of both drugs.
Beverages:	Decreases effect of fluoxetine.
Cocaine:	Decreases effect of fluoxetine.
Foods:	None expected.
Marijuana:	Decreases effect of fluoxetine.
Tobacco:	Decreases effect of fluoxetine.

*See Glossary

FLUPHENAZINE

BRAND NAMES

Apo-Fluphenazine	Permitil
Decanoate	Prolixin
Modecate	Prolixin Decanoate
Moditen	Prolixin Enanthate
Moditen Enanthate	

BASIC INFORMATION

Habit forming? No
Prescription needed? Yes
Available as generic? Yes
Drug class: Tranquilizer, antiemetic
(phenothiazine)

USES

- Stops nausea, vomiting, hiccups.
- Reduces anxiety, agitation.

DOSAGE & USAGE INFORMATION

How to take:
- Tablet or extended-release capsule—Swallow with liquid or food to lessen stomach irritation.
- Drops or liquid—Dilute dose in beverage.

When to take:
- Nervous and mental disorders—Take at the same times each day.
- Nausea and vomiting—Take as needed, no more often than every 4 hours.

If you forget a dose:
- Nervous and mental disorders—Take up to 2 hours late. If more than 2 hours, wait for next scheduled dose (don't double this dose).
- Nausea and vomiting—Take as soon as you remember. Wait 4 hours for next dose.

What drug does:
- Suppresses brain's vomiting center.
- Suppresses brain centers that control abnormal emotions and behavior.

Continued next column

OVERDOSE

SYMPTOMS:
Stupor, convulsions, coma.
WHAT TO DO:
- Dial 0 (operator) or 911 (emergency) for an ambulance or medical help. Then give first aid immediately.
- See emergency information on inside covers.

Time lapse before drug works:
- Nausea and vomiting—1 hour or less.
- Nervous and mental disorders—4 to 6 weeks.

Don't take with:
- Antacid or medicine for diarrhea.
- Non-prescription drug for cough, cold or allergy.
- See Interaction column and consult doctor.

POSSIBLE ADVERSE REACTIONS OR SIDE EFFECTS

SYMPTOMS	WHAT TO DO
Life-threatening:	
Uncontrollable movements of head, neck, arms, legs (neuroleptic malignant syndrome, rare).	Seek emergency treatment immediately.
Common:	
• Muscle spasms of face and neck, unsteady gait.	Discontinue. Seek emergency treatment.
• Restlessness, tremor, drowsiness.	Discontinue. Call doctor right away.
• Decreased sweating, dry mouth, runny nose, constipation.	Continue. Call doctor when convenient.
Infrequent:	
• Fainting.	Discontinue. Seek emergency treatment.
• Rash.	Discontinue. Call doctor right away.
• Painful or difficult urination, diminished sex drive, swollen breasts, menstrual irregularities.	Continue. Call doctor when convenient.
Rare:	
Vision changes, sore throat, fever, jaundice, abdominal pain, constipation.	Discontinue. Call doctor right away.

WARNINGS & PRECAUTIONS

Don't take if:
- You are allergic to any phenothiazine.
- You have a blood or bone-marrow disease.

Before you start, consult your doctor:
- If you will have surgery within 2 months, including dental surgery, requiring general or spinal anesthesia.
- If you have asthma, emphysema or other lung disorder, glaucoma, prostate trouble.
- If you take non-prescription ulcer medicine, asthma medicine or amphetamines.

Over age 60:
Adverse reactions and side effects may be more frequent and severe than in younger persons. More likely to develop involuntary movement of jaws, lips, tongue, chewing. Report this to your doctor immediately. Early treatment can help.

Pregnancy:
Risk to unborn child outweighs drug benefits. Don't use.

Breast-feeding:
Drug passes into milk. Avoid drug or discontinue nursing until you finish medicine. Consult doctor for advice on maintaining milk supply.

Infants & children:
Don't give to children younger than 2.

Prolonged use:
May lead to tardive dyskinesia (involuntary movement of jaws, lips, tongue, chewing).

Skin & sunlight:
May cause rash or intensify sunburn in areas exposed to sun or sunlamp. Skin may remain sensitive for 3 months after discontinuing.

Driving, piloting or hazardous work:
Don't drive or pilot aircraft until you learn how medicine affects you. Don't work around dangerous machinery. Don't climb ladders or work in high places. Danger increases if you drink alcohol or take medicine affecting alertness and reflexes.

Discontinuing:
- Nervous and mental disorders—Don't discontinue without doctor's advice until you complete prescribed dose, even though symptoms diminish or disappear.
- Nausea and vomiting—May be unnecessary to finish medicine. Follow doctor's instructions.

Others:
No problems expected.

POSSIBLE INTERACTION WITH OTHER DRUGS

GENERIC NAME OR DRUG CLASS	COMBINED EFFECT
Anticholinergics*	Increased anticholinergic effect.
Antidepressants, tricyclic (TCA)*	Increased fluphenazine effect.
Antihistamines*	Increased antihistamine effect.
Appetite suppressants*	Decreased suppressant effect.
Dronabinol	Increased effects of both drugs. Avoid.
Guanethidine	Decreased guanethidine effect.
Levodopa	Decreased levodopa effect.
Mind-altering drugs*	Increased effect of mind-altering drugs.
Molindone	Increased tranquilizer effect.
Nabilone	Greater depression of central nervous system.
Narcotics*	Increased narcotic effect.
Phenytoin	Increased phenytoin effect.
Procarbazine	Increased sedation.
Quinidine	Impaired heart function. Dangerous mixture.
Sedatives*	Increased sedation.
Tranquilizers, other*	Increased tranquilizer effect.

POSSIBLE INTERACTION WITH OTHER SUBSTANCES

INTERACTS WITH	COMBINED EFFECT
Alcohol:	Dangerous oversedation.
Beverages:	None expected.
Cocaine:	Decreased fluphenazine effect. Avoid.
Foods:	None expected.
Marijuana:	Drowsiness. May increase antinausea effect.
Tobacco:	None expected.

*See Glossary

FLUPREDNISOLONE

BRAND NAMES

Alphadrol

BASIC INFORMATION

Habit forming? No
Prescription needed? Yes
Available as generic? No
Drug class: Cortisone drug (adrenal corticosteroid)

 USES

- Reduces inflammation caused by many different medical problems.
- Treatment for some allergic diseases, blood disorders, kidney diseases, asthma and emphysema.
- Replaces corticosteroid deficiencies.

 DOSAGE & USAGE INFORMATION

How to take:
Tablet—Swallow with liquid or food to lessen stomach irritation. If you can't swallow whole, crumble tablet.

When to take:
At the same times each day. Take once-a-day or once-every-other-day doses in mornings.

If you forget a dose:
- Several-doses-per-day prescription—Take as soon as you remember up to 2 hours late. If more than 2 hours, wait for next scheduled dose (don't double this dose).
- Once-a-day dose or less—Wait for next dose. Double this dose.

What drug does:
Decreases inflammatory responses.

Time lapse before drug works:
2 to 4 days.

Don't take with:
See Interaction column and consult doctor.

 OVERDOSE

SYMPTOMS:
Headache, convulsions, heart failure.
WHAT TO DO:
- **Dial 0 (operator) or 911 (emergency) for an ambulance or medical help. Then give first aid immediately.**
- **See emergency information on inside covers.**

 POSSIBLE ADVERSE REACTIONS OR SIDE EFFECTS

SYMPTOMS	WHAT TO DO
Life-threatening:	
Hives, rash, intense itching, faintness soon after a dose (anaphylaxis).	Seek emergency treatment immediately.
Common:	
Acne, poor wound healing, thirst, indigestion, nausea, vomiting, decreased growth in children.	Continue. Call doctor when convenient.
Infrequent:	
• Black, bloody or tarry stools.	Discontinue. Seek emergency treatment.
• Blurred vision; halos around lights; sore throat; fever; muscle cramps; swollen legs, feet.	Discontinue. Call doctor right away.
• Mood changes, insomnia, fatigue, restlessness, frequent urination, weight gain, round face, weakness, TB recurrence, menstrual irregularities.	Continue. Call doctor when convenient.
Rare:	
• Irregular heartbeat.	Discontinue. Seek emergency treatment.
• Rash, hallucinations, thrombophlebitis, pancreatitis, numbness or tingling in hands or feet, convulsions.	Discontinue. Call doctor right away.

 WARNINGS & PRECAUTIONS

Don't take if:
- You are allergic to any cortisone drug.
- You have tuberculosis or fungus infection.
- You have herpes infection of eyes, lips or genitals.

Before you start, consult your doctor:
- If you have had tuberculosis.
- If you have congestive heart failure.
- If you have diabetes, peptic ulcer, glaucoma, underactive thyroid, high blood pressure, myasthenia gravis, blood clots in legs or lungs.

Over age 60:
Adverse reactions and side effects may be more frequent and severe than in younger persons. Likely to aggravate edema, diabetes or ulcers. Likely to cause cataracts and osteoporosis (softening of the bones).

Pregnancy:
Risk to unborn child outweighs drug benefits. Don't use.

Breast-feeding:
Drug passes into milk. Avoid drug or discontinue nursing until you finish medicine. Consult doctor for advice on maintaining milk supply.

Infants & children:
Use only under medical supervision.

Prolonged use:
- Retards growth in children.
- Possible glaucoma, cataracts, diabetes, fragile bones and thin skin.
- Functional dependence.

Skin & sunlight:
No problems expected.

Driving, piloting or hazardous work:
No problems expected.

Discontinuing:
- Don't discontinue without doctor's advice until you complete prescribed dose, even though symptoms diminish or disappear.
- Drug affects your response to surgery, illness, injury or stress for 2 years after discontinuing. Tell anyone who takes medical care of you about this drug for 2 years after discontinuing.

Others:
Avoid immunizations if possible.

POSSIBLE INTERACTION WITH OTHER DRUGS

GENERIC NAME OR DRUG CLASS	COMBINED EFFECT
Amphotericin B	Potassium depletion.
Anticholinergics*	Possible glaucoma.
Anticoagulants, oral*	Decreased anti-coagulant effect.
Anticonvulsants, hydantoin*	Decreased fluprednisolone effect.
Antidiabetics, oral*	Decreased anti-diabetic effect.
Antihistamines*	Decreased fluprednisolone effect.
Aspirin	Increased fluprednisolone effect.
Attentuated virus vaccines*	Possible viral infection.
Barbiturates*	Decreased fluprednisolone effect. Oversedation.
Chloral hydrate	Decreased fluprednisolone effect.
Chlorthalidone	Potassium depletion.
Cholestyramine	Decreased fluprednisolone absorption effect.
Cholinergics*	Decreased cholinergic effect.
Colestipol	Decreased fluprednisolone absorption effect.
Contraceptives, oral*	Increased fluprednisolone effect.
Digitalis preparations*	Dangerous potassium depletion. Possible digitalis toxicity.
Diuretics, thiazide*	Potassium depletion.
Ephedrine	Decreased fluprednisolone effect.
Estrogens*	Increased fluprednisolone effect.
Ethacrynic acid	Potassium depletion.
Furosemide	Potassium depletion.
Glutethimide	Decreased fluprednisolone effect.
Indapamide	Possible excessive potassium loss, causing dangerous heartbeat irregularity.
Indomethacin	Increased fluprednisolone effect.
Insulin	Decreased insulin effect.
Isoniazid	Decreased isoniazid effect.
Mitotane	Decreased fluprednisolone effect.

Continued page 1087

POSSIBLE INTERACTION WITH OTHER SUBSTANCES

INTERACTS WITH	COMBINED EFFECT
Alcohol:	Risk of stomach ulcers.
Beverages:	No proven problems.
Cocaine:	Overstimulation. Avoid.
Foods:	No proven problems.
Marijuana:	Decreased immunity.
Tobacco:	Increased flu-prednisolone effect. Possible toxicity.

*See Glossary

FLURAZEPAM

BRAND NAMES

Apo-Flurazepam	Novoflupam
Dalmane	Somnal
Durapam	Som-Pam

BASIC INFORMATION

Habit forming? Yes
Prescription needed? Yes
Available as generic? Yes
Drug class: Tranquilizer (benzodiazepine)

 ## USES

Treatment for insomnia and tension.

 ## DOSAGE & USAGE INFORMATION

How to take:
Tablet or capsule—Swallow with liquid. If you can't swallow whole, crumble tablet or open capsule and take with liquid or food.

When to take:
At the same time each day, according to instructions on prescription label.

If you forget a dose:
Take as soon as you remember up to 2 hours late. If more than 2 hours, wait for next scheduled dose (don't double this dose).

What drug does:
Affects limbic system of brain—part that controls emotions. Induces near-normal sleep pattern.

Time lapse before drug works:
30 minutes.

Continued next column

 ## OVERDOSE

SYMPTOMS:
Drowsiness, weakness, tremor, stupor, coma.
WHAT TO DO:
- **Dial 0 (operator) or 911 (emergency) for an ambulance or medical help. Then give first aid immediately.**
- **If patient is unconscious and not breathing, give mouth-to-mouth breathing. If there is no heartbeat, use cardiac massage and mouth-to-mouth breathing (CPR). Don't try to make patient vomit. If you can't get help quickly, take patient to nearest emergency facility.**
- **See emergency information on inside covers.**

Don't take with:
See Interaction column and consult doctor.

 ## POSSIBLE ADVERSE REACTIONS OR SIDE EFFECTS

SYMPTOMS	WHAT TO DO
Life-threatening: None expected.	
Common: Clumsiness, drowsiness, dizziness.	Continue. Call doctor when convenient.
Infrequent: • Hallucinations, confusion, irritability, depression, rash, itch, change in vision.	Discontinue. Call doctor right away.
• Constipation or diarrhea, nausea, vomiting, painful or difficult urination.	Continue. Call doctor when convenient.
Rare: • Slow heartbeat, difficult breathing.	Discontinue. Seek emergency treatment.
• Mouth, throat ulcers, jaundice.	Discontinue. Call doctor right away.

WARNINGS & PRECAUTIONS

Don't take if:
- You are allergic to any benzodiazepine.
- You have myasthenia gravis.
- You are active or recovering alcoholic.
- Patient is younger than 6 months.

Before you start, consult your doctor:
- If you have liver, kidney or lung disease.
- If you have diabetes, epilepsy or porphyria.

Over age 60:
Adverse reactions and side effects may be more frequent and severe than in younger persons. May develop agitation, rage or "hangover" effect.

Pregnancy:
Risk to unborn child outweighs drug benefits. Don't use.

Breast-feeding:
Drug passes into milk. Avoid drug or discontinue nursing until you finish medicine. Consult doctor for advice on maintaining milk supply.

Infants & children:
Use only under medical supervision for children older than 6 months.

Prolonged use:
May impair liver function.

Skin & sunlight:
No problems expected.

Driving, piloting or hazardous work:
Don't drive or pilot aircraft until you learn how medicine affects you. Don't work around dangerous machinery. Don't climb ladders or work in high places. Danger increases if you drink alcohol or take medicine affecting alertness and reflexes.

Discontinuing:
Don't discontinue without doctor's advice until you complete prescribed dose, even though symptoms diminish or disappear.

Others:
- Hot weather, heavy exercise and profuse sweat may reduce excretion and cause overdose.
- "Hangover" effect may occur.
- Blood sugar may rise in diabetics, requiring insulin adjustment.

 ## POSSIBLE INTERACTION WITH OTHER DRUGS

GENERIC NAME OR DRUG CLASS	COMBINED EFFECT
Anticonvulsants*	Change in seizure frequency or severity.
Antidepressants*	Increased sedative effect of both drugs.
Antihistamines*	Increased sedative effect of both drugs.
Antihypertensives*	Excessively low blood pressure.
Cimetidine	Excess sedation.
Disulfiram	Increased flurazepam effect.
Dronabinol	Increased effects of both drugs. Avoid.
MAO inhibitors*	Convulsions, deep sedation, rage.
Molindone	Increased sedative effect.
Nabilone	Greater depression of central nervous system.
Narcotics*	Increased sedative effect of both drugs.
Nizatidine	Increased effect and toxicity of flurazepam.
Sedatives*	Increased sedative effect of both drugs.
Sleep inducers*	Increased sedative effect of both drugs.
Tranquilizers*	Increased sedative effect of both drugs.

 ## POSSIBLE INTERACTION WITH OTHER SUBSTANCES

INTERACTS WITH	COMBINED EFFECT
Alcohol:	Heavy sedation. Avoid.
Beverages:	None expected.
Cocaine:	Decreased flurazepam effect.
Foods:	None expected.
Marijuana:	Heavy sedation. Avoid.
Tobacco:	Decreased flurazepam effect.

FOLIC ACID (Vitamin B-9)

BRAND NAMES

Apo-Folic
Folvite
Novofolacid

Numerous other multiple vitamin-mineral supplements.

BASIC INFORMATION

Habit forming? No
Prescription needed?
  High strength: Yes
  Vitamin mixtures: No
Available as generic? Yes
Drug class: Vitamin supplement

 USES

- Dietary supplement to promote normal growth, development and good health.
- Treatment for anemias due to folic-acid deficiency occurring from alcoholism, liver disease, hemolytic anemia, sprue, infants on artificial formula, pregnancy, breast-feeding and oral-contraceptive use.

 DOSAGE & USAGE INFORMATION

How to take:
Tablet—Swallow with liquid or food to lessen stomach irritation. If you can't swallow whole, crumble tablet and take with liquid or food.

When to take:
At the same time each day.

If you forget a dose:
Take when you remember. Don't double next dose. Resume regular schedule.

What drug does:
Essential to normal red-blood-cell formation.

Time lapse before drug works:
Not determined.

Don't take with:
See Interaction column and consult doctor.

 OVERDOSE

SYMPTOMS:
None expected.
WHAT TO DO:
Overdose unlikely to threaten life.

 POSSIBLE ADVERSE REACTIONS OR SIDE EFFECTS

SYMPTOMS	WHAT TO DO
Life-threatening: None expected.	
Common: Large dose may produce yellow urine.	Continue. Tell doctor at next visit.
Infrequent: None expected.	
Rare: Rash, itching, bronchospasm.	Discontinue. Call doctor right away.

WARNINGS & PRECAUTIONS

Don't take if:
You are allergic to any B vitamin.

Before you start, consult your doctor:
- If you have liver disease.
- If you have pernicious anemia. (Folic acid corrects anemia, but nerve damage of pernicious anemia continues.)

Over age 60:
No problems expected.

Pregnancy:
No problems expected.

Breast-feeding:
No problems expected.

Infants & children:
No problems expected.

Prolonged use:
No problems expected.

Skin & sunlight:
No problems expected.

Driving, piloting or hazardous work:
No problems expected.

Discontinuing:
Don't discontinue without doctor's advice until you complete prescribed dose, even though symptoms diminish or disappear.

Others:
- Folic acid removed by kidney dialysis. Dialysis patients should increase intake to 300% of RDA.
- A balanced diet should provide all the folic acid a healthy person needs and make supplements unnecessary. Best sources are green, leafy vegetables; fruits; liver and kidney.

POSSIBLE INTERACTION WITH OTHER DRUGS

GENERIC NAME OR DRUG CLASS	COMBINED EFFECT
Analgesics*	Decreased effect of folic acid.
Anticonvulsants*	Decreased effect of folic acid. Possible increased seizure frequency.
Chloramphenicol	Possible decreased folic acid effect.
Contraceptives, oral*	Decreased effect of folic acid.
Cortisone drugs*	Decreased effect of folic acid.
Methotrexate	Decreased effect of folic acid.
Para-aminosalicylic acid (PAS)	Decreased effect of folic acid.
Pyrimethamine	Decreased effect of folic acid.
Sulfasalazine	Decreased dietary absorption of folic acid.
Triamterene	Decreased effect of folic acid.
Trimethoprim	Decreased effect of folic acid.
Zinc	Decreased zinc effect.

POSSIBLE INTERACTION WITH OTHER SUBSTANCES

INTERACTS WITH	COMBINED EFFECT
Alcohol:	None expected.
Beverages:	None expected.
Cocaine:	None expected.
Foods:	None expected.
Marijuana:	None expected.
Tobacco:	None expected.

*See Glossary

FUROSEMIDE

BRAND NAMES

Apo-Furosemide	Neo-Renal
Furoside	Novosemide
Lasix	SK-Furosemide
Lasix Special	Uritol

BASIC INFORMATION

Habit forming? No
Prescription needed? Yes
Available as generic? Yes
Drug class: Diuretic, antihypertensive

 ## USES

- Lowers high blood pressure.
- Decreases fluid retention.

 ## DOSAGE & USAGE INFORMATION

How to take:
Tablet or liquid—Swallow with liquid. If you can't swallow whole, crumble tablet and take with liquid or food.

When to take:
- 1 dose a day—Take after breakfast.
- More than 1 dose a day—Take last dose no later than 6 p.m. unless otherwise directed.

If you forget a dose:
- 1 dose a day—Take as soon as you remember up to 12 hours late. If more than 12 hours, wait for next scheduled dose (don't double this dose).
- More than 1 dose a day—Take as soon as you remember up to 2 hours late. If more than 2 hours, wait for next scheduled dose (don't double this dose).

What drug does:
Increases elimination of sodium and water from body. Decreased body fluid reduces blood pressure.

Continued next column

 ## OVERDOSE

SYMPTOMS:
Weakness, lethargy, dizziness, confusion, nausea, vomiting, leg-muscle cramps, thirst, stupor, deep sleep, weak and rapid pulse, cardiac arrest.
WHAT TO DO:
- **Dial 0 (operator) or 911 (emergency) for an ambulance or medical help. Then give first aid immediately.**
- **See emergency information on inside covers.**

Time lapse before drug works:
1 hour to increase water loss. Requires 2 to 3 weeks to lower blood pressure.

Don't take with:
- Non-prescription drugs with aspirin.
- See Interaction column and consult doctor.

 ## POSSIBLE ADVERSE REACTIONS OR SIDE EFFECTS

SYMPTOMS	WHAT TO DO
Life-threatening: None expected.	
Common: Dizziness.	Continue. Call doctor when convenient.
Infrequent: Mood change, fatigue, appetite loss, diarrhea, irregular heartbeat, muscle cramps, low blood pressure, abdominal pain, weakness.	Discontinue. Call doctor right away.
Rare: Rash or hives, yellow vision, ringing in ears, hearing loss, sore throat, fever, dry mouth, thirst, side or stomach pain, nausea, vomiting, unusual bleeding or bruising, joint pain, jaundice, numbness or tingling in hands or feet.	Discontinue. Call doctor right away.

 ## WARNINGS & PRECAUTIONS

Don't take if:
You are allergic to furosemide.

Before you start, consult your doctor:
- If you are allergic to any sulfa drug.
- If you have liver or kidney disease.
- If you have gout, diabetes or impaired hearing.
- If you will have surgery within 2 months, including dental surgery, requiring general or spinal anesthesia.

Over age 60:
Adverse reactions and side effects may be more frequent and severe than in younger persons.

Pregnancy:
Risk to unborn child outweighs drug benefits. Don't use.

Breast-feeding:
Drug filters into milk. May harm child. Avoid.

Infants & children:
Use only under medical supervision.

Prolonged use:
- Impaired balance of water, salt and potassium in blood and body tissues.
- Possible diabetes.

Skin & sunlight:
May cause rash or intensify sunburn in areas exposed to sun or sunlamp.

Driving, piloting or hazardous work:
No problems expected.

Discontinuing:
Don't discontinue without doctor's advice until you complete prescribed dose, even though symptoms diminish or disappear.

Others:
Frequent laboratory studies to monitor potassium level in blood recommended. Eat foods rich in potassium or take potassium supplements. Consult doctor.

POSSIBLE INTERACTION WITH OTHER DRUGS

GENERIC NAME OR DRUG CLASS	COMBINED EFFECT
ACE inhibitors: captopril, enalapril, lisinopril*	Possible excessive potassium in blood.
Allopurinol	Decreased allopurinol effect.
Amiodarone	Increased risk of heartbeat irregularity due to low potassium.
Anticoagulants*	Abnormal clotting.
Antidepressants, tricyclic (TCA)*	Excessive blood-pressure drop.
Antidiabetics, oral*	Decreased anti-diabetic effect.
Antihypertensives*	Increased antihypertensive effect. Dosages may require adjustment.
Barbiturates*	Low blood pressure.
Beta-adrenergic blockers*	Increased antihypertensive effect. Dosages may require adjustment.
Calcium supplements*	Decreased calcium in blood.
Carteolol	Increased antihypertensive effect.
Corticosteroids*	Decreased potassium.
Cortisone drugs*	Excessive potassium loss.
Digitalis preparations*	Excessive potassium loss could lead to serious heart rhythm disorders.
Digoxin	Increased possibility of digitalis toxicity.
Diuretics, other*	Increased diuretic effect.
Insulin	Decreased insulin effect.
Lithium	Increased lithium toxicity.
Narcotics*	Dangerous low blood pressure. Avoid.
Nicardipine	Blood-pressure drop. Dosages may require adjustment.
Nitrates*	Excessive blood-pressure drop.
Non-steroidal anti-inflammatory drugs (NSAIDs)*	Decreased furosemide effect.
Phenytoin	Decreased furosemide effect.
Potassium supplements*	Decreased potassium effect.
Probenecid	Decreased probenecid effect.
Salicylates* (including aspirin)	Dangerous salicylate retention.
Sedatives*	Increased furosemide effect.
Sotalol	Increased antihypertensive effect.
Terazosin	Decreases effectiveness of terazosin.

POSSIBLE INTERACTION WITH OTHER SUBSTANCES

INTERACTS WITH	COMBINED EFFECT
Alcohol:	Blood-pressure drop. Avoid.
Beverages:	None expected.
Cocaine:	Dangerous blood-pressure drop. Avoid.
Foods:	None expected.
Marijuana:	Increased thirst and urinary frequency, fainting.
Tobacco:	Decreased furosemide effect.

*See Glossary

GALLBLADDER X-RAY TEST DRUGS
(Cholecystographic Agents)

BRAND AND GENERIC NAMES

Bilivist	IPODATE
Bilopaque	Oragrafin Calcium
Cholebrine	Oragrafin Sodium
IOCETAMIC ACID	Telepaque
IOPANOIC ACID	TYROPANOATE

BASIC INFORMATION

Habit forming? No
Prescription needed? Yes
Available as generic? No
Drug class: Diagnostic aid, radiopaque

 USES

To check for problems with the gallbladder or the bile ducts.

 DOSAGE & USAGE INFORMATION

How to take:
- Take tablets or liquid as directed after the evening meal on the evening before special x-rays will be taken.
- Don't eat or drink anything (except water) after taking.

When to take:
As directed.

If you forget a dose:
Take as soon as you remember.

What drug does:
These are organic iodine compounds which get absorbed into the blood stream, get concentrated in a healthy gallbladder and make the gallbladder and gallstones (if present) visible on special x-rays.

Time lapse before drug works:
10 to 15 hours.

Continued next column

 OVERDOSE

SYMPTOMS:
Severe diarrhea, nausea or vomiting; difficult urination.
WHAT TO DO:
Not life-threatening. Discontinue and call doctor right away.

Don't take with:
- Other medicines unless directed by your doctor or x-ray specialist.
- If you take cholestyramine, discontinue it for 48 hours before taking the radiopaque drug.

 POSSIBLE ADVERSE REACTIONS OR SIDE EFFECTS

SYMPTOMS	WHAT TO DO
Life-threatening:	
Faintness; swelling of lips, hands, face; difficult breathing.	Discontinue. Seek emergency treatment.
Common:	
None expected.	
Infrequent:	
Abdominal cramps, diarrhea, dizziness, headache, indigestion, vomiting, nausea.	Discontinue. Call doctor right away.
Rare:	
Itching, unusual bleeding or bruising, hives or rash.	Discontinue. Call doctor right away.

GALLBLADDER X-RAY TEST DRUGS
(Cholecystographic Agents)

 WARNINGS & PRECAUTIONS

Don't take if:
You are allergic to any iodine compound or other radiopaque chemicals.

Before you start, consult your doctor:
If you are allergic to anything, including shellfish, cabbage, kale, turnips, iodized salt.

Over age 60:
Adverse reactions and side effects may be more frequent and severe than in younger persons. Ask doctor about smaller doses.

Pregnancy:
X-rays should not be taken unless absolutely necessary during pregnancy.

Breast-feeding:
No problems expected, but ask doctor.

Infants & children:
No problems expected, but ask doctor.

Prolonged use:
Not intended for prolonged use.

Skin & sunlight:
No problems expected.

Driving, piloting or hazardous work:
Don't drive or pilot aircraft until you learn how medicine affects you. Don't work around dangerous machinery. Don't climb ladders or work in high places. Danger increases if you drink alcohol or take medicine affecting alertness and reflexes, such as antihistamines, tranquilizers, sedatives, pain medicine, narcotics and mind-altering drugs.

Discontinuing:
No problems expected.

Others:
* Special diets and laxatives or enemas before x-rays may be ordered. Follow instructions.
* Tests on your thyroid gland may be made inaccurate for 8 weeks because of the iodine contained in radiopaque substances. Keep this in mind if your doctor orders thyroid tests.

 POSSIBLE INTERACTION WITH OTHER DRUGS

GENERIC NAME OR DRUG CLASS	COMBINED EFFECT
None expected.	

 POSSIBLE INTERACTION WITH OTHER SUBSTANCES

INTERACTS WITH	COMBINED EFFECT
Alcohol:	None expected.
Beverages:	None expected.
Cocaine:	None expected.
Foods:	None expected.
Marijuana:	None expected.
Tobacco:	None expected.

GEMFIBROZIL

BRAND NAMES

Lopid

BASIC INFORMATION

Habit forming? No
Prescription needed? Yes
Available as generic? No
Drug class: Antihyperlipidemic

 USES

Reduces fatty substances in the blood (triglycerides).

 DOSAGE & USAGE INFORMATION

How to take:
Capsule—Swallow with liquid or food to lessen stomach irritation.

When to take:
At the same times each day.

If you forget a dose:
Take as soon as you remember up to 2 hours late. If more than 2 hours, wait for next scheduled dose (don't double this dose).

What drug does:
Inhibits formation of fatty substances.

Time lapse before drug works:
3 months or more.

Don't take with:
See Interaction column and consult doctor.

 OVERDOSE

SYMPTOMS:
Diarrhea, headache, muscle pain.
WHAT TO DO:
Overdose unlikely to threaten life. If person takes much larger amount than prescribed, call doctor, poison-control center or hospital emergency room for instructions.

 POSSIBLE ADVERSE REACTIONS OR SIDE EFFECTS

SYMPTOMS	WHAT TO DO
Life-threatening: None expected.	
Common: None expected.	
Infrequent:	
• Chest pain, shortness of breath, irregular heartbeat, gallstones.	Discontinue. Call doctor right away.
• Nausea, vomiting, diarrhea, stomach pain.	Continue. Call doctor when convenient.
Rare:	
• Rash, itch; sores in mouth, on lips; sore throat; swollen feet, legs; blood in urine; painful urination; fever; chills.	Discontinue. Call doctor right away.
• Dizziness, headache, drowsiness, muscle cramps, dry skin, backache, hair loss, diminished sex drive.	Continue. Call doctor when convenient.

WARNINGS & PRECAUTIONS

Don't take if:
You are allergic to any antihyperlipidemic.

Before you start, consult your doctor:
• If you have had liver or kidney disease.
• If you have had peptic-ulcer disease.
• If you have diabetes.

Over age 60:
Adverse reactions and side effects may be more frequent and severe than in younger persons.

Pregnancy:
Risk to unborn child outweighs drug benefits. Don't use.

Breast-feeding:
May harm child. Avoid.

Infants & children:
Not recommended.

Prolonged use:
Periodic blood-cell counts and liver-function studies recommended if you take gemfibrozil for a long time.

Skin & sunlight:
No problems expected.

Driving, piloting or hazardous work:
Avoid if you feel drowsy or dizzy. Otherwise, no problems expected.

Discontinuing:
Don't discontinue without doctor's advice until you complete prescribed dose, even though symptoms diminish or disappear.

Others:
Some studies question effectiveness. Many studies warn against toxicity.

POSSIBLE INTERACTION WITH OTHER DRUGS

GENERIC NAME OR DRUG CLASS	COMBINED EFFECT
Anticoagulants, oral*	Increased anti-coagulant effect. Dose reduction of anticoagulant necessary.
Antidiabetics, oral*	Increased antidiabetic effect.
Contraceptives, oral*	Decreased gemfibrozil effect.
Estrogens*	Decreased gemfibrozil effect.
Furosemide	Possible toxicity of both drugs.
Insulin	Increased insulin effect.
Thyroid hormones*	Increased gemfibrozil effect.

POSSIBLE INTERACTION WITH OTHER SUBSTANCES

INTERACTS WITH	COMBINED EFFECT
Alcohol:	None expected.
Beverages:	None expected.
Cocaine:	Decreased effect of gemfibrozil. Avoid.
Foods: Fatty foods.	Decreased gemfibrozil effect.
Marijuana:	None expected.
Tobacco:	Decreased gemfibrozil absorption. Avoid.

GLIPIZIDE

BRAND NAMES

Glucotrol

BASIC INFORMATION

Habit forming? No
Prescription needed? Yes
Available as generic? No
Drug class: Antidiabetic (oral), sulfonurea

 ## USES

Treatment for diabetes insipidus and for diabetes in adults who can't control blood sugar by diet, weight loss and exercise.

 ## DOSAGE & USAGE INFORMATION

How to take:
Tablet—Swallow with liquid or food to lessen stomach irritation. If you can't swallow whole, crumble tablet and take with liquid or food.

When to take:
At the same times each day.

If you forget a dose:
Take as soon as you remember up to 2 hours late. If more than 2 hours, wait for next scheduled dose (don't double this dose).

What drug does:
Stimulates pancreas to produce more insulin. Insulin in blood forces cells to use sugar in blood.

Time lapse before drug works:
3 to 4 hours. May require 2 weeks for maximum benefit.

Don't take with:
See Interaction column and consult doctor.

 ## OVERDOSE

SYMPTOMS:
Excessive hunger, nausea, anxiety, cool skin, cold sweats, drowsiness, rapid heartbeat, weakness, unconsciousness, coma.
WHAT TO DO:
- **Dial 0 (operator) or 911 (emergency) for an ambulance or medical help. Then give first aid immediately.**
- **See emergency information on inside covers.**

 ## POSSIBLE ADVERSE REACTIONS OR SIDE EFFECTS

SYMPTOMS	WHAT TO DO
Life-threatening: None expected.	
Common:	
• Dizziness.	Discontinue. Call doctor right away.
• Diarrhea, appetite loss, nausea, stomach pain, heartburn.	Continue. Call doctor when convenient.
Infrequent: Low blood sugar (hunger, anxiety, cold sweats, rapid pulse), drowsiness, nervousness, headache, weakness, dizziness.	Discontinue. Seek emergency treatment.
Rare: Itching or rash, sore throat, fever, ringing in ears, unusual bleeding or bruising, fatigue, jaundice, edema, weakness, confusion.	Discontinue. Call doctor right away.

 ## WARNINGS & PRECAUTIONS

Don't take if:
- You are allergic to any sulfonurea.
- You have impaired kidney or liver function.

Before you start, consult your doctor:
- If you have a severe infection.
- If you have thyroid disease.
- If you take insulin.
- If you have heart disease.

Over age 60:
Dose usually smaller than for younger adults. Avoid "low-blood-sugar" episodes because repeated ones can damage brain permanently.

Pregnancy:
No proven harm to unborn child. Avoid if possible.

Breast-feeding:
Drug filters into milk. May lower baby's blood sugar. Avoid.

Infants & children:
Don't give to infants or children.

Prolonged use:
None expected.

Skin & sunlight:
May cause rash or intensify sunburn in areas exposed to sun or sunlamp.

Driving, piloting or hazardous work:
No problems expected unless you develop hypoglycemia (low blood sugar). If so, avoid driving or hazardous activity.

Discontinuing:
Don't discontinue without consulting doctor. Dose may require gradual reduction if you have taken drug for a long time. Doses of other drugs may also require adjustment.

Others:
Don't exceed recommended dose. Hypoglycemia (low blood sugar) may occur, even with proper dose schedule. You must balance medicine, diet and exercise.

 POSSIBLE INTERACTION WITH OTHER DRUGS

GENERIC NAME OR DRUG CLASS	COMBINED EFFECT
Androgens*	Increased glipizide effect.
Anticoagulants, oral*	Unpredictable prothrombin times.*
Anticonvulsants, hydantoin*	Decreased glipizide effect.
Aspirin	Increased glipizide effect.
Beta-adrenergic blockers*	Increased glipizide effect. May increase difficulty in regulating blood sugar.
Bismuth subsalicylate	Increased insulin effect. May required dosage adjustment.
Chloramphenicol	Increased glipizide effect.
Cimetidine	Possible increased glipizide effect.
Clofibrate	Increased glipizide effect.
Contraceptives, oral*	Decreased glipizide effect.
Cortisone drugs*	Decreased glipizide effect.
Digoxin	Possible decreased digoxin effect.
Diuretics, thiazide and loop*	Decreased glipizide effect.
Epinephrine	Decreased glipizide effect.
Estrogens*	Decreased glipizide effect.
Guanethidine	Unpredictable glipizide effect.
Insulin	Increased glipizide effect.
Labetalol	Increased antidiabetic effect, may mask hypoglycemia.
Nicotinic acid	Decreased glipizide effect.
Nizatidine	Increased effect and toxicity of glipizide.
Non-steroidal anti-inflammatory drugs (NSAIDs)*	Increased glipizide effect.
Phenothiazines*	Decreased glipizide effect.
Phenytoin	Decreased glipizide effect.
Ranitidine	Possible increased glipizide effect.
Rifampin	Decreased glipizide effect.

 POSSIBLE INTERACTION WITH OTHER SUBSTANCES

INTERACTS WITH	COMBINED EFFECT
Alcohol:	Disulfiram reaction.* Avoid.
Beverages:	None expected.
Cocaine:	No proven problems.
Foods:	None expected.
Marijuana:	Decreased glipizide effect. Avoid.
Tobacco:	None expected.

*See Glossary

GLYBURIDE

BRAND NAMES

DiaBeta   **Glibenclamide**
Euglucon   **Micronase**

BASIC INFORMATION

Habit forming? No
Prescription needed? Yes
Available as generic? No
Drug class: Antidiabetic (oral), sulfonurea

USES

Treatment for diabetes in adults who can't control blood sugar by diet, weight loss and exercise.

DOSAGE & USAGE INFORMATION

How to take:
Tablet—Swallow with liquid or food to lessen stomach irritation. If you can't swallow whole, crumble tablet and take with liquid or food.

When to take:
At the same times each day.

If you forget a dose:
Take as soon as you remember up to 2 hours late. If more than 2 hours, wait for next scheduled dose (don't double this dose).

What drug does:
Stimulates pancreas to produce more insulin. Insulin in blood forces cells to use sugar in blood.

Time lapse before drug works:
3 to 4 hours. May require 2 weeks for maximum benefit.

Don't take with:
See Interaction column and consult doctor.

OVERDOSE

SYMPTOMS:
Excessive hunger, nausea, anxiety, cool skin, cold sweats, drowsiness, rapid heartbeat, weakness, unconsciousness, coma.
WHAT TO DO:
- **Dial 0 (operator) or 911 (emergency) for an ambulance or medical help. Then give first aid immediately.**
- **See emergency information on inside covers.**

POSSIBLE ADVERSE REACTIONS OR SIDE EFFECTS

SYMPTOMS	WHAT TO DO
Life-threatening: None expected.	
Common:	
• Dizziness.	Discontinue. Call doctor right away.
• Diarrhea, appetite loss, nausea, stomach pain, heartburn.	Continue. Call doctor when convenient.
Infrequent: Low blood sugar (hunger, anxiety, cold sweats, rapid pulse), drowsiness, nervousness, headache, weakness, rapid heartbeat.	Discontinue. Seek emergency treatment.
Rare:	
• Itching or rash, sore throat, fever, ringing in ears, unusual bleeding or bruising, fatigue, jaundice, joint pain, numbness or tingling in hands or feet.	Discontinue. Call doctor right away.
• Excess urination at night.	Continue. Call doctor when convenient.

GLYBURIDE

WARNINGS & PRECAUTIONS

Don't take if:
- You are allergic to any sulfonurea.
- You have impaired kidney or liver function.

Before you start, consult your doctor:
- If you have a severe infection.
- If you have thyroid disease.
- If you take insulin.
- If you have heart disease.

Over age 60:
Dose usually smaller than for younger adults. Avoid "low-blood-sugar" episodes because repeated ones can damage brain permanently.

Pregnancy:
No proven harm to unborn child. Avoid if possible.

Breast-feeding:
Drug filters into milk. May lower baby's blood sugar. Avoid.

Infants & children:
Don't give to infants or children.

Prolonged use:
None expected.

Skin & sunlight:
May cause rash or intensify sunburn in areas exposed to sun or sunlamp.

Driving, piloting or hazardous work:
No problems expected unless you develop hypoglycemia (low blood sugar). If so, avoid driving or hazardous activity.

Discontinuing:
Don't discontinue without consulting doctor. Dose may require gradual reduction if you have taken drug for a long time. Doses of other drugs may also require adjustment.

Others:
Don't exceed recommended dose. Hypoglycemia (low blood sugar) may occur, even with proper dose schedule. You must balance medicine, diet and exercise.

POSSIBLE INTERACTION WITH OTHER DRUGS

GENERIC NAME OR DRUG CLASS	COMBINED EFFECT
Androgens*	Increased glyburide effect.
Anticoagulants, oral*	Unpredictable prothrombin times.*
Anticonvulsants, hydantoin*	Decreased glyburide effect.
Aspirin	Increased glyburide effect.
Beta-adrenergic blockers*	Increased glyburide effect. Possible increased difficulty in regulating blood-sugar levels.
Bismuth subsalicylate	Increased insulin effect. May require dosage adjustment.
Chloramphenicol	Increased glyburide effect.
Clofibrate	Increased glyburide effect.
Contraceptives, oral*	Decreased glyburide effect.
Cortisone drugs*	Decreased glyburide effect.
Diuretics, thiazide*	Decreased glyburide effect.
Epinephrine	Decreased glyburide effect.
Estrogens*	Increased glyburide effect.
Guanethidine	Unpredictable glyburide effect.
Labetalol	Increased antidiabetic effect, may mask hypoglycemia.
Non-steroidal anti-inflammatory drugs (NSAIDs)*	Increased glyburide effect.

POSSIBLE INTERACTION WITH OTHER SUBSTANCES

INTERACTS WITH	COMBINED EFFECT
Alcohol:	Disulfiram reaction.* Avoid.
Beverages:	None expected.
Cocaine:	No proven problems.
Foods:	None expected.
Marijuana:	Decreased glyburide effect. Avoid.
Tobacco:	None expected.

*See Glossary

GLYCOPYRROLATE

BRAND NAMES

Robinul   Robinul Forte

BASIC INFORMATION

Habit forming? No
Prescription needed? Yes
Available as generic? Yes
Drug class: Antispasmodic, anticholinergic

USES

- Reduces spasms of digestive system.
- Reduces production of saliva during dental procedures.

DOSAGE & USAGE INFORMATION

How to take:
Tablet—Swallow with liquid. If you can't swallow whole, crumble tablet and take with small amount of liquid or food.

When to take:
30 minutes before meals (unless directed otherwise by doctor).

If you forget a dose:
Wait for next scheduled dose (don't double this dose).

What drug does:
Blocks nerve impulses at parasympathetic nerve endings, preventing smooth (involuntary) muscle contractions and gland secretions of organs involved.

Time lapse before drug works:
15 to 30 minutes.

Don't take with:
See Interaction column and consult doctor.

OVERDOSE

SYMPTOMS:
Dry mouth, blurred vision, low blood pressure, decreased breathing rate, rapid heartbeat, flushed skin, drowsiness.
WHAT TO DO:
- **Dial 0 (operator) or 911 (emergency) for an ambulance or medical help. Then give first aid immediately.**
- **See emergency information on inside covers.**

POSSIBLE ADVERSE REACTIONS OR SIDE EFFECTS

SYMPTOMS	WHAT TO DO
Life-threatening: Hives, rash, intense itching, faintness soon after a dose (anaphylaxis).	Seek emergency treatment immediately.
Common: Dry mouth, loss of taste, constipation, difficult urination.	Continue. Call doctor when convenient.
Infrequent: • Confusion; dizziness; drowsiness; eye pain; headache; rash; sleep disturbance such as nightmares, frequent waking; nausea; vomiting; rapid heartbeat.	Discontinue. Call doctor right away.
• Insomnia, blurred vision, diminished sex drive, decreased sweating.	Continue. Call doctor when convenient.
Rare: Rash, hives.	Discontinue. Call doctor right away.

WARNINGS & PRECAUTIONS

Don't take if:
- You are allergic to any anticholinergic.
- You have trouble with stomach bloating.
- You have difficulty emptying your bladder completely.
- You have narrow-angle glaucoma.
- You have severe ulcerative colitis.

Before you start, consult your doctor:
- If you have open-angle glaucoma.
- If you have angina, chronic bronchitis or asthma, liver disease, hiatal hernia, enlarged prostate, myasthenia gravis, peptic ulcer.
- If you will have surgery within 2 months, including dental surgery, requiring general or spinal anesthesia.

Over age 60:
Adverse reactions and side effects may be more frequent and severe than in younger persons.

Pregnancy:
Studies inconclusive on harm to unborn child. Animal studies show fetal abnormalities. Decide with your doctor whether drug benefits justify risk to unborn child.

Breast-feeding:
Drug passes into milk and decreases milk flow. Avoid drug or discontinue nursing until you finish medicine. Consult doctor for advice on maintaining milk supply.

Infants & children:
Use only under medical supervision.

Prolonged use:
Chronic constipation, possible fecal impaction. Consult doctor immediately.

Skin & sunlight:
No problems expected.

Driving, piloting or hazardous work:
Use disqualifies you for piloting aircraft. Otherwise, no problems expected.

Discontinuing:
May be unnecessary to finish medicine. Follow doctor's instructions.

Others:
Heatstroke more likely if you become overheated during exertion.

POSSIBLE INTERACTION WITH OTHER DRUGS

GENERIC NAME OR DRUG CLASS	COMBINED EFFECT
Antacids*	Decreased glycopyrrolate absorption effect.
Amantadine	Increased glycopyrrolate effect.
Anticholinergics, other*	Increased glycopyrrolate effect.
Antidepressants, tricyclics (TCA)*	Increased glycopyrrolate effect.
Buclizine	Increased glycopyrrolate effect.
Cortisone drugs*	Increased internal-eye pressure.
Digitalis	Possible decreased absorption of digitalis.
Haloperidol	Increased internal-eye pressure.
MAO inhibitors*	Increased glycopyrrolate effect.
Meperidine	Increased glycopyrrolate effect.
Methylphenidate	Increased glycopyrrolate effect.
Molindone	Increased anti-cholinergic effect.

Nizatidine	Increased nizatidine effect.
Orphenadrine	Increased glycopyrrolate effect.
Phenothiazines*	Increased glycopyrrolate effect.
Pilocarpine	Increased glycopyrrolate effect. Loss of pilocarpine effect in glaucoma treatment.
Potassium chloride tabs	Increased side effects of potassium tablets.
Quinidine	Increased glycopyrrolate effect.
Retocunazole	Decreased absorption of both.
Vitamin C	Increased glycopyrrolate effect. Avoid large vitamin C doses.

POSSIBLE INTERACTION WITH OTHER SUBSTANCES

INTERACTS WITH	COMBINED EFFECT
Alcohol:	None expected.
Beverages:	None expected.
Cocaine:	Excessively rapid heartbeat. Avoid.
Foods:	None expected.
Marijuana:	Drowsiness and dry mouth.
Tobacco:	None expected.

*See Glossary

GOLD COMPOUNDS

BRAND AND GENERIC NAMES

AURANOFIN—oral
Aurothioglucose—
  injection
Gold Sodium
  Thiomalate
Myochrysine—
  injection

Myocrisin
Ridaura—oral
SODIUM
  AUROTHIO-
  MALATE
SOLGANAL—
  injection

BASIC INFORMATION

Habit forming? No
Prescription needed? Yes
Available as generic? No
Drug class: Gold compounds

USES

Treatment for rheumatoid arthritis.

DOSAGE & USAGE INFORMATION

How to take:
Capsules—Swallow with full glass of fluid. Follow prescription directions. Taking too much can cause serious adverse reactions.

When to take:
Once or twice daily, morning and night.

If you forget a dose:
Take as soon as you remember up to 6 hours late, then go back to usual schedule.

What drug does:
Modifies disease activity of rheumatoid arthritis by mechanisms not yet understood.

Time lapse before drug works:
3 to 6 months.

Don't take with:
See Interaction column and consult doctor.

OVERDOSE

SYMPTOMS:
Confusion, delirium, numbness and tingling in feet and hands.
WHAT TO DO:
- Induce vomiting with syrup of ipecac if available.
- Dial 0 (operator) or 911 (emergency) for an ambulance or medical help. Then give first aid immediately.
- See emergency information on inside covers.

POSSIBLE ADVERSE REACTIONS OR SIDE EFFECTS

SYMPTOMS	WHAT TO DO
Life-threatening:	
Hives, rash, intense itching, faintness soon after a dose (anaphylaxis).	Seek emergency treatment immediately.
Common:	
• Itch; hives; sores or white spots in mouth, throat; appetite loss; diarrhea; vomiting; protein in urine; skin rashes; fever.	Discontinue. Call doctor right away.
• Abdominal cramps.	Continue. Call doctor when convenient.
Infrequent:	
• Excessive fatigue; sore tongue, mouth or gums; metallic or odd taste; unusual bleeding or bruising; blood in urine; changes in white blood cells, platelets; vaginal discharge; flushing; fainting; dizziness; sweating after injection.	Discontinue. Call doctor right away.
• Hair loss; pain in muscles, bones and joints (with injections).	Continue. Call doctor when convenient.
Rare:	
• Blood in stool, difficult breathing, coughing, seizures.	Discontinue. Seek emergency treatment.
• Abdominal pain, jaundice, numbness or tingling in hands or feet, muscle weakness.	Discontinue. Call doctor right away.
• "Pink eye."	Continue. Call doctor when convenient.

WARNINGS & PRECAUTIONS

Don't take if:
- You have history of allergy to gold or other metals.
- You have any blood disorder.
- You have kidney disease.

Before you start, consult your doctor:
- If you are pregnant or may become pregnant.
- If you have lupus erythematosus.
- If you have Schogren's syndrome.
- If you have chronic skin disease.

Over age 60:
Adverse reactions and side effects may be more frequent and severe than in younger persons.

Pregnancy:
Avoid if possible. Animal studies show that gold compounds can cause birth defects.

Breast-feeding:
Drug may filter into milk, causing side effects in infants. Avoid.

Infants & children:
Not recommended. Safety and dosage have not been established.

Prolonged use:
Request periodic laboratory studies of blood counts, urine and liver function. These should be done before use and at least once a month during treatment.

Skin & sunlight:
- Skin rash may be aggravated by sunlight.
- Blue-gray pigmentation in photoexposed areas.

Driving, piloting or hazardous work:
Avoid if you have serious adverse reactions or side effects. Otherwise, no problems expected.

Discontinuing:
Don't discontinue without doctor's advice until you complete prescribed dose.

Others:
- Side effects and adverse reactions may appear during treatment or for many months after discontinuing.
- Gold has been shown to cause kidney tumors and kidney cancer in animals given excessive doses.

POSSIBLE INTERACTION WITH OTHER DRUGS

GENERIC NAME OR DRUG CLASS	COMBINED EFFECT
Cyclosporine	May increase risk of kidney toxicity.
Non-steroidal anti-inflammatory drugs (NSAIDs)*	Possible increased likelihood of kidney damage.
Penicillamine	Possible increased likelihood of kidney damage.
Phenytoin	Increased phenytoin blood levels. Phenytoin dosage may require adjustment.

POSSIBLE INTERACTION WITH OTHER SUBSTANCES

INTERACTS WITH	COMBINED EFFECT
Alcohol:	None expected.
Beverages:	None expected.
Cocaine:	None expected.
Foods:	None expected.
Marijuana:	None expected.
Tobacco:	None expected.

GRISEOFULVIN

BRAND NAMES

Fulvicin P/G
Fulvicin U/F
Grifulvin V
Gris-PEG

Grisactin
Grisactin Ultra
Grisovin-FP
grisOwen

BASIC INFORMATION

Habit forming? No
Prescription needed? Yes
Available as generic? Yes
Drug class: Antibiotic (antifungal)

USES

Treatment for fungal infections susceptible to griseofulvin.

DOSAGE & USAGE INFORMATION

How to take:
- Tablet or capsule—Swallow with liquid or food to lessen stomach irritation. If you can't swallow whole, crumble tablet or open capsule and take with liquid or food.
- Liquid—Follow label instructions.

When to take:
With or immediately after meals.

If you forget a dose:
Take as soon as you remember up to 2 hours late. If more than 2 hours, wait for next scheduled dose (don't double this dose).

What drug does:
Prevents fungi from growing and reproducing.

Time lapse before drug works:
2 to 10 days for skin infections. 2 to 4 weeks for infections of fingernails or toenails. Complete cure of either may require several months.

Don't take with:
See Interaction column and consult doctor.

OVERDOSE

SYMPTOMS:
Nausea, vomiting, diarrhea. In sensitive individuals, severe diarrhea may occur without overdosing.
WHAT TO DO:
Overdose unlikely to threaten life. If person takes much larger amount than prescribed, call doctor, poison-control center or hospital emergency room for instructions.

POSSIBLE ADVERSE REACTIONS OR SIDE EFFECTS

SYMPTOMS	WHAT TO DO
Life-threatening: None expected.	
Common: Headache.	Continue. Tell doctor at next visit.
Infrequent: • Confusion; rash, hives, itch; mouth or tongue irritation; soreness; nausea; vomiting; diarrhea; stomach pain.	Discontinue. Call doctor right away.
• Insomnia, tiredness.	Continue. Call doctor when convenient.
Rare: Sore throat, fever, numbness or tingling in hands or feet, cloudy urine, sensitivity to sunlight.	Discontinue. Call doctor right away.

WARNINGS & PRECAUTIONS

Don't take if:
- You are allergic to any antifungal medicine.
- You are allergic to penicillin.
- You have liver disease.
- You have porphyria.
- The infection is minor and will respond to less-potent drugs.

Before you start, consult your doctor:
- If you plan to become pregnant within medication period.
- If you have liver disease.
- If you have lupus.

Over age 60:
Adverse reactions and side effects may be more frequent and severe than in younger persons.

Pregnancy:
Risk to unborn child outweighs drug benefits. Don't use.

Breast-feeding:
No problems expected, but consult your doctor.

Infants & children:
Not recommended for children younger than 2.

Prolonged use:
You may become susceptible to infections caused by germs not responsive to griseofulvin.

Skin & sunlight:
May cause rash or intensify sunburn in areas exposed to sun or sunlamp.

Driving, piloting or hazardous work:
- Don't drive if you feel dizzy or have vision problems.
- Don't pilot aircraft.

Discontinuing:
Don't discontinue without doctor's advice until you complete prescribed dose, even though symptoms diminish or disappear.

Others:
Periodic laboratory blood studies and liver- and kidney-function tests recommended.

POSSIBLE INTERACTION WITH OTHER DRUGS

GENERIC NAME OR DRUG CLASS	COMBINED EFFECT
Anticoagulants, oral*	Decreased anti-anticoagulant effect.
Barbiturates*	Decreased griseofulvin effect.
Contraceptives, oral*	Decreased contra-ceptive effect.

POSSIBLE INTERACTION WITH OTHER SUBSTANCES

INTERACTS WITH	COMBINED EFFECT
Alcohol:	Increased intoxication. Possible disulfiram reaction.*
Beverages:	None expected.
Cocaine:	None expected.
Foods:	None expected; but foods high in fat will improve drug absorption.
Marijuana:	None expected.
Tobacco:	None expected.

GUAIFENESIN

BRAND NAMES

See complete list of brand names in the *Brand Name Directory*, page 1063.

BASIC INFORMATION

Habit forming? No
Prescription needed? No
Available as generic? Yes
Drug class: Cough/cold preparation

 USES

Loosens mucus in respiratory passages from allergies and infections (hay fever, cough, cold).

 DOSAGE & USAGE INFORMATION

How to take:
- Tablet, capsule or extended-release tablet—Swallow with liquid. If you can't swallow whole, crumble tablet or open capsule and take with liquid or food.
- Syrup or lozenge—Take as directed on label. Follow with 8 oz. water.

When to take:
As needed, no more often than every 3 hours.

If you forget a dose:
Take as soon as you remember. Wait 3 hours for next dose.

What drug does:
Increases production of watery fluids to thin mucus so it can be coughed out or absorbed.

Time lapse before drug works:
15 to 30 minutes. Regular use for 5 to 7 days necessary for maximum benefit.

Don't take with:
See Interaction column and consult doctor.

 OVERDOSE

SYMPTOMS:
Drowsiness, mild weakness, nausea, vomiting.
WHAT TO DO:
Overdose unlikely to threaten life. If person takes much larger amount than prescribed, call doctor, poison-control center or hospital emergency room for instructions.

 POSSIBLE ADVERSE REACTIONS OR SIDE EFFECTS

SYMPTOMS	WHAT TO DO
Life-threatening: None expected.	
Common: None expected.	
Infrequent:	
• Rash, stomach pain, diarrhea, nausea, vomiting.	Discontinue. Call doctor right away.
• Drowsiness.	Continue. Call doctor when convenient.
Rare: None expected.	

WARNINGS & PRECAUTIONS

Don't take if:
You are allergic to any cough or cold preparation containing guaifenesin.

Before you start, consult your doctor:
See Interaction column and consult doctor.

Over age 60:
Adverse reactions and side effects may be more frequent and severe than in younger persons. For drug to work, you must drink 8 to 10 glasses of fluid per day.

Pregnancy:
No proven harm to unborn child. Avoid if possible.

Breast-feeding:
No proven problems. Consult your doctor.

Infants & children:
No problems expected.

Prolonged use:
No problems expected.

Skin & sunlight:
No problems expected.

Driving, piloting or hazardous work:
Avoid if you feel drowsy. Otherwise, no problems expected.

Discontinuing:
May be unnecessary to finish medicine. Discontinue when symptoms disappear. If symptoms persist more than 1 week, consult doctor.

Others:
No problems expected.

POSSIBLE INTERACTION WITH OTHER DRUGS

GENERIC NAME OR DRUG CLASS	COMBINED EFFECT
Anticoagulants*	Possible risk of bleeding.

POSSIBLE INTERACTION WITH OTHER SUBSTANCES

INTERACTS WITH	COMBINED EFFECT
Alcohol:	No proven problems.
Beverages:	You must drink 8 to 10 glasses of fluid per day for drug to work.
Cocaine:	No proven problems.
Foods:	None expected.
Marijuana:	No proven problems.
Tobacco:	No proven problems.

*See Glossary

GUANABENZ

BRAND NAMES

Wytensin

BASIC INFORMATION

Habit forming? No
Prescription needed? Yes
Available as generic? No
Drug class: Antihypertensive (alpha adrenergic stimulant)

USES

Controls, but doesn't cure, high blood pressure.

DOSAGE & USAGE INFORMATION

How to take:
Tablet—Swallow with liquid or food to lessen stomach irritation. If you can't swallow whole, crumble tablet and take with liquid or food.

When to take:
At the same times each day.

If you forget a dose:
Take as soon as you remember up to 2 hours late. If more than 2 hours, wait for next scheduled dose (don't double this dose).

What drug does:
● Relaxes muscle cells of small arteries.
● Slows heartbeat.

Time lapse before drug works:
1 hour.

Don't take with:
See Interaction column and consult doctor.

OVERDOSE

SYMPTOMS:
Severe dizziness, slow heartbeat, pinpoint pupils, fainting, coma.
WHAT TO DO:
● Dial 0 (operator) or 911 (emergency) for an ambulance or medical help. Then give first aid immediately.
● If patient is unconscious and not breathing, give mouth-to-mouth breathing. If there is no heartbeat, use cardiac massage and mouth-to-mouth breathing (CPR). Don't try to make patient vomit. If you can't get help quickly, take patient to nearest emergency facility.
● See emergency information on inside covers.

POSSIBLE ADVERSE REACTIONS OR SIDE EFFECTS

SYMPTOMS	WHAT TO DO
Life-threatening: None expected.	
Common:	
● Nervousness, rapid heartbeat, paleness, dry mouth, drowsiness.	Continue. Call doctor when convenient.
● Insomnia.	Continue. Tell doctor at next visit.
Infrequent:	
● Irregular heartbeat, shakiness in hands.	Discontinue. Call doctor right away.
● Dizziness, appetite loss, nausea, vomiting, painful or difficult urination, diminished sex drive.	Continue. Call doctor when convenient.
Rare: None expected.	

WARNINGS & PRECAUTIONS

Don't take if:
You are allergic to any sympathomimetic drug.

Before you start, consult your doctor:
● If you have blood disease.
● If you have heart disease.
● If you have liver disease.
● If you have diabetes or overactive thyroid.
● If you will have surgery within 2 months, including dental surgery, requiring general or spinal anesthesia.

Over age 60:
Adverse reactions and side effects may be more frequent and severe than in younger persons. Hot weather may cause need to reduce dosage.

Pregnancy:
Risk to unborn child outweighs drug benefits. Don't use.

Breast-feeding:
Avoid nursing.

Infants & children:
Not recommended.

Prolonged use:
Side effects tend to diminish. Request uric-acid and kidney-function studies periodically.

Skin & sunlight:
No problems expected.

Driving, piloting or hazardous work:
Avoid if you feel dizzy; otherwise, no problems expected.

Discontinuing:
Don't discontinue without consulting doctor. Dose may require gradual reduction if you have taken drug for a long time. Doses of other drugs may also require adjustment. Abrupt discontinuing may cause anxiety, chest pain, salivation, headache, abdominal cramps, fast heartbeat.

Others:
Stay away from high sodium foods. Lose weight if you are overweight.

POSSIBLE INTERACTION WITH OTHER DRUGS

GENERIC NAME OR DRUG CLASS	COMBINED EFFECT
ACE Inhibitors: captopril, enalapril, lisinopril*	Possible excessive potassium in blood.
Antihypertensives, other*	Decreases blood pressure more than either alone. May be beneficial, but requires dosage adjustment.
Brain depressants* (sedatives,* sleeping pills,* tranquilizers,* antidepressants,* narcotics*)	Increased brain depression. Avoid.
Diuretics*	Decreases blood pressure more than either alone. May be beneficial, but requires dosage adjustment.
Ethinamate	Dangerous increased effects of ethinamate. Avoid combining.
Fluoxetine	Increased depressant effects of both drugs.
Guanfacine	May increase depressant effects of either drug.

Leucovorin	High alcohol content of leucovorin may cause adverse effects.
Methyprylon	Increased sedative effect, perhaps to dangerous level. Avoid.
Nabilone	Greater depression of central nervous system.
Nicardipine	Blood-pressure drop. Dosages may require adjustment.

POSSIBLE INTERACTION WITH OTHER SUBSTANCES

INTERACTS WITH	COMBINED EFFECT
Alcohol:	Oversedation. Avoid.
Beverages: Caffeine.	Overstimulation. Avoid.
Cocaine:	Overstimulation. Avoid.
Foods: Salt.	Decrease salt intake to increase beneficial effects of guanabenz.
Marijuana:	Overstimulation. Avoid.
Tobacco:	Decreased guanabenz effect.

GUANADREL

BRAND NAMES

Hylorel

BASIC INFORMATION

Habit forming? No
Prescription needed? Yes
Available as generic? No
Drug class: Antihypertensive

USES

Controls, but doesn't cure, high blood pressure.

DOSAGE & USAGE INFORMATION

How to take:
Tablet—Swallow with liquid or food to lessen stomach irritation. If you can't swallow whole, crumble tablet and take with liquid or food.

When to take:
At the same time each day.

If you forget a dose:
Take as soon as you remember up to 2 hours late. If more than 2 hours, wait for next scheduled dose (don't double this dose).

What drug does:
Relaxes muscle cells of small arteries.

Time lapse before drug works:
4 to 6 hours. May need to take for lifetime.

Don't take with:
See Interaction column and consult doctor.

OVERDOSE

SYMPTOMS:
Severe blood-pressure drop; fainting; slow, weak pulse; cold, sweaty skin; loss of consciousness.
WHAT TO DO:
- Dial 0 (operator) or 911 (emergency) for an ambulance or medical help. Then give first aid immediately.
- See emergency information on inside covers.

POSSIBLE ADVERSE REACTIONS OR SIDE EFFECTS

SYMPTOMS	WHAT TO DO
Life-threatening: None expected.	
Common:	
• Diarrhea, more bowel movements, fatigue, weakness.	Continue. Call doctor when convenient.
• Dizziness, headache, lower sex drive.	Continue. Tell doctor at next visit.
• Stuffy nose, dry mouth.	No action necessary.
Infrequent:	
• Rash, blurred vision, drooping eyelids, chest pain or shortness of breath, muscle pain or tremor.	Discontinue. Call doctor right away.
• Nausea or vomiting.	Continue. Call doctor when convenient.
• Impotence, nighttime urination.	Continue. Tell doctor at next visit.
Rare:	
Decreased white blood cells causing sore throat, fever, headache.	Discontinue. Call doctor right away.

WARNINGS & PRECAUTIONS

Don't take if:
- You are allergic to guanadrel.
- You have taken MAO inhibitors within 2 weeks.

Before you start, consult your doctor:
- If you have stroke or heart disease.
- If you have asthma.
- If you have had kidney disease.
- If you have peptic ulcer or chronic acid indigestion.
- If you will have surgery within 2 months, including dental surgery, requiring general or spinal anesthesia.

Over age 60:
Adverse reactions and side effects may be more frequent and severe than in younger persons. Start with small doses and monitor blood pressure frequently.

Pregnancy:
No proven harm to unborn child. Avoid if possible.

Breast-feeding:
No proven harm to nursing infant. Avoid if possible.

Infants & children:
Not recommended.

Prolonged use:
Due to drug's cumulative effect, dose will require adjustment to prevent wide fluctuations in blood pressure.

Skin & sunlight:
No problems expected.

Driving, piloting or hazardous work:
Don't drive or pilot aircraft until you learn how medicine affects you. Don't work around dangerous machinery. Don't climb ladders or work in high places. Danger increases if you drink alcohol or take medicine affecting alertness and reflexes, such as antihistamines, tranquilizers, sedatives, pain medicine, narcotics and mind-altering drugs.

Discontinuing:
Don't discontinue without consulting doctor. Dose may require gradual reduction if you have taken drug for a long time. Doses of other drugs may also require adjustment.

Others:
Hot weather further lowers blood pressure, particularly in patients over 60.

POSSIBLE INTERACTION WITH OTHER DRUGS

GENERIC NAME OR DRUG CLASS	COMBINED EFFECT
ACE inhibitors: captopril, enalapril, lisinopril*	Possible excessive potassium in blood.
Antidepressants, tricyclic (TCA)*	Decreased effect of guanadrel.
Antihypertensives, other*	Increased effect of guanadrel.
Beta-adrenergic blockers*	Increased likelihood of dizziness and fainting.
Carteolol	Increased antihypertensive effect.
Contraceptives, oral*	Increased side effects of oral contraceptives.
CNS depressants* (anticonvulsants,* antihistamines,* muscle relaxants,* narcotics,* sedatives,* tranquilizers*)	Decreased effect of guanadrel.
Diuretics*	Increased likelihood of dizziness and fainting.
Haloperidol	Decreased effect of guanadrel.

Insulin	Increased insulin effect.
Loxapine	Decreased effect of guanadrel.
MAO inhibitors*	Severe high blood pressure. Avoid.
Nicardipine	Blood-pressure drop. Dosages may require adjustment.
Phenothiazines*	Decreased effect of guanadrel.
Rauwolfia alkaloids*	Increased likelihood of dizziness and fainting.
Sotalol	Increased antihypertensive effect.
Sympathomimetics*	Decreased effect of guanadrel.
Terazosin	Decreases effectiveness of terazosin.

POSSIBLE INTERACTION WITH OTHER SUBSTANCES

INTERACTS WITH	COMBINED EFFECT
Alcohol:	Decreased effect of guanadrel. Avoid.
Beverages: Caffeine.	Decreased effect of guanadrel.
Cocaine:	Increased risk of heart block and high blood pressure.
Foods:	No problems expected.
Marijuana:	Higher blood pressure. Avoid.
Tobacco:	Higher blood pressure. Avoid.

*See Glossary

GUANETHIDINE

BRAND NAMES

Apo-Guanethidine   Ismelin
Esimil   Ismelin-Esidrix

BASIC INFORMATION

Habit forming? No
Prescription needed? Yes
Available as generic? Yes
Drug class: Antihypertensive

USES

Reduces high blood pressure.

DOSAGE & USAGE INFORMATION

How to take:
Tablet—Swallow with liquid. If you can't swallow tablet whole, crumble and take with liquid or food.

When to take:
At the same time each day.

If you forget a dose:
Take as soon as you remember up to 2 hours late. If more than 2 hours, wait for next scheduled dose (don't double this dose).

What drug does:
Displaces norepinephrine—hormone necessary to maintain small blood-vessel tone. Blood vessels relax and high blood pressure drops.

Time lapse before drug works:
Regular use for several weeks may be necessary to determine effectiveness.

Don't take with:
- Non-prescription drugs containing alcohol without consulting doctor.
- See Interaction column and consult doctor.

OVERDOSE

SYMPTOMS:
Severe blood-pressure drop; fainting; slow, weak pulse; cold, sweaty skin; loss of consciousness.
WHAT TO DO:
- **Dial 0 (operator) or 911 (emergency) for an ambulance or medical help. Then give first aid immediately.**
- **See emergency information on inside covers.**

POSSIBLE ADVERSE REACTIONS OR SIDE EFFECTS

SYMPTOMS	WHAT TO DO
Life-threatening:	
None expected.	
Common:	
• Unusually slow heartbeat.	Discontinue. Call doctor right away.
• Diarrhea; more bowel movements; swollen feet, legs; fatigue, weakness.	Continue. Call doctor when convenient.
• Dizziness, headache, lower sex drive.	Continue. Tell doctor at next visit.
• Stuffy nose, dry mouth.	No action necessary.
Infrequent:	
• Rash, blurred vision, drooping eyelids, chest pain or shortness of breath, muscle pain or tremor.	Discontinue. Call doctor right away.
• Nausea or vomiting.	Continue. Call doctor when convenient.
• Impotence, nighttime urination.	Continue. Tell doctor at next visit.
Rare:	
Decreased white blood cells causing sore throat, fever, headache.	Discontinue. Call doctor right away.

WARNINGS & PRECAUTIONS

Don't take if:
- You are allergic to guanethidine.
- You have taken MAO inhibitors within 2 weeks.

Before you start, consult your doctor:
- If you have had stroke or heart disease.
- If you have asthma.
- If you have had kidney disease.
- If you have peptic ulcer or chronic acid indigestion.
- If you will have surgery within 2 months, including dental surgery, requiring general or spinal anesthesia.

Over age 60:
Adverse reactions and side effects may be more frequent and severe than in younger persons. Start with small doses and monitor blood pressure frequently.

Pregnancy:
No proven harm to unborn child. Avoid if possible.

Breast-feeding:
No proven harm to nursing infant. Avoid if possible.

Infants & children:
Not recommended.

Prolonged use:
Due to drug's cumulative effect, dose will require adjustment to prevent wide fluctuations in blood pressure.

Skin & sunlight:
No problems expected.

Driving, piloting or hazardous work:
Don't drive or pilot aircraft until you learn how medicine affects you. Don't work around dangerous machinery. Don't climb ladders or work in high places. Danger increases if you drink alcohol or take medicine affecting alertness and reflexes, such as antihistamines, tranquilizers, sedatives, pain medicine, narcotics and mind-altering drugs.

Discontinuing:
Don't discontinue without consulting doctor. Dose may require gradual reduction if you have taken drug for a long time. Doses of other drugs may also require adjustment.

Others:
Hot weather further lowers blood pressure.

POSSIBLE INTERACTION WITH OTHER DRUGS

GENERIC NAME OR DRUG CLASS	COMBINED EFFECT
ACE inhibitors: captopril, enalapril, lisinopril*	Possible excessive potassium in blood.
Amphetamines*	Decreased guanethidine effect.
Antidepressants, tricyclic (TCA)*	Decreased guanethidine effect.
Antihistamines*	Decreased guanethidine effect.
Carteolol	Increased antihypertensive effect.
Contraceptives, oral*	Decreased guanethidine effect. Increased side effects of oral contraceptives.
Digitalis preparations*	Slower heartbeat.
Diuretics, thiazide*	Increased guanethidine effect.
Haloperidol	Decreased guanethidine effect.

Indapamide	Possible increased effects of both drugs. When monitored carefully, combination may be beneficial in controlling hypertension.
Insulin	Increased insulin effect.
Loxapine	Decreased effect of guanethidine.
MAO inhibitors*	Increased blood pressure.
Minoxidil	Dosage adjustments may be necessary to keep blood pressure at proper level.
Nicardipine	Blood-pressure drop. Dosages may require adjustment.
Phenothiazines*	Decreased guanethidine effect.
Rauwolfia alkaloids*	Excessively slow heartbeat. Weakness and faintness upon rising from chair or bed.
Sotalol	Increased antihypertensive effect.
Terazosin	Decreases effectiveness of terazosin.

POSSIBLE INTERACTION WITH OTHER SUBSTANCES

INTERACTS WITH	COMBINED EFFECT
Alcohol:	Use caution. Decreases blood pressure.
Beverages: Carbonated drinks.	Use sparingly. Sodium content increases blood pressure.
Cocaine:	Increased risk of heart block and high blood pressure.
Foods: Spicy or acid foods.	Avoid if subject to indigestion or peptic ulcer.
Marijuana:	Excessively low blood pressure. Avoid.
Tobacco:	Possible blood-pressure rise. Avoid.

GUANETHIDINE & HYDROCHLOROTHIAZIDE

BRAND NAMES

Esimil

BASIC INFORMATION

Habit forming? No
Prescription needed? Yes
Available as generic? No
Drug class: Antihypertensive-diuretic

 ## USES

- Controls, but doesn't cure, high blood pressure.
- Reduces fluid retention (edema).

 ## DOSAGE & USAGE INFORMATION

How to take:
Tablet—Swallow with liquid. If you can't swallow whole, crumble tablet and take with liquid or food.

When to take:
At the same time each day.

If you forget a dose:
Take as soon as you remember up to 2 hours late. If more than 2 hours, wait for next scheduled dose (don't double this dose).

What drug does:
- Forces sodium and water secretion, reducing body fluid.
- Displaces norepinephrine—hormone necessary to maintain small blood-vessel tone. Blood vessels relax and high blood pressure drops.

Time lapse before drug works:
Regular use for several weeks may be necessary to determine effectiveness.

Continued next column

 ## OVERDOSE

SYMPTOMS:
Cramps, weakness, drowsiness, weak pulse, severe blood-pressure drop, fainting, cold and sweaty skin, loss of consciousness, coma.
WHAT TO DO:
- **Dial 0 (operator) or 911 (emergency) for an ambulance or medical help. Then give first aid immediately.**
- **See emergency information on inside covers.**

Don't take with:
- Non-prescription drugs containing alcohol without consulting doctor.
- See Interaction column and consult doctor.

 ## POSSIBLE ADVERSE REACTIONS OR SIDE EFFECTS

SYMPTOMS	WHAT TO DO
Life-threatening:	
Chest pain, shortness of breath, irregular heartbeat.	Discontinue. Seek emergency treatment.
Common:	
• Slow heartbeat, swollen feet and ankles, fatigue, weakness.	Discontinue. Call doctor right away.
• Dizziness, headache, stuffy nose, dry mouth, diarrhea, diminished sex drive.	Continue. Call doctor when convenient.
Infrequent:	
• Mood change, rash or hives, blurred vision, drooping eyelids, muscle pain or tremors.	Discontinue. Call doctor right away.
• Increased nighttime urination, abdominal pain, vomiting, nausea, weakness.	Continue. Call doctor when convenient.
• Impotence.	Continue. Tell doctor at next visit.
Rare:	
• Decreased white blood cells causing sore throat, fever, headache; jaundice.	Discontinue. Call doctor right away.
• Weight gain or loss.	Continue. Call doctor when convenient.

 ## WARNINGS & PRECAUTIONS

Don't take if:
- You are allergic to any thiazide diuretic drug or guanethidine.
- You have taken MAO inhibitors within 2 weeks.

Before you start, consult your doctor:
- If you are allergic to any sulfa drug.
- If you have gout, asthma, liver, pancreas or kidney disorder, peptic ulcer or chronic acid indigestion.
- If you have had stroke or heart disease.
- If you will have surgery within 2 months, including dental surgery, requiring general or spinal anesthesia.

Over age 60:
Adverse reactions and side effects may be more frequent and severe than in younger persons, especially dizziness and excessive potassium loss.

Pregnancy:
Risk to unborn child outweighs drug benefits. Don't use.

Breast-feeding:
Drug passes into milk. Avoid drug or discontinue nursing until you finish medicine. Consult doctor for advice on maintaining milk supply.

Infants & children:
Not recommended.

Prolonged use:
Due to drug's cumulative effect, dose will require adjustment to prevent wide fluctuations in blood pressure.

Skin & sunlight:
May cause rash or intensify sunburn in areas exposed to sun or sunlamp.

Driving, piloting or hazardous work:
Don't drive or pilot aircraft until you learn how medicine affects you. Don't work around dangerous machinery. Don't climb ladders or work in high places. Danger increases if you drink alcohol or take medicine affecting alertness and reflexes, such as antihistamines, tranquilizers, sedatives, pain medicine, narcotics and mind-altering drugs.

Discontinuing:
Don't discontinue without consulting doctor. Dose may require gradual reduction if you have taken drug for a long time. Doses of other drugs may also require adjustment.

Others:
• Hot weather and fever may cause dehydration and drop in blood pressure. Dose may require temporary adjustment. Weigh daily and report any unexpected weight decreases to your doctor.
• May cause rise in uric acid, leading to gout.
• May cause blood-sugar rise in diabetics.

POSSIBLE INTERACTION WITH OTHER DRUGS

GENERIC NAME OR DRUG CLASS	COMBINED EFFECT
Allopurinol	Decreased allopurinol effect.
Amphetamines*	Decreased guanethidine effect.
Antidepressants, tricyclic (TCA)*	Dangerous drop in blood pressure. Avoid combination unless under medical supervision.

Antihistamines*	Decreased guanethidine effect.
Barbiturates*	Increased hydro-chlorothiazide effect.
Beta-adrenergic blockers*	Increased antihyper-tensive effect. Dosages of both drugs may require adjustments.
Carteolol	Increased antihyper-tensive effect.
Cholestyramine	Decreased hydro-chlorothiazide effect.
Contraceptives, oral*	Decreased guanethi-dine effect.
Cortisone drugs*	Excessive potassium loss that causes dan-gerous heart rhythms.
Digitalis preparations*	Excessive potassium loss that causes dan-gerous heart rhythms.

Continued page 1087

POSSIBLE INTERACTION WITH OTHER SUBSTANCES

INTERACTS WITH	COMBINED EFFECT
Alcohol:	Use caution. Decreases blood pressure.
Beverages: Carbonated drinks.	Use sparingly. Sodium content increases blood pressure.
Cocaine:	Raises blood pressure. Avoid.
Foods: Spicy or acid foods. Licorice.	Avoid if subject to indi-gestion or peptic ulcer. Excessive potassium loss that causes dan-gerous heart rhythms.
Marijuana:	Effect on blood pressure unpredictable.
Tobacco:	Possible blood-pressure rise. Avoid.

*See Glossary

GUANFACINE

BRAND NAMES

Tenex

BASIC INFORMATION

Habit forming? No
Prescription needed? Yes
Available as generic? No
Drug class: Antihypertensive

 ## USES

Treats high blood pressure, usually in combination with a diuretic drug.

 ## DOSAGE & USAGE INFORMATION

How to take:
Tablets—Swallow with liquid or food to lessen stomach irritation. If you can't swallow whole, crumble tablet and take with liquid or food.

When to take:
Usually at bedtime.

If you forget a dose:
Take as soon as you remember up to 2 hours late. If more than 2 hours, wait for next scheduled dose (don't double this dose).

What drug does:
- Decreases stimulating effects of the sympathetic nervous system on the heart, kidneys and arteries throughout the body.
- Decreases both systolic and diastolic blood pressure.

Time lapse before drug works:
Within 1 week.

Don't take with:
See Interaction column and consult doctor.

 ## OVERDOSE

SYMPTOMS:
Difficulty breathing, loss of consciousness, dizziness, very slow heartbeat.
WHAT TO DO:
- **Dial 0 (operator) or 911 (emergency) for an ambulance or medical help. Then give first aid immediately.**
- **See emergency information on inside covers.**

 ## POSSIBLE ADVERSE REACTIONS OR SIDE EFFECTS

SYMPTOMS	WHAT TO DO
Life-threatening:	
Shortness of breath (rare).	Seek emergency treatment immediately.
Common:	
• Constipation.	Discontinue. Call doctor right away.
• Decreased sexual function.	Continue. Call doctor when convenient.
• Increased dental problems because of dry mouth and less salivation.	Consult your dentist about a prevention program.
Infrequent:	
• Confusion.	Discontinue. Call doctor right away.
• Mental depression, eye irritation, insomnia, tiredness or weakness.	Continue. Call doctor when convenient.
Rare:	
May occur if medicine is abruptly discontinued: Anxiety, chest pain, heartbeat irregularities, excess salivation, sleep problems, nervousness, sweating.	Discontinue. Seek emergency treatment.

 ## WARNINGS & PRECAUTIONS

Don't take if:
You have had a recent heart attack.

Before you start, consult your doctor:
- If you have heart disease or liver disease.
- If you have coronary insufficiency.
- If you have mental depression.

Over age 60:
None expected.

Pregnancy:
No proven harm to unborn child, but avoid if possible.

Breast-feeding:
Effect not documented. Consult your pediatrician.

Infants & children:
Effect not documented. Consult your pediatrician.

Prolonged use:
No problems expected.

Skin & sunlight:
No problems expected.

Driving, piloting or hazardous work:
Don't drive or pilot aircraft until you learn how medicine affects you. Don't work around dangerous machinery. Don't climb ladders or work in high places. Danger increases if you drink alcohol or take medicine affecting alertness and reflexes.

Discontinuing:
- Don't discontinue without consulting doctor. Dose may require gradual reduction if you have taken drug for a long time. Doses of other drugs may also require adjustment.
- May occur if medicine is discontinued abruptly: anxiety, chest pain, heartbeat irregularities, excess salivation, sleep problems, nervousness, sweating.

Others:
- This medication works better if you attempt to reduce your weight to normal, exercise regularly, restrict salt in your diet and reduce stress wherever possible. Continue taking medicine even when you feel good.
- Adverse reactions are usually dose-related and diminish when dosage is reduced.

POSSIBLE INTERACTION WITH OTHER DRUGS

GENERIC NAME OR DRUG CLASS	COMBINED EFFECT
Antihypertensives, other*	May increase effects of guanfacine and other medicines.
Carteolol	Increased antihypertensive effect.
Central nervous system (CNS) depressants*	Increases depressant effect of both drugs.
Estrogens*	May decrease antihypertensive effects of guanfacine.
Ethinamate	Dangerous increased effects of ethinamate. Avoid combining.
Fluoxetine	Increased depressant effects of both drugs.

Leucovorin	High alcohol content of leucovorin may cause adverse effects.
Lisinopril	Increased antihypertensive effect. Dosage of each may require adjustment.
Methyprylon	Increased sedative effect, perhaps to dangerous level. Avoid.
Nabilone	Greater depression of central nervous system.
Nicardipine	Blood-pressure drop. Dosages may require adjustment.

Continued page 1087

POSSIBLE INTERACTION WITH OTHER SUBSTANCES

INTERACTS WITH	COMBINED EFFECT
Alcohol:	Excess use may lead to dangerous drop in blood pressure.
Beverages: Any containing caffeine, such as coffee, tea or cocoa.	May decrease antihypertensive effect of guanfacine.
Cocaine:	Increased risk of heart block and high blood pressure.
Foods:	None expected.
Marijuana:	May decrease antihypertensive effect of guanfacine.
Tobacco:	May decrease antihypertensive effect of guanfacine.

HALAZEPAM

BRAND NAMES

Paxipam

BASIC INFORMATION

Habit forming? Yes
Prescription needed? Yes
Available as generic? No
Drug class: Tranquilizer (benzodiazepine)

 USES

Treatment for nervousness or tension.

 DOSAGE & USAGE INFORMATION

How to take:
Tablet—Swallow with liquid. If you can't swallow whole, crumble tablet and take with liquid or food.

When to take:
At the same time each day, according to instructions on prescription label.

If you forget a dose:
Take as soon as you remember up to 2 hours late. If more than 2 hours, wait for next scheduled dose (don't double this dose).

What drug does:
Affects limbic system of brain—part that controls emotions.

Time lapse before drug works:
2 hours. May take 6 weeks for full benefit.

Don't take with:
See Interaction column and consult doctor.

 OVERDOSE

SYMPTOMS:
Drowsiness, weakness, tremor, stupor, coma.
WHAT TO DO:
- Dial 0 (operator) or 911 (emergency) for an ambulance or medical help. Then give first aid immediately.
- If patient is unconscious and not breathing, give mouth-to-mouth breathing. If there is no heartbeat, use cardiac massage and mouth-to-mouth breathing (CPR). Don't try to make patient vomit. If you can't get help quickly, take patient to nearest emergency facility.
- See emergency information on inside covers.

 POSSIBLE ADVERSE REACTIONS OR SIDE EFFECTS

SYMPTOMS	WHAT TO DO
Life-threatening: None expected.	
Common: Clumsiness, dizziness, drowsiness.	Continue. Call doctor when convenient.
Infrequent: • Hallucinations, confusion, irritability, depression, rash, itch, change in vision.	Discontinue. Call doctor right away.
• Constipation or diarrhea, nausea, vomiting, painful or difficult urination, vivid dreams.	Continue. Call doctor when convenient.
Rare: • Slow heartbeat, difficult breathing.	Discontinue. Seek emergency treatment.
• Mouth, throat ulcers; jaundice.	Discontinue. Call doctor right away.
• Decreased libido.	Continue. Call doctor when convenient.

 WARNINGS & PRECAUTIONS

Don't take if:
- You are allergic to any benzodiazepine.
- You have myasthenia gravis.
- You are active or recovering alcoholic.
- Patient is younger than 6 months.

Before you start, consult your doctor:
- If you have liver, kidney or lung disease.
- If you have diabetes, epilepsy or porphyria.

Over age 60:
Adverse reactions and side effects may be more frequent and severe than in younger persons. You need smaller doses for shorter periods of time. May develop agitation, rage or "hangover" effect.

Pregnancy:
Risk to unborn child outweighs drug benefits. Don't use.

Breast-feeding:
Drug passes into milk. Avoid drug or discontinue nursing until you finish medicine. Consult doctor for advice on maintaining milk supply.

Infants & children:
Use only under medical supervision for children older than 6 months.

Prolonged use:
May impair liver function.

Skin & sunlight:
No problems expected.

Driving, piloting or hazardous work:
Don't drive or pilot aircraft until you learn how medicine affects you. Don't work around dangerous machinery. Don't climb ladders or work in high places. Danger increases if you drink alcohol or take medicine affecting alertness and reflexes.

Discontinuing:
Don't discontinue without consulting doctor. Dose may require gradual reduction if you have taken drug for a long time. Doses of other drugs may also require adjustment.

Others:
- Hot weather, heavy exercise and profuse sweat may reduce excretion and cause overdose.
- Blood sugar may rise in diabetics, requiring insulin adjustment.

POSSIBLE INTERACTION WITH OTHER DRUGS

GENERIC NAME OR DRUG CLASS	COMBINED EFFECT
Antidepressants*	Increased sedative effect of both drugs.
Antihistamines*	Increased sedative effect of both drugs.
Antihypertensives*	Excessively low blood pressure.
Contraceptives, oral*	Increased halazepam effect.
Disulfiram	Increased halazepam effect.
Dronabinol	Increased effects of both drugs. Avoid.
Erythromycin	Increased halazepam effect.
Ketoconazole	Increased halazepam effect.

Levodopa	Possible decreased levodopa effect.
MAO Inhibitors*	Convulsions, deep sedation, rage.
Molindone	Increased tranquilizer effect.
Nabilone	Greater depression of central nervous system.
Narcotics*	Increased sedative effect of both drugs.
Probenecid	Increased halazepam effect.
Sedatives*	Increased sedative effect of both drugs.
Sleep inducers*	Increased sedative effect of both drugs.
Tranquilizers*	Increased sedative effect of both drugs.

POSSIBLE INTERACTION WITH OTHER SUBSTANCES

INTERACTS WITH	COMBINED EFFECT
Alcohol:	Heavy sedation. Avoid.
Beverages:	None expected.
Cocaine:	Decreased halazepam effect.
Foods:	None expected.
Marijuana:	Heavy sedation. Avoid.
Tobacco:	Decreased halazepam effect.

HALOPERIDOL

BRAND NAMES

Apo-Haloperidol
Haldol
Haldol Decanoate

Haldol LA
Novoperidol
Peridol

BASIC INFORMATION

Habit forming? No
Prescription needed? Yes
Available as generic? Yes
Drug class: Tranquilizer (antipsychotic)

 USES

Reduces severe anxiety, agitation and psychotic behavior.

 DOSAGE & USAGE INFORMATION

How to take:
- Tablet or extended-release capsule—Swallow with liquid. If you can't swallow whole, crumble tablet and take with liquid or food.
- Drops—Dilute dose in beverage before swallowing.

When to take:
At the same times each day.

If you forget a dose:
Take as soon as you remember up to 2 hours late. If more than 2 hours, wait for next scheduled dose (don't double this dose).

What drug does:
Corrects an imbalance in nerve impulses from brain.

Continued next column

 OVERDOSE

SYMPTOMS:
Weak, rapid pulse; shallow, slow breathing; very low blood pressure; convulsions; deep sleep ending in coma.
WHAT TO DO:
- Dial 0 (operator) or 911 (emergency) for an ambulance or medical help. Then give first aid immediately.
- If patient is unconscious and not breathing, give mouth-to-mouth breathing. If there is no heartbeat, use cardiac massage and mouth-to-mouth breathing (CPR). Don't try to make patient vomit. If you can't get help quickly, take patient to nearest emergency facility.
- See emergency information on inside covers.

Time lapse before drug works:
3 weeks to 2 months for maximum benefit.

Don't take with:
- Non-prescription drugs without consulting doctor.
- See Interaction column and consult doctor.

 POSSIBLE ADVERSE REACTIONS OR SIDE EFFECTS

SYMPTOMS	WHAT TO DO
Life-threatening: Uncontrolled muscle movements of tongue, face and other muscles (neuroleptic malignant syndrome, rare).	Discontinue. Seek emergency treatment.
Common:	
• Blurred vision.	Discontinue. Call doctor right away.
• Shuffling, stiffness, jerkiness, shakiness, constipation.	Continue. Call doctor when convenient.
• Dry mouth.	No action necessary.
Infrequent:	
• Rash, circling motions of tongue.	Discontinue. Call doctor right away.
• Dizziness, faintness, drowsiness, difficult urination, decreased sexual ability, nausea or vomiting.	Continue. Call doctor when convenient.
Rare:	
Sore throat, fever, jaundice, abdominal pain, constipation.	Discontinue. Call doctor right away.

 WARNINGS & PRECAUTIONS

Don't take if:
- You have ever been allergic to haloperidol.
- You are depressed.
- You have Parkinson's disease.
- Patient is younger than 3 years old.

Before you start, consult your doctor:
- If you take sedatives, sleeping pills, tranquilizers, antidepressants, antihistamines, narcotics or mind-altering drugs.
- If you have a history of mental depression.
- If you have had kidney or liver problems.
- If you have diabetes, epilepsy, glaucoma, high blood pressure or heart disease, prostate trouble.
- If you drink alcoholic beverages frequently.

Over age 60:
Adverse reactions and side effects may be more frequent and severe than in younger persons.

Pregnancy:
Risk to unborn child outweighs drug benefits. Don't use.

Breast-feeding:
No proven harm to nursing infant. Avoid if possible.

Infants & children:
Not recommended.

Prolonged use:
May develop tardive dyskinesia (involuntary movements of jaws, lips and tongue).

Skin & sunlight:
May cause rash or intensify sunburn in areas exposed to sun or sunlamp.

Driving, piloting or hazardous work:
Don't drive or pilot aircraft until you learn how medicine affects you. Don't work around dangerous machinery. Don't climb ladders or work in high places. Danger increases if you drink alcohol or take medicine affecting alertness and reflexes.

Discontinuing:
Don't discontinue without consulting doctor. Dose may require gradual reduction if you have taken drug for a long time. Doses of other drugs may also require adjustment.

Others:
No problems expected.

POSSIBLE INTERACTION WITH OTHER DRUGS

GENERIC NAME OR DRUG CLASS	COMBINED EFFECT
Anticholinergics*	Increased anti-cholinergic effect. May cause pressure within the eye.
Anticonvulsants*	Changed seizure pattern.
Antidepressants*	Excessive sedation.
Antihistamines*	Excessive sedation.
Antihypertensives*	May cause severe blood-pressure drop.
Barbiturates*	Excessive sedation.
Dronabinol	Increased effects of both drugs. Avoid.
Ethinamate	Dangerous increased effects of ethinamate. Avoid combining.
Fluoxetine	Increased depressant effects of both drugs.
Guanethidine	Decreased guanethidine effect.
Guanfacine	May increase depressant effects of either drug.
Loxapine	May increase toxic effects of both drugs.
Leucovorin	High alcohol content of leucovorin may cause adverse effects.
Levodopa	Decreased levodopa effect.
Lithium	Increased toxicity.
Methyldopa	Possible psychosis.
Methyprylon	Increased sedative effect, perhaps to dangerous level. Avoid.
Nabilone	Greater depression of central nervous system.
Narcotics*	Excessive sedation.
Phenindione	Decreased anticoagulant effect.
Procarbazine	Increased sedation.
Sedatives*	Excessive sedation.
Tranquilizers*	Excessive sedation.

POSSIBLE INTERACTION WITH OTHER SUBSTANCES

INTERACTS WITH	COMBINED EFFECT
Alcohol:	Excessive sedation and depressed brain function. Avoid.
Beverages:	None expected.
Cocaine:	Decreased effect of haloperidol. Avoid.
Foods:	None expected.
Marijuana:	Occasional use— Increased sedation. Frequent use— Possible toxic psychosis.
Tobacco:	None expected.

*See Glossary

HYDRALAZINE

BRAND NAMES

Apresoline	Ser-Ap-Es
Dralzine	Serpasil-Apresoline
H-H-R	Unipes
Hydralazide	Uniserp
Rolazine	

BASIC INFORMATION

Habit forming? No
Prescription needed? Yes
Available as generic? Yes
Drug class: Antihypertensive

 USES

Treatment for high blood pressure and congestive heart failure.

 DOSAGE & USAGE INFORMATION

How to take:
Tablet—Swallow with liquid. If you can't swallow whole, crumble tablet and take with liquid or food.

When to take:
At the same time each day.

If you forget a dose:
Take as soon as you remember up to 2 hours late. If more than 2 hours, wait for next scheduled dose (don't double this dose).

What drug does:
Relaxes and expands blood-vessel walls, lowering blood pressure.

Continued next column

 OVERDOSE

SYMPTOMS:
Rapid and weak heartbeat, fainting, extreme weakness, cold and sweaty skin, flushing.
WHAT TO DO:
- **Dial 0 (operator) or 911 (emergency) for an ambulance or medical help. Then give first aid immediately.**
- **If patient is unconscious and not breathing, give mouth-to-mouth breathing. If there is no heartbeat, use cardiac massage and mouth-to-mouth breathing (CPR). Don't try to make patient vomit. If you can't get help quickly, take patient to nearest emergency facility.**
- **See emergency information on inside covers.**

Time lapse before drug works:
Regular use for several weeks may be necessary to determine drug's effectiveness.

Don't take with:
- Non-prescription drugs containing alcohol without consulting doctor.
- See Interaction column and consult doctor.

 POSSIBLE ADVERSE REACTIONS OR SIDE EFFECTS

SYMPTOMS	WHAT TO DO
Life-threatening: None expected.	
Common:	
• Nausea or vomiting, rapid or irregular heartbeat.	Discontinue. Call doctor right away.
• Headache, diarrhea, appetite loss, painful or difficult urination.	Continue. Tell doctor at next visit.
Infrequent:	
• Hives or rash, flushed face, sore throat, fever, chest pain, swelling of lymph gland.	Discontinue. Call doctor right away.
• Confusion, dizziness, anxiety, depression, joint pain, general discomfort or weakness, fever, muscle pain, chest pain.	Continue. Call doctor when convenient.
• Watery eyes and irritation, constipation.	Continue. Tell doctor at next visit.
Rare:	
• Weakness and faintness when arising from bed or chair, edema, jaundice.	Discontinue. Call doctor right away.
• Numbness or tingling in hands or feet, nasal congestion, impotence.	Continue. Call doctor when convenient.

WARNINGS & PRECAUTIONS

Don't take if:
- You are allergic to hydralazine or tartrazine dye.
- You have history of coronary-artery disease or rheumatic heart disease.

Before you start, consult your doctor:
- If you feel pain in chest, neck or arms on physical exertion.
- If you have had lupus.
- If you have had a stroke.
- If you have had kidney disease or impaired kidney function.
- If you will have surgery within 2 months, including dental surgery, requiring general or spinal anesthesia.

Over age 60:
Adverse reactions and side effects may be more frequent and severe than in younger persons.

Pregnancy:
Risk to unborn child outweighs drug benefits. Don't use.

Breast-feeding:
Drug filters into milk. May harm child. Avoid.

Infants & children:
Not recommended.

Prolonged use:
- May cause lupus (arthritis-like illness).
- Possible psychosis.
- May cause numbness, tingling in hands or feet.

Skin & sunlight:
No problems expected.

Driving, piloting or hazardous work:
Don't drive or pilot aircraft until you learn how medicine affects you. Don't work around dangerous machinery. Don't climb ladders or work in high places. Danger increases if you drink alcohol or take medicine affecting alertness and reflexes, such as antihistamines, tranquilizers, sedatives, pain medicine, narcotics and mind-altering drugs.

Discontinuing:
Don't discontinue without doctor's advice until you complete prescribed dose, even though symptoms diminish or disappear.

Others:
- Vitamin B-6 diet supplement may be advisable. Consult doctor.
- Some products contain tartrazine dye. Avoid, especially if you are allergic to aspirin.

POSSIBLE INTERACTION WITH OTHER DRUGS

GENERIC NAME OR DRUG CLASS	COMBINED EFFECT
Amphetamines*	Decreased hydralazine effect.
Antihypertensives, other*	Increased antihypertensive effect.
Carteolol	Increased antihypertensive effect.
Diazoxide	Increased antihypertensive effect.
Diuretics, oral*	Increased effects of both drugs. When monitored carefully, combination may be beneficial in controlling hypertension.
Guanfacine	Increased effects of both drugs.
Lisinopril	Increased antihypertensive effect. Dosage of each may require adjustment.
MAO Inhibitors*	Increased hydralazine effect.
Nicardipine	Blood-pressure drop. Dosages may require adjustment.
Non-steroidal anti-inflammatory drugs (NSAIDs)*	Decreased effect of hydralazine.
Sotalol	Increased antihypertensive effect.
Terazosin	Decreases effectiveness of terazosin.

POSSIBLE INTERACTION WITH OTHER SUBSTANCES

INTERACTS WITH	COMBINED EFFECT
Alcohol:	May lower blood pressure excessively. Use extreme caution.
Beverages:	None expected.
Cocaine:	Increased risk of heart block and high blood pressure.
Foods:	Increased hydralazine absorption.
Marijuana:	Weakness on standing.
Tobacco:	Possible angina attacks.

*See Glossary

HYDRALAZINE & HYDROCHLOROTHIAZIDE

BRAND NAMES

Apresazide
Apresodez

Apresoline-Esidrix
Hydral

BASIC INFORMATION

Habit forming? No
Prescription needed? Yes
Available as generic? Yes
Drug class: Antihypertensive-diuretic

 ## USES

- Controls, but doesn't cure, high blood pressure.
- Reduces fluid retention (edema).

 ## DOSAGE & USAGE INFORMATION

How to take:
Tablet or capsule—Swallow with liquid. If you can't swallow whole, crumble tablet or open capsule and take with liquid or food.

When to take:
At the same time each day.

If you forget a dose:
Take as soon as you remember up to 2 hours late. If more than 2 hours, wait for next scheduled dose (don't double this dose).

What drug does:
- Forces sodium and water excretion, reducing body fluid.
- Relaxes and expands blood-vessel walls, lowering blood pressure.

Continued next column

 ## OVERDOSE

SYMPTOMS:
Cramps, drowsiness, weak pulse, rapid and weak heartbeat, fainting, extreme weakness, cold and sweaty skin, coma.
WHAT TO DO:
- Dial 0 (operator) or 911 (emergency) for an ambulance or medical help. Then give first aid immediately.
- If patient is unconscious and not breathing, give mouth-to-mouth breathing. If there is no heartbeat, use cardiac massage and mouth-to-mouth breathing (CPR). Don't try to make patient vomit. If you can't get help quickly, take patient to nearest emergency facility.
- See emergency information on inside covers.

- Reduced body fluid and relaxed arteries lower blood pressure.

Time lapse before drug works:
Regular use for several weeks may be necessary to determine drug's effectiveness.

Don't take with:
- Non-prescription drugs containing alcohol without consulting doctor.
- See Interaction column and consult doctor.

 ## POSSIBLE ADVERSE REACTIONS OR SIDE EFFECTS

SYMPTOMS	WHAT TO DO
Life-threatening: Chest pain, irregular and fast heartbeat, weak pulse.	Discontinue. Seek emergency treatment.
Common:	
• Nausea, vomiting.	Discontinue. Call doctor right away.
• Headache, diarrhea, appetite loss, frequent urination, dry mouth, thirst.	Continue. Call doctor when convenient.
Infrequent:	
• Rash; black, bloody or tarry stool; red or flushed face; sore throat, fever, mouth sores; constipation; lymph glands swelling; blurred vision.	Discontinue. Call doctor right away.
• Dizziness; confusion; watery eyes; weight gain or loss; joint, muscle or chest pain; depression; anxiety; fever.	Continue. Call doctor when convenient.
Rare:	
• Weakness and faintness when arising from bed or chair, edema, jaundice.	Discontinue. Call doctor right away.
• Numbness or tingling in hands or feet, nasal congestion, impotence.	Continue. Call doctor when convenient.

 ## WARNINGS & PRECAUTIONS

Don't take if:
- You are allergic to hydralazine, any thiazide diuretic drug or tartrazine dye.
- You have history of coronary-artery disease or rheumatic heart disease.

HYDRALAZINE & HYDROCHLOROTHIAZIDE

Before you start, consult your doctor:
- If you feel pain in chest, neck or arms on physical exertion.
- If you are allergic to any sulfa drug.
- If you have had lupus or a stroke.
- If you have gout, liver, pancreas or kidney disorder.
- If you will have surgery within 2 months, including dental surgery, requiring general or spinal anesthesia.

Over age 60:
Adverse reactions and side effects may be more frequent and severe than in younger persons, especially dizziness and excessive potassium loss.

Pregnancy:
Risk to unborn child outweighs drug benefits. Don't use.

Breast-feeding:
Drug passes into milk. Avoid drug or discontinue nursing until you finish medicine. Consult doctor for advice on maintaining milk supply.

Infants & children:
Not recommended.

Prolonged use:
- May cause lupus (arthritis-like illness).
- Possible psychosis.
- May cause numbness, tingling in hands or feet.

Skin & sunlight:
May cause rash or intensify sunburn in areas exposed to sun or sunlamp.

Driving, piloting or hazardous work:
Don't drive or pilot aircraft until you learn how medicine affects you. Don't work around dangerous machinery. Don't climb ladders or work in high places. Danger increases if you drink alcohol or take medicine affecting alertness and reflexes, such as antihistamines, tranquilizers, sedatives, pain medicine, narcotics and mind-altering drugs.

Discontinuing:
Don't discontinue without consulting doctor's advice until you complete prescribed dose, even though symptoms diminish or disappear.

Others:
- Vitamin B-6 diet supplement may be advisable. Consult doctor.
- Hot weather and fever may cause dehydration and drop in blood pressure. Dose may require temporary adjustment. Weigh daily and report any unexpected weight decreases to your doctor.
- May cause rise in uric acid, leading to gout.
- May cause blood-sugar rise in diabetics.

POSSIBLE INTERACTION WITH OTHER DRUGS

GENERIC NAME OR DRUG CLASS	COMBINED EFFECT
Acebutolol	Decreased anti-hypertensive effect of acebutolol.
Allopurinol	Decreased allopurinol effect.
Amphetamines*	Decreased hydralazine effect.
Antidepressants, tricyclic (TCA)*	Dangerous drop in blood pressure. Avoid combination unless under medical supervision.
Antihypertensives, other*	Increased antihypertensive effect.
Barbiturates*	Increased hydrochlorothiazide effect.
Carteolol	Decreased anti-hypertensive effect.
Cholestyramine	Decreased hydrochlorothiazide effect.
Cortisone drugs*	Excessive potassium loss that causes dangerous heart rhythms.
Diazoxide	Increased antihypertensive effect.

Continued page 1087

POSSIBLE INTERACTION WITH OTHER SUBSTANCES

INTERACTS WITH	COMBINED EFFECT
Alcohol:	May lower blood pressure excessively. Use extreme caution.
Beverages:	None expected.
Cocaine:	Dangerous blood-pressure rise. Avoid.
Foods: Licorice.	Excessive potassium loss that causes dangerous heart rhythms.
Marijuana:	Weakness on standing. May increase blood pressure.
Tobacco:	Possible angina attacks.

*See Glossary

HYDROCHLOROTHIAZIDE

BRAND NAMES

See complete list of brand names in the *Brand Name Directory*, page 1063.

BASIC INFORMATION

Habit forming? No
Prescription needed? Yes
Available as generic? Yes
Drug class: Antihypertensive, diuretic (thiazide)

USES

- Controls, but doesn't cure, high blood pressure.
- Reduces fluid retention (edema).

DOSAGE & USAGE INFORMATION

How to take:
Tablet or liquid—Swallow with liquid. If you can't swallow whole, crumble tablet and take with liquid or food.

When to take:
At the same time each day.

If you forget a dose:
Take as soon as you remember up to 2 hours late. If more than 2 hours, wait for next scheduled dose (don't double this dose).

What drug does:
- Forces sodium and water excretion, reducing body fluid.
- Relaxes muscle cells of small arteries.
- Reduced body fluid and relaxed arteries lower blood pressure.

Time lapse before drug works:
4 to 6 hours. May require several weeks to lower blood pressure.

Continued next column

OVERDOSE

SYMPTOMS:
Cramps, weakness, drowsiness, weak pulse, coma.
WHAT TO DO:
- **Dial 0 (operator) or 911 (emergency) for an ambulance or medical help. Then give first aid immediately.**
- **See emergency information on inside covers.**

Don't take with:
- Non-prescription drugs without consulting doctor.
- See Interaction column and consult doctor.

POSSIBLE ADVERSE REACTIONS OR SIDE EFFECTS

SYMPTOMS	WHAT TO DO
Life-threatening: None expected.	
Common: None expected.	
Infrequent:	
• Blurred vision, severe abdominal pain, nausea, vomiting, irregular heartbeat, weak pulse.	Discontinue. Call doctor right away.
• Dizziness, mood change, headache, weakness, tiredness, weight changes.	Continue. Call doctor when convenient.
• Dry mouth, thirst.	Continue. Tell doctor at next visit.
Rare:	
• Rash or hives.	Discontinue. Seek emergency treatment.
• Sore throat, fever, jaundice.	Discontinue. Call doctor right away.

WARNINGS & PRECAUTIONS

Don't take if:
You are allergic to any thiazide diuretic drug.

Before you start, consult your doctor:
- If you are allergic to any sulfa drug.
- If you have gout.
- If you have liver, pancreas or kidney disorder.

Over age 60:
Adverse reactions and side effects may be more frequent and severe than in younger persons, especially dizziness and excessive potassium loss.

Pregnancy:
Risk to unborn child outweighs drug benefits. Don't use.

Breast-feeding:
Drug passes into milk. Avoid drug or discontinue nursing.

Infants & children:
No problems expected.

Prolonged use:
You may need medicine to treat high blood pressure for the rest of your life.

Skin & sunlight:
May cause rash or intensify sunburn in areas exposed to sun or sunlamp.

Driving, piloting or hazardous work:
Don't drive or pilot aircraft until you learn how medicine affects you. Don't work around dangerous machinery. Don't climb ladders or work in high places. Danger increases if you drink alcohol or take medicine affecting alertness and reflexes, such as antihistamines, tranquilizers, sedatives, pain medicine, narcotics and mind-altering drugs.

Discontinuing:
Don't discontinue without medical advice.

Others:
- Hot weather and fever may cause dehydration and drop in blood pressure. Dose may require temporary adjustment. Weigh daily and report any unexpected weight decreases to your doctor.
- May cause rise in uric acid, leading to gout.
- May cause blood-sugar rise in diabetics.

POSSIBLE INTERACTION WITH OTHER DRUGS

GENERIC NAME OR DRUG CLASS	COMBINED EFFECT
ACE inhibitors: captopril, enalapril, lisinopril*	Decreased blood pressure.
Allopurinol	Decreased allopurinol effect.
Amiodarone	Increased risk of heartbeat irregularity due to low potassium.
Amphotericin B	Increased potassium.
Antidepressants, tricyclic (TCA)*	Dangerous drop in blood pressure. Avoid combination unless under medical supervision.
Antidiabetic agents, oral*	Increased blood sugar.
Antihypertensives*	Increased hypertensive effect.
Barbiturates*	Increased hydrochlorothiazide effect.
Beta-adrenergic blockers*	Increased antihypertensive effect. Dosages of both drugs may require adjustments.
Calcium supplements*	Increased calcium in blood.

Carteolol	Increased antihypertensive effect.
Cholestyramine	Decreased hydrochlorothiazide effect.
Colestipol	Decreased hydrochlorothiazide effect.
Cortisone drugs*	Excessive potassium loss that causes dangerous heart rhythms.
Digitalis preparations*	Excessive potassium loss that causes dangerous heart rhythms.
Diuretics, thiazide*	Increased effect of other thiazide diuretics.
Indapamide	Increased diuretic effect.
Indomethacin	Decreased hydrochlorothiazide effect.
Labetalol	Increased antihypertensive effects.
Lithium	Increased effect of lithium.
MAO inhibitors*	Increased hydrochlorothiazide effect.
Nicardipine	Blood-pressure drop. Dosages may require adjustment.
Nitrates*	Excessive blood-pressure drop.

Continued page 1088

POSSIBLE INTERACTION WITH OTHER SUBSTANCES

INTERACTS WITH	COMBINED EFFECT
Alcohol:	Dangerous blood-pressure drop.
Beverages:	None expected.
Cocaine:	Increased risk of heart block and high blood pressure.
Foods: Licorice.	Excessive potassium loss that causes dangerous heart rhythms.
Marijuana:	May increase blood pressure.
Tobacco:	None expected.

*See Glossary

HYDROCORTISONE (Cortisol)

BRAND NAMES

See complete list of brand names in the *Brand Name Directory*, page 1064.

BASIC INFORMATION

Habit forming? No
Prescription needed? Yes
Available as generic? Yes
Drug class: Cortisone drug (adrenal corticosteroid)

 ## USES

- Reduces inflammation caused by many different medical problems.
- Treatment for some allergic diseases, blood disorders, kidney diseases, asthma and emphysema.
- Replaces corticosteroid deficiencies.

 ## DOSAGE & USAGE INFORMATION

How to take:
- Tablet or liquid—Swallow with liquid or food to lessen stomach irritation. If you can't swallow whole, crumble tablet.
- Other forms—Follow label instructions.

When to take:
At the same times each day. Take once-a-day or once-every-other-day doses in mornings.

If you forget a dose:
- Several-doses-per-day prescription—Take as soon as you remember up to 2 hours late. If more than 2 hours, wait for next scheduled dose (don't double this dose).
- Once-a-day dose or less—Wait for next dose. Double this dose.

What drug does:
Decreases inflammatory responses.

Time lapse before drug works:
2 to 4 days.

Don't take with:
See Interaction column and consult doctor.

 ## OVERDOSE

SYMPTOMS:
Headache, convulsions, heart failure.
WHAT TO DO:
- **Dial 0 (operator) or 911 (emergency) for an ambulance or medical help. Then give first aid immediately.**
- **See emergency information on inside covers.**

 ## POSSIBLE ADVERSE REACTIONS OR SIDE EFFECTS

SYMPTOMS	WHAT TO DO
Life-threatening:	
Hives, rash, intense itching, faintness soon after a dose (anaphylaxis).	Seek emergency treatment immediately.
Common:	
Acne, poor wound healing, thirst, indigestion, nausea, vomiting, decreased growth in children.	Continue. Call doctor when convenient.
Infrequent:	
• Black, bloody or tarry stools.	Discontinue. Seek emergency treatment.
• Blurred vision; halos around lights; sore throat; fever; muscle cramps; swollen legs, feet.	Discontinue. Call doctor right away.
• Mood change, insomnia, fatigue, restlessness, frequent urination, weight gain, round face, weakness, TB recurrence, irregular menstrual periods.	Continue. Tell doctor at next visit.
Rare:	
• Irregular heartbeat.	Discontinue. Seek emergency treatment.
• Rash, hallucinations, thrombophlebitis, pancreatitis, numbness or tingling in hands or feet, pancreatitis, convulsions.	Discontinue. Call doctor right away.

 ## WARNINGS & PRECAUTIONS

Don't take if:
- You are allergic to any cortisone drug.
- You have tuberculosis or fungus infection.
- You have herpes infection of eyes, lips or genitals.

Before you start, consult your doctor:
- If you have had tuberculosis.
- If you have congestive heart failure.
- If you have diabetes, peptic ulcer, glaucoma, underactive thyroid, high blood pressure, myasthenia gravis, blood clots in legs or lungs.

Over age 60:
Adverse reactions and side effects may be more frequent and severe than in younger persons. Likely to aggravate edema, diabetes or ulcers. Likely to cause cataracts and osteoporosis (softening of the bones).

Pregnancy:
Risk to unborn child outweighs drug benefits.
Don't use.

Breast-feeding:
Drug passes into milk. Avoid drug or discontinue
nursing until you finish medicine. Consult doctor
for advice on maintaining milk supply.

Infants & children:
Use only under medical supervision.

Prolonged use:
- Retards growth in children.
- Possible glaucoma, cataracts, diabetes, fragile
  bones and thin skin.
- Functional dependence.

Skin & sunlight:
No problems expected.

Driving, piloting or hazardous work:
No problems expected.

Discontinuing:
- Don't discontinue without doctor's advice until
  you complete prescribed dose, even though
  symptoms diminish or disappear.
- Drug affects your response to surgery, illness,
  injury or stress for 2 years after discontinuing.
  Tell anyone who takes medical care of you
  about the drug for up to 2 years after
  discontinuing.

Others:
Avoid immunizations if possible.

POSSIBLE INTERACTION WITH OTHER DRUGS

GENERIC NAME OR DRUG CLASS	COMBINED EFFECT
Amphotericin B	Potassium depletion.
Anticholinergics*	Possible glaucoma.
Anticoagulants, oral*	Decreased anticoagulant effect.
Anticonvulsants, hydantoin*	Decreased hydrocortisone effect.
Antidiabetics, oral*	Decreased antidiabetic effect.
Antihistamines*	Decreased hydrocortisone effect.
Aspirin	Increased hydrocortisone effect.
Attentuated virus vaccines*	Possible viral infection.
Barbiturates*	Decreased hydrocortisone effect. Oversedation.
Chloral hydrate	Decreased hydrocortisone effect.
Chlorthalidone	Potassium depletion.
Cholestyramine	Decreased hydrocortisone absorption effect.
Cholinergics*	Decreased cholinergic effect.
Colestipol	Decreased hydrocortisone absorption effect.
Contraceptives, oral*	Increased hydrocortisone effect.
Cyclosporine	Increased risk of infection.
Digitalis preparations*	Dangerous potassium depletion. Possible digitalis toxicity.
Diuretics, thiazide*	Potassium depletion.
Ephedrine	Decreased hydrocortisone effect.
Estrogens*	Increased hydrocortisone effect.
Ethacrynic acid	Potassium depletion.
Furosemide	Potassium depletion.
Glutethimide	Decreased hydrocortisone effect.
Indapamide	Possible excessive potassium loss, causing dangerous heartbeat irregularity.
Indomethacin	Increased hydrocortisone effect.

Continued page 1088

POSSIBLE INTERACTION WITH OTHER SUBSTANCES

INTERACTS WITH	COMBINED EFFECT
Alcohol:	Risk of stomach ulcers.
Beverages:	No proven problems.
Cocaine:	Overstimulation. Avoid.
Foods:	No proven problems.
Marijuana:	Decreased immunity.
Tobacco:	Increased hydrocortisone effect. Possible toxicity.

HYDROCORTISONE (Rectal)

BRAND AND GENERIC NAMES

Anusol-H.C.
Cort-Done
Corticaine
Cortiment
Dermolate

HYDROCORTISONE,
BISMUTH,
BENZYL,
BENZOATE,
PERUVIAN
BALSAM &
ZINC OXIDE
Rectocort

BASIC INFORMATION

Habit forming? No
Prescription needed? Yes
Available as generic? No
Drug class: Anti-inflammatory, anesthetic
   (rectal)

 USES

In or around the rectum to relieve swelling, itching and pain for hemorrhoids (piles) and other rectal conditions. Frequently used after hemorrhoid surgery.

 DOSAGE & USAGE INFORMATION

How to use:
- Follow instructions in package.
- Rectal cream or ointment—Apply to surface of rectum with fingers. Insert applicator into rectum no farther than 1/2 and apply inside. Wash applicator with warm soapy water or discard.
- Suppository—Remove wrapper and moisten with water. Lie on side. Push blunt end of suppository into rectum with finger. If suppository is too soft, run cold water over it or put in refrigerator for 15 to 45 minutes before using.
- Aerosol foam—Read patient instructions. Don't insert into rectum. Use the special applicator and wash carefully after using.

When to use:
Follow instructions in package or when needed.

Continued next column

 OVERDOSE

SYMPTOMS:
None expected.
WHAT TO DO:
Not intended for internal use. If child accidentally swallows, call poison-control center.

If you forget a dose:
Use as soon as you remember.

What drug does:
- Reduces inflammation.
- Relieves pain and itching.

Time lapse before drug works:
5 to 15 minutes.

Don't use with:
Other rectal medicines without consulting your doctor.

 POSSIBLE ADVERSE REACTIONS OR SIDE EFFECTS

SYMPTOMS	WHAT TO DO
Life-threatening None expected.	
Common None expected.	
Infrequent • Nervousness, trembling, hives, rash, itch, inflammation or tenderness not present before application, slow heartbeat.	Discontinue. Call doctor right away.
• Dizziness, blurred vision, swollen feet.	Continue. Call doctor when convenient.
Rare • Blood in urine.	Discontinue. Call doctor right away.
• Increased or painful urination.	Continue. Call doctor when convenient.

WARNINGS & PRECAUTIONS

Don't use if:
You are allergic to any topical anesthetic.

Before you start, consult your doctor:
* If you have skin infection at site of treatment.
* If you have had severe or extensive skin disorders such as eczema or psoriasis.
* If you have bleeding hemorrhoids.

Over age 60:
Adverse reactions and side effects may be more frequent and severe than in younger persons.

Pregnancy:
No proven harm to unborn child. Avoid if possible.

Breast-feeding:
No problems expected.

Infants & children:
Don't use without careful medical supervision. Too much may be absorbed into the blood stream and affect growth.

Prolonged use:
Possible excess absorption. Don't use longer than 3 days for any one problem.

Skin & sunlight:
No problems expected.

Driving, piloting or hazardous work:
No problems expected.

Discontinuing:
May be unnecessary to finish medicine. Follow doctor's instructions.

Others:
* Report any rectal bleeding to your doctor.
* Keep cool, but don't freeze.

POSSIBLE INTERACTION WITH OTHER DRUGS

GENERIC NAME OR DRUG CLASS	COMBINED EFFECT
Sulfa drugs*	Decreased anti-infective effect of sulfa drugs.

POSSIBLE INTERACTION WITH OTHER SUBSTANCES

INTERACTS WITH	COMBINED EFFECT
Alcohol:	None expected.
Beverages:	None expected.
Cocaine:	Possible nervous-system toxicity. Avoid.
Foods:	None expected.
Marijuana:	None expected.
Tobacco:	None expected.

HYDROFLUMETHIAZIDE

BRAND NAMES

Diucardin
Hydro-Fluserpine
#1 & #2

Saluron
Salutensin

BASIC INFORMATION

Habit forming? No
Prescription needed? Yes
Available as generic? Yes
Drug class: Antihypertensive, diuretic
(thiazide)

USES

- Controls, but doesn't cure, high blood pressure.
- Reduces fluid retention (edema) caused by conditions such as heart disorders and liver disease.

DOSAGE & USAGE INFORMATION

How to take:
Tablet—Swallow with liquid. If you can't swallow whole, crumble tablet and take with liquid or food. Don't exceed dose.

When to take:
At the same time each day.

If you forget a dose:
Take as soon as you remember up to 2 hours late. If more than 2 hours, wait for next scheduled dose (don't double this dose).

What drug does:
- Forces sodium and water excretion, reducing body fluid.
- Relaxes muscle cells of small arteries.
- Reduced body fluid and relaxed arteries lower blood pressure.

Continued next column

OVERDOSE

SYMPTOMS:
Cramps, weakness, drowsiness, weak pulse, coma.
WHAT TO DO:
- Dial 0 (operator) or 911 (emergency) for an ambulance or medical help. Then give first aid immediately.
- See emergency information on inside covers.

Time lapse before drug works:
4 to 6 hours. May require several weeks to lower blood pressure.

Don't take with:
- Non-prescription drugs without consulting doctor.
- See Interaction column and consult doctor.

POSSIBLE ADVERSE REACTIONS OR SIDE EFFECTS

SYMPTOMS	WHAT TO DO
Life-threatening: None expected.	
Common: None expected.	
Infrequent:	
• Blurred vision, severe abdominal pain, nausea, vomiting, irregular heartbeat, weak pulse.	Discontinue. Call doctor right away.
• Dizziness, mood change, headache, weakness, tiredness, weight changes.	Continue. Call doctor when convenient.
• Dry mouth, thirst.	Continue. Tell doctor at next visit.
Rare:	
• Rash or hives.	Discontinue. Seek emergency treatment.
• Sore throat, fever, jaundice.	Discontinue. Call doctor right away.

WARNINGS & PRECAUTIONS

Don't take if:
You are allergic to any thiazide diuretic drug.

Before you start, consult your doctor:
- If you are allergic to any sulfa drug.
- If you have gout.
- If you have liver, pancreas or kidney disorder.

Over age 60:
Adverse reactions and side effects may be more frequent and severe than in younger persons, especially dizziness and excessive potassium loss.

Pregnancy:
Risk to unborn child outweighs drug benefits. Don't use.

Breast-feeding:
Drug passes into milk. Avoid drug or discontinue nursing.

Infants & children:
No problems expected.

Prolonged use:
You may need medicine to treat high blood pressure for the rest of your life.

Skin & sunlight:
May cause rash or intensify sunburn in areas exposed to sun or sunlamp.

Driving, piloting or hazardous work:
Don't drive or pilot aircraft until you learn how medicine affects you. Don't work around dangerous machinery. Don't climb ladders or work in high places. Danger increases if you drink alcohol or take medicine affecting alertness and reflexes, such as antihistamines, tranquilizers, sedatives, pain medicine, narcotics and mind-altering drugs.

Discontinuing:
Don't discontinue without medical advice.

Others:
- Hot weather and fever may cause dehydration and drop in blood pressure. Dose may require temporary adjustment. Weigh daily and report any unexpected weight decreases to your doctor.
- May cause rise in uric acid, leading to gout.
- May cause blood-sugar rise in diabetics.

 ## POSSIBLE INTERACTION WITH OTHER DRUGS

GENERIC NAME OR DRUG CLASS	COMBINED EFFECT
ACE inhibitors: captopril, enalapril, lisinopril*	Decreased blood pressure.
Allopurinol	Decreased allopurinol effect.
Amiodarone	Increased risk of heartbeat irregularity due to low potassium.
Amphotericin B	Increased potassium.
Antidepressants, tricyclic (TCA)*	Dangerous drop in blood pressure. Avoid combination unless under medical supervision.
Antidiabetic agents, oral*	Increased blood sugar.
Antihypertensives*	Increased hypertensive effect.
Barbiturates*	Increased hydroflumethiazide effect.
Beta-adrenergic blockers*	Increased antihypertensive effect. Dosages of both drugs may require adjustments.

Calcium supplements*	Increased calcium in blood.
Carteolol	Increased antihypertensive effect.
Cholestyramine	Decreased hydroflumethiazide effect.
Colestipol	Decreased hydroflumethiazide effect.
Cortisone drugs*	Excessive potassium loss that causes dangerous heart rhythms.
Digitalis preparations*	Excessive potassium loss that causes dangerous heart rhythms.
Diuretics, thiazide*	Increased effect of other thiazide diuretics.
Indapamide	Increased diuretic effect.
Indomethacin	Decreased hydroflumethiazide effect.
Lithium	Increased effect of lithium.
MAO inhibitors*	Increased hydroflumethiazide effect.
Nicardipine	Blood-pressure drop. Dosages may require adjustment.
Nitrates*	Excessive blood-pressure drop.
Opiates*	Dizziness or weakness when standing up after sitting or lying down.

Continued page 1088

 ## POSSIBLE INTERACTION WITH OTHER SUBSTANCES

INTERACTS WITH	COMBINED EFFECT
Alcohol:	Dangerous blood-pressure drop.
Beverages:	None expected.
Cocaine:	Increased risk of heart block and high blood pressure.
Foods: Licorice.	Excessive potassium loss that causes dangerous heart rhythms.
Marijuana:	May increase blood pressure.
Tobacco:	None expected.

*See Glossary

HYDROXYCHLOROQUINE

BRAND NAMES

Plaquenil

BASIC INFORMATION

Habit forming? No
Prescription needed? Yes
Available as generic? No
Drug class: Antiprotozoal, antirheumatic

USES

- Treatment for protozoal infections, such as malaria and amebiasis.
- Treatment for some forms of arthritis and lupus.

DOSAGE & USAGE INFORMATION

How to take:
Tablet—Swallow with food or milk to lessen stomach irritation.

When to take:
- Depends on condition. Is adjusted during treatment.
- Malaria prevention—Begin taking medicine 2 weeks before entering areas with malaria.

If you forget a dose:
- 1 or more doses a day—Take as soon as you remember up to 2 hours late. If more than 2 hours, wait for next scheduled dose (don't double this dose).
- 1 dose weekly—Take as soon as possible, then return to regular dosing schedule.

What drug does:
- Inhibits parasite multiplication.
- Decreases inflammatory response in diseased joint.

Time lapse before drug works:
1 to 2 hours.

Don't take with:
See Interaction column and consult doctor.

OVERDOSE

SYMPTOMS:
Severe breathing difficulty, drowsiness, faintness, headache, seizures.
WHAT TO DO:
- **Dial 0 (operator) or 911 (emergency) for an ambulance or medical help. Then give first aid immediately.**
- **See emergency information on inside covers.**

POSSIBLE ADVERSE REACTIONS OR SIDE EFFECTS

SYMPTOMS	WHAT TO DO
Life-threatening: None expected.	
Common: Headache.	Continue. Tell doctor at next visit.
Infrequent: • Blurred vision, changes in vision.	Discontinue. Call doctor right away.
• Rash or itch, diarrhea, nausea, vomiting.	Continue. Call doctor when convenient.
Rare: • Mood or mental changes, seizures, sore throat, fever, unusual bleeding or bruising, muscle weakness, convulsions.	Discontinue. Call doctor right away.
• Ringing or buzzing in ears, hearing loss, headache.	Continue. Call doctor when convenient.

508

WARNINGS & PRECAUTIONS

Don't take if:
You are allergic to chloroquine or hydroxychloroquine.

Before you start, consult your doctor:
- If you plan to become pregnant within the medication period.
- If you have blood disease.
- If you have eye or vision problems.
- If you have a G6PD deficiency.
- If you have liver disease.
- If you have nerve or brain disease (including seizure disorders).
- If you have porphyria.
- If you have psoriasis.
- If you have stomach or intestinal disease.
- If you drink more than 3 oz. of alcohol daily.

Over age 60:
Adverse reactions and side effects may be more frequent and severe than in younger persons.

Pregnancy:
Risk to unborn child outweighs drug benefits. Don't use.

Breast-feeding:
Drug passes into milk. Avoid drug or discontinue nursing.

Infants & children:
Not recommended. Dangerous.

Prolonged use:
Permanent damage to the retina (back part of the eye) or nerve deafness.

Skin & sunlight:
May cause rash or intensify sunburn in areas exposed to sun or sunlamp.

Driving, piloting or hazardous work:
Don't drive or pilot aircraft until you learn how medicine affects you. Don't work around dangerous machinery. Don't climb ladders or work in high places. Danger increases if you drink alcohol or take medicine affecting alertness and reflexes.

Discontinuing:
Don't discontinue without doctor's advice until you complete prescribed dose, even though symptoms diminish or disappear.

Others:
- Periodic physical and blood examinations recommended.
- If you are in a malaria area for a long time, you may need to change to another preventive drug every 2 years.

 POSSIBLE INTERACTION WITH OTHER DRUGS

GENERIC NAME OR DRUG CLASS	COMBINED EFFECT
Estrogens*	Possible liver toxicity.
Gold compounds*	Risk of severe rash and itch.
Kaolin	Decreased absorption of hydroxychloroquine.
Magnesium trisilicate	Decreased absorption of hydroxychloroquine.
Penicillamine	Possible blood or kidney toxicity.

 POSSIBLE INTERACTION WITH OTHER SUBSTANCES

INTERACTS WITH	COMBINED EFFECT
Alcohol:	Possible liver toxicity. Avoid.
Beverages:	None expected.
Cocaine:	None expected.
Foods:	None expected.
Marijuana:	None expected.
Tobacco:	None expected.

*See Glossary

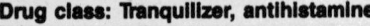

HYDROXYZINE

BRAND NAMES

See complete list of brand names in the *Brand Name Directory*, page 1064.

BASIC INFORMATION

Habit forming? No
Prescription needed? Yes
Available as generic? Yes
Drug class: Tranquilizer, antihistamine

 ## USES

- Treatment for anxiety, tension and agitation.
- Relieves itching from allergic reactions.

 ## DOSAGE & USAGE INFORMATION

How to take:
- Tablet, syrup or capsule—Swallow with liquid. If you can't swallow whole, crumble tablet or open capsule and take with liquid or food.
- Liquid—If desired, dilute dose in beverage before swallowing.

When to take:
At the same times each day.

If you forget a dose:
Take as soon as you remember up to 2 hours late. If more than 2 hours, wait for next scheduled dose (don't double this dose).

What drug does:
May reduce activity in areas of the brain that influence emotional stability.

Time lapse before drug works:
15 to 30 minutes.

Don't take with:
- Non-prescription drugs without consulting doctor.
- See Interaction column and consult doctor.

 ## OVERDOSE

SYMPTOMS:
Drowsiness, unsteadiness, agitation, purposeless movements, tremor, convulsions.
WHAT TO DO:
- **Dial 0 (operator) or 911 (emergency) for an ambulance or medical help. Then give first aid immediately.**
- **See emergency information on inside covers.**

 ## POSSIBLE ADVERSE REACTIONS OR SIDE EFFECTS

SYMPTOMS	WHAT TO DO
Life-threatening: None expected.	
Common: Drowsiness, difficult urination, dry mouth.	Continue. Tell doctor at next visit.
Infrequent: Headache.	Continue. Tell doctor at next visit.
Rare: Tremor, rash.	Discontinue. Call doctor right away.

 ## WARNINGS & PRECAUTIONS

Don't take if:
You are allergic to any antihistamine.

Before you start, consult your doctor:
- If you have epilepsy.
- If you will have surgery within 2 months, including dental surgery, requiring general or spinal anesthesia.

Over age 60:
Adverse reactions and side effects may be more frequent and severe than in younger persons. Drug likely to increase urination difficulty caused by enlarged prostate gland.

Pregnancy:
Studies inconclusive on harm to unborn child. Animal studies show fetal abnormalities. Decide with your doctor whether drug benefits justify risk to unborn child.

Breast-feeding:
Drug passes into milk. Avoid drug or discontinue nursing until you finish medicine. Consult doctor for advice on maintaining milk supply.

Infants & children:
Use only under medical supervision.

Prolonged use:
Tolerance develops and reduces effectiveness.

Skin & sunlight:
No problems expected.

Driving, piloting or hazardous work:
Don't drive or pilot aircraft until you learn how medicine affects you. Don't work around dangerous machinery. Don't climb ladders or work in high places. Danger increases if you drink alcohol or take medicine affecting alertness and reflexes, such as antihistamines, tranquilizers, sedatives, pain medicine, narcotics and mind-altering drugs.

Discontinuing:
Don't discontinue without consulting doctor. Dose may require gradual reduction if you have taken drug for a long time. Doses of other drugs may also require adjustment.

Others:
No problems expected.

 POSSIBLE INTERACTION
WITH OTHER DRUGS

GENERIC NAME OR DRUG CLASS	COMBINED EFFECT
Antidepressants, tricyclic (TCA)*	Increased effect of both drugs.
Antihistamines*	Increased hydroxyzine effect.
Carteolol	Decreased antihistamine effect.
Dronabinol	Increased effects of both drugs. Avoid.
Ethinamate	Dangerous increased effects of ethinamate. Avoid combining.
Fluoxetine	Increased depressant effects of both drugs.
Guanfacine	May increase depressant effects of either drug.
Leucovorin	High alcohol content of leucovorin may cause adverse effects.

Methyprylon	Increased sedative effect, perhaps to dangerous level. Avoid.
Nabilone	Greater depression of central nervous system.
Narcotics*	Increased effect of both drugs.
Pain relievers*	Increased effect of both drugs.
Sedatives*	Increased effect of both drugs.
Sleep inducers*	Increased effect of both drugs.
Sotalol	Increased antihistamine effect.
Tranquilizers*	Increased effect of both drugs.

 POSSIBLE INTERACTION
WITH OTHER SUBSTANCES

INTERACTS WITH	COMBINED EFFECT
Alcohol:	Increased sedation and intoxication. Use with caution.
Beverages: Caffeine drinks.	Decreased tranquilizer effect of hydroxyzine.
Cocaine:	Decreased hydroxyzine effect. Avoid.
Foods:	None expected.
Marijuana:	None expected.
Tobacco:	None expected.

HYOSCYAMINE

BRAND NAMES

See complete list of brand names in the *Brand Name Directory*, page 1064.

BASIC INFORMATION

Habit forming? No
Prescription needed?
  Low strength: No
  High strength: Yes
Available as generic? No
Drug class: Antispasmodic, anticholinergic

USES

Reduces spasms of digestive system, bladder and urethra.

DOSAGE & USAGE INFORMATION

How to take:
* Tablet or liquid—Swallow with liquid or food to lessen stomach irritation. You may chew or crush tablets.
* Extended-release capsules—Swallow each dose whole.
* Drops—Dilute dose in beverage before swallowing.

When to take:
30 minutes before meals (unless directed otherwise by doctor).

If you forget a dose:
Take as soon as you remember up to 2 hours late. If more than 2 hours, wait for next scheduled dose (don't double this dose).

What drug does:
Blocks nerve impulses at parasympathetic nerve endings, preventing muscle contractions and gland secretions of organs involved.

Continued next column

OVERDOSE

SYMPTOMS:
Dilated pupils, rapid pulse and breathing, dizziness, fever, hallucinations, confusion, slurred speech, agitation, flushed face, convulsions, coma.
WHAT TO DO:
* **Dial 0 (operator) or 911 (emergency) for an ambulance or medical help. Then give first aid immediately.**
* **See emergency information on inside covers.**

Time lapse before drug works:
15 to 30 minutes.

Don't take with:
See Interaction column and consult doctor.

POSSIBLE ADVERSE REACTIONS OR SIDE EFFECTS

SYMPTOMS	WHAT TO DO
Life-threatening: None expected.	
Common:	
• Confusion, delirium, rapid heartbeat.	Discontinue. Call doctor right away.
• Nausea, vomiting, decreased sweating.	Continue. Call doctor when convenient.
• Constipation.	Continue. Tell doctor at next visit.
• Dryness in ears, nose, throat.	No action necessary.
Infrequent: Headache, painful or difficult urination.	Continue. Call doctor when convenient.
Rare: Rash or hives, pain, blurred vision.	Discontinue. Call doctor right away.

WARNINGS & PRECAUTIONS

Don't take if:
- You are allergic to any anticholinergic.
- You have trouble with stomach bloating.
- You have difficulty emptying your bladder completely.
- You have narrow-angle glaucoma.
- You have severe ulcerative colitis.

Before you start, consult your doctor:
- If you have open-angle glaucoma.
- If you have angina.
- If you have chronic bronchitis or asthma.
- If you have hiatal hernia.
- If you have liver disease.
- If you have enlarged prostate.
- If you have myasthenia gravis.
- If you have peptic ulcer.
- If you will have surgery within 2 months, including dental surgery, requiring general or spinal anesthesia.

Over age 60:
Adverse reactions and side effects may be more frequent and severe than in younger persons.

Pregnancy:
Studies inconclusive on harm to unborn child. Animal studies show fetal abnormalities. Decide with your doctor whether drug benefits justify risk to unborn child.

Breast-feeding:
Drug passes into milk and decreases milk flow. Avoid drug or discontinue nursing until you finish medicine. Consult doctor for advice on maintaining milk supply.

Infants & children:
Use only under medical supervision.

Prolonged use:
Chronic constipation, possible fecal impaction. Consult doctor immediately.

Skin & sunlight:
No problems expected.

Driving, piloting or hazardous work:
Use disqualifies you for piloting aircraft. Otherwise, no problems expected.

Discontinuing:
May be unnecessary to finish medicine. Follow doctor's instructions.

Others:
No problems expected.

POSSIBLE INTERACTION WITH OTHER DRUGS

GENERIC NAME OR DRUG CLASS	COMBINED EFFECT
Amantadine	Increased hyoscyamine effect.
Anticholinergics, other*	Increased hyoscyamine effect.
Antidepressants, tricyclic (TCA)*	Increased hyoscyamine effect.
Antihistamines*	Increased hyoscyamine effect.
Cortisone drugs*	Increased internal-eye pressure.
Haloperidol	Increased internal-eye pressure.
MAO inhibitors*	Increased hyoscyamine effect.
Meperidine	Increased hyoscyamine effect.
Methylphenidate	Increased hyoscyamine effect.
Molindone	Increased anti-cholinergic effect.
Nizatidine	Increased nizatidine effect.
Orphenadrine	Increased hyoscyamine effect.
Phenothiazines*	Increased hyoscyamine effect.
Pilocarpine	Loss of pilocarpine effect in glaucoma treatment.
Vitamin C	Decreased hyoscyamine effect. Avoid large doses of vitamin C.

POSSIBLE INTERACTION WITH OTHER SUBSTANCES

INTERACTS WITH	COMBINED EFFECT
Alcohol:	None expected.
Beverages:	None expected.
Cocaine:	Excessively rapid heartbeat. Avoid.
Foods:	None expected.
Marijuana:	Drowsiness and dry mouth.
Tobacco:	None expected.

*See Glossary

IBUPROFEN

BRAND NAMES

Advil	Midol 200
Amersol	Motrin
Apo-Ibuprofen	Neuvil
Apsifen	Novoprofen
Apsifen-F	Nuprin
Brufen	Pamprin IB
Haltran	Rufen
Ifen	Trendar
Medipren	

BASIC INFORMATION

Habit forming? No
Prescription needed? Yes, for some brands at higher strength
Available as generic? Yes
Drug class: Anti-inflammatory (non-steroid)

USES

- Treatment for joint pain, stiffness, inflammation and swelling of arthritis and gout.
- Pain reliever.
- Treatment for dysmenorrhea (painful or difficult menstruation).
- Treats juvenile rheumatoid arthritis.

DOSAGE & USAGE INFORMATION

How to take:
Tablet or capsule—Swallow with liquid or food to lessen stomach irritation. If you can't swallow whole, crumble tablet and take with liquid or food.

When to take:
At the same times each day.

If you forget a dose:
Take as soon as you remember up to 2 hours late. If more than 2 hours, wait for next scheduled dose (don't double this dose).

Continued next column

OVERDOSE

SYMPTOMS:
Confusion, agitation, incoherence, convulsions, possible hemorrhage from stomach or intestine, coma.
WHAT TO DO:
- **Dial 0 (operator) or 911 (emergency) for an ambulance or medical help. Then give first aid immediately.**
- **See emergency information on inside covers.**

What drug does:
Reduces tissue concentration of prostaglandins (hormones which produce inflammation and pain).

Time lapse before drug works:
Begins in 4 to 24 hours. May require 3 weeks regular use for maximum benefit.

Don't take with:
See Interaction column and consult doctor.

POSSIBLE ADVERSE REACTIONS OR SIDE EFFECTS

SYMPTOMS	WHAT TO DO
Life-threatening: Hives, rash, intense itching, faintness soon after a dose (anaphylaxis in aspirin-sensitive persons).	Seek emergency treatment immediately.
Common:	
• Dizziness, nausea, pain.	Continue. Call doctor when convenient.
• Headache.	Continue. Tell doctor at next visit.
Infrequent: Depression; drowsiness; ringing in ears; swollen feet, legs; constipation or diarrhea; vomiting.	Continue. Call doctor when convenient.
Rare:	
• Convulsions; confusion; rash, hives or itch; blurred vision; black, bloody, tarry stool; difficult breathing; tightness in chest; rapid heartbeat; unusual bleeding or bruising; blood in urine; jaundice; psychosis; frequent, painful urination; severe abdominal pain.	Discontinue. Call doctor right away.
• Fatigue; weakness; impotence; menstrual irregularities; swollen breasts in males.	Continue. Call doctor when convenient.

WARNINGS & PRECAUTIONS

Don't take if:
- You are allergic to aspirin or any non-steroid, anti-inflammatory drug.
- You have gastritis, peptic ulcer, enteritis, ileitis, ulcerative colitis, asthma, heart failure, high blood pressure or bleeding problems.
- Patient is younger than 15.

Before you start, consult your doctor:
- If you have epilepsy.
- If you have Parkinson's disease.
- If you have been mentally ill.
- If you have had kidney disease or impaired kidney function.

Over age 60:
Adverse reactions and side effects may be more frequent and severe than in younger persons.

Pregnancy:
Studies inconclusive on harm to unborn child. Decide with your doctor whether drug benefits justify risk to unborn child.

Breast-feeding:
May harm child. Avoid.

Infants & children:
Not recommended for anyone younger than 15. Use only under medical supervision.

Prolonged use:
- Eye damage.
- Reduced hearing.
- Sore throat, fever.
- Weight gain.

Skin & sunlight:
Possible increased sensitivity to sunlight.

Driving, piloting or hazardous work:
Don't drive or pilot aircraft until you learn how medicine affects you. Don't work around dangerous machinery. Don't climb ladders or work in high places. Danger increases if you drink alcohol or take medicine affecting alertness and reflexes, such as antihistamines, tranquilizers, sedatives, pain medicine, narcotics and mind-altering drugs.

Discontinuing:
Don't discontinue without consulting doctor. Dose may require gradual reduction if you have taken drug for a long time. Doses of other drugs may also require adjustment.

Others:
No problems expected.

 ## POSSIBLE INTERACTION WITH OTHER DRUGS

GENERIC NAME OR DRUG CLASS	COMBINED EFFECT
ACE inhibitors: captopril, enalapril, lisinopril*	May decrease ACE inhibitor effect.
Anticoagulants, oral*	Increased risk of bleeding.
Aspirin	Increased risk of stomach ulcer.
Beta-adrenergic blockers*	Decreased antihypertensive effect.
Carteolol	Decreased antihypertensive effect of carteolol.
Cortisone drugs*	Increased risk of stomach ulcer.
Diuretics*	May decrease diuretic effect.
Lithium	Possible increase in effect and toxicity.
Methotrexate	May increase toxicity.
Minoxidil	Decreased minoxidil effect.
Oxyphenbutazone	Possible stomach ulcer.
Phenylbutazone	Possible stomach ulcer.
Probenecid	Increased ibuprofen effect.
Sotalol	Decreased antihypertensive effect of sotalol.
Terazosin	Decreases effectiveness of terazosin. Causes sodium and fluid retention.
Thyroid hormones*	Rapid heartbeat, blood-pressure rise.

 ## POSSIBLE INTERACTION WITH OTHER SUBSTANCES

INTERACTS WITH	COMBINED EFFECT
Alcohol:	Possible stomach ulcer or bleeding.
Beverages:	None expected.
Cocaine:	None expected.
Foods:	None expected.
Marijuana:	Increased pain relief from ibuprofen.
Tobacco:	None expected.

*See Glossary

INDAPAMIDE

BRAND NAMES

Lozide   Lozol

BASIC INFORMATION

Habit forming? No
Prescription needed? Yes
Available as generic? No
Drug class: Antihypertensive, diuretic

USES

- Controls, but doesn't cure, high blood pressure.
- Reduces fluid retention (edema) caused by conditions such as heart disorders.

DOSAGE & USAGE INFORMATION

How to take:
Tablet—Swallow with liquid or food to lessen stomach irritation.

When to take:
At the same times each day, usually at bedtime.

If you forget a dose:
Bedtime dose—If you forget your once-a-day bedtime dose, don't take it more than 3 hours late. Never double dose.

What drug does:
Forces kidney to excrete more sodium and causes excess salt and fluid to be excreted.

Time lapse before drug works:
2 hours for effect to begin. May require 1 to 4 weeks for full effects.

Continued next column

OVERDOSE

SYMPTOMS:
Nausea, vomiting, diarrhea, very dry mouth, thirst, weakness, excessive fatigue, very rapid heart rate, weak pulse.
WHAT TO DO:
- **Dial 0 (operator) or 911 (emergency) for an ambulance or medical help. Then give first aid immediately.**
- **If patient is unconscious and not breathing, give mouth-to-mouth breathing. If there is no heartbeat, use cardiac massage and mouth-to-mouth breathing (CPR). Don't try to make patient vomit. If you can't get help quickly, take patient to nearest emergency facility.**
- **See emergency information on inside covers.**

Don't take with:
See Interaction column and consult doctor.

POSSIBLE ADVERSE REACTIONS OR SIDE EFFECTS

SYMPTOMS	WHAT TO DO
Life-threatening: None expected.	
Common: • Excessive tiredness or weakness, muscle cramps.	Discontinue. Call doctor right away.
• Frequent urination.	Continue. Tell doctor at next visit.
Infrequent: • Gouty arthritis.	Discontinue. Call doctor right away.
• Insomnia, mood change, dizziness on changing position, headache, excessive thirst, diarrhea, appetite loss, nausea.	Continue. Call doctor when convenient.
Rare: • Weak pulse.	Discontinue. Seek emergency treatment.
• Itching, rash, hives, irregular heartbeat.	Discontinue. Call doctor right away.

WARNINGS & PRECAUTIONS

Don't take if:
- You are allergic to indapamide or to any sulfa drug or thiazide diuretic. *
- You have severe kidney disease.

Before you start, consult your doctor:
- If you have severe kidney disease.
- If you have diabetes.
- If you have gout.
- If you have liver disease.
- If you will have surgery within 2 months, including dental surgery, requiring general or spinal anesthesia.
- If you have lupus erythematosus.
- If you are pregnant or plan to become pregnant.

Over age 60:
Adverse reactions and side effects may be more frequent and severe than in younger persons.

Pregnancy:
Risk to unborn child outweighs drug benefits. Don't use.

Breast-feeding:
Unknown effect on child. Consult doctor.

Infants & children:
Use only under close medical supervision.

Prolonged use:
Request laboratory studies for blood sugar, BUN, uric acid and serum electrolytes (potassium and sodium).

Skin & sunlight:
May cause rash or intensify sunburn in areas exposed to sun or sunlamp.

Driving, piloting or hazardous work:
Don't drive or pilot aircraft until you learn how medicine affects you. Don't work around dangerous machinery. Don't climb ladders or work in high places. Danger increases if you drink alcohol or take medicine affecting alertness and reflexes, such as antihistamines, tranquilizers, sedatives, pain medicine, narcotics and mind-altering drugs.

Discontinuing:
Don't discontinue without consulting doctor. Dose may require gradual reduction if you have taken drug for a long time. Doses of other drugs may also require adjustment.

Others:
No problems expected.

 POSSIBLE INTERACTION WITH OTHER DRUGS

GENERIC NAME OR DRUG CLASS	COMBINED EFFECT
ACE Inhibitors: captopril, enalapril, lisinopril*	Decreased blood pressure. Possible excessive potassium in blood.
Allopurinol	Decreased allopurinol effect.
Amiodarone	Increased risk of heartbeat irregularity due to low potassium.
Amphotericin B	Increased potassium.
Antidepressants, tricyclic (TCA)*	Dangerous drop in blood pressure.
Antidiabetic agents, oral*	Increased blood sugar.
Antihypertensives, other*	Increased antihypertensive effect.
Barbiturates*	Increased indapamide effect.
Beta-adrenergic blockers*	Increased effect of indapamide.
Calcium supplements*	Increased calcium in blood.
Carteolol	Increased antihypertensive effect.

Cholestyramine	Decreased indapamide effect.
Colestipol	Decreased indapamide effect.
Cortisone drugs*	Excessive potassium loss that may cause dangerous heart rhythms.
Digitalis preparations*	Excessive potassium loss that may cause dangerous heart rhythms.
Diuretics, thiazide*	Increased effect of thiazide diuretics.
Indomethacin	Decreased indapamide effect.
Lithium	High risk of lithium toxicity.
MAO inhibitors*	Increased indapamide effect.
Nicardipine	Dangerous blood-pressure drop. Dosages may require adjustment.
Opiates*	Weakness and faintness when arising from bed or chair.
Probenecid	Decreased probenecid effect.
Sotalol	Increased antihypertensive effect.
Terazosin	Decreases effectiveness of terazosin.

 POSSIBLE INTERACTION WITH OTHER SUBSTANCES

INTERACTS WITH	COMBINED EFFECT
Alcohol:	Dangerous blood-pressure drop. Avoid.
Beverages:	No problems expected.
Cocaine:	Increased risk of heart block and high blood pressure.
Foods: Licorice.	Excessive potassium loss that may cause dangerous heart rhythms.
Marijuana:	Reduced effectiveness of indapamide. Avoid.
Tobacco:	Reduced effectiveness of indapamide. Avoid.

*See Glossary

INDOMETHACIN

BRAND NAMES

Apo-Indomethacin	Indocin-SR
Imbrilon	Indolar SR
Indocid	Indo-Lemmon
Indocid R	Indometacin
Indocid-SR	Novomethacin
Indocin	Zendole

BASIC INFORMATION

Habit forming? No
Prescription needed? Yes
Available as generic? Yes
Drug class: Anti-inflammatory (non-steroid)

 ## USES

- Treatment for joint pain, stiffness, inflammation and swelling of arthritis and gout.
- Pain reliever.
- Treatment for dysmenorrhea (painful or difficult menstruation).
- Treats juvenile rheumatoid arthritis.

 ## DOSAGE & USAGE INFORMATION

How to take:
- Capsule or suspension—Swallow with liquid or food to lessen stomach irritation. If you can't swallow whole, open capsule and take with liquid or food.
- Extended-release capsules—Swallow whole with liquid or food to lessen stomach irritation.
- Suppositories—Remove wrapper and insert blunt end into rectum.

When to take:
At the same times each day.

If you forget a dose:
Take as soon as you remember up to 2 hours late. If more than 2 hours, wait for next scheduled dose (don't double this dose).

Continued next column

 ## OVERDOSE

SYMPTOMS:
Confusion, agitation, incoherence, convulsions, possible hemorrhage from stomach or intestine, coma.
WHAT TO DO:
- Dial 0 (operator) or 911 (emergency) for an ambulance or medical help. Then give first aid immediately.
- See emergency information on inside covers.

What drug does:
Reduces tissue concentration of prostaglandins (hormones which produce inflammation and pain).

Time lapse before drug works:
Begins in 4 to 24 hours. May require 3 weeks regular use for maximum benefit.

Don't take with:
See Interaction column and consult doctor.

 ## POSSIBLE ADVERSE REACTIONS OR SIDE EFFECTS

SYMPTOMS	WHAT TO DO
Life-threatening: Hives, rash, intense itching, faintness soon after a dose (anaphylaxis in aspirin-sensitive persons).	Seek emergency treatment immediately.
Common: • Dizziness, nausea, pain.	Continue. Call doctor when convenient.
• Headache.	Continue. Tell doctor at next visit.
Infrequent: Depression; drowsiness; ringing in ears; constipation or diarrhea; vomiting; swollen feet, legs.	Continue. Call doctor when convenient.
Rare: • Convulsions; confusion; rash, hives or itch; blurred vision; black, bloody, tarry stool; difficult breathing; tightness in chest; rapid heartbeat; unusual bleeding or bruising; blood in urine; jaundice; severe abdominal pain; psychosis.	Discontinue. Call doctor right away.
• Frequent, painful or difficult urination; fatigue; weakness; rectal pain or irritation (with suppository); may worsen Parkinsonism and epilepsy; swollen breasts in males; impotence; menstrual irregularities.	Continue. Call doctor when convenient.

WARNINGS & PRECAUTIONS

Don't take if:
- You are allergic to aspirin or any non-steroid, anti-inflammatory drug.
- You have gastritis, peptic ulcer, enteritis, ileitis, ulcerative colitis, asthma, heart failure, high blood pressure or bleeding problems.
- Patient is younger than 15.

Before you start, consult your doctor:
- If you have epilepsy.
- If you have Parkinson's disease.
- If you have been mentally ill.
- If you have had kidney disease or impaired kidney function.

Over age 60:
Adverse reactions and side effects may be more frequent and severe than in younger persons.

Pregnancy:
Studies inconclusive on harm to unborn child. Decide with your doctor whether drug benefits justify risk to unborn child.

Breast-feeding:
May harm child. Avoid.

Infants & children:
Not recommended for anyone younger than 15. Use only under medical supervision.

Prolonged use:
- Eye damage.
- Reduced hearing.
- Sore throat, fever.
- Weight gain.

Skin & sunlight:
Increased sensitivity to sunlight.

Driving, piloting or hazardous work:
Don't drive or pilot aircraft until you learn how medicine affects you. Don't work around dangerous machinery. Don't climb ladders or work in high places. Danger increases if you drink alcohol or take medicine affecting alertness and reflexes, such as antihistamines, tranquilizers, sedatives, pain medicine, narcotics and mind-altering drugs.

Discontinuing:
Don't discontinue without consulting doctor. Dose may require gradual reduction if you have taken drug for a long time. Doses of other drugs may also require adjustment.

Others:
No problems expected.

POSSIBLE INTERACTION WITH OTHER DRUGS

GENERIC NAME OR DRUG CLASS	COMBINED EFFECT
ACE inhibitors: captopril, enalapril, lisinopril*	May decrease ACE inhibitor effect.
Anticoagulants, oral*	Increased risk of bleeding.
Aspirin	Increased risk of stomach ulcer.
Beta-adrenergic blockers*	Decreased antihypertensive effect.
Carteolol	Decreased effect of carteolol.
Cortisone drugs*	Increased risk of stomach ulcer.
Diuretics*	May decrease diuretic effect.
Lithium	Possible increased lithium effect and toxicity.
Methotrexate	May increase toxicity.
Minoxidil	Reduced minoxidil effect.
Oxyphenbutazone	Possible stomach ulcer.
Phenylbutazone	Possible stomach ulcer.
Phenylpropanolamine	Possible hypertension.
Probenecid	Increased indomethacin effect.
Sotalol	Decreased effect of sotalol.
Terazosin	Decreases effectiveness of terazosin. Causes sodium and fluid retention.
Thyroid hormones*	Rapid heartbeat, blood-pressure rise.

POSSIBLE INTERACTION WITH OTHER SUBSTANCES

INTERACTS WITH	COMBINED EFFECT
Alcohol:	Possible stomach ulcer or bleeding.
Beverages:	None expected.
Cocaine:	None expected.
Foods:	None expected.
Marijuana:	Increased pain relief from indomethacin.
Tobacco:	None expected.

*See Glossary

INSULIN

BRAND NAMES

See complete list of brand names in the *Brand Name Directory*, page 1064.

BASIC INFORMATION

Habit forming? No
Prescription needed? No
Available as generic? No
Drug class: Antidiabetic

 ## USES

Controls diabetes, a complex metabolic disorder, in which the body does not manufacture insulin.

 ## DOSAGE & USAGE INFORMATION

How to take:
Must be taken by injection under the skin. Use disposable, sterile needles. Rotate injection sites.

When to take:
At the same time each day.

If you forget a dose:
Take as soon as you remember. Wait at least 4 hours for next dose. Resume regular schedule.

What drug does:
Facilitates passage of blood sugar through cell membranes so sugar is usable.

Continued next column

 ## OVERDOSE

SYMPTOMS:
Low blood sugar (hypoglycemia)—Anxiety; chills, cold sweats, pale skin; drowsiness; excess hunger; headache; nausea; nervousness; fast heartbeat; shakiness; unusual tiredness or weakness.
WHAT TO DO:
- **Eat some type of sugar immediately, such as orange juice, honey, sugar cubes, crackers, sandwich.**
- **If patient loses consciousness, give glucagon if you have it and know how to use it.**
- **Otherwise, dial 0 (operator) or 911 (emergency) for an ambulance or medical help. Then give first aid immediately.**
- **See emergency information on inside covers.**

Time lapse before drug works:
30 minutes to 8 hours, depending on type of insulin used.

Don't take with:
See Interaction column and consult doctor.

 ## POSSIBLE ADVERSE REACTIONS OR SIDE EFFECTS

SYMPTOMS	WHAT TO DO
Life-threatening:	
Hives, rash, intense itching, faintness soon after a dose (anaphylaxis).	Seek emergency treatment immediately.
Common: None expected.	
Infrequent:	
• Hives.	Discontinue. Call doctor right away.
• Swelling, redness, itch at injection site.	Continue. Call doctor when convenient.
Rare: None expected.	

WARNINGS & PRECAUTIONS

Don't take if:
- Your diagnosis and dose schedule is not established.
- You don't know how to deal with overdose emergencies.

Before you start, consult your doctor:
- If you are allergic to insulin.
- If you take MAO inhibitors.
- If you have liver or kidney disease or low thyroid function.

Over age 60:
Guard against hypoglycemia. Repeated episodes can cause permanent confusion and abnormal behavior.

Pregnancy:
Possible drug benefits outweigh risk to unborn child. Adhere rigidly to diabetes treatment program.

Breast-feeding:
No problems expected.

Infants & children:
Use only under medical supervision.

Prolonged use:
No problems expected.

Skin & sunlight:
No problems expected.

Driving, piloting or hazardous work:
No problems expected after dose is established.

Discontinuing:
Don't discontinue without doctor's advice until you complete prescribed dose, even though symptoms diminish or disappear.

Others:
- Diet and exercise affect how much insulin you need. Work with your doctor to determine accurate dose.
- Notify your doctor if you skip a dose, overeat, have fever or infection.
- Notify doctor if you develop symptoms of high blood sugar: drowsiness, dry skin, orange fruit-like odor to breath, increased urination, appetite loss, unusual thirst.

POSSIBLE INTERACTION WITH OTHER DRUGS

GENERIC NAME OR DRUG CLASS	COMBINED EFFECT
Anticonvulsants, hydantoin*	Decreased insulin effect.
Antidiabetics, oral*	Increased antibiabetic effect.
Beta-adrenergic blockers*	Possible increased difficulty in regulating blood-sugar levels.
Bismuth subsalicylate	Increased insulin effect. May require dosage adjustment.
Carteolol	Hypoglycemic effects may be prolonged.
Contraceptives, oral*	Decreased insulin effect.
Cortisone drugs*	Decreased insulin effect.
Diuretics*	Decreased insulin effect.
Furosemide	Decreased insulin effect.
MAO inhibitors*	Increased insulin effect.
Nicotine gum and other smoking deterrents	Increased insulin effect.
Oxyphenbutazone	Increased insulin effect.
Phenylbutazone	Increased insulin effect.
Salicylates*	Increased insulin effect.
Sotalol	Hypoglycemic effects may be prolonged.
Sulfa drugs*	Increased insulin effect.
Tetracyclines*	Increased insulin effect.
Thyroid hormones*	Decreased insulin effect.

POSSIBLE INTERACTION WITH OTHER SUBSTANCES

INTERACTS WITH	COMBINED EFFECT
Alcohol:	Increased insulin effect. May cause hypoglycemia and brain damage.
Beverages:	None expected.
Cocaine:	May cause brain damage.
Foods:	None expected.
Marijuana:	Possible increase in blood sugar.
Tobacco:	None expected.

*See Glossary

IODOQUINOL

BRAND NAMES

Diiodohydroxyquin
Diodoquin

Diquinol
Yodoxin

BASIC INFORMATION

Habit forming? No
Prescription needed? Yes
Available as generic? Yes
Drug class: Antiprotozoal

USES

Treatment for intestinal amebiasis.

DOSAGE & USAGE INFORMATION

How to take:
Tablets—Mix with applesauce or chocolate syrup if unable to swallow tablets.

When to take:
Three times daily after meals for 20 days. Treatment may be repeated after 2 to 3 weeks.

If you forget a dose:
Take as soon as you remember up to 2 hours late. If more than 2 hours, wait for next scheduled dose (don't double this dose).

What drug does:
Kills amoeba (microscopic parasites) in intestinal tract.

Time lapse before drug works:
May require full course of treatment (20 days) to cure.

Don't take with:
See Interaction column and consult doctor.

OVERDOSE

SYMPTOMS:
- Prolonged dosing at high level may produce blurred vision, muscle pain, eye pain, numbness and tingling in hands or feet.
- Single overdosage unlikely to threaten life.

WHAT TO DO:
If person takes much larger amount than prescribed, call doctor, poison-control center or hospital emergency room for instructions.

POSSIBLE ADVERSE REACTIONS OR SIDE EFFECTS

SYMPTOMS	WHAT TO DO
Life-threatening: None expected.	
Common: Diarrhea, nausea, vomiting, stomach pain.	Discontinue. Call doctor right away.
Infrequent: Clumsiness, rash, hives, itching, blurred vision, muscle pain, numbness or tingling in hands or feet, chills, fever, weakness.	Discontinue. Call doctor right away.
Rare: Dizziness, headache.	Discontinue. Call doctor right away.

WARNINGS & PRECAUTIONS

Don't take if:
You have kidney or liver disease.

Before you start, consult your doctor:
If you have optic atrophy thyroid disease.

Over age 60:
Adverse reactions and side effects may be more frequent and severe than in younger persons.

Pregnancy:
No proven problems, but avoid if possible.

Breast-feeding:
No proven problems, but avoid if possible. Discontinue nursing until you finish medicine. Consult doctor for advice on maintaining milk supply.

Infants & children:
Not recommended. Safety and dosage has not been established.

Prolonged use:
Not recommended.

Skin & sunlight:
No problems expected.

Driving, piloting or hazardous work:
No problems expected.

Discontinuing:
Don't discontinue without consulting doctor.

Others:
Thyroid tests may be inaccurate for as long as 6 months after discontinuing iodoquinol treatment.

POSSIBLE INTERACTION WITH OTHER DRUGS

GENERIC NAME OR DRUG CLASS	COMBINED EFFECT
None expected.	

POSSIBLE INTERACTION WITH OTHER SUBSTANCES

INTERACTS WITH	COMBINED EFFECT
Alcohol:	None expected.
Beverages:	None expected.
Cocaine:	None expected.
Foods:	Taking with food may decrease gastrointestinal side effects.
Marijuana:	None expected.
Tobacco:	None expected.

IRON-POLYSACCHARIDE

BRAND NAMES

Hytinic	Nu-Iron
Niferex	Nu-Iron 150
Niferex-150	

BASIC INFORMATION

Habit forming? No
Prescription needed?
  With folic acid: Yes
  Without folic acid: No
Available as generic? No
Drug class: Mineral supplement (iron)

USES

Treatment for dietary iron deficiency or iron-deficiency anemia from other causes.

DOSAGE & USAGE INFORMATION

How to take:
Tablet, capsule or liquid—Swallow with liquid or food to lessen stomach irritation. If you can't swallow whole, crumble tablet or open capsule and take with liquid or food. Place medicine far back on tongue to avoid staining teeth.

When to take:
1 hour before or 2 hours after meals.

If you forget a dose:
Take up to 2 hours late. If more than 2 hours, wait for next dose (don't double this dose).

What drug does:
Stimulates bone-marrow production of hemoglobin (red-blood-cell pigment that carries oxygen to body cells).

Time lapse before drug works:
3 to 7 days. May require 3 weeks for maximum benefit.

Don't take with:
- Multiple vitamin and mineral supplements.
- See Interaction column and consult doctor.

OVERDOSE

SYMPTOMS:
Weakness, collapse; pallor, blue lips, hands and fingernails; weak, rapid heartbeat; shallow breathing; convulsions; coma.
WHAT TO DO:
- **Dial 0 (operator) or 911 (emergency) for an ambulance or medical help. Then give first aid immediately.**
- **See emergency information on inside covers.**

POSSIBLE ADVERSE REACTIONS OR SIDE EFFECTS

SYMPTOMS	WHAT TO DO
Life-threatening: Weak, rapid heartbeat.	Seek emergency treatment immediately.
Common: Stained teeth with liquid iron.	No action necessary.
Always: Gray or black stool.	No action necessary.
Infrequent: • Constipation or diarrhea, heartburn, nausea, vomiting.	Discontinue. Call doctor right away.
• Fatigue, weakness.	Continue. Call doctor when convenient.
• Dark urine.	Continue. Tell doctor at next visit.
Rare: • Throat or chest pain on swallowing, pain, cramps, blood in stool.	Discontinue. Call doctor right away.
• Drowsiness.	Continue. Call doctor when convenient.

WARNINGS & PRECAUTIONS

Don't take if:
- You are allergic to any iron supplement or tartrazine dye.
- You take iron injections.
- Your daily iron intake is high.
- You plan to take this supplement for a long time.
- You have acute hepatitis.
- You have hemosiderosis or hemochromatosis (conditions involving excess iron in body).
- You have hemolytic anemia.

Before you start, consult your doctor:
- If you plan to become pregnant within medication period.
- If you have had stomach surgery.
- If you have had peptic ulcer disease, enteritis or colitis.
- If you have had pancreatitis or hepatitis.

Over age 60:
May cause hemochromatosis (iron storage disease) with bronze skin, liver damage, diabetes, heart problems and impotence.

Pregnancy:
No proven harm to unborn child. Avoid if possible. Take only if your doctor prescribes supplement during last half of pregnancy.

Breast-feeding:
No problems expected. Take only if your doctor confirms you have a dietary deficiency or an iron-deficiency anemia.

Infants & children:
Use only under medical supervision. Overdose common and dangerous. Keep out of children's reach.

Prolonged use:
May cause hemochromatosis (iron storage disease) with bronze skin, liver damage, diabetes, heart problems and impotence.

Skin & sunlight:
No problems expected.

Driving, piloting or hazardous work:
No problems expected.

Discontinuing:
May be unnecessary to finish medicine. Follow doctor's instructions.

Others:
- Liquid form stains teeth. Mix with water or juice to lessen the effect. Brush with baking soda or hydrogen peroxide to help remove stain.
- Some products contain tartrazine dye. Avoid, especially if you are allergic to aspirin.

POSSIBLE INTERACTION WITH OTHER DRUGS

GENERIC NAME OR DRUG CLASS	COMBINED EFFECT
Allopurinol	Possible excess iron storage in liver.
Antacids*	Poor iron absorption.
Calcium supplements*	Decreased iron effect.
Chloramphenicol	Decreased effect of iron. Interferes with red-blood-cell and hemoglobin formation.
Cholestyramine	Decreased iron effect.
Iron supplements, other*	Possible excess iron storage in liver.
Penicillamine	Decreased penicillamine effect.
Tetracyclines*	Decreased tetracycline effect. Take iron 3 hours before or 2 hours after taking tetracycline.
Vitamin C	Increased iron effect.

POSSIBLE INTERACTION WITH OTHER SUBSTANCES

INTERACTS WITH	COMBINED EFFECT
Alcohol:	Increased iron absorption. May cause organ damage. Avoid or use in moderation.
Beverages: Milk, tea.	Decreased iron effect.
Cocaine:	None expected.
Foods: Dairy foods, eggs, whole-grain bread and cereal.	Decreased iron effect.
Marijuana:	None expected.
Tobacco:	None expected.

ISOETHARINE

BRAND NAMES

Arm-a-Med
  Isoetharine
Beta-2
Bisorine
Bronkometer
Bronkosol
Dey-Dose
  Isoetharine

Dey-Dose
  Isoetharine S/F
Dey-Lute
  Isoetharine
Dilabron
Disorine
Dispos-a Med
  Isoetharine

BASIC INFORMATION

Habit forming? No
Prescription needed? Yes
Available as generic? Yes
Drug class: Sympathomimetic
  (bronchodilator)

 ## USES

Eases breathing difficulty from bronchial asthma
attacks, bronchitis and emphysema.

 ## DOSAGE & USAGE
INFORMATION

How to take:
Aerosol—Use only as directed on label. Don't
inhale medicine more than twice per dose
unless otherwise directed by doctor.

When to take:
As needed, no more often than every 3 hours.

If you forget a dose:
Take as soon as you remember if you need it.
Never double dose.

Continued next column

 ## OVERDOSE

SYMPTOMS:
Nervousness, anxiety, dizziness,
palpitations, tremor, rapid heartbeat, spasm
of bronchial tubes, cardiac arrest.
WHAT TO DO:
• Dial 0 (operator) or 911 (emergency) for
  an ambulance or medical help. Then give
  first aid immediately.
• If patient is unconscious and not
  breathing, give mouth-to-mouth
  breathing. If there is no heartbeat, use
  cardiac massage and mouth-to-mouth
  breathing (CPR). Don't try to make patient
  vomit. If you can't get help quickly, take
  patient to nearest emergency facility.
• See emergency information on inside
  covers.

What drug does:
Dilates constricted bronchial tubes so air can
pass.

Time lapse before drug works:
1 to 2 minutes.

Don't take with:
• Non-prescription drugs containing caffeine
  without consulting doctor.
• See Interaction column and consult doctor.

 ## POSSIBLE
ADVERSE REACTIONS
OR SIDE EFFECTS

SYMPTOMS	WHAT TO DO
Life-threatening: None expected.	
Common: Dizziness, agitation, headache, insomnia, nausea, fast or pounding heartbeat.	Continue. Call doctor when convenient.
Infrequent: • Constriction of bronchial tubes, particularly after overuse.	Discontinue. Call doctor right away.
• Weakness.	Continue. Call doctor when convenient.
Rare: None expected.	

WARNINGS & PRECAUTIONS

Don't take if:
- You are allergic to any sympathomimetic drug.
- You have a heart-rhythm disorder.
- You have taken MAO inhibitors in past 2 weeks.

Before you start, consult your doctor:
- If you use epinephrine for asthma.
- If you have diabetes.
- If you have an overactive thyroid gland.
- If you take a digitalis preparation, have high blood pressure or heart disease.

Over age 60:
- If you have hardening of the arteries, use with caution.
- If you have enlarged prostate gland, drug may increase urination difficulty.
- If you have Parkinson's disease, drug may temporarily increase rigidity and tremor in extremities.

Pregnancy:
No proven harm to unborn child. Avoid if possible.

Breast-feeding:
No problems expected, but consult doctor.

Infants & children:
Don't give to infants younger than 2. For older children, use only under medical supervision.

Prolonged use:
No problems expected.

Skin & sunlight:
No problems expected.

Driving, piloting or hazardous work:
No problems expected. Use caution if you feel nervous or dizzy.

Discontinuing:
Discontinue if drug fails to provide relief. Don't increase dose or frequency.

Others:
May increase blood- and urine-sugar levels, particularly in diabetics.

POSSIBLE INTERACTION WITH OTHER DRUGS

GENERIC NAME OR DRUG CLASS	COMBINED EFFECT
Antidepressants, tricyclic (TCA)*	Increased isoetharine effect.
Beta-adrenergic blockers*	Decreased effects of both drugs.
Carteolol	Decreased beta-agonist effect.
Ephedrine	Increased ephedrine effect. Excessive heart stimulation.
Epinephrine	Excessive heart stimulation.
Isoproterenol	Excessive heart stimulation.
MAO inhibitors*	Dangerous mixture. Avoid.
Nitrates*	Possible decreased effects of both drugs.
Sotalol	Decreased beta-agonist effect.
Theophylline	Possible increased effect and toxicity of both drugs.

POSSIBLE INTERACTION WITH OTHER SUBSTANCES

INTERACTS WITH	COMBINED EFFECT
Alcohol:	None expected.
Beverages: Caffeine drinks.	May cause irregular or fast heartbeat.
Cocaine:	Excessive stimulation. Avoid.
Foods: Chocolates.	May cause irregular or fast heartbeat.
Marijuana:	Improves drug's antiasthmatic effect.
Tobacco:	None expected.

ISOMETHEPTENE, DICHLORALPHENAZONE & ACETAMINOPHEN

BRAND NAMES

Isocom   Midrin

BASIC INFORMATION

Habit forming? No
Prescription needed? Yes
Available as generic? No
Drug class: Analgesic, sedative

 ## USES

Treatment of vascular (throbbing or migraine type) and tension headaches.

 ## DOSAGE & USAGE INFORMATION

How to take:
Capsules—Take with fluid. Usual dose—2 capsules at start, then 1 every hour until fully relieved. Don't exceed 5 capsules in 12 hours.

When to take:
At first sign of headache.

If you forget a dose:
Use as soon as you remember.

What drug does:
Causes blood vessels in head to constrict or become narrower. Acetaminophen relieves pain by effects on hypothalamus—the part of the brain that helps regulate body heat and receives body's pain messages.

Time lapse before drug works:
30-60 minutes.

Continued next column

 ## OVERDOSE

SYMPTOMS:
Stomach upsets, irritability, sweating, anorexia, convulsions, coma.
WHAT TO DO:
- **Dial 0 (operator) or 911 (emergency) for an ambulance or medical help. Then give first aid immediately.**
- **See emergency information on inside covers.**

Don't take with:
- Any medicine that will decrease mental alertness or reflexes, such as alcohol, other mind-altering drugs, cough/cold medicines, antihistamines, allergy medicine, sedatives, tranquilizers (sleeping pills or "downers") barbiturates, seizure medicine, narcotics, other prescription medicine for pain, muscle relaxants, anesthetics.
- See Interaction column and consult doctor.

 ## POSSIBLE ADVERSE REACTIONS OR SIDE EFFECTS

SYMPTOMS	WHAT TO DO
Life-threatening: Fast heartbeat.	Discontinue. Seek emergency treatment.
Common: Dizziness.	Continue. Call doctor when convenient.
Infrequent: Diarrhea, vomiting, nausea, abdominal cramps.	Discontinue. Call doctor right away.
Rare: Rash; itchy skin; sore throat, fever, mouth sores; unusual bleeding or bruising; weakness; jaundice.	Discontinue. Call doctor right away.

ISOMETHEPTENE, DICHLORALPHENAZONE & ACETAMINOPHEN

WARNINGS & PRECAUTIONS

Don't take if:
- You are allergic to acetaminophen or any other component of this combination medicine.
- Your symptoms don't improve after 2 days use. Call your doctor.

Before you start, consult your doctor:
If you have kidney disease, liver damage, glaucoma, heart or blood vessel disorder, hypertension.

Over age 60:
Don't exceed recommended dose. You can't eliminate drug as efficiently as younger persons.

Pregnancy:
No proven harm to unborn child. Avoid if possible.

Breast-feeding:
No proven harm to nursing infant.

Infants & children:
Not recommended.

Prolonged use:
May affect blood system and cause anemia. Limit use to 5 days for children 12 and under, and 10 days for adults.

Skin & sunlight:
No problems expected.

Driving, piloting or hazardous work:
Avoid if you feel drowsy. Otherwise, no restrictions.

Discontinuing:
Discontinue in 2 days if symptoms don't improve.

Others:
No problems expected.

POSSIBLE INTERACTION WITH OTHER DRUGS

GENERIC NAME OR DRUG CLASS	COMBINED EFFECT
Anticoagulants, oral*	May increase anticoagulant effect. If combined frequently, prothrombin time should be monitored.
Aspirin or other salicylates*	Long-term combined effect (3 years or longer) increases chance of damage to kidney, including malignancy.
Beta-adrenergic blockers*	Narrowed arteries in heart if taken in large doses.
MAO inhibitors*	Sudden increase in blood pressure.
Non-steroidal anti-inflammatory drugs (NSAIDs)*	Long-term combined effect (3 years or longer) increases chance of damage to kidney, including malignancy.
Phenacetin	Long-term combined effect (3 years or longer) increases chance of damage to kidney, including malignancy.
Phenobarbital	Quicker elimination and decreased effect of acetaminophen.
Tetracyclines* (effervescent granules or tablets)	May slow tetracycline absorption. Space doses 2 hours apart.
Zidovudine (AZT)	Increased toxic effect of zidovudine.

POSSIBLE INTERACTION WITH OTHER SUBSTANCES

INTERACTS WITH	COMBINED EFFECT
Alcohol:	Drowsiness. Toxicity to liver.
Beverages:	None expected.
Cocaine:	None expected. However, cocaine may slow body's recovery. Avoid.
Foods:	None expected.
Marijuana:	Increased pain relief. However, marijuana may slow body's recovery. Avoid.
Tobacco:	May decrease effectiveness of Midrin.

*See Glossary

ISONIAZID

BRAND NAMES

DOW-Isoniazid
Ethionamide
INH
Isotamine
Laniazid
Laniazid C.P.

Nydrazid
PMS Isoniazid
Rifamate
Rimifon
Trecator-SC

BASIC INFORMATION

Habit forming? No
Prescription needed? Yes
Available as generic? Yes
Drug class: Antitubercular (antimicrobial)

USES

Kills tuberculosis germs.

DOSAGE & USAGE INFORMATION

How to take:
- Tablet—Swallow with liquid to lessen stomach irritation.
- Syrup—Follow label directions.

When to take:
At the same time each day.

If you forget a dose:
Take as soon as you remember up to 12 hours late. If more than 12 hours, wait for next scheduled dose (don't double this dose).

What drug does:
Interferes with TB germ metabolism. Eventually destroys the germ.

Continued next column

OVERDOSE

SYMPTOMS:
Difficult breathing, convulsions, coma.
WHAT TO DO:
- Dial 0 (operator) or 911 (emergency) for an ambulance or medical help. Then give first aid immediately.
- If patient is unconscious and not breathing, give mouth-to-mouth breathing. If there is no heartbeat, use cardiac massage and mouth-to-mouth breathing (CPR). Don't try to make patient vomit. If you can't get help quickly, take patient to nearest emergency facility.
- See emergency information on inside covers.

Time lapse before drug works:
3 to 6 months. You may need to take drug as long as 2 years.

Don't take with:
See Interaction column and consult doctor.

POSSIBLE ADVERSE REACTIONS OR SIDE EFFECTS

SYMPTOMS	WHAT TO DO
Life-threatening:	
None expected.	
Common:	
• Muscle pain and pain in joints, tingling or numbness in extremities, jaundice.	Discontinue. Call doctor right away.
• Confusion, unsteady walk.	Continue. Call doctor when convenient.
Infrequent:	
• Swollen glands, nausea, indigestion, vomiting, appetite loss.	Discontinue. Call doctor right away.
• Dizziness, increase in blood sugar.	Continue. Call doctor when convenient.
Rare:	
• Rash, fever, impaired vision, anemia with fatigue, weakness, fever, sore throat, unusual bleeding or bruising.	Discontinue. Call doctor right away.
• Breast enlargement or discomfort.	Continue. Tell doctor at next visit.

WARNINGS & PRECAUTIONS

Don't take if:
You are allergic to isoniazid.

Before you start, consult your doctor:
- If you plan to become pregnant within medication period.
- If you are allergic to athionamide, pyrazinamide or nicotinic acid.
- If you drink alcohol.
- If you have liver or kidney disease.
- If you have epilepsy, diabetes or lupus.

Over age 60:
Adverse reactions and side effects, especially jaundice, may be more frequent and severe than in younger persons. Kidneys may be less efficient.

Pregnancy:
No proven harm to unborn child. Avoid if possible, especially in the first 6 months of pregnancy. Consult doctor about use in last 3 months.

Breast-feeding:
Drug passes into milk. Avoid drug or discontinue nursing until you finish medicine. Consult doctor for advice on maintaining milk supply.

Infants & children:
Use only under medical supervision.

Prolonged use:
Numbness and tingling of hands and feet.

Skin & sunlight:
No problems expected.

Driving, piloting or hazardous work:
Avoid if you feel dizzy. Otherwise, no problems expected.

Discontinuing:
Don't discontinue without doctor's advice until you complete prescribed dose, even though symptoms diminish or disappear.

Others:
- Diabetic patients may have false blood-sugar tests.
- Periodic liver-function tests and laboratory blood studies recommended.
- Prescription for vitamin B-6 (pyridoxine) recommended to prevent nerve damage.

POSSIBLE INTERACTION WITH OTHER DRUGS

GENERIC NAME OR DRUG CLASS	COMBINED EFFECT
Antacids* (aluminum-containing)	Decreased absorption of isoniazid.
Anticholinergics*	May increase pressure within eyeball.
Anticoagulants*	Increased anticoagulant effect.
Antidiabetics*	Increased antidiabetic effect.
Antihypertensives*	Increased antihypertensive effect.
Cyclosporine	Increased risk of central nervous system effects.
Disulfiram	Increased effect of disulfiram.
Laxatives*	Decreased absorption and effect of isoniazid.
Narcotics*	Increased narcotic effect.
Niacin	Decreased niacin effect.
Phenytoin	Increased phenytoin effect.
Pyridoxine (Vitamin B-6)	Decreased chance of nerve damage in extremities.
Rifampin	Increased isoniazid toxicity to liver.
Sedatives*	Increased sedative effect.
Stimulants*	Increased stimulant effect.

POSSIBLE INTERACTION WITH OTHER SUBSTANCES

INTERACTS WITH	COMBINED EFFECT
Alcohol:	Increased incidence of liver disease.
Beverages:	None expected.
Cocaine:	None expected.
Foods:	Decreased absorption of isoniazid.
Marijuana:	No interactions expected, but marijuana may slow body's recovery.
Tobacco:	No interactions expected, but tobacco may slow body's recovery.

ISOPROPAMIDE

BRAND NAMES

Allergine
Allernade
Capade
Combid
Darbid

Oraminic
Ornade
Prochlor-Iso
Pro-Iso

BASIC INFORMATION

Habit forming? No
Prescription needed?
  Low strength: No
  High strength: Yes
Available as generic? No
Drug class: Antispasmodic, anticholinergic

 ## USES

Reduces spasms of digestive system, bladder and urethra.

 ## DOSAGE & USAGE INFORMATION

How to take:
Tablet—Swallow with liquid or food to lessen stomach irritation.

When to take:
30 minutes before meals (unless directed otherwise by doctor).

If you forget a dose:
Take as soon as you remember up to 2 hours late. If more than 2 hours, wait for next scheduled dose (don't double this dose).

What drug does:
Blocks nerve impulses at parasympathetic nerve endings, preventing muscle contractions and gland secretions of organs involved.

Time lapse before drug works:
15 to 30 minutes.

Don't take with:
See Interaction column and consult doctor.

 ## OVERDOSE

SYMPTOMS:
Dilated pupils, blurred vision, rapid pulse and breathing, dizziness, fever, hallucinations, confusion, slurred speech, agitation, flushed face, convulsions, coma.
WHAT TO DO:
- Dial 0 (operator) or 911 (emergency) for an ambulance or medical help. Then give first aid immediately.
- See emergency information on inside covers.

 ## POSSIBLE ADVERSE REACTIONS OR SIDE EFFECTS

SYMPTOMS	WHAT TO DO
Life-threatening:	
Hives, rash, intense itching, faintness soon after a dose (anaphylaxis).	Seek emergency treatment immediately.
Common:	
• Confusion, delirium, rapid heartbeat.	Discontinue. Call doctor right away.
• Nausea, vomiting, decreased sweating.	Continue. Call doctor when convenient.
• Constipation, loss of taste.	Continue. Tell doctor at next visit.
• Dryness in ears, nose, throat.	No action necessary.
Infrequent:	
Headache, difficult urination.	Continue. Call doctor when convenient.
Rare:	
Rash or hives, pain, blurred vision.	Discontinue. Call doctor right away.

 ## WARNINGS & PRECAUTIONS

Don't take if:
- You are allergic to any anticholinergic or iodine.
- You have trouble with stomach bloating.
- You have difficulty emptying your bladder completely.
- You have narrow-angle glaucoma.
- You have severe ulcerative colitis.

Before you start, consult your doctor:
- If you have open-angle glaucoma.
- If you have angina.
- If you have chronic bronchitis or asthma.
- If you have hiatal hernia.
- If you have liver disease.
- If you have enlarged prostate.
- If you have myasthenia gravis.
- If you have peptic ulcer.
- If you will have surgery within 2 months, including dental surgery, requiring general or spinal anesthesia.

Over age 60:
Adverse reactions and side effects may be more frequent and severe than in younger persons.

Pregnancy:
Studies inconclusive on harm to unborn child. Animal studies show fetal abnormalities. Decide with your doctor whether drug benefits justify risk to unborn child.

Breast-feeding:
Drug passes into milk and decreases milk flow. Avoid drug or discontinue nursing until you finish medicine. Consult doctor for advice on maintaining milk supply.

Infants & children:
Use only under medical supervision.

Prolonged use:
Chronic constipation, possible fecal impaction. Consult doctor immediately.

Skin & sunlight:
No problems expected.

Driving, piloting or hazardous work:
Use disqualifies you for piloting aircraft. Otherwise, no problems expected.

Discontinuing:
May be unnecessary to finish medicine. Follow doctor's instructions.

Others:
No problems expected.

 POSSIBLE INTERACTION WITH OTHER DRUGS

GENERIC NAME OR DRUG CLASS	COMBINED EFFECT
Amantadine	Increased isopropamide effect.
Antacids*	Decreased isopropamide effect.
Anticholinergics, other*	Increased isopropamide effect
Antidepressants, tricyclic (TCA)*	Increased atropine effect. Increased sedation.
Antihistamines*	Increased isopropamide effect.
Buclizine	Increased isopropamide effect.
Cortisone drugs*	Increased internal-eye pressure.
Digitalis	Possible decreased absorption of digitalis.
Haloperidol	Increased internal-eye pressure.
MAO inhibitors*	Increased isopropamide effect.
Meperidine	Increased isopropamide effect.
Methylphenidate	Increased isopropamide effect.

Nitrates*	Increased internal-eye pressure.
Nizatidine	Increased nizatidine effect.
Orphenadrine	Increased isopropamide effect.
Phenothiazines*	Increased isopropamide effect.
Pilocarpine	Loss of pilocarpine effect in glaucoma treatment.
Potassium supplements*	Possible intestinal ulcers with oral potassium tablets.
Quinidine	Increased isopropamide effect.
Vitamin C	Decreased isopropamide effect. Avoid large doses of vitamin C.

 POSSIBLE INTERACTION WITH OTHER SUBSTANCES

INTERACTS WITH	COMBINED EFFECT
Alcohol:	None expected.
Beverages:	None expected.
Cocaine:	Excessively rapid heartbeat. Avoid.
Foods:	None expected.
Marijuana:	Drowsiness and dry mouth.
Tobacco:	None expected.

*See Glossary

ISOPROTERENOL

BRAND NAMES

Aerolone	Isuprel
Brondilate	Isuprel Mistometer
Dey-Dose	Medihaler-Iso
Isoproterenol	Norisodrine
Dispose-a-Med	Norisodrine
Isoproterenol	Aerotrol
Duo-Medihaler	Proternol
Iprenol	Vapo-Iso

BASIC INFORMATION

Habit forming? No
Prescription needed? Yes
Available as generic? Yes
Drug class: Sympathomimetic, bronchodilator

USES

Treatment for breathing difficulty from acute asthma, bronchitis and emphysema.

DOSAGE & USAGE INFORMATION

How to take:
- Sublingual tablets—Dissolve under tongue.
- Aerosol inhaler—Don't inhale more than twice per dose.

When to take:
As needed, no more often than every 4 hours.

If you forget a dose:
Take as soon as you remember. Wait 4 hours for next dose.

What drug does:
- Dilates constricted bronchial tubes, improving air flow.
- Stimulates heart muscle and dilates blood vessels.

Continued next column

OVERDOSE

SYMPTOMS:
Nervousness, rapid or irregular heartbeat, fainting, sweating, headache, tremor, vomiting, chest pain, blood-pressure drop.
WHAT TO DO:
- Dial 0 (operator) or 911 (emergency) for an ambulance or medical help. Then give first aid immediately.
- See emergency information on inside covers.

Time lapse before drug works:
2 to 4 minutes.

Don't take with:
See Interaction column and consult doctor.

POSSIBLE ADVERSE REACTIONS OR SIDE EFFECTS

SYMPTOMS	WHAT TO DO
Life-threatening: None expected.	
Common:	
• Nervousness, insomnia.	Continue. Call doctor when convenient.
• Dry mouth, dry throat.	Continue. Tell doctor at next visit.
Infrequent:	
• Chest pain; irregular, fast or pounding heartbeat; unusual sweating.	Discontinue. Call doctor right away.
• Dizziness, headache, shakiness, weakness, flushed face, nausea, vomiting.	Continue. Call doctor when convenient.
Rare: None expected.	

WARNINGS & PRECAUTIONS

Don't take if:
- You are allergic to any sympathomimetic, including some diet pills.
- You have serious heart-rhythm disorder.
- You have taken MAO inhibitors in past 2 weeks.

Before you start, consult your doctor:
- If you are sensitive to sympathomimetics.
- If you use epinephrine.
- If you have high blood pressure, heart disease, or take a digitalis preparation.
- If you have diabetes.
- If you have overactive thyroid.
- If your heartbeat is faster than 100 beats per minute.

Over age 60:
You may be more sensitive to drug's stimulant effects. Use with caution if you have hardening of the arteries.

Pregnancy:
Studies inconclusive on harm to unborn child. Animal studies show fetal abnormalities. Decide with your doctor whether drug benefits justify risk to unborn child.

Breast-feeding:
Drug does not appear in milk. Consult doctor.

Infants & children:
Not recommended.

Prolonged use:
- Salivary glands may swell.
- Mouth ulcers (sublingual tablets).

Skin & sunlight:
No problems expected.

Driving, piloting or hazardous work:
Use caution if you feel dizzy or nervous.

Discontinuing:
Discontinue if drug fails to provide relief after 2 or 3 days. Consult doctor.

Others:
No problems expected.

POSSIBLE INTERACTION WITH OTHER DRUGS

GENERIC NAME OR DRUG CLASS	COMBINED EFFECT
Albuterol	Increased effect of both drugs, especially harmful side effects.
Antidepressants, tricyclic (TCA)*	Increased effect of both drugs.
Beta-adrenergic blockers*	Decreased effects of both drugs.
Carteolol	Decreased beta-agonist effect.
Ephedrine	Increased ephedrine effect.
Epinephrine	Increased chance of serious heart disturbances.
MAO inhibitors*	Possible increased blood pressure.
Nitrates*	Possible decreased effects of both drugs.
Sympathomimetics, other*	Increased effect of both drugs, especially harmful side effects.
Sotalol	Decreased beta-agonist effect.
Terazosin	Decreases effectiveness of terazosin.
Theophylline	Possible increased effect and toxicity of both drugs

POSSIBLE INTERACTION WITH OTHER SUBSTANCES

INTERACTS WITH	COMBINED EFFECT
Alcohol:	Decreased isoproterenol effect.
Beverages: Caffeine drinks.	Overstimulation. Avoid.
Cocaine:	High risk of heartbeat irregularities and high blood pressure. Overstimulation of brain. Avoid.
Foods:	None expected.
Marijuana:	Increased antiasthmatic effect of isoproterenol.
Tobacco:	None expected.

*See Glossary

ISOPROTERENOL & PHENYLEPHRINE

BRAND NAMES

Duo-Medihaler

BASIC INFORMATION

Habit forming? No
Prescription needed? Yes
Available as generic? No
Drug class: Sympathomimetic, bronchodilator

 USES

- Temporary relief of congestion of nose, sinuses and throat caused by allergies, colds or sinusitis.
- Treatment for breathing difficulty from acute asthma, bronchitis and emphysema.

 DOSAGE & USAGE INFORMATION

How to take:
Aerosol inhaler—Don't inhale more than twice per dose. Follow package instructions.

When to take:
As needed, no more often than every 4 hours.

If you forget a dose:
Take as soon as you remember. Wait 4 hours for next dose. Don't double this dose.

What drug does:
- Dilates constricted bronchial tubes, improving air flow.
- Stimulates heart muscle and dilates blood vessels.

Time lapse before drug works:
2 to 4 minutes.

Continued next column

 OVERDOSE

SYMPTOMS:
Headache, blood-pressure rise, slow and forceful pulse, nervousness, rapid or irregular heartbeat, fainting, sweating, tremor, vomiting, chest pain, convulsions, coma.
WHAT TO DO:
- **Dial 0 (operator) or 911 (emergency) for an ambulance or medical help. Then give first aid immediately.**
- **See emergency information on inside covers.**

Don't take with:
Non-prescription drugs for asthma, cough, cold, allergy, appetite suppressants, sleeping pills or drugs containing caffeine without consulting doctor.

 POSSIBLE ADVERSE REACTIONS OR SIDE EFFECTS

SYMPTOMS	WHAT TO DO
Life-threatening: None expected.	
Common: Chest pain; irregular, fast heartbeat; dry mouth.	Discontinue. Call doctor right away.
Infrequent: • Increased sweating.	Discontinue. Call doctor right away.
• Nervousness, insomnia, dizziness, headache, shakiness, weakness, red or flushed face, vomiting, nausea, pale skin.	Continue. Call doctor when convenient.
Rare: None expected.	

 WARNINGS & PRECAUTIONS

Don't take if:
- You are allergic to any sympathomimetic, including some diet pills.
- You have serious heart-rhythm disorder.
- You have taken MAO inhibitors in past 2 weeks.

Before you start, consult your doctor:
- If you have high blood pressure, heart disease, or take a digitalis preparation.
- If you have diabetes or overactive thyroid.
- If you have taken MAO inhibitors in past 2 weeks.
- If you are sensitive to sympathomimetics.
- If you use epinephrine.
- If your heartbeat is faster than 100 beats per minute.

Over age 60:
You may be more sensitive to drug's stimulant effects. Use with caution if you have hardening of the arteries.

ISOPROTERENOL & PHENYLEPHRINE

Pregnancy:
Risk to unborn child outweighs drug benefits. Don't use.

Breast-feeding:
Drug passes into milk. Avoid drug or discontinue nursing until you finish medicine. Consult doctor for advice on maintaining milk supply.

Infants & children:
Use only under close supervision.

Prolonged use:
- May cause functional dependence.
- Salivary glands may swell.

Skin & sunlight:
No problems expected.

Driving, piloting or hazardous work:
Use caution if you feel dizzy or nervous.

Discontinuing:
Discontinue if drug fails to provide relief after 2 or 3 days. Consult doctor.

Others:
No problems expected.

POSSIBLE INTERACTION WITH OTHER DRUGS

GENERIC NAME OR DRUG CLASS	COMBINED EFFECT
Acebutolol	Decreased effect of both drugs.
Amphetamines*	Increased nervousness.
Antiasthmatics*	Nervous stimulation.
Antidepressants*	Increased effect of both drugs.
Antihypertensives*	Increased antihypertensive effect.
Beta-adrenergic blockers*	Decreased effect of both drugs.
Ephedrine	Increased ephedrine effect.
Epinephrine	Increased chance of serious heart disturbances.

MAO inhibitors*	Dangerous blood-pressure rise.
Nitrates*	Possible decreased effect of both drugs.
Oxprenolol	Decreased effect of both drugs.
Sedatives*	Decreased sedative effect.
Sympathomimetics, other*	Increased effect of both drugs, especially harmful side effects.
Terazosin	Decreases effectiveness of terazosin.
Theophylline	Possible increased effect and toxicity of both drugs.
Tranquilizers*	Decreased tranquilizer effect.

POSSIBLE INTERACTION WITH OTHER SUBSTANCES

INTERACTS WITH	COMBINED EFFECT
Alcohol:	Decreased isoproterenol effect.
Beverages: Caffeine drinks.	Overstimulation. Avoid.
Cocaine:	High risk of heartbeat irregularities and high blood pressure. Overstimulation of brain. Avoid.
Foods:	None expected.
Marijuana:	Increased antiasthmatic effect of isoproterenol.
Tobacco:	None expected.

*See Glossary

ISOTRETINOIN

BRAND NAMES

Accutane

BASIC INFORMATION

Habit forming? No
Prescription needed? Yes
Available as generic? No
Drug classification: Antiacne

 USES

- Decreases cystic acne formation in severe cases.
- Certain other skin disorders involving an overabundance of outer skin layer.

 DOSAGE & USAGE INFORMATION

How to take:
Capsule—Swallow with liquid or food to lessen stomach irritation. If you can't swallow whole, open capsule and take with liquid or food.

When to take:
Twice a day. Follow prescription directions.

If you forget a dose:
Take as soon as you remember up to 2 hours late. If more than 2 hours, wait for next scheduled dose and double dose.

What drug does:
Reduces sebaceous gland activity and size.

Time lapse before drug works:
May require 15 to 20 weeks to experience full benefit.

Don't take with:
Vitamin A or supplements containing Vitamin A.

 OVERDOSE

SYMPTOMS:
None reported.
WHAT TO DO:
Overdose unlikely to threaten life. If person takes much larger amount than prescribed, call doctor, poison-control center or hospital emergency room for instructions.

 POSSIBLE ADVERSE REACTIONS OR SIDE EFFECTS

SYMPTOMS	WHAT TO DO
Life-threatening: None expected.	
Common:	
• Burning, red, itching eyes; lip scaling; burning pain.	Discontinue. Call doctor right away.
• Itchy skin.	Continue. Call doctor when convenient.
Frequent: Dry mouth.	Continue. Tell doctor at next visit. (Suck ice or chew gum.)
Infrequent:	
• Rash, infection, nausea, vomiting.	Discontinue. Call doctor right away.
• Headache; pain in muscles, bones, joints; hair thinning, tiredness.	Continue. Call doctor when convenient.
Rare: Abdominal pain, bleeding gums, blurred vision, diarrhea, headache, moodiness, vomiting, eye pain, rectal bleeding, yellow skin or eyes.	Discontinue. Call doctor right away.

ISOTRETINOIN

WARNINGS & PRECAUTIONS

Don't take if:
- You are allergic to isotretinoin.
- You are pregnant or plan pregnancy.
- *You are even able to bear children. Read, understand and follow the patient information enclosure with your prescription.*

Before you start, consult your doctor:
- If you have diabetes.
- If you or any member of family have high triglyceride levels in blood.

Over age 60:
Adverse reactions and side effects may be more frequent and severe than in younger persons.

Pregnancy:
Causes birth defects in fetus. Don't use.

Breast-feeding:
Drug filters into milk. May harm child. Avoid.

Infants & children:
Not recommended.

Prolonged use:
Possible damage to cornea.

Skin & sunlight:
May cause rash or intensify sunburn in areas exposed to sun or sunlamp.

Driving, piloting or hazardous work:
No problems expected.

Discontinuing:
Single course of treatment is usually all that's needed. If second course required, wait 8 weeks after completing first course.

Others:
Use only for severe cases of cystic acne that have not responded to less hazardous forms of acne treatment.

POSSIBLE INTERACTION WITH OTHER DRUGS

GENERIC NAME OR DRUG CLASS	COMBINED EFFECT
Etretinate	Increased chance of toxicity of each drug.
Vitamin A	Additive toxic effect of each. Avoid.

POSSIBLE INTERACTION WITH OTHER SUBSTANCES

INTERACTS WITH	COMBINED EFFECT
Alcohol:	Significant increase in triglycerides in blood. Avoid.
Beverages:	No problems expected.
Cocaine:	Increased chance of toxicity of isotretinoin. Avoid.
Foods:	No problems expected.
Marijuana:	Increased chance of toxicity of isotretinoin. Avoid.
Tobacco:	May decrease absorption of medicine. Avoid tobacco while in treatment.

*See Glossary

ISOXSUPRINE

BRAND NAMES

Vasodilan   Vasoprine

BASIC INFORMATION

Habit forming? No
Prescription needed? Yes
Available as generic? Yes
Drug class: Vasodilator

USES

May improve poor blood circulation.

DOSAGE & USAGE INFORMATION

How to take:
Tablet—Swallow with liquid or food to lessen stomach irritation. If you can't swallow whole, crumble tablet and take with liquid or food.

When to take:
At the same times each day.

If you forget a dose:
Take as soon as you remember up to 2 hours late. If more than 2 hours, wait for next scheduled dose (don't double this dose).

What drug does:
Expands blood vessels, increasing flow and permitting distribution of oxygen and nutrients.

Time lapse before drug works:
1 hour.

Don't take with:
See Interaction column and consult doctor.

OVERDOSE

SYMPTOMS:
Headache, dizziness, flush, vomiting, weakness, sweating, fainting, shortness of breath, coma.
WHAT TO DO:
- Dial 0 (operator) or 911 (emergency) for an ambulance or medical help. Then give first aid immediately.
- If patient is unconscious and not breathing, give mouth-to-mouth breathing. If there is no heartbeat, use cardiac massage and mouth-to-mouth breathing (CPR). Don't try to make patient vomit. If you can't get help quickly, take patient to nearest emergency facility.
- See emergency information on inside covers.

POSSIBLE ADVERSE REACTIONS OR SIDE EFFECTS

SYMPTOMS	WHAT TO DO
Life-threatening: None expected.	
Common: ● Appetite loss, nausea, vomiting.	Discontinue. Call doctor right away.
● Dizziness, faintness, flushing.	Continue. Call doctor when convenient.
● Weakness, lethargy.	Continue. Tell doctor at next visit.
Infrequent: Rash.	Discontinue. Call doctor right away.
Rare: Rapid or irregular heartbeat.	Discontinue. Call doctor right away.

WARNINGS & PRECAUTIONS

Don't take if:
- You are allergic to any vasodilator.
- You have any bleeding disease.

Before you start, consult your doctor:
- If you have high blood pressure, hardening of the arteries or heart disease.
- If you plan to become pregnant within medication period.
- If you have glaucoma.

Over age 60:
Adverse reactions and side effects may be more frequent and severe than in younger persons.

Pregnancy:
Studies inconclusive on harm to unborn child. Decide with your doctor whether drug benefits justify risk to unborn child.

Breast-feeding:
No problems expected, but consult doctor.

Infants & children:
Not recommended.

Prolonged use:
No problems expected.

Skin & sunlight:
No problems expected.

Driving, piloting or hazardous work:
Avoid if you feel dizzy or faint. Otherwise, no problems expected.

Discontinuing:
Don't discontinue without doctor's advice until you complete prescribed dose, even though symptoms diminish or disappear.

Others:
Be cautious when arising from lying or sitting position, when climbing stairs, or if dizziness occurs.

POSSIBLE INTERACTION WITH OTHER DRUGS

GENERIC NAME OR DRUG CLASS	COMBINED EFFECT
None expected.	

POSSIBLE INTERACTION WITH OTHER SUBSTANCES

INTERACTS WITH	COMBINED EFFECT
Alcohol:	None expected.
Beverages: Milk.	Decreased stomach irritation.
Cocaine:	Decreased blood circulation to extremities. Avoid.
Foods:	None expected.
Marijuana:	Rapid heartbeat.
Tobacco:	Decreased isoxsuprine effect.

KAOLIN & PECTIN

BRAND NAMES

Donnagel-MB
Donnagel-PG
Kao-Con
Kaopectate
Kapectolin
Kaypectol

K-C
K-P
K-Pek
Parepectolin
Pecto Kay

BASIC INFORMATION

Habit forming? No
Prescription needed? No
Available as generic? No
Drug class: Antidiarrheal

 USES

Reduces intestinal cramps and diarrhea.

 DOSAGE & USAGE INFORMATION

How to take:
Liquid—Swallow prescribed dosage (without diluting) after each loose bowel movement.

When to take:
After each loose bowel movement.

If you forget a dose:
Take when you remember.

What drug does:
Makes loose stools less watery, but may not prevent loss of fluids.

Time lapse before drug works:
15 to 30 minutes.

Don't take with:
See Interaction column and consult doctor.

 OVERDOSE

SYMPTOMS:
Fecal impaction.
WHAT TO DO:
Overdose unlikely to threaten life. If person takes much larger amount than prescribed, call doctor, poison-control center or hospital emergency room for instructions.

 POSSIBLE ADVERSE REACTIONS OR SIDE EFFECTS

SYMPTOMS	WHAT TO DO
Life-threatening: None expected.	
Common: None expected.	
Infrequent: None expected.	
Rare: Constipation (mild).	Continue. Call doctor when convenient.

WARNINGS & PRECAUTIONS

Don't take if:
You are allergic to kaolin or pectin.

Before you start, consult your doctor:
- If patient is child or infant.
- If you have any chronic medical problem with heart disease, peptic ulcer, asthma or others.
- If you have fever over 101F.

Over age 60:
Fluid loss caused by diarrhea, especially if taking other medicines, may lead to serious disability. Consult doctor.

Pregnancy:
No problems expected.

Breast-feeding:
No problems expected.

Infants & children:
Fluid loss caused by diarrhea in infants and children can cause serious dehydration. Consult doctor before giving any medicine for diarrhea.

Prolonged use:
Not recommended.

Skin & sunlight:
No problems expected.

Driving, piloting or hazardous work:
No problems expected.

Discontinuing:
May be unnecessary to finish medicine. Follow doctor's instructions.

Others:
Consult doctor about fluids, diet and rest.

POSSIBLE INTERACTION WITH OTHER DRUGS

GENERIC NAME OR DRUG CLASS	COMBINED EFFECT
Digoxin	Decreases absorption of digoxin. Separate doses by at least 2 hours.
Lincomycin	Decreases absorption of lincomycin. Separate doses by at least 2 hours.
All other oral medicines	May decrease absorption of other medicines. Separate doses by at least 2 hours.

POSSIBLE INTERACTION WITH OTHER SUBSTANCES

INTERACTS WITH	COMBINED EFFECT
Alcohol:	Increased diarrhea. Prevents action of kaolin and pectin.
Beverages:	No problems expected.
Cocaine:	Aggravates underlying disease. Avoid.
Foods:	No problems expected.
Marijuana:	Aggravates underlying disease. Avoid.
Tobacco:	Aggravates underlying disease. Avoid.

*See Glossary

KAOLIN, PECTIN, BELLADONNA & OPIUM

BRAND NAMES

Amogel PG	Kaodonna-PG
Donnagel-PG	Kapectolin PG
Kaodene with	Quiagel PG
Paregoric	

BASIC INFORMATION

Habit forming? Yes
Prescription needed? Yes
Available as generic? No
Drug class: Narcotic, antidiarrheal, antispasmodic

USES

Reduces intestinal cramps and diarrhea.

DOSAGE & USAGE INFORMATION

How to take:
Liquid—Swallow prescribed dosage (without diluting) after each loose bowel movement.

When to take:
As needed for diarrhea, no more often than every 4 hours.

If you forget a dose:
Take when you remember.

What drug does:
- Blocks nerve impulses at parasympathetic nerve endings, preventing muscle contractions and gland secretions of organs involved.

Continued next column

OVERDOSE

SYMPTOMS:
Fecal impaction, rapid pulse, dizziness, fever, hallucinations, confusion, slurred speech, agitation, flushed face, convulsions, deep sleep, slow breathing, slow pulse, warm skin, constricted pupils, coma.
WHAT TO DO:
- **Dial 0 (operator) or 911 (emergency) for an ambulance or medical help. Then give first aid immediately.**
- **If patient is unconscious and not breathing, give mouth-to-mouth breathing. If there is no heartbeat, use cardiac massage and mouth-to-mouth breathing (CPR). Don't try to make patient vomit. If you can't get help quickly, take patient to nearest emergency facility.**
- **See emergency information on inside covers.**

- Makes loose stools less watery, but may not prevent loss of fluids.
- Anesthetizes surface membranes of intestines and blocks nerve impulses.

Time lapse before drug works:
15 to 30 minutes.

Don't take with:
See Interaction column and consult doctor.

POSSIBLE ADVERSE REACTIONS OR SIDE EFFECTS

SYMPTOMS	WHAT TO DO
Life-threatening: Unusually rapid heartbeat (over 100), difficult breathing, slow heartbeat (under 50/minute).	Discontinue. Seek emergency treatment.
Common: (with large dosage) Weakness, increased sweating, red or flushed face, lightheadedness, headache, dry mouth, dry skin, drowsiness, dizziness, frequent urination, decreased sweating, constipation, confusion.	Continue. Call doctor when convenient.
Infrequent: • Taste sense reduced, nervousness, sunlight hurts eyes, blurred vision.	Discontinue. Call doctor right away.
• Diminished sex drive.	Continue. Call doctor when convenient.
Rare: Bloating, abdominal cramps and vomiting, eye pain, hallucinations, shortness of breath, rash, itchy skin.	Discontinue. Call doctor right away.

WARNINGS & PRECAUTIONS

Don't take if:
- You are allergic to any anticholinergic, narcotic, kaolin or pectin.
- You have trouble with stomach bloating, difficulty emptying your bladder completely, narrow-angle glaucoma, severe ulcerative colitis.

KAOLIN, PECTIN, BELLADONNA & OPIUM

Before you start, consult your doctor:
- If you have open-angle glaucoma, angina, chronic bronchitis or asthma, hiatal hernia, liver disease, enlarged prostate, myasthenia gravis, peptic ulcer, impaired liver or kidney function, fever over 101°F, any chronic medical problem with heart disease, peptic ulcer, asthma or others.
- If patient is child or infant.
- If you will have surgery within 2 months, including dental surgery, requiring general or spinal anesthesia.

Over age 60:
- Adverse reactions and side effects may be more frequent and severe than in younger persons.
- More likely to be drowsy, dizzy, unsteady or constipated.
- Fluid loss caused by diarrhea, especially if taking other medicines, may lead to serious disability. Consult doctor.

Pregnancy:
No proven harm to unborn child. Avoid if possible.

Breast-feeding:
Drug passes into milk. Avoid drug or discontinue nursing until you finish medicine. Consult doctor for advice on maintaining milk supply.

Infants & children:
Fluid loss caused by diarrhea in infants and children can cause serious dehydration. Consult doctor before giving any medicine for diarrhea.

Prolonged use:
Causes psychological and physical dependence. Not recommended.

Skin & sunlight:
No problems expected.

Driving, piloting or hazardous work:
Don't drive or pilot aircraft until you learn how medicine affects you. Don't work around dangerous machinery. Don't climb ladders or work in high places. Danger increases if you drink alcohol or take medicine affecting alertness and reflexes, such as antihistamines, tranquilizers, sedatives, pain medicine, narcotics and mind-altering drugs.

Discontinuing:
May be unnecessary to finish medicine. Follow doctor's instructions.

Others:
- Great potential for abuse.
- Consult doctor about fluids, diet and rest.

POSSIBLE INTERACTION WITH OTHER DRUGS

GENERIC NAME OR DRUG CLASS	COMBINED EFFECT
Amantadine	Increased belladonna effect.
Analgesics*	Increased analgesic effect.
Antidepressants*	Increased sedative effect.
Antihistamines*	Increased sedative effect.
Carteolol	Increased narcotic effect. Dangerous sedation.
Cortisone drugs*	Increased internal-eye pressure.
Digoxin	Decreases absorption of digoxin. Separate doses by at least 2 hours.
Haloperidol	Increased internal-eye pressure.
Lincomycin	Decreases absorption of lincomycin. Separate doses by at least 2 hours.
MAO inhibitors*	Increased belladonna effect.
Meperidine	Increased belladonna effect.

Continued page 1088

POSSIBLE INTERACTION WITH OTHER SUBSTANCES

INTERACTS WITH	COMBINED EFFECT
Alcohol:	Increases alcohol's intoxicating effect, increased diarrhea, prevents action of kaolin and pectin. Avoid.
Beverages:	No problems expected.
Cocaine:	Aggravates underlying disease. Avoid.
Foods:	No problems expected.
Marijuana:	Impairs physical and mental performance, aggravates underlying disease. Avoid.
Tobacco:	Aggravates underlying disease. Avoid.

*See Glossary

KAOLIN, PECTIN & PAREGORIC

BRAND NAMES

Donnagel-PG   Parepectolin
Kapectolin with
  Paregoric and
  Parepectolin

BASIC INFORMATION

Habit forming? Yes
Prescription needed? Yes
Available as generic? No
Drug class: Narcotic, antidiarrheal,
  antispasmodic

USES

- Reduces intestinal cramps and diarrhea.
- Relieves pain.

DOSAGE & USAGE INFORMATION

How to take:
Liquid—Swallow prescribed dosage (without diluting) after each loose bowel movement.

When to take:
After each loose bowel movement. No more often then every 4 hours.

If you forget a dose:
Take when you remember.

What drug does:
Makes loose stools less watery, but may not prevent loss of fluids.

Time lapse before drug works:
15 to 30 minutes.

Don't take with:
See Interaction column and consult doctor.

OVERDOSE

SYMPTOMS:
Deep sleep; slow breathing; slow pulse; flushed, warm skin.
WHAT TO DO:
- **Dial 0 (operator) or 911 (emergency) for an ambulance or medical help. Then give first aid immediately.**
- **If patient is unconscious and not breathing, give mouth-to-mouth breathing. If there is no heartbeat, use cardiac massage and mouth-to-mouth breathing (CPR). Don't try to make patient vomit. If you can't get help quickly, take patient to nearest emergency facility.**
- **See emergency information on inside covers.**

POSSIBLE ADVERSE REACTIONS OR SIDE EFFECTS

SYMPTOMS	WHAT TO DO
Life-threatening: Unusually rapid heartbeat (over 100), difficult breathing, slow heartbeat (under 50/minute).	Discontinue. Seek emergency treatment.
Common: (with large dosage) Weakness, increased sweating, red or flushed face, lightheadedness, headache, dry mouth, dry skin, drowsiness, dizziness, frequent urination, decreased sweating, constipation, confusion.	Continue. Call doctor when convenient.
Infrequent: • Taste sense reduced, nervousness, sunlight hurts eyes, blurred vision.	Discontinue. Call doctor right away.
• Diminished sex drive.	Continue. Call doctor when convenient.
Rare: Bloating, abdominal cramps and vomiting, eye pain, hallucinations, shortness of breath, rash, itchy skin.	Discontinue. Call doctor right away.

WARNINGS & PRECAUTIONS

Don't take if:
You are allergic to any narcotic, kaolin or pectin.

Before you start, consult your doctor:
- If you have impaired liver or kidney function, chronic medical problem with heart disease, peptic ulcer, asthma or others, fever over 101F.
- If patient is child or infant.
- If you will have surgery within 2 months, including dental surgery, requiring general or spinal anesthesia.

Over age 60:
Fluid loss caused by diarrhea, especially if taking other medicines, may lead to serious disability. Consult doctor.

Pregnancy:
Abuse by pregnant woman will result in addicted newborn. Withdrawal of newborn can be life-threatening.

Breast-feeding:
Drug filters into milk. May harm child. Avoid.

Infants & children:
Fluid loss caused by diarrhea in infants and children can cause serious dehydration. Consult doctor before giving any medicine for diarrhea.

Prolonged use:
Causes psychological and physical dependence. Not recommended.

Skin & sunlight:
May cause rash or intensify sunburn in areas exposed to sun or sunlamp.

Driving, piloting or hazardous work:
Don't drive or pilot aircraft until you learn how medicine affects you. Don't work around dangerous machinery. Don't climb ladders or work in high places. Danger increases if you drink alcohol or take medicine affecting alertness and reflexes, such as antihistamines, tranquilizers, sedatives, pain medicine, narcotics and mind-altering drugs.

Discontinuing:
May be unnecessary to finish medicine. Follow doctor's instructions.

Others:
Consult doctor about fluids, diet and rest.

POSSIBLE INTERACTION WITH OTHER DRUGS

GENERIC NAME OR DRUG CLASS	COMBINED EFFECT
Analgesics, other*	Increased analgesic effect.
Antidepressants*	Increased sedative effect.
Antihistamines*	Increased sedative effect.
Carteolol	Increased narcotic effect. Dangerous sedation.
Digoxin	Decreases absorption of digoxin. Separate doses by at least 2 hours.
Lincomycin	Decreases absorption of lincomycin. Separate doses by at least 2 hours.
Mind-altering drugs*	Increased sedative effect.
Narcotics, other*	Increased narcotic effect.
Phenothiazines*	Increased phenothiazine effect.
Sedatives*	Increased sedative effect.
Sleep inducers*	Increased sedative effect.
Sotalol	Increased narcotic effect. Dangerous sedation.
Tranquilizers*	Increased sedative effect.
All other oral medicines	Decreases absorption of other medicines. Separate doses by at least 2 hours.

POSSIBLE INTERACTION WITH OTHER SUBSTANCES

INTERACTS WITH	COMBINED EFFECT
Alcohol:	Increases alcohol's intoxicating effect, increased diarrhea, prevents action of kaolin and pectin. Avoid.
Beverages:	No problems expected.
Cocaine:	Increased cocaine toxic effects, aggravates underlying disease. Avoid.
Foods:	No problems expected.
Marijuana:	Aggravates underlying disease. Avoid.
Tobacco:	Aggravates underlying disease. Avoid.

KETOCONAZOLE

BRAND NAMES

Nizoral

BASIC INFORMATION

Habit forming? No
Prescription needed? Yes
Available as generic? No
Drug class: Antifungal

 USES

Treatment of fungus infections susceptible to ketoconazole.

 DOSAGE & USAGE INFORMATION

How to take:
Tablet or oral suspension—Swallow with liquid or food to lessen stomach irritation. If you can't swallow whole, crumble tablet and take with liquid or food.

When to take:
At same time once a day.

If you forget a dose:
Take as soon as you remember up to 2 hours late. If more than 2 hours, wait for next scheduled dose (don't double this dose).

What drug does:
Prevents fungi from growing and reproducing.

Time lapse before drug works:
8 to 10 months or longer.

Don't take with:
See Interaction column and consult doctor.

 OVERDOSE

SYMPTOMS:
Nausea, vomiting, diarrhea.
WHAT TO DO:
Overdose unlikely to threaten life. If person takes much larger amount than prescribed, call doctor, poison-control center or hospital emergency room for instructions.

 POSSIBLE ADVERSE REACTIONS OR SIDE EFFECTS

SYMPTOMS	WHAT TO DO
Life-threatening: None expected.	
Common: Nausea or vomiting.	Discontinue. Call doctor right away.
Infrequent: • Rash or itchy skin, increased sensitivity to light.	Discontinue. Call doctor right away.
• Drowsiness, insomnia, diarrhea.	Continue. Call doctor when convenient.
Rare: • Pale stools, abdominal pain, dark or amber urine.	Discontinue. Call doctor right away.
• Diminished sex drive in males, swollen breasts in males, tiredness, weakness.	Continue. Call doctor when convenient.

 WARNINGS & PRECAUTIONS

Don't take if:
You are allergic to ketoconazole.

Before you start, consult your doctor:
• If you have absence of stomach acid (achlorhydria).
• If you have liver disease.

Over age 60:
Adverse reactions and side effects may be more frequent and severe than in younger persons.

Pregnancy:
Risk to unborn child outweighs drug benefits. Don't use.

Breast-feeding:
Drug passes into milk. Avoid drug or discontinue nursing until you finish medicine. Consult doctor for advice on maintaining milk supply.

Infants & children:
Only under close medical supervision.

Prolonged use:
Request liver-function studies.

Skin & sunlight:
No problems expected.

Driving, piloting or hazardous work:
Don't drive or pilot aircraft until you learn how medicine affects you. Don't work around dangerous machinery. Don't climb ladders or work in high places. Danger increases if you drink alcohol or take medicine affecting alertness and reflexes, such as antihistamines, tranquilizers, sedatives, pain medicine, narcotics and mind-altering drugs.

Discontinuing:
May be unnecessary to finish medicine. Follow doctor's instructions.

Others:
No problems expected.

POSSIBLE INTERACTION WITH OTHER DRUGS

GENERIC NAME OR DRUG CLASS	COMBINED EFFECT
Antacids*	Decreased absorption of ketoconazole.
Anticoagulants*	Increased anticoagulant effect.
Anticholinergics*	Decreased absorption of ketoconazole.
Atropine	Decreased absorption of ketoconazole.
Belladonna	Decreased absorption of ketoconazole.
Cimetidine	Decreased absorption of ketoconazole.
Clidinium	Decreased absorption of ketoconazole.
Cyclosporine	Increased risk of toxicity to kidney.
Famotidine	Reduced absorption of ketoconazole. Take famatodine at least 2 hours after any dose of ketoconazole.
Glycopyrrolate	Decreased absorption of ketoconazole.
Hyoscyamine	Decreased absorption of ketoconazole.
Hypoglycemics, oral*	Increased effect of oral hypoglycemics.
Isoniazid	Decreased effect of ketoconazole.
Methscopolamine	Decreased absorption of ketoconazole.
Methylprednisolone	Increased effect of methylprednisolone.
Nizatidine	Decreased absorption of ketoconazole.
Phenytoin	May alter effect of both drugs.
Propantheline	Decreased absorption of ketoconazole.
Ranitidine	Decreased absorption of ketoconazole.
Rifampin	Decreased effect of ketoconazole.
Scopolamine	Decreased absorption of ketoconazole.

POSSIBLE INTERACTION WITH OTHER SUBSTANCES

INTERACTS WITH	COMBINED EFFECT
Alcohol:	Increased chance of liver damage and disulfiram reaction.*
Beverages:	No problems expected.
Cocaine:	Decreased ketoconazole effect. Avoid.
Foods:	No problems expected.
Marijuana:	Decreased ketoconazole effect. Avoid.
Tobacco:	Decreased ketoconazole effect. Avoid.

KETOPROFEN

BRAND NAMES

Alrheumat	Orudis-E
Orudis	Profenid

BASIC INFORMATION

Habit forming? No
Prescription needed? Yes
Available as generic? No
Drug class: Analgesic, antidysmenorreal (non-steroidal antiinflammatory analgesic [NSAIA])

USES

- Treatment of pain.
- Treatment of soft-tissue athletic injuries.
- Treats dysmenorrhea and juvenile rheumatoid arthritis.

DOSAGE & USAGE INFORMATION

How to take:
- Tablets—Swallow dose whole with liquid or food to lessen stomach irritation.
- Suppositories—Remove wrapper and moisten suppository with water. Gently insert into rectum, large end first. If suppository is too soft, chill in refrigerator or cool water before removing wrapper.

When to take:
At the same times each day.

If you forget a dose:
Take as soon as you remember up to 2 hours late. If more than 2 hours, wait for next scheduled dose (don't double this dose).

What drug does:
Reduces tissue concentration of prostaglandins (hormones which produce inflammation and pain).

Continued next column

OVERDOSE

SYMPTOMS:
Confusion, agitation, incoherence, convulsions, possible hemorrhage from stomach or intestine, coma.
WHAT TO DO:
- Dial 0 (operator) or 911 (emergency) for an ambulance or medical help. Then give first aid immediately.
- See emergency information on inside covers.

Time lapse before drug works:
Begins in 4 to 24 hours. May require 3 weeks regular use for maximum benefit.

Don't take with:
- Large doses of acetaminophen. Combination increases possibility of kidney damage.
- See Interaction column and consult doctor.

POSSIBLE ADVERSE REACTIONS OR SIDE EFFECTS

SYMPTOMS	WHAT TO DO
Life-threatening: Hives, rash, intense itching, faintness soon after a dose (anaphylaxis); breathing difficulty; tightness in chest; rapid heartbeat.	Discontinue. Seek emergency treatment.
Common: Dizziness, headache, nausea, pain, ringing in ears, depression, drowsiness.	Continue. Call doctor when convenient.
Infrequent: • Flank pain.	Discontinue. Call doctor right away.
• Constipation or diarrhea, vomiting.	Continue. Call doctor when convenient.
Rare: • Bloody or black, tarry stools; rash, hives or itch; convulsions; confusion; blurred vision; unusual bleeding or bruising; jaundice; blood in urine; difficult, painful or frequent urination; severe abdominal pain, psychosis.	Discontinue. Call doctor right away.
• Fatigue, weakness. swollen breasts in males, impotence, menstrual irregularities.	Continue. Call doctor when convenient.

WARNINGS & PRECAUTIONS

Don't take if:
- You are allergic to ketoprofen, aspirin or any non-steroid, anti-inflammatory drug.
- You have gastritis, peptic ulcer, enteritis, ileitis, ulcerative colitis, asthma, heart failure, high blood pressure or bleeding problems.
- Patient is younger than 15.

Before you start, consult your doctor:
- If you have epilepsy or Parkinson's disease.
- If you have been mentally ill.
- If you have had kidney disease or impaired kidney function.

Over age 60:
Adverse reactions and side effects may be more frequent and severe than in younger persons.

Pregnancy:
Studies inconclusive on harm to unborn child. Decide with your doctor whether drug benefits justify risk to unborn child.

Breast-feeding:
May harm child. Avoid.

Infants & children:
Not recommended for anyone younger than 15. Use only under medical supervision.

Prolonged use:
- Eye damage.
- Reduced hearing.
- Sore throat, fever.
- Weight gain.

Skin & sunlight:
Increased sensitivity to sunlight.

Driving, piloting or hazardous work:
Don't drive or pilot aircraft until you learn how medicine affects you. Don't work around dangerous machinery. Don't climb ladders or work in high places. Danger increases if you drink alcohol or take medicine affecting alertness and reflexes, such as antihistamines, tranquilizers, sedatives, pain medicine, narcotics and mind-altering drugs.

Discontinuing:
Don't discontinue without consulting doctor. Dose may require gradual reduction if you have taken drug for a long time. Doses of other drugs may also require adjustment.

Others:
No problems expected.

POSSIBLE INTERACTION WITH OTHER DRUGS

GENERIC NAME OR DRUG CLASS	COMBINED EFFECT
ACE inhibitors: captopril, enalapril, lisinopril*	May decrease ACE inhibitor effect.
Anticoagulants, oral*	Increased risk of bleeding.
Non-steroidal, anti-inflammatory analgesics (NSAIAs), other*	Increased possibility of internal bleeding.
Aspirin	Increased risk of stomach ulcer.
Beta-adrenergic blockers*	Decreased antihypertensive effect.
Cortisone drugs*	Increased risk of stomach ulcer and bleeding.
Diuretics*	May decrease diuretic effect.
Lithium	Possible increased lithium effect and toxicity.
Methotrexate	May increase toxicity.
Minoxidil	Decreased minoxidil effect.
Nifedipine	Increases chance of nifedipine toxicity.
Oxyphenbutazone	Possible stomach ulcer.
Phenylbutazone	Possible stomach ulcer.
Probenecid	Increased ketoprofen effect.
Thyroid hormones*	Rapid heartbeat, blood-pressure rise.
Verapamil	Increases chance of verapamil toxicity.

POSSIBLE INTERACTION WITH OTHER SUBSTANCES

INTERACTS WITH	COMBINED EFFECT
Alcohol:	Possible stomach ulcer or bleeding. Avoid.
Beverages:	None expected.
Cocaine:	None expected.
Foods:	None expected.
Marijuana:	Increased pain relief from ketoprofen.
Tobacco:	None expected.

LABETALOL

BRAND NAMES

Normodyne   Trandate

BASIC INFORMATION

Habit forming? No
Prescription needed? Yes
Available as generic? No
Drug class: Antihypertensive (beta- and alpha-adrenergic blocker)

USES

Controls, but doesn't cure, high blood pressure.

DOSAGE & USAGE INFORMATION

How to take:
Tablets—Swallow whole with liquid or food to lessen stomach irritation.

When to take:
With meals or milk at same times each day.

If you forget a dose:
Take as soon as you remember up to 3 hours late. If more than 3 hours, wait for next scheduled dose (don't double this dose).

What drug does:
- Blocks transmission of impulses in sympathetic nervous system.
- Slows nerve impulses through heart.

Time lapse before drug works:
1 to 4 hours.

Don't take with:
See Interaction column and consult doctor.

OVERDOSE

SYMPTOMS:
Fainting, bradycardia, convulsions, coma.
WHAT TO DO:
- Dial 0 (operator) or 911 (emergency) for an ambulance or medical help. Then give first aid immediately.
- See emergency information on inside covers.

POSSIBLE ADVERSE REACTIONS OR SIDE EFFECTS

SYMPTOMS	WHAT TO DO
Life-threatening: Congestive heart failure (weight gain, rapid pulse, breathlessness on exertion, swelling of feet and abdomen).	Discontinue. Seek emergency treatment.
Common: None expected.	
Infrequent: Taste change, skin rash, diminished sex drive, dizziness, drowsiness, headache, itchy skin, skin and scalp numbness and tingling, abdominal pain, stuffy nose, vomiting.	Discontinue. Call doctor right away.
Rare: • Drug-induced systemic lupus erythematosus.	Discontinue. Seek emergency treatment.
• Jaundice, fever, dry eyes, weakness and faintness when arising from bed or chair, bronchospasm.	Discontinue. Call doctor right away.
• Difficult urination, diarrhea.	Continue. Call doctor when convenient.

WARNINGS & PRECAUTIONS

Don't take if:
- You are allergic to any alpha- or beta-blocking agent.
- You have asthma, congestive heart failure, heart block.

Before you start, consult your doctor:
- If you have allergies, coronary artery disease, liver disease, overactive thyroid function, chronic kidney disease.
- If you will have surgery within 2 months, including dental surgery, requiring general or spinal anesthesia.

Over age 60:
Adverse reactions and side effects may be more frequent and severe than in younger persons. Ask doctor about smaller doses.

Pregnancy:
Risk to unborn child outweighs drug benefits. Don't use.

Breast-feeding:
Risk to unborn child outweighs drug benefits. Don't use.

Infants & children:
Use only under close medical supervision.

Prolonged use:
Weakens heart muscle contractions.

Skin & sunlight:
No problems expected.

Driving, piloting or hazardous work:
Don't drive or pilot aircraft until you learn how medicine affects you. Don't work around dangerous machinery. Don't climb ladders or work in high places. Danger increases if you drink alcohol or take medicine affecting alertness and reflexes, such as antihistamines, tranquilizers, sedatives, pain medicine, narcotics and mind-altering drugs.

Discontinuing:
- Don't discontinue without consulting doctor. Dose may require gradual reduction if you have taken drug for a long time. Doses of other drugs may also require adjustment.
- These symptoms may occur if you stop taking labetalol abruptly—Chest pain, headache, sweating, weakness, trembling, fast or irregular heartbeat.

Others:
- You may need to take some form of antihypertensive treatment for the remainder of your life.
- May mask hypoglycemia.
- Get up slowly after sitting or lying to prevent fainting or dizziness.

POSSIBLE INTERACTION WITH OTHER DRUGS

GENERIC NAME OR DRUG CLASS	COMBINED EFFECT
Antidiabetics*	Increased antidiabetic effect, may mask hypoglycemia.
Antidepressants, tricyclic (TCA)*	Tremor.
Antihypertensives*	Increased labetalol effect.
Beta-agonists*	Decreased labetalol effect.
Cimetidine	Increased antihypertensive effect of labetalol.

Clonidine	May cause precipitous change in blood pressure if clonidine and labetalol are discontinued simultaneously.
Diuretics*	Increased antihypertensive effect.
Insulin	Increased antidiabetic effect, may mask hypoglycemia.
Lisinopril	Increased antihypertensive effect. Dosage of each may require adjustment.
Nitroglycerin	Increased antihypertensive effect.
Nicardipine	Blood-pressure drop. Dosages may require adjustment.
Nizatidine	Increased antihypertensive effect.
Phentolamine	Increased antihypertensive effect.

POSSIBLE INTERACTION WITH OTHER SUBSTANCES

INTERACTS WITH	COMBINED EFFECT
Alcohol:	Excessive blood pressure drop. Avoid.
Beverages:	No problems expected.
Cocaine:	Irregular heartbeat, unusual anxiety. Avoid.
Foods:	No problems expected.
Marijuana:	Daily use—Impaired circulation to hands and feet.
Tobacco:	Irregular heartbeat. Avoid.

LACTULOSE

BRAND NAMES

Cephalac   Chronulac

BASIC INFORMATION

Habit forming? No
Prescription needed? No
Available as generic? No
Drug class: Laxative (hyperosmotic)

 ## USES

- Constipation relief.
- Treats brain changes caused by liver disease.

 ## DOSAGE & USAGE INFORMATION

How to take:
Liquid—Dilute dose in beverage before swallowing.

When to take:
Usually once a day, preferably in the morning.

If you forget a dose:
Take as soon as you remember up to 8 hours before bedtime. If later, wait for next scheduled dose (don't double this dose). Don't take at bedtime.

What drug does:
Draws water into bowel from other body tissues. Causes distention through fluid accumulation, which promotes soft stool and accelerates bowel motion.

Time lapse before drug works:
30 minutes to 3 hours.

Don't take with:
Another medicine. Space 2 hours apart.

 ## OVERDOSE

SYMPTOMS:
Fluid depletion, weakness, vomiting, fainting.
WHAT TO DO:
Overdose unlikely to threaten life. If person takes much larger amount than prescribed, call doctor, poison-control center or hospital emergency room for instructions.

 ## POSSIBLE ADVERSE REACTIONS OR SIDE EFFECTS

SYMPTOMS	WHAT TO DO
Life-threatening: None expected.	
Common: Increased thirst, cramps, nausea, diarrhea, gaseousness.	Continue. Tell doctor at next visit.
Infrequent: Irregular heartbeat.	Discontinue. Call doctor right away.
Rare: Dizziness, confusion, fatigue, weakness.	Continue. Call doctor when convenient.

WARNINGS & PRECAUTIONS

Don't take if:
- You are allergic to any hyperosmotic laxative.
- You have symptoms of appendicitis, inflamed bowel or intestinal blockage.
- You have missed a bowel movement for only 1 or 2 days.

Before you start, consult your doctor:
- If you have congestive heart disease.
- If you have diabetes.
- If you have high blood pressure.
- If you have a colostomy or ileostomy.
- If you have kidney disease.
- If you have a laxative habit.
- If you have rectal bleeding.
- If you take another laxative.
- If you require a low-galactose diet.

Over age 60:
Adverse reactions and side effects may be more frequent and severe than in younger persons.

Pregnancy:
No proven problems. Avoid if possible.

Breast-feeding:
No problems expected.

Infants & children:
Use only under medical supervision.

Prolonged use:
Don't take for more than 1 week unless under a doctor's supervision. May cause laxative dependence.

Skin & sunlight:
No problems expected.

Driving, piloting or hazardous work:
No problems expected.

Discontinuing:
May be unnecessary to finish medicine. Follow doctor's instructions.

Others:
Don't take to "flush out" your system or as a "tonic."

POSSIBLE INTERACTION WITH OTHER DRUGS

GENERIC NAME OR DRUG CLASS	COMBINED EFFECT
Laxatives, other*	Diarrhea.
Neomycin	Increased effect of both in brain changes caused by liver disease.

POSSIBLE INTERACTION WITH OTHER SUBSTANCES

INTERACTS WITH	COMBINED EFFECT
Alcohol:	None expected.
Beverages:	None expected.
Cocaine:	None expected.
Foods:	None expected.
Marijuana:	None expected.
Tobacco:	None expected.

*See Glossary

LEUCOVORIN

BRAND NAMES

Citrocovorin Calcium   Folinic Acid
Citrovorum Factor   Wellcoverin

BASIC INFORMATION

Habit forming? No
Prescription needed? Yes
Available as generic? No
Drug class: Antianemic

USES

- Antidote to folic acid antagonists.
- Treats anemia.

DOSAGE & USAGE INFORMATION

How to take:
- Oral solution—Take after meals with liquid to decrease stomach irritation.
- Tablets—Swallow with liquid or food to lessen stomach irritation. If you can't swallow whole, crumble tablet and take with liquid or food.

When to take:
At the same time each day, according to instructions on prescription label.

If you forget a dose:
Take as soon as you remember up to 2 hours late. If more than 2 hours, wait for next scheduled dose (don't double this dose).

What drug does:
Favors development of DNA, RNA and protein synthesis.

Time lapse before drug works:
20 to 30 minutes.

Don't take with:
See Interaction column and consult doctor.

OVERDOSE

SYMPTOMS:
Unlikely to threaten life. If overdose is suspected, follow instructions below.
WHAT TO DO:
- Dial 0 (operator) or 911 (emergency) for an ambulance or medical help. Then give first aid immediately.
- See emergency information on inside covers.

POSSIBLE ADVERSE REACTIONS OR SIDE EFFECTS

SYMPTOMS	WHAT TO DO
Life-threatening: Wheezing.	Seek emergency treatment immediately.
Common: None expected.	
Infrequent: None expected.	
Rare: Skin rash, hives.	Discontinue. Call doctor right away.

WARNINGS & PRECAUTIONS

Don't take if:
- You have pernicious anemia.
- You have vitamin B-12 deficiency.

Before you start, consult your doctor:
- If you have acid urine, acites, dehydration.
- If you have kidney function impairment.

Over age 60:
Adverse reactions and side effects may be more frequent and severe than in younger persons. You may need smaller doses for shorter periods of time.

Pregnancy:
Recommended for treatment of megaloblastic anemia caused by pregnancy.

Breast-feeding:
No problems expected.

Infants & children:
May increase frequency of seizures. Avoid if possible.

Prolonged use:
No problems expected.

Skin & sunlight:
No problems expected.

Driving, piloting or hazardous work:
Don't drive or pilot aircraft until you learn how medicine affects you. Don't work around dangerous machinery. Don't climb ladders or work in high places. Danger increases if you drink alcohol or take medicine affecting alertness and reflexes.

Discontinuing:
Don't discontinue without consulting doctor. Dose may require gradual reduction if you have taken drug for a long time. Doses of other drugs may also require adjustment.

Others:
No problems expected.

POSSIBLE INTERACTION WITH OTHER DRUGS

GENERIC NAME OR DRUG CLASS	COMBINED EFFECT
Anticonvulsants, barbiturate and hydantoin*	Large doses of leucovorin may counteract the effects of these medicines.
Central nervous system (CNS) depressants*	High alcohol content of leucovorin may cause adverse effects.
Primidone	Large doses of leucovorin may counteract the effects of both drugs.

POSSIBLE INTERACTION WITH OTHER SUBSTANCES

INTERACTS WITH	COMBINED EFFECT
Alcohol:	Increased adverse reactions of both drugs.
Beverages:	None expected.
Cocaine:	Increased adverse reactions of both drugs.
Foods:	None expected.
Marijuana:	Increased adverse reactions of both drugs.
Tobacco:	Increased adverse reactions of both drugs.

*See Glossary

LEVOCARNITINE

BRAND NAMES

Carnitor   Vita Carn

BASIC INFORMATION

Habit forming? No
Prescription needed? Yes
Available as generic? No
Drug class: Nutritional supplement

 USES

Treats carnitine deficiency, a genetic impairment preventing normal utilization from diet.

 DOSAGE & USAGE INFORMATION

How to take:
- Oral solution—Take after meals with liquid to decrease stomach irritation.
- Tablets—Swallow with liquid or food to lessen stomach irritation. If you can't swallow whole, crumble tablet and take with liquid or food.

When to take:
Immediately or following meals to reduce stomach irritation.

If you forget a dose:
Take as soon as you remember up to 2 hours late. If more than 2 hours, wait for next scheduled dose (don't double this dose).

What drug does:
Facilitates normal use of fat to produce energy. Dietary source is meat and milk.

Time lapse before drug works:
Immediate action.

Don't take with:
See Interaction column and consult doctor.

 OVERDOSE

SYMPTOMS:
Severe muscle weakness.
WHAT TO DO:
- Dial 0 (operator) or 911 (emergency) for an ambulance or medical help. Then give first aid immediately.
- See emergency information on inside covers.

 POSSIBLE ADVERSE REACTIONS OR SIDE EFFECTS

SYMPTOMS	WHAT TO DO
Life-threatening: None expected.	
Common: Changed body odor.	Continue. Call doctor when convenient.
Infrequent: Diarrhea, abdominal pain, nausea, vomiting.	Discontinue. Call doctor right away.
Rare: None expected.	

WARNINGS & PRECAUTIONS

Don't take if:
No contraindications.

Before you start, consult your doctor:
No documented reasons not to take.

Over age 60:
No problems expected.

Pregnancy:
No proven harm to unborn child, but avoid if possible.

Breast-feeding:
No problems expected.

Infants & children:
No problems expected. Deficiency can cause impaired growth and development.

Prolonged use:
No problems expected.

Skin & sunlight:
No problems expected.

Driving, piloting or hazardous work:
No problems expected.

Discontinuing:
Don't discontinue without consulting doctor. Dose may require gradual reduction if you have taken drug for a long time. Doses of other drugs may also require adjustment.

Others:
Health food store "vitamin B-T" contains dextro- and levo-carnitine which completely negates the effectiveness of levocarnitine (L-carnitine). Only the L-carnitine form is effective in levocarnitine deficiency.

POSSIBLE INTERACTION WITH OTHER DRUGS

GENERIC NAME OR DRUG CLASS	COMBINED EFFECT
Valproic acid	Decreased levocarnitine effect. Patients taking valproic acid may need to take the supplement levocarnitine.

POSSIBLE INTERACTION WITH OTHER SUBSTANCES

INTERACTS WITH	COMBINED EFFECT
Alcohol:	None expected.
Beverages:	None expected.
Cocaine:	None expected.
Foods:	None expected.
Marijuana:	None expected.
Tobacco:	None expected.

LEVODOPA

BRAND NAMES

Bendopa
Dopar
Larodopa

Levopa
Sinemet

BASIC INFORMATION

Habit forming? No
Prescription needed? Yes
Available as generic? Yes
Drug class: Antiparkinsonism

 USES

Controls Parkinson's disease symptoms such as
rigidity, tremor and unsteady gait.

 DOSAGE & USAGE INFORMATION

How to take:
Tablet or capsule—Swallow with liquid or food to
lessen stomach irritation. If you can't swallow
whole, crumble tablet or open capsule and take
with liquid or food.

When to take:
At the same times each day.

If you forget a dose:
Take as soon as you remember up to 2 hours
late. If more than 2 hours, wait for next
scheduled dose (don't double this dose).

What drug does:
Restores chemical balance necessary for normal
nerve impulses.

Continued next column

 OVERDOSE

SYMPTOMS:
**Muscle twitch, spastic eyelid closure,
nausea, vomiting, diarrhea, irregular and
rapid pulse, weakness, fainting, confusion,
agitation, hallucination, coma.**
WHAT TO DO:
- **Dial 0 (operator) or 911 (emergency) for
an ambulance or medical help. Then give
first aid immediately.**
- **If patient is unconscious and not
breathing, give mouth-to-mouth
breathing. If there is no heartbeat, use
cardiac massage and mouth-to-mouth
breathing (CPR). Don't try to make patient
vomit. If you can't get help quickly, take
patient to nearest emergency facility.**
- **See emergency information on inside
covers.**

Time lapse before drug works:
2 to 3 weeks to improve; 6 weeks or longer for
maximum benefit.

Don't take with:
See Interaction column and consult doctor.

 POSSIBLE ADVERSE REACTIONS OR SIDE EFFECTS

SYMPTOMS	WHAT TO DO
Life-threatening:	
None expected.	
Common:	
• Mood change, uncontrollable body movements, diarrhea.	Continue. Call doctor when convenient.
• Dry mouth, body odor.	No action necessary.
Infrequent:	
• Fainting, severe dizziness, headache, insomnia, nightmares, itchy skin, rash, nausea, vomiting, irregular heartbeat.	Discontinue. Call doctor right away.
• Flushed face, muscle twitching, discolored or dark urine, difficult urination, blurred vision.	Continue. Call doctor when convenient.
• Constipation, tiredness.	Continue. Tell doctor at next visit.
Rare:	
• High blood pressure.	Discontinue. Call doctor right away.
• Duodenal ulcer, anemia.	Continue. Call doctor when convenient.

WARNINGS & PRECAUTIONS

Don't take if:
- You are allergic to levodopa or carbidopa.
- You have taken MAO inhibitors in past 2 weeks.
- You have glaucoma (narrow-angle type).

Before you start, consult your doctor:
- If you have diabetes or epilepsy.
- If you have had high blood pressure, heart or lung disease.
- If you have had liver or kidney disease.
- If you have a peptic ulcer.
- If you have malignant melanoma.
- If you will have surgery within 2 months, including dental surgery, requiring general or spinal anesthesia.

Over age 60:
Adverse reactions and side effects may be more frequent and severe than in younger persons.

Pregnancy:
Risk to unborn child outweighs drug benefits. Don't use.

Breast-feeding:
Drug filters into milk. May harm child. Avoid.

Infants & children:
Not recommended.

Prolonged use:
May lead to uncontrolled movements of head, face, mouth, tongue, arms or legs.

Skin & sunlight:
No problems expected.

Driving, piloting or hazardous work:
Don't drive or pilot aircraft until you learn how medicine affects you. Don't work around dangerous machinery. Don't climb ladders or work in high places. Danger increases if you drink alcohol or take medicine affecting alertness and reflexes, such as antihistamines, tranquilizers, sedatives, pain medicine, narcotics and mind-altering drugs.

Discontinuing:
Don't discontinue without doctor's advice until you complete prescribed dose, even though symptoms diminish or disappear.

Others:
Expect to start with small dose and increase gradually to lessen frequency and severity of adverse reactions.

POSSIBLE INTERACTION WITH OTHER DRUGS

GENERIC NAME OR DRUG CLASS	COMBINED EFFECT
Albuterol	Increased risk of heartbeat irregularity.
Antidepressants, tricyclic (TCA) *	Decreased blood pressure. Weakness and faintness when arising from bed or chair.
Antihypertensives *	Decreased blood pressure and levodopa effect.
Antiparkinsonism drugs, other *	Increased levodopa effect.
Guanfacine	Increased effects of both drugs.
Haloperidol	Decreased levodopa effect.
MAO inhibitors *	Dangerous rise in blood pressure.
Methyldopa	Decreased levodopa effect.
Molindone	Decreased levodopa effect.
Papaverine	Decreased levodopa effect.
Phenothiazines *	Decreased levodopa effect.
Phenytoin	Decreased levodopa effect.
Pyridoxine (Vitamin B-6)	Decreased levodopa effect.
Rauwolfia alkaloids *	Decreased levodopa effect.

POSSIBLE INTERACTION WITH OTHER SUBSTANCES

INTERACTS WITH	COMBINED EFFECT
Alcohol:	None expected.
Beverages:	None expected.
Cocaine:	Increased risk of heartbeat irregularity.
Foods:	None expected.
Marijuana:	Increased fatigue, lethargy, fainting.
Tobacco:	None expected.

*See Glossary

LINCOMYCIN

BRAND AND GENERIC NAMES

Lincocin   LINCOMYCIN

BASIC INFORMATION

Habit forming? No
Prescription needed? Yes
Available as generic? No
Drug class: Antibiotic (lincomycin)

USES

Treatment of bacterial infections that are susceptible to lincomycin.

DOSAGE & USAGE INFORMATION

How to take:
Capsule or liquid—Swallow with liquid 1 hour before or 2 hours after eating.

When to take:
At the same times each day.

If you forget a dose:
Take as soon as you remember up to 2 hours late. If more than 2 hours, wait for next scheduled dose (don't double this dose).

What drug does:
Destroys susceptible bacteria. Does not kill viruses.

Time lapse before drug works:
3 to 5 days.

Don't take with:
See Interaction column and consult doctor.

OVERDOSE

SYMPTOMS:
Severe nausea, vomiting, diarrhea.
WHAT TO DO:
Overdose unlikely to threaten life. If person takes much larger amount than prescribed, call doctor, poison-control center or hospital emergency room for instructions.

POSSIBLE ADVERSE REACTIONS OR SIDE EFFECTS

SYMPTOMS	WHAT TO DO
Life-threatening:	
None expected.	
Common:	
None expected.	
Infrequent:	
Unusual thirst; vomiting; stomach cramps; severe and watery diarrhea with blood or mucus; painful, swollen joints; jaundice; fever; tiredness; weakness; weight loss; rash; itch around groin, rectum or armpits; white patches in mouth; vaginal discharge, itching.	Discontinue. Call doctor right away.
Rare:	
None expected.	

WARNINGS & PRECAUTIONS

Don't take if:
- You are allergic to lincomycins.
- You have had ulcerative colitis.
- Prescribed for infant under 1 month old.

Before you start, consult your doctor:
- If you have had yeast infections of mouth, skin or vagina.
- If you will have surgery within 2 months, including dental surgery, requiring general or spinal anesthesia.
- If you have kidney or liver disease.
- If you have allergies of any kind.

Over age 60:
Adverse reactions and side effects may be more frequent and severe than in younger persons.

Pregnancy:
Risk to unborn child outweighs drug benefits. Don't use.

Breast-feeding:
Drug passes into milk. Avoid drug or discontinue nursing until you finish medicine. Consult doctor for advice on maintaining milk supply.

Infants & children:
Don't give to infants younger than 1 month. Use for children only under medical supervision.

Prolonged use:
- Severe colitis with diarrhea and bleeding.
- You may become more susceptible to infections caused by germs not responsive to lincomycin.

Skin & sunlight:
No problems expected.

Driving, piloting or hazardous work:
No problems expected.

Discontinuing:
Don't discontinue without doctor's advice until you complete prescribed dose, even though symptoms diminish or disappear.

Others:
No problems expected.

POSSIBLE INTERACTION WITH OTHER DRUGS

GENERIC NAME OR DRUG CLASS	COMBINED EFFECT
Antidiarrheal preparations*	Decreased lincomycin effect.
Chloramphenicol	Decreased lincomycin effect.
Diphenoxylate	May delay removal of toxins from colon in cases of diarrhea caused by side effects of lincomycin.
Erythromycin	Decreased lincomycin effect.
Loperamide	May delay removal of toxins from colon in cases of diarrhea caused by side effects of lincomycin.

POSSIBLE INTERACTION WITH OTHER SUBSTANCES

INTERACTS WITH	COMBINED EFFECT
Alcohol:	None expected.
Beverages:	None expected.
Cocaine:	None expected.
Foods:	None expected.
Marijuana:	None expected.
Tobacco:	None expected.

*See Glossary

LIOTHYRONINE

BRAND NAMES

Cytomel   Tertroxin
Ro-Thyronine

BASIC INFORMATION

Habit forming? No
Prescription needed? Yes
Available as generic? No
Drug class: Thyroid hormone

 USES

Replacement for thyroid hormone deficiency.

DOSAGE & USAGE INFORMATION

How to take:
Tablet—Swallow with liquid.

When to take:
At the same time each day before a meal or on awakening.

If you forget a dose:
Take as soon as you remember up to 12 hours late. If more than 12 hours, wait for next scheduled dose (don't double this dose).

What drug does:
Increases cell metabolism rate.

Time lapse before drug works:
48 hours.

Don't take with:
See Interaction column and consult doctor.

 OVERDOSE

SYMPTOMS:
"Hot" feeling, heart palpitations, nervousness, sweating, hand tremors, insomnia, rapid and irregular pulse, headache, irritability, diarrhea, weight loss, muscle cramps.
WHAT TO DO:
Overdose unlikely to threaten life. If person takes much larger amount than prescribed, call doctor, poison-control center or hospital emergency room for instructions.

POSSIBLE ADVERSE REACTIONS OR SIDE EFFECTS

SYMPTOMS	WHAT TO DO
Life-threatening: None expected.	
Common: • Tremor, headache, irritability, insomnia.	Discontinue. Call doctor right away.
• Appetite change, diarrhea, leg cramps, menstrual irregularities, fever, heat sensitivity, unusual sweating, weight loss.	Continue. Call doctor when convenient.
Infrequent: Hives, rash, chest pain, rapid and irregular heartbeat, shortness of breath, vomiting.	Discontinue. Call doctor right away.
Rare: None expected.	

WARNINGS & PRECAUTIONS

Don't take if:
- You have had a heart attack within 6 weeks.
- You have no thyroid deficiency, but use this to lose weight.

Before you start, consult your doctor:
- If you have heart disease or high blood pressure.
- If you have diabetes.
- If you have Addison's disease, have had adrenal gland deficiency or use epinephrine, ephedrine or isoproterenol for asthma.

Over age 60:
More sensitive to thyroid hormone. May need smaller doses.

Pregnancy:
Considered safe if for thyroid deficiency only.

Breast-feeding:
Present in milk. Considered safe if dose is correct.

Infants & children:
Use only under medical supervision.

Prolonged use:
No problems expected, if dose is correct.

Skin & sunlight:
No problems expected.

Driving, piloting or hazardous work:
No problems expected.

Discontinuing:
Don't discontinue without consulting doctor. Dose may require gradual reduction if you have taken drug for a long time. Doses of other drugs may also require adjustment.

Others:
Digestive upsets, tremors, cramps, nervousness, insomnia or diarrhea may indicate need for dose adjustment.

POSSIBLE INTERACTION WITH OTHER DRUGS

GENERIC NAME OR DRUG CLASS	COMBINED EFFECT
Amphetamines*	Increased amphetamine effect.
Anticoagulants, oral*	Increased anti-coagulant effect.
Antidepressants, tricyclic (TCA)*	Irregular heartbeat.
Antidiabetics*	Antidiabetic may require adjustment.
Aspirin (large doses, continuous use)	Increased liothyronine effect.
Barbiturates*	Decreased barbiturate effect.
Cholestyramine	Decreased liothyronine effect.
Contraceptives, oral*	Decreased liothyronine effect.
Cortisone drugs*	Requires dose adjustment to prevent cortisone deficiency.
Diclofenac	Rapid heartbeat, blood-pressure rise.
Digitalis preparations*	Increased digitalis effect.
Ephedrine	Increased ephedrine effect.
Epinephrine	Increased epinephrine effect.
Methylphenidate	Increased methylphenidate effect.
Phenytoin	Increased liothyronine effect.

POSSIBLE INTERACTION WITH OTHER SUBSTANCES

INTERACTS WITH	COMBINED EFFECT
Alcohol:	None expected.
Beverages:	None expected.
Cocaine:	Excess stimulation. Avoid.
Foods: Soybeans.	Heavy consumption interferes with thyroid function.
Marijuana:	None expected.
Tobacco:	None expected.

*See Glossary

LIOTRIX

BRAND NAMES

Euthroid   Thyrolar

BASIC INFORMATION

Habit forming? No
Prescription needed? Yes
Available as generic? No
Drug class: Thyroid hormone

 USES

Replacement for thyroid hormone deficiency.

 DOSAGE & USAGE INFORMATION

How to take:
Tablet—Swallow with liquid.

When to take:
At the same time each day before a meal or on awakening.

If you forget a dose:
Take as soon as you remember up to 12 hours late. If more than 12 hours, wait for next scheduled dose (don't double this dose).

What drug does:
Increases cell metabolism rate.

Time lapse before drug works:
48 hours.

Don't take with:
See Interaction column and consult doctor.

 OVERDOSE

SYMPTOMS:
"Hot" feeling, heart palpitations, nervousness, sweating, hand tremors, insomnia, rapid and irregular pulse, headache, irritability, diarrhea, weight loss, muscle cramps, angina, congestive heart failure possible.
WHAT TO DO:
Overdose unlikely to threaten life. If person takes much larger amount than prescribed, call doctor, poison-control center or hospital emergency room for instructions.

 POSSIBLE ADVERSE REACTIONS OR SIDE EFFECTS

SYMPTOMS	WHAT TO DO
Life-threatening: None expected.	
Common:	
• Tremor, headache, irritability, insomnia.	Discontinue. Call doctor right away.
• Appetite change, diarrhea, leg cramps, menstrual irregularities, fever, heat sensitivity, unusual sweating, weight loss.	Continue. Call doctor when convenient.
Infrequent: Hives, itchy skin, vomiting, chest pain, rapid and irregular heartbeat, shortness of breath.	Discontinue. Call doctor right away.
Rare: None expected.	

WARNINGS & PRECAUTIONS

Don't take if:
- You have had a heart attack within 6 weeks.
- You have no thyroid deficiency, but use this to lose weight.

Before you start, consult your doctor:
- If you have heart disease or high blood pressure.
- If you have diabetes.
- If you have Addison's disease, have had adrenal gland deficiency or use epinephrine, ephedrine or isoproterenol for asthma.

Over age 60:
More sensitive to thyroid hormone. May need smaller doses.

Pregnancy:
Considered safe if for thyroid deficiency only.

Breast-feeding:
Present in milk. Considered safe if dose is correct.

Infants & children:
Use only under medical supervision.

Prolonged use:
No problems expected, if dose is correct.

Skin & sunlight:
No problems expected.

Driving, piloting or hazardous work:
No problems expected.

Discontinuing:
Don't discontinue without consulting doctor. Dose may require gradual reduction if you have taken drug for a long time. Doses of other drugs may also require adjustment.

Others:
- Digestive upsets, tremors, cramps, nervousness, insomnia or diarrhea may indicate need for dose adjustment.
- Different brands can result in different results. Don't change brands without consulting doctor.

POSSIBLE INTERACTION WITH OTHER DRUGS

GENERIC NAME OR DRUG CLASS	COMBINED EFFECT
Amphetamines*	Increased amphetamine effect.
Anticoagulants, oral*	Increased anti-coagulant effect.
Antidepressants, tricyclic (TCA)*	Irregular heartbeat.
Antidiabetics*	Antidiabetic may require adjustment.
Aspirin (large doses, continuous use)	Increased liotrix effect.
Barbiturates*	Decreased barbiturate effect.
Beta-adrenergic blockers*	Decreased effect of beta-blockers.
Cholestyramine	Decreased liotrix effect.
Colestipol	Decreased liotrix effect.
Contraceptives, oral*	Decreased liotrix effect.
Cortisone drugs*	Requires dose adjustment to prevent cortisone deficiency.
Digitalis preparations*	Decreased digitalis effect.
Ephedrine	Increased ephedrine effect.
Epinephrine	Increased epinephrine effect.
Estrogens*	Decreased liotrix effect.
Methylphenidate	Increased methyl-phenidate effect.

POSSIBLE INTERACTION WITH OTHER SUBSTANCES

INTERACTS WITH	COMBINED EFFECT
Alcohol:	None expected.
Beverages:	None expected.
Cocaine:	Excess stimulation. Avoid.
Foods: Soybeans.	Heavy consumption interferes with thyroid function.
Marijuana:	None expected.
Tobacco:	None expected.

*See Glossary

LISINOPRIL

BRAND NAMES

Priniril   Zestril

BASIC INFORMATION

Habit forming? No
Prescription needed? Yes
Available as generic? No
Drug class: Angiotensin-Converting Enzyme
(ACE) inhibitor, antihypertensive

USES

Treatment for high blood pressure and
congestive heart failure.

DOSAGE & USAGE INFORMATION

How to take:
Tablet—Swallow with liquid. These are long-
acting tablets. Food does not alter normal
absorption from the gastrointestinal tract.

When to take:
Usually once a day, sometimes twice a day.
Follow doctor's instructions.

If you forget a dose:
Take as soon as you remember up to 8 hours
late. If more than 8 hours, wait for next
scheduled dose (don't double this dose).

What drug does:
- Reduces resistance in arteries.
- Strengthens heartbeat.

Time lapse before drug works:
60 to 90 minutes.

Don't take with:
See Interaction column and consult doctor.

OVERDOSE

SYMPTOMS:
Fever, chills, sore throat, fainting,
convulsions, coma.
WHAT TO DO:
- Dial 0 (operator) or 911 (emergency) for
an ambulance or medical help. Then give
first aid immediately.
- See emergency information on inside
covers.

POSSIBLE ADVERSE REACTIONS OR SIDE EFFECTS

SYMPTOMS	WHAT TO DO
Life-threatening: None expected.	
Common: Rash, loss of taste.	Discontinue. Call doctor right away.
Infrequent: • Swelling of face, hands, mouth or feet.	Discontinue. Seek emergency treatment.

• Dizziness, fainting,
  chest pain, fast or
  irregular heartbeat.
	Discontinue. Call
	doctor right away.

Rare: • Sore throat, cloudy urine, fever, chills.	Discontinue. Call doctor right away.

• Nausea, vomiting,
  indigestion,
  abdominal pain.
	Continue. Call doctor
	when convenient.

WARNINGS & PRECAUTIONS

Don't take if:
- If you are allergic to enalapril, lisinopril or captopril.
- You have any autoimmune disease, including
AIDS or lupus.
- You are receiving blood from a blood bank.
- You take drugs for cancer.
- You will have surgery within 2 months,
including dental surgery, requiring general or
spinal anesthesia.

Before you start, consult your doctor:
- If you have had a stroke.
- If you have angina, heart or blood-vessel
disease, a high level of potassium in blood,
kidney disease, lupus.
- If you are on severe salt-restricted diet.

Over age 60:
Adverse reactions and side effects may be more frequent and severe than in younger persons.

Pregnancy:
Risk to unborn child outweighs drug benefits. Don't use.

Breast-feeding:
Drug passes into milk. Avoid drug or discontinue nursing until you finish medicine. Consult doctor for advice on maintaining milk supply.

Infants & children:
Not recommended.

Prolonged use:
May decrease white cells in blood or cause protein loss in urine. Request periodic laboratory blood counts and urine tests.

Skin & sunlight:
No problems expected.

Driving, piloting or hazardous work:
Avoid if you become dizzy or faint. Otherwise, no problems expected.

Discontinuing:
Don't discontinue without consulting doctor. Dose may require gradual reduction if you have taken drug for a long time. Doses of other drugs may also require adjustment.

Others:
- Stop taking diuretics or increase salt intake 1 week before starting lisinopril.
- Avoid exercising in hot weather.

POSSIBLE INTERACTION WITH OTHER DRUGS

GENERIC NAME OR DRUG CLASS	COMBINED EFFECT
Amiloride	Possible excessive potassium in blood.
Antihypertensives, other*	Increased antihypertensive effect. Dosage of each may require adjustment.
Beta-adrenergic blockers*	Increased antihypertensive effect. Dosage of each may require adjustment.
Carteolol	Increased antihypertensive effects of both drugs. Dosages may require adjustment.
Chloramphenicol	Possible blood disorders.
Diuretics*	Possible severe blood-pressure drop with first dose.
Guanfacine	Increased effect of both drugs.
Nicardipine	Possible excessive potassium in blood. Dosages may require adjustment.
Nitrates*	Possible excessive blood-pressure drop.
Non-steroidal anti-inflammatory drugs (NSAIDs)*	Decreased lisinopril effect.
Potassium supplements*	Possible increased potassium in blood.
Sotalol	Increased antihypertensive effects of both drugs. Dosages may require adjustment.
Spironolactone	Possible excessive potassium in blood.
Triamterene	Possible excessive potassium in blood.

POSSIBLE INTERACTION WITH OTHER SUBSTANCES

INTERACTS WITH	COMBINED EFFECT
Alcohol:	Possible excessive blood-pressure drop.
Beverages: Low-salt milk.	Possible excessive potassium in blood.
Cocaine:	Increased dizziness and chest pain.
Foods: Salt substitutes.	Possible excessive potassium.
Marijuana:	Increased dizziness.
Tobacco:	May decrease lisinopril effect.

LITHIUM

BRAND NAMES

Carbolith	Lithizine
Cibalith-S	Lithobid
Duralith	Lithonate
Eskalith	Lithotabs
Eskalith CR	Pfi-Lithium
Lithane	

BASIC INFORMATION

Habit forming? No
Prescription needed? Yes
Available as generic? Yes
Drug class: Tranquilizer

 ## USES

- Normalizes mood and behavior in manic-depressive illness.
- Treats alcohol toxicity and addiction.
- Treats schizoid personality disorders.

 ## DOSAGE & USAGE INFORMATION

How to take:
- Tablet or capsule—Swallow with liquid or food to lessen stomach irritation. If you can't swallow whole, crumble tablet or open capsule and take with liquid or food. Drink 2 or 3 quarts liquid per day.
- Extended-release tablets—Swallow each dose whole.
- Syrup—Take at mealtime. Follow with 8 oz. water.

When to take:
At the same times each day, preferably mealtime.

If you forget a dose:
Take as soon as you remember up to 2 hours late. If more than 2 hours, wait for next scheduled dose (don't double this dose).

Continued next column

 ## OVERDOSE

SYMPTOMS:
Moderate overdose increases some side effects and may cause diarrhea, nausea. Large overdose may cause vomiting, muscle weakness, convulsions, stupor and coma.
WHAT TO DO:
- Dial 0 (operator) or 911 (emergency) for an ambulance or medical help. Then give first aid immediately.
- See emergency information on inside covers.

What drug does:
May correct chemical imbalance in brain's transmission of nerve impulses that influence mood and behavior.

Time lapse before drug works:
1 to 3 weeks. May require 3 months before depressive phase of illness improves.

Don't take with:
See Interaction column and consult doctor.

 ## POSSIBLE ADVERSE REACTIONS OR SIDE EFFECTS

SYMPTOMS	WHAT TO DO
Life-threatening: None expected.	
Common:	
• Dizziness, diarrhea, nausea, vomiting, shakiness, tremor.	Continue. Call doctor when convenient.
• Dry mouth, thirst, decreased sexual ability, increased urination, anorexia.	Continue. Tell doctor at next visit.
Infrequent:	
• Rash, stomach pain.	Discontinue. Call doctor right away.
• Swollen hands, feet; slurred speech; thyroid impairment (coldness, dry, puffy skin); muscle aches; headache; weight gain; fatigue; menstrual irregularities, acne-like eruptions.	Continue. Call doctor when convenient.
• Drowsiness, confusion, weakness.	Continue. Tell doctor at next visit.
Rare:	
• Blurred vision.	Discontinue. Call doctor right away.
• Jerking of arms and legs, worsening of psoriasis, hair loss.	Continue. Call doctor when convenient.

 ## WARNINGS & PRECAUTIONS

Don't take if:
- You are allergic to lithium or tartrazine dye.
- You have kidney or heart disease.
- Patient is younger than 12.

Before you start, consult your doctor:
- About all medications you take.
- If you plan to become pregnant within medication period.
- If you have diabetes, low thyroid function, epilepsy or any significant medical problem.

- If you are on a low-salt diet or drink more than 4 cups of coffee per day.
- If you plan surgery within 2 months.

Over age 60:
Adverse reactions and side effects may be more frequent and severe than in younger persons.

Pregnancy:
Risk to unborn child outweighs drug benefits. Don't use.

Breast-feeding:
Drug passes into milk. Avoid drug or discontinue nursing until you finish medicine. Consult doctor for advice on maintaining milk supply.

Infants & children:
Don't give to children younger than 12.

Prolonged use:
Enlarged thyroid with possible impaired function.

Skin & sunlight:
No problems expected.

Driving, piloting or hazardous work:
Don't drive or pilot aircraft until you learn how medicine affects you. Don't work around dangerous machinery. Don't climb ladders or work in high places. Danger increases if you drink alcohol or take medicine affecting alertness and reflexes.

Discontinuing:
Don't discontinue without consulting doctor. Dose may require gradual reduction if you have taken drug for a long time. Doses of other drugs may also require adjustment.

Others:
- Regular checkups, periodic blood tests, and tests of lithium levels and thyroid function recommended.
- Avoid exercise in hot weather and other activities that cause heavy sweating. This contributes to lithium poisoning.
- Some products contain tartrazine dye. Avoid, especially if allergic to aspirin.

POSSIBLE INTERACTION WITH OTHER DRUGS

GENERIC NAME OR DRUG CLASS	COMBINED EFFECT
Acetazolamide	Decreased lithium effect.
Antihistamines*	Possible excessive sedation.
Carbamazepine	Increased lithium effect.
Diazepam	Possible hypothermia.
Diclofenac	Possible increase in effect and toxicity.
Diuretics*	Increased lithium effect.
Dronabinol	Increased effects of both drugs. Avoid.
Haloperidol	Increased toxicity of both drugs.
Indomethacin	Increased lithium effect.
Iodide salts	Increased lithium effects on thyroid function.
Ketoprofen	May increase lithium in blood.
Methyldopa	Increased lithium effect.
Molindone	Brain changes.
Muscle relaxants, skeletal*	Increased skeletal-muscle relaxation.
Nicardipine	Possible decreased lithium effect.
Non-steroidal anti-inflammatory drugs (NSAIDs)*	Increased lithium toxicity.
Oxyphenbutazone	Increased lithium effect.
Phenothiazines*	Decreased lithium effect.
Phentyoin	Increased lithium effect.
Phenylbutazone	Increased lithium effect.
Potassium iodide	Increased potassium iodide effect.
Sodium bicarbonate	Decreased lithium effect.
Tetracyclines*	Increased lithium effect.
Theophylline	Decreased lithium effect.
Verapamil	Decreased lithium effect.

POSSIBLE INTERACTION WITH OTHER SUBSTANCES

INTERACTS WITH	COMBINED EFFECT
Alcohol:	Possible lithium poisoning.
Beverages: Caffeine drinks.	Decreased lithium effect.
Cocaine:	Possible psychosis.
Foods: Salt.	High intake could decrease lithium effect. Low intake could increase lithium effect. *Don't* restrict intake.
Marijuana:	Increased tremor and possible psychosis.
Tobacco:	None expected.

LOPERAMIDE

BRAND NAMES

Imodium

BASIC INFORMATION

Habit forming? No, unless taken in high
doses for long periods.
Prescription needed? No
Available as generic? No
Drug class: Antidiarrheal

 ## USES

Relieves diarrhea and reduces volume of
discharge from ileostomies and colostomies.

 ## DOSAGE & USAGE
INFORMATION

How to take:
- Capsule—Swallow with food to lessen
  stomach irritation.
- Liquid—Follow label instructions and use
  marked dropper.

When to take:
No more often than directed on label.

If you forget a dose:
Take as soon as you remember up to 2 hours
late. If more than 2 hours, wait for next
scheduled dose (don't double this dose).

What drug does:
Blocks digestive tract's nerve supply, which
reduces irritability and contractions in intestinal
tract.

Time lapse before drug works:
1 to 2 hours.

Don't take with:
See Interaction column and consult doctor.

 ## OVERDOSE

SYMPTOMS:
Constipation, lethargy, drowsiness or
unconsciousness.
WHAT TO DO:
Overdose unlikely to threaten life. If person
takes much larger amount than prescribed,
call doctor, poison-control center or hospital
emergency room for instructions.

 ## POSSIBLE
ADVERSE REACTIONS
OR SIDE EFFECTS

SYMPTOMS	WHAT TO DO
Life-threatening: None expected.	
Common: None expected.	
Infrequent:	
• Rash.	Discontinue. Call doctor right away.
• Drowsiness, dry mouth, bloating, constipation, appetite loss, stomach pain.	Continue. Call doctor when convenient.
Rare: Unexplained fever.	Discontinue. Call doctor right away.

WARNINGS & PRECAUTIONS

Don't take if:
- You have severe colitis.
- You have colitis resulting from antibiotic treatment or infection.

Before you start, consult your doctor:
- If you are dehydrated from fluid loss caused by diarrhea.
- If you have liver disease.

Over age 60:
Adverse reactions and side effects may be more frequent and severe than in younger persons.

Pregnancy:
No proven harm. Avoid if possible.

Breast-feeding:
No proven problems, but avoid if possible or discontinue nursing until you finish medicine. Consult doctor for advice on maintaining milk supply.

Infants & children:
Don't give to infants or toddlers. Use only under doctor's supervision for children older than 2.

Prolonged use:
Habit forming at high dose.

Skin & sunlight:
No problems expected.

Driving, piloting or hazardous work:
Don't drive or pilot aircraft until you learn how medicine affects you. Don't work around dangerous machinery. Don't climb ladders or work in high places. Danger increases if you drink alcohol or take medicine affecting alertness and reflexes.

Discontinuing:
- May be unnecessary to finish medicine. Follow doctor's instructions.
- After discontinuing, consult doctor if you experience muscle cramps, nausea, vomiting, trembling, stomach cramps or unusual sweating.

Others:
If acute diarrhea lasts longer than 48 hours, discontinue and call doctor. In chronic diarrhea, loperamide is unlikely to be effective if diarrhea doesn't improve in 10 days.

POSSIBLE INTERACTION WITH OTHER DRUGS

GENERIC NAME OR DRUG CLASS	COMBINED EFFECT
Antibiotics* (cephalosporins, clindamycin, lincomycins, penicillins)	May delay removal of toxins from colon in cases of diarrhea caused by side effects of these antibiotics.

POSSIBLE INTERACTION WITH OTHER SUBSTANCES

INTERACTS WITH	COMBINED EFFECT
Alcohol:	Depressed brain function. Avoid.
Beverages:	None expected.
Cocaine:	Decreased loperamide effect.
Foods:	None expected.
Marijuana:	None expected.
Tobacco:	None expected.

---

*See Glossary

LORAZEPAM

BRAND NAMES

Alzapam
Apo-Lorazepam
Ativan

Loraz
Novolorazem

BASIC INFORMATION

Habit forming? Yes
Prescription needed? Yes
Available as generic? Yes
Drug class: Tranquilizer (benzodiazepine)

 ## USES

Treatment for nervousness or tension.

 ## DOSAGE & USAGE INFORMATION

How to take:
Tablet—Swallow with liquid. If you can't swallow whole, crumble tablet and take with liquid or food.

When to take:
At the same time each day, according to instructions on prescription label.

If you forget a dose:
Take as soon as you remember up to 2 hours late. If more than 2 hours, wait for next scheduled dose (don't double this dose).

What drug does:
Affects limbic system of brain—part that controls emotions.

Time lapse before drug works:
2 hours. May take 6 weeks for full benefit.

Don't take with:
See Interaction column and consult doctor.

 ## OVERDOSE

SYMPTOMS:
Drowsiness, weakness, tremor, stupor, coma.
WHAT TO DO:
- **Dial 0 (operator) or 911 (emergency) for an ambulance or medical help. Then give first aid immediately.**
- **If patient is unconscious and not breathing, give mouth-to-mouth breathing. If there is no heartbeat, use cardiac massage and mouth-to-mouth breathing (CPR). Don't try to make patient vomit. If you can't get help quickly, take patient to nearest emergency facility.**
- **See emergency information on inside covers.**

 ## POSSIBLE ADVERSE REACTIONS OR SIDE EFFECTS

SYMPTOMS	WHAT TO DO
Life-threatening: None expected.	
Common: Clumsiness, drowsiness, dizziness.	Continue. Call doctor when convenient.
Infrequent: • Hallucinations, confusion, depression, irritability, itchy skin, rash, change in vision.	Discontinue. Call doctor right away.
• Constipation or diarrhea, nausea, vomiting, difficult urination, vivid dreams.	Continue. Call doctor when convenient.
Rare: • Slow heartbeat, difficult breathing.	Discontinue. Seek emergency treatment.
• Mouth, throat ulcers; jaundice.	Discontinue. Call doctor right away.
• Decreased libido.	Continue. Call doctor when convenient.

WARNINGS & PRECAUTIONS

Don't take if:
- You are allergic to any benzodiazepine.
- You have myasthenia gravis.
- You are active or recovering alcoholic.
- Patient is younger than 6 months.

Before you start, consult your doctor:
- If you have liver, kidney or lung disease.
- If you have diabetes, epilepsy or porphyria.

Over age 60:
Adverse reactions and side effects may be more frequent and severe than in younger persons. You need smaller doses for shorter periods of time. May develop agitation, rage or "hangover" effect.

Pregnancy:
Risk to unborn child outweighs drug benefits. Don't use.

Breast-feeding:
Drug passes into milk. Avoid drug or discontinue nursing until you finish medicine. Consult doctor for advice on maintaining milk supply.

Infants & children:
Use only under medical supervision for children older than 6 months.

Prolonged use:
May impair liver function.

Skin & sunlight:
No problems expected.

Driving, piloting or hazardous work:
Don't drive or pilot aircraft until you learn how medicine affects you. Don't work around dangerous machinery. Don't climb ladders or work in high places. Danger increases if you drink alcohol or take medicine affecting alertness and reflexes.

Discontinuing:
Don't discontinue without consulting doctor. Dose may require gradual reduction if you have taken drug for a long time. Doses of other drugs may also require adjustment.

Others:
- Hot weather, heavy exercise and profuse sweat may reduce excretion and cause overdose.
- Blood sugar may rise in diabetics, requiring insulin adjustment.

POSSIBLE INTERACTION WITH OTHER DRUGS

GENERIC NAME OR DRUG CLASS	COMBINED EFFECT
Antidepressants*	Increased sedative effect of both drugs.
Antihistamines*	Increased sedative effect of both drugs.
Antihypertensives*	Excessively low blood pressure.
Contraceptives, oral*	Increased lorazepam effect.
Disulfiram	Increased lorazepam effect.
Dronabinol	Increased effects of both drugs. Avoid.
Levodopa	Possible decreased levodopa effect.
MAO inhibitors*	Convulsions, deep sedation, rage.
Molindone	Increased tranquilizer effect.
Nabilone	Greater depression of central nervous system.
Narcotics*	Increased sedative effect of both drugs.
Probenecid	Increased lorazepam effect.
Sedatives*	Increased sedative effect of both drugs.
Sleep inducers*	Increased sedative effect of both drugs.
Tranquilizers*	Increased sedative effect of both drugs.

POSSIBLE INTERACTION WITH OTHER SUBSTANCES

INTERACTS WITH	COMBINED EFFECT
Alcohol:	Heavy sedation. Avoid.
Beverages:	None expected.
Cocaine:	Decreased lorazepam effect.
Foods:	None expected.
Marijuana:	Heavy sedation. Avoid.
Tobacco:	Decreased lorazepam effect.

*See Glossary

LOVASTATIN

BRAND NAMES

Mevacor

BASIC INFORMATION

Habit forming? No
Prescription needed? Yes
Available as generic? No
Drug class: Antihyperlipidemic (lowers high blood fats)

USES

Lowers blood cholesterol levels caused by low-density cholesterol (LDL) in persons who haven't improved by exercising, dieting or using other measures.

DOSAGE & USAGE INFORMATION

How to take:
Tablet—Swallow with liquid. If you can't swallow whole, crumble tablet and take with liquid or food.

When to take:
With the evening meal.

If you forget a dose:
Take as soon as you remember up to 2 hours late. If more than 2 hours, wait for next scheduled dose (don't double this dose).

What drug does:
Inhibits an enzyme in the liver.

Time lapse before drug works:
Within 2 weeks.

Don't take with:
- A high-fat diet.
- See Interaction column and consult doctor.

OVERDOSE

SYMPTOMS:
None expected.
WHAT TO DO:
Overdose not expected to threaten life. If person takes much larger amount than prescribed, call doctor, poison-control center or hospital emergency room for instructions.

POSSIBLE ADVERSE REACTIONS OR SIDE EFFECTS

SYMPTOMS	WHAT TO DO
Life-threatening: None expected.	
Common: None expected.	
Infrequent: • Aching muscles, fever, blurred vision.	Discontinue. Call doctor right away.
• Constipation, nausea, tiredness, weakness, dizziness, skin rash.	Continue. Call doctor when convenient.
Rare: Muscle pain.	Discontinue. Call doctor right away.

WARNINGS & PRECAUTIONS

Don't take if:
You are allergic to lovastatin.

Before you start, consult your doctor:
- If you take immunosuppressive drugs, particularly following a heart transplant.
- If you have low blood pressure.
- If you have hormone abnormalities
- If you have an active infection.
- If you have active liver disease.
- If you have a seizure disorder.
- If you have had a recent major accident.

Over age 60:
Likely to be more sensitive to drug.

Pregnancy:
Studies inconclusive on harm to unborn child. Decide with your doctor whether drug benefits justify risk to unborn child.

Breast-feeding:
No problems expected. Consult your doctor.

Infants & children:
Not recommended for children.

Prolonged use:
No special problems expected.

Skin & sunlight:
No problems expected.

Driving, piloting or hazardous work:
No special problems expected.

Discontinuing:
Don't discontinue without consulting doctor. Dose may require gradual reduction if you have taken drug for a long time. Doses of other drugs may also require adjustment.

Others:
Request liver function tests and eye examinations before beginning this medicine and repeat every 2 to 6 months.

POSSIBLE INTERACTION WITH OTHER DRUGS

GENERIC NAME OR DRUG CLASS	COMBINED EFFECT
Cyclosporine or other drugs to suppress the immune system	Increased heart and kidney damage.

POSSIBLE INTERACTION WITH OTHER SUBSTANCES

INTERACTS WITH	COMBINED EFFECT
Alcohol:	None expected.
Beverages:	None expected.
Cocaine:	None expected.
Foods:	None expected.
Marijuana:	None expected.
Tobacco:	None expected.

LOXAPINE

BRAND NAMES

Loxapac
Loxitane

Loxitane C
Loxitane M

BASIC INFORMATION

Habit forming? No
Prescription needed? Yes
Available as generic? No
Drug class: Antianxiety, antidepressant

 ## USES

* Treats serious mental illness.
* Treats anxiety and depression.

 ## DOSAGE & USAGE INFORMATION

How to take:
* Oral solution—Take after meals with liquid to decrease stomach irritation.
* Tablets—Swallow with liquid or food to lessen stomach irritation. If you can't swallow whole, crumble tablet and take with liquid or food.
* Capsules—Swallow with liquid or food to lessen stomach irritation. If you can't swallow whole, open capsule and take with liquid or food.

When to take:
At the same time each day, according to instructions on prescription label.

If you forget a dose:
Take as soon as you remember up to 2 hours late. If more than 2 hours, wait for next scheduled dose (don't double this dose).

What drug does:
Probably blocks the effects of dopamine in the brain.

Time lapse before drug works:
1/2 to 3 hours.

Don't take with:
See Interaction column and consult doctor.

 ## OVERDOSE

SYMPTOMS:
Dizziness, drowsiness, severe shortness of breath, muscle spasms, coma.
WHAT TO DO:
* Dial 0 (operator) or 911 (emergency) for an ambulance or medical help. Then give first aid immediately.
* See emergency information on inside covers.

 ## POSSIBLE ADVERSE REACTIONS OR SIDE EFFECTS

SYMPTOMS	WHAT TO DO
Life-threatening: Severe shortness of breath, skin rash, convulsions (rare).	Seek emergency treatment immediately.
Common: Increased dental problems because of dry mouth and less salivation.	Consult your dentist about a prevention program.
Infrequent: • Chewing movements with lip smacking, loss of balance, shuffling walk, tremor of fingers and hands.	Discontinue. Call doctor right away.
• Constipation, difficult urination, blurred vision, confusion, loss of sex drive, headache, insomnia, menstrual irregularities, weight gain.	Continue. Call doctor when convenient.
Rare: Rapid heartbeat, fever, sore throat, jaundice.	Discontinue. Call doctor right away.

 ## WARNINGS & PRECAUTIONS

Don't take if:
* You are an alcoholic.
* You have liver disease.

Before you start, consult your doctor:
* If you have a seizure disorder.
* If you have an enlarged prostate, glaucoma, Parkinson's disease, heart disease.

Over age 60:
Adverse reactions and side effects may be more frequent and severe than in younger persons. You may need smaller doses for shorter periods of time.

Pregnancy:
Risk to unborn child outweighs drug benefits. Don't use.

Breast-feeding:
Drug passes into milk. Avoid drug or discontinue nursing until you finish medicine. Consult doctor for advice on maintaining milk supply.

Infants & children:
Not recommended.

Prolonged use:
Increased possibility of infections.

Skin & sunlight:
Increased sensitivity to sunlight.

Driving, piloting or hazardous work:
Don't drive or pilot aircraft until you learn how medicine affects you. Don't work around dangerous machinery. Don't climb ladders or work in high places. Danger increases if you drink alcohol or take medicine affecting alertness and reflexes.

Discontinuing:
- Don't discontinue without consulting doctor. Dose may require gradual reduction if you have taken drug for a long time. Doses of other drugs may also require adjustment.
- These symptoms may occur after medicine has been discontinued: dizziness; nausea; abdominal pain; uncontrolled movements of mouth, tongue and jaw.

Others:
Use careful oral hygiene.

 POSSIBLE INTERACTION WITH OTHER DRUGS

GENERIC NAME OR DRUG CLASS	COMBINED EFFECT
Anticonvulsants*	Decreased effect of anticonvulsants.
Antidepressants, tricyclic (TCA)*	May increase toxic effects of both drugs.
Epinephrine	Rapid heart rate and severe drop in blood pressure.
Ethinamate	Dangerous increased effects of ethinamate. Avoid combining.
Fluoxetine	Increased depressant effects of both drugs.
Guanadrel	Decreased effect of guanadrel.
Guanethidine	Decreased effect of guanethidine.
Guanfacine	Increased effect of both drugs.
Haloperidol	May increase toxic effects of both drugs.
Leucovorin	High alcohol content of leucovorin may cause adverse effects.
Methyldopa	May increase toxic effects of both drugs.

Methyprylon	Increased sedative effect, perhaps to dangerous level. Avoid.
Metoclopramide	May increase toxic effects of both drugs.
Metyrosine	May increase toxic effects of both drugs.
Molindone	May increase toxic effects of both drugs.
Nabilone	Greater depression of central nervous system.
Pemoline	May increase toxic effects of both drugs.
Phenothiazines*	May increase toxic effects of both drugs.
Pimozide	May increase toxic effects of both drugs.
Rauwolfia	May increase toxic effects of both drugs.
Thioxanthenes*	May increase toxic effects of both drugs.

 POSSIBLE INTERACTION WITH OTHER SUBSTANCES

INTERACTS WITH	COMBINED EFFECT
Alcohol:	May decrease effect of loxapine. Avoid.
Beverages:	None expected.
Cocaine:	May increase toxicity of both drugs. Avoid.
Foods:	None expected.
Marijuana:	May increase toxicity of both drugs. Avoid.
Tobacco:	May increase toxicity of both drugs. Avoid.

*See Glossary

MAGNESIUM CARBONATE

BRAND NAMES

Alkets
Bisodol
Calcitrel
De Witt's
Di-Gel
Estomul-M
Gaviscon

Liquimint
Magnagel
Marblen
Noralac
Osti-Derm
Silain-Gel
Spastosed

BASIC INFORMATION

Habit forming? No
Prescription needed? No
Available as generic? Yes
Drug class: Antacid, laxative

USES

- Treatment for hyperacidity in upper gastrointestinal tract, including stomach and esophagus. Symptoms may be heartburn or acid indigestion. Diseases include peptic ulcer, gastritis, esophagitis, hiatal hernia.
- Constipation relief.

DOSAGE & USAGE INFORMATION

How to take:
- Tablet—Swallow with liquid.
- Chewable tablets or wafers—Chew well before swallowing.
- Liquid—Shake well and take undiluted.
- Powder—Mix with water and drink all liquid.

When to take:
1 to 3 hours after meals unless directed otherwise by your doctor.

If you forget a dose:
Take as soon as you remember.

What drug does:
- Neutralizes some of the hydrochloric acid in the stomach.
- Reduces action of pepsin, a digestive enzyme.
- Stimulates muscles in lower bowel wall.

Continued next column

OVERDOSE

SYMPTOMS:
Dry mouth, diarrhea, shallow breathing, stupor.
WHAT TO DO:
- **Dial 0 (operator) or 911 (emergency) for an ambulance or medical help. Then give first aid immediately.**
- **See emergency information on inside covers.**

Time lapse before drug works:
15 minutes.

Don't take with:
Other medicines at the same time. Decreases absorption of other drugs.

POSSIBLE ADVERSE REACTIONS OR SIDE EFFECTS

SYMPTOMS	WHAT TO DO
Life-threatening: None expected.	
Common: Constipation, appetite loss.	Continue. Call doctor when convenient.
Infrequent: • Lower abdominal pain and swelling, bone pain, muscle weakness, swollen wrists or ankles.	Discontinue. Call doctor right away.
• Weight loss, mood change, nausea, vomiting.	Continue. Call doctor when convenient.
Rare: Unusual weakness or tiredness.	Discontinue. Call doctor right away.

WARNINGS & PRECAUTIONS

Don't take if:
You are allergic to any antacid.

Before you start, consult your doctor:
- If you have kidney disease.
- If you have chronic constipation, colitis or diarrhea.
- If you have symptoms of appendicitis.
- If you have stomach or intestinal bleeding.

Over age 60:
Adverse reactions and side effects may be more frequent and severe than in younger persons. Diarrhea or constipation particularly likely.

Pregnancy:
Risk to unborn child outweighs drug benefits. Don't use.

Breast-feeding:
Drug passes into milk. Avoid drug or discontinue nursing until you finish medicine. Consult doctor for advice on maintaining milk supply.

Infants & children:
Use only under medical supervision.

Prolonged use:
No problems expected.

Skin & sunlight:
No problems expected.

Driving, piloting or hazardous work:
No problems expected.

Discontinuing:
May be unnecessary to finish medicine. Follow doctor's instructions.

Others:
Don't take longer than 2 weeks unless under medical supervision.

POSSIBLE INTERACTION WITH OTHER DRUGS

GENERIC NAME OR DRUG CLASS	COMBINED EFFECT
Anticoagulants*	Increased anticoagulant effect.
Chlorpromazine	Decreased chlorpromazine effect.
Ciprofloxacin	May cause kidney dysfunction.
Digitalis preparations*	Decreased digitalis effect.
Flecainide	Decreased flecainide effect.
Iron supplements*	Decreased iron effect.
Isoniazid	Decreased isoniazid effect.
Levodopa	Increased levodopa effect.
Meperidine	Increased meperidine effect.
Mexiletine	May slow elimination of mexiletine and cause need to adjust dosage.
Nalidixic acid	Decreased effect of nalidixic acid.
Nitrofurantoin	Decreased nitrofurantoin effect.
Nizatidine	Decreased nizatidine absorption.
Oxyphenbutazone	Decreased oxyphenbutazone effect.
Para-aminosalicylic acid (PAS)	Decreased PAS effect.
Penicillamine	May decrease penicillamine effect.
Penicillins*	Decreased penicillin effect.
Pentobarbital	Decreased pentobarbital effect.
Phenothiazines*	Decreased phenothiazine effect.
Phenylbutazone	Decreased phenylbutazone effect.
Pseudoephedrine	Increased pseudoephedrine effect.
Sodium polystyrene sulfonate	Decreased sodium sulfonate effect.
Sulfa drugs*	Decreased sulfa effect.
Tetracyclines*	Decreased tetracycline effect.
Vitamins A and C	Decreased vitamin effect.

POSSIBLE INTERACTION WITH OTHER SUBSTANCES

INTERACTS WITH	COMBINED EFFECT
Alcohol:	Decreased antacid effect.
Beverages:	No proven problems.
Cocaine:	No proven problems.
Foods:	Decreased antacid effect if taken with food. Wait 1 hour after eating.
Marijuana:	No proven problems.
Tobacco:	Decreased antacid effect.

*See Glossary

MAGNESIUM CITRATE

BRAND NAMES

Citrate of Magnesia
Citro-Mag
Citro-Nesia
Citroma

Evac-Q-Kit
Evac-Q-Kwik
National

BASIC INFORMATION

Habit forming? No
Prescription needed? No
Available as generic? Yes
Drug class: Laxative (hyperosmotic)

USES

Constipation relief.

DOSAGE & USAGE INFORMATION

How to take:
Liquid—Dilute dose in beverage before swallowing.

When to take:
Usually once a day, preferably in the morning.

If you forget a dose:
Take as soon as you remember up to 8 hours before bedtime. If later, wait for next scheduled dose (don't double this dose). Don't take at bedtime.

What drug does:
Draws water into bowel from other body tissues. Causes distention through fluid accumulation, which promotes soft stool and accelerates bowel motion.

Time lapse before drug works:
30 minutes to 3 hours.

Don't take with:
See Interaction column and consult doctor.

OVERDOSE

SYMPTOMS:
Fluid depletion, weakness, vomiting, fainting.
WHAT TO DO:
Overdose unlikely to threaten life. If person takes much larger amount than prescribed, call doctor, poison-control center or hospital emergency room for instructions.

POSSIBLE ADVERSE REACTIONS OR SIDE EFFECTS

SYMPTOMS	WHAT TO DO
Life-threatening: None expected.	
Common: None expected.	
Infrequent: • Irregular heartbeat.	Discontinue. Call doctor right away.
• Increased thirst, cramps, nausea, diarrhea, gaseousness.	Continue. Tell doctor at next visit.
Rare: Dizziness, confusion, tiredness or weakness.	Continue. Call doctor when convenient.

WARNINGS & PRECAUTIONS

Don't take if:
- You are allergic to any hyperosmotic laxative.
- You have symptoms of appendicitis, inflamed bowel or intestinal blockage.
- You have missed a bowel movement for only 1 or 2 days.

Before you start, consult your doctor:
- If you have congestive heart disease.
- If you have diabetes.
- If you have high blood pressure.
- If you have a colostomy or ileostomy.
- If you have kidney disease.
- If you have a laxative habit.
- If you have rectal bleeding.
- If you take another laxative.

Over age 60:
Adverse reactions and side effects may be more frequent and severe than in younger persons.

Pregnancy:
Salt content may cause fluid retention and swelling. Avoid if possible.

Breast-feeding:
No problems expected.

Infants & children:
Use only under medical supervision.

Prolonged use:
Don't take for more than 1 week unless under a doctor's supervision. May cause laxative dependence.

Skin & sunlight:
No problems expected.

Driving, piloting or hazardous work:
No problems expected.

Discontinuing:
May be unnecessary to finish medicine. Follow doctor's instructions.

Others:
- Don't take to "flush out" your system or as a "tonic."
- Don't take within 2 hours of taking another medicine.

POSSIBLE INTERACTION WITH OTHER DRUGS

GENERIC NAME OR DRUG CLASS	COMBINED EFFECT
Antidepressants, tricyclic (TCA)*	Decreased TCA effect.
Chlordiazepoxide	Decreased chlordiazepoxide effect.
Chlorpromazine	Decreased chlorpromazine effect.
Dicumarol	Decreased dicumarol effect.
Digoxin	Decreased digoxin effect.
Isoniazid	Decreased isoniazid effect.
Mexiletine	May slow elimination of mexiletine and cause need to adjust dosage.
Tetracyclines*	Possible intestinal blockage.

POSSIBLE INTERACTION WITH OTHER SUBSTANCES

INTERACTS WITH	COMBINED EFFECT
Alcohol:	None expected.
Beverages:	None expected.
Cocaine:	None expected.
Foods:	None expected.
Marijuana:	None expected.
Tobacco:	None expected.

MAGNESIUM HYDROXIDE

BRAND NAMES

See complete list of brand names in the *Brand Name Directory*, page 1065.

BASIC INFORMATION

Habit forming? No
Prescription needed? No
Available as generic? Yes
Drug class: Antacid, laxative

 ## USES

- Treatment for hyperacidity in upper gastrointestinal tract, including stomach and esophagus. Symptoms may be heartburn or acid indigestion. Diseases include peptic ulcer, gastritis, esophagitis, hiatal hernia.
- Constipation relief.

 ## DOSAGE & USAGE INFORMATION

How to take:
- Tablet—Swallow with liquid.
- Liquid—Shake well and take undiluted.

When to take:
1 to 3 hours after meals unless directed otherwise by your doctor.

If you forget a dose:
Take as soon as you remember.

What drug does:
- Neutralizes some of the hydrochloric acid in the stomach.
- Reduces action of pepsin, a digestive enzyme.
- Stimulates muscles in lower bowel wall.

Time lapse before drug works:
15 minutes.

Don't take with:
Other medicines at the same time. Decreases absorption of other drugs.

 ## OVERDOSE

SYMPTOMS:
Dry mouth, shallow breathing, diarrhea, stupor.
WHAT TO DO:
- **Dial 0 (operator) or 911 (emergency) for an ambulance or medical help. Then give first aid immediately.**
- **See emergency information on inside covers.**

 ## POSSIBLE ADVERSE REACTIONS OR SIDE EFFECTS

SYMPTOMS	WHAT TO DO
Life-threatening:	
None expected.	
Common:	
Constipation, appetite loss.	Continue. Call doctor when convenient.
Infrequent:	
• Lower abdominal pain and swelling, bone pain, muscle weakness, swollen wrists or ankles.	Discontinue. Call doctor right away.
• Mood change, nausea, vomiting, weight loss.	Continue. Call doctor when convenient.
Rare:	
None expected.	

 ## WARNINGS & PRECAUTIONS

Don't take if:
You are allergic to any antacid.

Before you start, consult your doctor:
- If you have kidney disease.
- If you have chronic constipation, colitis or diarrhea.
- If you have symptoms of appendicitis.
- If you have stomach or intestinal bleeding.

Over age 60:
Adverse reactions and side effects may be more frequent and severe than in younger persons. Diarrhea or constipation particularly likely.

Pregnancy:
Risk to unborn child outweighs drug benefits. Don't use.

Breast-feeding:
Drug passes into milk. Avoid drug or discontinue nursing until you finish medicine. Consult doctor for advice on maintaining milk supply.

Infants & children:
Use only under medical supervision.

Prolonged use:
No problems expected.

Skin & sunlight:
No problems expected.

Driving, piloting or hazardous work:
No problems expected.

Discontinuing:
May be unnecessary to finish medicine. Follow doctor's instructions.

Others:
Don't take longer than 2 weeks unless under medical supervision.

POSSIBLE INTERACTION WITH OTHER DRUGS

GENERIC NAME OR DRUG CLASS	COMBINED EFFECT
Chlorpromazine	Decreased chlorpromazine effect.
Ciprofloxacin	May cause kidney dysfunction.
Digitalis preparations*	Decreased digitalis effect.
Flecainide	Increased flecainide effect.
Iron supplements*	Decreased iron effect.
Isoniazid	Decreased isoniazid effect.
Ketoconazole	Decreased ketoconazole effect.
Levodopa	Possible increased levodopa effect.
Lithium	Decreased lithium effect.
Meperidine	Increased meperidine effect.
Methenamine	Decreased methenamine effect.
Mexiletine	May slow elimination of mexiletine and cause need to adjust dosage.
Nalidixic acid	Decreased effect of nalidixic acid.
Nitrofurantoin	Possible decreased nitrofurantoin effect.
Nizatidine	Decreased nizatidine absorption.
Norfloxacin	Decreased effect of norfloxacin.
Oxyphenbutazone	Decreased oxyphenbutazone effect.
Para-aminosalicylic acid (PAS)	Decreased PAS effect.
Penicillamine	Decreased penicillamine effect.
Penicillins*	Decreased penicillin effect.
Pentobarbital	Decreased pentobarbital effect.
Phenylbutazone	Decreased phenylbutazone effect.
Pseudoephedrine	Increased pseudoephedrine effect.
Sodium polystyrene sulfonate	Decreased sodium sulfonate effect.
Sulfa drugs*	Decreased sulfa effect.
Tetracyclines*	Decreased tetracycline effect.
Vitamins A and C	Decreased vitamin effect.

POSSIBLE INTERACTION WITH OTHER SUBSTANCES

INTERACTS WITH	COMBINED EFFECT
Alcohol:	Decreased antacid effect.
Beverages:	No proven problems.
Cocaine:	No proven problems.
Foods:	Decreased antacid effect if taken with food. Wait 1 hour after eating.
Marijuana:	No proven problems.
Tobacco:	Decreased antacid effect.

MAGNESIUM SULFATE

BRAND NAMES

Bilagog
Eldercaps
Eldertonic

Epsom Salts
Glutofac
Vicon

BASIC INFORMATION

Habit forming? No
Prescription needed? No
Available as generic? Yes
Drug class: Laxative (hyperosmotic)

USES

Constipation relief.

DOSAGE & USAGE INFORMATION

How to take:
- Tablet—Swallow with liquid.
- Powder or solid form—Dilute dose in beverage before swallowing. Solid form must be dissolved.

When to take:
Usually once a day, preferably in the morning.

If you forget a dose:
Take as soon as you remember up to 8 hours before bedtime. If later, wait for next scheduled dose (don't double this dose). Don't take at bedtime.

What drug does:
Draws water into bowel from other body tissues. Causes distention through fluid accumulation, which promotes soft stool and accelerates bowel motion.

Time lapse before drug works:
30 minutes to 3 hours.

Don't take with:
See Interaction column and consult doctor.

OVERDOSE

SYMPTOMS:
Fluid depletion, weakness, vomiting, fainting.
WHAT TO DO:
Overdose unlikely to threaten life. If person takes much larger amount than prescribed, call doctor, poison-control center or hospital emergency room for instructions.

POSSIBLE ADVERSE REACTIONS OR SIDE EFFECTS

SYMPTOMS	WHAT TO DO
Life-threatening: None expected.	
Common: None expected.	
Infrequent:	
• Irregular heartbeat.	Discontinue. Call doctor right away.
• Increased thirst, cramps, nausea, diarrhea, gaseousness.	Continue. Tell doctor at next visit.
Rare: Dizziness, confusion, tiredness or weakness.	Continue. Call doctor when convenient.

WARNINGS & PRECAUTIONS

Don't take if:
- You are allergic to any hyperosmotic laxative.
- You have symptoms of appendicitis, inflamed bowel or intestinal blockage.
- You have missed a bowel movement for only 1 or 2 days.

Before you start, consult your doctor:
- If you have congestive heart disease.
- If you have diabetes.
- If you have high blood pressure.
- If you have a colostomy or ileostomy.
- If you have kidney disease.
- If you have a laxative habit.
- If you have rectal bleeding.
- If you take another laxative.

Over age 60:
Adverse reactions and side effects may be more frequent and severe than in younger persons.

Pregnancy:
Salt content may cause fluid retention and swelling. Avoid if possible.

Breast-feeding:
No problems expected.

Infants & children:
Use only under medical supervision.

Prolonged use:
Don't take for more than 1 week unless under a doctor's supervision. May cause laxative dependence.

Skin & sunlight:
No problems expected.

Driving, piloting or hazardous work:
No problems expected.

Discontinuing:
May be unnecessary to finish medicine. Follow doctor's instructions.

Others:
- Don't take to "flush out" your system or as a "tonic."
- Don't take within 2 hours of taking another medicine.

POSSIBLE INTERACTION WITH OTHER DRUGS

GENERIC NAME OR DRUG CLASS	COMBINED EFFECT
Antidepressants, tricyclic (TCA)*	Decreased antidepressant effect.
Chlordiazepoxide	Decreased chlordiazepoxide effect.
Chlorpromazine	Decreased chlorpromazine effect.
Dicumarol	Decreased dicumarol effect.
Digoxin	Decreased digoxin effect.
Isoniazid	Decreased isoniazid effect.
Mexiletine	May slow elimination of mexiletine and cause need to adjust dosage.
Tetracyclines*	Possible intestinal blockage.

POSSIBLE INTERACTION WITH OTHER SUBSTANCES

INTERACTS WITH	COMBINED EFFECT
Alcohol:	None expected.
Beverages:	None expected.
Cocaine:	None expected.
Foods:	None expected.
Marijuana:	None expected.
Tobacco:	None expected.

MAGNESIUM TRISILICATE

BRAND NAMES

A-M-T
Alma-Mag
Gaviscon
Gelusil
Gelusil-M

Magnatril
Mucotin
Neutrocomp
Sterazolidin
Trisogel

BASIC INFORMATION

Habit forming? No
Prescription needed? No
Available as generic? Yes
Drug class: Antacid, laxative

 ## USES

- Treatment for hyperacidity in upper gastrointestinal tract, including stomach and esophagus. Symptoms may be heartburn or acid indigestion. Diseases include peptic ulcer, gastritis, esophagitis, hiatal hernia.
- Constipation relief.

 ## DOSAGE & USAGE INFORMATION

How to take:
- Tablet or capsule—Swallow with liquid.
- Chewable tablets or wafers—Chew well before swallowing.
- Liquid—Shake well and take undiluted.

When to take:
1 to 3 hours after meals unless directed otherwise by your doctor.

If you forget a dose:
Take as soon as you remember.

What drug does:
- Neutralizes some of the hydrochloric acid in the stomach.
- Reduces action of pepsin, a digestive enzyme.
- Stimulates muscles in lower bowel wall.

Continued next column

 ## OVERDOSE

SYMPTOMS:
Dry mouth, diarrhea, shallow breathing, stupor.
WHAT TO DO:
- Dial 0 (operator) or 911 (emergency) for an ambulance or medical help. Then give first aid immediately.
- See emergency information on inside covers.

Time lapse before drug works:
15 minutes.

Don't take with:
Other medicines at the same time. Decreases absorption of other drugs.

 ## POSSIBLE ADVERSE REACTIONS OR SIDE EFFECTS

SYMPTOMS	WHAT TO DO
Life-threatening: None expected.	
Common: Constipation, appetite loss.	Continue. Call doctor when convenient.
Infrequent: • Lower abdominal pain and swelling, bone pain, muscle weakness, swollen wrists or ankles.	Discontinue. Call doctor right away.
• Mood change, nausea, vomiting, weight loss.	Continue. Call doctor when convenient.
Rare: None expected.	

 ## WARNINGS & PRECAUTIONS

Don't take if:
You are allergic to any antacid.

Before you start, consult your doctor:
- If you have kidney disease.
- If you have chronic constipation, colitis or diarrhea.
- If you have symptoms of appendicitis.
- If you have stomach or intestinal bleeding.

Over age 60:
Adverse reactions and side effects may be more frequent and severe than in younger persons. Diarrhea or constipation particularly likely.

Pregnancy:
Risk to unborn child outweighs drug benefits. Don't use.

Breast-feeding:
Drug passes into milk. Avoid drug or discontinue nursing until you finish medicine. Consult doctor for advice on maintaining milk supply.

Infants & children:
Use only under medical supervision.

Prolonged use:
No problems expected.

MAGNESIUM TRISILICATE

Skin & sunlight:
No problems expected.

Driving, piloting or hazardous work:
No problems expected.

Discontinuing:
May be unnecessary to finish medicine. Follow doctor's instructions.

Others:
Don't take longer than 2 weeks unless under medical supervision.

 ## POSSIBLE INTERACTION WITH OTHER DRUGS

GENERIC NAME OR DRUG CLASS	COMBINED EFFECT
Chlorpromazine	Decreased chlorpromazine effect.
Ciprofloxacin	May cause kidney dysfunction.
Digitalis preparations*	Decreased digitalis effect.
Flecainide	Increased flecainide effect.
Iron supplements*	Decreased iron effect.
Isoniazid	Decreased isoniazid effect.
Ketoconazole	Decreased ketoconazole effect.
Levodopa	Increased levodopa effect.
Lithium	Decreased lithium effect.
Meperidine	Increased meperidine effect.
Methenamine	Decreased methenamine effect.
Mexiletine	May slow elimination of mexiletine and cause need to adjust dosage.
Nalidixic acid	Decreased effect of nalidixic acid.
Nitrofurantoin	Possible decreased nitrofurantoin effect.
Nizatidine	Decreased nizatidine absorption.
Norfloxacin	Decreased effect of norfloxacin.
Oxyphenbutazone	Decreased oxyphenbutazone effect.
Para-aminosalicylic acid (PAS)	Decreased PAS effect.
Penicillamine	Decreased penicillamine effect.
Penicillins*	Decreased penicillin effect.
Pentobarbital	Decreased pentobarbital effect.
Phenylbutazone	Decreased phenylbutazone effect.
Pseudoephedrine	Increased pseudoephedrine effect.
Sodium polystyrene sulfonate	Decreased effect of sodium polystyrene sulfonate.
Sulfa drugs*	Decreased sulfa effect.
Tetracyclines*	Decreased tetracycline effect.
Vitamins A and C	Decreased vitamin effect.

 ## POSSIBLE INTERACTION WITH OTHER SUBSTANCES

INTERACTS WITH	COMBINED EFFECT
Alcohol:	Decreased antacid effect.
Beverages:	No proven problems.
Cocaine:	No proven problems.
Foods:	Decreased antacid effect if taken with food. Wait 1 hour after eating.
Marijuana:	No proven problems.
Tobacco:	Decreased antacid effect.

MALT SOUP EXTRACT

BRAND NAMES

Maltsupex

BASIC INFORMATION

Habit forming? No
Prescription needed? No
Available as generic? No
Drug class: Laxative (bulk-forming)

 USES

Relieves constipation and prevents straining for bowel movement.

 DOSAGE & USAGE INFORMATION

How to take:
- Liquid or powder—Dilute dose in 8 oz. cold water or fruit juice.
- Tablets—Swallow with 8 oz. cold liquid. Drink 6 to 8 glasses of water each day in addition to the one with each dose.

When to take:
At the same time each day, preferably morning.

If you forget a dose:
Take as soon as you remember. Resume regular schedule.

What drug does:
Absorbs water, stimulating the bowel to form a soft, bulky stool.

Time lapse before drug works:
May require 2 or 3 days to begin, then works in 12 to 24 hours.

Don't take with:
- Don't take within 2 hours of taking another medicine.
- See Interaction column and consult doctor.

 OVERDOSE

SYMPTOMS:
None expected.
WHAT TO DO:
Overdose unlikely to threaten life. If person takes much larger amount than prescribed, call doctor, poison-control center or hospital emergency room for instructions.

 POSSIBLE ADVERSE REACTIONS OR SIDE EFFECTS

SYMPTOMS	WHAT TO DO
Life-threatening: None expected.	
Common: None expected.	
Infrequent: Swallowing difficulty, "lump in throat" sensation, nausea, vomiting, diarrhea.	Continue. Call doctor when convenient.
Rare: Itchy skin, rash, asthma, intestinal blockage.	Discontinue. Call doctor right away.

MALT SOUP EXTRACT

WARNINGS & PRECAUTIONS

Don't take if:
- You are allergic to any bulk-forming laxative.
- You have symptoms of appendicitis, inflamed bowel or intestinal blockage.
- You have missed a bowel movement for only 1 or 2 days.

Before you start, consult your doctor:
- If you have diabetes.
- If you have a laxative habit.
- If you have rectal bleeding.
- If you have difficulty swallowing.
- If you take other laxatives.

Over age 60:
Adverse reactions and side effects may be more frequent and severe than in younger persons.

Pregnancy:
Most bulk-forming laxatives contain sodium or sugars which may cause fluid retention. Avoid if possible.

Breast-feeding:
No problems expected.

Infants & children:
Use only under medical supervision.

Prolonged use:
Don't take for more than 1 week unless under a doctor's supervision. May cause laxative dependence.

Skin & sunlight:
No problems expected.

Driving, piloting or hazardous work:
No problems expected.

Discontinuing:
May be unnecessary to finish medicine. Follow doctor's instructions.

Others:
Don't take to "flush out" your system or as a "tonic."

POSSIBLE INTERACTION WITH OTHER DRUGS

GENERIC NAME OR DRUG CLASS	COMBINED EFFECT
Antibiotics*	Possible decreased antibiotic effect.
Digitalis preparations*	Decreased digitalis effect.
Salicylates* (including aspirin)	Decreased salicylate effect.

POSSIBLE INTERACTION WITH OTHER SUBSTANCES

INTERACTS WITH	COMBINED EFFECT
Alcohol:	None expected.
Beverages:	None expected.
Cocaine:	None expected.
Foods:	None expected.
Marijuana:	None expected.
Tobacco:	None expected.

MAPROTILINE

BRAND NAMES

Ludiomil

BASIC INFORMATION

Habit forming? No
Prescription needed? Yes
Available as generic? No
Drug class: Antidepressant

 ## USES

Treatment for depression or anxiety associated with depression.

 ## DOSAGE & USAGE INFORMATION

How to take:
Tablet—Swallow with liquid.

When to take:
At the same time each day, usually bedtime.

If you forget a dose:
Bedtime dose—If you forget your once-a-day bedtime dose, don't take it more than 3 hours late. If more than 3 hours, wait for next scheduled dose. Don't double this dose.

What drug does:
Probably affects part of brain that controls messages between nerve cells.

Time lapse before drug works:
Begins in 1 to 2 weeks. May require 4 to 6 weeks for maximum benefit.

Don't take with:
- Non-prescription drugs without consulting doctor.
- See Interaction column and consult doctor.

 ## OVERDOSE

SYMPTOMS:
Respiratory failure, fever, cardiac arrhythmia, hallucinations, convulsions, coma.
WHAT TO DO:
- Dial 0 (operator) or 911 (emergency) for an ambulance or medical help. Then give first aid immediately.
- If patient is unconscious and not breathing, give mouth-to-mouth breathing. If there is no heartbeat, use cardiac massage and mouth-to-mouth breathing (CPR). Don't try to make patient vomit. If you can't get help quickly, take patient to nearest emergency facility.
- See emergency information on inside covers.

 ## POSSIBLE ADVERSE REACTIONS OR SIDE EFFECTS

SYMPTOMS	WHAT TO DO
Life-threatening: Seizures.	Seek emergency treatment immediately.
Common: • Tremor.	Discontinue. Call doctor right away.
• Headache, dry mouth or unpleasant taste, constipation or diarrhea, nausea, indigestion, fatigue, weakness, drowsiness, nervousness, anxiety, excessive sweating.	Continue. Call doctor when convenient.
• Insomnia, craving sweets.	Continue. Tell doctor at next visit.
Infrequent: • Convulsions.	Discontinue. Seek emergency treatment.
• Hallucinations, shakiness, dizziness, fainting, blurred vision, eye pain, vomiting, irregular heartbeat or slow pulse, inflamed tongue, abdominal pain, jaundice, hair loss, rash, fever, chills, joint pain, palpitations, hiccups, vision changes.	Discontinue. Call doctor right away.
• Painful or difficult urination; fatigue; decreased libido; abnormal dreams; nasal congestion; back pain; muscle aches; frequent urination; painful, absent or irregular menstruation.	Continue. Call doctor when convenient.
Rare: Itchy skin; rash; sore throat; jaundice; fever; involuntary movements of jaw, lips and tongue; nightmares; confusion; swollen breasts in men.	Discontinue. Call doctor right away.

WARNINGS & PRECAUTIONS

Don't take if:
- You are allergic to any tricyclic antidepressant.
- You drink alcohol.
- You have had a heart attack within 6 weeks.
- You have glaucoma.
- You have taken MAO inhibitors within 2 weeks.
- Patient is younger than 12.

Before you start, consult your doctor:
- If you will have surgery within 2 months, including dental surgery, requiring general or spinal anesthesia.
- If you have an enlarged prostate, heart disease or high blood pressure, stomach or intestinal problems, overactive thyroid, asthma, liver disease.

Over age 60:
More likely to develop urination difficulty and side effects such as hallucinations, shakiness, dizziness, fainting, headache or insomnia.

Pregnancy:
Studies inconclusive on harm to unborn child. Animal studies show fetal abnormalities. Decide with your doctor whether drug benefits justify risk to unborn child.

Breast-feeding:
Drug passes into milk. Avoid drug or discontinue nursing until you finish medicine. Consult doctor for advice on maintaining milk supply.

Infants & children:
Don't give to children younger than 12.

Prolonged use:
Request blood cell counts, liver-function studies, monitor blood pressure closely.

Skin & sunlight:
May cause rash or intensify sunburn in areas exposed to sun or sunlamp.

Driving, piloting or hazardous work:
Don't drive or pilot aircraft until you learn how medicine affects you. Don't work around dangerous machinery. Don't climb ladders or work in high places. Danger increases if you drink alcohol or take medicine affecting alertness and reflexes.

Discontinuing:
Don't discontinue without consulting doctor. Dose may require gradual reduction if you have taken drug for a long time. Doses of other drugs may also require adjustment.

Others:
No problems expected.

POSSIBLE INTERACTION WITH OTHER DRUGS

GENERIC NAME OR DRUG CLASS	COMBINED EFFECT
Anticoagulants*	Increased anticoagulant effect.
Anticholinergics*	Increased sedation.
Antihistamines*	Increased antihistamine effect.
Barbiturates*	Decreased anti-depressant effect.
Benzodiazepine	Increased sedation.
Cimetidine	Possible increased antidepressant effect and toxicity.
Clonidine	Decreased clonidine effect.
Disulfiram	Delirium.
Diuretics, thiazide*	Increased maprotiline effect.
Ethchlorvynol	Delirium.
Ethinamate	Dangerous increased effects of ethinamate. Avoid combining.
Fluoxetine	Increased depressant effects of both drugs.
Guanabenz	Possible decreased clonidine effect.
Guanethidine	Decreased guanethidine effect.

Continued page 1089

POSSIBLE INTERACTION WITH OTHER SUBSTANCES

INTERACTS WITH	COMBINED EFFECT
Alcohol: Beverages or medicines with alcohol.	Excessive intoxication. Avoid.
Beverages:	None expected.
Cocaine:	Excessive intoxication. Avoid.
Foods:	None expected.
Marijuana:	Excessive drowsiness. Avoid.
Tobacco:	May decrease absorption of maprotiline. Avoid.

*See Glossary

MEBENDAZOLE

BRAND NAMES

Mebendacin	Sirben
Mebutar	Vermirax
Nemasole	Vermox
Pantelmin	

BASIC INFORMATION

Habit forming? No
Prescription needed? Yes
Available as generic? No
Drug class: Antihelminthic

USES

Treatment of roundworms, pinworms, whipworms, hookworms and other intestinal parasites.

DOSAGE & USAGE INFORMATION

How to take:
Chewable tablets—May be chewed, swallowed whole or mixed with food.

When to take:
Morning and evening with food to increase uptake.

If you forget a dose:
Skip dose and begin treatment again.

What drug does:
Kills parasites by blocking their uptake of glucose.

Time lapse before drug works:
2 to 5 hours.

Don't take with:
See Interaction column and consult doctor.

OVERDOSE

SYMPTOMS:
None expected.
WHAT TO DO:
Overdose unlikely to threaten life.

POSSIBLE ADVERSE REACTIONS OR SIDE EFFECTS

SYMPTOMS	WHAT TO DO
Life-threatening: None expected.	
Common: None expected.	
Infrequent: Abdominal pain, diarrhea, dizziness, fever, headache, nausea.	Continue. Call doctor when convenient.
Rare: Skin rash, itching.	Discontinue. Call doctor right away.

594

WARNINGS & PRECAUTIONS

Don't take if:
- You have Crohn's disease.
- You have ulcerative colitis.

Before you start, consult your doctor:
If you have liver disease.

Over age 60:
Adverse reactions and side effects may be more frequent and severe than in younger persons. You may need smaller doses for shorter periods of time.

Pregnancy:
High dose may cause slight maternal toxicity. Avoid if possible.

Breast-feeding:
No problems expected.

Infants & children:
No problems expected.

Prolonged use:
Not intended for long term use.

Skin & sunlight:
No problems expected.

Driving, piloting or hazardous work:
No problems expected.

Discontinuing:
No problems expected.

Others:
- Take full course of treatment. Repeat course may be necessary if follow-up examinations reveal persistent infection.
- Wash all bedding after treatment to prevent re-infection.

POSSIBLE INTERACTION WITH OTHER DRUGS

GENERIC NAME OR DRUG CLASS	COMBINED EFFECT
Carbamazapine	Decreased effect of mebendazole.

POSSIBLE INTERACTION WITH OTHER SUBSTANCES

INTERACTS WITH	COMBINED EFFECT
Alcohol:	Decreased mebendazole effect. Avoid.
Beverages:	None expected.
Cocaine:	None expected.
Foods:	None expected.
Marijuana:	None expected.
Tobacco:	None expected.

MECLIZINE

BRAND NAMES

Antivert
Bonamine
Bonine

Motion Cure
Ru-Vert-M
Wehvert

BASIC INFORMATION

Habit forming? No
Prescription needed?
U.S.—Tablets: No
     Liquid: Yes
Canada: Yes
Available as generic? Yes
Drug class: Antihistamine, antiemetic

USES

Prevents motion sickness.

DOSAGE & USAGE INFORMATION

How to take:
Tablet—Swallow with liquid or food to lessen stomach irritation. If you can't swallow whole, crumble tablet and chew or take with liquid or food.

When to take:
30 minutes to 1 hour before traveling.

If you forget a dose:
Take as soon as you remember. Wait 4 hours for next dose.

What drug does:
Reduces sensitivity of nerve endings in inner ear, blocking messages to brain's vomiting center.

Time lapse before drug works:
30 to 60 minutes.

Don't take with:
See Interaction column and consult doctor.

OVERDOSE

SYMPTOMS:
Drowsiness, confusion, incoordination, stupor, coma, weak pulse, shallow breathing, hallucinations.
WHAT TO DO:
- Dial 0 (operator) or 911 (emergency) for an ambulance or medical help. Then give first aid immediately.
- See emergency information on inside covers.

POSSIBLE ADVERSE REACTIONS OR SIDE EFFECTS

SYMPTOMS	WHAT TO DO
Life-threatening: None expected.	
Common: Drowsiness.	Continue. Tell doctor at next visit.
Infrequent: • Headache, diarrhea or constipation, fast heartbeat.	Continue. Call doctor when convenient.
• Dry mouth, nose, throat.	Continue. Tell doctor at next visit.
Rare: • Rash, hives.	Discontinue. Call doctor right away.
• Restlessness, excitement, insomnia, blurred vision, frequent and difficult urination, hallucinations.	Continue. Call doctor when convenient.
• Appetite loss, nausea.	Continue. Tell doctor at next visit.

WARNINGS & PRECAUTIONS

Don't take if:
- You are allergic to meclizine, buclizine or cyclizine.
- You have taken MAO inhibitors in the past 2 weeks.

Before you start, consult your doctor:
- If you have glaucoma.
- If you have prostate enlargement.
- If you have reacted badly to any antihistamine.

Over age 60:
Adverse reactions and side effects may be more frequent and severe than in younger persons, especially impaired urination from enlarged prostate gland.

Pregnancy:
Studies inconclusive on harm to unborn child. Animal studies show fetal abnormalities. Decide with your doctor whether drug benefits justify risk to unborn child.

Breast-feeding:
Drug passes into milk. Avoid drug or discontinue nursing until you finish medicine. Consult doctor for advice on maintaining milk supply.

Infants & children:
Safety not established. Avoid if under age 12.

Prolonged use:
No problems expected.

Skin & sunlight:
No problems expected.

Driving, piloting or hazardous work:
Don't fly aircraft. Don't drive until you learn how medicine affects you. Don't work around dangerous machinery. Don't climb ladders or work in high places. Danger increases if you drink alcohol or take medicine affecting alertness and reflexes, such as antihistamines, tranquilizers, sedatives, pain medicine, narcotics and mind-altering drugs.

Discontinuing:
No problems expected.

Others:
Some products contain tartrazine dye. Avoid, especially if you are allergic to aspirin.

POSSIBLE INTERACTION WITH OTHER DRUGS

GENERIC NAME OR DRUG CLASS	COMBINED EFFECT
Amphetamines*	May decrease drowsiness caused by meclizine.
Anticholinergics*	Increased effect of both drugs.
Antidepressants, tricyclic (TCA)*	Increased effect of both drugs.
Carteolol	Decreased antihistamine effect.
Dronabinol	Increases meclizine effect.
Ethinamate	Dangerous increased effects of ethinamate. Avoid combining.
Fluoxetine	Increased depressant effects of both drugs.
Guanfacine	May increase depressant effects of either drug.
Leucovorin	High alcohol content of leucovorin may cause adverse effects.
MAO inhibitors*	Increased meclizine effect.

	COMBINED EFFECT
Methyprylon	Increased sedative effect, perhaps to dangerous level. Avoid.
Nabilone	Greater depression of central nervous system.
Narcotics*	Increased effect of both drugs.
Pain relievers*	Increased effect of both drugs.
Sedatives*	Increased effect of both drugs.
Sleep inducers*	Increased effect of both drugs.
Sotalol	Increased antihistamine effect.
Tranquilizers*	Increased effect of both drugs.

POSSIBLE INTERACTION WITH OTHER SUBSTANCES

INTERACTS WITH	COMBINED EFFECT
Alcohol:	Increased sedation. Avoid.
Beverages: Caffeine drinks.	May decrease drowsiness.
Cocaine:	None expected.
Foods:	None expected.
Marijuana:	Increased drowsiness, dry mouth.
Tobacco:	None expected.

MECLOFENAMATE

BRAND NAMES

Meclomen

BASIC INFORMATION

Habit forming? No
Prescription needed? Yes
Available as generic? Yes
Drug class: Anti-inflammatory (non-steroid)

USES

- Treatment for joint pain, stiffness, inflammation and swelling of arthritis and gout.
- Treats juvenile rheumatoid arthritis.

DOSAGE & USAGE INFORMATION

How to take:
Capsule—Swallow with liquid or food to lessen stomach irritation. If you can't swallow whole, open capsule and take with liquid or food.

When to take:
At the same times each day.

If you forget a dose:
Take as soon as you remember up to 2 hours late. If more than 2 hours, wait for next scheduled dose (don't double this dose).

What drug does:
Reduces tissue concentration of prostaglandins (hormones which produce inflammation and pain).

Time lapse before drug works:
Begins in 4 to 24 hours. May require 3 weeks regular use for maximum benefit.

Don't take with:
See Interaction column and consult doctor.

OVERDOSE

SYMPTOMS:
Confusion, agitation, incoherence, convulsions, possible hemorrhage from stomach or intestine, coma.
WHAT TO DO:
- Dial 0 (operator) or 911 (emergency) for an ambulance or medical help. Then give first aid immediately.
- See emergency information on inside covers.

POSSIBLE ADVERSE REACTIONS OR SIDE EFFECTS

SYMPTOMS	WHAT TO DO
Life-threatening:	
Hives, rash, intense itching, faintness soon after a dose (anaphylaxis in aspirin-sensitive persons).	Seek emergency treatment immediately.
Common:	
• Dizziness, nausea, diarrhea, pain.	Continue. Call doctor when convenient.
• Headache.	Continue. Tell doctor at next visit.
Infrequent:	
Depression; drowsiness; ringing in ears; constipation; vomiting; swollen feet, legs.	Continue. Call doctor when convenient.
Rare:	
• Convulsions; confusion; rash, hives or itchy skin; blurred vision; black, bloody or tarry stool; difficult breathing; tightness in chest; rapid heartbeat; unusual bleeding or bruising; blood in urine; jaundice; severe abdominal pain, psychosis.	Discontinue. Call doctor right away.
• Frequent, painful or difficult urination; fatigue, weakness, swollen breasts in males; impotence; menstrual irregularities.	Continue. Call doctor when convenient.

WARNINGS & PRECAUTIONS

Don't take if:
- You are allergic to aspirin or any non-steroid, anti-inflammatory drug.
- You have gastritis, peptic ulcer, enteritis, ileitis, ulcerative colitis, asthma, heart failure, high blood pressure or bleeding problems.
- Patient is younger than 15.

Before you start, consult your doctor:
- If you have epilepsy.
- If you have Parkinson's disease.
- If you have been mentally ill.
- If you have had kidney disease or impaired kidney function.

Over age 60:
Adverse reactions and side effects may be more frequent and severe than in younger persons.

Pregnancy:
Studies inconclusive on harm to unborn child. Decide with your doctor whether drug benefits justify risk to unborn child.

Breast-feeding:
May harm child. Avoid.

Infants & children:
Not recommended for anyone younger than 15. Use only under medical supervision.

Prolonged use:
- Eye damage.
- Reduced hearing.
- Sore throat, fever.
- Weight gain.

Skin & sunlight:
Increased sensitivity to sunlight.

Driving, piloting or hazardous work:
Don't drive or pilot aircraft until you learn how medicine affects you. Don't work around dangerous machinery. Don't climb ladders or work in high places. Danger increases if you drink alcohol or take medicine affecting alertness and reflexes, such as antihistamines, tranquilizers, sedatives, pain medicine, narcotics and mind-altering drugs.

Discontinuing:
Don't discontinue without consulting doctor. Dose may require gradual reduction if you have taken drug for a long time. Doses of other drugs may also require adjustment.

Others:
No problems expected.

POSSIBLE INTERACTION WITH OTHER DRUGS

GENERIC NAME OR DRUG CLASS	COMBINED EFFECT
ACE inhibitors: captopril, enalapril, lisinopril*	May decrease ACE inhibitor effect.
Anticoagulants, oral*	Increased risk of bleeding.
Aspirin	Increased risk of stomach ulcer.
Beta-adrenergic blockers*	Decreased antihypertensive effect.
Carteolol	Decreased antihypertensive effect of carteolol.
Cortisone drugs*	Increased risk of stomach ulcer.
Diuretics*	May decrease diuretic effect.
Lithium	Possible increased lithium effect and toxicity.
Methotrexate	May increase toxicity.
Minoxidil	Decreased minoxidil effect.
Oxyphenbutazone	Possible stomach ulcer.
Phenylbutazone	Possible stomach ulcer.
Probenecid	Increased meclofenamate effect.
Sotalol	Decreased antihypertensive effect of sotalol.
Terazosin	Decreases effectiveness of terazosin. Causes sodium and fluid retention.
Thyroid hormones*	Rapid heartbeat, blood-pressure rise.

POSSIBLE INTERACTION WITH OTHER SUBSTANCES

INTERACTS WITH	COMBINED EFFECT
Alcohol:	Possible stomach ulcer or bleeding.
Beverages:	None expected.
Cocaine:	None expected.
Foods:	None expected.
Marijuana:	Increased pain relief from meclofenamate.
Tobacco:	None expected.

MEDROXYPROGESTERONE

BRAND NAMES

Amen
Curretab

Depo-Provera
Provera

BASIC INFORMATION

Habit forming? No
Prescription needed? Yes
Available as generic? Yes
Drug class: Female sex hormone (progestin)

 USES

- Treatment for menstrual or uterine disorders caused by progestin imbalance.
- Contraceptive.
- Treatment for cancer of breast and uterus.
- Treatment for toxic sleep apnea.

 DOSAGE & USAGE INFORMATION

How to take:
- Tablet—Swallow with liquid or food to lessen stomach irritation. You may crumble tablet.
- Injection—Take under doctor's supervision.

When to take:
At the same time each day.

If you forget a dose:
- Menstrual disorders—Take up to 2 hours late. If more than 2 hours, wait for next dose (don't double this dose).
- Contraceptive—Consult your doctor. You may need to use another birth-control method until next period.

What drug does:
- Creates a uterine lining similar to pregnancy that prevents bleeding.
- Suppresses a pituitary gland hormone responsible for ovulation.
- Stimulates cervical mucus, which stops sperm penetration and prevents pregnancy.

Continued next column

 OVERDOSE

SYMPTOMS:
Nausea, vomiting, fluid retention, breast discomfort or enlargement, vaginal bleeding.
WHAT TO DO:
Overdose unlikely to threaten life. If person takes much larger amount than prescribed, call doctor, poison-control center or hospital emergency room for instructions.

Time lapse before drug works:
- Menstrual disorders—24 to 48 hours.
- Contraception—3 weeks.
- Cancer—May require 2 to 3 months regular use for maximum benefit.

Don't take with:
See Interaction column and consult doctor.

 POSSIBLE ADVERSE REACTIONS OR SIDE EFFECTS

SYMPTOMS	WHAT TO DO
Life-threatening:	
Blood clot in leg, brain or lung; hives, rash, intense itching, faintness soon after a dose (anaphylaxis).	Seek emergency treatment immediately.
Common:	
Appetite or weight changes, swollen feet or ankles, unusual tiredness or weakness.	Continue. Tell doctor at next visit.
Infrequent:	
• Prolonged vaginal bleeding.	Discontinue. Call doctor right away.
• Depression.	Continue. Call doctor when convenient.
• Acne, increased facial or body hair, nausea, tender breasts.	Continue. Tell doctor at next visit.
Rare:	
• Rash, stomach or side pain, jaundice, fever, excess hair growth, voice change, enlarged clitoris in women.	Discontinue. Call doctor right away.
• Amenorrhea, hair loss, insomnia.	Continue. Call doctor when convenient.

WARNINGS & PRECAUTIONS

Don't take if:
- You are allergic to any progestin hormone.
- You may be pregnant.
- You have liver or gallbladder disease.
- You have had thrombophlebitis, embolism or stroke.
- You have unexplained vaginal bleeding.
- You have had breast or uterine cancer.

Before you start, consult your doctor:
- If you have heart or kidney disease.
- If you have diabetes.
- If you have a seizure disorder.
- If you suffer migraines.
- If you are easily depressed.

Over age 60:
Not recommended.

Pregnancy:
May harm child. Discontinue at first sign of pregnancy.

Breast-feeding:
Drug passes into milk. Avoid drug or discontinue nursing until you finish medicine. Consult doctor for advice on maintaining milk supply.

Infants & children:
Use only for female children under medical supervision.

Prolonged use:
No problems expected.

Skin & sunlight:
No problems expected.

Driving, piloting or hazardous work:
No problems expected.

Discontinuing:
Consult doctor. This medicine stays in the body and causes fetal abnormalities. Wait at least 3 months before becoming pregnant.

Others:
- Patients with diabetes must be monitored closely.
- Symptoms of blood clot in leg, brain or lung are: chest, groin, leg pain; sudden, severe headache; loss of coordination; vision change; shortness of breath; slurred speech.

POSSIBLE INTERACTION WITH OTHER DRUGS

GENERIC NAME OR DRUG CLASS	COMBINED EFFECT
Hypoglycemics, oral*	Decreased effect of oral hypoglycemics.
Insulin	Decreased effect of insulin.
Oxyphenbutazone	Decreased medroxy-progesterone effect.
Phenobarbital	Decreased medroxy-progesterone effect.
Phenothiazines*	Increased pheno-thiazine effect.
Phenylbutazone	Decreased medroxy-progesterone effect.
Rifampin	Decreased contraceptive effect.

POSSIBLE INTERACTION WITH OTHER SUBSTANCES

INTERACTS WITH	COMBINED EFFECT
Alcohol:	None expected.
Beverages:	None expected.
Cocaine:	Decreased medroxy-progesterone effect.
Foods: Salt.	Fluid retention.
Marijuana:	Possible menstrual irregularities or bleeding between periods.
Tobacco: All forms.	Possible blood clots in lung, brain, legs. Avoid.

MEFENAMIC ACID

BRAND NAMES

Ponstan   Ponstel

BASIC INFORMATION

Habit forming? No
Prescription needed? Yes
Available as generic? No
Drug class: Anti-inflammatory (non-steroid)

USES

- Pain reliever.
- Treatment for dysmenorrhea (painful or difficult menstruation).
- Treats juvenile rheumatoid arthritis.

DOSAGE & USAGE INFORMATION

How to take:
Capsule—Swallow with liquid or food to lessen stomach irritation. If you can't swallow whole, open capsule and take with liquid or food.

When to take:
At the same times each day.

If you forget a dose:
Take as soon as you remember up to 2 hours late. If more than 2 hours, wait for next scheduled dose (don't double this dose).

What drug does:
Reduces tissue concentration of prostaglandins (hormones which produce inflammation and pain).

Time lapse before drug works:
Begins in 4 to 24 hours. May require 3 weeks regular use for maximum benefit.

Don't take with:
See Interaction column and consult doctor.

OVERDOSE

SYMPTOMS:
Confusion, agitation, incoherence, convulsions, possible hemorrhage from stomach or intestine, coma.
WHAT TO DO:
- Dial 0 (operator) or 911 (emergency) for an ambulance or medical help. Then give first aid immediately.
- See emergency information on inside covers.

POSSIBLE ADVERSE REACTIONS OR SIDE EFFECTS

SYMPTOMS	WHAT TO DO
Life-threatening: Hives, rash, intense itching, faintness soon after a dose (anaphylaxis in aspirin-sensitive persons).	Seek emergency treatment immediately.
Common: • Dizziness, nausea, pain.	Continue. Call doctor when convenient.
• Headache.	Continue. Tell doctor at next visit.
Infrequent: Depression, drowsiness, ringing in ears, constipation or diarrhea, vomiting, swollen feet or legs.	Continue. Call doctor when convenient.
Rare: • Convulsions; confusion; rash, hives or itchy skin; blurred vision; black, bloody or tarry stool; difficult breathing; tightness in chest; rapid heartbeat; unusual bleeding or bruising; blood in urine; jaundice; severe abdominal pain, psychosis.	Discontinue. Call doctor right away.
• Frequent, painful or difficult urination; fatigue, weakness; swollen breasts in males; impotence; menstrual irregularities.	Continue. Call doctor when convenient.

WARNINGS & PRECAUTIONS

Don't take if:
- You are allergic to aspirin or any non-steroid, anti-inflammatory drug.
- You have gastritis, peptic ulcer, enteritis, ileitis, ulcerative colitis, asthma, heart failure, high blood pressure or bleeding problems.
- Patient is younger than 15.

Before you start, consult your doctor:
- If you have epilepsy.
- If you have Parkinson's disease.
- If you have been mentally ill.
- If you have had kidney disease or impaired kidney function.

Over age 60:
Adverse reactions and side effects may be more frequent and severe than in younger persons.

Pregnancy:
Studies inconclusive on harm to unborn child. Decide with your doctor whether drug benefits justify risk to unborn child.

Breast-feeding:
May harm child. Avoid.

Infants & children:
Not recommended for anyone younger than 15. Use only under medical supervision.

Prolonged use:
- Eye damage.
- Reduced hearing.
- Sore throat, fever.
- Weight gain.

Skin & sunlight:
Increased sensitivity to sunlight.

Driving, piloting or hazardous work:
Don't drive or pilot aircraft until you learn how medicine affects you. Don't work around dangerous machinery. Don't climb ladders or work in high places. Danger increases if you drink alcohol or take medicine affecting alertness and reflexes, such as antihistamines, tranquilizers, sedatives, pain medicine, narcotics and mind-altering drugs.

Discontinuing:
Don't discontinue without consulting doctor. Dose may require gradual reduction if you have taken drug for a long time. Doses of other drugs may also require adjustment.

Others:
Don't take for more than 1 week.

POSSIBLE INTERACTION WITH OTHER DRUGS

GENERIC NAME OR DRUG CLASS	COMBINED EFFECT
ACE inhibitors: captopril, enalapril, lisinopril *	May decrease ACE inhibitor effect.
Anticoagulants, oral *	Increased risk of bleeding.
Aspirin	Increased risk of stomach ulcer.

Beta-adrenergic blockers *	Decreased antihypertensive effect.
Carteolol	Decreased antihypertensive effect of carteolol.
Cortisone drugs *	Increased risk of stomach ulcer.
Diuretics *	May decrease diuretic effect.
Lithium	Possible increased lithium effect and toxicity.
Methotrexate	May increase toxicity.
Minoxidil	Decreased minoxidil effect.
Oxyphenbutazone	Possible stomach ulcer.
Phenylbutazone	Possible stomach ulcer.
Probenecid	Increased effect of mefenamic acid.
Sotalol	Decreased antihypertensive effect of sotalol.
Terazosin	Decreases effectiveness of terazosin. Causes sodium and fluid retention.
Thyroid hormones *	Rapid heartbeat, blood-pressure rise.

POSSIBLE INTERACTION WITH OTHER SUBSTANCES

INTERACTS WITH	COMBINED EFFECT
Alcohol:	Possible stomach ulcer or bleeding.
Beverages:	None expected.
Cocaine:	None expected.
Foods:	None expected.
Marijuana:	Increased pain relief from mefenamic acid.
Tobacco:	None expected.

MELPHALAN (PAM, L-PAM, Phenylalanine Mustard)

BRAND NAMES

Alkeran
L-PAM

Phenylalanine
Mustard

BASIC INFORMATION

Habit forming? No
Prescription needed? Yes
Available as generic? No
Drug class: Antineoplastic,
immunosuppressant

 ## USES

- Treatment for some kinds of cancer.
- Suppresses immune response after transplant and in immune disorders.

 ## DOSAGE & USAGE INFORMATION

How to take:
Tablet—Swallow with liquid after light meal. Don't drink fluids with meals. Drink extra fluids between meals. Avoid sweet or fatty foods.

When to take:
At the same time each day.

If you forget a dose:
Take as soon as you remember. Don't ever double dose.

What drug does:
Inhibits abnormal cell reproduction. May suppress immune system.

Continued next column

 ## OVERDOSE

SYMPTOMS:
Bleeding, chills, fever, collapse, stupor, seizure.
WHAT TO DO:
- Dial 0 (operator) or 911 (emergency) for an ambulance or medical help. Then give first aid immediately.
- If patient is unconscious and not breathing, give mouth-to-mouth breathing. If there is no heartbeat, use cardiac massage and mouth-to-mouth breathing (CPR). Don't try to make patient vomit. If you can't get help quickly, take patient to nearest emergency facility.
- See emergency information on inside covers.

Time lapse before drug works:
Up to 6 weeks for full effect.

Don't take with:
See Interaction column and consult doctor.

 ## POSSIBLE ADVERSE REACTIONS OR SIDE EFFECTS

SYMPTOMS	WHAT TO DO
Life-threatening: None expected.	
Common:	
• Unusual bleeding or bruising, mouth sores with sore throat, chills and fever, black stools, sores in mouth and lips, menstrual irregularities.	Discontinue. Call doctor right away.
• Hair loss, joint pain.	Continue. Call doctor when convenient.
• Nausea, vomiting, diarrhea (unavoidable), tiredness, weakness.	Continue. Tell doctor at next visit.
Infrequent:	
• Skin rash.	Discontinue. Call doctor right away.
• Mental confusion, shortness of breath, may increase chance of developing leukemia.	Continue. Call doctor when convenient.
• Cough.	Continue. Tell doctor at next visit.
Rare: Jaundice.	Discontinue. Call doctor right away.

MELPHALAN (PAM, L-PAM, Phenylalanine Mustard)

WARNINGS & PRECAUTIONS

Don't take if:
- You have had hypersensitivity to alkylating antineoplastic drugs.
- Your physician has not explained serious nature of your medical problem and risks of taking this medicine.

Before you start, consult your doctor:
- If you have gout.
- If you have had kidney stones.
- If you have active infection.
- If you have impaired kidney or liver function.
- If you have taken other antineoplastic drugs or had radiation treatment in last 3 weeks.

Over age 60:
Adverse reactions and side effects may be more frequent and severe than in younger persons.

Pregnancy:
Consult doctor. Risk to child is significant.

Breast-feeding:
Drug passes into milk. Don't nurse.

Infants & children:
Use only under special medical supervision at center experienced in anticancer drugs.

Prolonged use:
Adverse reactions more likely the longer drug is required.

Skin & sunlight:
No problems expected.

Driving, piloting or hazardous work:
No problems expected.

Discontinuing:
Don't discontinue without doctor's advice until you complete prescribed dose, even though symptoms diminish or disappear. Some side effects may follow discontinuing. Report to doctor blurred vision, convulsions, confusion, persistent headache.

Others:
May cause sterility.

POSSIBLE INTERACTION WITH OTHER DRUGS

GENERIC NAME OR DRUG CLASS	COMBINED EFFECT
Antigout drugs*	Decreased antigout effect.
Antineoplastic drugs, other*	Increased effect of all drugs (may be beneficial).
Chloramphenicol	Increased likelihood of toxic effects of both drugs.
Lovastatin	Increased heart and kidney damage.

POSSIBLE INTERACTION WITH OTHER SUBSTANCES

INTERACTS WITH	COMBINED EFFECT
Alcohol:	May increase chance of intestinal bleeding.
Beverages:	No problems expected.
Cocaine:	Increases chance of toxicity.
Foods:	Reduces irritation in stomach.
Marijuana:	No problems expected.
Tobacco:	Increases lung toxicity.

*See Glossary

MEPHENYTOIN

BRAND NAMES

Mesantoin   Methoin

BASIC INFORMATION

Habit forming? No
Prescription needed? Yes
Available as generic? No
Drug class: Anticonvulsant (hydantoin)

 ## USES

- Prevents epileptic seizures.
- Stabilizes irregular heartbeat.

 ## DOSAGE & USAGE INFORMATION

How to take:
- Tablet—Swallow with liquid.
- Chewable tablets—Chew well before swallowing.
- Suspension—Shake well before taking with liquid.

When to take:
At the same time each day.

If you forget a dose:
- If drug taken 1 time per day—Take as soon as you remember up to 12 hours late. If more than 12 hours, wait for next scheduled dose (don't double this dose).
- If taken several times per day—Take as soon as possible, then return to regular schedule.

What drug does:
Promotes sodium loss from nerve fibers. This lessens excitability and inhibits spread of nerve impulses.

Time lapse before drug works:
7 to 10 days continual use.

Don't take with:
See Interaction column and consult doctor.

 ## OVERDOSE

SYMPTOMS:
Jerky eye movements; stagger; slurred speech; imbalance; drowsiness; blood-pressure drop; slow, shallow breathing; coma.
WHAT TO DO:
- **Dial 0 (operator) or 911 (emergency) for an ambulance or medical help. Then give first aid immediately.**
- **See emergency information on inside covers.**

 ## POSSIBLE ADVERSE REACTIONS OR SIDE EFFECTS

SYMPTOMS	WHAT TO DO
Life-threatening: None expected.	
Common: Mild dizziness, drowsiness, nausea, constipation, vomiting.	Continue. Call doctor when convenient.
Infrequent: • Hallucinations, confusion, slurred speech, stagger, rash, change in vision.	Discontinue. Call doctor right away.
• Headache, sleeplessness, diarrhea, muscle twitching.	Continue. Call doctor when convenient.
• Increased body and facial hair.	Continue. Tell doctor at next visit.
Rare: Sore throat, fever, stomach pain, unusual bleeding or bruising, jaundice, swollen lymph glands.	Discontinue. Call doctor right away.

 ## WARNINGS & PRECAUTIONS

Don't take if:
You are allergic to any hydantoin anticonvulsant.

Before you start, consult your doctor:
- If you have had impaired liver function or disease.
- If you will have surgery within 2 months, including dental surgery, requiring general or spinal anesthesia.

Over age 60:
Adverse reactions and side effects may be more frequent and severe than in younger persons.

Pregnancy:
Risk to unborn child outweighs drug benefits. Don't use.

Breast-feeding:
Drug passes into milk. Avoid drug or discontinue nursing until you finish medicine. Consult doctor for advice on maintaining milk supply.

Infants & children:
Use only under medical supervision.

Prolonged use:
- Weakened bones.
- Lymph gland enlargement.
- Possible liver damage.
- Numbness and tingling of hands and feet.
- Continual back-and-forth eye movements.
- Bleeding, swollen or tender gums.

Skin & sunlight:
May cause rash or intensify sunburn in areas exposed to sun or sunlamp.

Driving, piloting or hazardous work:
Don't drive or pilot aircraft until you learn how medicine affects you. Don't work around dangerous machinery. Don't climb ladders or work in high places. Danger increases if you drink alcohol or take medicine affecting alertness and reflexes.

Discontinuing:
Don't discontinue without consulting doctor. Dose may require gradual reduction if you have taken drug for a long time. Doses of other drugs may also require adjustment.

Others:
No problems expected.

POSSIBLE INTERACTION WITH OTHER DRUGS

GENERIC NAME OR DRUG CLASS	COMBINED EFFECT
Anticoagulants*	Increased effect of both drugs.
Antidepressants, tricyclic (TCA)*	Need to adjust mephenytoin dose.
Barbiturates*	Changed seizure pattern.
Carbamazepine	Possible increased mephenytoin metabolism.
Carbonic anhydrase inhibitors*	Increased chance of bone disease.
Chloramphenicol	Increased mephenytoin effect.
Cimetidine	Increased mephenytoin toxicity.
Contraceptives, oral*	Increased seizures.
Cortisone drugs*	Decreased cortisone effect.
Cyclosporine	May decrease cyclosporine effect.
Digitalis preparations*	Decreased digitalis effect.
Disopyramide	Decreased disopyramide effect.
Disulfiram	Increased mephenytoin effect.
Estrogens*	Increased estrogen effect.
Furosemide	Decreased furosemide effect.
Glutethimide	Decreased mephenytoin effect.
Griseofulvin	Increased griseofulvin effect.
Hypoglycemics, other*	Possible decreased hypoglycemic effect.
Isoniazid	Increased mephenytoin effect.
Methadone	Decreased methadone effect.
Methotrexate	Increased methotrexate effect.
Methylphenidate	Increased mephenytoin effect.
Nicardipine	Increased anti-convulsant effect.
Oxyphenbutazone	Increased mephenytoin effect.
Para-aminosalicylic acid (PAS)	Increased mephenytoin effect.
Phenothiazines*	Increased mephenytoin effect.
Phenylbutazone	Increased mephenytoin effect.
Propranolol	Increased propranolol effect.
Quinidine	Increased quinidine effect.

Continued page 1089

POSSIBLE INTERACTION WITH OTHER SUBSTANCES

INTERACTS WITH	COMBINED EFFECT
Alcohol:	Possible decreased anticonvulsant effect. Use with caution.
Beverages:	None expected.
Cocaine:	Possible seizures.
Foods:	None expected.
Marijuana:	Drowsiness, unsteadiness, decreased anticonvulsant effect.
Tobacco:	None expected.

*See Glossary

MEPHOBARBITAL

BRAND NAMES

Mebaral

BASIC INFORMATION

Habit forming? Yes
Prescription needed? Yes
Available as generic? No
Drug class: Sedative, hypnotic (barbiturate)

 USES

- Reduces anxiety or nervous tension (low dose).
- Prevents seizures in epilepsy.

 DOSAGE & USAGE INFORMATION

How to take:
Tablet—Swallow with liquid or food to lessen stomach irritation. If you can't swallow whole, crumble tablet and take with liquid or food.

When to take:
At the same times each day.

If you forget a dose:
Take as soon as you remember up to 2 hours late. If more than 2 hours, wait for next scheduled dose (don't double this dose).

What drug does:
May partially block nerve impulses at nerve-cell connections.

Time lapse before drug works:
60 minutes.

Continued next column

 OVERDOSE

SYMPTOMS:
Deep sleep, weak pulse, coma.
WHAT TO DO:
- **Dial 0 (operator) or 911 (emergency) for an ambulance or medical help. Then give first aid immediately.**
- **If patient is unconscious and not breathing, give mouth-to-mouth breathing. If there is no heartbeat use cardiac massage and mouth-to-mouth breathing (CPR). Don't try to make patient vomit. If you can't get help quickly, take patient to nearest emergency facility.**
- **See emergency information on inside covers.**

Don't take with:
- Non-prescription drugs without consulting doctor.
- See Interaction column and consult doctor.

 POSSIBLE ADVERSE REACTIONS OR SIDE EFFECTS

SYMPTOMS	WHAT TO DO
Life-threatening: None expected.	
Common: Dizziness, drowsiness, "hangover" effect.	Continue. Call doctor when convenient.
Infrequent: • Rash or hives; face, lip or eyelid swelling; sore throat; fever.	Discontinue. Call doctor right away.
• Depression, confusion, diarrhea, nausea, vomiting, joint or muscle pain, slurred speech.	Continue. Call doctor when convenient.
Rare: • Agitation, slow heartbeat, difficult breathing, jaundice.	Discontinue. Call doctor right away.
• Unexplained bleeding or bruising.	Continue. Call doctor when convenient.

 WARNINGS & PRECAUTIONS

Don't take if:
- You are allergic to any barbiturate.
- You have porphyria.

Before you start, consult your doctor:
- If you have epilepsy.
- If you have kidney or liver damage.
- If you have asthma.
- If you have anemia.
- If you have chronic pain.
- If you will have surgery within 2 months, including dental surgery, requiring general or spinal anesthesia.

Over age 60:
Adverse reactions and side effects may be more frequent and severe than in younger persons. Use small doses.

Pregnancy:
Risk to unborn child outweighs drug benefits. Don't use.

Breast-feeding:
Drug passes into milk. Avoid drug or discontinue nursing until you finish medicine. Consult doctor for advice on maintaining milk supply.

Infants & children:
Use only under doctor's supervision.

Prolonged use:
- May cause addiction, anemia, chronic intoxication.
- May lower body temperature, making exposure to cold temperatures hazardous.

Skin & sunlight:
May cause rash or intensify sunburn in areas exposed to sun or sunlamp.

Driving, piloting or hazardous work:
Don't drive or pilot aircraft until you learn how medicine affects you. Don't work around dangerous machinery. Don't climb ladders or work in high places. Danger increases if you drink alcohol or take medicine affecting alertness and reflexes.

Discontinuing:
May be unnecessary to finish medicine. Follow doctor's instructions. If you develop withdrawal symptoms of hallucinations, agitation or sleeplessness after discontinuing, call doctor right away.

Others:
No problems expected.

 POSSIBLE INTERACTION WITH OTHER DRUGS

GENERIC NAME OR DRUG CLASS	COMBINED EFFECT
Anticoagulants, oral*	Decreased effect of anticoagulant.
Anticonvulsants*	Changed seizure patterns.
Antidepressants, tricyclics (TCA)*	Decreased anti-depressant effect. Possible dangerous oversedation.
Antidiabetics, oral*	Increased effect of mephobarbital.
Antihistamines*	Dangerous sedation. Avoid.
Aspirin	Decreased aspirin effect.
Beta-adrenergic blockers*	Decreased effect of beta-adrenergic blocker.
Carteolol	Increased barbiturate effect. Dangerous sedation.
Contraceptives, oral*	Decreased contraceptive effect.
Cortisone drugs*	Decreased cortisone effect.
Digitoxin	Decreased digitoxin effect.
Doxycycline	Decreased doxycycline effect.
Dronabinol	Increased effects of both drugs. Avoid.
Griseofulvin	Decreased griseofulvin effect.
Indapamide	Increased indapamide effect.
MAO inhibitors*	Increased mephobarbital effect.
Mind-altering drugs*	Dangerous sedation. Avoid.
Molindone	Increased sedative effect.
Nabilone	Greater depression of central nervous system.
Narcotics*	Dangerous sedation. Avoid.
Non-steroidal anti-inflammatory drugs (NSAIDs)*	Decreased anti-inflammatory effect.
Pain relievers*	Dangerous sedation. Avoid.
Sedatives*	Dangerous sedation. Avoid.
Sleep inducers*	Dangerous sedation. Avoid.
Sotalol	Increased barbiturate effect. Dangerous sedation.
Tranquilizers*	Dangerous sedation. Avoid.
Valproic acid	Increased mephobarbital effect.

 POSSIBLE INTERACTION WITH OTHER SUBSTANCES

INTERACTS WITH	COMBINED EFFECT
Alcohol:	Possible fatal oversedation. Avoid.
Beverages:	None expected.
Cocaine:	Decreased mephobarbital effect.
Foods:	None expected.
Marijuana:	Excessive sedation. Avoid.
Tobacco:	None expected.

*See Glossary

MEPROBAMATE

BRAND NAMES

See complete list of brand names in the *Brand Name Directory*, page 1065.

BASIC INFORMATION

Habit forming? Yes
Prescription needed? Yes
Available as generic? Yes
Drug class: Tranquilizer

 USES

Reduces mild anxiety, tension and insomnia.

 DOSAGE & USAGE INFORMATION

How to take:
- Tablet—Swallow with liquid.
- Extended-release capsules—Swallow each dose whole.

When to take:
At the same time each day.

If you forget a dose:
Take as soon as you remember up to 2 hours late. If more than 2 hours, wait for next scheduled dose (don't double this dose).

What drug does:
Sedates brain centers which control behavior and emotions.

Time lapse before drug works:
1 to 2 hours.

Don't take with:
- Non-prescription drugs containing alcohol or caffeine without consulting doctor.
- See Interaction column and consult doctor.

 OVERDOSE

SYMPTOMS:
Dizziness, slurred speech, stagger, depressed breathing and heart function, stupor, coma.
WHAT TO DO:
- **Dial 0 (operator) or 911 (emergency) for an ambulance or medical help. Then give first aid immediately.**
- **See emergency information on inside covers.**

 POSSIBLE ADVERSE REACTIONS OR SIDE EFFECTS

SYMPTOMS	WHAT TO DO
Life-threatening:	
Hives, rash, intense itching, faintness soon after a dose (anaphylaxis).	Seek emergency treatment immediately.
Common:	
Dizziness, confusion, agitation, drowsiness, unsteadiness, fatigue, weakness.	Continue. Tell doctor at next visit.
Infrequent:	
• Rash, hives, itchy skin; change in vision; diarrhea, nausea or vomiting.	Discontinue. Call doctor right away.
• False sense of well-being, headache, slurred speech.	Continue. Call doctor when convenient.
Rare:	
Sore throat; fever; rapid, pounding, unusually slow or irregular heartbeat; difficult breathing; unusual bleeding or bruising.	Discontinue. Call doctor right away.

 WARNINGS & PRECAUTIONS

Don't take if:
- You are allergic to meprobamate, tybamate, carbromal or carisoprodol.
- You have had porphyria.
- Patient is younger than 6.

Before you start, consult your doctor:
- If you have epilepsy.
- If you have impaired liver or kidney function.
- If you have tartrazine dye allergy.

Over age 60:
Adverse reactions and side effects may be more frequent and severe than in younger persons.

Pregnancy:
Risk to unborn child outweighs drug benefits. Don't use.

Breast-feeding:
Drug filters into milk. May harm child. Avoid.

Infants & children:
Not recommended.

Prolonged use:
- Habit forming.
- May impair blood-cell production.

Skin & sunlight:
No problems expected.

Driving, piloting or hazardous work:
Don't drive or pilot aircraft until you learn how medicine affects you. Don't work around dangerous machinery. Don't climb ladders or work in high places. Danger increases if you drink alcohol or take medicine affecting alertness and reflexes, such as antihistamines, tranquilizers, sedatives, pain medicine, narcotics and mind-altering drugs.

Discontinuing:
Don't discontinue without consulting doctor. Dose may require gradual reduction if you have taken drug for a long time. Doses of other drugs may also require adjustment.

Others:
No problems expected.

POSSIBLE INTERACTION WITH OTHER DRUGS

GENERIC NAME OR DRUG CLASS	COMBINED EFFECT
Anticoagulants*	Decreased anticoagulant effect.
Anticonvulsants*	Change in seizure pattern.
Antidepressants, tricyclic (TCA)*	Increased antidepressant effect.
Antihistamines*	Possible excessive sedation.
Contraceptives, oral*	Decreased contraceptive effect.
Dronabinol	Increased effects of both drugs. Avoid.
Estrogens*	Decreased estrogen effect.
Ethinamate	Dangerous increased effects of ethinamate. Avoid combining.
Fluoxetine	Increased depressant effects of both drugs.
Guanfacine	May increase depressant effects of either drug.
Leucovorin	High alcohol content of leucovorin may cause adverse effects.
MAO Inhibitors*	Increased meprobamate effect.
Methyprylon	Increased sedative effect, perhaps to dangerous level. Avoid.
Molindone	Increased tranquilizer effect.
Nabilone	Greater depression of central nervous system.
Narcotics*	Increased narcotic effect.
Sedatives*	Increased sedative effect.
Sleep Inducers*	Increased effect of sleep inducer.
Tranquilizers*	Increased tranquilizer effect.

POSSIBLE INTERACTION WITH OTHER SUBSTANCES

INTERACTS WITH	COMBINED EFFECT
Alcohol:	Dangerous increased effect of meprobamate.
Beverages: Caffeine drinks.	Decreased calming effect of meprobamate.
Cocaine:	Decreased meprobamate effect.
Foods:	None expected.
Marijuana:	Increased sedative effect of meprobamate.
Tobacco:	None expected.

MEPROBAMATE & ASPIRIN

BRAND NAMES

Equagesic
Equazine-M
Meprogestic Q

Micrainin
Tranquigesic

BASIC INFORMATION

Habit forming? Yes
Prescription needed? Yes
Available as generic? No
Drug class: Anti-inflammatory, analgesic, tranquilizer

USES

- Reduces mild anxiety, tension and insomnia.
- Reduces pain, fever, inflammation.
- Relieves swelling, stiffness, joint pain.
- Antiplatelet effect.

DOSAGE & USAGE INFORMATION

How to take:
- Tablet—Swallow with liquid.
- Effervescent tablets—Dissolve in water.

When to take:
Pain, fever, inflammation—As needed, no more often than every 4 hours.

If you forget a dose:
Take as soon as you remember up to 2 hours late. If more than 2 hours, wait for next scheduled dose (don't double this dose).

What drug does:
- Sedates brain centers which control behavior and emotions.
- Affects hypothalamus, the part of the brain which regulates temperature by dilating small blood vessels in skin.

Continued next column

OVERDOSE

SYMPTOMS:
Dizziness; slurred speech; stagger; depressed heart function; ringing in ears; nausea; vomiting; fever; deep, rapid breathing; hallucinations; convulsions; stupor; coma.
WHAT TO DO:
- **Dial 0 (operator) or 911 (emergency) for an ambulance or medical help. Then give first aid immediately.**
- **See emergency information on inside covers.**

- Prevents clumping of platelets (small blood cells) so blood vessels remain open.
- Decreases prostaglandin effect.
- Suppresses body's pain messages.

Time lapse before drug works:
1 to 2 hours.

Don't take with:
- Tetracyclines.
- Non-prescription drugs containing alcohol or caffeine without consulting doctor.
- See Interaction column and consult doctor.

POSSIBLE ADVERSE REACTIONS OR SIDE EFFECTS

SYMPTOMS	WHAT TO DO
Life-threatening:	
Hives, rash, intense itching, faintness soon after a dose (anaphylaxis); difficulty breathing.	Seek emergency treatment immediately.
Common:	
• Nausea, vomiting.	Discontinue. Call doctor right away.
• Dizziness, confusion, agitation, drowsiness, unsteadiness, fatigue, weakness, ears ringing, heartburn, indigestion.	Continue. Call doctor when convenient.
Infrequent:	
None expected.	
Rare:	
• Black, bloody or tarry stool; vomiting blood or black material; blood in urine.	Discontinue. Seek emergency treatment.
• Rash, hives, itchy skin, change in vision, fever, jaundice, mental confusion.	Discontinue. Call doctor right away.

WARNINGS & PRECAUTIONS

Don't take if:
- You are allergic to meprobamate, tybamate, carbromal or carisoprodol.
- You are sensitive to aspirin.
- You have had porphyria.
- You have a peptic ulcer of stomach or duodenum or a bleeding disorder.
- Patient is younger than 6.

Before you start, consult your doctor:
- If you have epilepsy, impaired liver or kidney function, asthma or nasal polyps.
- If you are allergic to tartrazine dye.
- If you have had gout, stomach or duodenal ulcers.

Over age 60:
Adverse reactions and side effects may be more frequent and severe than in younger persons. More likely to cause hidden bleeding in stomach or intestines. Watch for dark stools.

Pregnancy:
Risk to unborn child outweighs drug benefits. Don't use.

Breast-feeding:
Drug passes into milk. Avoid drug or discontinue nursing until you finish medicine. Consult doctor for advice on maintaining milk supply.

Infants & children:
Not recommended.

Prolonged use:
- Habit forming.
- May impair blood-cell production.
- Kidney damage. Periodic kidney-function test recommended.

Skin & sunlight:
Aspirin combined with sunscreen may decrease sunburn.

Driving, piloting or hazardous work:
Don't drive or pilot aircraft until you learn how medicine affects you. Don't work around dangerous machinery. Don't climb ladders or work in high places. Danger increases if you drink alcohol or take medicine affecting alertness and reflexes, such as antihistamines, tranquilizers, sedatives, pain medicine, narcotics and mind-altering drugs.

Discontinuing:
Don't discontinue without consulting doctor. Dose may require gradual reduction if you have taken drug for a long time. Doses of other drugs may also require adjustment.

Others:
- Aspirin can complicate surgery; illness; pregnancy, labor and delivery.
- Urine tests for blood sugar may be inaccurate.

POSSIBLE INTERACTION WITH OTHER DRUGS

GENERIC NAME OR DRUG CLASS	COMBINED EFFECT
Acebutolol	Decreased antihypertensive effect of acebutolol.
ACE inhibitors: captopril, enalapril, lisinopril*	Decreased effect of inhibitors.
Allopurinol	Decreased allopurinol effect.
Antacids*	Decreased aspirin effect.
Anticoagulants*	Increased anticoagulant effect. Abnormal bleeding.
Anticonvulsants*	Change in seizure pattern.
Antidepressants, tricyclic (TCA)*	Increased antidepressant effect.
Antidiabetics, oral*	Low blood sugar.
Aspirin, other	Likely aspirin toxicity.
Bumetanide	Possible aspirin toxicity.
Contraceptives, oral*	Decreased contraceptive effect.
Cortisone drugs*	Increased cortisone effect. Risk of ulcers and stomach bleeding.
Dronabinol	Increased effect of both drugs.
Estrogens*	Decreased estrogen effect.
Ethacrynic acid	Possible aspirin toxicity.
Furosemide	Possible aspirin toxicity. May decrease furosemide effect.
Gold compounds*	Increased likelihood of kidney damage.
Indomethacin	Risk of stomach bleeding and ulcers.

Continued page 1089

POSSIBLE INTERACTION WITH OTHER SUBSTANCES

INTERACTS WITH	COMBINED EFFECT
Alcohol:	Possible stomach irritation and bleeding. Dangerous increased effect of meprobamate. Avoid.
Beverages: Caffeine drinks.	Decreased calming effect of meprobamate.
Cocaine:	Decreased meprobamate effect.
Foods:	None expected.
Marijuana:	Possible increased pain relief, but marijuana may slow body's recovery. Avoid.
Tobacco:	None expected.

MERCAPTOPURINE

BRAND NAMES

Purinethol   6-MP

BASIC INFORMATION

Habit forming? No
Prescription needed? Yes
Available as generic? No
Drug class: Antineoplastic,
   Immunosuppressant

USES

- Treatment for some kinds of cancer.
- Treatment for regional enteritis and ulcerative colitis and other immune disorders.

DOSAGE & USAGE INFORMATION

How to take:
Tablet—Swallow with liquid.

When to take:
At the same time each day.

If you forget a dose:
Skip the missed dose. Don't double the next dose.

What drug does:
Inhibits abnormal-cell reproduction.

Time lapse before drug works:
May require 6 weeks for maximum effect.

Don't take with:
See Interaction column and consult doctor.

OVERDOSE

SYMPTOMS:
Headache, stupor, seizures.
WHAT TO DO:
- Dial 0 (operator) or 911 (emergency) for an ambulance or medical help. Then give first aid immediately.
- If patient is unconscious and not breathing, give mouth-to-mouth breathing. If there is no heartbeat, use cardiac massage and mouth-to-mouth breathing (CPR). Don't try to make patient vomit. If you can't get help quickly, take patient to nearest emergency facility.
- See emergency information on inside covers.

POSSIBLE ADVERSE REACTIONS OR SIDE EFFECTS

SYMPTOMS	WHAT TO DO
Life-threatening:	
None expected.	
Common:	
• Black stools or bloody vomit.	Discontinue. Seek emergency treatment.
• Mouth sores, sore throat, fever, chills, unusual bleeding or bruising.	Discontinue. Call doctor right away.
• Stomach pain, nausea, vomiting.	Continue. Call doctor when convenient.
Infrequent:	
• Seizures.	Discontinue. Seek emergency treatment.
• Diarrhea, headache, confusion, blurred vision, shortness of breath, joint pain, blood in urine, jaundice.	Discontinue. Call doctor right away.
• Cough.	Continue. Call doctor when convenient.
• Acne, boils, hair loss, itchy skin.	Continue. Tell doctor at next visit.
Rare:	
Fever.	Discontinue. Call doctor right away.

WARNINGS & PRECAUTIONS

Don't take if:
You are allergic to any antineoplastic.

Before you start, consult your doctor:
- If you are alcoholic.
- If you have blood, liver or kidney disease.
- If you have colitis or peptic ulcer.
- If you have gout.
- If you have an infection.
- If you plan to become pregnant within 3 months.

Over age 60:
Adverse reactions and side effects may be more frequent and severe than in younger persons.

Pregnancy:
Consult doctor.

Breast-feeding:
Drug passes into milk. Avoid drug or discontinue nursing.

Infants & children:
Use only under special medical supervision.

Prolonged use:
Adverse reactions more likely the longer drug is required.

Skin & sunlight:
No problems expected.

Driving, piloting or hazardous work:
Avoid if you feel dizzy, drowsy or confused. Otherwise, no problems expected.

Discontinuing:
Don't discontinue without doctor's advice until you complete prescribed dose, even though symptoms diminish or disappear. Some side effects may follow discontinuing. Report to doctor blurred vision, convulsions, confusion, persistent headache.

Others:
- Drink more water than usual to cause frequent urination.
- Don't give this medicine to anyone else for any purpose. It is a strong drug that requires close medical supervision.
- Report for frequent medical follow-up and laboratory studies.

POSSIBLE INTERACTION WITH OTHER DRUGS

GENERIC NAME OR DRUG CLASS	COMBINED EFFECT
Acetaminophen	Increased likelihood of liver toxicity.
Allopurinol	Increased toxic effect of mercaptopurine.
Anticoagulants, oral*	May increase or decrease anticoagulant effect.
Antineoplastic drugs, other*	Increased effect of both (may be desirable) or increased toxicity of each.
Chloramphenicol	Increased toxicity of each.
Cyclosporine	May increase risk of infection.
Isoniazid	Increased likelihood of liver toxicity.
Lovastatin	Increased heart and kidney damage.

POSSIBLE INTERACTION WITH OTHER SUBSTANCES

INTERACTS WITH	COMBINED EFFECT
Alcohol:	May increase chance of intestinal bleeding.
Beverages:	No problems expected.
Cocaine:	Increases chance of toxicity.
Foods:	Reduced irritation in stomach.
Marijuana:	No problems expected.
Tobacco:	Increases lung toxicity.

MESALAMINE (Rectal)

BRAND NAMES

Mesalazine

BASIC INFORMATION

Habit forming? No
Prescription needed? Yes
Available as generic? No
Drug class: Anti-inflammatory

USES

- Treats ulcerative colitis.
- Reduces inflammatory conditions of the lower colon and rectum.

DOSAGE & USAGE INFORMATION

How to use:
Use as an enema. Insert the tip of the pre-packaged medicine container into the rectum. Squeeze container to empty contents. Retain in rectum all night or as long as possible.

When to use:
Each night, preferably after a bowel movement. Continue for 3 to 6 weeks according to your doctor's instructions.

If you forget a dose:
Take as soon as you remember up to 2 hours late. If more than 2 hours, wait for next scheduled dose (don't double this dose).

What drug does:
Decreases production of arachidonic acid forms which are increased in patients with chronic inflammatory bowel disease.

Time lapse before drug works:
3 to 21 days.

Don't take with:
- Oral sulfasalazine concurrently. To do so may increase chances of kidney damage.
- See Interaction column and consult doctor.

OVERDOSE

SYMPTOMS:
None expected.
WHAT TO DO:
No action needed.

POSSIBLE ADVERSE REACTIONS OR SIDE EFFECTS

SYMPTOMS	WHAT TO DO
Life-threatening: None expected.	
Common: None expected.	
Infrequent: Hair loss.	Continue. Call doctor when convenient.
Rare:	
• Abdominal pain.	Discontinue. Call doctor right away.
• Gaseousness, nausea, headache.	Continue. Call doctor when convenient.

WARNINGS & PRECAUTIONS

Don't take if:
You are allergic to any medication containing sulfasalazine (such as Azulfidine) or mesalamine.

Before you start, consult your doctor:
If you have had chronic kidney disease.

Over age 60:
More sensitive to drug. Aggravates symptoms of enlarged prostate. Causes impaired thinking, hallucinations, nightmares. Consult doctor about any of these.

Pregnancy:
Studies inconclusive on harm to unborn child. Decide with your doctor whether drug benefits justify risk to unborn child.

Breast-feeding:
No problems expected. Consult your doctor.

Infants & children:
Not recommended for children 3 and younger. Use for older children only under doctor's supervision.

Prolonged use:
Possible glaucoma.

Skin & sunlight:
No problems expected.

Driving, piloting or hazardous work:
Don't drive or pilot aircraft until you learn how medicine affects you. Don't work around dangerous machinery. Don't climb ladders or work in high places. Danger increases if you drink alcohol or take medicine affecting alertness and reflexes.

Discontinuing:
Don't discontinue without consulting doctor. Dose may require gradual reduction if you have taken drug for a long time. Doses of other drugs may also require adjustment.

Others:
* Internal eye pressure should be measured regularly.
* Avoid becoming overheated.

POSSIBLE INTERACTION WITH OTHER DRUGS

GENERIC NAME OR DRUG CLASS	COMBINED EFFECT
None expected.	

POSSIBLE INTERACTION WITH OTHER SUBSTANCES

INTERACTS WITH	COMBINED EFFECT
Alcohol:	None expected.
Beverages:	None expected.
Cocaine:	None expected.
Foods:	None expected.
Marijuana:	None expected.
Tobacco:	None expected.

MESORIDAZINE

BRAND NAMES

Serentil

BASIC INFORMATION

Habit forming? No
Prescription needed? Yes
Available as generic? No
Drug class: Tranquilizer, antiemetic
(phenothiazine)

USES

- Stops nausea, vomiting, hiccups.
- Reduces anxiety, agitation.

DOSAGE & USAGE INFORMATION

How to take:
- Tablet or extended-release capsule—Swallow with liquid or food to lessen stomach irritation.
- Drops or liquid—Dilute dose in beverage.

When to take:
- Nervous and mental disorders—Take at the same times each day.
- Nausea and vomiting—Take as needed, no more often than every 4 hours.

If you forget a dose:
- Nervous and mental disorders—Take up to 2 hours late. If more than 2 hours, wait for next scheduled dose (don't double this dose).
- Nausea and vomiting—Take as soon as you remember. Wait 4 hours for next dose.

What drug does:
- Suppresses brain's vomiting center.
- Suppresses brain centers that control abnormal emotions and behavior.

Time lapse before drug works:
- Nausea and vomiting—1 hour or less.
- Nervous and mental disorders—4-6 weeks.

Continued next column

OVERDOSE

SYMPTOMS:
Stupor, convulsions, coma.
WHAT TO DO:
- Dial 0 (operator) or 911 (emergency) for an ambulance or medical help. Then give first aid immediately.
- See emergency information on inside covers.

Don't take with:
- Antacid or medicine for diarrhea.
- Non-prescription drug for cough, cold or allergy.
- See Interaction column and consult doctor.

POSSIBLE ADVERSE REACTIONS OR SIDE EFFECTS

SYMPTOMS	WHAT TO DO
Life-threatening:	
Uncontrolled muscle movements of tongue, face and other muscles (neuroleptic malignant syndrome, rare); unsteady gait.	Discontinue. Seek emergency treatment.
Common:	
• Muscle spasms of face and neck, unsteady gait.	Discontinue. Seek emergency treatment.
• Restlessness, tremor, drowsiness.	Discontinue. Call doctor right away.
• Decreased sweating, dry mouth, runny nose, constipation.	Continue. Call doctor when convenient.
Infrequent:	
• Fainting.	Discontinue. Seek emergency treatment.
• Rash.	Discontinue. Call doctor right away.
• Difficult urination, diminished sex drive, swollen breasts, menstrual irregularities.	Continue. Call doctor when convenient.
Rare:	
Change in vision, jaundice, sore throat, fever, abdominal pain.	Discontinue. Call doctor right away.

618

WARNINGS & PRECAUTIONS

Don't take if:
- You are allergic to any phenothiazine.
- You have a blood or bone-marrow disease.

Before you start, consult your doctor:
- If you will have surgery within 2 months, including dental surgery, requiring general or spinal anesthesia.
- If you have asthma, emphysema or other lung disorder, glaucoma, prostate trouble.
- If you take non-prescription ulcer medicine, asthma medicine or amphetamines.

Over age 60:
Adverse reactions and side effects may be more frequent and severe than in younger persons. More likely to develop involuntary movement of jaws, lips, tongue, chewing. Report this to your doctor immediately. Early treatment can help.

Pregnancy:
Risk to unborn child outweighs drug benefits. Don't use.

Breast-feeding:
Drug passes into milk. Avoid drug or discontinue nursing until you finish medicine. Consult doctor for advice on maintaining milk supply.

Infants & children:
Don't give to children younger than 2.

Prolonged use:
May lead to tardive dyskinesia (involuntary movement of jaws, lips, tongue, chewing).

Skin & sunlight:
May cause rash or intensify sunburn in areas exposed to sun or sunlamp. Skin may remain sensitive for 3 months after discontinuing.

Driving, piloting or hazardous work:
Don't drive or pilot aircraft until you learn how medicine affects you. Don't work around dangerous machinery. Don't climb ladders or work in high places. Danger increases if you drink alcohol or take medicine affecting alertness and reflexes.

Discontinuing:
- Nervous and mental disorders—Don't discontinue without doctor's advice until you complete prescribed dose, even though symptoms diminish or disappear.
- Nausea and vomiting—May be unnecessary to finish medicine. Follow doctor's instructions.

Others:
No problems expected.

POSSIBLE INTERACTION WITH OTHER DRUGS

GENERIC NAME OR DRUG CLASS	COMBINED EFFECT
Anticholinergics*	Increased anti-cholinergic effect.
Antidepressants, tricyclic (TCA)*	Increased mesoridazine effect.
Antihistamines*	Increased antihistamine effect.
Appetite suppressants*	Decreased suppressant effect.
Dronabinol	Increased effects of both drugs. Avoid.
Guanethidine	Decreased guanethidine effect.
Levodopa	Decreased levodopa effect.
Mind-altering drugs*	Increased effect of mind-altering drugs.
Molindone	Increased tranquilizer effect.
Nabilone	Greater depression of central nervous system.
Narcotics*	Increased narcotic effect.
Phenytoin	Increased phenytoin effect.
Procarbazine	Increased sedation.
Quinidine	Impaired heart function. Dangerous mixture.
Sedatives*	Increased sedation.
Tranquilizers, other*	Increased tranquilizer effect.

POSSIBLE INTERACTION WITH OTHER SUBSTANCES

INTERACTS WITH	COMBINED EFFECT
Alcohol:	Dangerous oversedation.
Beverages:	None expected.
Cocaine:	Decreased effect of mesoridazine. Avoid.
Foods:	None expected.
Marijuana:	Drowsiness. May increase antinausea effect.
Tobacco:	None expected.

METAPROTERENOL

BRAND NAMES

Alupent   Metaprel

BASIC INFORMATION

Habit forming? No
Prescription needed? Yes
Available as generic? No
Drug class: Bronchodilator,
   sympathomimetic

 USES

Relieves wheezing and shortness of breath in
bronchial asthma attacks, bronchitis and
emphysema.

 DOSAGE & USAGE INFORMATION

How to take:
- Tablet or liquid—Swallow with liquid or food to
  lessen stomach irritation.
- Inhaler—Follow instructions on package.

When to take:
When needed, according to doctor's
instructions. Don't take more than 2 doses 1
hour apart.

If you forget a dose:
Take when you remember. Wait 2 hours for next
dose.

What drug does:
Relaxes smooth muscles to relieve constriction of
bronchial tubes.

Time lapse before drug works:
5 to 30 minutes.

Don't take with:
See Interaction column and consult doctor.

 OVERDOSE

SYMPTOMS:
Chest pain, irregular heartbeat, convulsions,
coma.
WHAT TO DO:
- Dial 0 (operator) or 911 (emergency) for
  an ambulance or medical help. Then give
  first aid immediately.
- If patient is unconscious and not
  breathing, give mouth-to-mouth
  breathing. If there is no heartbeat, use
  cardiac massage and mouth-to-mouth
  breathing (CPR). Don't try to make patient
  vomit. If you can't get help quickly, take
  patient to nearest emergency facility.
- See emergency information on inside covers.

 POSSIBLE ADVERSE REACTIONS OR SIDE EFFECTS

SYMPTOMS	WHAT TO DO
Life-threatening: None expected.	
Common:	
• Rapid or pounding heartbeat.	Discontinue. Call doctor right away.
• Nervousness, restlessness, dizziness, weakness, headache, shakiness.	Continue. Call doctor when convenient.
Infrequent: Chest pain; muscle cramps in arms, hands, legs; unusual sweating; paleness; bad taste in mouth; nausea or vomiting.	Discontinue. Call doctor right away.
Rare: None expected.	

WARNINGS & PRECAUTIONS

Don't take if:
You are allergic to any sympathomimetic.

Before you start, consult your doctor:
- If you have irregular or rapid heartbeat, congestive heart failure, coronary-artery disease or high blood pressure.
- If you have diabetes.
- If you have overactive thyroid.

Over age 60:
Adverse reactions and side effects may be more frequent and severe than in younger persons.

Pregnancy:
Risk to unborn child outweighs drug benefits. Don't use.

Breast-feeding:
Drug passes into milk. Avoid drug or discontinue nursing until you finish medicine. Consult doctor for advice on maintaining milk supply.

Infants & children:
Use only under medical supervision.

Prolonged use:
No problems expected.

Skin & sunlight:
No problems expected.

Driving, piloting or hazardous work:
Don't drive or pilot aircraft until you learn how medicine affects you. Don't work around dangerous machinery. Don't climb ladders or work in high places. Danger increases if you drink alcohol or take medicine affecting alertness and reflexes, such as antihistamines, tranquilizers, sedatives, pain medicine, narcotics and mind-altering drugs.

Discontinuing:
No problems expected.

Others:
Consult doctor immediately if breathing difficulty continues or worsens after using metaproterenol.

POSSIBLE INTERACTION WITH OTHER DRUGS

GENERIC NAME OR DRUG CLASS	COMBINED EFFECT
Albuterol	Increased effect of both drugs, especially harmful side effects.
Antidepressants, tricyclic (TCA)*	Increased effect of both drugs.
Beta-adrenergic blockers*	Decreased effects of both drugs.
MAO inhibitors*	Possible increased blood pressure.
Nitrates*	Possible decreased effects of both drugs.
Sympathomimetics, other*	Increased effect of both drugs, especially harmful side effects.
Terazosin	Decreases effectiveness of terazosin.
Theophylline	Possible increased response and toxicity to both drugs.

POSSIBLE INTERACTION WITH OTHER SUBSTANCES

INTERACTS WITH	COMBINED EFFECT
Alcohol:	Decreased metaproterenol effect.
Beverages:	None expected.
Cocaine:	High risk of heartbeat irregularities and high blood pressure. Possible metaproterenol toxicity.
Foods:	None expected.
Marijuana:	Overstimulation. Avoid.
Tobacco:	No proven problems.

METAXALONE

BRAND NAMES

Skelaxin

BASIC INFORMATION

Habit forming? Possibly
Prescription needed? Yes
Available as generic? No
Drug class: Muscle relaxant (skeletal)

 ## USES

Adjunctive treatment to rest, analgesics and
physical therapy for muscle spasms.

 ## DOSAGE & USAGE INFORMATION

How to take:
Tablet—Swallow with liquid.

When to take:
As needed, no more often than every 4 hours.

If you forget a dose:
Take as soon as you remember. Wait 4 hours for
next dose.

What drug does:
Blocks body's pain messages to brain. Also
causes sedation.

Time lapse before drug works:
60 minutes.

Don't take with:
See Interaction column and consult doctor.

 ## OVERDOSE

SYMPTOMS:
**Nausea, vomiting, diarrhea, headache. May
progress to severe weakness, difficult
breathing, sensation of paralysis, coma.**
WHAT TO DO:
- **Dial 0 (operator) or 911 (emergency) for
  an ambulance or medical help. Then give
  first aid immediately.**
- **If patient is unconscious and not
  breathing, give mouth-to-mouth
  breathing. If there is no heartbeat, use
  cardiac massage and mouth-to-mouth
  breathing (CPR). Don't try to make patient
  vomit. If you can't get help quickly, take
  patient to nearest emergency facility.**
- **See emergency information on inside
  covers.**

 ## POSSIBLE ADVERSE REACTIONS OR SIDE EFFECTS

SYMPTOMS	WHAT TO DO
Life-threatening:	
Extreme weakness; transient paralysis; temporary loss of vision; hives, rash, intense itching, faintness soon after a dose (anaphylaxis).	Seek emergency treatment immediately.
Common:	
• Drowsiness, fainting, dizziness.	Continue. Call doctor when convenient.
• Orange or red-purple urine.	No action necessary.
Infrequent:	
Agitation, headache, constipation or diarrhea, nausea, cramps, vomiting, wheezing, shortness of breath, depression.	Discontinue. Call doctor right away.
Rare:	
• Black, bloody or tarry stools.	Discontinue. Seek emergency treatment.
• Rash, hives or itch; sore throat; fever; jaundice; tiredness; weakness; hiccups.	Discontinue. Call doctor right away.

WARNINGS & PRECAUTIONS

Don't take if:
- You are allergic to any skeletal-muscle relaxant.
- You have porphyria.

Before you start, consult your doctor:
- If you have had liver or kidney disease.
- If you plan pregnancy within medication period.
- If you are allergic to tartrazine dye.

Over age 60:
Adverse reactions and side effects may be more frequent and severe than in younger persons.

Pregnancy:
Safety not proven. Avoid if possible.

Breast-feeding:
Drug passes into milk. Avoid drug or discontinue nursing until you finish medicine. Consult doctor for advice on maintaining milk supply.

Infants & children:
Not recommended.

Prolonged use:
Periodic liver-function tests recommended if you use this drug for a long time.

Skin & sunlight:
No problems expected.

Driving, piloting or hazardous work:
Don't drive or pilot aircraft until you learn how medicine affects you. Don't work around dangerous machinery. Don't climb ladders or work in high places. Danger increases if you drink alcohol or take medicine affecting alertness and reflexes, such as antihistamines, tranquilizers, sedatives, pain medicine, narcotics and mind-altering drugs.

Discontinuing:
Don't discontinue without doctor's advice until you complete prescribed dose, even though symptoms diminish or disappear.

Others:
No problems expected.

POSSIBLE INTERACTION WITH OTHER DRUGS

GENERIC NAME OR DRUG CLASS	COMBINED EFFECT
Antidepressants*	Increased sedation.
Antihistamines*	Increased sedation.
Dronabinol	Increased effect of dronabinol on central nervous system. Avoid combination.
Mind-altering drugs*	Increased sedation.
Muscle relaxants, other*	Increased sedation.
Narcotics*	Increased sedation.
Sedatives*	Increased sedation.
Sleep inducers*	Increased sedation.
Tranquilizers*	Increased sedation.

POSSIBLE INTERACTION WITH OTHER SUBSTANCES

INTERACTS WITH	COMBINED EFFECT
Alcohol:	Increased sedation.
Beverages:	None expected.
Cocaine:	Lack of coordination, increased sedation.
Foods:	None expected.
Marijuana:	Lack of coordination, drowsiness, fainting.
Tobacco:	None expected.

*See Glossary

METHAMPHETAMINE

BRAND NAMES

Desoxyn   Methampex

BASIC INFORMATION

Habit forming? Yes
Prescription needed? Yes
Available as generic? Yes
Drug class: Central nervous system
  stimulant (amphetamine)

USES

- Prevents narcolepsy (attacks of uncontrollable sleepiness).
- Controls hyperactivity in children.

DOSAGE & USAGE INFORMATION

How to take:
- Tablet—Swallow with liquid.
- Extended-release tablets—Swallow each dose whole with liquid.

When to take:
- At the same times each day.
- Short-acting form—Don't take later than 6 hours before bedtime.
- Long-acting form—Take on awakening.

If you forget a dose:
- Short-acting form—Take up to 2 hours late. If more than 2 hours, wait for next dose (don't double this dose).
- Long-acting form—Take as soon as you remember. Wait 20 hours for next dose.

What drug does:
- Narcolepsy—Apparently affects brain centers to decrease fatigue or sleepiness and increase alertness and motor activity.
- Hyperactive children—Calms children, opposite to effect on narcoleptic adults.

Continued next column

OVERDOSE

SYMPTOMS:
Rapid heartbeat, hyperactivity, high fever, hallucinations, suicidal or homicidal feelings, convulsions, coma.
WHAT TO DO:
- **Dial 0 (operator) or 911 (emergency) for an ambulance or medical help. Then give first aid immediately.**
- **See emergency information on inside covers.**

Time lapse before drug works:
15 to 30 minutes.

Don't take with:
See Interaction column and consult doctor.

POSSIBLE ADVERSE REACTIONS OR SIDE EFFECTS

SYMPTOMS	WHAT TO DO
Life-threatening: None expected.	
Common: • Irritability, insomnia, nervousness.	Continue. Call doctor when convenient.
• Dry mouth.	Continue. Tell doctor at next visit.
Infrequent: • Dizziness; lack of alertness; blurred vision; fast, pounding heartbeat; unusual sweating.	Discontinue. Call doctor right away.
• Headache.	Continue. Call doctor when convenient.
• Diarrhea or constipation, appetite loss, stomach pain, nausea, vomiting, weight loss, diminished sex drive, impotence.	Continue. Tell doctor at next visit.
Rare: • Pancytopenia (reduced blood cells of all kinds, causing weakness, paleness, sore throat and fever).	Discontinue. Seek emergency treatment.
• Rash; hives; chest pain or irregular heartbeat; uncontrollable movements of head, neck, arms, legs.	Discontinue. Call doctor right away.
• Swollen breasts, mood change.	Continue. Call doctor when convenient.

624

WARNINGS & PRECAUTIONS

Don't take if:
- You are allergic to any methamphetamine.
- You will have surgery within 2 months, including dental surgery, requiring general or spinal anesthesia.

Before you start, consult your doctor:
- If you plan to become pregnant within medication period.
- If you have glaucoma.
- If you have heart or blood-vessel disease, or high blood pressure.
- If you have overactive thyroid, anxiety or tension.
- If you have a severe mental illness (especially children).

Over age 60:
Adverse reactions and side effects may be more frequent and severe than in younger persons.

Pregnancy:
Risk to unborn child outweighs drug benefits. Don't use.

Breast-feeding:
Drug passes into milk. Avoid drug or discontinue nursing.

Infants & children:
Not recommended for children under 12.

Prolonged use:
Habit forming.

Skin & sunlight:
No problems expected.

Driving, piloting or hazardous work:
Don't drive or pilot aircraft until you learn how medicine affects you. Don't work around dangerous machinery. Don't climb ladders or work in high places. Danger increases if you drink alcohol or take medicine affecting alertness and reflexes.

Discontinuing:
May be unnecessary to finish medicine. Follow doctor's instructions.

Others:
- This is a dangerous drug and must be closely supervised. Don't use for appetite control or depression. Potential for damage and abuse.
- During withdrawal phase, may cause prolonged sleep of several days.

POSSIBLE INTERACTION WITH OTHER DRUGS

GENERIC NAME OR DRUG CLASS	COMBINED EFFECT
Anesthesias, general*	Irregular heartbeat.
Antidepressants, tricyclic (TCA)*	Decreased methamphetamine effect.
Antihypertensives*	Decreased antihypertensive effect.
Barbiturates*	Decreased methamphetamine effect.
Carbonic anhydrase inhibitors*	Increased methamphetamine effect.
Guanadrel	Decreased guanadrel effect. Insulin requirements may change.
Guanethidine	Decreased guanethidine effect. Insulin requirements may change.
Haloperidol	Decreased methamphetamine effect.
MAO inhibitors*	May severely increase blood pressure.
Nabilone	Greater depression of central nervous system.
Phenothiazines*	Decreased methamphetamine effect.
Sodium bicarbonate	Increased methamphetamine effect.

POSSIBLE INTERACTION WITH OTHER SUBSTANCES

INTERACTS WITH	COMBINED EFFECT
Alcohol:	Decreased methamphetamine effect. Avoid.
Beverages: Caffeine drinks.	Overstimulation. Avoid.
Cocaine:	Dangerous stimulation of nervous system. Avoid.
Foods:	None expected.
Marijuana:	Frequent use— Severely impaired mental function.
Tobacco:	None expected.

*See Glossary

METHARBITAL

BRAND NAMES

Gemonil

BASIC INFORMATION

Habit forming? Yes
Prescription needed? Yes
Available as generic? No
Drug class: Sedative, hypnotic (barbiturate)

 ## USES

Prevents convulsions.

 ## DOSAGE & USAGE INFORMATION

How to take:
Tablet—Swallow with liquid or food to lessen
stomach irritation. If you can't swallow whole,
crumble tablet and take with liquid or food.

When to take:
At the same times each day.

If you forget a dose:
Take as soon as you remember up to 2 hours
late. If more than 2 hours, wait for next
scheduled dose (don't double this dose).

What drug does:
May partially block nerve impulses at nerve-cell
connections.

Time lapse before drug works:
60 minutes.

Don't take with:
- Non-prescription drugs without consulting
  doctor.
- See Interaction column and consult doctor.

 ## OVERDOSE

SYMPTOMS:
Deep sleep, weak pulse, coma.
WHAT TO DO:
- **Dial 0 (operator) or 911 (emergency) for
  an ambulance or medical help. Then give
  first aid immediately.**
- **If patient is unconscious and not
  breathing, give mouth-to-mouth
  breathing. If there is no heartbeat use
  cardiac massage and mouth-to-mouth
  breathing (CPR). Don't try to make patient
  vomit. If you can't get help quickly, take
  patient to nearest emergency facility.**
- **See emergency information on inside
  covers.**

 ## POSSIBLE ADVERSE REACTIONS OR SIDE EFFECTS

SYMPTOMS	WHAT TO DO
Life-threatening:	
Hives, rash, intense itching, faintness soon after a dose (anaphylaxis).	Seek emergency treatment immediately.
Common:	
Dizziness, drowsiness, "hangover" effect.	Continue. Call doctor when convenient.
Infrequent:	
• Rash or hives; fever; face, lip or eyelid swelling; sore throat.	Discontinue. Call doctor right away.
• Depression, confusion, slurred speech, diarrhea, nausea, vomiting, joint or muscle pain.	Continue. Call doctor when convenient.
Rare:	
• Agitation, slow heartbeat, difficult breathing, jaundice.	Discontinue. Call doctor right away.
• Unusual bleeding or bruising.	Continue. Call doctor when convenient.

 ## WARNINGS & PRECAUTIONS

Don't take if:
- You are allergic to any barbiturate.
- You have porphyria.

Before you start, consult your doctor:
- If you have epilepsy.
- If you have kidney or liver damage.
- If you have asthma.
- If you have anemia.
- If you have chronic pain.
- If you will have surgery within 2 months,
  including dental surgery, requiring general or
  spinal anesthesia.

Over age 60:
Adverse reactions and side effects may be more
frequent and severe than in younger persons.
Use small doses.

Pregnancy:
Risk to unborn child outweighs drug benefits.
Don't use.

Breast-feeding:
Drug passes into milk. Avoid drug or discontinue
nursing until you finish medicine. Consult doctor
for advice on maintaining milk supply.

Infants & children:
Use only under doctor's supervision.

Prolonged use:
- May cause addiction, anemia, chronic intoxication.
- May lower body temperature, making exposure to cold temperatures hazardous.

Skin & sunlight:
May cause rash or intensify sunburn in areas exposed to sun or sunlamp.

Driving, piloting or hazardous work:
Don't drive or pilot aircraft until you learn how medicine affects you. Don't work around dangerous machinery. Don't climb ladders or work in high places. Danger increases if you drink alcohol or take medicine affecting alertness and reflexes.

Discontinuing:
May be unnecessary to finish medicine. Follow doctor's instructions. If you develop withdrawal symptoms of hallucinations, agitation or sleeplessness after discontinuing, call doctor right away.

Others:
Great potential for abuse.

POSSIBLE INTERACTION WITH OTHER DRUGS

GENERIC NAME OR DRUG CLASS	COMBINED EFFECT
Anticoagulants, oral*	Decreased anticoagulant effect.
Anticonvulsants*	Changed seizure patterns.
Antidepressants, tricyclics (TCA)*	Decreased antidepressant effect. Possible dangerous oversedation.
Antidiabetics, oral*	Increased metharbital effect.
Antihistamines*	Dangerous sedation. Avoid.
Aspirin	Decreased aspirin effect.
Beta-adrenergic blockers*	Decreased effect of beta-adrenergic blocker.
Carteolol	Increased barbiturate effect. Dangerous sedation.
Contraceptives, oral*	Decreased contraceptive effect.
Cortisone drugs*	Decreased cortisone effect.
Digitoxin	Decreased digitoxin effect.
Disulfiram	Possible increased metharbital effect.
Doxycycline	Decreased doxycycline effect.
Dronabinol	Increased effects of both drugs. Avoid.
Estrogen	Decreased estrogen effect.
Griseofulvin	Possible decreased griseofulvin effect.
Indapamide	Increased indapamide effect.
MAO inhibitors*	Increased metharbital effect.
Metronidazole	Possible decreased metronidazole effect.
Mind-altering drugs*	Dangerous sedation. Avoid.
Nabilone	Greater depression of central nervous system.
Narcotics*	Dangerous sedation. Avoid.
Non-steroidal anti-inflammatory drugs (NSAIDs)*	Decreased anti-inflammatory effect.
Pain relievers*	Dangerous sedation. Avoid.
Rifampin	Possible decreased metharbital effect.
Sedatives*	Dangerous sedation. Avoid.

Continued page 1090

POSSIBLE INTERACTION WITH OTHER SUBSTANCES

INTERACTS WITH	COMBINED EFFECT
Alcohol:	Possible fatal oversedation. Avoid.
Beverages:	None expected.
Cocaine:	Decreased metharbital effect.
Foods:	None expected.
Marijuana:	Excessive sedation. Avoid.
Tobacco:	None expected.

*See Glossary

METHENAMINE

BRAND NAMES

Azo-Mandelamine
Hexamine
Hip-Rex
Hiprex
Mandelamine
Mandelets
Methandine
Prov-U-Sep

Renalgin
Sterine
Trac 2X
Urex
Urised
Uro-phosphate
Uroblue
Uroquid-Acid

BASIC INFORMATION

Habit forming? No
Prescription needed? Yes
Available as generic? Yes
Drug class: Anti-infective (urinary)

USES

Suppresses chronic urinary-tract infections.

DOSAGE & USAGE INFORMATION

How to take:
• Tablet—Swallow with liquid or food to lessen stomach irritation. If you can't swallow whole, crumble tablet and take with liquid or food.
• Liquid form—Use a measuring spoon to ensure correct dose.
• Granules—Dissolve dose in 4 oz. of water. Drink all the liquid.

When to take:
At the same times each day.

If you forget a dose:
Take as soon as you remember up to 8 hours late. If more than 8 hours, wait for next scheduled dose (don't double this dose).

What drug does:
A chemical reaction in the urine changes methenamine into formaldehyde, which destroys certain bacteria.

Continued next column

OVERDOSE

SYMPTOMS:
Bloody urine, weakness, deep breathing, stupor, coma.
WHAT TO DO:
• Dial 0 (operator) or 911 (emergency) for an ambulance or medical help. Then give first aid immediately.
• See emergency information on inside covers.

Time lapse before drug works:
Continual use for 3 to 6 months.

Don't take with:
See Interaction column and consult doctor.

POSSIBLE ADVERSE REACTIONS OR SIDE EFFECTS

SYMPTOMS	WHAT TO DO
Life-threatening: None expected.	
Common:	
• Rash.	Discontinue. Call doctor right away.
• Nausea, difficult urination.	Continue. Call doctor when convenient.
Infrequent:	
• Blood in urine.	Discontinue. Call doctor right away.
• Burning on urination, lower back pain.	Continue. Call doctor when convenient.
Rare: None expected.	

WARNINGS & PRECAUTIONS

Don't take if:
- You are allergic to methenamine.
- You have a severe impairment of kidney or liver function.
- The urine cannot or should not be acidified (check with your doctor).

Before you start, consult your doctor:
- If you have had kidney or liver disease.
- If you plan to become pregnant within medication period.
- If you have had gout.

Over age 60:
Don't exceed recommended dose.

Pregnancy:
Studies inconclusive on harm to unborn child. Avoid if possible, especially first 3 months.

Breast-feeding:
Drug passes into milk in small amounts. Consult doctor.

Infants & children:
Use only under medical supervision.

Prolonged use:
No problems expected.

Skin & sunlight:
No problems expected.

Driving, piloting or hazardous work:
No problems expected.

Discontinuing:
Don't discontinue without doctor's advice until you complete prescribed dose, even though symptoms diminish or disappear.

Others:
Requires an acid urine to be effective. Eat more protein foods, cranberries, cranberry juice with vitamin C, plums, prunes.

POSSIBLE INTERACTION WITH OTHER DRUGS

GENERIC NAME OR DRUG CLASS	COMBINED EFFECT
Antacids*	Decreased methenamine effect.
Carbonic anhydrase inhibitors*	Decreased methenamine effect.
Citrates*	Decreases effects of methenamine.
Diuretics, thiazide*	Decreased urine acidity.
Sodium bicarbonate	Decreased methenamine effect.
Sulfa drugs*	Possible kidney damage.
Vitamin C (1 to 4 grams per day)	Increased effect of methenamine, contributing to urine's acidity.

POSSIBLE INTERACTION WITH OTHER SUBSTANCES

INTERACTS WITH	COMBINED EFFECT
Alcohol:	Possible brain depression. Avoid or use with caution.
Beverages: Milk.	Decreased methenamine effect.
Cocaine:	None expected.
Foods:	None expected.
Marijuana:	Drowsiness, muscle weakness or blood-pressure drop.
Tobacco:	None expected.

METHICILLIN

BRAND NAMES

Azapen   Staphcillin
Celbenin

BASIC INFORMATION

Habit forming? No
Prescription needed? Yes
Available as generic? No
Drug class: Antibiotic (penicillin)

USES

Treatment of bacterial infections that are
susceptible to methicillin.

DOSAGE & USAGE INFORMATION

How to take:
By injection only.

When to take:
Follow doctor's instructions.

If you forget a dose:
Consult doctor.

What drug does:
Destroys susceptible bacteria. Does not kill
viruses.

Time lapse before drug works:
May be several days before medicine affects
infection.

Don't take with:
See Interaction column and consult doctor.

OVERDOSE

SYMPTOMS:
Severe diarrhea, nausea or vomiting.
WHAT TO DO:
Overdose unlikely to threaten life. If person
takes much larger amount than prescribed,
call doctor, poison-control center or hospital
emergency room for instructions.

POSSIBLE ADVERSE REACTIONS OR SIDE EFFECTS

SYMPTOMS	WHAT TO DO
Life-threatening: Hives, rash, intense itching, faintness soon after a dose (anaphylaxis).	Seek emergency treatment immediately.
Common: Dark or discolored tongue.	Continue. Tell doctor at next visit.
Infrequent: Mild nausea, vomiting, diarrhea.	Continue. Call doctor when convenient.
Rare: Unexplained bleeding.	Discontinue. Call doctor right away.

WARNINGS & PRECAUTIONS

Don't take if:
You are allergic to methicillin, cephalosporin antibiotics, other penicillins or penicillamine. Life-threatening reaction may occur.

Before you start, consult your doctor:
If you are allergic to any substance or drug.

Over age 60:
You may have skin reactions, particularly around genitals and anus.

Pregnancy:
Studies inconclusive on harm to unborn child. Animal studies show fetal abnormalities. Decide with your doctor whether drug benefits justify risk to unborn child.

Breast-feeding:
Drug passes into milk. Child may become sensitive to penicillins and have allergic reactions to penicillin drugs. Avoid methicillin or discontinue nursing until you finish medicine. Consult doctor for advice on maintaining milk supply.

Infants & children:
No problems expected.

Prolonged use:
- You may become more susceptible to infections caused by germs not responsive to methicillin.
- May cause kidney damage. Laboratory studies to detect damage recommended if you take for a long time.

Skin & sunlight:
No problems expected.

Driving, piloting or hazardous work:
Usually not dangerous. Most hazardous reactions likely to occur a few minutes after taking methicillin.

Discontinuing:
Don't discontinue without doctor's advice until you complete prescribed dose, even though symptoms diminish or disappear.

Others:
No problems expected.

POSSIBLE INTERACTION WITH OTHER DRUGS

GENERIC NAME OR DRUG CLASS	COMBINED EFFECT
Beta-adrenergic blockers*	Increased chance of anaphylaxis (see emergency information on inside front cover).
Chloramphenicol	Decreased effect of both drugs.
Erythromycins*	Decreased effect of both drugs.
Loperamide	Decreased methicillin effect.
Paromomycin	Decreased effect of both drugs.
Tetracyclines*	Decreased effect of both drugs.
Troleandomycin	Decreased effect of both drugs.

POSSIBLE INTERACTION WITH OTHER SUBSTANCES

INTERACTS WITH	COMBINED EFFECT
Alcohol:	Occasional stomach irritation.
Beverages:	None expected.
Cocaine:	No proven problems.
Foods:	None expected.
Marijuana:	No proven problems.
Tobacco:	None expected.

*See Glossary

METHOCARBAMOL

BRAND NAMES

Delaxin	Robamol
Forbaxin	Robaxin
Marbaxin	Robaxisal
Marbaxin-750	Spinaxin
Metho-500	Tumol

BASIC INFORMATION

Habit forming? Possibly
Prescription needed? Yes
Available as generic? Yes
Drug class: Muscle relaxant (skeletal)

USES

Adjunctive treatment to rest, analgesics and physical therapy for muscle spasms.

DOSAGE & USAGE INFORMATION

How to take:
Tablet—Swallow with liquid. If you can't swallow whole, crumble tablet and take with liquid or food.

When to take:
As directed on label.

If you forget a dose:
Take as soon as you remember up to 2 hours late. If more than 2 hours, wait for next scheduled dose (don't double this dose).

What drug does:
Blocks reflex nerve impulses in brain and spinal cord.

Continued next column

OVERDOSE

SYMPTOMS:
Unsteadiness, lack of coordination, extreme weakness, paralysis, weak and rapid pulse, shallow breathing, cold and sweaty skin.
WHAT TO DO:
- Dial 0 (operator) or 911 (emergency) for an ambulance or medical help. Then give first aid immediately.
- If patient is unconscious and not breathing, give mouth-to-mouth breathing. If there is no heartbeat, use cardiac massage and mouth-to-mouth breathing (CPR). Don't try to make patient vomit. If you can't get help quickly, take patient to nearest emergency facility.
- See emergency information on inside covers.

Time lapse before drug works:
30 to 45 minutes.

Don't take with:
- Non-prescription drugs containing alcohol without consulting doctor.
- See Interaction column and consult doctor.

POSSIBLE ADVERSE REACTIONS OR SIDE EFFECTS

SYMPTOMS	WHAT TO DO
Life-threatening: Extreme weakness; transient paralysis; temporary loss of vision; hives, rash, intense itching, faintness soon after a dose (anaphylaxis).	Seek emergency treatment immediately.
Common: • Blurred or double vision.	Discontinue. Call doctor right away.
• Dizziness, drowsiness, lightheadedness.	Continue. Call doctor when convenient.
Infrequent: • Rash, itchy skin.	Discontinue. Call doctor right away.
• Headache, bloodshot eyes, metallic taste, fever, agitation, depression.	Continue. Call doctor when convenient.
• Stuffy nose, nausea.	Continue. Tell doctor at next visit.
Rare: Hiccups.	Discontinue. Call doctor right away.

METHOCARBAMOL

WARNINGS & PRECAUTIONS

Don't take if:
You are allergic to any muscle relaxant.

Before you start, consult your doctor:
- If you have epilepsy.
- If you have myasthenia gravis.
- If you have impaired kidney function.
- If you are allergic to tartrazine dye.

Over age 60:
Adverse reactions and side effects may be more frequent and severe than in younger persons.

Pregnancy:
Safety not established. Avoid if possible.

Breast-feeding:
Drug filters into milk. May harm child. Avoid.

Infants & children:
Not recommended.

Prolonged use:
No problems expected.

Skin & sunlight:
No problems expected.

Driving, piloting or hazardous work:
Don't drive or pilot aircraft until you learn how medicine affects you. Don't work around dangerous machinery. Don't climb ladders or work in high places. Danger increases if you drink alcohol or take medicine affecting alertness and reflexes, such as antihistamines, tranquilizers, sedatives, pain medicine, narcotics and mind-altering drugs.

Discontinuing:
May be unnecessary to finish medicine. Follow doctor's instructions.

Others:
No problems expected.

POSSIBLE INTERACTION WITH OTHER DRUGS

GENERIC NAME OR DRUG CLASS	COMBINED EFFECT
Antidepressants, tricyclic (TCA)*	Increased effect of both drugs.
Antimyasthenics*	Decreased anti-myasthenic effect.
Dronabinol	Increased effect of dronabinol on central nervous system. Avoid combination.
Narcotics*	Increased sedative effect.
Sedatives*	Increased sedative effect.
Sleep inducers*	Increased effect of sleep inducer.
Tranquilizers*	Increased tranquilizer effect.

POSSIBLE INTERACTION WITH OTHER SUBSTANCES

INTERACTS WITH	COMBINED EFFECT
Alcohol:	Depressed brain function. Avoid.
Beverages:	None expected.
Cocaine:	May increase muscle spasms.
Foods:	None expected.
Marijuana:	Drowsiness, muscle weakness, lack of coordination, fainting.
Tobacco:	None expected.

METHOTREXATE

BRAND NAMES

Folex	Mexate
Folex PFS	Mexate AQ

BASIC INFORMATION

Habit forming? No
Prescription needed? Yes
Available as generic? Yes
Drug class: Antimetabolite, antipsoriatic

 USES

- Treatment for some kinds of cancer.
- Treatment for psoriasis in patients with severe problems.
- Treatment for severe rheumatoid arthritis.

 DOSAGE & USAGE INFORMATION

How to take:
Tablet—Swallow with liquid.

When to take:
At the same time each day.

If you forget a dose:
Skip the missed dose. Don't double the next dose.

What drug does:
Inhibits abnormal-cell reproduction.

Time lapse before drug works:
May require 6 weeks for maximum effect.

Don't take with:
See Interaction column and consult doctor.

 OVERDOSE

SYMPTOMS:
Headache, stupor, seizures.
WHAT TO DO:
- Dial 0 (operator) or 911 (emergency) for an ambulance or medical help. Then give first aid immediately.
- If patient is unconscious and not breathing, give mouth-to-mouth breathing. If there is no heartbeat, use cardiac massage and mouth-to-mouth breathing (CPR). Don't try to make patient vomit. If you can't get help quickly, take patient to nearest emergency facility.
- See emergency information on inside covers.

 POSSIBLE ADVERSE REACTIONS OR SIDE EFFECTS

SYMPTOMS	WHAT TO DO
Life-threatening:	
Hives, rash, intense itching, faintness soon after a dose (anaphylaxis).	Seek emergency treatment immediately.
Common:	
• Black stools or bloody vomit.	Discontinue. Seek emergency treatment.
• Sore throat, fever, mouth sores; chills; unusual bleeding or bruising.	Discontinue. Call doctor right away.
• Stomach pain, nausea, vomiting.	Continue. Call doctor when convenient.
Infrequent:	
• Seizures.	Discontinue. Seek emergency treatment.
• Dizziness when standing after sitting or lying, drowsiness, headache, confusion, blurred vision, shortness of breath, joint pain, blood in urine, jaundice.	Discontinue. Call doctor right away.
• Cough, rash.	Continue. Call doctor when convenient.
• Acne, boils, hair loss, itchy skin.	Continue. Tell doctor at next visit.
Rare:	
None expected.	

WARNINGS & PRECAUTIONS

Don't take if:
You are allergic to any antimetabolite.

Before you start, consult your doctor:
- If you are alcoholic.
- If you have blood, liver or kidney disease.
- If you have colitis or peptic ulcer.
- If you have gout.
- If you have an infection.
- If you plan to become pregnant within 3 months.

Over age 60:
Adverse reactions and side effects may be more frequent and severe than in younger persons.

Pregnancy:
- Psoriasis—Risk to unborn child outweighs drug benefits. Don't use.
- Cancer—Consult doctor.

Breast-feeding:
Drug passes into milk. Avoid drug or discontinue nursing.

Infants & children:
Use only under special medical supervision.

Prolonged use:
Adverse reactions more likely the longer drug is required.

Skin & sunlight:
Increased sensitivity to sunlight.

Driving, piloting or hazardous work:
Avoid if you feel dizzy, drowsy or confused. Otherwise, no problems expected.

Discontinuing:
Don't discontinue without doctor's advice until you complete prescribed dose, even though symptoms diminish or disappear. Some side effects may follow discontinuing. Report to doctor blurred vision, convulsions, confusion, persistent headache.

Others:
- Drink more water than usual to cause frequent urination.
- Don't give this medicine to anyone else for any purpose. It is a strong drug that requires close medical supervision.
- Report for frequent medical follow-up and laboratory studies.

POSSIBLE INTERACTION WITH OTHER DRUGS

GENERIC NAME OR DRUG CLASS	COMBINED EFFECT
Anticoagulants, oral*	Increased anti-coagulant effect.
Anticonvulsants, hydantoin*	Possible methotrexate toxicity.
Antigout drugs*	Decreased antigout effect.
Asparaginase	Decreased methotrexate effect.
Diclofenac	May increase toxicity.
Etretinate	Increased chance of toxicity to liver.
Fluorouracil	Decreased methotrexate effect.
Folic acid	Possible decreased methotrexate effect.
Leukovorin calcium	Decreased methotrexate toxicity.
Non-steroidal anti-inflammatory drugs (NSAIDs)*	Possible increased methotrexate toxicity.
Oxyphenbutazone	Possible methotrexate toxicity.
Phenylbutazone	Possible methotrexate toxicity.
Phenytoin	Possible increased methotrexate toxicity.
Probenecid	Possible methotrexate toxicity.
Pyrimethamine	Increased toxic effect of methotrexate.
Salicylates* (including aspirin)	Possible methotrexate toxicity.
Sulfa drugs*	Possible methotrexate toxicity.
Tetracyclines*	Possible methotrexate toxicity.

POSSIBLE INTERACTION WITH OTHER SUBSTANCES

INTERACTS WITH	COMBINED EFFECT
Alcohol:	Likely liver damage. Avoid.
Beverages:	Extra fluid intake decreases chance of methotrexate toxicity.
Cocaine:	Increased chance of methotrexate adverse reactions. Avoid.
Foods:	None expected.
Marijuana:	None expected.
Tobacco:	None expected.

*See Glossary

METHSUXIMIDE

BRAND NAMES

Celontin

BASIC INFORMATION

Habit forming? No
Prescription needed? Yes
Available as generic? No
Drug class: Anticonvulsant (succinimide)

 USES

Controls seizures in treatment of epilepsy.

 DOSAGE & USAGE INFORMATION

How to take:
Capsule—Swallow with liquid or food to lessen stomach irritation.

When to take:
Every day in regularly spaced doses, according to prescription.

If you forget a dose:
Take as soon as you remember up to 2 hours late. If more than 2 hours, wait for next scheduled dose (don't double this dose).

What drug does:
Depresses nerve transmissions in part of brain that controls muscles.

Time lapse before drug works:
3 hours.

Don't take with:
See Interaction column and consult doctor.

 OVERDOSE

SYMPTOMS:
Coma
WHAT TO DO:
- Dial 0 (operator) or 911 (emergency) for an ambulance or medical help. Then give first aid immediately.
- If patient is unconscious and not breathing, give mouth-to-mouth breathing. If there is no heartbeat, use cardiac massage and mouth-to-mouth breathing (CPR). Don't try to make patient vomit. If you can't get help quickly, take patient to nearest emergency facility.
- See emergency information on inside covers.

 POSSIBLE ADVERSE REACTIONS OR SIDE EFFECTS

SYMPTOMS	WHAT TO DO
Life-threatening: None expected.	
Common: Nausea, vomiting, stomach cramps, appetite loss, dizziness, drowsiness.	Continue. Call doctor when convenient.
Infrequent: Headache, irritability mood change, blurred vision.	Continue. Call doctor when convenient.
Rare: • Rash, sore throat, fever, unusual bleeding or bruising, depression, confusion, eye or gum swelling, blood in urine, vaginal bleeding.	Discontinue. Call doctor right away.
• Swollen lymph glands.	Continue. Call doctor when convenient.

WARNINGS & PRECAUTIONS

Don't take if:
You are allergic to any succinimide anticonvulsant.

Before you start, consult your doctor:
- If you plan to become pregnant within medication period.
- If you take other anticonvulsants.
- If you have blood disease.
- If you have kidney or liver disease.

Over age 60:
Adverse reactions and side effects may be more frequent and severe than in younger persons.

Pregnancy:
Risk to unborn child outweighs drug benefits. Don't use.

Breast-feeding:
Drug passes into milk. Avoid drug or discontinue nursing.

Infants & children:
Use only under medical supervision.

Prolonged use:
No problems expected.

Skin & sunlight:
No problems expected.

Driving, piloting or hazardous work:
Don't drive or pilot aircraft until you learn how medicine affects you. Don't work around dangerous machinery. Don't climb ladders or work in high places. Danger increases if you drink alcohol or take medicine affecting alertness and reflexes, such as antihistamines, tranquilizers, sedatives, pain medicine, narcotics and mind-altering drugs.

Discontinuing:
Don't discontinue without doctor's advice until you complete prescribed dose, even though symptoms diminish or disappear.

Others:
- Your response to medicine should be checked regularly by your doctor. Dose and schedule may have to be altered frequently to fit individual needs.
- Periodic blood-cell counts, kidney- and liver-function studies recommended.
- May discolor urine pink to red-brown. No action necessary.

POSSIBLE INTERACTION WITH OTHER DRUGS

GENERIC NAME OR DRUG CLASS	COMBINED EFFECT
Anticonvulsants, other*	Increased effect of both drugs.
Antidepressants, tricyclic (TCA)*	May provoke seizures.
Antipsychotics*	May provoke seizures.

POSSIBLE INTERACTION WITH OTHER SUBSTANCES

INTERACTS WITH	COMBINED EFFECT
Alcohol:	May provoke seizures.
Beverages:	None expected.
Cocaine:	May provoke seizures.
Foods:	None expected.
Marijuana:	May provoke seizures.
Tobacco:	None expected.

METHYCLOTHIAZIDE

BRAND NAMES

Aquatensen
Diutensen
Duretic

Enduron
Enduronyl

BASIC INFORMATION

Habit forming? No
Prescription needed? Yes
Available as generic? Yes
Drug class: Antihypertensive, diuretic (thiazide)

USES

- Controls, but doesn't cure, high blood pressure.
- Reduces fluid retention (edema) caused by conditions such as heart disorders and liver disease.

DOSAGE & USAGE INFORMATION

How to take:
Tablet—Swallow with liquid. If you can't swallow whole, crumble tablet and take with liquid or food. Don't exceed dose.

When to take:
At the same time each day.

If you forget a dose:
Take as soon as you remember up to 2 hours late. If more than 2 hours, wait for next scheduled dose (don't double this dose).

What drug does:
- Forces sodium and water excretion, reducing body fluid.
- Relaxes muscle cells of small arteries.
- Reduced body fluid and relaxed arteries lower blood pressure.

Continued next column

OVERDOSE

SYMPTOMS:
Cramps, weakness, drowsiness, weak pulse, coma.
WHAT TO DO:
- Dial 0 (operator) or 911 (emergency) for an ambulance or medical help. Then give first aid immediately.
- See emergency information on inside covers.

Time lapse before drug works:
4 to 6 hours. May require several weeks to lower blood pressure.

Don't take with:
- Non-prescription drugs without consulting doctor.
- See Interaction column and consult doctor.

POSSIBLE ADVERSE REACTIONS OR SIDE EFFECTS

SYMPTOMS	WHAT TO DO
Life-threatening: None expected.	
Common: None expected.	
Infrequent:	
• Blurred vision, severe abdominal pain, nausea, vomiting, irregular heartbeat, weak pulse.	Discontinue. Call doctor right away.
• Dizziness, mood change, headache, weakness, tiredness, weight changes.	Continue. Call doctor when convenient.
• Dry mouth, thirst.	Continue. Tell doctor at next visit.
Rare:	
• Rash or hives.	Discontinue. Seek emergency treatment.
• Jaundice, sore throat, fever.	Discontinue. Call doctor right away.

WARNINGS & PRECAUTIONS

Don't take if:
You are allergic to any thiazide diuretic drug.

Before you start, consult your doctor:
- If you are allergic to any sulfa drug.
- If you have gout.
- If you have liver, pancreas or kidney disorder.

Over age 60:
Adverse reactions and side effects may be more frequent and severe than in younger persons, especially dizziness and excessive potassium loss.

Pregnancy:
Risk to unborn child outweighs drug benefits. Don't use.

Breast-feeding:
Drug passes into milk. Avoid drug or discontinue nursing.

Infants & children:
No problems expected.

Prolonged use:
You may need medicine to treat high blood pressure for the rest of your life.

Skin & sunlight:
May cause rash or intensify sunburn in areas exposed to sun or sunlamp.

Driving, piloting or hazardous work:
Don't drive or pilot aircraft until you learn how medicine affects you. Don't work around dangerous machinery. Don't climb ladders or work in high places. Danger increases if you drink alcohol or take medicine affecting alertness and reflexes, such as antihistamines, tranquilizers, sedatives, pain medicine, narcotics and mind-altering drugs.

Discontinuing:
Don't discontinue without medical advice.

Others:
- Hot weather and fever may cause dehydration and drop in blood pressure. Dose may require temporary adjustment. Weigh daily and report any unexpected weight decreases to your doctor.
- May cause rise in uric acid, leading to gout.
- May cause blood-sugar rise in diabetics.

POSSIBLE INTERACTION WITH OTHER DRUGS

GENERIC NAME OR DRUG CLASS	COMBINED EFFECT
ACE inhibitors: captopril, enalapril, lisinopril*	Decreased blood pressure. Possible excessive potassium in blood.
Allopurinol	Decreased allopurinol effect.
Amiodarone	Increased risk of heartbeat irregularity due to low potassium.
Amphotericin B	Increased potassium.
Antidiabetic agents, oral*	Increased blood sugar.
Antidepressants, tricyclic (TCA)*	Dangerous drop in blood pressure. Avoid combination unless under medical supervision.
Barbiturates*	Increased methyclothiazide effect.
Beta-adrenergic blockers*	Increased antihypertensive effect. Dosages of both drugs may require adjustment.

Calcium supplements*	Increased calcium in blood.
Carteolol	Increased antihypertensive effect.
Cholestyramine	Decreased methyclothiazide effect.
Colestipol	Decreased methyclothiazide effect.
Cortisone drugs*	Excessive potassium loss that causes dangerous heart rhythms.
Digitalis preparations*	Excessive potassium loss that causes dangerous heart rhythms.
Diuretics, thiazide*	Increased effect of other thiazide diuretics.
Indapamide	Increased diuretic effect.
Indomethacin	Decreased methyclothiazide effect.
Lithium	Increased effect of lithium.
MAO inhibitors*	Increased metolazone effect.
Nicardipine	Blood-pressure drop. Dosages may require adjustment.
Nitrates*	Excessive blood-pressure drop.
Opiates*	Weakness and faintness when arising from bed or chair.

Continued page 1090

POSSIBLE INTERACTION WITH OTHER SUBSTANCES

INTERACTS WITH	COMBINED EFFECT
Alcohol:	Dangerous blood-pressure drop.
Beverages:	None expected.
Cocaine:	Increased risk of heart block and high blood pressure.
Foods: Licorice.	Excessive potassium loss that causes dangerous heart rhythms.
Marijuana:	May increase blood pressure.
Tobacco:	None expected.

*See Glossary

METHYLCELLULOSE

BRAND NAMES

Anorex-CCK	Gonio-Gel
Cellothyl	Hydrolose
Citrucel	Lacril
Cologel	Murocel

BASIC INFORMATION

Habit forming? No
Prescription needed? No
Available as generic? Yes
Drug class: Laxative (bulk-forming)

USES

Relieves constipation and prevents straining for bowel movement.

DOSAGE & USAGE INFORMATION

How to take:
Tablet, liquid, powder, flakes, granules—Dilute dose in 8 oz. cold water or fruit juice. Drink 6 to 8 glasses of water each day in addition to the one with each dose.

When to take:
At the same time each day, preferably morning.

If you forget a dose:
Take as soon as you remember. Resume regular schedule.

What drug does:
Absorbs water, stimulating the bowel to form a soft, bulky stool.

Time lapse before drug works:
May require 2 or 3 days to begin, then works in 12 to 24 hours.

Don't take with:
- See Interaction column and consult doctor.
- Don't take within 2 hours of taking another medicine. Laxative interferes with medicine absorption.

OVERDOSE

SYMPTOMS:
None expected.
WHAT TO DO:
Overdose unlikely to threaten life. If person takes much larger amount than prescribed, call doctor, poison-control center or hospital emergency room for instructions.

POSSIBLE ADVERSE REACTIONS OR SIDE EFFECTS

SYMPTOMS	WHAT TO DO
Life-threatening: None expected.	
Common: None expected.	
Infrequent: Swallowing difficulty, "lump in throat" sensation, nausea, vomiting, diarrhea.	Continue. Call doctor when convenient.
Rare: Itchy skin, rash, intestinal blockage, asthma.	Discontinue. Call doctor right away.

WARNINGS & PRECAUTIONS

Don't take if:
- You are allergic to any bulk-forming laxative.
- You have symptoms of appendicitis, inflamed bowel or intestinal blockage.
- You have missed a bowel movement for only 1 or 2 days.

Before you start, consult your doctor:
- If you have diabetes.
- If you have a laxative habit.
- If you have rectal bleeding.
- If you have difficulty swallowing.
- If you take other laxatives.

Over age 60:
Adverse reactions and side effects may be more frequent and severe than in younger persons.

Pregnancy:
Most bulk-forming laxatives contain sodium or sugars which may cause fluid retention. Avoid if possible.

Breast-feeding:
No problems expected.

Infants & children:
Use only under medical supervision.

Prolonged use:
Don't take for more than 1 week unless under a doctor's supervision. May cause laxative dependence.

Skin & sunlight:
No problems expected.

Driving, piloting or hazardous work:
No problems expected.

Discontinuing:
May be unnecessary to finish medicine. Follow doctor's instructions.

Others:
Don't take to "flush out" your system or as a "tonic."

POSSIBLE INTERACTION WITH OTHER DRUGS

GENERIC NAME OR DRUG CLASS	COMBINED EFFECT
Digitalis preparations*	Decreased digitalis effect.
Salicylates* (including aspirin)	Decreased salicylate effect.

POSSIBLE INTERACTION WITH OTHER SUBSTANCES

INTERACTS WITH	COMBINED EFFECT
Alcohol:	None expected.
Beverages:	None expected.
Cocaine:	None expected.
Foods:	None expected.
Marijuana:	None expected.
Tobacco:	None expected.

METHYLDOPA

BRAND NAMES

Aldoclor
Aldomet
Aldoril D30
Aldoril D50
Aldoril-15
Aldoril-25

Apo-Methyldopa
Dopamet
Medimet
Novomedopa
PMS Dopazide

BASIC INFORMATION

Habit forming? No
Prescription needed? Yes
Available as generic? Yes
Drug class: Antihypertensive

 ## USES

Reduces high blood pressure.

 ## DOSAGE & USAGE INFORMATION

How to take:
Liquid or tablet—Swallow with liquid. If you can't swallow whole, crumble tablet and take with liquid or food.

When to take:
At the same times each day.

If you forget a dose:
Take as soon as you remember up to 2 hours late. If more than 2 hours, wait for next scheduled dose (don't double this dose).

What drug does:
Relaxes walls of small arteries to decrease blood pressure.

Continued next column

 ## OVERDOSE

SYMPTOMS:
Drowsiness; exhaustion; stupor; confusion; slow, weak pulse.
WHAT TO DO:
- Dial 0 (operator) or 911 (emergency) for an ambulance or medical help. Then give first aid immediately.
- If patient is unconscious and not breathing, give mouth-to-mouth breathing. If there is no heartbeat, use cardiac massage and mouth-to-mouth breathing (CPR). Don't try to make patient vomit. If you can't get help quickly, take patient to nearest emergency facility.
- See emergency information on inside covers.

Time lapse before drug works:
Continual use for 2 to 4 weeks may be necessary to determine effectiveness.

Don't take with:
See Interaction column and consult doctor.

 ## POSSIBLE ADVERSE REACTIONS OR SIDE EFFECTS

SYMPTOMS	WHAT TO DO
Life-threatening: None expected.	
Common: Depression, sedation, nightmares, headache, drowsiness, weakness, stuffy nose, dry mouth, fluid retention, swollen feet or legs.	Continue. Call doctor when convenient.
Infrequent: • Fast heartbeat.	Discontinue. Call doctor right away.
• Insomnia, nausea, vomiting, diarrhea, constipation.	Continue. Call doctor when convenient.
• Swollen breasts, diminished sex drive.	Continue. Tell doctor at next visit.
Rare: Rash; jaundice; unexplained fever; sore or "black" tongue; severe abdominal pain; decreased mental activity and memory impairment; facial paralysis; slow heartbeat; chest pain; swollen abdomen; drug-induced systemic lupus erythematosus.	Discontinue. Call doctor right away.

 ## WARNINGS & PRECAUTIONS

Don't take if:
You will have surgery within 2 months, including dental surgery, requiring general or spinal anesthesia.

Before you start, consult your doctor:
If you have liver disease.

Over age 60:
- Increased susceptibility to dizziness, unsteadiness, fainting, falling.
- Drug can produce or intensify Parkinson's disease.

Pregnancy:
No proven problems. Consult doctor.

Breast-feeding:
No proven problems. Consult doctor.

Infants & children:
Not used.

Prolonged use:
- May cause anemia.
- Severe edema (fluid retention).

Skin & sunlight:
No problems expected.

Driving, piloting or hazardous work:
Don't drive or pilot aircraft until you learn how medicine affects you. Don't work around dangerous machinery. Don't climb ladders or work in high places. Danger increases if you drink alcohol or take medicine affecting alertness and reflexes, such as antihistamines, tranquilizers, sedatives, pain medicine, narcotics and mind-altering drugs.

Discontinuing:
Don't discontinue without consulting doctor. Dose may require gradual reduction if you have taken drug for a long time. Doses of other drugs may also require adjustment.

Others:
Avoid heavy exercise, exertion, sweating.

 ## POSSIBLE INTERACTION WITH OTHER DRUGS

GENERIC NAME OR DRUG CLASS	COMBINED EFFECT
ACE inhibitors: captopril, enalapril, lisinopril*	Possible excessive potassium in blood.
Amphetamines*	Decreased methyldopa effect.
Anticoagulants, oral*	Increased anticoagulant effect.
Antidepressants, tricyclic (TCA)*	Dangerous blood-pressure rise. Decreased methyldopa effect.
Antihypertensives*	Increased antihypertensive effect.
Carteolol	Increased antihypertensive effect.
Digitalis preparations*	Excessively slow heartbeat.
Diuretics, thiazide*	Increased methyldopa effect.
Ethinamate	Dangerous increased effects of ethinamate. Avoid combining.

Fluoxetine	Increased depressant effects of both drugs.
Guanfacine	May increase depressant effects of either drug.
Haloperidol	Increased sedation. Possibly dementia.
Leucovorin	High alcohol content of leucovorin may cause adverse effects.
Levodopa	Increased effect of both drugs.
Loxapine	May increase toxic effects of both drugs.
MAO inhibitors*	Dangerous blood-pressure rise.
Methyprylon	Increased sedative effect, perhaps to dangerous level. Avoid.
Nabilone	Greater depression of central nervous system.
Nicardipine	Blood-pressure drop. Dosages may require adjustment.
Phenoxybenzamine	Urinary retention.
Propranolol	Increased blood pressure (rarely).
Sotalol	Increased antihypertensive effect.
Terazosin	Decreases effectiveness of terazosin.
Tolbutamide	Increased tolbutamide effect.

 ## POSSIBLE INTERACTION WITH OTHER SUBSTANCES

INTERACTS WITH	COMBINED EFFECT
Alcohol:	Increased sedation. Excessive blood-pressure drop. Avoid.
Beverages:	None expected.
Cocaine:	Increased risk of heart block and high blood pressure.
Foods:	None expected.
Marijuana:	Possible fainting.
Tobacco:	Possible increased blood pressure.

METHYLDOPA & THIAZIDE DIURETICS

BRAND NAMES

Aldomet
Aldoril
Dopamet
Medimet-250

Novodoparil
Novomedopa
PMS Dopazide

BASIC INFORMATION

Habit forming? No
Prescription needed? Yes
Available as generic? Yes
Drug class: Antihypertensive, diuretic
  (thiazide)

 USES

- Controls, but doesn't cure, high blood pressure.
- Reduces fluid retention (edema).

 DOSAGE & USAGE INFORMATION

How to take:
Tablet—Swallow with liquid. If you can't swallow whole, crumble tablet and take with liquid or food.

When to take:
At the same times each day.

If you forget a dose:
Take as soon as you remember up to 2 hours late. If more than 2 hours, wait for next scheduled dose (don't double this dose).

Continued next column

 OVERDOSE

SYMPTOMS:
Drowsiness; exhaustion; cramps; weakness; stupor; confusion; slow, weak pulse; coma.
WHAT TO DO:
- Dial 0 (operator) or 911 (emergency) for an ambulance or medical help. Then give first aid immediately.
- If patient is unconscious and not breathing, give mouth-to-mouth breathing. If there is no heartbeat, use cardiac massage and mouth-to-mouth breathing (CPR). Don't try to make patient vomit. If you can't get help quickly, take patient to nearest emergency facility.
- See emergency information on inside covers.

What drug does:
- Relaxes walls of small arteries to decrease blood pressure.
- Forces sodium and water excretion, reducing body fluid.
- Reduced body fluid and relaxed arteries lower blood pressure.

Time lapse before drug works:
Continual use for 2 to 4 weeks may be necessary to determine effectiveness.

Don't take with:
- Non-prescription drugs without consulting doctor.
- See Interaction column and consult doctor.

 POSSIBLE ADVERSE REACTIONS OR SIDE EFFECTS

SYMPTOMS	WHAT TO DO
Life-threatening: Irregular heartbeat, weak pulse.	Discontinue. Seek emergency treatment.
Common: Depression, nightmares, drowsiness, weakness, stuffy nose, dry mouth, swollen feet and ankles, dizziness, sedation.	Continue. Call doctor when convenient.
Infrequent: • Fast heartbeat, change in vision, abdominal pain, nervousness.	Discontinue. Call doctor right away.
• Insomnia, nausea, vomiting, diarrhea, headache, constipation.	Continue. Call doctor when convenient.
Rare: • Rash; jaundice; hives; sore throat, fever, mouth sores; sore or "black" tongue; severe abdominal pain; decreased mental activity; memory impairment; facial paralysis; slow heartbeat; chest pain; drug-induced systemic lupus erythematosus.	Discontinue. Call doctor right away.
• Weight gain or loss.	Continue. Call doctor when convenient.

METHYLDOPA & THIAZIDE DIURETICS

 ## WARNINGS & PRECAUTIONS

Don't take if:
- You are allergic to any thiazide diuretic drug.
- If you will have surgery within 2 months, including dental surgery, requiring general or spinal anesthesia.

Before you start, consult your doctor:
- If you are allergic to any sulfa drug.
- If you have gout, liver, pancreas or kidney disorder.

Over age 60:
- Increased susceptibility to dizziness, unsteadiness, fainting, falling.
- Drug can produce or intensify Parkinson's disease.

Pregnancy:
Risk to unborn child outweighs drug benefits. Don't use.

Breast-feeding:
Drug passes into milk. Avoid drug or discontinue nursing until you finish medicine. Consult doctor for advice on maintaining milk supply.

Infants & children:
Not recommended.

Prolonged use:
- May cause anemia.
- Severe edema (fluid retention).

Skin & sunlight:
May cause rash or intensify sunburn in areas exposed to sun or sunlamp.

Driving, piloting or hazardous work:
Don't drive or pilot aircraft until you learn how medicine affects you. Don't work around dangerous machinery. Don't climb ladders or work in high places. Danger increases if you drink alcohol or take medicine affecting alertness and reflexes, such as antihistamines, tranquilizers, sedatives, pain medicine, narcotics and mind-altering drugs.

Discontinuing:
Don't discontinue without consulting doctor. Dose may require gradual reduction if you have taken drug for a long time. Doses of other drugs may also require adjustment.

Others:
- Hot weather and fever may cause dehydration and drop in blood pressure. Dose may require temporary adjustment. Weigh daily and report any unexpected weight decreases to your doctor.
- May cause rise in uric acid, leading to gout.
- May cause blood-sugar rise in diabetics.
- Avoid heavy exercise, exertion, sweating.

 ## POSSIBLE INTERACTION WITH OTHER DRUGS

GENERIC NAME OR DRUG CLASS	COMBINED EFFECT
Acebutolol	Increased antihypertensive effect. Dosages of both drugs may require adjustments.
ACE inhibitors: captopril, enalapril, lisinopril*	Possible excessive potassium in blood.
Allopurinol	Decreased allopurinol effect.
Amphetamines*	Decreased methyldopa effect.
Anticoagulants, oral*	Increased anticoagulant effect.
Antidepressants, tricyclic (TCA)*	Dangerous changes in blood pressure. Avoid combination unless under medical supervision.
Antihypertensives*	Increased antihypertensive effect.
Barbiturates*	Increased hydrochlorothiazide effect.
Carteolol	Increased antihypertensive effect.
Cholestyamine	Decreased hydrochlorothiazide effect.

Continued page 1090

 ## POSSIBLE INTERACTION WITH OTHER SUBSTANCES

INTERACTS WITH	COMBINED EFFECT
Alcohol:	Increased sedation. Excessive blood-pressure drop. Avoid.
Beverages:	None expected.
Cocaine:	Increased risk of heart block and high blood pressure.
Foods: Licorice.	Excessive potassium loss that causes dangerous heart rhythms.
Marijuana:	May increase blood pressure.
Tobacco:	Possible increased blood pressure.

*See Glossary

METHYLERGONOVINE

BRAND NAMES

Methergine   Methylergometrine
Methylergobasine-
  Sandoz

BASIC INFORMATION

Habit forming? No
Prescription needed? Yes
Available as generic? No
Drug class: Ergot preparation (uterine
  stimulant)

 ## USES

Retards excessive post-delivery bleeding.

 ## DOSAGE & USAGE INFORMATION

How to take:
Tablet—Swallow with liquid or food to lessen
stomach irritation.

When to take:
At the same times each day.

If you forget a dose:
Don't take missed dose and don't double next
one. Wait for next scheduled dose.

What drug does:
Causes smooth-muscle cells of uterine wall to
contract and surround bleeding blood vessels of
relaxed uterus.

Time lapse before drug works:
Tablets—20 to 30 minutes.

Don't take with:
See Interaction column and consult doctor.

 ## OVERDOSE

SYMPTOMS:
**Vomiting, diarrhea, weak pulse, low blood
pressure, dyspnea, angina, convulsions.**
WHAT TO DO:
- **Dial 0 (operator) or 911 (emergency) for
an ambulance or medical help. Then give
first aid immediately.**
- **If patient is unconscious and not
breathing, give mouth-to-mouth
breathing. If there is no heartbeat, use
cardiac massage and mouth-to-mouth
breathing (CPR). Don't try to make patient
vomit. If you can't get help quickly, take
patient to nearest emergency facility.**
- **See emergency information on inside
covers.**

 ## POSSIBLE ADVERSE REACTIONS OR SIDE EFFECTS

SYMPTOMS	WHAT TO DO
Life-threatening: None expected.	
Common: Nausea, vomiting.	Discontinue. Call doctor right away.

Infrequent:
• Confusion, ringing
  in ears, diarrhea,
  muscle cramps.
	Discontinue. Call
	doctor right away.

• Unusual sweating.	Continue. Call doctor when convenient.
Rare: Sudden, severe headache; shortness of breath; chest pain; numb, cold hands and feet.	Discontinue. Seek emergency treatment.

WARNINGS & PRECAUTIONS

Don't take if:
You are allergic to any ergot preparation.

Before you start, consult your doctor:
- If you have coronary-artery or blood-vessel disease.
- If you have liver or kidney disease.
- If you have high blood pressure.
- If you have postpartum infection.

Over age 60:
Not recommended.

Pregnancy:
Risk to unborn child outweighs drug benefits. Don't use.

Breast-feeding:
Drug passes into milk. Avoid drug or discontinue nursing until you finish medicine. Consult doctor for advice on maintaining milk supply.

Infants & children:
Not recommended.

Prolonged use:
Not recommended.

Skin & sunlight:
No problems expected.

Driving, piloting or hazardous work:
No problems expected.

Discontinuing:
May be unnecessary to finish medicine. Follow doctor's instructions.

Others:
Drug should be used for short time only following childbirth or miscarriage.

 ## POSSIBLE INTERACTION WITH OTHER DRUGS

GENERIC NAME OR DRUG CLASS	COMBINED EFFECT
Beta-adrenergic blockers*	Possible vasospasm (peripheral and cardiac)
Ergot preparations, other*	Increased methyl-ergonovine effect.

 ## POSSIBLE INTERACTION WITH OTHER SUBSTANCES

INTERACTS WITH	COMBINED EFFECT
Alcohol:	None expected.
Beverages:	None expected.
Cocaine:	None expected.
Foods:	None expected.
Marijuana:	None expected.
Tobacco:	None expected.

METHYLPHENIDATE

BRAND NAMES

Methidate   Ritalin SR
Ritalin

BASIC INFORMATION

Habit forming? Yes
Available as generic? Yes
Prescription needed? Yes
Drug class: Sympathomimetic

 USES

- Treatment for hyperactive children.
- Treatment for narcolepsy (uncontrollable attacks of sleepiness).

 DOSAGE & USAGE INFORMATION

How to take:
Tablet or extended-release tablet—Swallow with liquid or food to lessen stomach irritation. If you can't swallow whole, crumble tablet and take with liquid or food.

When to take:
At the same times each day.

If you forget a dose:
Take as soon as you remember up to 2 hours late. If more than 2 hours, wait for next scheduled dose (don't double this dose).

Continued next column

 OVERDOSE

SYMPTOMS:
Rapid heartbeat, fever, confusion, vomiting, agitation, hallucinations, convulsions, coma.
WHAT TO DO:
- Dial 0 (operator) or 911 (emergency) for an ambulance or medical help. Then give first aid immediately.
- If patient is unconscious and not breathing, give mouth-to-mouth breathing. If there is no heartbeat, use cardiac massage and mouth-to-mouth breathing (CPR). Don't try to make patient vomit. If you can't get help quickly, take patient to nearest emergency facility.
- See emergency information on inside covers.

What drug does:
Stimulates brain to improve alertness, concentration and attention span. Calms the hyperactive child.

Time lapse before drug works:
- 1 month or more for maximum effect on child.
- 30 minutes to stimulate adults.

Don't take with:
See Interaction column and consult doctor.

 POSSIBLE ADVERSE REACTIONS OR SIDE EFFECTS

SYMPTOMS	WHAT TO DO
Life-threatening: None expected.	
Common:	
• Mood change.	Continue. Call doctor when convenient.
• Nervousness, insomnia, dizziness, headache, appetite loss.	Continue. Tell doctor at next visit.
Infrequent:	
• Rash or hives; chest pain; fast, irregular heartbeat; unusual bruising; joint pain; psychosis; uncontrollable movements; unexplained fever.	Discontinue. Call doctor right away.
• Nausea, abdominal pain.	Continue. Call doctor when convenient.
Rare:	
• Blurred vision, sore throat, fever, red spots under skin.	Discontinue. Call doctor right away.
• Unusual tiredness.	Continue. Call doctor when convenient.

WARNINGS & PRECAUTIONS

Don't take if:
- You are allergic to methylphenidate.
- You have glaucoma.
- Patient is younger than 6.

Before you start, consult your doctor:
- If you have epilepsy.
- If you have high blood pressure.
- If you take MAO inhibitors.

Over age 60:
Adverse reactions and side effects may be more frequent and severe than in younger persons.

Pregnancy:
No proven harm to unborn child. Avoid if possible.

Breast-feeding:
No proven problems. Consult doctor.

Infants & children:
Use only under medical supervision for children 6 or older.

Prolonged use:
Rare possibility of physical growth retardation.

Skin & sunlight:
No problems expected.

Driving, piloting or hazardous work:
No problems expected.

Discontinuing:
Don't discontinue abruptly. Don't discontinue without doctor's advice until you complete prescribed dose, even though symptoms diminish or disappear.

Others:
Dose must be carefully adjusted by doctor.

POSSIBLE INTERACTION WITH OTHER DRUGS

GENERIC NAME OR DRUG CLASS	COMBINED EFFECT
Acebutolol	Decreased effects of both drugs.
Anticholinergics*	Increased anticholinergic effect.
Anticoagulants, oral*	Increased anticoagulant effect.
Anticonvulsants*	Increased anticonvulsant effect.
Antidepressants, tricyclic (TCA)*	Increased antidepressant effect. Decreased methylphenidate effect.
Antihypertensives*	Decreased antihypertensive effect.
Guanadrel	Decreased guanadrel effect.
Guanethidine	Decreased guanethidine effect.
MAO inhibitors*	Dangerous rise in blood pressure.
Minoxidil	Decreased minoxidil effect.
Nitrates*	Possible decreased effects of both drugs.
Oxprenolol	Decreased effects of both drugs.
Oxyphenbutazone	Increased oxyphenbutazone effect.
Phenylbutazone	Increased phenylbutazone effect.
Terazosin	Decreases effectiveness of terazosin.

POSSIBLE INTERACTION WITH OTHER SUBSTANCES

INTERACTS WITH	COMBINED EFFECT
Alcohol:	None expected.
Beverages: Caffeine drinks.	May raise blood pressure.
Cocaine:	High risk of heartbeat irregularities and high blood pressure.
Foods: Foods containing tyramine*	May raise blood pressure.
Marijuana:	None expected.
Tobacco:	None expected.

METHYLPREDNISOLONE

BRAND NAMES

See complete list of brand names in the
Brand Name Directory, page 1065.

BASIC INFORMATION

Habit forming? No
Prescription needed? Yes
Available as generic? Yes
**Drug class: Cortisone drug (adrenal
corticosteroid)**

 ## USES

- Reduces inflammation caused by many
  different medical problems.
- Treatment for some allergic diseases, blood
  disorders, kidney diseases, asthma and
  emphysema.
- Replaces corticosteroid deficiencies.

 ## DOSAGE & USAGE
INFORMATION

How to take:
- Tablet—Swallow with liquid or food to lessen
  stomach irritation. If you can't swallow whole,
  crumble tablet and take with liquid or food.
- Injection—Take under doctor's supervision.

When to take:
At the same times each day. Take once-a-day or
once-every-other-day doses in mornings.

If you forget a dose:
- Several-doses-per-day prescription—Take as
  soon as you remember up to 2 hours late. If
  more than 2 hours, wait for next scheduled
  dose (don't double this dose).
- Once-a-day dose or less—Wait for next dose.
  Double this dose.

What drug does:
Decreases inflammatory responses.

Time lapse before drug works:
2 to 4 days.

Don't take with:
See Interaction column and consult doctor.

 ## OVERDOSE

SYMPTOMS:
Headache, convulsions, heart failure.
WHAT TO DO:
- **Dial 0 (operator) or 911 (emergency) for
  an ambulance or medical help. Then give
  first aid immediately.**
- **See emergency information on inside
  covers.**

 ## POSSIBLE
ADVERSE REACTIONS
OR SIDE EFFECTS

SYMPTOMS	WHAT TO DO
Life-threatening:	
Hives, rash, intense itching, faintness soon after a dose (anaphylaxis).	Seek emergency treatment immediately.
Common:	
Acne, poor wound healing, thirst, indigestion, nausea, vomiting, decreased growth in children.	Continue. Call doctor when convenient.
Infrequent:	
• Black, bloody or tarry stools.	Discontinue. Seek emergency treatment.
• Blurred vision, halos around lights, sore throat, fever, muscle cramps, swollen legs or feet.	Discontinue. Call doctor right away.
• Mood change, insomnia, fatigue, restlessness, frequent urination, weight gain, round face, weakness, TB recurrence, irregular menstrual periods.	Continue. Call doctor when convenient.
Rare:	
• Irregular heartbeat.	Discontinue. Seek emergency treatment.
• Rash, numbness or tingling in hands or feet, pancreatitis, thrombophlebitis, hallucinations, convulsions.	Discontinue. Call doctor right away.

 ## WARNINGS &
PRECAUTIONS

Don't take if:
- You are allergic to any cortisone drug.
- You have tuberculosis or fungus infection.
- You have herpes infection of eyes, lips or
  genitals.

Before you start, consult your doctor:
- If you have had tuberculosis.
- If you have congestive heart failure.
- If you have diabetes, peptic ulcer, glaucoma,
  underactive thyroid, high blood pressure,
  myasthenia gravis, blood clots in legs or
  lungs.

Over age 60:
Adverse reactions and side effects may be more frequent and severe than in younger persons. Likely to aggravate edema, diabetes or ulcers. Likely to cause cataracts and osteoporosis (softening of the bones).

Pregnancy:
Risk to unborn child outweighs drug benefits. Don't use.

Breast-feeding:
Drug passes into milk. Avoid drug or discontinue nursing until you finish medicine. Consult doctor for advice on maintaining milk supply.

Infants & children:
Use only under medical supervision.

Prolonged use:
- Retards growth in children.
- Possible glaucoma, cataracts, diabetes, fragile bones and thin skin.
- Functional dependence.

Skin & sunlight:
No problems expected.

Driving, piloting or hazardous work:
No problems expected.

Discontinuing:
- Don't discontinue without doctor's advice until you complete prescribed dose, even though symptoms diminish or disappear.
- Drug affects your response to surgery, illness, injury or stress for 2 years after discontinuing. Tell anyone who takes medical care of you within 2 years about drug.

Others:
Avoid immunizations if possible.

 ## POSSIBLE INTERACTION WITH OTHER DRUGS

GENERIC NAME OR DRUG CLASS	COMBINED EFFECT
Amphotericin B	Potassium depletion.
Anticholinergics*	Possible glaucoma.
Anticoagulants, oral*	Decreased anti-coagulant effect.
Anticonvulsants, hydantoin*	Decreased methyl-prednisolone effect.
Antidiabetics, oral*	Decreased anti-diabetic effect.
Antihistamines*	Decreased methyl-prednisolone effect.
Aspirin	Increased methyl-prednisolone effect.

	COMBINED EFFECT
Attentuated virus vaccines*	Possible viral infection.
Barbiturates*	Decreased methyl-prednisolone effect. Oversedation.
Chloral hydrate	Decreased methyl-prednisolone effect.
Chlorthalidone	Potassium depletion.
Cholestyramine	Decreased methyl-prednisolone absorption.
Cholinergics*	Decreased cholinergic effect.
Colestipol	Decreased methyl-prednisolone absorption.
Contraceptives, oral*	Increased methyl-prednisolone effect.
Digitalis preparations*	Dangerous potassium depletion. Possible digitalis toxicity.
Diuretics, thiazide*	Potassium depletion.
Ephedrine	Decreased methyl-prednisolone effect.
Estrogens*	Increased methyl-prednisolone effect.
Ethacrynic acid	Potassium depletion.
Furosemide	Potassium depletion.
Glutethimide	Decreased methyl-prednisolone effect.
Indapamide	Possible excessive potassium loss, causing dangerous heartbeat irregularity.

Continued page 1091

 ## POSSIBLE INTERACTION WITH OTHER SUBSTANCES

INTERACTS WITH	COMBINED EFFECT
Alcohol:	Risk of stomach ulcers.
Beverages:	No proven problems.
Cocaine:	Overstimulation. Avoid.
Foods:	No proven problems.
Marijuana:	Decreased immunity.
Tobacco:	Increased methyl-prednisolone effect. Possible toxicity.

METHYPRYLON

BRAND NAMES

Noludar

BASIC INFORMATION

Habit forming? Yes
Prescription needed? Yes
Available as generic? No
Drug class: Sedative-hypnotic

 USES

Treats insomnia.

 DOSAGE & USAGE INFORMATION

How to take:
Capsules—Swallow with liquid or food to lessen
stomach irritation. If you can't swallow whole,
open capsule and take with liquid or food.

When to take:
At bedtime.

If you forget a dose:
Take as soon as you remember up to 2 hours
late. If more than 2 hours, wait for next
scheduled dose (don't double this dose).

What drug does:
Increases threshold of arousal centers in the
midbrain.

Time lapse before drug works:
Within 45 minutes.

Don't take with:
- Any other medicine that will affect alertness or
  reflexes.
- See Interaction column and consult doctor.

 OVERDOSE

SYMPTOMS:
Confusion, difficulty breathing, slow
heartbeat, staggering, severe weakness,
convulsions, coma.
WHAT TO DO:
- **Dial 0 (operator) or 911 (emergency) for**
  an ambulance or medical help. Then give
  first aid immediately.
- **See emergency information on inside**
  covers.

 POSSIBLE ADVERSE REACTIONS OR SIDE EFFECTS

SYMPTOMS	WHAT TO DO
Life-threatening:	
Coma.	Seek emergency treatment immediately.
Common:	
Dizziness, headache, daytime drowsiness.	Continue. Call doctor when convenient.
Infrequent:	
Diarrhea, nausea, vomiting, skin rash, unusual excitement.	Discontinue. Call doctor right away.
Rare:	
Mouth ulcers, unusual bleeding or bruising.	Discontinue. Call doctor right away.

WARNINGS & PRECAUTIONS

Don't take if:
You have a history of drug abuse.

Before you start, consult your doctor:
- If you have liver disease.
- If you have intermittent porphyria.
- If you have significant kidney disease.

Over age 60:
Adverse reactions and side effects may be more frequent and severe than in younger persons. You may need smaller doses for shorter periods of time.

Pregnancy:
Risk to unborn child outweighs drug benefits. Don't use.

Breast-feeding:
Drug passes into milk. Avoid drug or discontinue nursing until you finish medicine. Consult doctor for advice on maintaining milk supply.

Infants & children:
Not recommended. Avoid.

Prolonged use:
Not intended for prolonged use.

Skin & sunlight:
No problems expected.

Driving, piloting or hazardous work:
Don't drive or pilot aircraft until you learn how medicine affects you. Don't work around dangerous machinery. Don't climb ladders or work in high places. Danger increases if you drink alcohol or take medicine affecting alertness and reflexes.

Discontinuing:
These symptoms may occur after medicine has been discontinued: confusion, seizures, hallucinations, increased dreaming, vomiting, nightmares, restlessness, trembling, insomnia, weakness.

Others:
No problems expected.

POSSIBLE INTERACTION WITH OTHER DRUGS

GENERIC NAME OR DRUG CLASS	COMBINED EFFECT
Central nervous system (CNS) depressants*	Increased sedative effect, perhaps to dangerous level. Avoid.
Ethinamate	Dangerous increased effects of ethinamate. Avoid combining.
Fluoxetine	Increased depressant effects of both drugs.
Guanfacine	May increase depressant effects of either drug.
Leucovorin	High alcohol content of leucovorin may cause adverse effects.
Nabilone	Greater depression of central nervous system.
Other addictive medicines	Increased risk of habituation.

POSSIBLE INTERACTION WITH OTHER SUBSTANCES

INTERACTS WITH	COMBINED EFFECT
Alcohol:	Excess sedation. Avoid.
Beverages: Caffeine drinks.	Decreased methyprylon effect. Avoid.
Cocaine:	Decreased methyprylon effect.
Foods:	None expected.
Marijuana:	Decreased methyprylon effect.
Tobacco:	None expected.

*See Glossary

METHYSERGIDE

BRAND NAMES

Sansert

BASIC INFORMATION

Habit forming? Yes
Prescription needed? Yes
Available as generic? No
Drug class: Vasoconstrictor (antiserotonin)

 USES

Prevents migraine and other recurring vascular headaches. Not for acute attack.

 DOSAGE & USAGE INFORMATION

How to take:
Tablet—Swallow with liquid or with food to lessen stomach irritation. If you can't swallow whole, crumble tablet and take with liquid or food.

When to take:
At the same times each day.

If you forget a dose:
Don't take missed dose. Wait for next scheduled dose (don't double this dose).

What drug does:
Blocks the action of serotonin, a chemical that constricts blood vessels.

Time lapse before drug works:
About 3 weeks.

Don't take with:
See Interaction column and consult doctor.

 OVERDOSE

SYMPTOMS:
Nausea, vomiting, abdominal pain, severe diarrhea, lack of coordination, extreme thirst.
WHAT TO DO:
Overdose unlikely to threaten life. If person takes much larger amount than prescribed, call doctor, poison-control center or hospital emergency room for instructions.

 POSSIBLE ADVERSE REACTIONS OR SIDE EFFECTS

SYMPTOMS	WHAT TO DO
Life-threatening: None expected.	
Common:	
• Itchy skin.	Discontinue. Call doctor right away.
• Nausea, vomiting, diarrhea, numbness or tingling of extremities, leg weakness.	Continue. Call doctor when convenient.
• Drowsiness, constipation.	Continue. Tell doctor at next visit.
Infrequent:	
• Anxiety, agitation, hallucinations, unusually fast or slow heartbeat.	Discontinue. Call doctor right away.
• Change in vision.	Continue. Call doctor when convenient.
Rare:	
• Extreme thirst, chest pain, shortness of breath, fever, pale or swollen extremities, leg cramps, lower back pain, side or groin pain, appetite loss, joint and muscle pain, rash, facial flush.	Discontinue. Call doctor right away.
• Painful or difficult urination.	Continue. Call doctor when convenient.
• Weight change, hair loss, swollen feet and ankles.	Continue. Tell doctor at next visit.

WARNINGS & PRECAUTIONS

Don't take if:
- You are allergic to any antiserotonin.
- You plan to become pregnant within medication period.
- You have an infection.
- You have a heart or blood-vessel disease.
- You have a chronic lung disease.
- You have a collagen (connective tissue) disorder.
- You have impaired liver or kidney function.

Before you start, consult your doctor:
- If you have been allergic to any ergot preparation.
- If you have had a peptic ulcer.

Over age 60:
Adverse reactions and side effects may be more frequent and severe than in younger persons.

Pregnancy:
Manufacturer suggests risk to unborn child outweighs drug benefits, even though studies are inconclusive.

Breast-feeding:
Drug probably passes into milk. Avoid drug or discontinue nursing until you finish medicine. Consult doctor for advice on maintaining milk supply.

Infants & children:
Not recommended.

Prolonged use:
Possible fibrosis, a condition in which scar tissue is deposited on heart valves, in lung tissue, blood vessels and internal organs. After 6 months, decrease dose over 2 to 3 weeks. Then discontinue for at least 2 months for re-evaluation.

Skin & sunlight:
No problems expected.

Driving, piloting or hazardous work:
Avoid if you feel drowsy or dizzy. Otherwise, no problems expected.

Discontinuing:
- Don't discontinue without consulting doctor. Dose may require gradual reduction if you have taken drug for a long time. Doses of other drugs may also require adjustment.
- Probably should discontinue drug if you don't improve after 3 weeks use.

Others:
- Periodic laboratory tests for liver function and blood counts recommended.
- Potential for abuse.
- Some products contain tartrazine dye. Avoid, especially if you are allergic to aspirin.

POSSIBLE INTERACTION WITH OTHER DRUGS

GENERIC NAME OR DRUG CLASS	COMBINED EFFECT
Ergot preparations*	Unpredictable increased or decreased effect of either drug.
Narcotics*	Decreased narcotic effect.

POSSIBLE INTERACTION WITH OTHER SUBSTANCES

INTERACTS WITH	COMBINED EFFECT
Alcohol:	None expected. However, alcohol may trigger a migraine headache.
Beverages: Caffeine drinks.	Decreased methysergide effect.
Cocaine:	May make headache worse.
Foods:	None expected. Avoid foods to which you are allergic.
Marijuana:	No proven problems.
Tobacco:	Blood-vessel constriction. Makes headache worse.

METOCLOPRAMIDE

BRAND NAMES

Clopa	Maxolon
Emex	Reclomide
Maxeran	Reglan

BASIC INFORMATION

Habit forming? No
Prescription needed? Yes
Available as generic? Yes
Drug class: Antiemetic; dopaminergic blocker

USES

- Relieves nausea and vomiting caused by chemotherapy and drug related postoperative factors.
- Relieves symptoms of esophagitis and stomach swelling in people with diabetes.

DOSAGE & USAGE INFORMATION

How to take:
Tablet or syrup—Swallow with liquid or food to lessen stomach irritation.

When to take:
30 minutes before symptoms expected, up to 4 times a day.

If you forget a dose:
Take as soon as you remember up to 2 hours late. If more than 2 hours, wait for next scheduled dose (don't double this dose).

What drug does:
- Prevents smooth muscle in stomach from relaxing.
- Affects vomiting center in brain.

Continued next column

OVERDOSE

SYMPTOMS:
Severe drowsiness, mental confusion, trembling, seizure, coma.
WHAT TO DO:
- Dial 0 (operator) or 911 (emergency) for an ambulance or medical help. Then give first aid immediately.
- If patient is unconscious and not breathing, give mouth-to-mouth breathing. If there is no heartbeat, use cardiac massage and mouth-to-mouth breathing (CPR). Don't try to make patient vomit. If you can't get help quickly, take patient to nearest emergency facility.
- See emergency information on inside covers.

Time lapse before drug works:
30 to 60 minutes.

Don't take with:
See Interaction column and consult doctor.

POSSIBLE ADVERSE REACTIONS OR SIDE EFFECTS

SYMPTOMS	WHAT TO DO
Life-threatening: None expected.	
Common: Drowsiness, restlessness.	Continue. Call doctor when convenient.
Frequent Rash.	Continue. Call doctor when convenient.
Infrequent: • Wheezing, shortness of breath.	Discontinue. Call doctor right away.
• Dizziness; headache; insomnia; tender, swollen breasts; increased milk flow.	Continue. Call doctor when convenient.
Rare: • Abnormal, involuntary movements of jaw, lips and tongue; depression; Parkinson syndrome.	Discontinue. Call doctor right away.
• Constipation, nausea, diarrhea.	Continue. Call doctor when convenient.

WARNINGS & PRECAUTIONS

Don't take if:
You are allergic to procaine, procainamide or metoclopramide.

Before you start, consult your doctor:
- If you have Parkinson's disease.
- If you have liver or kidney disease.
- If you have epilepsy.
- If you have bleeding from gastrointestinal tract or intestinal obstruction.
- If you will have surgery within 2 months, including dental surgery, requiring general or spinal anesthesia.

Over age 60:
Adverse reactions and side effects may be more frequent and severe than in younger persons.

Pregnancy:
No proven harm to unborn child. Avoid if possible.

Breast-feeding:
Unknown effect.

Infants & children:
Adverse reactions more likely to occur than in adults.

Prolonged use:
Adverse reactions including muscle spasms and trembling hands more likely to occur.

Skin & sunlight:
No problems expected.

Driving, piloting or hazardous work:
Don't drive or pilot aircraft until you learn how medicine affects you. Don't work around dangerous machinery. Don't climb ladders or work in high places. Danger increases if you drink alcohol or take medicine affecting alertness and reflexes, such as antihistamines, tranquilizers, sedatives, pain medicine, narcotics and mind-altering drugs.

Discontinuing:
May be unnecessary to finish medicine. Follow doctor's instructions.

Others:
No problems expected.

 ## POSSIBLE INTERACTION WITH OTHER DRUGS

GENERIC NAME OR DRUG CLASS	COMBINED EFFECT
Acetaminophen	Increased absorption of acetaminophen.
Anticholinergics*	Decreased metoclopramide effect.
Aspirin	Increased absorption of aspirin.
Bromocriptine	Decreased bromocriptine effect.
Butyophenone	Increased chance of muscle spasm and trembling.
Central nervous system depressants* (antidepressants,* antihistamines,* muscle relaxants,* narcotics,* sedatives,* sleeping pills,* tranquilizers*)	Excess sedation.
Digitalis preparations*	Decreased absorption of digitalis.
Ethinamate	Dangerous increased effects of ethinamate. Avoid combining.
Fluoxetine	Increased depressant effects of both drugs.

Guanfacine	May increase depressant effects of either drug.
Insulin	Unpredictable changes in blood glucose. Dosages may require adjustment.
Leucovorin	High alcohol content of leucovorin may cause adverse effects.
Levodopa	Increased absorption of levodopa.
Lithium	Increased absorption of lithium.
Loxapine	May increase toxic effects of both drugs.
Methyprylon	Increased sedative effect, perhaps to dangerous level. Avoid.
Nabilone	Greater depression of central nervous system.
Narcotics*	Decreased metoclopramide effect.
Nizatidine	Decreased nizatidine absorption.
Phenothiazines*	Increased chance of muscle spasm and trembling.
Tetracyclines*	Slow stomach emptying.
Thiothixines*	Increased chance of muscle spasm and trembling.

 ## POSSIBLE INTERACTION WITH OTHER SUBSTANCES

INTERACTS WITH	COMBINED EFFECT
Alcohol:	Excess sedation. Avoid.
Beverages: Coffee.	Decreased metoclopramide effect.
Cocaine:	Decreased metoclopramide effect.
Foods:	No problems expected.
Marijuana:	Decreased metoclopramide effect.
Tobacco:	Decreased metoclopramide effect.

*See Glossary

METOLAZONE

BRAND NAMES

Diulo   **Zaroxolyn**

BASIC INFORMATION

Habit forming? No
Prescription needed? Yes
Available as generic? No
Drug class: Antihypertensive, diuretic
(thiazide)

USES

- Controls, but doesn't cure, high blood pressure.
- Reduces fluid retention (edema) caused by conditions such as heart disorders and liver disease.

DOSAGE & USAGE INFORMATION

How to take:
Tablet—Swallow with 8 oz. of liquid. If you can't swallow whole, crumble tablet and take with liquid or food. Don't exceed dose.

When to take:
At the same time each day.

If you forget a dose:
Take as soon as you remember up to 2 hours late. If more than 2 hours, wait for next scheduled dose (don't double this dose).

What drug does:
- Forces sodium and water excretion, reducing body fluid.
- Relaxes muscle cells of small arteries.
- Reduced body fluid and relaxed arteries lower blood pressure.

Time lapse before drug works:
4 to 6 hours. May require several weeks to lower blood pressure.

Continued next column

OVERDOSE

SYMPTOMS:
Cramps, weakness, drowsiness, weak pulse, coma.
WHAT TO DO:
- **Dial 0 (operator) or 911 (emergency) for an ambulance or medical help. Then give first aid immediately.**
- **See emergency information on inside covers.**

Don't take with:
- See Interaction column and consult doctor.
- Non-prescription drugs without consulting doctor.

POSSIBLE ADVERSE REACTIONS OR SIDE EFFECTS

SYMPTOMS	WHAT TO DO
Life-threatening: None expected.	
Common: None expected.	
Infrequent:	
• Blurred vision, severe abdominal pain, nausea, vomiting, irregular heartbeat, weak pulse.	Discontinue. Call doctor right away.
• Dizziness, mood change, headache, weakness, tiredness, weight changes.	Continue. Call doctor when convenient.
• Dry mouth, thirst.	Continue. Tell doctor at next visit.
Rare:	
• Rash or hives.	Discontinue. Seek emergency treatment.
• Jaundice, sore throat, fever.	Discontinue. Call doctor right away.

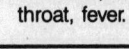

WARNINGS & PRECAUTIONS

Don't take if:
You are allergic to any thiazide diuretic drug.

Before you start, consult your doctor:
- If you are allergic to any sulfa drug.
- If you have gout.
- If you have liver, pancreas or kidney disorder.

Over age 60:
Adverse reactions and side effects may be more frequent and severe than in younger persons, especially dizziness and excessive potassium loss.

Pregnancy:
Risk to unborn child outweighs drug benefits. Don't use.

Breast-feeding:
Drug passes into milk. Avoid this medicine or discontinue nursing.

Infants & children:
No problems expected.

Prolonged use:
You may need medicine to treat high blood pressure for the rest of your life.

Skin & sunlight:
May cause rash or intensify sunburn in areas exposed to sun or sunlamp.

Driving, piloting or hazardous work:
Don't drive or pilot aircraft until you learn how medicine affects you. Don't work around dangerous machinery. Don't climb ladders or work in high places. Danger increases if you drink alcohol or take medicine affecting alertness and reflexes, such as antihistamines, tranquilizers, sedatives, pain medicine, narcotics and mind-altering drugs.

Discontinuing:
Don't discontinue without medical advice.

Others:
* Hot weather and fever may cause dehydration and drop in blood pressure. Dose may require temporary adjustment. Weigh daily and report any unexpected weight decreases to your doctor.
* May cause rise in uric acid, leading to gout.
* May cause blood-sugar rise in diabetics.

POSSIBLE INTERACTION WITH OTHER DRUGS

GENERIC NAME OR DRUG CLASS	COMBINED EFFECT
ACE inhibitors: captopril, enalapril, lisinopril*	Decreased blood pressure. Possible excessive potassium in blood.
Allopurinol	Decreased allopurinol effect.
Amiodarone	Increased risk of heartbeat irregularity due to low potassium.
Amphotericin B	Increased potassium.
Antidepressants, tricyclic (TCA)*	Dangerous drop in blood pressure. Avoid combination unless under medical supervision.
Antidiabetic agents, oral*	Increased blood sugar.
Antihypertensives*	Increased hypertensive effect.
Barbiturates*	Increased metolazone effect.
Beta-adrenergic blockers*	Increased antihypertensive effect. Dosages of both drugs may require adjustment.
Calcium supplements*	Increased calcium in blood.

Carteolol	Increased antihypertensive effect.
Cholestyramine	Decreased metolazone effect.
Colestipol	Decreased metolazone effect.
Cortisone drugs*	Excessive potassium loss that causes dangerous heart rhythms.
Digitalis preparations*	Excessive potassium loss that causes dangerous heart rhythms.
Diuretics, thiazide*	Increased effect of other thiazide diuretics.
Indapamide	Increased diuretic effect.
Indomethacin	Decreased metolazone effect.
Lithium	Increased effect of lithium.
MAO inhibitors*	Increased metolazone effect.
Nicardipine	Blood-pressure drop. Dosages may require adjustment.
Nitrates*	Excessive blood-pressure drop.
Opiates*	Weakness and faintness when arising from bed or chair.

Continued page 1091

POSSIBLE INTERACTION WITH OTHER SUBSTANCES

INTERACTS WITH	COMBINED EFFECT
Alcohol:	Dangerous blood-pressure drop.
Beverages:	None expected.
Cocaine:	Increased risk of heart block and high blood pressure.
Foods: Licorice.	Excessive potassium loss that causes dangerous heart rhythms.
Marijuana:	May increase blood pressure.
Tobacco:	None expected.

*See Glossary

METOPROLOL

BRAND NAMES

Apo-metoprolol	Lopressor
Betaloc	Lopressor SR
Betaloc Durules	Novometoprol
Lopresor	

BASIC INFORMATION

Habit forming? No
Prescription needed? Yes
Available as generic? No
Drug class: Beta-adrenergic blocker

USES

- Reduces angina attacks.
- Stabilizes irregular heartbeat.
- Lowers blood pressure.
- Reduces frequency of migraine headaches. (Does not relieve headache pain.)
- Other uses prescribed by your doctor.

DOSAGE & USAGE INFORMATION

How to take:
Tablet or extended-release tablet—Swallow with liquid. If you can't swallow whole, crumble tablet and take with liquid or food.

When to take:
With meals or immediately after.

If you forget a dose:
Take as soon as you remember. Return to regular schedule, but allow 3 hours between doses.

What drug does:
- Blocks certain actions of sympathetic nervous system.
- Lowers heart's oxygen requirements.
- Slows nerve impulses through heart.
- Reduces blood vessel contraction in heart, scalp and other body parts.

Continued next column

OVERDOSE

SYMPTOMS:
Weakness, slow or weak pulse, blood-pressure drop, difficulty breathing, fainting, convulsions, cold and sweaty skin.
WHAT TO DO:
- Dial 0 (operator) or 911 (emergency) for an ambulance or medical help. Then give first aid immediately.
- See emergency information on inside covers.

Time lapse before drug works:
1 to 4 hours.

Don't take with:
Non-prescription drugs or drugs in Interaction column without consulting doctor.

POSSIBLE ADVERSE REACTIONS OR SIDE EFFECTS

SYMPTOMS	WHAT TO DO
Life-threatening:	
Congestive heart failure.	Discontinue. Seek emergency treatment.
Common:	
• Pulse slower than 50 beats per minute.	Discontinue. Call doctor right away.
• Drowsiness, fatigue, numbness or tingling of fingers or toes, dizziness, diarrhea, nausea, weakness.	Continue. Call doctor when convenient.
• Cold hands, feet; dry mouth, eyes, skin.	Continue. Tell doctor at next visit.
Infrequent:	
• Hallucinations, nightmares, insomnia, headache, difficult breathing, joint pain, anxiety.	Discontinue. Call doctor right away.
• Confusion, reduced alertness, depression.	Continue. Call doctor when convenient.
• Constipation.	Continue. Tell doctor at next visit.
Rare:	
• Rash, sore throat, fever, breathing difficulty.	Discontinue. Call doctor right away.
• Unusual bleeding and bruising; dry, burning eyes; impotence.	Continue. Call doctor when convenient.

WARNINGS & PRECAUTIONS

Don't take if:
- You are allergic to any beta-adrenergic blocker.
- You have asthma or hay fever symptoms.
- You have taken MAO inhibitors in past 2 weeks.

Before you start, consult your doctor:
- If you have heart disease or poor circulation to the extremities.
- If you have hay fever, asthma, chronic bronchitis, emphysema.
- If you have overactive thyroid function.
- If you have impaired liver or kidney function.

- If you will have surgery within 2 months, including dental surgery, requiring general or spinal anesthesia.
- If you have diabetes or hypoglycemia.

Over age 60:
Adverse reactions and side effects may be more frequent and severe than in younger persons.

Pregnancy:
Risk to unborn child outweighs drug benefits. Don't use.

Breast-feeding:
Drug passes into milk. Avoid drug or discontinue nursing until you finish medicine. Consult doctor for advice on maintaining milk supply.

Infants & children:
Not recommended.

Prolonged use:
Weakens heart muscle contractions.

Skin & sunlight:
No problems expected.

Driving, piloting or hazardous work:
Don't drive or pilot aircraft until you learn how medicine affects you. Don't work around dangerous machinery. Don't climb ladders or work in high places. Danger increases if you drink alcohol or take medicine affecting alertness and reflexes.

Discontinuing:
Don't discontinue without consulting doctor. Dose may require gradual reduction if you have taken drug for a long time. Doses of other drugs may also require adjustment.

Others:
May mask hypoglycemia.

 ## POSSIBLE INTERACTION WITH OTHER DRUGS

GENERIC NAME OR DRUG CLASS	COMBINED EFFECT
ACE inhibitors: captopril, enalapril, lisinopril*	Increased antihypertensive effects of both drugs. Dosages may require adjustment.
Antidiabetics*	Increased antidiabetic effect.
Antihistamines*	Decreased antihistamine effect.
Antihypertensives*	Increased antihypertensive effect.
Barbiturates*	Increased barbiturate effect. Dangerous sedation.
Beta-agonists*	Decreased beta-agonist effect.
Betaxolol eyedrops	Possible increased metoprolol effect.
Digitalis preparations*	Can either increase or decrease heart rate. Improves irregular heartbeat.
Encainide	Increased effect of toxicity on the heart muscle.
Indapamide	Increased effects of both drugs. Can help control high blood pressure.
Indomethacin	Decreased metoprolol effect.
Insulin	Hypoglycemic effects may be prolonged.
Levobunolol eyedrops	Possible increased metoprolol effect.
Molindone	Increased tranquilizer effect.
Narcotics*	Increased narcotic effect. Dangerous sedation.
Nicardipine	Possible irregular heartbeat and congestive heart failure.
Nitrates*	Possible decreased blood pressure.
Nizatidine	Increased effect and toxicity of metoprolol.
Non-steroidal anti-inflammatory drugs (NSAIDs)*	Decreased antihypertensive effect of metoprolol.

Continued page 1091

 ## POSSIBLE INTERACTION WITH OTHER SUBSTANCES

INTERACTS WITH	COMBINED EFFECT
Alcohol:	Excessive blood-pressure drop. Avoid.
Beverages:	None expected.
Cocaine:	Irregular heartbeat. Avoid.
Foods:	None expected.
Marijuana:	Daily use—Impaired circulation to hands and feet.
Tobacco:	Possible irregular heartbeat.

METRONIDAZOLE

BRAND NAMES

Apo-Metronidazole	Metryl IV
Flagyl	Neo-Metric
Flagyl I.V.	Neo-Tric
Flagyl I.V. RTU	Novonidazol
Metizol	PMS Metronidazole
Metric 21	Protostat
Metro I.V.	Satric
Metronid	SK-Metronidazole
Metryl	Trikacide

BASIC INFORMATION

Habit forming? No
Prescription needed? Yes
Available as generic? Yes
Drug class: Antiprotozoal

USES

Treatment for infections susceptible to metronidazole, such as trichomoniasis and amebiasis.

DOSAGE & USAGE INFORMATION

How to take:
Tablet—Swallow with liquid or food to lessen stomach irritation. If you can't swallow whole, crumble tablet and take with liquid or food.

When to take:
At the same times each day.

If you forget a dose:
Take as soon as you remember up to 2 hours late. If more than 2 hours, wait for next scheduled dose (don't double this dose).

What drug does:
Kills organisms causing the infection.

Continued next column

OVERDOSE

SYMPTOMS:
Weakness, nausea, vomiting, diarrhea, confusion, seizures.
WHAT TO DO:
Overdose unlikely to threaten life. If person takes much larger amount than prescribed, call doctor, poison-control center or hospital emergency room for instructions.

Time lapse before drug works:
Begins in 1 hour. May require regular use for 10 days to cure infection.

Don't take with:
* Non-prescription medicines containing alcohol.
* See Interaction column and consult doctor.

POSSIBLE ADVERSE REACTIONS OR SIDE EFFECTS

SYMPTOMS	WHAT TO DO
Life-threatening: None expected.	
Common:	
• Appetite loss, nausea, stomach pain, diarrhea, vomiting.	Discontinue. Call doctor right away.
• Unpleasant taste.	Continue. Tell doctor at next visit.
Infrequent:	
• Dizziness; headache; rash; hives; skin redness; itchy skin; mouth irritation, soreness or infection; sore throat; fever.	Discontinue. Call doctor right away.
• Vaginal irritation, discharge, dryness; fatigue; weakness.	Continue. Call doctor when convenient.
• Constipation.	Continue. Tell doctor at next visit.
Rare:	
• Mood change; unsteadiness; numbness, tingling, weakness or pain in hands or feet.	Discontinue. Call doctor right away.
• Metallic taste.	Continue. Call doctor when convenient.

WARNINGS & PRECAUTIONS

Don't take if:
- You are allergic to metronidazole.
- You have had a blood-cell or bone-marrow disorder.

Before you start, consult your doctor:
- If you plan to become pregnant within medication period.
- If you have a brain or nervous-system disorder.
- If you have liver or heart disease.
- If you drink alcohol.

Over age 60:
Adverse reactions and side effects may be more frequent and severe than in younger persons.

Pregnancy:
Risk to unborn child outweighs drug benefits. Manufacturer advises against use during first 3 months and only limited use after that. Don't use.

Breast-feeding:
Drug passes into milk. Avoid drug or discontinue nursing until you finish medicine. Consult doctor for advice on maintaining milk supply.

Infants & children:
Use in children for amoeba infection only under close medical supervision.

Prolonged use:
No problems expected.

Skin & sunlight:
No problems expected.

Driving, piloting or hazardous work:
Avoid if you feel dizzy or unsteady. Otherwise, no problems expected.

Discontinuing:
Don't discontinue without doctor's advice until you complete prescribed dose, even though symptoms diminish or disappear.

Others:
Avoid alcohol 12 hours before and *at least* 24 hours after treatment period with metronidazole.

POSSIBLE INTERACTION WITH OTHER DRUGS

GENERIC NAME OR DRUG CLASS	COMBINED EFFECT
Anticoagulants, oral*	Increased anti-coagulant effect. Possible bleeding or bruising.
Cimetidine	Prolongs increased serum levels.
Disulfiram	Disulfiram reaction.* Avoid.
Nizatidine	Increased effect and toxicity of metoprolol.
Oxytetracycline	Decreased metronidazole effect.
Phenobarbital	Decreased effect of metronidazole.
Phenytoin	Decreased effect of metronidazole.

POSSIBLE INTERACTION WITH OTHER SUBSTANCES

INTERACTS WITH	COMBINED EFFECT
Alcohol:	Possible disulfiram reaction.* Avoid alcohol in *any* form or amount.
Beverages:	None expected.
Cocaine:	Decreased metronidazole effect. Avoid.
Foods:	None expected.
Marijuana:	None expected.
Tobacco:	None expected.

MEXILETINE

BRAND NAMES

Mexitil

BASIC INFORMATION

Habit forming? No
Prescription needed? Yes
Available as generic? No
Drug class: Antiarrhythmic

 ## USES

Stabilizes irregular heartbeat.

 ## DOSAGE & USAGE INFORMATION

How to take:
Capsules—Swallow whole with food, milk or antacid to lessen stomach irritation.

When to take:
At the same times each day as directed by your doctor.

If you forget a dose:
Take as soon as you remember up to 4 hours late. If more than 4 hours, wait for next scheduled dose (don't double this dose).

What drug does:
Blocks the fast sodium channel in heart tissue.

Time lapse before drug works:
30 minutes to 2 hours.

Don't take with:
See Interaction column and consult doctor.

 ## OVERDOSE

SYMPTOMS:
Nausea, vomiting, seizures, convulsions, cardiac arrest.
WHAT TO DO:
- **Dial 0 (operator) or 911 (emergency) for an ambulance or medical help. Then give first aid immediately.**
- **See emergency information on inside covers.**

 ## POSSIBLE ADVERSE REACTIONS OR SIDE EFFECTS

SYMPTOMS	WHAT TO DO
Life-threatening:	
Chest pain, shortness of breath, irregular or fast heartbeat.	Discontinue. Seek emergency treatment.
Common:	
Dizziness, anxiety, shakiness, unsteadiness when walking, heartburn, nausea, vomiting.	Discontinue. Call doctor right away.
Infrequent:	
• Sore throat, fever, mouth sores; blurred vision; confusion; constipation; diarrhea; headache; numbness or tingling in hands or feet; ringing in ears; unexplained bleeding or bruising; rash; slurred speech; insomnia; weakness; difficult swallowing.	Discontinue. Call doctor right away.
• Loss of taste.	Continue. Call doctor when convenient.
Rare:	
• Seizures.	Discontinue. Seek emergency treatment.
• Hallucinations, psychosis, memory loss, difficult breathing, swollen feet and ankles, hiccups, systemic lupus erythematosus, jaundice.	Discontinue. Call doctor right away.
• Hair loss, impotence.	Continue. Call doctor when convenient.

WARNINGS & PRECAUTIONS

Don't take if:
- If you are allergic to mexiletine, lidocaine or tocainide.
- If you take other heart medicine such as digitalis.

Before you start, consult your doctor:
- If you have had liver or kidney disease or impaired kidney function.
- If you have had lupus.
- If you have a history of seizures.
- If you will have surgery within 2 months, including dental surgery, requiring general or spinal anesthesia.

Over age 60:
Adverse reactions and side effects may be more frequent and severe than in younger persons. Ask doctor about smaller doses.

Pregnancy:
Risk to unborn child outweighs drug benefits. Don't use.

Breast-feeding:
Drug passes into milk. Avoid drug or discontinue nursing until you finish medicine. Consult doctor for advice on maintaining milk supply.

Infants & children:
Use only under close medical supervision.

Prolonged use:
May possibly cause lupus-like illness.

Skin & sunlight:
No problems expected.

Driving, piloting or hazardous work:
Use caution if you feel dizzy or weak. Otherwise, no problems expected.

Discontinuing:
Don't discontinue without consulting doctor. Dose may require gradual reduction if you have taken drug for a long time. Doses of other drugs may also require adjustment.

Others:
No problems expected.

POSSIBLE INTERACTION WITH OTHER DRUGS

GENERIC NAME OR DRUG CLASS	COMBINED EFFECT
Cimetidine	Increased mexiletine effect and toxicity.
Encainide	Increased effect of toxicity on the heart muscle.
Nicardipine	Possible increased effect and toxicity of each drug.
Phenobarbital	Decreased mexiletine effect.
Phenytoin	Decreased mexiletine effect.
Rifampin	Decreased mexiletine effect.
Urinary acidifiers* (ammonium chloride, ascorbic acid, potassium or sodium phosphate)	May decrease effectiveness of medicine.
Urinary alkalizers* (acetazolamide, antacids with calcium or magnesium, citric acid, dichlorphenamide, methazolamide, potassium citrate, sodium bicarbonate, sodium citrate)	May slow elimination of mexiletine and cause need to adjust dosage.

POSSIBLE INTERACTION WITH OTHER SUBSTANCES

INTERACTS WITH	COMBINED EFFECT
Alcohol:	Causes irregular effectiveness of mexiletine. Avoid.
Beverages: Caffeine drinks, iced drinks.	Irregular heartbeat.
Cocaine:	Decreased mexiletine effect.
Foods:	None expected.
Marijuana:	Irregular heartbeat. Avoid.
Tobacco:	Dangerous combination. May lead to liver problems and reduce effectiveness of mexiletine.

*See Glossary

MINOXIDIL

BRAND NAMES

Loniten

BASIC INFORMATION

Habit forming? No
Prescription needed? Yes
Available as generic? Yes
Drug class: Antihypertensive

 USES

- Treatment for high blood pressure in conjunction with other drugs, such as beta-adrenergic blockers and diuretics.
- Treatment for congestive heart failure.
- Can stimulate hair growth.

 DOSAGE & USAGE INFORMATION

How to take:
Tablet—Swallow with liquid. If you can't swallow whole, crumble tablet and take with liquid or food.

When to take:
At the same time each day, according to instructions on prescription label.

If you forget a dose:
Take as soon as you remember up to 2 hours late. If more than 2 hours, wait for next scheduled dose (don't double this dose).

What drug does:
Relaxes small blood vessels (arterioles) so blood can pass through more easily.

Time lapse before drug works:
2 to 3 hours for effect to begin; 3 to 7 days of continuous use may be necessary for maximum blood-pressure response.

Don't take with:
See Interaction column and consult doctor.

 OVERDOSE

SYMPTOMS:
Low blood pressure, fainting, coma.
WHAT TO DO:
- Dial 0 (operator) or 911 (emergency) for an ambulance or medical help. Then give first aid immediately.
- See emergency information on inside covers.

 POSSIBLE ADVERSE REACTIONS OR SIDE EFFECTS

SYMPTOMS	WHAT TO DO
Life-threatening: None expected.	
Common: Excessive hair growth.	Continue. Call doctor when convenient.
Frequent: Flushed skin or redness.	Continue. Call doctor when convenient.
Infrequent: • Chest pain, irregular or slow heartbeat, shortness of breath, swollen feet or legs, rapid weight gain.	Discontinue. Call doctor right away.
• Numbness of hands, feet, or face; headache; tender breasts; darkening of skin.	Continue. Call doctor when convenient.
Rare: Rash.	Discontinue. Call doctor right away.

WARNINGS & PRECAUTIONS

Don't take if:
You are allergic to minoxidil.

Before you start, consult your doctor:
- If you have had recent stroke, heart attack or angina pectoris in past 3 weeks.
- If you have impaired kidney function.

Over age 60:
Adverse reactions and side effects may be more frequent and severe than in younger persons.

Pregnancy:
Human studies not available. Avoid if possible.

Breast-feeding:
Human studies not available. Avoid if possible.

Infants & children:
Not recommended. Safety and dosage have not been established.

Prolonged use:
Request periodic blood examinations that include potassium levels.

Skin & sunlight:
No problems expected.

Driving, piloting or hazardous work:
Avoid if you become dizzy or faint. Otherwise, no problems expected.

Discontinuing:
Don't discontinue without consulting doctor. Dose may require gradual reduction if you have taken drug for a long time. Doses of other drugs may also require adjustment.

Others:
- Check pulse regularly. If it exceeds 20 or more beats per minute over your normal rate, consult doctor immediately.
- Check blood pressure frequently.

POSSIBLE INTERACTION WITH OTHER DRUGS

GENERIC NAME OR DRUG CLASS	COMBINED EFFECT
Anesthesia	Drastic drop in blood pressure.
Antihypertensives, other*	Dosage adjustments may be necessary to keep blood pressure at desired level.
Carteolol	Increased antihypertensive effect.
Diuretics*	Dosage adjustments may be necessary to keep blood pressure at desired level.
Guanadrel	Weakness and faintness when arising from bed or chair.
Guanethidine	Weakness and faintness when arising from bed or chair.
Lisinopril	Increased antihypertensive effect. Dosage of each may require adjustment.
Nicardipine	Blood-pressure drop. Dosages may require adjustment.
Nitrates*	Drastic drop in blood pressure.
Sotalol	Increased antihypertensive effect.
Sympathomimetics*	Possible decreased minoxidil effect.
Terazosin	Decreases effectiveness of terazosin.

POSSIBLE INTERACTION WITH OTHER SUBSTANCES

INTERACTS WITH	COMBINED EFFECT
Alcohol:	Possible excessive blood-pressure drop.
Beverages:	None expected.
Cocaine:	Increased risk of heart block and high blood pressure.
Foods: Salt substitutes.	Possible excessive potassium levels in blood.
Marijuana:	Increased dizziness.
Tobacco:	May decrease minoxidil effect. Avoid.

MINOXIDIL (Topical)

BRAND NAMES

Rogaine

BASIC INFORMATION

Habit forming? No
Prescription needed? Yes
Available as generic? No
Drug class: Hair growth stimulant

 ## USES

Hair loss on scalp from male pattern baldness (alopecia androgenetica).

 ## DOSAGE & USAGE INFORMATION

How to use:
- Topical solution—Apply only to dry hair and scalp. With the provided applicator, apply the amount prescribed to the scalp area being treated. Begin in center of the treated area.
- Wash hands immediately after use.
- Don't use a blow dryer.
- If you are using at bedtime, wait 30 minutes after applying before retiring.

When to use:
Twice a day or as directed.

If you forget a dose:
Use as soon as you remember. No need to ever double the dose.

What drug does:
Stimulates hair growth by possibly dilating small blood capillaries, thereby providing more blood to hair follicles.

Time lapse before drug works:
Varies with individuals.

Don't use with:
See Interaction column and consult doctor.

Continued next column

 ## OVERDOSE

SYMPTOMS:
None expected.
WHAT TO DO:
Not for internal use. If child accidentally swallows, call poison-control center.

 ## POSSIBLE ADVERSE REACTIONS OR SIDE EFFECTS

SYMPTOMS	WHAT TO DO
Life-threatening	
Fast, irregular heartbeat (rare; represents too much absorbed into body).	Discontinue. Seek emergency treatment.
Common	
None expected.	
Infrequent	
Itching scalp; flaking, reddened skin.	Continue. Call doctor when convenient.
Rare	
Burning scalp, skin rash, swollen face, headache, dizziness or fainting, hands and feet numb or tingling, rapid weight gain.	Discontinue. Call doctor right away.

WARNINGS & PRECAUTIONS

Don't use if:
You are allergic to minoxidil.

Before you start, consult your doctor:
If you are allergic to anything.

Over age 60:
No problems expected.

Pregnancy:
Don't use.

Breast-feeding:
Don't use.

Infants & children:
Don't use.

Prolonged use:
No problems expected.

Skin & sunlight:
No problems expected.

Driving, piloting or hazardous work:
No problems expected.

Discontinuing:
No problems expected.

Others:
- Keep away from eyes, nose and mouth. Flush with plain water if accident occurs.
- New hair will drop out when you stop using minoxidil.
- Keep cool, but don't freeze.

 POSSIBLE INTERACTION WITH OTHER DRUGS

GENERIC NAME OR DRUG CLASS	COMBINED EFFECT
None expected.	

 POSSIBLE INTERACTION WITH OTHER SUBSTANCES

INTERACTS WITH	COMBINED EFFECT
Alcohol:	None expected.
Beverages:	None expected.
Cocaine:	None expected.
Foods:	None expected.
Marijuana:	None expected.
Tobacco:	None expected.

MITOTANE

BRAND NAMES

Lysodren   O.p-DDD

BASIC INFORMATION

Habit forming? No
Prescription needed? Yes
Available as generic? No
Drug class: Antineoplastic

USES

- Treatment for some kinds of cancer.
- Treatment of Cushing's disease.

DOSAGE & USAGE INFORMATION

How to take:
Tablet—Take with liquid after light meal. Don't drink fluid with meals. Drink extra fluids between meals. Avoid sweet and fatty foods.

When to take:
At the same time each day.

If you forget a dose:
Take as soon as you remember. Don't ever double dose.

What drug does:
Suppresses adrenal cortex to prevent manufacture of excess cortisone.

Time lapse before drug works:
2 to 3 weeks for full effect.

Don't take with:
See Interaction column and consult doctor.

OVERDOSE

SYMPTOMS:
Headache, vomiting blood, stupor, seizure.
WHAT TO DO:
- Dial 0 (operator) or 911 (emergency) for an ambulance or medical help. Then give first aid immediately.
- If patient is unconscious and not breathing, give mouth-to-mouth breathing. If there is no heartbeat, use cardiac massage and mouth-to-mouth breathing (CPR). Don't try to make patient vomit. If you can't get help quickly, take patient to nearest emergency facility.
- See emergency information on inside covers.

POSSIBLE ADVERSE REACTIONS OR SIDE EFFECTS

SYMPTOMS	WHAT TO DO
Life-threatening:	
None expected.	
Common:	
• Darkened skin, appetite loss, nausea, vomiting.	Continue. Call doctor when convenient.
• Mental depression, drowsiness.	Continue. Tell doctor at next visit.
Infrequent:	
• Fever, chills, sore throat.	Discontinue. Seek emergency treatment.
• Unusual bleeding or bruising.	Discontinue. Call doctor right away.
• Rash, hair loss, blurred vision, difficult breathing, purple bands on nails, seeing double, cough, numbness or tingling in feet and toes, tiredness, weakness, dizziness when standing after sitting or lying down.	Continue. Call doctor when convenient.
Rare:	
Blood in urine.	Continue. Call doctor when convenient.

670

WARNINGS & PRECAUTIONS

Don't take if:
You are allergic to mitotane, adrenocorticosteroids or any antineoplastic drug.

Before you start, consult your doctor:
- If you have liver disease.
- If you have infection.

Over age 60:
Adverse reactions and side effects may be more frequent and severe than in younger persons.

Pregnancy:
Consult doctor. Risk to child is significant.

Breast-feeding:
Drug passes into milk. Don't nurse.

Infants & children:
Use only under care of medical supervisors who are experienced in anticancer drugs.

Prolonged use:
Adverse reactions more likely the longer drug is required.

Skin & sunlight:
No problems expected.

Driving, piloting or hazardous work:
No problems expected.

Discontinuing:
- Don't discontinue without consulting doctor. Dose may require gradual reduction if you have taken drug for a long time. Doses of other drugs may also require adjustment.
- Some side effects may follow discontinuing. Report any new symptoms.

Others:
No problems expected.

POSSIBLE INTERACTION WITH OTHER DRUGS

GENERIC NAME OR DRUG CLASS	COMBINED EFFECT
Antidepressants*	Increased central nervous system depression.
Antihistamines*	Increased central nervous system depression.
Corticosteroids*	Decreased effect of corticosteroid.
Ethinamate	Dangerous increased effects of ethinamate. Avoid combining.
Fluoxetine	Increased depressant effects of both drugs.
Guanfacine	May increase depressant effects of either drug.
Leucovorin	High alcohol content of leucovorin may cause adverse effects.
Methyprylon	Increased sedative effect, perhaps to dangerous level. Avoid.
Mind-altering drugs*	Increased central nervous system depression.
Nabilone	Greater depression of central nervous system.
Narcotics*	Increased central nervous system depression.
Phenytoin	Possible increased metabolism.
Sedatives*	Increased central nervous system depression.
Sleeping pills*	Increased central nervous system depression.
Spironolactone	Decreased mitotane effect.
Tranquilizers*	Increased central nervous system depression.
Warfarin	Possible increased metabolism.

POSSIBLE INTERACTION WITH OTHER SUBSTANCES

INTERACTS WITH	COMBINED EFFECT
Alcohol:	Increased depression. Avoid.
Beverages:	No problems expected.
Cocaine:	Increased toxicity. Avoid.
Foods:	Reduced irritation in stomach.
Marijuana:	No problems expected.
Tobacco:	Increased possibility of lung toxicity.

*See Glossary

MOLINDONE

BRAND NAMES

Moban

BASIC INFORMATION

Habit forming? No
Prescription needed? Yes
Available as generic? No
Drug class: Antipsychotic

 ## USES

Treats severe emotional, mental or nervous problems.

 ## DOSAGE & USAGE INFORMATION

How to take:
Tablet—Swallow with liquid or food to lessen stomach irritation. If you can't swallow whole, crumble tablet and take with food or liquid.

When to take:
Follow instructions on prescription label or side of package. Doses should be evenly spaced. For example, 4 times a day means every 6 hours.

If you forget a dose:
Take as soon as you remember up to 2 hours late. If more than 2 hours, wait for next scheduled dose (don't double this dose).

What drug does:
Corrects an imbalance in nerve impulses from the brain.

Time lapse before drug works:
- Nausea and vomiting—1 hour or less.
- Nervous and mental disorders—4 to 6 weeks.

Don't take with:
- Antacid or medicine for diarrhea.
- Non-prescription drugs for cough, cold or allergy.
- See Interaction column and consult doctor.

 ## OVERDOSE

SYMPTOMS:
Stupor, convulsions, coma.
WHAT TO DO:
- Dial 0 (operator) or 911 (emergency) for an ambulance or medical help. Then give first aid immediately.
- See emergency information on inside covers.

 ## POSSIBLE ADVERSE REACTIONS OR SIDE EFFECTS

SYMPTOMS	WHAT TO DO
Life-threatening:	
Uncontrolled muscle movements of tongue, face and other muscles (neuroleptic malignant syndrome, rare); unsteady gait.	Discontinue. Seek emergency treatment.
Common:	
• Muscle spasms of face and neck, unsteady gait.	Discontinue. Seek emergency treatment.
• Restlessness, tremor, drowsiness.	Discontinue. Call doctor right away.
• Decreased sweating, dry mouth, runny nose, constipation.	Continue. Call doctor when convenient.
Infrequent:	
• Fainting.	Discontinue. Seek emergency treatment.
• Rash.	Discontinue. Call doctor right away.
• Frequent urination, diminished sex drive, swollen breasts, menstrual irregularities.	Continue. Call doctor when convenient.
Rare:	
Change in vision, sore throat, fever, jaundice, abdominal pain.	Discontinue. Call doctor right away.

 ## WARNINGS & PRECAUTIONS

Don't take if:
- You are allergic to any phenothiazine.
- You have a blood or bone-marrow disease.

Before you start, consult your doctor:
- If you will have surgery within 2 months, including dental surgery, requiring general or spinal anesthesia.
- If you have asthma, emphysema or other lung disorder, glaucoma, prostate trouble.
- If you take non-prescription ulcer medicine, asthma medicine or amphetamines.

Over age 60:
Adverse reactions and side effects may be more frequent and severe than in younger persons. More likely to develop involuntary movement of jaws, lips, tongue, chewing. Report this to your doctor immediately. Early treatment can help.

Pregnancy:
Risk to unborn child outweighs drug benefits.
Don't use.

Breast-feeding:
Drug passes into milk. Avoid drug or discontinue
nursing until you finish medicine. Consult doctor
for advice on maintaining milk supply.

Infants & children:
Don't give to children younger than 2.

Prolonged use:
May lead to tardive dyskinesia (involuntary
movement of jaws, lips, tongue, chewing).

Skin & sunlight:
May cause rash or intensify sunburn in areas
exposed to sun or sunlamp. Skin may remain
sensitive for 3 months after discontinuing.

Driving, piloting or hazardous work:
Don't drive or pilot aircraft until you learn how
medicine affects you. Don't work around
dangerous machinery. Don't climb ladders or
work in high places. Danger increases if you
drink alcohol or take medicine affecting alertness
and reflexes.

Discontinuing:
- Nervous and mental disorders—Don't
  discontinue without doctor's advice until you
  complete prescribed dose, even though
  symptoms diminish or disappear.
- Nausea and vomiting—May be unnecessary
  to finish medicine. Follow doctor's instructions.

Others:
No problems expected.

POSSIBLE INTERACTION
WITH OTHER DRUGS

GENERIC NAME OR DRUG CLASS	COMBINED EFFECT
Anticholinergics*	Increased anticholinergic effect.
Antidepressants, tricyclic (TCA)*	Increased molindone effect.
Antihistamines*	Increased antihistamine effect.
Appetite suppressants*	Decreased suppressant effect.
Carteolol	Increased tranquilizer effect.
Dronabinol	Increased effects of both drugs. Avoid.
Ethinamate	Dangerous increased effects of ethinamate. Avoid combining.
Fluoxetine	Increased depressant effects of both drugs.
Guanethidine	Decreased guanethidine effect.
Guanfacine	May increase depressant effects of either drug.
Leucovorin	High alcohol content of leucovorin may cause adverse effects.
Levodopa	Decreased levodopa effect.
Loxapine	May increase toxic effects of both drugs.
Methyprylon	Increased sedative effect, perhaps to dangerous level. Avoid.
Mind-altering drugs*	Increased effect of mind-altering drugs.
Nabilone	Greater depression of central nervous system.
Narcotics*	Increased narcotic effect.
Phenytoin	Increased phenytoin effect.
Procarbazine	Increased sedation.
Quinidine	Impaired heart function. Dangerous mixture.
Sedatives*	Increased sedative effect.
Sotalol	Increased tranquilizer effect.
Tetracyclines*	May decrease absorption of both drugs.
Tranquilizers, other*	Increased tranquilizer effect.

POSSIBLE INTERACTION
WITH OTHER SUBSTANCES

INTERACTS WITH	COMBINED EFFECT
Alcohol:	Dangerous oversedation.
Beverages:	None expected.
Cocaine:	Decreased molindone effect. Avoid.
Foods:	None expected.
Marijuana:	Drowsiness. May increase antinausea effect.
Tobacco:	None expected.

MONAMINE OXIDASE (MAO) INHIBITORS

BRAND AND GENERIC NAMES

Eutonyl	PARGYLINE
ISOCARBOXAZID	Parnate
Marplan	PHENELZINE
Nardil	TRANYLCYPROMINE

BASIC INFORMATION

Habit forming? No
Prescription needed? Yes
Available as generic? No
Drug class: MAO (monamine oxidase)
  inhibitor, antidepressant

USES

- Treatment for depression.
- Pargyline sometimes used to lower blood pressure.

DOSAGE & USAGE INFORMATION

How to take:
Tablet—Swallow with liquid. If you can't swallow whole, crumble tablet and take with liquid or food.

When to take:
At the same times each day.

If you forget a dose:
Take as soon as you remember up to 2 hours late. If more than 2 hours, wait for next scheduled dose (don't double this dose).

What drug does:
Inhibits nerve transmissions in brain that may cause depression.

Time lapse before drug works:
4 to 6 weeks for maximum effect.

Continued next column

OVERDOSE

SYMPTOMS:
Restlessness, agitation, excitement, fever, convulsions, coma.
WHAT TO DO:
- Dial 0 (operator) or 911 (emergency) for an ambulance or medical help. Then give first aid immediately.
- See emergency information on inside covers.

Don't take with:
- Non-prescription diet pills, nose drops, medicine for asthma, cough, cold or allergy, or medicine containing caffeine or alcohol.
- See Interaction column and consult doctor.

POSSIBLE ADVERSE REACTIONS OR SIDE EFFECTS

SYMPTOMS	WHAT TO DO
Life-threatening: None expected.	
Common:	
• Fatigue, weakness.	Continue. Call doctor when convenient.
• Dizziness when changing position, restlessness, tremors, dry mouth, constipation, difficult urination.	Continue. Tell doctor at next visit.
Infrequent:	
• Fainting.	Discontinue. Seek emergency treatment.
• Severe headache, chest pain.	Discontinue. Call doctor right away.
• Hallucinations, insomnia, nightmares, diarrhea, rapid or pounding heartbeat, swollen feet or legs, joint pain.	Continue. Call doctor when convenient.
• Diminished sex drive.	Continue. Tell doctor at next visit.
Rare: Rash, nausea, vomiting, stiff neck, jaundice, fever, increased sweating.	Discontinue. Call doctor right away.

WARNINGS & PRECAUTIONS

Don't take if:
- You are allergic to any MAO inhibitor.
- You have heart disease, congestive heart failure, heart-rhythm irregularities or high blood pressure.
- You have liver or kidney disease.

Before you start, consult your doctor:
- If you are alcoholic.
- If you have had a stroke.
- If you have diabetes, epilepsy, asthma, overactive thyroid, schizophrenia, Parkinson's disease, adrenal-gland tumor.
- If you will have surgery within 2 months, including dental surgery, requiring general or spinal anesthesia.

Over age 60:
Not recommended.

Pregnancy:
No proven harm to unborn child. Avoid if possible.

Breast-feeding:
Safety not established. Consult doctor.

Infants & children:
Not recommended.

Prolonged use:
May be toxic to liver.

Skin & sunlight:
May cause rash or intensify sunburn in areas exposed to sun or sunlamp.

Driving, piloting or hazardous work:
Don't drive or pilot aircraft until you learn how medicine affects you. Don't work around dangerous machinery. Don't climb ladders or work in high places. Danger increases if you drink alcohol or take medicine affecting alertness and reflexes.

Discontinuing:
- Don't discontinue without doctor's advice until you complete prescribed dose, even though symptoms diminish or disappear.
- Follow precautions regarding foods, drinks and other medicines for 2 weeks after discontinuing.

Others:
- May affect blood-sugar levels in patients with diabetes.
- Fever may indicate that MAO inhibitor dose requires adjustment.

POSSIBLE INTERACTION WITH OTHER DRUGS

GENERIC NAME OR DRUG CLASS	COMBINED EFFECT
Amphetamines*	Blood-pressure rise to life-threatening level.
Anticholinergics*	Increased anticholinergic effect.
Anticonvulsants*	Changed seizure pattern.
Antidepressants, tricyclic (TCA)*	Blood-pressure rise to life-threatening level. Possible fever, convulsions, delirium.
Antidiabetics, oral and insulin*	Excessively low blood sugar.
Antihypertensives*	Excessively low blood pressure.

Beta-adrenergic blockers*	Possible blood-pressure rise if MAO inhibitor is discontinued after simultaneous use with acebutolol.
Caffeine	Irregular heartbeat or high blood pressure.
Carbamazepine	Fever, seizures. Avoid.
Cyclobenzaprine	Fever, seizures. Avoid.
Diuretics*	Excessively low blood pressure.
Ephedrine	Increased blood pressure.
Ethinamate	Dangerous increased effects of ethinamate. Avoid combining.
Fluoxetine	Increased depressant effects of both drugs.
Guanethidine	Blood-pressure rise to life-threatening level.
Guanfacine	May increase depressant effects of either drug.
Hypoglycemics, oral*	Increased hypoglycemic effect.
Indapamide	Increased indapamide effect.
Insulin	Increased hypoglycemic effect.

Continued page 1091

POSSIBLE INTERACTION WITH OTHER SUBSTANCES

INTERACTS WITH	COMBINED EFFECT
Alcohol:	Increased sedation to dangerous level.
Beverages: Caffeine drinks.	Irregular heartbeat or high blood pressure.
Drinks containing tyramine*	Blood-pressure rise to life-threatening level.
Cocaine:	Overstimulation. Possibly fatal.
Foods: Foods containing tyramine*	Blood-pressure rise to life-threatening level.
Marijuana:	Overstimulation. Avoid.
Tobacco:	No proven problems.

*See Glossary

675

NABILONE

BRAND NAMES

Cesamet

BASIC INFORMATION

Habit forming? No
Prescription needed? Yes
Available as generic? No
Drug class: Anti-emetic

USES

- Treats nausea and vomiting.
- Prevents nausea and vomiting in patients receiving cancer chemotherapy.

DOSAGE & USAGE INFORMATION

How to take:
Capsule—Swallow with liquid. If you can't swallow whole, open capsule and take with liquid or food.

When to take:
At the same each day, according to instructions on prescription label.

If you forget a dose:
Take as soon as you remember up to 2 hours late. If more than 2 hours, wait for next scheduled dose (don't double this dose).

What drug does:
Chemically related to marijuana, it probably regulates the vomiting control center in the brain.

Continued next column

OVERDOSE

SYMPTOMS:
Mood changes; confusion and delusions; hallucinations; mental depression; nervousness; breathing difficulty; fast, slow or pounding heartbeat; fainting.
WHAT TO DO:
- Dial 0 (operator) or 911 (emergency) for an ambulance or medical help. Then give first aid immediately.
- If patient is unconscious and not breathing, give mouth-to-mouth breathing. If there is no heartbeat, use cardiac massage and mouth-to-mouth breathing (CPR). Don't try to make patient vomit. If you can't get help quickly, take patient to nearest emergency facility.
- See emergency information on inside covers.

Time lapse before drug works:
2 hours.

Don't take with:
Alcohol or any drug that depresses the central nervous system. (See Central Nervous System [CNS] Depression-Producing Medications in the Glossary.)

POSSIBLE ADVERSE REACTIONS OR SIDE EFFECTS

SYMPTOMS	WHAT TO DO
Life-threatening: Mood changes; fainting; hallucinations; fast, slow or pounding heartbeat; confusion and delusions; mental depression; nervousness; breathing difficulty.	Discontinue. Call doctor right away.
Common: Dry mouth.	Continue. Call doctor when convenient.
Infrequent: Clumsiness, mental changes, drowsiness, headache, false sense of well-being.	Discontinue. Call doctor right away.
Rare: Blurred vision, dizziness on standing, appetite loss, muscle pain.	Discontinue. Call doctor right away.

WARNINGS & PRECAUTIONS

Don't take if:
- You are allergic to nabilone or marijuana.
- You have schizophrenic, manic or depressive states.

Before you start, consult your doctor:
- If you have abused drugs or are dependent on them, including alcohol.
- If you have had high blood pressure or heart disease.
- If you have had impaired liver function.

Over age 60:
Adverse reactions and side effects may be more frequent and severe than in younger persons. You may need smaller doses for shorter periods of time.

Pregnancy:
Studies inconclusive on harm to unborn child. Decide with your doctor whether drug benefits justify risk to unborn child.

Breast-feeding:
Drug passes into milk. Avoid drug or discontinue nursing until you finish medicine. Consult doctor for advice on maintaining milk supply.

Infants & children:
Not recommended for children 18 and younger. Use only under doctor's supervision.

Prolonged use:
Avoid prolonged use. This medicine is intended to be used only during a cycle of cancer chemotherapy.

Skin & sunlight:
No problems expected.

Driving, piloting or hazardous work:
Don't drive or pilot aircraft until you learn how medicine affects you. Don't work around dangerous machinery. Don't climb ladders or work in high places. Danger increases if you drink alcohol or take medicine affecting alertness and reflexes.

Discontinuing:
No problems expected.

Others:
- Blood pressure should be measured regularly.
- Learn to count and recognize changes in your pulse.
- Get up from bed or chair slowly to avoid fainting.

POSSIBLE INTERACTION WITH OTHER DRUGS

GENERIC NAME OR DRUG CLASS	COMBINED EFFECT
Apomorphine	Decreases effect of apomorphine.
Central nervous system depressants, other*	Greater depression of the central nervous system.

POSSIBLE INTERACTION WITH OTHER SUBSTANCES

INTERACTS WITH	COMBINED EFFECT
Alcohol:	Dangerous depression of the central nervous system. Avoid.
Beverages:	None expected.
Cocaine:	Decreased nabilone effect. Avoid.
Foods:	None expected.
Marijuana:	None expected.
Tobacco:	None expected.

*See Glossary

NADOLOL

BRAND NAMES

Corgard   Corzide

BASIC INFORMATION

Habit forming? No
Prescription needed? Yes
Available as generic? No
Drug class: Beta-adrenergic blocker

 ## USES

- Reduces angina attacks.
- Stabilizes irregular heartbeat.
- Lowers blood pressure.
- Reduces frequency of migraine headaches. (Does not relieve headache pain.)
- Other uses prescribed by your doctor.

 ## DOSAGE & USAGE INFORMATION

How to take:
Tablet—Swallow with liquid. If you can't swallow whole, crumble tablet and take with liquid or food.

When to take:
With meals or immediately after.

If you forget a dose:
Take as soon as you remember. Return to regular schedule, but allow 3 hours between doses.

What drug does:
- Blocks certain actions of sympathetic nervous system.
- Lowers heart's oxygen requirements.
- Slows nerve impulses through heart.
- Reduces blood vessel contraction in heart, scalp and other body parts.

Time lapse before drug works:
1 to 4 hours.

Continued next column

 ## OVERDOSE

SYMPTOMS:
Weakness, slow or weak pulse, blood-pressure drop, difficulty breathing, fainting, convulsions, cold and sweaty skin.
WHAT TO DO:
- Dial 0 (operator) or 911 (emergency) for an ambulance or medical help. Then give first aid immediately.
- See emergency information on inside covers.

Don't take with:
Non-prescription drugs or drugs in Interaction column without consulting doctor.

 ## POSSIBLE ADVERSE REACTIONS OR SIDE EFFECTS

SYMPTOMS	WHAT TO DO
Life-threatening:	
Congestive heart failure.	Discontinue. Seek emergency treatment.
Common:	
• Pulse lower than 50 beats per minute.	Discontinue. Call doctor right away.
• Drowsiness, numbness or tingling in fingers or toes, dizziness, nausea, diarrhea, fatigue, weakness.	Continue. Call doctor when convenient.
• Cold hands, feet; dry mouth, eyes, skin.	Continue. Tell doctor at next visit.
Infrequent:	
• Hallucinations, nightmares, insomnia, headache, difficult breathing, joint pain, anxiety.	Discontinue. Call doctor right away.
• Confusion, reduced alertness, depression.	Continue. Call doctor when convenient.
• Constipation.	Continue. Tell doctor at next visit.
Rare:	
• Rash, sore throat, fever.	Discontinue. Call doctor right away.
• Unusual bleeding or bruising; impotence; dry, burning eyes.	Continue. Call doctor when convenient.

 ## WARNINGS & PRECAUTIONS

Don't take if:
- You are allergic to any beta-adrenergic blocker.
- You have asthma or hay fever symptoms.
- You have taken MAO inhibitors in past 2 weeks.

Before you start, consult your doctor:
- If you have heart disease or poor circulation to the extremities.
- If you have hay fever, asthma, chronic bronchitis, emphysema.
- If you have overactive thyroid function.
- If you have impaired liver or kidney function.
- If you will have surgery within 2 months, including dental surgery, requiring general or spinal anesthesia.
- If you have diabetes or hypoglycemia.

678

Over age 60:
Adverse reactions and side effects may be more frequent and severe than in younger persons.

Pregnancy:
Risk to unborn child outweighs drug benefits. Don't use.

Breast-feeding:
Drug passes into milk. Avoid drug or discontinue nursing until you finish medicine. Consult doctor for advice on maintaining milk supply.

Infants & children:
Not recommended.

Prolonged use:
Weakens heart muscle contractions.

Skin & sunlight:
No problems expected.

Driving, piloting or hazardous work:
Don't drive or pilot aircraft until you learn how medicine affects you. Don't work around dangerous machinery. Don't climb ladders or work in high places. Danger increases if you drink alcohol or take medicine affecting alertness and reflexes.

Discontinuing:
Don't discontinue without consulting doctor. Dose may require gradual reduction if you have taken drug for a long time. Doses of other drugs may also require adjustment.

Others:
May mask hypoglycemia.

POSSIBLE INTERACTION WITH OTHER DRUGS

GENERIC NAME OR DRUG CLASS	COMBINED EFFECT
ACE inhibitors: captopril, enalapril, lisinopril*	Increased antihypertensive effects of both drugs. Dosages may require adjustment.
Antidiabetics*	Increased antidiabetic effect.
Antihistamines*	Decreased antihistamine effect.
Antihypertensives*	Increased antihypertensive effect.
Barbiturates*	Increased barbiturate effect. Dangerous sedation.
Beta-adrenergic blockers*	Increased antihypertensive effects of both drugs. Dosages may require adjustment.
Beta-agonists*	Decreased effect of nadolol.

Betaxolol eyedrops	Possible increased nadolol effect.
Digitalis preparations*	Increased or decreased heart rate. Improves irregular heartbeat.
Encainide	Increased effect of toxicity on the heart muscle.
Indomethacin	Decreased nadolol effect.
Insulin	May prolong hypoglycemic effects.
Levobunolol eyedrops	Possible increased nadolol effect.
Narcotics*	Increased narcotic effect. Dangerous sedation.
Nicardipine	Possible irregular heartbeat and congestive heart failure.
Nitrates*	Possible excessive blood-pressure drop.
Non-steroidal anti-inflammatory drugs (NSAIDs)*	Decreased hypertensive effect of nadolol.
Phenytoin	Decreased nadolol effect.
Quinidine	Slows heart excessively.
Reserpine	Increased reserpine effect. Oversedation, depression.
Rifampin	Decreased nadolol effect.
Sympathomimetics*	Decreased effect of nadolol.

Continued page 1092

POSSIBLE INTERACTION WITH OTHER SUBSTANCES

INTERACTS WITH	COMBINED EFFECT
Alcohol:	Excessive blood-pressure drop. Avoid.
Beverages:	None expected.
Cocaine:	Irregular heartbeat. Avoid.
Foods:	None expected.
Marijuana:	Daily use—Impaired circulation to hands and feet.
Tobacco:	Possible irregular heartbeat.

*See Glossary

NAFCILLIN

BRAND NAMES

Nafcil   Unipen
Nallpen

BASIC INFORMATION

Habit forming? No
Prescription needed? Yes
Available as generic? No
Drug class: Antibiotic (penicillin)

USES

Treatment of bacterial infections that are susceptible to nafcillin.

DOSAGE & USAGE INFORMATION

How to take:
- Tablets or capsules—Swallow with liquid on an empty stomach 1 hour before or 2 hours after eating.
- Liquid—Take with cold beverage. Liquid form is perishable and effective for only 7 days at room temperature. Effective for 14 days if stored in refrigerator. Don't freeze.

When to take:
Follow instructions on prescription label or side of package. Doses should be evenly spaced. For example, 4 times a day means every 6 hours.

If you forget a dose:
Take as soon as you remember. Continue regular schedule.

What drug does:
Destroys susceptible bacteria. Does not kill viruses.

Time lapse before drug works:
May be several days before medicine affects infection.

Don't take with:
See Interaction column and consult doctor.

OVERDOSE

SYMPTOMS:
Severe diarrhea, nausea or vomiting.
WHAT TO DO:
Overdose unlikely to threaten life. If person takes much larger amount than prescribed, call doctor, poison-control center or hospital emergency room for instructions.

POSSIBLE ADVERSE REACTIONS OR SIDE EFFECTS

SYMPTOMS	WHAT TO DO
Life-threatening:	
Hives, rash, intense itching, faintness soon after a dose (anaphylaxis).	Seek emergency treatment immediately.
Common:	
Dark or discolored tongue.	Continue. Tell doctor at next visit.
Infrequent:	
Mild nausea, vomiting, diarrhea.	Continue. Call doctor when convenient.
Rare:	
Unexplained bleeding.	Discontinue. Call doctor right away.

WARNINGS & PRECAUTIONS

Don't take if:
You are allergic to nafcillin, cephalosporin antibiotics, other penicillins or penicillamine. Life-threatening reaction may occur.

Before you start, consult your doctor:
If you are allergic to any substance or drug.

Over age 60:
You may have skin reactions, particularly around genitals and anus.

Pregnancy:
Studies inconclusive on harm to unborn child. Animal studies show fetal abnormalities. Decide with your doctor whether drug benefits justify risk to unborn child.

Breast-feeding:
Drug passes into milk. Child may become sensitive to penicillins and have allergic reactions to penicillin drugs. Avoid nafcillin or discontinue nursing until you finish medicine. Consult doctor for advice on maintaining milk supply.

Infants & children:
No problems expected.

Prolonged use:
You may become more susceptible to infections caused by germs not responsive to nafcillin.

Skin & sunlight:
No problems expected.

Driving, piloting or hazardous work:
Usually not dangerous. Most hazardous reactions likely to occur a few minutes after taking nafcillin.

Discontinuing:
Don't discontinue without doctor's advice until you complete prescribed dose, even though symptoms diminish or disappear.

Others:
Absorption of this drug in oral form is unpredictable. Injections are more reliable.

POSSIBLE INTERACTION WITH OTHER DRUGS

GENERIC NAME OR DRUG CLASS	COMBINED EFFECT
Beta-adrenergic blockers*	Increased chance of anaphylaxis (see emergency information on inside front cover).
Chloramphenicol	Decreased effect of both drugs.
Erythromycins*	Decreased effect of both drugs.
Loperamide	Decreased nafcillin effect.
Paromomycin	Decreased effect of both drugs.
Tetracyclines*	Decreased effect of both drugs.
Troleandomycin	Decreased effect of both drugs.

POSSIBLE INTERACTION WITH OTHER SUBSTANCES

INTERACTS WITH	COMBINED EFFECT
Alcohol:	Occasional stomach irritation.
Beverages:	None expected.
Cocaine:	No proven problems.
Foods:	None expected.
Marijuana:	No proven problems.
Tobacco:	None expected.

NALIDIXIC ACID

BRAND NAMES

NegGram

BASIC INFORMATION

Habit forming? No
Prescription needed? Yes
Available as generic? No
Drug class: Antimicrobial

 ## USES

Treatment for urinary-tract infections.

 ## DOSAGE & USAGE INFORMATION

How to take:
- Tablet—Swallow with food or milk to lessen stomach irritation. If you can't swallow whole, crumble tablet and take with liquid or food.
- Liquid—Take with liquid or food.

When to take:
At the same times each day.

If you forget a dose:
Take as soon as you remember up to 2 hours late. If more than 2 hours, wait for next scheduled dose (don't double this dose).

What drug does:
Destroys bacteria susceptible to nalidixic acid.

Time lapse before drug works:
1 to 2 weeks.

Don't take with:
See Interaction column and consult doctor.

 ## OVERDOSE

SYMPTOMS:
Lethargy, stomach upset, behavioral changes, hyperglycemia, psychosis, convulsions and stupor.
WHAT TO DO:
- Dial 0 (operator) or 911 (emergency) for an ambulance or medical help. Then give first aid immediately.
- If patient is unconscious and not breathing, give mouth-to-mouth breathing. If there is no heartbeat, use cardiac massage and mouth-to-mouth breathing (CPR). Don't try to make patient vomit. If you can't get help quickly, take patient to nearest emergency facility.
- See emergency information on inside covers.

 ## POSSIBLE ADVERSE REACTIONS OR SIDE EFFECTS

SYMPTOMS	WHAT TO DO
Life-threatening: Hives, rash, intense itching, faintness soon after a dose (anaphylaxis).	Seek emergency treatment immediately.
Common: Rash; itchy skin; decreased, blurred or double vision; halos around lights or excess brightness; changes in color vision; nausea; vomiting; diarrhea.	Discontinue. Call doctor right away.
Infrequent: Dizziness, drowsiness.	Continue. Call doctor when convenient.
Rare: • Paleness, sore throat or fever, severe stomach pain, pale stool, unusual bleeding or bruising, jaundice, fatigue, weakness, seizures, psychosis, joint pain, numbness or tingling in hands or feet.	Discontinue. Call doctor right away.
• Dizziness, headache.	Continue. Call doctor when convenient.

WARNINGS & PRECAUTIONS

Don't take if:
- You are allergic to nalidixic acid.
- You have a seizure disorder (epilepsy, convulsions).

Before you start, consult your doctor:
- If you plan to become pregnant within medication period.
- If you have or have had kidney or liver disease.
- If you have impaired circulation of the brain (hardened arteries).
- If you have Parkinson's disease.
- If you have diabetes (it may affect urine-sugar tests).

Over age 60:
Adverse reactions and side effects may be more frequent and severe than in younger persons.

Pregnancy:
Risk to unborn child outweighs drug benefits. Don't use, especially during first 3 months.

Breast-feeding:
No problems expected, unless you have impaired kidney function. Consult doctor.

Infants & children:
Don't give to infants younger than 3 months.

Prolonged use:
No problems expected.

Skin & sunlight:
May cause rash or intensify sunburn in areas exposed to sun or sunlamp.

Driving, piloting or hazardous work:
Avoid if you feel drowsy, dizzy or have vision problems. Otherwise, no problems expected.

Discontinuing:
Don't discontinue without consulting doctor. Dose may require gradual reduction if you have taken drug for a long time. Doses of other drugs may also require adjustment.

Others:
Periodic blood counts and liver- and kidney-function tests recommended.

POSSIBLE INTERACTION WITH OTHER DRUGS

GENERIC NAME OR DRUG CLASS	COMBINED EFFECT
Antacids*	Decreased absorption of nalidixic acid.
Anticoagulants, oral*	Increased anticoagulant effect.
Calcium supplements*	Decreased effect of nalidixic acid.
Nitrofurantoin	Decreased effect of nalidixic acid.
Probenecid	Decreased effect of nalidixic acid.
Vitamin C (in large doses)	Increased effect of nalidixic acid.

POSSIBLE INTERACTION WITH OTHER SUBSTANCES

INTERACTS WITH	COMBINED EFFECT
Alcohol:	Impaired alertness, judgment and coordination.
Beverages:	None expected.
Cocaine:	Impaired judgment and coordination.
Foods:	None expected.
Marijuana:	Impaired alertness, judgment and coordination.
Tobacco:	None expected.

*See Glossary

NALTREXONE

BRAND NAMES

Trexan

BASIC INFORMATION

Habit forming? No
Prescription needed? Yes
Available as generic? No
Drug class: Narcotic antagonist

 ## USES

Treats detoxified former narcotic addicts. It helps maintain a drug-free state.

 ## DOSAGE & USAGE INFORMATION

How to take:
- *Don't take at all until detoxification has been accomplished.*
- Tablets—Swallow with liquid or food to lessen stomach irritation. If you can't swallow whole, crumble tablet and take with liquid or food.

When to take:
At the same time every day or every other day as directed.

If you forget a dose:
Follow detailed instructions from the one who prescribed for you.

What drug does:
Binds to opiod receptors in the central nervous system and prohibits the effects of narcotic drugs.

Time lapse before drug works:
1 hour.

Don't take with:
- Narcotics.
- See Interaction column and consult doctor.

 ## OVERDOSE

SYMPTOMS:
Seizures, coma.
WHAT TO DO:
- Dial 0 (operator) or 911 (emergency) for an ambulance or medical help. Then give first aid immediately.
- See emergency information on inside covers.

 ## POSSIBLE ADVERSE REACTIONS OR SIDE EFFECTS

SYMPTOMS	WHAT TO DO
Life-threatening:	
Hallucinations, very fast heartbeat, fainting.	Seek emergency treatment immediately.
Common:	
Skin rash, chills, constipation, appetite loss, irritability.	Continue. Call doctor when convenient.
Infrequent:	
• Nosebleeds.	Discontinue. Call doctor right away.
• Abdominal pain, blurred vision, confusion, earache, fever, hallucinations, depression.	Continue. Call doctor when convenient.
Rare:	
• Pain, tenderness or color change in feet.	Discontinue. Call doctor right away.
• Ringing in ears, swollen glands.	Continue. Call doctor when convenient.

WARNINGS & PRECAUTIONS

Don't take if:
- You don't have close medical supervision.
- You are currently dependent on drugs.
- You have severe liver disease.

Before you start, consult your doctor:
If you have mild liver disease.

Over age 60:
Adverse reactions and side effects may be more frequent and severe than in younger persons. You may need smaller doses for shorter periods of time.

Pregnancy:
Risk to unborn child outweighs drug benefits. Don't use.

Breast-feeding:
Drug passes into milk. Avoid drug or discontinue nursing until you finish medicine. Consult doctor for advice on maintaining milk supply.

Infants & children:
Not recommended.

Prolonged use:
Not recommended.

Skin & sunlight:
No problems expected.

Driving, piloting or hazardous work:
Don't drive or pilot aircraft until you learn how medicine affects you. Don't work around dangerous machinery. Don't climb ladders or work in high places. Danger increases if you drink alcohol or take medicine affecting alertness and reflexes.

Discontinuing:
Don't discontinue without consulting doctor. Dose may require gradual reduction if you have taken drug for a long time. Doses of other drugs may also require adjustment.

Others:
- Probably not effective in treating people addicted to substances other than opium or morphine derivatives.
- Must be given under close supervision by people experienced in using naltrexone to treat addicts.
- Attempting to use narcotics to overcome effects of naltrexone may lead to coma and death.
- Withdraw several days prior to expected surgery.

POSSIBLE INTERACTION WITH OTHER DRUGS

GENERIC NAME OR DRUG CLASS	COMBINED EFFECT
Carteolol	Increased narcotic effect. Dangerous sedation.
Narcotic medicines* (butorphenal, codeine, heroin, hydrocodone, hydromorphone, levorphanol, morphine, nalbuphine, opium, oxycodone, oxymorphone, paregoric, pentazocine, propoxyphene)	Precipitates withdrawal symptoms. May lead to arrest, coma and death.
Sotalol	Increased narcotic effect. Dangerous sedation.

POSSIBLE INTERACTION WITH OTHER SUBSTANCES

INTERACTS WITH	COMBINED EFFECT
Alcohol:	Unpredictable effects. Avoid.
Beverages:	None expected.
Cocaine:	Unpredictable effects. Avoid.
Foods:	None expected.
Marijuana:	Unpredictable effects. Avoid.
Tobacco:	None expected.

NAPROXEN

BRAND NAMES

Anaprox	Naxen
Apo-Nan	Novonaprox
Naprosyn	Synflex

BASIC INFORMATION

Habit forming? No
Prescription needed? Yes
Available as generic? No
Drug class: Anti-inflammatory (non-steroid)

USES

- Treatment for joint pain, stiffness, inflammation and swelling of arthritis and gout.
- Pain reliever.
- Treatment for dysmenorrhea (painful or difficult menstruation).
- Treatment for juvenile rheumatoid arthritis.

DOSAGE & USAGE INFORMATION

How to take:
- Tablet or oral suspension—Swallow with liquid or food to lessen stomach irritation. If you can't swallow whole, crumble tablet and take with liquid or food.
- Suppositories—Remove wrapper and moisten suppository with water. Gently insert larger end into rectum. Push well into rectum with finger.

When to take:
At the same times each day.

If you forget a dose:
Take as soon as you remember up to 2 hours late. If more than 2 hours, wait for next scheduled dose (don't double this dose).

What drug does:
Reduces tissue concentration of prostaglandins (hormones which produce inflammation and pain).

Continued next column

OVERDOSE

SYMPTOMS:
Confusion, agitation, incoherence, convulsions, possible hemorrhage from stomach or intestine, coma.
WHAT TO DO:
- Dial 0 (operator) or 911 (emergency) for an ambulance or medical help. Then give first aid immediately.
- See emergency information on inside covers.

Time lapse before drug works:
Begins in 4 to 24 hours. May require 3 weeks regular use for maximum benefit.

Don't take with:
See Interaction column and consult doctor.

POSSIBLE ADVERSE REACTIONS OR SIDE EFFECTS

SYMPTOMS	WHAT TO DO
Life-threatening: Hives, rash, intense itching, faintness soon after a dose (anaphylaxis in aspirin-sensitive persons).	Seek emergency treatment immediately.
Common: • Dizziness, nausea, pain. • Headache.	Continue. Call doctor when convenient. Continue. Tell doctor at next visit.
Infrequent: Depression, drowsiness, ringing in ears, constipation or diarrhea, vomiting, swollen feet or legs.	Continue. Call doctor when convenient.
Rare: • Convulsions; confusion; rash, hives or itchy skin; blurred vision; black, bloody or tarry stool; difficult breathing; tightness in chest; rapid heartbeat; unusual bleeding or bruising; blood in urine; jaundice; severe abdominal pain, psychosis.	Discontinue. Call doctor right away.
• Urgent, frequent, painful or difficult urination; fatigue; weakness; swollen breasts in males; impotence; menstrual irregularities.	Continue. Call doctor when convenient.

WARNINGS & PRECAUTIONS

Don't take if:
- You are allergic to aspirin or any non-steroid, anti-inflammatory drug.
- You have gastritis, peptic ulcer, enteritis, ileitis, ulcerative colitis, asthma, heart failure, high blood pressure or bleeding problems.
- You have had recent rectal bleeding and suppository form has been prescribed.
- Patient is younger than 15.

Before you start, consult your doctor:
- If you have epilepsy.
- If you have Parkinson's disease.
- If you have been mentally ill.
- If you have had kidney disease or impaired kidney function.

Over age 60:
Adverse reactions and side effects may be more frequent and severe than in younger persons.

Pregnancy:
Studies inconclusive on harm to unborn child. Decide with your doctor whether drug benefits justify risk to unborn child.

Breast-feeding:
May harm child. Avoid.

Infants & children:
Not recommended for anyone younger than 15. Use only under medical supervision.

Prolonged use:
- Eye damage.
- Reduced hearing.
- Sore throat, fever.
- Weight gain.

Skin & sunlight:
Increased sensitivity to sunlight.

Driving, piloting or hazardous work:
Don't drive or pilot aircraft until you learn how medicine affects you. Don't work around dangerous machinery. Don't climb ladders or work in high places. Danger increases if you drink alcohol or take medicine affecting alertness and reflexes, such as antihistamines, tranquilizers, sedatives, pain medicine, narcotics and mind-altering drugs.

Discontinuing:
Don't discontinue without consulting doctor. Dose may require gradual reduction if you have taken drug for a long time. Doses of other drugs may also require adjustment.

Others:
No problems expected.

POSSIBLE INTERACTION WITH OTHER DRUGS

GENERIC NAME OR DRUG CLASS	COMBINED EFFECT
ACE inhibitors: captopril, enalapril, lisinopril*	May decrease ACE inhibitor effect.
Anticoagulants, oral*	Increased risk of bleeding.
Aspirin	Increased risk of stomach ulcer.
Beta-adrenergic blockers*	Decreased antihypertensive effect.
Carteolol	Decreased antihypertensive effect of carteolol.
Cortisone drugs*	Increased risk of stomach ulcer.
Diuretics*	May decrease diuretic effect.
Lithium	Possible increased lithium effect and toxicity.
Methotrexate	May increase toxicity.
Minoxidil	Decreased minoxidil effect.
Oxyphenbutazone	Possible stomach ulcer.
Phenylbutazone	Possible stomach ulcer.
Probenecid	Increased naproxen effect.
Sotalol	Decreased antihypertensive effect of sotalol.

Continued page 1092

POSSIBLE INTERACTION WITH OTHER SUBSTANCES

INTERACTS WITH	COMBINED EFFECT
Alcohol:	Possible stomach ulcer or bleeding.
Beverages:	None expected.
Cocaine:	None expected.
Foods:	None expected.
Marijuana:	Increased pain relief from naproxen.
Tobacco:	None expected.

*See Glossary

NARCOTIC & ACETAMINOPHEN

BRAND NAMES

See complete list of brand names in the *Brand Name Directory*, page 1065.

BASIC INFORMATION

Habit forming? Yes
Prescription needed? Yes
Available as generic? Yes
Drug class: Narcotic, analgesic, fever-reducer

 ## USES

Relieves pain.

 ## DOSAGE & USAGE INFORMATION

How to take:
- Tablet or capsule—Swallow with liquid. If you can't swallow whole, crumble tablet or open capsule and take with liquid or food.
- Drops or liquid—Dilute dose in beverage before swallowing.

When to take:
When needed. No more often than every 4 hours.

If you forget a dose:
Take as soon as you remember. Wait 4 hours for next dose.

Continued next column

 ## OVERDOSE

SYMPTOMS:
Stomach upset; irritability; sweating, convulsions; deep sleep; slow breathing; slow pulse; flushed, warm skin; constricted pupils; coma.
WHAT TO DO:
- **Dial 0 (operator) or 911 (emergency) for an ambulance or medical help. Then give first aid immediately.**
- **If patient is unconscious and not breathing, give mouth-to-mouth breathing. If there is no heartbeat, use cardiac massage and mouth-to-mouth breathing (CPR). Don't try to make patient vomit. If you can't get help quickly, take patient to nearest emergency facility.**
- **See emergency information on inside covers.**

What drug does:
- May affect hypothalamus—the part of the brain that helps regulate body heat and receives body's pain messages.
- Blocks pain messages to brain and spinal cord.
- Reduces sensitivity of brain's cough-control center.

Time lapse before drug works:
15 to 30 minutes. May last 4 hours.

Don't take with:
- Other drugs with acetaminophen. Too much acetaminophen can damage liver and kidneys.
- See Interaction column and consult doctor.

 ## POSSIBLE ADVERSE REACTIONS OR SIDE EFFECTS

SYMPTOMS	WHAT TO DO
Life-threatening: Irregular or slow heartbeat, difficult breathing.	Discontinue. Seek emergency treatment.
Common: Dizziness, agitation, tiredness.	Continue. Call doctor when convenient.
Infrequent: Abdominal pain, constipation, vomiting.	Discontinue. Call doctor right away.
Rare: • Fatigue; itchy skin; rash; sore throat, fever, mouth sores; bruising and bleeding increased; painful or difficult urination; blood in urine; anemia; blurred vision.	Discontinue. Call doctor right away.
• Depression.	Continue. Call doctor when convenient.

 ## WARNINGS & PRECAUTIONS

Don't take if:
- You are allergic to any narcotic or acetaminophen.
- Your symptoms don't improve after 2 days use. Call your doctor.

Before you start, consult your doctor:
- If you have bronchial asthma, kidney disease or liver damage.
- If you will have surgery within 2 months, including dental surgery, requiring general or spinal anesthesia.

Over age 60:
More likely to be drowsy, dizzy, unsteady or constipated. Don't exceed recommended dose. You can't eliminate drug as efficiently as younger persons. Use only if absolutely necessary.

Pregnancy:
Decide with your doctor whether drug benefits justify risk to unborn child. Abuse by pregnant woman will result in addicted newborn. Withdrawal of newborn can be life-threatening.

Breast-feeding:
Drug filters into milk. May harm child. Avoid.

Infants & children:
Not recommended.

Prolonged use:
- Causes psychological and physical dependence (addiction).
- May affect blood stream and cause anemia. Limit use to 5 days for children 12 and under, and 10 days for adults.

Skin & sunlight:
May cause rash or intensify sunburn in areas exposed to sun or sunlamp.

Driving, piloting or hazardous work:
Don't drive or pilot aircraft until you learn how medicine affects you. Don't work around dangerous machinery. Don't climb ladders or work in high places. Danger increases if you drink alcohol or take medicine affecting alertness and reflexes, such as antihistamines, tranquilizers, sedatives, pain medicine, narcotics and mind-altering drugs.

Discontinuing:
Discontinue in 2 days if symptoms don't improve.

Others:
No problems expected.

POSSIBLE INTERACTION WITH OTHER DRUGS

GENERIC NAME OR DRUG CLASS	COMBINED EFFECT
Analgesics, other*	Increased analgesic effect.
Anticoagulants, other*	May increase anticoagulant effect. Prothrombin times should be monitored.
Anticholinergics*	Increased anticholinergic effect.
Antidepressants*	Increased sedative effect.
Antihistamines*	Increased sedative effect.
Carteolol	Increased narcotic effect. Dangerous sedation.
Mind-altering drugs*	Increased sedative effect.
Narcotics, other*	Increased narcotic effect.
Nitrates*	Excessive blood-pressure drop.
Phenobarbital and other barbiturates*	Quicker elimination and decreased effect of acetaminophen.
Phenothiazines*	Increased phenothiazine effect.
Sedatives*	Increased sedative effect.
Sleep inducers*	Increased sedative effect.
Sotalol	Increased narcotic effect. Dangerous sedation.
Terfenadine	Possible oversedation.
Tetracyclines*	May slow tetracycline absorption. Space doses 2 hours apart.
Tranquilizers*	Increased sedative effect.
Zidovudine	Increased toxicity of zidovudine.

POSSIBLE INTERACTION WITH OTHER SUBSTANCES

INTERACTS WITH	COMBINED EFFECT
Alcohol:	Increases alcohol's intoxicating effect. Long-term use may cause toxic effect in liver. Avoid.
Beverages:	None expected.
Cocaine:	Increased toxic effects of cocaine. Avoid.
Foods:	None expected.
Marijuana:	Impairs physical and mental performance. Avoid.
Tobacco:	None expected.

*See Glossary

NARCOTIC ANALGESICS

BRAND AND GENERIC NAMES

See complete list of brand names in the *Brand Name Directory*, page 1065.

BASIC INFORMATION

Habit forming? Yes
Prescription needed? Yes
Available as generic? Yes
Drug class: Narcotic

 ## USES

Relieves pain and diarrhea; suppresses cough.

 ## DOSAGE & USAGE INFORMATION

How to take:
- Tablet, capsule or extended-release tablet— Swallow with liquid. If you can't swallow whole, crumble tablet or open capsule and take with liquid or food.
- Drops or liquid—Dilute dose in beverage before swallowing.

When to take:
When needed. No more often than every 4 hours.

If you forget a dose:
Take as soon as you remember. Wait 4 hours for next dose.

What drug does:
- Blocks pain messages to brain and spinal cord.
- Reduces sensitivity of brain's cough-control center.

Continued next column

 ## OVERDOSE

SYMPTOMS:
Deep sleep, slow breathing; slow pulse; respiratory arrest; flushed, warm skin; constricted pupils.
WHAT TO DO:
- **Dial 0 (operator) or 911 (emergency) for an ambulance or medical help. Then give first aid immediately.**
- **If patient is unconscious and not breathing, give mouth-to-mouth breathing. If there is no heartbeat, use cardiac massage and mouth-to-mouth breathing (CPR). Don't try to make patient vomit. If you can't get help quickly, take patient to nearest emergency facility.**
- **See emergency information on inside covers.**

Time lapse before drug works:
30 minutes.

Don't take with:
See Interaction column and consult doctor.

 ## POSSIBLE ADVERSE REACTIONS OR SIDE EFFECTS

SYMPTOMS	WHAT TO DO
Life-threatening: Hives, rash, intense itching, faintness soon after a dose (anaphylaxis); morphine by injection.	Seek emergency treatment immediately.
Common: Dizziness, flushed face, difficult urination, unusual tiredness.	Continue. Call doctor when convenient.
Infrequent: Severe constipation, abdominal pain, vomiting, nausea.	Discontinue. Call doctor right away.
Rare: • Hives, rash, itchy skin, face swelling, slow heartbeat, irregular breathing, hallucinations, disorientation, fainting.	Discontinue. Call doctor right away.
• Depression, blurred vision, decreased mental performance, anxiety, insomnia, weakness and faintness when arising from bed or chair, euphoria.	Continue. Call doctor when convenient.

 ## WARNINGS & PRECAUTIONS

Don't take if:
- You are allergic to any narcotic.
- Diarrhea is due to toxic effect of drugs or poisons.

Before you start, consult your doctor:
- If you have impaired liver or kidney function.
- If you will have surgery within 2 months, including dental surgery, requiring general or spinal anesthesia.
- If you have asthma.

Over age 60:
More likely to be drowsy, dizzy, unsteady or constipated. Use only if absolutely necessary.

Pregnancy:
Decide with your doctor whether drug benefits justify risk to unborn child. Abuse by pregnant woman will result in addicted newborn. Withdrawal of newborn can be life-threatening.

Breast-feeding:
Drug filters into milk. May harm child. Avoid.

Infants & children:
Not recommended.

Prolonged use:
Causes psychological and physical dependence (addiction).

Skin & sunlight:
May cause rash or intensify sunburn in areas exposed to sun or sunlamp.

Driving, piloting or hazardous work:
Don't drive or pilot aircraft until you learn how medicine affects you. Don't work around dangerous machinery. Don't climb ladders or work in high places. Danger increases if you drink alcohol or take medicine affecting alertness and reflexes, such as antihistamines, tranquilizers, sedatives, pain medicine, narcotics and mind-altering drugs.

Discontinuing:
May be unnecessary to finish medicine. Follow doctor's instructions.

Others:
Some products contain tartrazine dye. Avoid, especially if you are allergic to aspirin.

POSSIBLE INTERACTION WITH OTHER DRUGS

GENERIC NAME OR DRUG CLASS	COMBINED EFFECT
Analgesics, other*	Increased analgesic effect.
Anticoagulants, oral*	Possible increased anticoagulant effect.
Anticholinergics*	Increased anticholinergic effect.
Antidepressants*	Increased sedative effect.
Antihistamines*	Increased sedative effect.
Butorphanol	Possibly precipitates withdrawal with chronic narcotic use.
Carbamazepine	Increased carbamazepine effect with propoxyphene possible.
Carteolol	Increased narcotic effect. Dangerous sedation.

Cimetidine	Possible increased narcotic effect and toxicity.
Ethinamate	Dangerous increased effects of ethinamate. Avoid combining.
Fluoxetine	Increased depressant effects of both drugs.
Guanfacine	May increase depressant effects of either drug.
Leucovorin	High alcohol content of leucovorin may cause adverse effects.
MAO inhibitors*	Serious toxicity (including death).
Methyprylon	Increased sedative effect, perhaps to dangerous level. Avoid.
Mind-altering drugs*	Increased sedative effect.
Molindone	Increased narcotic effect.
Nabilone	Greater depression of central nervous system.
Nalbuphine	Possibly precipitates withdrawal with chronic narcotic use.
Naltrexone	Precipitates withdrawal symptoms. May lead to respiratory arrest, coma and death.
Narcotics, other*	Increased narcotic effect.

Continued page 1092

POSSIBLE INTERACTION WITH OTHER SUBSTANCES

INTERACTS WITH	COMBINED EFFECT
Alcohol:	Increases alcohol's intoxicating effect. Avoid.
Beverages:	None expected.
Cocaine:	Increased cocaine toxic effects. Avoid.
Foods:	None expected.
Marijuana:	Impairs physical and mental performance. Avoid.
Tobacco:	None expected.

*See Glossary

NARCOTIC & ASPIRIN

BRAND NAMES

See complete list of brand names in the *Brand Name Directory,* page 1066.

BASIC INFORMATION

Habit forming? Yes
Prescription needed? Yes
Available as generic? Yes
Drug class: Narcotic, analgesic,
   anti-inflammatory

 ## USES

Reduces pain, fever, inflammation.

 ## DOSAGE & USAGE INFORMATION

How to take:
Tablet or capsule—Swallow with liquid. If you can't swallow whole, crumble tablet or open capsule and take with liquid or food.

When to take:
When needed. No more often than every 4 hours.

If you forget a dose:
Take as soon as you remember. Wait 4 hours for next dose.

What drug does:
- Affects hypothalamus, the part of the brain which regulates temperature by dilating small blood vessels in skin.

Continued next column

 ## OVERDOSE

SYMPTOMS:
Ringing in ears; nausea; vomiting; dizziness; fever; deep sleep; slow breathing; slow pulse; flushed, warm skin; constricted pupils; hallucinations; convulsions; coma.
WHAT TO DO:
- **Dial 0 (operator) or 911 (emergency) for an ambulance or medical help. Then give first aid immediately.**
- **If patient is unconscious and not breathing, give mouth-to-mouth breathing. If there is no heartbeat, use cardiac massage and mouth-to-mouth breathing (CPR). Don't try to make patient vomit. If you can't get help quickly, take patient to nearest emergency facility.**
- **See emergency information on inside covers.**

- Prevents clumping of platelets (small blood cells) so blood vessels remain open.
- Decreases prostaglandin effect.
- Suppresses body's pain messages.
- Reduces sensitivity of brain's cough-control center.

Time lapse before drug works:
30 minutes.

Don't take with:
- Tetracyclines. Space doses 1 hour apart.
- See Interaction column and consult doctor.

 ## POSSIBLE ADVERSE REACTIONS OR SIDE EFFECTS

SYMPTOMS	WHAT TO DO
Life-threatening:	
Hives, rash, intense itching, faintness soon after a dose (anaphylaxis); difficulty breathing.	Seek emergency treatment immediately.
Clot or pain over blood vessel; cold hands, feet.	Discontinue. Seek emergency treatment.
Common:	
Nausea, abdominal cramps or pain.	Discontinue. Call doctor right away.
Dizziness, red or flushed face, ringing in ears, unusual tiredness, frequent urination, heartburn, indigestion.	Continue. Call doctor when convenient.
Infrequent:	
Constipation, abdominal pain or cramps, vomiting.	Discontinue. Call doctor right away.
Rare:	
Slow heartbeat; change in vision; black, bloody or tarry stool; blood in urine; jaundice; mental confusion.	Discontinue. Call doctor right away.
Depression, blurred vision.	Continue. Call doctor when convenient.

WARNINGS & PRECAUTIONS

Don't take if:
- You are allergic to any narcotic or subject to any substance abuse.
- You have a peptic ulcer of stomach or duodenum or a bleeding disorder.

Before you start, consult your doctor:
- If you have impaired liver or kidney function, asthma or nasal polyps.
- If you have had stomach or duodenal ulcers, gout.
- If you will have surgery within 2 months, including dental surgery, requiring general or spinal anesthesia.

Over age 60:
- More likely to be drowsy, dizzy, unsteady or constipated. Use only if absolutely necessary.
- More likely to cause hidden bleeding in stomach or intestines. Watch for dark stools.

Pregnancy:
Risk to unborn child outweighs drug benefits. Don't use.

Breast-feeding:
Drug passes into milk and may harm child. Avoid drug or discontinue nursing until you finish medicine. Consult doctor for advice on maintaining milk supply.

Infants & children:
Not recommended.

Prolonged use:
- Causes psychological and physical dependence (addiction).
- Kidney damage. Periodic kidney-function test recommended.

Skin & sunlight:
May cause rash or intensify sunburn in areas exposed to sun or sunlamp.

Driving, piloting or hazardous work:
Don't drive or pilot aircraft until you learn how medicine affects you. Don't work around dangerous machinery. Don't climb ladders or work in high places. Danger increases if you drink alcohol or take medicine affecting alertness and reflexes, such as antihistamines, tranquilizers, sedatives, pain medicine, narcotics and mind-altering drugs.

Discontinuing:
May be unnecessary to finish medicine. Follow doctor's instructions.

Others:
- Aspirin can complicate surgery; illness; pregnancy, labor and delivery.
- Urine tests for blood sugar may be inaccurate.

POSSIBLE INTERACTION WITH OTHER DRUGS

GENERIC NAME OR DRUG CLASS	COMBINED EFFECT
Acebutolol	Decreased anti-hypertensive effect of acebutolol.
ACE inhibitors: captopril, enalapril, lisinopril*	Decreased effect of ACE inhibitors.
Allopurinol	Decreased allopurinol effect.
Antacids*	Decreased aspirin effect.
Anticoagulants*	Increased anti-coagulant effect. Abnormal bleeding.
Antidepressants*	Increased sedative effect.
Antidiabetics, oral*	Low blood sugar.
Aspirin, other	Likely aspirin toxicity.
Bumetanide	Possible aspirin toxicity.
Carteolol	Increased narcotic effect. Dangerous sedation.
Cortisone drugs*	Increased cortisone effect. Risk of ulcers and stomach bleeding.
Ethacrynic acid	Possible aspirin toxicity.

Continued page 1092

POSSIBLE INTERACTION WITH OTHER SUBSTANCES

INTERACTS WITH	COMBINED EFFECT
Alcohol:	Possible stomach irritation and bleeding. Increases alcohol's intoxicating effect. Avoid.
Beverages:	None expected.
Cocaine:	Decreased cocaine toxic effects. Avoid.
Foods:	None expected.
Marijuana:	Impairs physical and mental performance. Avoid.
Tobacco:	None expected.

*See Glossary

NATAMYCIN (Ophthalmic)

BRAND NAMES

Natacyn   Pimaricin

BASIC INFORMATION

Habit forming? No
Prescription needed? Yes
Available as generic? No
Drug class: Antifungal (ophthalmic).
Note: Limited availability. Must be ordered directly from manufacturer.

 ## USES

Treats fungus infections of the eye.

 ## DOSAGE & USAGE INFORMATION

How to use:
Eye drops
- Wash hands.
- Apply pressure to inside corner of eye with middle finger.
- Tilt head backward. Pull lower lid away from eye with index finger of the same hand.
- Drop eye drops into pouch and close eye. Don't blink.
- Continue pressure for 1 minute after placing medicine in eye.
- Keep eyes closed for 1 to 2 minutes.
- Don't touch applicator tip to any surface (including the eye). If you accidentally touch tip, clean with warm soap and water.
- Keep container tightly closed.
- Keep cool, but don't freeze.
- Wash hands immediately after using.

When to use:
As directed. Usually 1 drop in eye every 1 or 2 hours for 3 or 4 days, then every 3 to 4 hours.

If you forget a dose:
Use as soon as you remember.

What drug does:
Changes cell membrane of fungus causing loss of essential constituents of fungus cell.

Continued next column

 ## OVERDOSE

SYMPTOMS:
None expected.
WHAT TO DO:
Not intended for internal use. If child accidentally swallows, call poison-control center.

Time lapse before drug works:
Starts to work immediately. May require 2 weeks or more to cure infection.

Don't use with:
Other eye drops without consulting your eye doctor.

 ## POSSIBLE ADVERSE REACTIONS OR SIDE EFFECTS

SYMPTOMS	WHAT TO DO
Life-threatening: None expected.	
Common: None expected.	
Infrequent: Eye irritation not present before using natamycin.	Discontinue. Call doctor right away.
Rare: None expected.	

WARNINGS & PRECAUTIONS

Don't use if:
You are allergic to natamycin or any antifungal medicine.

Before you start, consult your doctor:
If you have allergies to any substance.

Over age 60:
No problems expected.

Pregnancy:
No problems expected, but check with doctor.

Breast-feeding:
No problems expected, but check with doctor.

Infants & children:
No problems expected.

Prolonged use:
May cause eye irritation.

Skin & sunlight:
No problems expected.

Driving, piloting or hazardous work:
No problems expected.

Discontinuing:
Don't discontinue without consulting your eye doctor.

Others:
- Keep cool, but don't freeze.
- Notify doctor if condition doesn't improve within 1 week.

POSSIBLE INTERACTION WITH OTHER DRUGS

GENERIC NAME OR DRUG CLASS	COMBINED EFFECT
Clinically significant interactions with oral or injected medicines unlikely.	

POSSIBLE INTERACTION WITH OTHER SUBSTANCES

INTERACTS WITH	COMBINED EFFECT
Alcohol:	None expected.
Beverages:	None expected.
Cocaine:	None expected.
Foods:	None expected.
Marijuana:	None expected.
Tobacco:	None expected.

NEOMYCIN (Oral)

BRAND NAMES

Myclfradin **Neobiotic**

BASIC INFORMATION

Habit forming? No
Prescription needed? Yes
Available as generic? Yes
Drug class: Antibiotic

 USES

- Clears intestinal tract of germs prior to surgery.
- Treats some causes of diarrhea.
- Lowers blood cholesterol.
- Lessens symptoms of hepatic coma.

 DOSAGE & USAGE INFORMATION

How to take:
Tablet—Swallow with liquid or food to lessen stomach irritation. If you can't swallow whole, crumble tablet and take with liquid or food.

When to take:
According to directions on prescription.

If you forget a dose:
Take as soon as you remember up to 2 hours late. If more than 2 hours, wait for next scheduled dose (don't double this dose).

What drug does:
Kills germs susceptible to neomycin.

Time lapse before drug works:
2 to 3 days.

Continued next column

 OVERDOSE

SYMPTOMS:
Loss of hearing, difficulty breathing, respiratory paralysis.
WHAT TO DO:
- **Dial 0 (operator) or 911 (emergency) for an ambulance or medical help. Then give first aid immediately.**
- **If patient is unconscious and not breathing, give mouth-to-mouth breathing. If there is no heartbeat, use cardiac massage and mouth-to-mouth breathing (CPR). Don't try to make patient vomit. If you can't get help quickly, take patient to nearest emergency facility.**
- **See emergency information on inside covers.**

Don't take with:
See Interaction column and consult doctor.

 POSSIBLE ADVERSE REACTIONS OR SIDE EFFECTS

SYMPTOMS	WHAT TO DO
Life-threatening: None expected.	
Common: Sore mouth, nausea, vomiting.	Continue. Call doctor when convenient.
Infrequent: None expected.	
Rare: Clumsiness, dizziness, rash, hearing loss, ringing or noises in ear, frothy stools, gaseousness, decreased frequency of urination.	Discontinue. Call doctor right away.

WARNINGS & PRECAUTIONS

Don't take if:
You are allergic to neomycin or any aminoglycoside. (See Interactions column.)

Before you start, consult your doctor:
- If you will have surgery within 2 months, including dental surgery, requiring general or spinal anesthesia.
- If you have hearing loss or loss of balance secondary to 8th cranial nerve disease.
- If you have intestinal obstruction.
- If you have myasthenia gravis, Parkinson's disease, kidney disease, ulcers in intestines.

Over age 60:
Adverse reactions and side effects may be more frequent and severe than in younger persons.

Pregnancy:
No proven harm to unborn child. Avoid if possible.

Breast-feeding:
Avoid if possible.

Infants & children:
Only under close medical supervision.

Prolonged use:
Adverse effects more likely.

Skin & sunlight:
No problems expected.

Driving, piloting or hazardous work:
No problems expected.

Discontinuing:
May be unnecessary to finish medicine. Follow doctor's instructions.

Others:
No problems expected.

POSSIBLE INTERACTION WITH OTHER DRUGS

GENERIC NAME OR DRUG CLASS	COMBINED EFFECT
Aminoglycosides* (amikacin, gentamicin, kanamycin, streptomycin, tobramycin)	Increases chance of toxic effect on hearing, kidney, muscles.
Capreomycin Cisplatin Ethacrynic acid Furosemide Mercaptomerin Vancomycin	Increases chance of toxic effects on hearing, kidneys.
Cephalothin	Increased chance of toxic effect on kidneys.

POSSIBLE INTERACTION WITH OTHER SUBSTANCES

INTERACTS WITH	COMBINED EFFECT
Alcohol:	Increased chance of toxicity. Avoid.
Beverages:	No problems expected.
Cocaine:	Increased chance of toxicity. Avoid.
Foods:	No problems expected.
Marijuana:	Increased chance of toxicity. Avoid.
Tobacco:	No problems expected.

*See Glossary

NEOSTIGMINE

BRAND NAMES

Prostigmin

BASIC INFORMATION

Habit forming? No
Prescription needed? Yes
Available as generic? Yes
Drug class: Cholinergic (anticholinesterase)

 USES

- Treatment of myasthenia gravis.
- Treatment of urinary retention and abdominal distention.
- Antidote to adverse effects of muscle relaxants used in surgery.

 DOSAGE & USAGE INFORMATION

How to take:
Tablet—Swallow with liquid or food to lessen stomach irritation.

When to take:
As directed, usually 3 or 4 times a day.

If you forget a dose:
Take as soon as you remember up to 2 hours late. If more than 2 hours, wait for next scheduled dose (don't double this dose).

What drug does:
Inhibits the chemical activity of an enzyme (cholinesterase) so nerve impulses can cross the junction of nerves and muscles.

Time lapse before drug works:
3 hours.

Don't take with:
See Interaction column and consult doctor.

 OVERDOSE

SYMPTOMS:
Muscle weakness, cramps, twitching or clumsiness; severe diarrhea, nausea, vomiting, stomach cramps or pain; breathing difficulty; confusion, irritability, nervousness, restlessness, fear; unusually slow heartbeat; seizures.
WHAT TO DO:
- Dial 0 (operator) or 911 (emergency) for an ambulance or medical help. Then give first aid immediately.
- See emergency information on inside covers.

 POSSIBLE ADVERSE REACTIONS OR SIDE EFFECTS

SYMPTOMS	WHAT TO DO
Life-threatening: None expected.	
Common:	
• Mild diarrhea, nausea, vomiting, stomach cramps or pain.	Discontinue. Call doctor right away.
• Excess saliva, unusual sweating.	Continue. Call doctor when convenient.
Infrequent:	
• Confusion, irritability.	Discontinue. Seek emergency treatment.
• Constricted pupils, watery eyes, lung congestion, frequent urge to urinate.	Continue. Call doctor when convenient.
Rare:	
Bronchospasm, slow heartbeat, weakness.	Discontinue. Call doctor right away.

WARNINGS & PRECAUTIONS

Don't take if:
- You are allergic to any cholinergic or bromide.
- You take mecamylamine.

Before you start, consult your doctor:
- If you plan to become pregnant within medication period.
- If you have bronchial asthma.
- If you have heartbeat irregularities.
- If you have urinary obstruction or urinary-tract infection.

Over age 60:
Adverse reactions and side effects may be more frequent and severe than in younger persons.

Pregnancy:
No proven harm to unborn child. Avoid if possible. May increase uterus contractions close to delivery.

Breast-feeding:
No problems expected, but consult doctor.

Infants & children:
Not recommended.

Prolonged use:
Medication may lose effectiveness. Discontinuing for a few days may restore effect.

Skin & sunlight:
No problems expected.

Driving, piloting or hazardous work:
Don't drive or pilot aircraft until you learn how medicine affects you. Don't work around dangerous machinery. Don't climb ladders or work in high places. Danger increases if you drink alcohol or take medicine affecting alertness and reflexes, such as antihistamines, tranquilizers, sedatives, pain medicine, narcotics and mind-altering drugs.

Discontinuing:
Don't discontinue without doctor's advice until you complete prescribed dose, even though symptoms diminish or disappear.

Others:
No problems expected.

POSSIBLE INTERACTION WITH OTHER DRUGS

GENERIC NAME OR DRUG CLASS	COMBINED EFFECT
Anesthetics, local or general*	Decreased neostigmine effect.
Antiarrhythmics*	Decreased neostigmine effect.
Anticholinergics*	Decreased neostigmine effect. May mask severe side effects.
Cholinergics, other*	Reduced intestinal-tract function. Possible brain and nervous-system toxicity.
Mecamylamine	Decreased neostigmine effect.
Nitrates*	Decreased neostigmine effect.
Quinidine	Decreased neostigmine effect.

POSSIBLE INTERACTION WITH OTHER SUBSTANCES

INTERACTS WITH	COMBINED EFFECT
Alcohol:	No proven problems with small doses.
Beverages:	None expected.
Cocaine:	Decreased neostigmine effect. Avoid.
Foods:	None expected.
Marijuana:	No proven problems.
Tobacco:	No proven problems.

NIACIN (Nicotinic Acid)

BRAND NAMES

See complete list of brand names in the *Brand Name Directory*, page 1066.

There are numerous other multiple vitamin-mineral supplements available.

BASIC INFORMATION

Habit forming? No
Prescription needed?
  Tablets: No
  Liquid, capsules: Yes
Available as generic? Yes
Drug class: Vitamin supplement, vasodilator, antihyperlipidemic

USES

- Replacement for niacin deficiency caused by inadequate diet.
- Treatment for vertigo (dizziness) and ringing in ears.
- Prevention of premenstrual headache.
- Reduction of blood levels of cholesterol and triglycerides.
- Treatment for pellagra.

DOSAGE & USAGE INFORMATION

How to take:
- Tablet, capsule or liquid—Swallow with liquid or food to lessen stomach irritation.
- Extended-release tablets or capsules—Swallow each dose whole.

When to take:
At the same times each day.

If you forget a dose:
Take as soon as you remember. Wait 4 hours for next dose.

Continued next column

OVERDOSE

SYMPTOMS:
Body flush, nausea, vomiting, abdominal cramps, diarrhea, weakness, lightheadedness, fainting, sweating.
WHAT TO DO:
Overdose unlikely to threaten life. If person takes much larger amount than prescribed, call doctor, poison-control center or hospital emergency room for instructions.

What drug does:
- Corrects niacin deficiency.
- Dilates blood vessels.
- In large doses, decreases cholesterol production.

Time lapse before drug works:
15 to 20 minutes.

Don't take with:
See Interaction column and consult doctor.

POSSIBLE ADVERSE REACTIONS OR SIDE EFFECTS

SYMPTOMS	WHAT TO DO
Life-threatening: None expected.	
Common: None expected.	
Infrequent:	
• Upper abdominal pain.	Discontinue. Call doctor right away.
• Headache, dizziness, faintness, temporary numbness and tingling in hands and feet.	Continue. Call doctor when convenient.
• "Hot" feeling, flush.	No action necessary.
Rare: Rash, itching, jaundice, double vision, weakness and faintness when arising from bed or chair.	Discontinue. Call doctor right away.

WARNINGS & PRECAUTIONS

Don't take if:
- You are allergic to niacin or any niacin-containing vitamin mixtures.
- You have impaired liver function.
- You have active peptic ulcer.

Before you start, consult your doctor:
- If you have sensitivity to tartrazine dye.
- If you have diabetes.
- If you have gout.
- If you have gallbladder or liver disease.

Over age 60:
Response to drug cannot be predicted. Dose must be individualized.

Pregnancy:
Risk to unborn child outweighs drug benefits. Don't use.

Breast-feeding:
Studies inconclusive. Consult doctor.

Infants & children:
- Use only under supervision.
- Keep vitamin-mineral supplements out of children's reach.

Prolonged use:
Possible impaired liver function.

Skin & sunlight:
No problems expected.

Driving, piloting or hazardous work:
Avoid if you feel dizzy or faint. Otherwise, no problems expected.

Discontinuing:
May be unnecessary to finish medicine. Follow doctor's instructions.

Others:
- A balanced diet should provide all the niacin a healthy person needs and make supplements unnecessary. Best sources are meat, eggs and dairy products.
- Store in original container in cool, dry, dark place. Bathroom medicine chest too moist.
- Obesity reduces effectiveness.
- Some nicotinic acid products contain tartrazine dye. Read labels carefully if sensitive to tartrazine.

POSSIBLE INTERACTION WITH OTHER DRUGS

GENERIC NAME OR DRUG CLASS	COMBINED EFFECT
Antidiabetics*	Decreased anti-diabetic effect.
Beta-adrenergic blockers*	Excessively low blood pressure.
Guanethidine	Increased guanethidine effect.
Isoniazid	Decreased niacin effect.
Mecamylamine	Excessively low blood pressure.
Methyldopa	Excessively low blood pressure.
Pargyline	Excessively low blood pressure.
Probenecid	Decreased effect of probenecid.
Sulfinpyrazone	Decreased effect of sulfinpyrazone.

POSSIBLE INTERACTION WITH OTHER SUBSTANCES

INTERACTS WITH	COMBINED EFFECT
Alcohol:	Excessively low blood pressure. Use caution.
Beverages:	None expected.
Cocaine:	Increased flushing.
Foods:	None expected.
Marijuana:	None expected.
Tobacco:	Decreased niacin effect.

NICARDIPINE

BRAND NAMES

Cardene

BASIC INFORMATION

Habit forming? No
Prescription needed? Yes
Available as generic? Yes
Drug class: Calcium-channel blocker, antiarrhythmic, antianginal

USES

- Prevents angina attacks.
- Stabilizes irregular heartbeat.
- Treats high blood pressure.

DOSAGE & USAGE INFORMATION

How to take:
Extended-release tablet—Swallow with liquid.

When to take:
At the same times each day 1 hour before or 2 hours after eating.

If you forget a dose:
Take as soon as you remember up to 2 hours late. If more than 2 hours, wait for next scheduled dose (don't double this dose).

What drug does:
- Reduces work that heart must perform.
- Reduces blood pressure.
- Increases oxygen to heart muscle.

Time lapse before drug works:
1 to 2 hours.

Don't take with:
See Interaction column and consult doctor.

OVERDOSE

SYMPTOMS:
Unusually fast or unusually slow heartbeat, loss of consciousness, cardiac arrest.
WHAT TO DO:
- Dial 0 (operator) or 911 (emergency) for an ambulance or medical help. Then give first aid immediately.
- If patient is unconscious and not breathing, give mouth-to-mouth breathing. If there is no heartbeat, use cardiac massage and mouth-to-mouth breathing (CPR). Don't try to make patient vomit. If you can't get help quickly, take patient to nearest emergency facility.
- See emergency information on inside covers.

POSSIBLE ADVERSE REACTIONS OR SIDE EFFECTS

SYMPTOMS	WHAT TO DO
Life-threatening: None expected.	
Common: Tiredness.	Continue. Tell doctor at next visit.
Infrequent:	
• Unusually fast or unusually slow heartbeat, wheezing, cough, shortness of breath.	Discontinue. Call doctor right away.
• Dizziness; numbness or tingling in hands and feet; swollen feet, ankles or legs; difficult urination.	Continue. Call doctor when convenient.
• Nausea, constipation.	Continue. Tell doctor at next visit.
Rare:	
• Fainting, depression, psychosis, rash, jaundice.	Discontinue. Call doctor right away.
• Headache, insomnia, vivid dreams, hair loss.	Continue. Tell doctor at next visit.

WARNINGS & PRECAUTIONS

Don't take if:
- You are allergic to nicardipine.
- You have very low blood pressure.

Before you start, consult your doctor:
- If you have kidney or liver disease.
- If you have high blood pressure.
- If you have heart disease other than coronary-artery disease.

Over age 60:
Adverse reactions and side effects may be more frequent and severe than in younger persons.

Pregnancy:
No proven harm to unborn child. Avoid if possible.

Breast-feeding:
Safety not established. Avoid if possible.

Infants & children:
Not recommended.

Prolonged use:
No problems expected.

Skin & sunlight:
No problems expected.

Driving, piloting or hazardous work:
Avoid if you feel dizzy. Otherwise, no problems expected.

Discontinuing:
Don't discontinue without doctor's advice until you complete prescribed dose, even though symptoms diminish or disappear.

Others:
Learn to check your own pulse rate. If it drops to 50 beats per minute or lower, don't take nicardipine until your consult your doctor.

POSSIBLE INTERACTION WITH OTHER DRUGS

GENERIC NAME OR DRUG CLASS	COMBINED EFFECT
ACE inhibitors: captopril, enalapril, lisinopril*	Possible excessive potassium in blood. Dosages may require adjustment.
Antiarrhythmics*	Possible increased effect and toxicity of each drug.
Anticoagulants, oral*	Possible increased anticoagulant effect.
Anticonvulsants, hydantoin*	Increased anticonvulsant effect.
Antihypertensives*	Blood-pressure drop. Dosages may require adjustment.
Beta-adrenergic blockers*	Possible irregular heartbeat and congestive heart failure.
Calcium (large doses)	Possible decreased nicardipine effect.
Carbamazepine	May increase carbamazepine effect and toxicity.
Cimetidine	Possible increased nicardipine effect and toxicity.
Digitalis preparations*	Increased digitalis effect. May need to reduce dose.
Disopyramide	May cause dangerously slow, fast or irregular heartbeat.
Diuretics*	Dangerous blood-pressure drop. Dosages may require adjustment.
Encainide	Increased effect of toxicity on heart muscle.
Lithium	Possible decreased lithium effect.
Nitrates*	Reduced angina attacks.
Quinidine	Increased quinidine effect.
Rifampin	Decreased nicardipine effect.
Theophylline	May increase theophylline effect and toxicity.
Phenytoin	Possible decreased nicardipine effect.
Vitamin D (large doses)	Decreased nicardipine effect.

POSSIBLE INTERACTION WITH OTHER SUBSTANCES

INTERACTS WITH	COMBINED EFFECT
Alcohol:	Dangerously low blood pressure. Avoid.
Beverages:	None expected.
Cocaine:	Possible irregular heartbeat. Avoid.
Foods:	None expected.
Marijuana:	Possible irregular heartbeat. Avoid.
Tobacco:	Possible rapid heartbeat. Avoid.

NICOTINE RESIN COMPLEX

BRAND NAMES

Nicorette

BASIC INFORMATION

Habit forming? Yes
Prescription needed? Yes
Available as generic? No
Drug class: Antismoking agent

 USES

Treats smoking addiction.

 DOSAGE & USAGE INFORMATION

How to take:
• Follow detailed instructions on patient instruction sheet provided with prescription.
• Chewing gum tablets—Chew gum pieces slowly for best effect.

When to take:
Follow detailed instructions on patient instruction sheet provided with prescription.

If you forget a dose:
Follow detailed instructions on patient instruction sheet provided with prescription.

What drug does:
Satisfies physical craving for nicotine in addicted persons and avoids peaks in blood nicotine level resulting from smoking.

Time lapse before drug works:
30 minutes.

Don't take with:
See Interaction column and consult doctor.

 OVERDOSE

SYMPTOMS:
Vomiting, irregular heartbeat.
WHAT TO DO:
Overdose unlikely to threaten life. If person takes much larger amount than prescribed, call doctor, poison-control center or hospital emergency room for instructions.

 POSSIBLE ADVERSE REACTIONS OR SIDE EFFECTS

SYMPTOMS	WHAT TO DO
Life-threatening: None expected.	
Frequent: Increased irritability causing heartbeat irregularity.	Continue. Call doctor when convenient.
Common:	
• Injury to loose teeth, jaw muscle ache.	Continue. Call doctor when convenient.
• Belching, mouth irritation or tingling, excessive salivation.	Continue. Tell doctor at next visit.
Infrequent:	
• Nausea and vomiting, abdominal pain.	Discontinue. Call doctor right away.
• Lightheadedness, headache, hiccups.	Continue. Call doctor when convenient.
Rare: None expected.	

NICOTINE RESIN COMPLEX

 ## WARNINGS & PRECAUTIONS

Don't take if:
- You are a non-smoker.
- You are pregnant or intend to become pregnant.
- You recently suffered a heart attack.

Before you start, consult your doctor:
- If you have coronary artery disease.
- If you have active temperomandibular joint disease.
- If you have severe angina.
- If you have peptic ulcer.

Over age 60:
Adverse reactions and side effects may be more frequent and severe than in younger persons.

Pregnancy:
Risk to unborn child outweighs drug benefits. Don't use.

Breast-feeding:
Drug passes into milk. Avoid drug or discontinue nursing until you finish medicine. Consult doctor for advice on maintaining milk supply.

Infants & children:
Don't use.

Prolonged use:
May cause addiction and greater likelihood of toxicity.

Skin & sunlight:
No problems expected.

Driving, piloting or hazardous work:
No problems expected.

Discontinuing:
May be unnecessary to finish medicine. Follow doctor's instructions.

Others:
- Children are very susceptible to toxic effects of nicotine; low doses can be fatal.
- Can cause tooth fillings to be pulled out.

 ## POSSIBLE INTERACTION WITH OTHER DRUGS

GENERIC NAME OR DRUG CLASS	COMBINED EFFECT
Beta-adrenergic blockers*	Decreased blood pressure (slight).
Caffeine	Increased effect of caffeine.
Cortisone drugs*	Increased cortisone circulating in blood.
Furosemide	Increased effect of furosemide.
Glutethimide	Increased absorption of glutethimide.
Imipramine	Increased effect of imipramine.
Pentazocine	Increased effect of pentazocine.
Phenacetin	Increased effect of phenacetin.
Propoxyphene	Decreased blood level of propoxyphene.
Theophylline	Increased effect of theophylline.

 ## POSSIBLE INTERACTION WITH OTHER SUBSTANCES

INTERACTS WITH	COMBINED EFFECT
Alcohol:	Increased cardiac irritability. Avoid.
Beverages: Caffeine.	Increased cardiac irritability. Avoid any beverage with caffeine.
Cocaine:	Increased cardiac irritability. Avoid.
Foods:	No problems expected.
Marijuana:	Increased toxic effects. Avoid.
Tobacco:	Increased toxic effects. Avoid.

NIFEDIPINE

BRAND NAMES

Adalat   Procardia

BASIC INFORMATION

Habit forming? No
Prescription needed? Yes
Available as generic? No
Drug class: Calcium-channel blocker,
  antiarrhythmic, antianginal

USES

- Prevents angina attacks.
- Treats Reynaud's disease.
- Treats high blood pressure.
- Treats spasm of the esophagus.

DOSAGE & USAGE INFORMATION

How to take:
Capsule or extended-release tablet—Swallow
with liquid.

When to take:
At the same times each day 1 hour before or 2
hours after eating.

If you forget a dose:
Take as soon as you remember up to 2 hours
late. If more than 2 hours, wait for next
scheduled dose (don't double this dose).

What drug does:
- Reduces work that heart must perform.
- Reduces normal artery pressure.
- Increases oxygen to heart muscle.

Continued next column

OVERDOSE

SYMPTOMS:
**Unusually fast or unusually slow heartbeat,
loss of consciousness, cardiac arrest.**
WHAT TO DO:
- **Dial 0 (operator) or 911 (emergency) for
  an ambulance or medical help. Then give
  first aid immediately.**
- **If patient is unconscious and not
  breathing, give mouth-to-mouth
  breathing. If there is no heartbeat, use
  cardiac massage and mouth-to-mouth
  breathing (CPR). Don't try to make patient
  vomit. If you can't get help quickly, take
  patient to nearest emergency facility.**
- **See emergency information on inside
  covers.**

Time lapse before drug works:
1 to 2 hours.

Don't take with:
See Interaction column and consult doctor.

POSSIBLE ADVERSE REACTIONS OR SIDE EFFECTS

SYMPTOMS	WHAT TO DO
Life-threatening: None expected.	
Common: Tiredness, flushing, swelling of feet, ankles and abdomen.	Continue. Tell doctor at next visit.
Infrequent: • Unusually fast or unusually slow heartbeat, wheezing, cough, shortness of breath.	Discontinue. Call doctor right away.
• Dizziness; numbness or tingling in hands or feet; swelling of ankles, feet, legs; difficult urination.	Continue. Call doctor when convenient.
• Nausea, constipation.	Continue. Tell doctor at next visit.
Rare: • Transient blindness, increased angina.	Discontinue. Seek emergency treatment.
• Fainting, chest pain, fever, rash, jaundice, depression, psychosis.	Discontinue. Call doctor right away.
• Arthritis, hair loss, vivid dreams.	Continue. Call doctor when convenient.
• Headache.	Continue. Tell doctor at next visit.

WARNINGS & PRECAUTIONS

Don't take if:
- You are allergic to nifedipine.
- You have very low blood pressure.

Before you start, consult your doctor:
- If you have kidney or liver disease.
- If you have high blood pressure.
- If you have heart disease other than coronary-artery disease.

Over age 60:
Adverse reactions and side effects may be more
frequent and severe than in younger persons.

Pregnancy:
No proven harm to unborn child. Avoid if
possible.

Breast-feeding:
Safety not established. Avoid if possible.

Infants & children:
Not recommended.

Prolonged use:
No problems expected.

Skin & sunlight:
Increased sensitivity to sunlight.

Driving, piloting or hazardous work:
Avoid if you feel dizzy. Otherwise, no problems expected.

Discontinuing:
Don't discontinue without doctor's advice until you complete prescribed dose, even though symptoms diminish or disappear.

Others:
- Learn to check your own pulse rate. If it drops to 50 beats per minute or lower, don't take nifedipine until you consult your doctor.
- Drug may lower blood-sugar level if daily dose is more than 60 mg.

 ## POSSIBLE INTERACTION WITH OTHER DRUGS

GENERIC NAME OR DRUG CLASS	COMBINED EFFECT
ACE inhibitors: captopril, enalapril, lisinopril*	Possible excessive potassium in blood. Dosages may need adjustment.
Antiarrhythmics*	Possible increased effect and toxicity of each drug.
Anticoagulants, oral*	Possible increased anticoagulant effect.
Anticonvulsants, hydantoin*	Increased anticonvulsant effect.
Antihypertensives*	Dangerous blood-pressure drop. Dosage may need adjustment.
Beta-adrenergic blockers*	Possible irregular heartbeat. May worsen congestive heart failure.
Calcium (large doses)	Possible decreased nifedipine effect.
Carbamazepine	May increase carbamazepine effect and toxicity.
Cimetidine	Possible increased nifedipine effect and toxicity.
Disopyramide	May cause dangerously slow, fast or irregular heartbeat.
Diuretics*	Dangerous blood-pressure drop.
Lithium	Possible decreased lithium effect.
Nicardipine	Possible increased effect and toxicity of each drug.
Nitrates*	Reduced angina attacks.
Phenytoin	Possible decreased nifedipine effect.
Quinidine	Increased quinidine effect.
Rifampin	Decreased nifedipine effect.
Theophylline	May increase theophylline effect and toxicity.
Tocainide	Increased likelihood of adverse reactions from either drug.
Vitamin D (large doses)	Decreased nifedipine effect.

POSSIBLE INTERACTION WITH OTHER SUBSTANCES

INTERACTS WITH	COMBINED EFFECT
Alcohol:	Dangerously low blood pressure. Avoid.
Beverages:	None expected.
Cocaine:	Possible irregular heartbeat. Avoid.
Foods:	None expected.
Marijuana:	Possible irregular heartbeat. Avoid.
Tobacco:	Possible rapid heartbeat. Avoid.

*See Glossary

NITRATES

BRAND NAMES

See complete list of brand names in the *Brand Name Directory,* page 1066.

BASIC INFORMATION

Habit forming? No
Prescription needed? Yes
Available as generic? Yes
Drug class: Antianginal (nitrate)

USES

- Reduces frequency and severity of angina attacks.
- Treats congestive heart failure.

DOSAGE & USAGE INFORMATION

How to take:
- Extended-release tablets or capsules—Swallow each dose whole with liquid.
- Chewable tablet—Chew tablet at earliest sign of angina, and hold in mouth for 2 minutes.
- Regular tablet or capsule—Swallow whole with liquid. Don't crush, chew or open.
- Buccal tablets (Nitrogard)—Allow to dissolve in side of mouth.
- Translingual spray (nitrolingual)—Spray under tongue according to instructions enclosed with prescription.
- Ointment—Apply as directed.
- Patches—Apply to skin according to package instructions.
- Sublingual tablets—Place under tongue every 3 to 5 minutes at earliest sign of angina. If you don't have complete relief with 3 or 4 tablets, call doctor.

Continued next column

OVERDOSE

SYMPTOMS:
Dizziness; blue fingernails and lips; fainting; shortness of breath; weak, fast heartbeat; convulsions.
WHAT TO DO:
- **Dial 0 (operator) or 911 (emergency) for an ambulance or medical help. Then give first aid immediately.**
- **See emergency information on inside covers.**

When to take:
- Swallowed tablets—Take at the same times each day, 1 or 2 hours after meals.
- Sublingual tablets or spray—At onset of angina.
- Ointment—Follow prescription directions.
- Patches—According to physician's instructions.

If you forget a dose:
Take as soon as you remember up to 2 hours late. If more than 2 hours, wait for next scheduled dose (don't double this dose).

What drug does:
Relaxes blood vessels, increasing blood flow to heart muscle.

Time lapse before drug works:
- Sublingual tablets and spray—1 to 3 minutes.
- Other forms—15 to 30 minutes. Will not stop an attack, but may prevent attacks.

Don't take with:
See Interaction column and consult doctor.

POSSIBLE ADVERSE REACTIONS OR SIDE EFFECTS

SYMPTOMS	WHAT TO DO
Life-threatening: None expected.	
Common: Headache, flushed face and neck, dry mouth, nausea, vomiting, rapid heartbeat.	Continue. Tell doctor at next visit.
Infrequent:	
• Fainting.	Discontinue. Call doctor right away.
• Restlessness, blurred vision.	Continue. Call doctor when convenient.
Rare:	
• Rash.	Discontinue. Call doctor right away.
• Severe irritation, peeling.	Continue. Call doctor when convenient.

WARNINGS & PRECAUTIONS

Don't take if:
You are allergic to nitrates, including nitroglycerin.

Before you start, consult your doctor:
- If you are taking non-prescription drugs.
- If you plan to become pregnant within medication period.
- If you have glaucoma.
- If you have reacted badly to any vasodilator drug.
- If you drink alcoholic beverages or smoke marijuana.

Over age 60:
Adverse reactions and side effects may be more frequent and severe than in younger persons.

Pregnancy:
No proven harm to unborn child. Avoid if possible.

Breast-feeding:
No problems expected. Consult your doctor.

Infants & children:
Not recommended.

Prolonged use:
Drug may become less effective and require higher doses.

Skin & sunlight:
No problems expected.

Driving, piloting or hazardous work:
Don't drive or pilot aircraft until you learn how medicine affects you. Don't work around dangerous machinery. Don't climb ladders or work in high places. Danger increases if you drink alcohol or take medicine affecting alertness and reflexes.

Discontinuing:
Except for sublingual tablets, don't discontinue without doctor's advice until you complete prescribed dose, even though symptoms diminish or disappear.

Others:
- If discomfort is not caused by angina, nitrate medication will not bring relief. Call doctor if discomfort persists.
- Periodic urine and laboratory blood studies of white cell counts recommended if you take nitrates.
- Keep sublingual tablets in original container. Always carry them with you, but keep from body heat if possible.
- Sublingual tablets produce a burning, stinging sensation when placed under the tongue. Replace supply if no burning or stinging is noted.

POSSIBLE INTERACTION WITH OTHER DRUGS

GENERIC NAME OR DRUG CLASS	COMBINED EFFECT
Anticholinergics*	Increased internal-eye pressure.
Antidepressants, tricyclic (TCA)*	Excessive blood-pressure drop.
Antihypertensives*	Excessive blood-pressure drop.
Beta-adrenergic blockers*	Excessive blood-pressure drop.
Calcium channel blockers*	Decreased blood pressure.
Carteolol	Possible excessive blood-pressure drop.
Cholinergics*	Decreased cholinergic effect.
Ephedrine	Decreased nitrate effect.
Guanfacine	Increased effects of both drugs.
Lisinopril	Possible excessive blood-pressure drop.
Narcotics*	Excessive blood-pressure drop.
Nicardipine	Reduced angina attacks.
Phenothiazines*	May decrease blood pressure.
Sotalol	Possible excessive blood-pressure drop.
Sympathomimetics*	Possible reduced effects of both medicines.

POSSIBLE INTERACTION WITH OTHER SUBSTANCES

INTERACTS WITH	COMBINED EFFECT
Alcohol:	Excessive blood-pressure drop.
Beverages:	None expected.
Cocaine:	Reduced effectiveness of nitrates.
Foods:	None expected.
Marijuana:	Decreased nitrate effect.
Tobacco:	Decreased nitrate effect.

NITROFURANTOIN

BRAND NAMES

Apo-Nitrofurantoin	Nephronex
Cyantin	Nifuran
Furadantin	Nitrex
Furalan	Nitrodan
Furaloid	Novofuran
Furantoin	Sarodant
Furatine	Trantoin
Macrodantin	Urotoin

BASIC INFORMATION

Habit forming? No
Prescription needed? Yes
Available as generic? Yes
Drug class: Antimicrobial

 ## USES

Treatment for urinary-tract infections.

 ## DOSAGE & USAGE INFORMATION

How to take:
- Tablet or capsule—Swallow with food or milk to lessen stomach irritation. If you can't swallow whole, crumble tablet or open capsule and take with liquid or food.
- Liquid—Shake well and take with food. Use a measuring spoon to ensure accuracy.

When to take:
At the same times each day.

If you forget a dose:
Take as soon as you remember up to 2 hours late. If more than 2 hours, wait for next scheduled dose (don't double this dose).

What drug does:
Prevents susceptible bacteria in the urinary tract from growing and multiplying.

Time lapse before drug works:
1 to 2 weeks.

Don't take with:
See Interaction column and consult doctor.

 ## OVERDOSE

SYMPTOMS:
Nausea, vomiting, abdominal pain, diarrhea.
WHAT TO DO:
Overdose unlikely to threaten life. If person takes much larger amount than prescribed, call doctor, poison-control center or hospital emergency room for instructions.

 ## POSSIBLE ADVERSE REACTIONS OR SIDE EFFECTS

SYMPTOMS	WHAT TO DO
Life-threatening:	
Hives, rash, intense itching, faintness soon after a dose (anaphylaxis).	Seek emergency treatment immediately.
Common:	
• Diarrhea, appetite loss, nausea, vomiting, chest pain, cough, difficult breathing, chills or unexplained fever.	Discontinue. Call doctor right away.
• Rusty colored or brown urine.	No action necessary.
Infrequent:	
• Rash, itchy skin, numbness, tingling or burning of face or mouth, fatigue, weakness.	Discontinue. Call doctor right away.
• Dizziness, headache, drowsiness, paleness (in children), discolored teeth (from liquid form).	Continue. Call doctor when convenient.
Rare:	
Jaundice.	Discontinue. Call doctor right away.

WARNINGS & PRECAUTIONS

Don't take if:
- You are allergic to nitrofurantoin.
- You have impaired kidney function.
- You drink alcohol.

Before you start, consult your doctor:
- If you are prone to allergic reactions.
- If you are pregnant and within 2 weeks of delivery.
- If you have had kidney disease, lung disease, anemia, nerve damage, or G6PD deficiency (a metabolic deficiency).
- If you have diabetes. Drug may affect urine sugar tests.

Over age 60:
Adverse reactions and side effects may be more frequent and severe than in younger persons.

Pregnancy:
Risk to unborn child outweighs drug benefits, especially in last month of pregnancy. Don't use.

Breast-feeding:
Drug passes into milk. Avoid drug or discontinue nursing until you finish medicine. Consult doctor for advice on maintaining milk supply.

Infants & children:
Don't give to infants younger than 1 month. Use only under medical supervision for older children.

Prolonged use:
Chest pain, cough, shortness of breath.

Skin & sunlight:
No problems expected.

Driving, piloting or hazardous work:
Avoid if you feel dizzy or drowsy. Otherwise, no problems expected.

Discontinuing:
Don't discontinue without consulting doctor. Dose may require gradual reduction if you have taken drug for a long time. Doses of other drugs may also require adjustment.

Others:
Periodic blood counts, liver-function tests, and chest X-rays recommended.

POSSIBLE INTERACTION WITH OTHER DRUGS

GENERIC NAME OR DRUG CLASS	COMBINED EFFECT
Nalidixic acid	Decreased nitrofurantoin effect.
Phenobarbital	Decreased nitrofurantoin effect.
Probenecid	Increased nitrofurantoin effect.
Sulfinpyrazone	Possible nitrofurantoin toxicity.

POSSIBLE INTERACTION WITH OTHER SUBSTANCES

INTERACTS WITH	COMBINED EFFECT
Alcohol:	Possible disulfiram reaction. * Avoid.
Beverages:	None expected.
Cocaine:	No proven problems.
Foods:	None expected.
Marijuana:	None expected.
Tobacco:	None expected.

NIZATIDINE

BRAND NAMES

Axid

BASIC INFORMATION

Habit forming? No
Prescription needed? Yes
Available as generic? No
Drug class: Histamine H-2 antagonist

 ## USES

Treatment for duodenal ulcers and other
conditions in which stomach produces excess
hydrochloric acid.

 ## DOSAGE & USAGE INFORMATION

How to take:
Tablet or liquid—Swallow with liquid.

When to take:
- 1 dose per day—Take at bedtime.
- 2 or more doses per day—Take at the same
  times each day.

If you forget a dose:
Take as soon as you remember up to 2 hours
late. If more than 2 hours, wait for next
scheduled dose (don't double this dose).

What drug does:
Blocks histamine release so stomach secretes
less acid.

Time lapse before drug works:
Begins in 30 minutes. May require several days
to relieve pain.

Don't take with:
See Interaction column and consult doctor.

 ## OVERDOSE

SYMPTOMS:
Confusion, slurred speech, breathing
difficulty, rapid heartbeat, delirium.
WHAT TO DO:
Overdose unlikely to threaten life. If person
takes much larger amount than prescribed,
call doctor, poison-control center or hospital
emergency room for instructions.

 ## POSSIBLE ADVERSE REACTIONS OR SIDE EFFECTS

SYMPTOMS	WHAT TO DO
Life-threatening: None expected.	
Common: None expected.	
Infrequent:	
• Diarrhea, jaundice.	Discontinue. Call doctor right away.
• Dizziness or headache, diarrhea, decreased sperm production.	Continue. Call doctor when convenient.
• Diminished sex drive, breast swelling and soreness in males, unusual milk flow in females, hair loss.	Continue. Tell doctor at next visit.
Rare: Confusion; rash, hives; sore throat, fever; slow, fast or irregular heartbeat; unusual bleeding or bruising; muscle cramps or pain; fatigue; weakness; peripheral neuritis; chronic kidney disease.	Discontinue. Call doctor right away.

 ## WARNINGS & PRECAUTIONS

Don't take if:
You are allergic to nizatidine or other histamine
H-2 antagonists.

Before you start, consult your doctor:
- If you plan to become pregnant during
  medication period.
- If you take aspirin. Aspirin may irritate
  stomach.

Over age 60:
Adverse reactions and side effects may be more
frequent and severe than in younger persons.

Pregnancy:
No proven harm to unborn child. Avoid if
possible.

Breast-feeding:
No problems expected.

Infants & children:
Not recommended.

Prolonged use:
Possible liver damage.

Skin & sunlight:
No problems expected.

Driving, piloting or hazardous work:
Don't drive or pilot aircraft until you learn how medicine affects you. Don't work around dangerous machinery. Don't climb ladders or work in high places. Danger increases if you drink alcohol or take medicine affecting alertness and reflexes, such as antihistamines, tranquilizers, sedatives, pain medicine, narcotics and mind-altering drugs.

Discontinuing:
Don't discontinue without consulting doctor. Dose may require gradual reduction if you have taken drug for a long time. Doses of other drugs may also require adjustment.

Others:
Patients on kidney dialysis—Take at end of dialysis treatment.

 POSSIBLE INTERACTION WITH OTHER DRUGS

GENERIC NAME OR DRUG CLASS	COMBINED EFFECT
Alprazolam	Increased effect and toxicity of alprazolam.
Antacids*	Decreased nizatidine absorption.
Anticoagulants, oral*	Increased anti-anticoagulant effect.
Anticholinergics*	Increased nizatidine effect.
Carbamazepine	Increased effect and toxicity of carbamazepine.
Carmustine (BCNU)	Severe impairment of red-blood-cell production; some interference with white-blood-cell formation.
Chlordiazepoxide	Increased effect and toxicity of chlordiazepoxide.
Diazepam	Increased effect and toxicity of diazepam.
Digitalis preparations*	Increased digitalis effect.
Encainide	Increased effect of nizatidine.
Flurazepam	Increased effect and toxicity of flurazepam.
Glipizide	Increased effect and toxicity of glipizide.

Ketoconazole	Decreased ketoconazole absorption.
Labetalol	Increased antihypertensive effects.
Methadone	Increased effect and toxicity of methadone.
Metoclopramide	Decreased nizatidine absorption.
Metoprolol	Increased effect and toxicity of metoprolol.
Metronidazole	Increased effect and toxicity of metronidazole.
Morphine	Increased effect and toxicity of morphine.
Phenytoin	Increased effect and toxicity of phenytoin.
Procainamide	Increased effect and toxicity of procainamide.

 POSSIBLE INTERACTION WITH OTHER SUBSTANCES

INTERACTS WITH	COMBINED EFFECT
Alcohol:	No interactions expected, but alcohol may slow body's recovery. Avoid.
Beverages: Milk.	Enhanced effectiveness. Small amounts useful for taking medication.
Caffeine drinks.	May increase acid secretion and delay healing.
Cocaine:	Decreased nizatidine effect.
Foods:	Enhanced effectiveness. Protein-rich foods should be eaten in moderation to minimize secretion of stomach acid.
Marijuana:	Increased chance of low sperm count. Marijuana may slow body's recovery. Avoid.
Tobacco:	Reverses nizatidine effect. Tobacco may slow body's recovery. Avoid.

*See Glossary

NORETHINDRONE

BRAND NAMES

Micronor
Modicon 21
Norinyl 1+35
21-Day Tablets
Norlestrin
Norlutate

Norlutin
Nor-Q.D.
Ortho-Novum 1/35
Ovcon
Tri-Norinyl

BASIC INFORMATION

Habit forming? No
Prescription needed? Yes
Available as generic? No
Drug class: Female sex hormone (progestin)

 USES

- Treatment for menstrual or uterine disorders caused by progestin imbalance.
- Contraceptive.

 DOSAGE & USAGE INFORMATION

How to take:
Tablet—Swallow with liquid or food to lessen stomach irritation. You may crumble tablet.

When to take:
At the same time each day.

If you forget a dose:
- Menstrual disorders—Take up to 2 hours late. If more than 2 hours, wait for next dose (don't double this dose).
- Contraceptive—Consult your doctor. You may need to use another birth-control method until next period.

What drug does:
- Creates a uterine lining similar to pregnancy that prevents bleeding.
- Suppresses a pituitary gland hormone responsible for ovulation.
- Stimulates cervical mucus, which stops sperm penetration and prevents pregnancy.

Continued next column

 OVERDOSE

SYMPTOMS:
Nausea, vomiting, fluid retention, breast discomfort or enlargement, vaginal bleeding.
WHAT TO DO:
Overdose unlikely to threaten life. If person takes much larger amount than prescribed, call doctor, poison-control center or hospital emergency room for instructions.

Time lapse before drug works:
- Menstrual disorders—24 to 48 hours.
- Contraception—3 weeks.

Don't take with:
See Interaction column and consult doctor.

 POSSIBLE ADVERSE REACTIONS OR SIDE EFFECTS

SYMPTOMS	WHAT TO DO
Life-threatening:	
Blood clot in leg, brain or lung; hives, rash, intense itching, faintness soon after a dose (anaphylaxis).	Seek emergency treatment immediately.
Common:	
Appetite or weight changes, swollen ankles or feet, unusual tiredness or weakness.	Continue. Tell doctor at next visit.
Infrequent:	
• Prolonged vaginal bleeding.	Discontinue. Call doctor right away.
• Depression.	Continue. Call doctor when convenient.
• Acne, increased facial or body hair, nausea, breast tenderness.	Continue. Tell doctor at next visit.
Rare:	
• Rash, stomach or side pain, jaundice, fever.	Discontinue. Call doctor right away.
• Insomnia, hair loss, amenorrhea.	Continue. Call doctor when convenient.

WARNINGS & PRECAUTIONS

Don't take if:
- You are allergic to any progestin hormone.
- You may be pregnant.
- You have liver or gallbladder disease.
- You have had thrombophlebitis, embolism or stroke.
- You have unexplained vaginal bleeding.
- You have had breast or uterine cancer.

Before you start, consult your doctor:
- If you have heart or kidney disease.
- If you have diabetes.
- If you have a seizure disorder.
- If you suffer migraines.
- If you are easily depressed.

Over age 60:
Not recommended.

Pregnancy:
May harm child. Discontinue at first sign of pregnancy.

Breast-feeding:
Drug passes into milk. Avoid drug or discontinue nursing until you finish medicine. Consult doctor for advice on maintaining milk supply.

Infants & children:
Use only for female children under medical supervision.

Prolonged use:
No problems expected.

Skin & sunlight:
No problems expected.

Driving, piloting or hazardous work:
No problems expected.

Discontinuing:
Consult doctor. This medicine stays in the body and causes fetal abnormalities. Wait at least 3 months before becoming pregnant.

Others:
- Patients with diabetes must be monitored closely.
- Symptoms of blood clot in leg, brain or lung are: chest, groin, leg pain; sudden, severe headache; loss of coordination; vision change; shortness of breath; slurred speech.

POSSIBLE INTERACTION WITH OTHER DRUGS

GENERIC NAME OR DRUG CLASS	COMBINED EFFECT
Insulin	Decreased effect of insulin.
Hypoglycemics, oral*	Decreased effect of oral hypoglycemics.
Oxyphenbutazone	Decreased norethindrone effect.
Phenobarbital	Decreased norethindrone effect.
Phenothiazines*	Increased phenothiazine effect.
Phenylbutazone	Decreased norethindrone effect.
Ursodiol	Decreased effect of ursodiol.

POSSIBLE INTERACTION WITH OTHER SUBSTANCES

INTERACTS WITH	COMBINED EFFECT
Alcohol:	None expected.
Beverages:	None expected.
Cocaine:	Decreased norethindrone effect.
Foods: Salt.	Fluid retention.
Marijuana:	Possible menstrual irregularities or bleeding between periods.
Tobacco:	Possible blood clots in lung, brain, legs. Avoid.

*See Glossary

NORETHINDRONE ACETATE

BRAND NAMES

Aygestin
Micronor
Norlutate

Norlutate Acetate
Norlutin
Nor-O.-D.

BASIC INFORMATION

Habit forming? No
Prescription needed? Yes
Available as generic? No
Drug class: Female sex hormone (progestin)

USES

- Treatment for menstrual or uterine disorders caused by progestin imbalance.
- Contraceptive.
- Treatment for cancer of breast and uterus.

DOSAGE & USAGE INFORMATION

How to take:
Tablet—Swallow with liquid or food to lessen stomach irritation. You may crumble tablet.

When to take:
At the same time each day.

If you forget a dose:
- Menstrual disorders—Take up to 2 hours late. If more than 2 hours, wait for next dose (don't double this dose).
- Contraceptive—Consult your doctor. You may need to use another birth-control method until next period.

What drug does:
- Creates a uterine lining similar to pregnancy that prevents bleeding.
- Suppresses a pituitary gland hormone responsible for ovulation.
- Stimulates cervical mucus, which stops sperm penetration and prevents pregnancy.

Continued next column

OVERDOSE

SYMPTOMS:
Nausea, vomiting, fluid retention, breast discomfort or enlargement, vaginal bleeding.
WHAT TO DO:
Overdose unlikely to threaten life. If person takes much larger amount than prescribed, call doctor, poison-control center or hospital emergency room for instructions.

Time lapse before drug works:
- Menstrual disorders—24 to 48 hours.
- Contraception—3 weeks.
- Cancer—May require 2 to 3 months.

Don't take with:
See Interaction column and consult doctor.

POSSIBLE ADVERSE REACTIONS OR SIDE EFFECTS

SYMPTOMS	WHAT TO DO
Life-threatening: Blood clot in leg, brain or lung; hives, rash, intense itching, faintness soon after a dose (anaphylaxis).	Seek emergency treatment immediately.
Common: Appetite or weight changes, swollen ankles or feet, unusual tiredness or weakness.	Continue. Tell doctor at next visit.
Infrequent: • Prolonged vaginal bleeding.	Discontinue. Call doctor right away.
• Depression.	Continue. Call doctor when convenient.
• Acne, increased facial or body hair, nausea, breast tenderness.	Continue. Tell doctor at next visit.
Rare: • Rash, stomach or side pain, jaundice, fever.	Discontinue. Call doctor right away.
• Insomnia, hair loss, amenorrhea.	Continue. Call doctor when convenient.

NORETHINDRONE ACETATE

WARNINGS & PRECAUTIONS

Don't take if:
- You are allergic to any progestin hormone.
- You may be pregnant.
- You have liver or gallbladder disease.
- You have had thrombophlebitis, embolism or stroke.
- You have unexplained vaginal bleeding.
- You have had breast or uterine cancer.

Before you start, consult your doctor:
- If you have heart or kidney disease.
- If you have diabetes.
- If you have a seizure disorder.
- If you suffer migraines.
- If you are easily depressed.

Over age 60:
Not recommended.

Pregnancy:
May harm child. Discontinue at first sign of pregnancy.

Breast-feeding:
Drug passes into milk. Avoid drug or discontinue nursing until you finish medicine. Consult doctor for advice on maintaining milk supply.

Infants & children:
Use only for female children under medical supervision.

Prolonged use:
No problems expected.

Skin & sunlight:
No problems expected.

Driving, piloting or hazardous work:
No problems expected.

Discontinuing:
Consult doctor. This medicine stays in the body and causes fetal abnormalities. Wait at least 3 months before becoming pregnant.

Others:
- Patients with diabetes must be monitored closely.
- Symptoms of blood clot in leg, brain or lung are: chest, groin, leg pain; sudden, severe headache; loss of coordination; vision change; shortness of breath; slurred speech.

POSSIBLE INTERACTION WITH OTHER DRUGS

GENERIC NAME OR DRUG CLASS	COMBINED EFFECT
Insulin	Decreased effect of insulin.
Hypoglycemics, oral*	Decreased effect of oral hypoglycemics.
Oxyphenbutazone	Decreased norethindrone acetate effect.
Phenobarbital	Decreased norethindrone acetate effect.
Phenothiazines*	Increased phenothiazine effect.
Phenylbutazone	Decreased norethindrone acetate effect.
Ursodiol	Decreased effect of ursodiol.

POSSIBLE INTERACTION WITH OTHER SUBSTANCES

INTERACTS WITH	COMBINED EFFECT
Alcohol:	None expected.
Beverages:	None expected.
Cocaine:	Decreased norethindrone acetate effect.
Foods: Salt.	Fluid retention.
Marijuana:	Possible menstrual irregularities or bleeding between periods.
Tobacco:	Possible blood clots in lung, brain, legs. Avoid.

NORFLOXACIN

BRAND NAMES

Noroxin

BASIC INFORMATION

Habit forming? No
Prescription needed? Yes
Available as generic? No
Drug class: Antibacterial, fluoroquinolones

USES

- Treats infections of the kidney, ureter, bladder and urethra.
- Treats traveler's diarrhea, bacterial gastroenteritis.

DOSAGE & USAGE INFORMATION

How to take:
Tablet—On an empty stomach 1 hour before or 2 hours after meals. Take with lots of water.

When to take:
As directed. Usually every 12 hours on empty stomach.

If you forget a dose:
Take as soon as you remember up to 6 hours late. If more than 6 hours, wait for next scheduled dose (don't double this dose).

What drug does:
Interferes with nutrient necessary for growth and reproduction of bacteria. Will not kill viruses.

Time lapse before drug works:
2 hours to peak level in blood. May require 7 to 21 days of treatment to cure infections.

Don't take with:
- Food, antacids.
- See Interaction column and consult doctor.

OVERDOSE

SYMPTOMS:
Seizures
WHAT TO DO:
- Dial 0 (operator) or 911 (emergency) for an ambulance or medical help. Then give first aid immediately.
- See emergency information on inside covers.

POSSIBLE ADVERSE REACTIONS OR SIDE EFFECTS

SYMPTOMS	WHAT TO DO
Life-threatening: None expected.	
Common: None expected.	
Infrequent: Nausea, abdominal pains, heartburn, insomnia, diarrhea, dizziness, fatigue, rash, vulvar irritation, crystals in urine.	Discontinue. Call doctor right away.
Rare:	
• Seizures.	Discontinue. Seek emergency treatment.
• Anemia, joint pain, joint swelling, fever.	Discontinue. Call doctor right away.
• Dry mouth.	Continue. Call doctor when convenient.

WARNINGS & PRECAUTIONS

Don't take if:
You are allergic to any quinolone antibiotics.

Before you start, consult your doctor:
If you have chronic kidney disease with loss of kidney function.

Over age 60:
Adverse reactions and side effects may be more frequent and severe than in younger persons. Ask doctor about smaller doses.

Pregnancy:
Safety to unborn child unestablished. Avoid if possible.

Breast-feeding:
Drug passes into milk. Avoid drug or discontinue nursing until you finish medicine. Consult doctor for advice on maintaining milk supply.

Infants & children:
Not recommended if under 17 years old. Use only under close medical supervision.

Prolonged use:
No problems expected.

Skin & sunlight:
No problems expected.

Driving, piloting or hazardous work:
Avoid if you feel drowsy or dizzy.

Discontinuing:
No problems expected.

Others:
No problems expected.

POSSIBLE INTERACTION WITH OTHER DRUGS

GENERIC NAME OR DRUG CLASS	COMBINED EFFECT
Antacids*	Decreased absorption of norfloxacin.
Nitrofurantoin	Decreased norfloxacin effect.
Probenecid	Decreased effect of norfloxacin.
Theophylline	Increased effect and toxicity of theophylline.
Warfarin	Possible increased effect of warfarin.

POSSIBLE INTERACTION WITH OTHER SUBSTANCES

INTERACTS WITH	COMBINED EFFECT
Alcohol:	Decreased effect of norfloxacin.
Beverages:	None expected.
Cocaine:	Decreased effect of norfloxacin.
Foods:	None expected.
Marijuana:	Decreased effect of norfloxacin.
Tobacco:	May stimulate irritated gastrointestinal tract. Avoid.

NORGESTREL

BRAND NAMES

Lo-Ovral   Ovrette
Ovral

BASIC INFORMATION

Habit forming? No
Prescription needed? Yes
Available as generic? No
Drug class: Female sex hormone (progestin)

 USES

Contraceptive.

 DOSAGE & USAGE INFORMATION

How to take:
Tablet—Swallow with liquid or food to lessen stomach irritation. You may crumble tablet.

When to take:
At the same time each day.

If you forget a dose:
Consult your doctor. You may need to use another birth-control method until next period, then resume norgestrel.

What drug does:
- Creates a uterine lining similar to pregnancy that prevents bleeding.
- Suppresses a pituitary gland hormone responsible for ovulation.
- Stimulates cervical mucus, which stops sperm penetration and prevents pregnancy.

Time lapse before drug works:
3 weeks. Use another method of birth control until then.

Don't take with:
See Interaction column and consult doctor.

 OVERDOSE

SYMPTOMS:
Nausea, vomiting, fluid retention, breast discomfort or enlargement, vaginal bleeding.
WHAT TO DO:
Overdose unlikely to threaten life. If person takes much larger amount than prescribed, call doctor, poison-control center or hospital emergency room for instructions.

 POSSIBLE ADVERSE REACTIONS OR SIDE EFFECTS

SYMPTOMS	WHAT TO DO
Life-threatening:	
Blood clot in leg, brain or lung; hives, rash, intense itching, faintness soon after a dose (anaphylaxis).	Seek emergency treatment immediately.
Common:	
Appetite or weight changes, swollen ankles or feet, unusual tiredness or weakness.	Continue. Tell doctor at next visit.
Infrequent:	
• Prolonged vaginal bleeding.	Discontinue. Call doctor right away.
• Depression.	Continue. Call doctor when convenient.
• Acne, increased facial or body hair, nausea, breast tenderness.	Continue. Tell doctor at next visit.
Rare:	
• Rash, stomach or side pain, jaundice, fever.	Discontinue. Call doctor right away.
• Insomnia, hair loss, amenorrhea.	Continue. Call doctor when convenient.

WARNINGS & PRECAUTIONS

Don't take if:
- You are allergic to any progestin hormone.
- You may be pregnant.
- You have liver or gallbladder disease.
- You have had thrombophlebitis, embolism or stroke.
- You have unexplained vaginal bleeding.
- You have had breast or uterine cancer.

Before you start, consult your doctor:
- If you have heart or kidney disease.
- If you have diabetes.
- If you have a seizure disorder.
- If you suffer migraines.
- If you are easily depressed.

Over age 60:
Not recommended.

Pregnancy:
May harm child. Discontinue at first sign of pregnancy.

Breast-feeding:
Drug passes into milk. Avoid drug or discontinue nursing until you finish medicine. Consult doctor for advice on maintaining milk supply.

Infants & children:
Use only for female children under medical supervision.

Prolonged use:
No problems expected.

Skin & sunlight:
No problems expected.

Driving, piloting or hazardous work:
No problems expected.

Discontinuing:
Consult doctor. This medicine stays in the body and causes fetal abnormalities. Wait at least 3 months before becoming pregnant.

Others:
- Patients with diabetes must be monitored closely.
- Symptoms of blood clot in leg, brain or lung are: chest, groin, leg pain; sudden, severe headache; loss of coordination; vision change; shortness of breath; slurred speech.

POSSIBLE INTERACTION WITH OTHER DRUGS

GENERIC NAME OR DRUG CLASS	COMBINED EFFECT
Insulin	Decreased effect of insulin.
Hypoglycemics, oral *	Decreased effect of oral hypoglycemics.
Oxyphenbutazone	Decreased norgestrel effect.
Phenobarbital	Decreased norgestrel effect.
Phenothiazines *	Increased phenothiazine effect.
Phenylbutazone	Decreased norgestrel effect.
Ursodiol	Decreased effect of ursodiol.

POSSIBLE INTERACTION WITH OTHER SUBSTANCES

INTERACTS WITH	COMBINED EFFECT
Alcohol:	None expected.
Beverages:	None expected.
Cocaine:	Decreased norgestrel effect.
Foods: Salt.	Fluid retention.
Marijuana:	Possible menstrual irregularities or bleeding between periods.
Tobacco:	Possible blood clots in lung, brain, legs. Avoid.

NYLIDRIN

BRAND NAMES

Arlidin
Arlidin Forte
Circlidrin

Pervadil
PMS Nylidrin
Rolidrin

BASIC INFORMATION

Habit forming? No
Prescription needed? Yes
Available as generic? No
Drug class: Vasodilator

 ## USES

- May improve poor circulation in extremities.
- Reduces dizziness caused by poor circulation in inner ear.

 ## DOSAGE & USAGE INFORMATION

How to take:
Tablet—Swallow with liquid or food to lessen stomach irritation. If you can't swallow whole, crumble tablet and take with liquid or food.

When to take:
At the same times each day.

If you forget a dose:
Take as soon as you remember up to 2 hours late. If more than 2 hours, wait for next scheduled dose (don't double this dose).

What drug does:
Stimulates nerves that dilate blood vessels, increasing oxygen and nutrients.

Continued next column

 ## OVERDOSE

SYMPTOMS:
Blood-pressure drop; nausea, vomiting; rapid, irregular heartbeat, chest pain; blurred vision; metallic taste.
WHAT TO DO:
- Dial 0 (operator) or 911 (emergency) for an ambulance or medical help. Then give first aid immediately.
- If patient is unconscious and not breathing, give mouth-to-mouth breathing. If there is no heartbeat, use cardiac massage and mouth-to-mouth breathing (CPR). Don't try to make patient vomit. If you can't get help quickly, take patient to nearest emergency facility.
- See emergency information on inside covers.

Time lapse before drug works:
10 to 30 minutes.

Don't take with:
See Interaction column and consult doctor.

 ## POSSIBLE ADVERSE REACTIONS OR SIDE EFFECTS

SYMPTOMS	WHAT TO DO
Life-threatening: None expected.	
Common:	
• Chest pain.	Discontinue. Call doctor right away.
• Blurred vision, fever, low blood pressure on standing, decreased or difficult urination.	Continue. Call doctor when convenient.
• Metallic taste.	Continue. Tell doctor at next visit.
Infrequent:	
• Rapid or irregular heartbeat.	Discontinue. Call doctor right away.
• Dizziness, weakness, tiredness.	Continue. Call doctor when convenient.
Rare:	
• Shakiness, chills.	Discontinue. Call doctor right away.
• Headache, nausea, vomiting, flushed face, nervousness.	Continue. Call doctor when convenient.

WARNINGS & PRECAUTIONS

Don't take if:
- You are allergic to any vasodilator drugs.
- You have had a heart attack or stroke within 4 weeks.
- You have an active peptic ulcer.

Before you start, consult your doctor:
- If you have had heart disease, heart-rhythm disorders (especially rapid heartbeat), a stroke or poor circulation to the brain.
- If you have glaucoma.
- If you have an overactive thyroid gland.
- If you plan to become pregnant within medication period.
- If you use tobacco.

Over age 60:
Adverse reactions and side effects may be more frequent and severe than in younger persons.

Pregnancy:
No proven harm to unborn child. Avoid if possible.

Breast-feeding:
No proven problems. Consult doctor.

Infants & children:
Not recommended.

Prolonged use:
No problems expected.

Skin & sunlight:
No problems expected.

Driving, piloting or hazardous work:
Don't drive or pilot aircraft until you learn how medicine affects you. Don't work around dangerous machinery. Don't climb ladders or work in high places. Danger increases if you drink alcohol or take medicine affecting alertness and reflexes, such as antihistamines, tranquilizers, sedatives, pain medicine, narcotics and mind-altering drugs.

Discontinuing:
Don't discontinue without consulting doctor. If your condition worsens, contact your doctor immediately. Dose may require gradual reduction if you have taken drug for a long time. Doses of other drugs may also require adjustment.

Others:
No problems expected.

POSSIBLE INTERACTION WITH OTHER DRUGS

GENERIC NAME OR DRUG CLASS	COMBINED EFFECT
Beta-adrenergic blockers*	Decreased effect of nylidrin.
Phenothiazines*	Increased blood level of phenothiazines.

POSSIBLE INTERACTION WITH OTHER SUBSTANCES

INTERACTS WITH	COMBINED EFFECT
Alcohol:	Possible increased stomach-acid secretion. Use with caution.
Beverages:	None expected.
Cocaine:	Increased adverse effects of nylidrin.
Foods:	None expected.
Marijuana:	None expected.
Tobacco:	Decreased nylidrin effect. Worsens circulation. Avoid.

NYSTATIN

BRAND NAMES

Achrostatin V	Mytrex
Candex	Nadostine
Declostatin	Nilstat
Korostatin	Nyaderm
Mycolog	Nystaform
Mycostatin	Nystex
Myco-Triacet	O-V statin
Mykinac	Terrastatin

BASIC INFORMATION

Habit forming? No
Prescription needed? Yes
Available as generic? Yes
Drug class: Antifungal

 ## USES

Treatment of fungus infections susceptible to nystatin.

 ## DOSAGE & USAGE INFORMATION

How to take:
- Tablet—Swallow with liquid. If you can't swallow whole, crumble tablet and take with liquid or food.
- Suppositories—Remove wrapper and moisten suppository with water. Gently insert larger end into vagina. Push well into vagina with finger.
- Ointment, cream or lotion—Use as directed by doctor and label.
- Liquid—Take as directed. Instruction varies by preparation.
- Lozenges—Take as directed on label.

When to take:
At the same time each day.

If you forget a dose:
Take as soon as you remember up to 2 hours late. If more than 2 hours, wait for next scheduled dose (don't double this dose).

Continued next column

 ## OVERDOSE

SYMPTOMS:
Mild overdose may cause nausea, vomiting, diarrhea.
WHAT TO DO:
Overdose unlikely to threaten life. If person takes much larger amount than prescribed, call doctor, poison-control center or hospital emergency room for instructions.

What drug does:
Prevents growth and reproduction of fungus.

Time lapse before drug works:
Begins immediately. May require 3 weeks for maximum benefit, depending on location and severity of infection.

Don't take with:
See Interaction column and consult doctor.

 ## POSSIBLE ADVERSE REACTIONS OR SIDE EFFECTS

SYMPTOMS	WHAT TO DO
Life-threatening: None expected.	
Common: (at high doses) Nausea, stomach pain, vomiting, diarrhea.	Discontinue. Call doctor right away.
Infrequent: Mild irritation, itch at application site.	Discontinue. Call doctor right away.
Rare: None expected.	

WARNINGS & PRECAUTIONS

Don't take if:
You are allergic to nystatin.

Before you start, consult your doctor:
If you plan to become pregnant within medication period.

Over age 60:
No problems expected.

Pregnancy:
No proven harm to unborn child. Avoid if possible.

Breast-feeding:
No proven problems. Consult doctor.

Infants & children:
No problems expected.

Prolonged use:
No problems expected.

Skin & sunlight:
No problems expected.

Driving, piloting or hazardous work:
No problems expected.

Discontinuing:
Don't discontinue without doctor's advice until you complete prescribed dose, even though symptoms diminish or disappear.

Others:
No problems expected.

POSSIBLE INTERACTION WITH OTHER DRUGS

GENERIC NAME OR DRUG CLASS	COMBINED EFFECT
None	

POSSIBLE INTERACTION WITH OTHER SUBSTANCES

INTERACTS WITH	COMBINED EFFECT
Alcohol:	None expected.
Beverages:	None expected.
Cocaine:	None expected.
Foods:	None expected.
Marijuana:	None expected.
Tobacco:	None expected.

ORPHENADRINE

BRAND NAMES

Banflex	Neocyten
Disipal	Norflex
Flexoject	O-Flex
Flexon	Orflagen
K-Flex	Orphenate
Marflex	Ro-Orphena
Myolin	Tega-Flex
Myotrol	X-Otag

BASIC INFORMATION

Habit forming? Possibly
Prescription needed?
    U.S.: Yes
    Canada: No
Available as generic? Yes
Drug class: Muscle relaxant, anticholinergic, antihistamine, antiparkinsonism

USES

- Reduces muscle-strain discomfort.
- Relieves symptoms of Parkinson's disease.
- Adjunctive treatment to rest, analgesics and physical therapy for muscle spasms.

DOSAGE & USAGE INFORMATION

How to take:
Tablet or extended-release tablet—Swallow with liquid. If you can't swallow whole, crumble tablet and take with liquid or food.

When to take:
At the same times each day.

If you forget a dose:
Take as soon as you remember up to 6 hours late. If more than 6 hours, wait for next scheduled dose (don't double this dose).

Continued next column

OVERDOSE

SYMPTOMS:
Fainting, confusion, blurred vision, difficulty swallowing, difficulty breathing, decreased urination, widely dilated pupils, rapid heartbeat, rapid pulse, paralysis, convulsions, coma.
WHAT TO DO:
- Dial 0 (operator) or 911 (emergency) for an ambulance or medical help. Then give first aid immediately.
- See emergency information on inside covers.

What drug does:
Sedative and analgesic effects reduce spasm and pain in skeletal muscles.

Time lapse before drug works:
1 to 2 hours.

Don't take with:
See Interaction column and consult doctor.

POSSIBLE ADVERSE REACTIONS OR SIDE EFFECTS

SYMPTOMS	WHAT TO DO
Life-threatening: Extreme weakness; transient paralysis; temporary loss of vision; hives, rash, intense itching, faintness soon after a dose (anaphylaxis).	Seek emergency treatment immediately.
Common: None expected.	
Infrequent: • Weakness, headache, dizziness, agitation, drowsiness, tremor, confusion, rapid or pounding heartbeat, depression.	Discontinue. Call doctor right away.
• Dry mouth, nausea, vomiting, constipation, urinary hesitancy or retention.	Continue. Call doctor when convenient.
Rare: Rash, itchy skin, blurred vision, dilated pupils, mental confusion, hiccups.	Discontinue. Call doctor right away.

726

WARNINGS & PRECAUTIONS

Don't take if:
- You are allergic to orphenadrine.
- You are allergic to tartrazine dye.

Before you start, consult your doctor:
- If you have glaucoma.
- If you have myasthenia gravis.
- If you have difficulty emptying bladder.
- If you have had heart disease or heart-rhythm disturbance.
- If you have had a peptic ulcer.
- If you have prostate enlargement.

Over age 60:
Adverse reactions and side effects may be more frequent and severe than in younger persons.

Pregnancy:
Safety not established. Avoid if possible.

Breast-feeding:
No proven problems. Consult doctor.

Infants & children:
Not recommended for children younger than 12.

Prolonged use:
Increased internal-eye pressure.

Skin & sunlight:
No problems expected.

Driving, piloting or hazardous work:
Don't drive or pilot aircraft until you learn how medicine affects you. Don't work around dangerous machinery. Don't climb ladders or work in high places. Danger increases if you drink alcohol or take medicine affecting alertness and reflexes, such as antihistamines, tranquilizers, sedatives, pain medicine, narcotics and mind-altering drugs.

Discontinuing:
May be unnecessary to finish medicine. Follow doctor's instructions.

Others:
No problems expected.

POSSIBLE INTERACTION WITH OTHER DRUGS

GENERIC NAME OR DRUG CLASS	COMBINED EFFECT
Anticholinergics*	Increased anti-cholinergic effect.
Antidepressants, tricyclic (TCA)*	Increased sedation.
Antihistamines*	Increased sedation.
Carteolol	Decreased antihistamine effect.
Chlorpromazine	Hypoglycemia (low blood sugar).
Contraceptives, oral*	Decreased contraceptive effect.
Griseofulvin	Decreased griseofulvin effect.
Levodopa	Increased effect of levodopa. (Improves effectiveness in treating Parkinson's disease.)
Nabilone	Greater depression of central nervous system.
Nitrates*	Increased internal-eye pressure.
Nizatidine	Increased nizatidine effect.
Phenylbutazone	Decreased phenyl-butazone effect.
Potassium supplements*	Increased possibility of intestinal ulcers with oral potassium tablets.
Propoxyphene	Possible confusion, nervousness, tremors.
Sotalol	Increased antihistamine effect.

POSSIBLE INTERACTION WITH OTHER SUBSTANCES

INTERACTS WITH	COMBINED EFFECT
Alcohol:	Increased drowsiness. Avoid.
Beverages:	None expected.
Cocaine:	Decreased orphenadrine effect. Avoid.
Foods:	None expected.
Marijuana:	Increased drowsiness, mouth dryness, muscle weakness, fainting.
Tobacco:	None expected.

ORPHENADRINE, ASPIRIN & CAFFEINE

BRAND NAMES

Back-Ese
Norgesic

Norgesic Forte

BASIC INFORMATION

Habit forming? Yes
Prescription needed? Yes
Available as generic? No
**Drug class: Stimulant, vasoconstrictor,
muscle relaxant, analgesic, anti-inflammatory**

USES

- Reduces muscle-strain discomfort.
- Reduces pain, fever, inflammation.
- Relieves swelling, stiffness, joint pain.
- Treatment for drowsiness and fatigue.

DOSAGE & USAGE INFORMATION

How to take:
Tablet—Swallow with liquid. If you can't swallow whole, crumble tablet and take with liquid or food.

When to take:
At the same times each day.

If you forget a dose:
Take as soon as you remember up to 2 hours late. If more than 2 hours, wait for next scheduled dose (don't double this dose).

What drug does:
- Sedative and analgesic effects reduce spasm and pain in skeletal muscles.
- Affects hypothalamus, the part of the brain which regulates temperature by dilating small blood vessels in skin.
- Prevents clumping of platelets (small blood cells) so blood vessels remain open.
- Decreases prostaglandin effect.
- Suppresses body's pain messages.

Continued next column

OVERDOSE

SYMPTOMS:
Fainting, confusion, widely dilated pupils, rapid pulse, ringing in ears, nausea, vomiting, dizziness, fever, deep and rapid breathing, excitement, rapid heartbeat, hallucinations, coma.
WHAT TO DO:
- **Dial 0 (operator) or 911 (emergency) for an ambulance or medical help. Then give first aid immediately.**
- **See emergency information on inside covers.**

- Constricts blood-vessel walls.
- Stimulates central nervous system.

Time lapse before drug works:
1 hour.

Don't take with:
- Tetracyclines. Space doses 1 hour apart.
- Non-prescription drugs without consulting doctor.
- See Interaction column and consult doctor.

POSSIBLE ADVERSE REACTIONS OR SIDE EFFECTS

SYMPTOMS	WHAT TO DO
Life-threatening: Hives, rash, intense itching, faintness soon after a dose (anaphylaxis).	Seek emergency treatment immediately.
Common: • Nausea, vomiting, abdominal cramps, nervousness, urgent urination, low blood sugar (hunger, anxiety, cold sweats, rapid pulse).	Discontinue. Call doctor right away.
• Ringing in ears, indigestion, heartburn, insomnia.	Continue. Call doctor when convenient.
Infrequent: • Weakness, headache, dizziness, drowsiness, agitation, tremor, confusion, irregular heartbeat.	Discontinue. Call doctor right away.
• Dry mouth, constipation.	Continue. Call doctor when convenient.
Rare: • Black or bloody vomit.	Discontinue. Seek emergency treatment.
• Change in vision; blurred vision; black, bloody or tarry stool; bloody urine; jaundice; dilated pupils.	Discontinue. Call doctor right away.
• Drowsiness.	Continue. Call doctor when convenient.

WARNINGS & PRECAUTIONS

Don't take if:
- You need to restrict sodium in your diet. Buffered effervescent tablets and sodium salicylate are high in sodium.
- Aspirin has a strong vinegar-like odor, which means it has decomposed.
- You have a peptic ulcer of stomach or duodenum, a bleeding disorder, heart disease.
- You are allergic to any stimulant or orphenadrine.

ORPHENADRINE, ASPIRIN & CAFFEINE

Before you start, consult your doctor:
- If you have had stomach or duodenal ulcers, gout, heart disease or heart-rhythm disturbance, peptic ulcer.
- If you have asthma, nasal polyps, irregular heartbeat, hypoglycemia (low blood sugar), epilepsy, glaucoma, myasthenia gravis, difficulty emptying bladder, prostate enlargement.

Over age 60:
- More likely to cause hidden bleeding in stomach or intestines. Watch for dark stools.
- Adverse reactions and side effects may be more frequent and severe than in younger persons.

Pregnancy:
Risk to unborn child outweighs drug benefits. Don't use.

Breast-feeding:
Drug passes into milk. Avoid drug or discontinue nursing until you finish medicine. Consult doctor for advice on maintaining milk supply.

Infants & children:
- Overdose frequent and severe. Keep bottles out of children's reach.
- Consult doctor before giving to persons under age 18 who have fever and discomfort of viral illness, especially chicken pox and influenza. Probably increases risk of Reye's syndrome.
- Not recommended for children younger than 12.

Prolonged use:
- Kidney damage. Periodic kidney-function test recommended.
- Stomach ulcers more likely.
- Increased internal-eye pressure.

Skin & sunlight:
Aspirin combined with sunscreen may decrease sunburn.

Driving, piloting or hazardous work:
Don't drive or pilot aircraft until you learn how medicine affects you. Don't work around dangerous machinery. Don't climb ladders or work in high places. Danger increases if you drink alcohol or take medicine affecting alertness and reflexes, such as antihistamines, tranquilizers, sedatives, pain medicine, narcotics and mind-altering drugs.

Discontinuing:
- For chronic illness—Don't discontinue without doctor's advice until you complete prescribed dose, even though symptoms diminish or disappear.
- May be unnecessary to finish medicine if you take it for a short-term illness. Follow doctor's instructions.

Others:
- Aspirin can complicate surgery; illness; pregnancy, labor and delivery.
- For arthritis, don't change dose without consulting doctor.
- Urine tests for blood sugar may be inaccurate.
- May produce or aggravate fibrocystic breast disease in women.

POSSIBLE INTERACTION WITH OTHER DRUGS

GENERIC NAME OR DRUG CLASS	COMBINED EFFECT
Acebutolol	Decreased antihypertensive effect of acebutolol.
Allopurinol	Decreased allopurinol effect.
Antacids*	Decreased aspirin effect.
Anticholinergics*	Increased anticholinergic effect.
Anticoagulants*	Increased anticoagulant effect. Abnormal bleeding.

Continued page 1093

POSSIBLE INTERACTION WITH OTHER SUBSTANCES

INTERACTS WITH	COMBINED EFFECT
Alcohol:	Possible stomach irritation and bleeding, increased drowsiness. Avoid.
Beverages: Caffeine drinks.	Increased caffeine effect.
Cocaine:	Decreased orphenadrine effect. Overstimulation. Avoid.
Foods:	No proven problems.
Marijuana:	Increased effect of drugs. May lead to dangerous, rapid heartbeat. Increased dry mouth. Avoid.
Tobacco:	Increased heartbeat. Avoid.

*See Glossary

OXACILLIN

BRAND NAMES

Bactocill   Prostaphlin

BASIC INFORMATION

Habit forming? No
Prescription needed? Yes
Available as generic? Yes
Drug class: Antibiotic (penicillin)

 USES

Treatment of bacterial infections that are
susceptible to oxacillin.

 **DOSAGE & USAGE
INFORMATION**

How to take:
- Capsules—Swallow with liquid on an empty
  stomach 1 hour before or 2 hours after
  eating.
- Liquid—Take with cold beverage. Liquid form
  is perishable and effective for only 7 days at
  room temperature. Effective for 14 days if
  stored in refrigerator. Don't freeze.

When to take:
Follow instructions on prescription label or side
of package. Doses should be evenly spaced.
For example, 4 times a day means every 6
hours.

If you forget a dose:
Take as soon as you remember. Continue
regular schedule.

What drug does:
Destroys susceptible bacteria. Does not kill
viruses.

Time lapse before drug works:
May be several days before medicine affects
infection.

Don't take with:
See Interaction column and consult doctor.

 OVERDOSE

SYMPTOMS:
Severe diarrhea, nausea or vomiting.
WHAT TO DO:
Overdose unlikely to threaten life. If person
takes much larger amount than prescribed,
call doctor, poison-control center or hospital
emergency room for instructions.

 **POSSIBLE
ADVERSE REACTIONS
OR SIDE EFFECTS**

SYMPTOMS	WHAT TO DO
Life-threatening: Hives, rash, intense itching, faintness soon after a dose (anaphylaxis).	Seek emergency treatment immediately.
Common: Dark or discolored tongue.	Continue. Tell doctor at next visit.
Infrequent: Mild nausea, vomiting, diarrhea.	Continue. Call doctor when convenient.
Rare: Unexplained bleeding.	Discontinue. Call doctor right away.

WARNINGS & PRECAUTIONS

Don't take if:
You are allergic to oxacillin, cephalosporin antibiotics, or other penicillins. Life-threatening reaction may occur.

Before you start, consult your doctor:
If you are allergic to any substance or drug.

Over age 60:
You may have skin reactions, particularly around genitals and anus.

Pregnancy:
Studies inconclusive on harm to unborn child. Animal studies show fetal abnormalities. Decide with your doctor whether drug benefits justify risk to unborn child.

Breast-feeding:
Drug passes into milk. Child may become sensitive to penicillins and have allergic reactions to penicillin drugs. Avoid oxacillin or discontinue nursing until you finish medicine. Consult doctor for advice on maintaining milk supply.

Infants & children:
No problems expected.

Prolonged use:
You may become more susceptible to infections caused by germs not responsive to oxacillin.

Skin & sunlight:
No problems expected.

Driving, piloting or hazardous work:
Usually not dangerous. Most hazardous reactions likely to occur a few minutes after taking oxacillin.

Discontinuing:
Don't discontinue without doctor's advice until you complete prescribed dose, even though symptoms diminish or disappear.

Others:
No problems expected.

POSSIBLE INTERACTION WITH OTHER DRUGS

GENERIC NAME OR DRUG CLASS	COMBINED EFFECT
Beta-adrenergic blockers*	Increased chance of anaphylaxis (see emergency information on inside front cover).
Chloramphenicol	Decreased effect of both drugs.
Erythromycins*	Decreased effect of both drugs.
Loperamide	Decreased oxacillin effect.
Paromomycin	Decreased effect of both drugs.
Tetracyclines*	Decreased effect of both drugs.
Troleandomycin	Decreased effect of both drugs.

POSSIBLE INTERACTION WITH OTHER SUBSTANCES

INTERACTS WITH	COMBINED EFFECT
Alcohol:	Occasional stomach irritation.
Beverages:	None expected.
Cocaine:	No proven problems.
Foods:	None expected.
Marijuana:	No proven problems.
Tobacco:	None expected.

*See Glossary

OXAZEPAM

BRAND NAMES

Apo-Oxazepam   Serax
Novoxapam   Zapex
Ox-Pam

BASIC INFORMATION

Habit forming? Yes
Prescription needed? Yes
Available as generic? Yes
Drug class: Tranquilizer (benzodiazepine)

 ## USES

Treatment for nervousness or tension.

 ## DOSAGE & USAGE INFORMATION

How to take:
Tablet or capsule—Swallow with liquid. If you can't swallow whole, crumble tablet or open capsule and take with liquid or food.

When to take:
At the same time each day, according to instructions on prescription label.

If you forget a dose:
Take as soon as you remember up to 2 hours late. If more than 2 hours, wait for next scheduled dose (don't double this dose).

What drug does:
Affects limbic system of brain—part that controls emotions.

Time lapse before drug works:
2 hours. May take 6 weeks for full benefit.

Don't take with:
See Interaction column and consult doctor.

 ## OVERDOSE

SYMPTOMS:
Drowsiness, weakness, tremor, stupor, coma.
WHAT TO DO:
- **Dial 0 (operator) or 911 (emergency) for an ambulance or medical help. Then give first aid immediately.**
- **If patient is unconscious and not breathing, give mouth-to-mouth breathing. If there is no heartbeat, use cardiac massage and mouth-to-mouth breathing (CPR). Don't try to make patient vomit. If you can't get help quickly, take patient to nearest emergency facility.**
- **See emergency information on inside covers.**

 ## POSSIBLE ADVERSE REACTIONS OR SIDE EFFECTS

SYMPTOMS	WHAT TO DO
Life-threatening: None expected.	
Common: Clumsiness, drowsiness, dizziness.	Continue. Call doctor when convenient.
Infrequent: • Hallucinations, confusion, irritability, depression, rash, itchy skin, change in vision.	Discontinue. Call doctor right away.
• Constipation or diarrhea, nausea, vomiting, difficult urination, vivid dreams.	Continue. Call doctor when convenient.
Rare: • Slow heartbeat, difficult breathing.	Discontinue. Seek emergency treatment.
• Mouth, throat ulcers; jaundice.	Discontinue. Call doctor right away.
• Decreased libido.	Continue. Call doctor when convenient.

WARNINGS & PRECAUTIONS

Don't take if:
- You are allergic to any benzodiazepine.
- You have myasthenia gravis.
- You are active or recovering alcoholic.
- Patient is younger than 6 months.

Before you start, consult your doctor:
- If you have liver, kidney or lung disease.
- If you have diabetes, epilepsy or porphyria.

Over age 60:
Adverse reactions and side effects may be more frequent and severe than in younger persons. You need smaller doses for shorter periods of time. May develop agitation, rage or "hangover" effect.

Pregnancy:
Risk to unborn child outweighs drug benefits. Don't use.

Breast-feeding:
Drug passes into milk. Avoid drug or discontinue nursing until you finish medicine. Consult doctor for advice on maintaining milk supply.

Infants & children:
Use only under medical supervision for children older than 6 months.

Prolonged use:
May impair liver function.

Skin & sunlight:
No problems expected.

Driving, piloting or hazardous work:
Don't drive or pilot aircraft until you learn how medicine affects you. Don't work around dangerous machinery. Don't climb ladders or work in high places. Danger increases if you drink alcohol or take medicine affecting alertness and reflexes.

Discontinuing:
Don't discontinue without consulting doctor. Dose may require gradual reduction if you have taken drug for a long time. Doses of other drugs may also require adjustment.

Others:
- Hot weather, heavy exercise and profuse sweat may reduce excretion and cause overdose.
- Blood sugar may rise in diabetics, requiring insulin adjustment.

POSSIBLE INTERACTION WITH OTHER DRUGS

GENERIC NAME OR DRUG CLASS	COMBINED EFFECT
Antidepressants, tricyclic (TCA)*	Increased sedative effect of both drugs.
Antihistamines*	Increased sedative effect of both drugs.
Antihypertensives*	Excessively low blood pressure.
Contraceptives, oral*	Increased oxazepam effect.
Disulfiram	Increased oxazepam effect.
Dronabinol	Increased effects of both drugs. Avoid.
Levodopa	Possible decreased levodopa effect.
MAO inhibitors*	Convulsions, deep sedation, rage.
Molindone	Increased tranquilizer effect.
Nabilone	Greater depression of central nervous system.
Narcotics*	Increased sedative effect of both drugs.
Probenecid	Increased oxazepam effect.
Sedatives*	Increased sedative effect of both drugs.
Sleep inducers*	Increased sedative effect of both drugs.
Tranquilizers*	Increased sedative effect of both drugs.

POSSIBLE INTERACTION WITH OTHER SUBSTANCES

INTERACTS WITH	COMBINED EFFECT
Alcohol:	Heavy sedation. Avoid.
Beverages:	None expected.
Cocaine:	Decreased oxazepam effect.
Foods:	None expected.
Marijuana:	Heavy sedation. Avoid.
Tobacco:	Decreased oxazepam effect.

*See Glossary

OXPRENOLOL

BRAND NAMES

Slow-trasicor Trasicor

BASIC INFORMATION

Habit forming? No
Prescription needed? Yes
Available as generic? No
Drug class: Beta-adrenergic blocker

USES

- Reduces frequency and severity of angina attacks.
- Stabilizes irregular heartbeat.
- Lowers blood pressure.
- Reduces frequency of migraine headaches. (Does not relieve headache pain.)

DOSAGE & USAGE INFORMATION

How to take:
Tablet, capsule or extended-release tablet—
Swallow with liquid. If you can't swallow whole, crumble tablet or open capsule and take with liquid or food. Don't crush capsule.

When to take:
With meals or immediately after.

If you forget a dose:
Take as soon as you remember. Return to regular schedule, but allow 3 hours between doses.

What drug does:
- Blocks actions of sympathetic nervous system.
- Lowers heart's oxygen requirements.
- Slows nerve impulses through heart.
- Reduces blood-vessel contraction in several major organs and glands.

Time lapse before drug works:
1 to 4 hours.

Continued next column

OVERDOSE

SYMPTOMS:
Weakness, slow or weak pulse, blood-pressure drop, fainting, difficulty breathing, convulsions, cold and sweaty skin.
WHAT TO DO:
- **Dial 0 (operator) or 911 (emergency) for an ambulance or medical help. Then give first aid immediately.**
- **See emergency information on inside covers.**

Don't take with:
Non-prescription drugs or drugs in interaction column without consulting doctor.

POSSIBLE ADVERSE REACTIONS OR SIDE EFFECTS

SYMPTOMS	WHAT TO DO
Life-threatening:	
Congestive heart failure.	Discontinue. Seek emergency treatment.
Common:	
• Pulse slower than 50 beats per minute.	Discontinue. Call doctor right away.
• Drowsiness, fatigue, numbness or tingling of fingers or toes, dizziness, diarrhea, nausea, weakness.	Continue. Call doctor when convenient.
• Dry skin, eyes or mouth; cold hands, feet.	Continue. Tell doctor at next visit.
Infrequent:	
• Hallucinations, nightmares, insomnia, headache, difficult breathing.	Discontinue. Call doctor right away.
• Confusion, reduced alertness, depression.	Continue. Call doctor when convenient.
• Constipation.	Continue. Tell doctor at next visit.
Rare:	
• Rash, sore throat, fever, breathing difficulty.	Discontinue. Call doctor right away.
• Unusual bleeding and bruising; dry, burning eyes; impotence.	Continue. Call doctor when convenient.

WARNINGS & PRECAUTIONS

Don't take if:
- You are allergic to any beta-adrenergic blocker.
- You have asthma.
- You have hay-fever symptoms.
- You have taken MAO inhibitors in past 2 weeks.

Before you start, consult your doctor:
- If you have heart disease or poor circulation to extremities.
- If you have hay fever, asthma, chronic bronchitis or emphysema.
- If you have overactive thyroid function.
- If you have impaired liver or kidney function.
- If you will have surgery within 2 months, including dental surgery, requiring general or spinal anesthesia.
- If you have diabetes or hypoglycemia.

Over age 60:
Adverse reactions and side effects may be more frequent and severe than in younger persons.

Pregnancy:
Risk to unborn child outweighs drug benefits. Don't use.

Breast-feeding:
Drug passes into milk. Avoid drug or discontinue nursing until you finish medicine. Consult doctor for advice on maintaining milk supply.

Infants & children:
Not recommended. Safety and dosage have not been established.

Prolonged use:
Weakens heart-muscle contractions.

Skin & sunlight:
No problems expected.

Driving, piloting or hazardous work:
Don't drive or pilot aircraft until you learn how medicine affects you. Don't work around dangerous machinery. Don't climb ladders or work in high places. Danger increases if you drink alcohol or take medicine affecting alertness and reflexes.

Discontinuing:
Don't discontinue without consulting doctor. Dose may require gradual reduction if you have taken drug for a long time. Doses of other drugs may also require adjustment.

Others:
May mask hypoglycemia.

 ## POSSIBLE INTERACTION WITH OTHER DRUGS

GENERIC NAME OR DRUG CLASS	COMBINED EFFECT
ACE inhibitors: captopril, enalapril, lisinopril*	Increased antihypertensive effects of both drugs. Dosages may require adjustment.
Anesthetics used in surgery	Increased antihypertensive effect.
Antidiabetics*	May make blood-sugar levels difficult to control.
Antihypertensives*	Increased antihypertensive effect.
Beta-agonists*	Decreased beta-agonist effect.
Betaxolol eyedrops	Possible increased oxprenolol effect.
Calcium-channel blockers*	May worsen congestive heart failure.
Clonidine	Possible blood-pressure rise once clonidine is discontinued.
Digitalis preparations*	Increased *or* decreased heart rate. Improves irregular heartbeat.
Diuretics*	Increased antihypertensive effect.
Encainide	Increased effect of toxicity on heart muscle.
Indomethacin	Decreased oxprenolol effect.
Insulin	Hypoglycemic effects may be prolonged.
Ketoprofen	Decreased antihypertensive effect of oxprenolol.
Levobunolol eyedrops	Possible increased oxprenolol effect.
MAO inhibitors*	Possible excessive blood-pressure rise once MAO inhibitor is discontinued.
Molindone	Increased tranquilizer effect.
Nicardipine	Possible irregular heartbeat and congestive heart failure.
Nitrates*	Possible decreased blood pressure.
Non-steroidal anti-inflammatory drugs (NSAIDs)*	Decreased antihypertensive effect of oxprenolol.

Continued page 1094

 ## POSSIBLE INTERACTION WITH OTHER SUBSTANCES

INTERACTS WITH	COMBINED EFFECT
Alcohol:	Excessive blood pressure drop. Avoid.
Beverages:	None expected.
Cocaine:	Irregular heartbeat. Avoid.
Foods:	None expected.
Marijuana:	Daily use—Impaired circulation to hands and feet.
Tobacco:	Possible irregular heartbeat.

*See Glossary

OXTRIPHYLLINE & GUAIFENESIN

BRAND NAMES

Brondecon   Brondelate

BASIC INFORMATION

Habit forming? No
Prescription needed? Yes
Available as generic? No
Drug class: Bronchodilator (xanthine),
  cough/cold preparation

USES

- Treatment for bronchial asthma symptoms.
- Loosens mucus in respiratory passages from allergies and infections.

DOSAGE & USAGE INFORMATION

How to take:
Tablet or elixir—Swallow with liquid. If you can't swallow whole, crumble tablet and take with liquid or food.

When to take:
Most effective taken on empty stomach 1 hour before or 2 hours after eating. However, may take with food to lessen stomach upset.

If you forget a dose:
Take as soon as you remember up to 2 hours late. If more than 2 hours, wait for next scheduled dose (don't double this dose).

What drug does:
- Relaxes and expands bronchial tubes.
- Increases production of watery fluids to thin mucus so it can be coughed out or absorbed.

Time lapse before drug works:
15 to 30 minutes.

Don't take with:
- Any stimulant.
- See Interaction column and consult doctor.

OVERDOSE

SYMPTOMS:
Restlessness, irritability, confusion, delirium, convulsions, rapid pulse, nausea, vomiting, coma.
WHAT TO DO:
- Dial 0 (operator) or 911 (emergency) for an ambulance or medical help. Then give first aid immediately.
- See emergency information on inside covers.

POSSIBLE ADVERSE REACTIONS OR SIDE EFFECTS

SYMPTOMS	WHAT TO DO
Life-threatening:	
Difficult breathing, irregular or fast heartbeat.	Discontinue. Seek emergency treatment.
Common:	
Headache, irritability, nervousness, restlessness, insomnia, nausea, vomiting, abdominal pain, drowsiness.	Continue. Call doctor when convenient.
Infrequent:	
• Hives, rash, red or flushed face, diarrhea.	Discontinue. Call doctor right away.
• Dizziness, lightheadedness, appetite loss.	Continue. Call doctor when convenient.
Rare:	
None expected.	

OXTRIPHYLLINE & GUAIFENESIN

WARNINGS & PRECAUTIONS

Don't take if:
- You are allergic to any cough or cold preparation containing guaifenesin or any bronchodilator.
- You have an active peptic ulcer.

Before you start, consult your doctor:
- If you have had impaired kidney or liver function.
- If you have gastritis, peptic ulcer, high blood pressure or heart disease.
- If you take medication for gout.

Over age 60:
Adverse reactions and side effects may be more frequent and severe than in younger persons. For drug to work, you must drink 8 to 10 glasses of fluid per day.

Pregnancy:
Risk to unborn child outweighs drug benefits. Don't use.

Breast-feeding:
Drug passes into milk. Avoid drug or discontinue nursing until you finish medicine. Consult doctor for advice on maintaining milk supply.

Infants & children:
Use only under medical supervision.

Prolonged use:
Stomach irritation.

Skin & sunlight:
No problems expected.

Driving, piloting or hazardous work:
Avoid if lightheaded or dizzy. Otherwise, no problems expected.

Discontinuing:
May be unnecessary to finish medicine. Follow doctor's instructions.

Others:
No problems expected.

POSSIBLE INTERACTION WITH OTHER DRUGS

GENERIC NAME OR DRUG CLASS	COMBINED EFFECT
Allopurinol	Decreased allopurinol effect.
Anticoagulants*	Possible risk of bleeding.
Ephedrine	Increased effect of both drugs.
Epinephrine	Increased effect of both drugs.
Erythromycin	Increased bronchodilator effect.
Furosemide	Increased furosemide effect.
Lincomycins*	Increased bronchodilator effect.
Lithium	Decreased lithium effect.
Probenecid	Decreased effect of both drugs.
Propranolol	Decreased bronchodilator effect.
Rauwolfia alkaloids*	Rapid heartbeat.
Sulfinpyrazone	Decreased sulfinpyrazone effect.
Troleandomycin	Increased bronchodilator effect.

POSSIBLE INTERACTION WITH OTHER SUBSTANCES

INTERACTS WITH	COMBINED EFFECT
Alcohol:	None expected.
Beverages: Caffeine drinks.	Nervousness and insomnia. You must drink 8 to 10 glasses of fluid per day for drug to work.
Cocaine:	Excess stimulation. Avoid.
Foods:	None expected.
Marijuana:	Slightly increased antiasthmatic effect of bronchodilator.
Tobacco:	Decreased bronchodilator effect and harmful for all conditions requiring bronchodilator treatment. Avoid.

OXYPHENBUTAZONE

BRAND NAMES

Oxalid   Tandearil
Oxybutazone

BASIC INFORMATION

Habit forming? No
Prescription needed? Yes
Available as generic? Yes
Drug class: Anti-inflammatory (non-steroid)

USES

- Treatment for joint pain, stiffness, inflammation and swelling of arthritis and gout.
- Pain reliever.
- Treatment for dysmenorrhea (painful or difficult menstruation).

DOSAGE & USAGE INFORMATION

How to take:
Tablet—Swallow with liquid or food to lessen stomach irritation. If you can't swallow whole, crumble tablet and take with liquid or food.

When to take:
At the same times each day.

If you forget a dose:
Take as soon as you remember up to 2 hours late. If more than 2 hours, wait for next scheduled dose (don't double this dose).

What drug does:
Reduces tissue concentration of prostaglandins (hormones which produce inflammation and pain).

Time lapse before drug works:
Begins in 4 to 24 hours. May require 3 weeks regular use for maximum benefit.

Don't take with:
See Interaction column and consult doctor.

OVERDOSE

SYMPTOMS:
Confusion, agitation, incoherence, convulsions, upper abdominal pain, nausea, vomiting, possible hemorrhage from stomach or intestine, coma.
WHAT TO DO:
- **Dial 0 (operator) or 911 (emergency) for an ambulance or medical help. Then give first aid immediately.**
- **See emergency information on inside covers.**

POSSIBLE ADVERSE REACTIONS OR SIDE EFFECTS

SYMPTOMS	WHAT TO DO
Life-threatening: Hives, rash, intense itching, faintness soon after a dose (anaphylaxis)	Seek emergency emergency treatment.
Common: • Dizziness, stomach upset.	Continue. Call doctor when convenient.
• Headache, swollen feet or legs.	Continue. Tell doctor at next visit.
Infrequent: Depression, drowsiness, ringing in ears, constipation or diarrhea, vomiting.	Continue. Call doctor when convenient.
Rare: • Convulsions; confusion; rash, hives or itchy skin; blurred vision; sore throat, fever, mouth ulcers; black stools; vomiting blood; stomach pain; difficulty breathing; tightness in chest; heartburn; unusual bleeding or bruising; blood in urine.	Discontinue. Call doctor right away.
• Urgent, frequent, painful or difficult urination; fatigue, weakness; weight gain.	Continue. Call doctor when convenient.

WARNINGS & PRECAUTIONS

Don't take if:
- You are allergic to aspirin or any non-steroid, anti-inflammatory drug.
- You have gastritis, peptic ulcer, enteritis, ileitis, ulcerative colitis.
- Patient is younger than 15.

Before you start, consult your doctor:
- If you have epilepsy.
- If you have Parkinson's disease.
- If you have been mentally ill.
- If you have had kidney disease or impaired kidney function, asthma, high blood pressure, heart failure, temporal arthritis, or polymyalgia rheumatica.

Over age 60:
Adverse reactions and side effects may be more frequent and severe than in younger persons.

Pregnancy:
Studies inconclusive on harm to unborn child.
Animal studies show fetal abnormalities. Decide
with your doctor whether drug benefits justify
risk to unborn child.

Breast-feeding:
Drug filters into milk. May harm child. Avoid.

Infants & children:
Not recommended for those younger than 15.
Use only under medical supervision.

Prolonged use:
- Eye damage.
- May cause rare bone-marrow damage,
  jaundice, reduced hearing.
- Periodic blood counts recommended if you
  use a long time.

Skin & sunlight:
No problems expected.

Driving, piloting or hazardous work:
Don't drive or pilot aircraft until you learn how
medicine affects you. Don't work around
dangerous machinery. Don't climb ladders or
work in high places. Danger increases if you
drink alcohol or take medicine affecting alertness
and reflexes, such as antihistamines,
tranquilizers, sedatives, pain medicine, narcotics
and mind-altering drugs.

Discontinuing:
Don't discontinue without consulting doctor.
Dose may require gradual reduction if you have
taken drug for a long time. Doses of other drugs
may also require adjustment.

Others:
No problems expected.

POSSIBLE INTERACTION
WITH OTHER DRUGS

GENERIC NAME OR DRUG CLASS	COMBINED EFFECT
Acebutolol	Decreased antihypertensive effect of acebutolol.
Anticoagulants, oral*	Increased anticoagulant effect.
Antidiabetics, oral*	Increased antidiabetic effect.
Antihypertensives*	May decrease antihypertensive effect.
Aspirin	Possible stomach ulcer.
Barbiturates*	Decreased oxyphenbutazone effect.
Beta-adrenergic blockers*	Decreased antihypertensive effect.

Carteolol	Decreased antihypertensive effect of carteolol.
Chloroquine	Possible skin toxicity.
Cholestyramine	Possible decreased oxyphenbutazone effect.
Colestipol	Possible decreased oxyphenbutazone effect.
Cortisone	Decreased cortisone effect.
Diclofenac	Possible stomach ulcer.
Digitoxin	Decreased digitoxin effect.
Gold compounds*	Possible increased likelihood of kidney damage.
Hydroxychloroquine	Possible skin toxicity.
Insulin	Decreased insulin effect. Dosages may require adjustment.
Ketoprofen	Increased possibility of internal bleeding.
Lisinopril	Decreased lisinopril effect.
Methotrexate	Increased toxicity of both drugs to bone marrow.
Minoxidil	Decreased minoxidil effect.

Continued page 1094

POSSIBLE INTERACTION
WITH OTHER SUBSTANCES

INTERACTS WITH	COMBINED EFFECT
Alcohol:	Possible stomach ulcer or bleeding. May increase sedation.
Beverages:	None expected.
Cocaine:	None expected.
Foods:	None expected.
Marijuana:	Increased pain relief from oxyphenbutazone.
Tobacco:	None expected.

PANCREATIN, PEPSIN, BILE SALTS, HYOSCYAMINE, ATROPINE, SCOPOLAMINE & PHENOBARBITAL

BRAND NAMES

Donnazyme

BASIC INFORMATION

Habit forming? Yes
Prescription needed? Yes
Available as generic? No
Drug class: Digestant, sedative, anticholinergic

USES

- Replaces deficient digestive enzymes.
- Sometimes used to relieve indigestion.

DOSAGE & USAGE INFORMATION

How to take:
Tablet—Swallow with liquid or food to lessen stomach irritation. If you can't swallow whole, crumble tablet and take with food or liquid.

When to take:
With or after meals.

If you forget a dose:
Skip it and resume schedule. Don't double-dose.

What drug does:
Blocks nerve impulses at parasympathetic nerve endings, preventing smooth muscle contraction and gland secretions.

Time lapse before drug works:
30 to 60 minutes.

Don't take with:
- Any medicine that will decrease mental alertness or reflexes, such as alcohol, other mind-altering drugs, cough/cold medicines,

Continued next column

OVERDOSE

SYMPTOMS:
Hallucinations, excitement, irregular heartbeat (too fast or too slow), fainting, collapse, coma.
WHAT TO DO:
- Dial 0 (operator) or 911 (emergency) for an ambulance or medical help. Then give first aid immediately.
- See emergency information on inside covers.

antihistamines, allergy medicine, sedatives, tranquilizers (sleeping pills or "downers") barbiturates, seizure medicine, narcotics, other prescription medicine for pain, muscle relaxants, anesthetics.
- See Interaction column and consult doctor.

POSSIBLE ADVERSE REACTIONS OR SIDE EFFECTS

SYMPTOMS	WHAT TO DO
Life-threatening: None expected.	
Common:	
• Constipation, decreased sweating, headache.	Discontinue. Call doctor right away.
• Drowsiness, dry mouth, frequent urination.	Continue. Call doctor when convenient.
Infrequent:	
• Blurred vision.	Discontinue. Call doctor right away.
• Diminished sex drive, swallowing difficulty, sensitivity to light, insomnia.	Continue. Call doctor when convenient.
Rare:	
• Jaundice; unusual bleeding or bruising; swollen feet and ankles; abdominal pain; sore throat, fever, mouth sores; rash; hives; vomiting; joint pain; eye pain; diarrhea; blood in urine.	Discontinue. Call doctor right away.
• Unusual tiredness.	Continue. Call doctor when convenient.

WARNINGS & PRECAUTIONS

Don't take if:
- You are allergic to any of the drugs in this combination.
- You have trouble with stomach bloating, difficulty emptying your bladder completely, narrow-angle glaucoma, severe ulcerative colitis, porphyria.

Before you start, consult your doctor:
- If you have open-angle glaucoma, angina, chronic bronchitis or asthma, liver disease, hiatal hernia, enlarged prostate, myasthenia gravis, epilepsy, kidney or liver damage, anemia, chronic pain.

PANCREATIN, PEPSIN, BILE SALTS, HYOSCYAMINE, ATROPINE, SCOPOLAMINE & PHENOBARBITAL

- If you will have surgery within 2 months, including dental surgery, requiring general or spinal anesthesia.

Over age 60:
Adverse reactions and side effects may be more frequent and severe than in younger persons

Pregnancy:
Risk to unborn child outweighs drug benefits. Don't use.

Breast-feeding:
Drug passes into milk. Avoid drug or discontinue nursing until you finish medicine. Consult doctor for advice on maintaining milk supply.

Infants & children:
Use only under medical supervision.

Prolonged use:
- Chronic constipation, possible fecal impaction.
- May cause addiction, anemia, chronic intoxication.
- May lower body temperature, making exposure to cold temperatures hazardous.

Skin & sunlight:
May cause rash or intensify sunburn in areas exposed to sun or sunlamp.

Driving, piloting or hazardous work:
Don't drive or pilot aircraft until you learn how medicine affects you. Don't work around dangerous machinery. Don't climb ladders or work in high places. Danger increases if you drink alcohol or take medicine affecting alertness and reflexes, such as antihistamines, tranquilizers, sedatives, pain medicine, narcotics and mind-altering drugs.

Discontinuing:
- May be unnecessary to finish medicine. Follow doctor's instructions.
- If you develop withdrawal symptoms of hallucinations, agitation or sleeplessness after discontinuing, call doctor right away.

Others:
- Potential for abuse.
- Enzyme deficiencies probably better treated with identified separate substances rather than a mixture of components.

 POSSIBLE INTERACTION WITH OTHER DRUGS

GENERIC NAME OR DRUG CLASS	COMBINED EFFECT
Amantadine	Increased atropine effect.
Antacids*	Decreased absorption of scopolamine.
Anticholinergics, other*	Increased anticholinergic effect.
Anticoagulants, oral*	Decreased anticoagulant effect.
Antidepressants, tricyclic (TCA)*	Decreased antidepressant effect. Possible dangerous oversedation.
Antidiabetics, oral*	Increased phenobarbital effect.
Antihistamines*	Increased atropine effect.
Aspirin	Decreased aspirin effect.
Beta-adrenergic blockers*	Decreased effect of beta-adrenergic blocker.
Buclizine	Increased scopolamine effect.
Contraceptives, oral*	Decreased contraceptive effect.
Cortisone drugs*	Decreased cortisone effect.
Digitalis	Possible decreased absorption of digitalis.
Disopyramide	Increased atropine effect.

Continued page 1094

 POSSIBLE INTERACTION WITH OTHER SUBSTANCES

INTERACTS WITH	COMBINED EFFECT
Alcohol:	Possible fatal oversedation. Avoid.
Beverages:	None expected.
Cocaine:	Excessively rapid heartbeat. Avoid.
Foods:	None expected.
Marijuana:	Excessive sedation, drowsiness and dry mouth.
Tobacco:	May increase stomach acidity, decreasing the effectiveness of Donnazyme. Avoid.

*See Glossary

PANCRELIPASE

BRAND NAMES

Cotazym
Cotazym E.C.S.
Cotazym-S
Festal II
Ilozyme

Ku-Zyme HP
Lipancreatin
Pancrease
Viokase

BASIC INFORMATION

Habit forming? No
Prescription needed? Yes
Available as generic? No
Drug class: Enzyme (pancreatic)

USES

- Replaces pancreatic enzyme deficiency caused by surgery or disease.
- Treats fatty stools (steatorrhea).

DOSAGE & USAGE INFORMATION

How to take:
- Tablets, capsules or delayed-release capsules—Swallow whole. Do not take with milk or milk products.
- Powder—Sprinkle on liquid or soft food.

When to take:
Before meals.

If you forget a dose:
Take as soon as you remember up to 2 hours late. If more than 2 hours, wait for next scheduled dose (don't double this dose).

What drug does:
Enhances digestion of proteins, carbohydrates and fats.

Time lapse before drug works:
30 minutes.

Don't take with:
See Interaction column and consult doctor.

OVERDOSE

SYMPTOMS:
Shortness of breath, wheezing, diarrhea.
WHAT TO DO:
Overdose unlikely to threaten life. If person takes much larger amount than prescribed, call doctor, poison-control center or hospital emergency room for instructions.

POSSIBLE ADVERSE REACTIONS OR SIDE EFFECTS

SYMPTOMS	WHAT TO DO
Life-threatening: None expected.	
Common: None expected.	
Infrequent: Diarrhea, asthma.	Discontinue. Call doctor right away.
Rare: • Rash, hives, blood in urine, swollen feet or legs, abdominal cramps.	Discontinue. Call doctor right away.
• Nausea, joint pain.	Continue. Call doctor when convenient.

WARNINGS & PRECAUTIONS

Don't take if:
You are allergic to pancreatin, pancrelipase, or pork.

Before you start, consult your doctor:
If you take any other medicines.

Over age 60:
Adverse reactions and side effects may be more frequent and severe than in younger persons.

Pregnancy:
Risk to unborn child outweighs drug benefits. Don't use.

Breast-feeding:
Drug passes into milk. Avoid drug or discontinue nursing until you finish medicine. Consult doctor for advice on maintaining milk supply.

Infants & children:
Under close medical supervision only.

Prolonged use:
No additional problems expected.

Skin & sunlight:
No problems expected.

Driving, piloting or hazardous work:
No problems expected.

Discontinuing:
Don't discontinue without consulting doctor. Dose may require gradual reduction if you have taken drug for a long time. Doses of other drugs may also require adjustment.

Others:
If you take powder form, avoid inhaling.

POSSIBLE INTERACTION WITH OTHER DRUGS

GENERIC NAME OR DRUG CLASS	COMBINED EFFECT
Calcium carbonate antacids*	Decreased effect of pancrelipase.
H2 receptor antagonists	Possible increased pancrelipase effect.
Magnesium hydroxide antacids*	Decreased effect of pancrelipase.

POSSIBLE INTERACTION WITH OTHER SUBSTANCES

INTERACTS WITH	COMBINED EFFECT
Alcohol:	Unknown.
Beverages: Milk.	Decreased effect of pancrelipase.
Cocaine:	Unknown.
Foods: Ice cream, milk products.	Decreased effect of pancrelipase.
Marijuana:	Decreased absorption of pancrelipase.
Tobacco:	Decreased absorption of pancrelipase.

PANTOTHENIC ACID (Vitamin B-5)

BRAND AND GENERIC NAMES

CALCIUM
  PATOTHENATE
Dexol T.D.

Durasil
Pantholin
PANTOTHENIC
ACID

Ingredients in numerous multiple vitamin-mineral supplements.

BASIC INFORMATION

Habit forming? No
Prescription needed? No
Available as generic? Yes
Drug class: Vitamin supplement

 ## USES

Prevents and treats vitamin B-5 deficiency.

 ## DOSAGE & USAGE INFORMATION

How to take:
Tablet—Swallow with liquid.

When to take:
At the same times each day.

If you forget a dose:
Take as soon as you remember, then resume regular schedule.

What drug does:
Acts as co-enzyme in carbohydrate, protein and fat metabolism.

Time lapse before drug works:
15 to 20 minutes.

Don't take with:
- Levodopa—Small amounts of pantothenic acid will nullify levodopa effect. Carbidopa-levodopa combination not affected by this interaction.
- See Interaction column and consult doctor.

 ## OVERDOSE

SYMPTOMS:
None expected.
WHAT TO DO:
Overdose unlikely to threaten life.

 ## POSSIBLE ADVERSE REACTIONS OR SIDE EFFECTS

SYMPTOMS	WHAT TO DO
Life-threatening: None expected.	
Common: Heartburn.	Discontinue. Seek emergency treatment.
Infrequent: Cramps.	Discontinue Call doctor right away.
Rare: Rash, hives, difficult breathing.	Discontinue. Seek emergency treatment.

PANTOTHENIC ACID (Vitamin B-5)

 ## WARNINGS & PRECAUTIONS

Don't take if:
You are allergic to pantothenic acid.

Before you start, consult your doctor:
If you have hemophilia.

Over age 60:
No problems expected.

Pregnancy:
Don't exceed recommended dose.

Breast-feeding:
Don't exceed recommended dose.

Infants & children:
Don't exceed recommended dose.

Prolonged use:
Large doses for more than 1 month may cause toxicity.

Skin & sunlight:
No problems expected.

Driving, piloting or hazardous work:
No problems expected.

Discontinuing:
No problems expected.

Others:
Regular pantothenic acid supplements are recommended if you take chloramphenicol, cycloserine, ethionamide, hydralazine, immunosuppressants, isoniazid or penicillamine. These decrease pantothenic acid absorption and can cause anemia or tingling and numbness in hands and feet.

 ## POSSIBLE INTERACTION WITH OTHER DRUGS

GENERIC NAME OR DRUG CLASS	COMBINED EFFECT
None expected.	

 ## POSSIBLE INTERACTION WITH OTHER SUBSTANCES

INTERACTS WITH	COMBINED EFFECT
Alcohol:	None expected.
Beverages:	None expected.
Cocaine:	None expected.
Foods:	None expected.
Marijuana:	None expected.
Tobacco:	May decrease pantothenic acid absorption. Decreased pantothenic acid effect.

PAPAVERINE

BRAND NAMES

See complete list of brand names in the *Brand Name Directory*, page 1067.

BASIC INFORMATION

Habit forming? No
Prescription needed? Yes
Available as generic? Yes
Drug class: Vasodilator

 ## USES

May improve poor circulation in the extremities or brain.

 ## DOSAGE & USAGE INFORMATION

How to take:
- Tablet—Swallow with liquid or food to lessen stomach irritation. If you can't swallow whole, crumble tablet and take with liquid or food.
- Extended-release capsules—Swallow whole with liquid.

When to take:
At the same times each day.

If you forget a dose:
Take as soon as you remember up to 2 hours late. If more than 2 hours, wait for next scheduled dose (don't double this dose).

What drug does:
Relaxes and expands blood-vessel walls, allowing better distribution of oxygen and nutrients.

Time lapse before drug works:
30 to 60 minutes.

Don't take with:
- Non-prescription drugs without consulting doctor.
- See Interaction column and consult doctor.

 ## OVERDOSE

SYMPTOMS:
Weakness, fainting, flush, sweating, stupor, irregular heartbeat.
WHAT TO DO:
- **Dial 0 (operator) or 911 (emergency) for an ambulance or medical help. Then give first aid immediately.**
- **See emergency information on inside covers.**

 ## POSSIBLE ADVERSE REACTIONS OR SIDE EFFECTS

SYMPTOMS	WHAT TO DO
Life-threatening:	
None expected.	
Common:	
• Drowsiness, dizziness, headache, flushed face, stomach irritation, indigestion, nausea, mild constipation, low blood pressure causing lethargy or dizziness (especially on change of position).	Continue. Call doctor when convenient.
• Dry mouth, throat.	Continue. Tell doctor at next visit.
Infrequent:	
• Rash, itchy skin, blurred or double vision, weakness, flushing.	Discontinue. Call doctor right away.
• Deep breathing, decreased heartbeat.	Continue. Call doctor when convenient.
Rare:	
Jaundice.	Discontinue. Call doctor right away.

WARNINGS & PRECAUTIONS

Don't take if:
You are allergic to papaverine.

Before you start, consult your doctor:
- If you plan to become pregnant within medication period.
- If you have had a heart attack, heart disease, angina or stroke.
- If you have Parkinson's disease.

Over age 60:
Adverse reactions and side effects may be more frequent and severe than in younger persons.

Pregnancy:
No proven harm to unborn child. Avoid if possible.

Breast-feeding:
Drug filters into milk. May harm child. Avoid.

Infants & children:
Not recommended.

Prolonged use:
No problems expected.

Skin & sunlight:
No problems expected.

Driving, piloting or hazardous work:
Don't drive or pilot aircraft until you learn how medicine affects you. Don't work around dangerous machinery. Don't climb ladders or work in high places. Danger increases if you drink alcohol or take medicine affecting alertness and reflexes, such as antihistamines, tranquilizers, sedatives, pain medicine, narcotics and mind-altering drugs.

Discontinuing:
May be unnecessary to finish medicine. If drug does not help in 1 to 2 weeks, consult doctor about discontinuing.

Others:
- Periodic liver-function tests recommended.
- Internal eye-pressure measurements recommended if you have glaucoma.

POSSIBLE INTERACTION WITH OTHER DRUGS

GENERIC NAME OR DRUG CLASS	COMBINED EFFECT
Levodopa	Decreased levodopa effect.
Narcotics*	Increased sedation.
Pain relievers*	Increased sedation.
Sedatives*	Increased sedation.
Tranquilizers*	Increased sedation.

POSSIBLE INTERACTION WITH OTHER SUBSTANCES

INTERACTS WITH	COMBINED EFFECT
Alcohol:	None expected.
Beverages:	None expected.
Cocaine:	Decreased papaverine effect.
Foods:	None expected.
Marijuana:	None expected.
Tobacco:	Decrease in papaverine's dilation of blood vessels.

PARA-AMINOSALICYLIC ACID (PAS)

BRAND NAMES

Nemasol

Parasal

P.A.S.

P.A.S. Acid

Pasna

Teebacin

BASIC INFORMATION

Habit forming? No
Prescription needed? Yes
Available as generic? No
Drug class: Antitubercular

USES

Treatment for tuberculosis.

DOSAGE & USAGE INFORMATION

How to take:
- Tablet—Swallow with liquid or food to lessen stomach irritation.
- Powder—Dissolve dose in water. Stir well and drink all liquid.

When to take:
At the same times each day.

If you forget a dose:
Take as soon as you remember up to 2 hours late. If more than 2 hours, wait for next scheduled dose (don't double this dose).

What drug does:
- Prevents growth of TB germs.
- Makes TB germs more susceptible to other antituberculosis drugs.

Time lapse before drug works:
6 months.

Don't take with:
See Interaction column and consult doctor.

OVERDOSE

SYMPTOMS:
Nausea, vomiting, diarrhea; rapid breathing; convulsions.
WHAT TO DO:
- Dial 0 (operator) or 911 (emergency) for an ambulance or medical help. Then give first aid immediately.
- See emergency information on inside covers.

POSSIBLE ADVERSE REACTIONS OR SIDE EFFECTS

SYMPTOMS	WHAT TO DO
Life-threatening:	
None expected.	
Common:	
• Painful urination, chills, low back pain. nausea, vomiting.	Discontinue. Call doctor right away.
• Diarrhea or stomach pain.	Continue. Call doctor when convenient.
Infrequent:	
• Confusion, blood in urine.	Discontinue. Call doctor right away.
• Headache; itchy, dry, puffy skin; rash; light sensitivity; sore throat; fever; constipation or vomiting; swelling in front of neck; decreased sex drive in men; fatigue; weakness; thrombocytopenia.	Continue. Call doctor when convenient.
• Menstrual irregularities.	Continue. Tell doctor at next visit.
Rare:	
Jaundice.	Discontinue. Call doctor right away.

PARA-AMINOSALICYLIC ACID (PAS)

 ## WARNINGS & PRECAUTIONS

Don't take if:
- You are allergic to PAS, aspirin or other salicylates.
- Tablets have turned brownish or purplish.

Before you start, consult your doctor:
- If you have ulcers in stomach or duodenum.
- If you have liver or kidney disease.
- If you have epilepsy.
- If you have adrenal insufficiency.
- If you have heart disease or congestive heart failure.
- If you have cancer.
- If you have overactive thyroid.

Over age 60:
Adverse reactions and side effects may be more frequent and severe than in younger persons.

Pregnancy:
Risk to unborn child outweighs drug benefits. Don't use.

Breast-feeding:
No proven problems. Consult doctor.

Infants & children:
Use only under medical supervision.

Prolonged use:
Enlarged thyroid gland and decreased function.

Skin & sunlight:
No problems expected.

Driving, piloting or hazardous work:
No problems expected.

Discontinuing:
No problems expected.

Others:
- Treatment may need to continue for several years or indefinitely.
- Periodic blood tests and liver- and kidney-function studies recommended.

 ## POSSIBLE INTERACTION WITH OTHER DRUGS

GENERIC NAME OR DRUG CLASS	COMBINED EFFECT
Aminobenzoic acid (PABA)	Decreased effect of PAS.
Anticoagulants, oral*	Increased anticoagulant effect.
Anticonvulsants, hydantoin*	Increased anticonvulsant effect.
Aspirin	Stomach irritation.
Barbiturates*	Oversedation.
Folic acid	Decreased effect of folic acid.
Probenecid	Increased PAS effect. Possible toxicity.
Rifampin	Decreased rifampin effect.
Sulfa drugs*	Decreased effect of sulfa drugs.
Sulfinpyrazone	Increased PAS effect. Possible toxicity.
Tetracyclines*	Reduced absorption of PAS. Space doses 3 hours apart.

 ## POSSIBLE INTERACTION WITH OTHER SUBSTANCES

INTERACTS WITH	COMBINED EFFECT
Alcohol:	Possible liver disease.
Beverages:	None expected
Cocaine:	None expected.
Foods:	None expected.
Marijuana:	None expected.
Tobacco:	None expected, but tobacco smoking may slow recovery. Avoid.

*See Glossary

PARAMETHASONE

BRAND NAMES

Haldrone

BASIC INFORMATION

Habit forming? No
Prescription needed? Yes
Available as generic? No
Drug class: Cortisone drug (adrenal corticosteroid)

 ## USES

- Reduces inflammation caused by many different medical problems.
- Treatment for some allergic diseases, blood disorders, kidney diseases, asthma and emphysema.
- Replaces corticosteroid deficiencies.

 ## DOSAGE & USAGE INFORMATION

How to take:
Tablet—Swallow with liquid or food to lessen stomach irritation. If you can't swallow whole, crumble tablet and take with liquid or food.

When to take:
At the same times each day. Take once-a-day or once-every-other-day doses in mornings.

If you forget a dose:
- Several-doses-per-day prescription—Take as soon as you remember up to 2 hours late. If more than 2 hours, wait for next scheduled dose (don't double this dose).
- Once-a-day dose or less—Wait for next dose. Double this dose.

What drug does:
Decreases inflammatory responses.

Time lapse before drug works:
2 to 4 days.

Don't take with:
See Interaction column and consult doctor.

 ## OVERDOSE

SYMPTOMS:
Headache, convulsions, heart failure.
WHAT TO DO:
- Dial 0 (operator) or 911 (emergency) for an ambulance or medical help. Then give first aid immediately.
- Additional emergency information on inside covers.

 ## POSSIBLE ADVERSE REACTIONS OR SIDE EFFECTS

SYMPTOMS	WHAT TO DO
Life-threatening:	
Rash, hives, intense itching, faintness soon after a dose (anaphylaxis).	Seek emergency treatment immediately.
Common:	
Acne, poor wound healing, indigestion, nausea, vomiting, thirst, decreased growth in children.	Continue. Call doctor when convenient.
Infrequent:	
• Black, bloody or tarry stool.	Discontinue. Seek emergency treatment.
• Blurred vision, halos around lights, sore throat, fever, muscle cramps.	Discontinue. Call doctor right away.
• Mood change, fatigue, frequent urination, weight gain, round face, weakness, TB recurrence, irregular menstrual periods, insomnia, restlessness.	Continue. Call doctor when convenient.
Rare:	
• Irregular heartbeat.	Discontinue. Seek emergency treatment.
• Rash, pancreatitis, numbness or tingling in hands or feet, thrombophlebitis, hallucinations, convulsions.	Discontinue. Call doctor right away.

 ## WARNINGS & PRECAUTIONS

Don't take if:
- You are allergic to any cortisone drug.
- You have tuberculosis or fungus infection.
- You have herpes infection of eyes, lips or genitals.

Before you start, consult your doctor:
- If you have had tuberculosis.
- If you have congestive heart failure, diabetes, peptic ulcer, glaucoma, underactive thyroid, high blood pressure, myasthenia gravis.
- If you have blood clots in legs or lungs.

Over age 60:
Adverse reactions and side effects may be more frequent and severe than in younger persons. Likely to aggravate edema, diabetes or ulcers. Likely to cause cataracts and osteoporosis (softening of the bones).

Pregnancy:
Risk to unborn child outweighs drug benefits.
Don't use.

Breast-feeding:
Drug passes into milk. Avoid drug or discontinue nursing until you finish medicine. Consult doctor for advice on maintaining milk supply.

Infants & children:
Use only under medical supervision.

Prolonged use:
- Retards growth in children.
- Possible glaucoma, cataracts, diabetes, fragile bones and thin skin.
- Functional dependence.

Skin & sunlight:
No problems expected.

Driving, piloting or hazardous work:
No problems expected.

Discontinuing:
- Don't discontinue without doctor's advice until you complete prescribed dose, even though symptoms diminish or disappear.
- Drug affects your response to surgery, illness, injury or stress for 2 years after discontinuing. Tell anyone who takes medical care of you within 2 years about drug.

Others:
Avoid immunizations if possible.

POSSIBLE INTERACTION WITH OTHER DRUGS

GENERIC NAME OR DRUG CLASS	COMBINED EFFECT
Amphotericin B	Potassium depletion.
Anticholinergics*	Possible glaucoma.
Anticoagulants, oral*	Decreased anti-coagulant effect.
Anticonvulsants, hydantoin*	Decreased para-methasone effect.
Antidiabetics, oral*	Decreased anti-diabetic effect.
Antihistamines*	Decreased para-methasone effect.
Aspirin	Increased para-methasone effect.
Attenuated virus vaccines*	Possible viral infection.
Barbiturates*	Decreased para-methasone effect. Oversedation.
Chloral hydrate	Decreased para-methasone effect.

Chlorthalidone	Potassium depletion.
Cholestyramine	Decreased para-methasone absorption.
Cholinergics*	Decreased cholinergic effect.
Colestipol	Decreased para-methasone absorption.
Contraceptives, oral*	Increased para-methasone effect.
Digitalis preparations*	Dangerous potassium depletion. Possible digitalis toxicity.
Diuretics, thiazide*	Potassium depletion.
Ephedrine	Decreased para-methasone effect.
Estrogens*	Increased para-methasone effect.
Ethacrynic acid	Potassium depletion.
Furosemide	Potassium depletion.
Glutethimide	Decreased para-methasone effect.
Indapamide	Possible excessive potassium loss, causing dangerous heartbeat irregularity.
Indomethacin	Increased para-methasone effect.
Insulin	Decreased insulin effect.
Isoniazid	Decreased isoniazid effect.

Continued page 1095

POSSIBLE INTERACTION WITH OTHER SUBSTANCES

INTERACTS WITH	COMBINED EFFECT
Alcohol:	Risk of stomach ulcers.
Beverages:	No proven problems.
Cocaine:	Overstimulation. Avoid.
Foods:	No proven problems.
Marijuana:	Decreased immunity.
Tobacco:	Increased para-methasone effect. Possible toxicity.

*See Glossary

PAREGORIC

BRAND NAMES

Brown Mixture	Kaoparin
CM with Paregoric	Opium Tincture
Diban	Parepectolin
Donnagel-PG	Pomalin

BASIC INFORMATION

Habit forming? Yes
Prescription needed? Yes
Available as generic? Yes
Drug class: Narcotic, antidiarrheal

USES

Reduces intestinal cramps and diarrhea.

DOSAGE & USAGE INFORMATION

How to take:
Drops or liquid—Dilute dose in beverage before swallowing.

When to take:
As needed for diarrhea, no more often than every 4 hours.

If you forget a dose:
Take as soon as you remember. Wait 4 hours for next dose.

What drug does:
Anesthetizes surface membranes of intestines and blocks nerve impulses.

Time lapse before drug works:
2 to 6 hours.

Don't take with:
See Interaction column and consult doctor.

OVERDOSE

SYMPTOMS:
Deep sleep; slow breathing; slow pulse; flushed, warm skin; constricted pupils.
WHAT TO DO:
- Dial 0 (operator) or 911 (emergency) for an ambulance or medical help. Then give first aid immediately.
- If patient is unconscious and not breathing, give mouth-to-mouth breathing. If there is no heartbeat, use cardiac massage and mouth-to-mouth breathing (CPR). Don't try to make patient vomit. If you can't get help quickly, take patient to nearest emergency facility.
- See emergency information on inside covers.

POSSIBLE ADVERSE REACTIONS OR SIDE EFFECTS

SYMPTOMS	WHAT TO DO
Life-threatening: None expected.	
Common: Dizziness, flushed face, unusual tiredness, difficult urination.	Continue. Call doctor when convenient.
Infrequent: Severe constipation, abdominal pain, vomiting.	Discontinue. Call doctor right away.
Rare: • Hives, rash, itchy skin, slow heartbeat, irregular breathing.	Discontinue. Call doctor right away.
• Depression.	Continue. Call doctor when convenient.

PAREGORIC

WARNINGS & PRECAUTIONS

Don't take if:
You are allergic to any narcotic.

Before you start, consult your doctor:
If you have impaired liver or kidney function.

Over age 60:
More likely to be drowsy, dizzy, unsteady or constipated.

Pregnancy:
No proven harm to unborn child. Avoid if possible.

Breast-feeding:
Drug filters into milk. May depress infant. Avoid.

Infants & children:
Use only under medical supervision.

Prolonged use:
Causes psychological and physical dependence.

Skin & sunlight:
No problems expected.

Driving, piloting or hazardous work:
Don't drive or pilot aircraft until you learn how medicine affects you. Don't work around dangerous machinery. Don't climb ladders or work in high places. Danger increases if you drink alcohol or take medicine affecting alertness and reflexes, such as antihistamines, tranquilizers, sedatives, pain medicine, narcotics and mind-altering drugs.

Discontinuing:
May be unnecessary to finish medicine. Follow doctor's instructions.

Others:
Great potential for abuse.

POSSIBLE INTERACTION WITH OTHER DRUGS

GENERIC NAME OR DRUG CLASS	COMBINED EFFECT
Analgesics*	Increased analgesic effect.
Antidepressants*	Increased sedation.
Antihistamines*	Increased sedation.
Carteolol	Increased narcotic effect. Dangerous sedation.
Ethinamate	Dangerous increased effects of ethinamate. Avoid combining.
Fluoxetine	Increased depressant effects of both drugs.
Guanfacine	May increase depressant effects of either medicine.
Leucovorin	High alcohol content of leucovorin may cause adverse effects.
Methyprylon	May increase sedative effect to dangerous level. Avoid.
Mind-altering drugs*	Increased sedation.
Nabilone	Greater depression of central nervous system.
Narcotics, other*	Increased narcotic effect.
Phenothiazines*	Increased sedative effect of paregoric.
Sedatives*	Excessive sedation.
Sleep inducers*	Increased effect of sleep inducers.
Sotalol	Increased narcotic effect. Dangerous sedation.
Tranquilizers*	Increased tranquilizer effect.

POSSIBLE INTERACTION WITH OTHER SUBSTANCES

INTERACTS WITH	COMBINED EFFECT
Alcohol:	Increases alcohol's intoxicating effect. Avoid.
Beverages:	None expected.
Cocaine:	None expected.
Foods:	None expected.
Marijuana:	Impairs physical and mental performance.
Tobacco:	None expected.

PARGYLINE & METHYCLOTHIAZIDE

BRAND NAMES

Eutron

BASIC INFORMATION

Habit forming? No
Prescription needed? Yes
Available as generic? No
Drug class: Antihypertensive, MAO inhibitor

USES

- Controls, but doesn't cure, high blood pressure.
- Reduces fluid retention (edema) caused by conditions such as heart disorders and liver disease.

DOSAGE & USAGE INFORMATION

How to take:
Tablet—Swallow with liquid. If you can't swallow whole, crumble tablet and take with liquid or food. Don't exceed dose.

When to take:
At the same times each day.

If you forget a dose:
Take as soon as you remember up to 2 hours late. If more than 2 hours, wait for next scheduled dose (don't double this dose).

What drug does:
- Forces sodium and water excretion, reducing body fluid.
- Relaxes muscle cells of small arteries.
- Reduced body fluid and relaxed arteries lower blood pressure.
- Inhibits nerve transmissions in brain that may cause hypertension.

Time lapse before drug works:
4 to 6 weeks for maximum effect.

Continued next column

OVERDOSE

SYMPTOMS:
Cramps, weakness, drowsiness, weak pulse, restlessness, agitation, fever, convulsions, coma.
WHAT TO DO:
- Dial 0 (operator) or 911 (emergency) for an ambulance or medical help. Then give first aid immediately.
- See emergency information on inside covers.

Don't take with:
- Non-prescription drugs without consulting doctor.
- Non-prescription diet pills, nose drops, medicine for asthma, cough, cold or allergy, or medicine containing caffeine or alcohol.
- See Interaction column and consult doctor.

POSSIBLE ADVERSE REACTIONS OR SIDE EFFECTS

SYMPTOMS	WHAT TO DO
Life-threatening:	
Irregular heartbeat, weak pulse, chest pain, fast heartbeat.	Discontinue. Seek emergency treatment.
Common:	
• Constipation, frequent urination.	Discontinue. Call doctor right away.
• Dry mouth, increased thirst, muscle cramps, muscle pain.	Continue. Call doctor when convenient.
Infrequent:	
• Fainting.	Discontinue. Seek emergency treatment.
• Blurred vision, abdominal pain, nausea, vomiting, swollen feet and ankles, chills.	Discontinue. Call doctor right away.
• Dizziness, headache, mood change, muscle cramps, weakness, tiredness, weight gain or loss, nightmares, shakiness, restlessness.	Continue. Call doctor when convenient.
Rare:	
Sore throat; jaundice; headache; nausea; vomiting; fever; hallucinations; joint pain; rash; hives; sore throat, fever, mouth sores; unusual bruising; stiff or sore neck.	Discontinue. Call doctor right away.

WARNINGS & PRECAUTIONS

Don't take if:
- You are allergic to any MAO inhibitor.
- You are allergic to any thiazide diuretic drug.

Before you start, consult your doctor:
- If you are alcoholic or allergic to any sulfa drug.
- If you have asthma, diabetes, epilepsy, overactive thyroid, schizophrenia, Parkinson's disease, adrenal-gland tumor, gout, liver, pancreas or kidney disorder.
- If you have had a stroke.
- If you will have surgery within 2 months, including dental surgery, requiring general or spinal anesthesia.

Over age 60:
Not recommended.

Pregnancy:
Risk to unborn child outweighs drug benefits. Don't use.

Breast-feeding:
Drug passes into milk. Avoid drug or discontinue nursing until you finish medicine. Consult doctor for advice on maintaining milk supply.

Infants & children:
Not recommended.

Prolonged use:
May be toxic to liver.

Skin & sunlight:
May cause rash or intensify sunburn in areas exposed to sun or sunlamp.

Driving, piloting or hazardous work:
Don't drive or pilot aircraft until you learn how medicine affects you. Don't work around dangerous machinery. Don't climb ladders or work in high places. Danger increases if you drink alcohol or take medicine affecting alertness and reflexes, such as antihistamines, tranquilizers, sedatives, pain medicine, narcotics and mind-altering drugs.

Discontinuing:
- Don't discontinue without doctor's advice until you complete prescribed dose, even though symptoms diminish or disappear.
- Follow precautions regarding foods, drinks and other medicines for 2 weeks after discontinuing.

Others:
- May affect blood-sugar levels in patients with diabetes.
- Hot weather and fever may cause dehydration and drop in blood pressure. Dose may require temporary adjustment. Weigh daily and report any unexpected weight decreases to your doctor.
- May cause rise in uric acid, leading to gout.

POSSIBLE INTERACTION WITH OTHER DRUGS

GENERIC NAME OR DRUG CLASS	COMBINED EFFECT
Allopurinol	Decreased allopurinol effect.
Amphetamines*	Blood-pressure rise to life-threatening level.
Anticholinergics*	Increased anticholinergic effect.
Anticonvulsants*	Changed seizure pattern.
Antidepressants, tricyclic (TCA)*	Blood-pressure rise to life-threatening level. Possible fever, convulsions, delirium.
Antidiabetics, oral and insulin*	Excessively low blood sugar.
Antihistamines*	Increased sedation.
Antihypertensives*	Excessively low blood pressure.
Barbiturates*	Increased methyclothiazide effect.

Continued page 1095

POSSIBLE INTERACTION WITH OTHER SUBSTANCES

INTERACTS WITH	COMBINED EFFECT
Alcohol:	Dangerous blood-pressure drop, increased sedation to dangerous level.
Beverages: Caffeine drinks.	Irregular heartbeat or high blood pressure.
Drinks containing tyramine*	Blood-pressure rise to life-threatening level.
Cocaine:	Overstimulation. Possibly fatal.
Foods: Foods containing tyramine* Licorice.	Blood-pressure rise to life-threatening level. Excessive potassium loss that causes dangerous heart rhythms.
Marijuana:	Overstimulation. May increase blood pressure. Avoid.
Tobacco:	No proven problems.

*See Glossary

PEDICULOSIDES (Topical)

BRAND AND GENERIC NAMES

Barc
Blue
GBH
G-well
Kwell
Kwellada
Kwildane
Licetrol
MALATHION
Prioderm

PYRETHRINS AND
  PIPERONYL
  BUTOXIDE
Pyrinyl
R&C
RID
Scabene
TISIT
TISIT BLue
Triple X
Z-200 Pyrinate

BASIC INFORMATION

Habit forming? No
Prescription needed? Yes
Available as generic? Yes, some
Drug class: Pediculoside, scabicide

USES

- Treats scabies and lice infections of skin or scalp.
- Cream and lotion treats scabies.
- Shampoo treats lice infections.
- Carefully read patient instructions contained in package.

DOSAGE & USAGE INFORMATION

How to use:
- Follow package directions.
- Wear plastic gloves when you apply.
- Bathe before applying.
- Use in well-ventilated room.
- Use care not to apply more than directed.

When to use:
As directed on package.

Continued next column

OVERDOSE

SYMPTOMS:
Rarely (toxic effects from too much absorbed through skin)—Vomiting, muscle cramps, dizziness, seizure, rapid heartbeat.
WHAT TO DO:
- Not for internal use. If child accidentally swallows, call poison-control center.
- Dial 0 (operator) or 911 (emergency) for an ambulance or medical help. Then give first aid immediately.
- See emergency information on inside covers.

If you forget a dose:
Use as soon as you remember.

What drug does:
Becomes absorbed into bodies of lice and scabies organisms, stimulates their central nervous system causing convulsions and death. Does not affect humans in this way.

Time lapse before drug works:
Cream or lotion requires 8 to 12 hours contact with skin.

Don't use with:
Other medicines for scabies or lice.

POSSIBLE ADVERSE REACTIONS OR SIDE EFFECTS

SYMPTOMS	WHAT TO DO
Life-threatening None expected.	
Common None expected.	
Infrequent None expected.	
Rare Skin irritation or rash.	Discontinue. Call doctor right away.

PEDICULOSIDES (Topical)

WARNINGS & PRECAUTIONS

Don't use if:
You are allergic to any medicine with lindane, pyrethrins or piperonyl butoxide.

Before you start, consult your doctor:
- If you are allergic to anything that touches your skin.
- If you are using any other medicines, creams, lotions or oils.

Over age 60:
Adverse reactions and side effects may be more frequent and severe than in younger persons. Ask doctor about smaller doses.

Pregnancy:
Avoid. May be absorbed through skin and harm baby.

Breast-feeding:
Drug filters into milk. May harm child. Avoid if possible.

Infants & children:
More likely to be toxic. Use only under close medical supervision.

Prolonged use:
Not recommended. Avoid.

Skin & sunlight:
No problems expected, but check with doctor.

Driving, piloting or hazardous work:
No problems expected, but check with doctor.

Discontinuing:
No problems expected, but check with doctor.

Others:
- Don't use on open sores or wounds.
- Put on freshly dry cleaned or washed clothing after treatment.
- After treatment, boil all bed sheets, covers and towels before using.
- Store items that can't be washed or cleaned in plastic bags for 2 weeks.
- Avoid inhaling or swallowing.
- Thoroughly clean house.
- Wash combs and hairbrushes in hot soapy water. Don't share with others.

POSSIBLE INTERACTION WITH OTHER DRUGS

GENERIC NAME OR DRUG CLASS	COMBINED EFFECT
None expected.	

POSSIBLE INTERACTION WITH OTHER SUBSTANCES

INTERACTS WITH	COMBINED EFFECT
Alcohol:	None expected.
Beverages:	None expected.
Cocaine:	None expected.
Foods:	None expected.
Marijuana:	None expected.
Tobacco:	None expected.

PEMOLINE

BRAND NAMES

Cylert

BASIC INFORMATION

Habit forming? Yes
Prescription needed? Yes
Available as generic? No
Drug class: Central nervous system
stimulant

 ## USES

- Decreases overactivity and lengthens attention span in hyperactive children.
- Treatment of minimal brain dysfunction.

 ## DOSAGE & USAGE INFORMATION

How to take:
- Tablet—Swallow with liquid or food to lessen stomach irritation. If you can't swallow whole, crumble tablet and take with liquid or food.
- Chewable tablets—Chew well before swallowing.

When to take:
At the same times each day.

If you forget a dose:
Take as soon as you remember up to 2 hours late. If more than 2 hours, wait for next scheduled dose (don't double this dose).

What drug does:
Stimulates brain to improve alertness, concentration and attention span. Calms the hyperactive child.

Continued next column

 ## OVERDOSE

SYMPTOMS:
Rapid heartbeat, hallucinations, fever, confusion, convulsions, coma.
WHAT TO DO:
- Dial 0 (operator) or 911 (emergency) for an ambulance or medical help. Then give first aid immediately.
- If patient is unconscious and not breathing, give mouth-to-mouth breathing. If there is no heartbeat, use cardiac massage and mouth-to-mouth breathing (CPR). Don't try to make patient vomit. If you can't get help quickly, take patient to nearest emergency facility.
- See emergency information on inside covers.

Time lapse before drug works:
- 1 month or more for maximum effect on child.
- 30 minutes to stimulate adults.

Don't take with:
See Interaction column and consult doctor.

 ## POSSIBLE ADVERSE REACTIONS OR SIDE EFFECTS

SYMPTOMS	WHAT TO DO
Life-threatening: None expected.	
Common: Insomnia.	Continue. Call doctor when convenient.
Infrequent: • Irritability, depression dizziness, headache, drowsiness, unusual movement of eyes, rapid heartbeat.	Discontinue. Call doctor right away.
• Rash, unusual movements of tongue, appetite loss, abdominal pain, nausea, weight loss.	Continue. Call doctor when convenient.
Rare: • Seizures.	Discontinue. Seek emergency treatment.
• Abnormal muscular movements, jaundice, hallucinations.	Discontinue. Call doctor right away.

758

WARNINGS & PRECAUTIONS

Don't take if:
You are allergic to pemoline.

Before you start, consult your doctor:
- If you have liver disease.
- If you have kidney disease.
- If patient younger than 6 years.
- If there is marked emotional instability.

Over age 60:
Adverse reactions and side effects may be more frequent and severe than in younger persons.

Pregnancy:
No proven harm to unborn child. Avoid if possible.

Breast-feeding:
No problems expected. Consult doctor.

Infants & children:
Use only under close medical supervision for children 6 or older.

Prolonged use:
Rare possibility of physical growth retardation.

Skin & sunlight:
No problems expected.

Driving, piloting or hazardous work:
Don't drive or pilot aircraft until you learn how medicine affects you. Don't work around dangerous machinery. Don't climb ladders or work in high places. Danger increases if you drink alcohol or take medicine affecting alertness and reflexes, such as antihistamines, tranquilizers, sedatives, pain medicine, narcotics and mind-altering drugs.

Discontinuing:
Don't discontinue without consulting doctor. Dose may require gradual reduction if you have taken drug for a long time. Doses of other drugs may also require adjustment.

Others:
Dose must be carefully adjusted by doctor.

POSSIBLE INTERACTION WITH OTHER DRUGS

GENERIC NAME OR DRUG CLASS	COMBINED EFFECT
Loxapine	May increase toxic effects of both drugs.
Nabilone	Greater depression of central nervous system.

POSSIBLE INTERACTION WITH OTHER SUBSTANCES

INTERACTS WITH	COMBINED EFFECT
Alcohol:	More chance of depression. Avoid.
Beverages: Caffeine drinks.	May raise blood pressure. Avoid.
Cocaine:	Convulsions or excessive nervousness.
Foods:	No problems expected.
Marijuana:	Unknown.
Tobacco:	Unknown.

PENICILLAMINE

BRAND NAMES

Cuprimine	Distamine
Depen	Pendramine

BASIC INFORMATION

Habit forming? No
Prescription needed? Yes
Available as generic? No
Drug class: Chelating agent, antirheumatic, antidote (heavy-metal)

USES

- Treatment for rheumatoid arthritis.
- Prevention of kidney stones.
- Treatment for heavy-metal poisoning.

DOSAGE & USAGE INFORMATION

How to take:
Tablets or capsules—With liquid on an empty stomach 1 hour before or 2 hours after eating.

When to take:
At the same times each day.

If you forget a dose:
- 1 dose a day—Take as soon as you remember up to 12 hours late. If more than 12 hours, wait for next scheduled dose (don't double this dose).
- More than 1 dose a day—Take as soon as you remember up to 2 hours late. If more than 2 hours, wait for next scheduled dose (don't double this dose).

What drug does:
- Combines with heavy metals so kidney can excrete them.
- Combines with cysteine (amino acid found in many foods) to prevent cysteine kidney stones.
- May improve protective function of some white-blood cells against rheumatoid arthritis.

Continued next column

OVERDOSE

SYMPTOMS:
Ulcers, sores, convulsions, coughing up blood, coma.
WHAT TO DO:
- **Dial 0 (operator) or 911 (emergency) for an ambulance or medical help. Then give first aid immediately.**
- **See emergency information on inside covers.**

Time lapse before drug works:
2 to 3 months.

Don't take with:
See Interaction column and consult doctor.

POSSIBLE ADVERSE REACTIONS OR SIDE EFFECTS

SYMPTOMS	WHAT TO DO
Life-threatening: None expected.	
Common: Rash, itchy skin, joint pain, fever, swollen lymph glands, appetite loss, nausea, diarrhea, vomiting, decreased taste.	Discontinue. Call doctor right away.
Infrequent: • Sore throat, fever, unusual bruising, swollen feet or legs, bloody or cloudy urine, weight gain, fatigue, weakness, low blood sugar, joint pain.	Discontinue. Call doctor right away.
• Hair loss.	Continue. Call doctor when convenient.
Rare: • Fever, joint pain, skin rash.	Discontinue. Seek emergency treatment.
• Double or blurred vision; pain; ringing in ears; ulcers, sores, white spots in mouth; difficult breathing; coughing up blood; jaundice.	Discontinue. Call doctor right away.

WARNINGS & PRECAUTIONS

Don't take if:
- You are allergic to penicillamine.
- You have severe anemia.

Before you start, consult your doctor:
- If you have kidney disease.
- If you are allergic to any pencillin antibiotic.

Over age 60:
More likely to damage blood cells and kidneys.

Pregnancy:
Risk to unborn child outweighs drug benefits. Don't use.

Breast-feeding:
Drug filters into milk. May harm child. Avoid.

Infants & children:
Use only under medical supervision.

Prolonged use:
May damage blood cells, kidney, liver.

Skin & sunlight:
No problems expected.

Driving, piloting or hazardous work:
No problems expected.

Discontinuing:
No problems expected.

Others:
Request laboratory studies on blood and urine every 2 weeks. Kidney- and liver-function studies recommended every 6 months.

POSSIBLE INTERACTION WITH OTHER DRUGS

GENERIC NAME OR DRUG CLASS	COMBINED EFFECT
Flecainide	Possible decreased blood-cell production in bone marrow.
Gold compounds*	Damage to blood cells and kidney.
Immuno-suppressants*	Damage to blood cells and kidney.
Iron supplements*	Decreased effect of penicillamine. Wait 2 hours between doses.
Oxyphenbutazone	Damage to blood cells and kidney.
Phenylbutazone	Damage to blood cells and kidney.
Quinine	Damage to blood cells and kidney.
Tocainide	Possible decreased blood-cell production in bone marrow.

POSSIBLE INTERACTION WITH OTHER SUBSTANCES

INTERACTS WITH	COMBINED EFFECT
Alcohol:	Increased side effects of penicillamine.
Beverages:	None expected.
Cocaine:	Increased side effects of penicillamine.
Foods:	Possible decreased penicillamine effect by decreased absorption.
Marijuana:	Increased side effects of penicillamine.
Tobacco:	None expected.

PENICILLIN G

BRAND NAMES

Ayercillin	P-50
Bicillin	Penioral
Bicillin L.A.	Pentids
Crystapen	Permapen
Crysticillin	Pfizerpen
Duracillin	Pfizerpen-AS
Duracillin A.S.	Pfizerpen G
Megacillin	SK-Penicillin G
Novopen-G	Wycillin

BASIC INFORMATION

Habit forming? No
Prescription needed? Yes
Available as generic? Yes
Drug class: Antibiotic (penicillin)

 ## USES

Treatment of bacterial infections that are susceptible to penicillin G.

 ## DOSAGE & USAGE INFORMATION

How to take:
- Tablet—Swallow with liquid on an empty stomach 1 hour before or 2 hours after eating.
- Liquid—Take with cold beverage. Liquid form is perishable and effective for only 7 days at room temperature. Effective for 14 days if stored in refrigerator. Don't freeze.

When to take:
Follow instructions on prescription label or side of package. Doses should be evenly spaced. For example, 4 times a day means every 6 hours.

If you forget a dose:
Take as soon as you remember. Continue regular schedule.

What drug does:
Destroys susceptible bacteria. Does not kill viruses.

Continued next column

 ## OVERDOSE

SYMPTOMS:
Severe diarrhea, nausea or vomiting.
WHAT TO DO:
Overdose unlikely to threaten life. If person takes much larger amount than prescribed, call doctor, poison-control center or hospital emergency room for instructions.

Time lapse before drug works:
May be several days before medicine affects infection.

Don't take with:
See Interaction column and consult doctor.

 ## POSSIBLE ADVERSE REACTIONS OR SIDE EFFECTS

SYMPTOMS	WHAT TO DO
Life-threatening: Hives, rash, intense itching, faintness soon after a dose (anaphylaxis).	Seek emergency treatment immediately.
Common: Dark or discolored tongue.	Continue. Tell doctor at next visit.
Infrequent: Mild nausea, vomiting, diarrhea.	Continue. Call doctor when convenient.
Rare: Unexplained bleeding.	Discontinue. Call doctor right away.

WARNINGS & PRECAUTIONS

Don't take if:
You are allergic to penicillin G, cephalosporin antibiotics, other penicillins. Life-threatening reaction may occur.

Before you start, consult your doctor:
If you are allergic to any substance or drug.

Over age 60:
You may have skin reactions, particularly around genitals and anus.

Pregnancy:
Studies inconclusive on harm to unborn child. Animal studies show fetal abnormalities. Decide with your doctor whether drug benefits justify risk to unborn child.

Breast-feeding:
Drug passes into milk. Child may become sensitive to penicillins and have allergic reactions to penicillin drugs. Avoid penicillin G or discontinue nursing until you finish medicine. Consult doctor for advice on maintaining milk supply.

Infants & children:
No problems expected.

Prolonged use:
You may become more susceptible to infections caused by germs not responsive to penicillin G.

Skin & sunlight:
No problems expected.

Driving, piloting or hazardous work:
Usually not dangerous. Most hazardous reactions likely to occur a few minutes after taking penicillin G.

Discontinuing:
Don't discontinue without doctor's advice until you complete prescribed dose, even though symptoms diminish or disappear.

Others:
Urine sugar test for diabetes may show false positive result.

POSSIBLE INTERACTION WITH OTHER DRUGS

GENERIC NAME OR DRUG CLASS	COMBINED EFFECT
Beta-adrenergic blockers*	Increased chance of anaphylaxis (see emergency information on inside front cover).
Calcium supplements*	Decreased penicillin effect.
Chloramphenicol	Decreased effect of both drugs.
Cholestyramine	May decrease penicillin effect.
Colestipol	May decrease penicillin effect.
Contraceptives, oral*	Possible decreased contraceptive effect.
Erythromycins*	Decreased effect of both drugs.
Paromomycin	Decreased effect of both drugs.
Probenecid	Possible decreased penicillin effect.
Tetracyclines*	Decreased effect of both drugs.
Troleandomycin	Decreased effect of both drugs.

POSSIBLE INTERACTION WITH OTHER SUBSTANCES

INTERACTS WITH	COMBINED EFFECT
Alcohol:	Occasional stomach irritation.
Beverages:	None expected.
Cocaine:	No proven problems.
Foods:	Decreased effect of penicillin G.
Marijuana:	No proven problems.
Tobacco:	None expected.

*See Glossary

PENICILLIN V

BRAND NAMES

Apo-Pen-VK
Beepen-VK
Betapen-VK
Compocillin VK
Ledercillin VK
Nadopen-V
Novapen V
Novopen-VK
Pen-Vee K

Penapar VK
Pfizerpen VK
Robicillin VK
SK-Penicillin VK
Uticillin VK
V-Cillin
V-Cillin K
VC-K
Veetids

BASIC INFORMATION

Habit forming? No
Prescription needed? Yes
Available as generic? Yes
Drug class: Antibiotic (penicillin)

USES

- Treatment of bacterial infections that are susceptible to penicillin V.
- Prevention of streptococcal infections in susceptible persons such as those with heart valves damaged by rheumatic fever.

DOSAGE & USAGE INFORMATION

How to take:
- Tablet—Swallow with liquid on an empty stomach 1 hour before meals or 2 hours after eating.
- Liquid—Take with cold beverage. Liquid form is perishable and effective for only 7 days at room temperature. Effective for 14 days if stored in refrigerator. Don't freeze.

When to take:
Follow instructions on prescription label or side of package. Doses should be evenly spaced. For example, 4 times a day means every 6 hours.

If you forget a dose:
Take as soon as you remember. Continue regular schedule.

Continued next column

OVERDOSE

SYMPTOMS:
Severe diarrhea, nausea or vomiting.
WHAT TO DO:
Overdose unlikely to threaten life. If person takes much larger amount than prescribed, call doctor, poison-control center or hospital emergency room for instructions.

What drug does:
Destroys susceptible bacteria. Does not kill viruses.

Time lapse before drug works:
May be several days before penicillin V affects infection.

Don't take with:
See Interaction column and consult doctor.

 POSSIBLE ADVERSE REACTIONS OR SIDE EFFECTS

SYMPTOMS	WHAT TO DO
Life-threatening: Hives, rash, intense itching, faintness soon after a dose (anaphylaxis).	Seek emergency treatment immediately.
Common: Dark or discolored tongue.	Continue. Tell doctor at next visit.
Infrequent: Mild nausea, vomiting, diarrhea.	Continue. Call doctor when convenient.
Rare: Unexplained bleeding.	Discontinue. Call doctor right away.

WARNINGS & PRECAUTIONS

Don't take if:
You are allergic to penicillin V, cephalosporin antibiotics, other penicillins or penicillamine. Life-threatening reaction may occur.

Before you start, consult your doctor:
If you are allergic to any substance or drug.

Over age 60:
You may have skin reactions, particularly around genitals and anus.

Pregnancy:
Studies inconclusive on danger to unborn child. Decide with your doctor whether drug benefits justify risk to unborn child.

Breast-feeding:
Drug passes into milk. Child may become sensitive to penicillin. Child more likely to have future allergic reactions to penicillin. Avoid penicillin V or discontinue nursing until you finish medicine. Consult doctor for advice on maintaining milk supply.

Infants & children:
No problems expected.

Prolonged use:
You may become more susceptible to infections caused by germs not responsive to penicillin V.

Skin & sunlight:
No problems expected.

Driving, piloting or hazardous work:
Usually not dangerous. Most hazardous reactions likely to occur a few minutes after taking penicillin V.

Discontinuing:
Don't discontinue without doctor's advice until you have finished prescribed dose, even if symptoms diminish or disappear.

Others:
No problems expected.

POSSIBLE INTERACTION WITH OTHER DRUGS

GENERIC NAME OR DRUG CLASS	COMBINED EFFECT
Beta-adrenergic blockers*	Increased chance of anaphylaxis (see emergency information on inside front cover).
Calcium supplements*	Decreased penicillin effect.
Chloramphenicol	Decreased effect of both drugs.
Cholestyramine	May decrease penicillin effect.
Colestipol	May decrease penicillin effect.
Contraceptives, oral*	Possible decreased contraceptive effect.
Erythromycins*	Decreased effect of both drugs.
Paromomycin	Decreased effect of both drugs.
Tetracyclines*	Decreased effect of both drugs.
Troleandomycin	Decreased effect of both drugs.

POSSIBLE INTERACTION WITH OTHER SUBSTANCES

INTERACTS WITH	COMBINED EFFECT
Alcohol:	Occasional stomach irritation.
Beverages:	None expected.
Cocaine:	No proven problems.
Foods:	Decreased effect of penicillin V.
Marijuana:	No proven problems.
Tobacco:	None expected.

PENTOBARBITAL

BRAND NAMES

Carbrital
Nembutal
Nova-Rectal
Novopentobarb

Pentogen
Quless
Wigraine-PB

BASIC INFORMATION

Habit forming? Yes
Prescription needed? Yes
Available as generic? Yes
Drug class: Sedative, hypnotic (barbiturate)

USES

Relieves insomnia (higher bedtime dose).

DOSAGE & USAGE INFORMATION

How to take:
- Capsule or liquid—Swallow with food or liquid to lessen stomach irritation. If you can't swallow whole, open capsule and take with liquid or food.
- Suppositories—Remove wrapper and moisten suppository with water. Gently insert larger end into rectum. Push well into rectum with finger.

When to take:
At the same times each day.

If you forget a dose:
Take as soon as you remember up to 2 hours late. If more than 2 hours, wait for next scheduled dose (don't double this dose).

What drug does:
May partially block nerve impulses at nerve-cell connections.

Time lapse before drug works:
60 minutes.

Don't take with:
- Non-prescription drugs without consulting doctor.
- See Interaction column and consult doctor.

OVERDOSE

SYMPTOMS:
Deep sleep, weak pulse, coma.
WHAT TO DO:
- Dial 0 (operator) or 911 (emergency) for an ambulance or medical help. Then give first aid immediately.
- See emergency information on inside covers.

POSSIBLE ADVERSE REACTIONS OR SIDE EFFECTS

SYMPTOMS	WHAT TO DO
Life-threatening: Hives, rash, intense itching, faintness soon after a dose (anaphylaxis).	Seek emergency treatment immediately.
Common: Dizziness, drowsiness, "hangover" effect.	Continue. Call doctor when convenient.
Infrequent: • Rash or hives; face, lip swelling; swollen eyelids; sore throat, fever.	Discontinue. Call doctor right away.
• Depression, confusion, slurred speech, diarrhea, nausea, vomiting, joint or muscle pain.	Continue. Call doctor when convenient.
Rare: • Agitation, slow heartbeat, difficult breathing, jaundice.	Discontinue. Call doctor right away.
• Unexplained bleeding or bruising.	Continue. Call doctor when convenient.

WARNINGS & PRECAUTIONS

Don't take if:
- You are allergic to any barbiturate.
- You have porphyria.

Before you start, consult your doctor:
- If you have epilepsy.
- If you have kidney or liver damage, asthma, anemia, chronic pain.
- If you will have surgery within 2 months, including dental surgery, requiring general or spinal anesthesia.

Over age 60:
Adverse reactions and side effects may be more frequent and severe than in younger persons. Use small doses.

Pregnancy:
Risk to unborn child outweighs drug benefits. Don't use.

Breast-feeding:
Drug passes into milk. Avoid drug or discontinue nursing until you finish medicine. Consult doctor for advice on maintaining milk supply.

Infants & children:
Use only under doctor's supervision.

Prolonged use:
- May cause addiction, anemia, chronic intoxication.
- May lower body temperature, making exposure to cold temperatures hazardous.

Skin & sunlight:
May cause rash or intensify sunburn in areas exposed to sun or sunlamp.

Driving, piloting or hazardous work:
Don't drive or pilot aircraft until you learn how medicine affects you. Don't work around dangerous machinery. Don't climb ladders or work in high places. Danger increases if you drink alcohol or take medicine affecting alertness and reflexes.

Discontinuing:
May be unnecessary to finish medicine. Follow doctor's instructions. If you develop withdrawal symptoms of hallucinations, agitation or sleeplessness after discontinuing, call doctor right away.

Others:
Great potential for abuse.

POSSIBLE INTERACTION WITH OTHER DRUGS

GENERIC NAME OR DRUG CLASS	COMBINED EFFECT
Anticoagulants, oral*	Decreased anticoagulant effect.
Anticonvulsants*	Changed seizure patterns.
Antidepressants, tricyclics (TCA)*	Decreased antidepressant effect. Possible dangerous oversedation.
Antidiabetics, oral*	Increased pentobarbital effect.
Antihistamines*	Dangerous sedation. Avoid.
Aspirin	Decreased aspirin effect.
Beta-adrenergic blockers*	Decreased effect of beta-blocker.
Carteolol	Increased barbiturate effect. Dangerous sedation.
Contraceptives, oral*	Decreased contraceptive effect.
Cortisone drugs*	Decreased cortisone effect.

Digitoxin	Decreased digitoxin effect.
Disulfiram	Possible increased pentobarbital effect.
Doxycycline	Decreased doxycycline effect.
Dronabinol	Increased effects of both drugs. Avoid.
Estrogens*	Decreased estrogen effect.
Griseofulvin	Decreased griseofulvin effect.
Indapamide	Increased indapamide effect.
MAO inhibitors*	Increased pentobarbital effect.
Metronidazole	Possible decreased metronidazole effect.
Mind-altering drugs*	Dangerous sedation. Avoid.
Molindone	Increased sedative effect.
Nabilone	Greater depression of central nervous system.
Narcotics*	Dangerous sedation. Avoid.
Non-steroidal anti-inflammatory drugs (NSAIDs)*	Decreased anti-inflammatory effect.
Pain relievers*	Dangerous sedation. Avoid.

Continued page 1096

POSSIBLE INTERACTION WITH OTHER SUBSTANCES

INTERACTS WITH	COMBINED EFFECT
Alcohol:	Possible fatal oversedation. Avoid.
Beverages:	None expected.
Cocaine:	Decreased pentobarbital effect.
Foods:	None expected.
Marijuana:	Excessive sedation. Avoid.
Tobacco:	None expected.

PENTOXIFYLLINE

BRAND NAMES

Trental

BASIC INFORMATION

Habit forming? No
Prescription needed? Yes
Available as generic? No
Drug class: Hemorrheologic agent*

 USES

Reduces pain in legs caused by poor circulation.

 DOSAGE & USAGE INFORMATION

How to take:
Extended-release tablets—Swallow whole with water and food.

When to take:
At mealtimes. Taking with food decreases the likelihood of irritating the stomach to cause nausea.

If you forget a dose:
Take as soon as you remember up to 3 hours late. If more than 3 hours, wait for next scheduled dose (don't double this dose).

What drug does:
- Reduces "stickiness" of red blood cells and improves flexibility of the red cells.
- Improves blood flow through blood vessels.

Time lapse before drug works:
1 hour. Several weeks for full effect on circulation.

Don't take with:
- Tobacco or medicines to treat hypertension.
- See Interaction column and consult doctor.

 OVERDOSE

SYMPTOMS:
Drowsiness, flushed face, fainting, nervousness, convulsions, coma.
WHAT TO DO:
- **Dial 0 (operator) or 911 (emergency) for an ambulance or medical help. Then give first aid immediately.**
- **See emergency information on inside covers.**

 POSSIBLE ADVERSE REACTIONS OR SIDE EFFECTS

SYMPTOMS	WHAT TO DO
Life-threatening: Chest pain, irregular heartbeat.	Discontinue. Seek emergency treatment.
Common: None expected.	
Infrequent: • Dizziness, headache, nausea, vomiting, low blood pressure, nose bleed, swollen feet and ankles, viral-like syndrome, nasal congestion, laryngitis, rash, itchy skin, blurred vision.	Discontinue. Call doctor right away.
• Insomnia, nervousness, red eyes.	Continue. Call doctor when convenient.
Rare: None expected.	

WARNINGS & PRECAUTIONS

Don't take if:
You are allergic to pentoxifylline.

Before you start, consult your doctor:
- If you are allergic to caffeine, theophylline, theobromine, aminophyllin, dyphyllin, oxtriphylline, theobromine.
- If you have angina.

Over age 60:
Adverse reactions and side effects may be more frequent and severe than in younger persons. Ask doctor about smaller doses.

Pregnancy:
Safety to unborn child unestablished. Avoid if possible.

Breast-feeding:
No problems expected, but ask doctor.

Infants & children:
Not recommended.

Prolonged use:
No problems expected.

Skin & sunlight:
No problems expected.

Driving, piloting or hazardous work:
Wait to see if drug causes drowsiness or dizziness. If none, no problems expected.

Discontinuing:
No problems expected.

Others:
Don't smoke.

POSSIBLE INTERACTION WITH OTHER DRUGS

GENERIC NAME OR DRUG CLASS	COMBINED EFFECT
Anticoagulants, oral*	Possible decreased effect of anticoagulant.
Antihypertensives* (acebutolol, aiseroxylen, amiloride, atenolol, butmetanide, captopril, chlorothiazide, chlorthalidone, clonidine, cyclothiazide, guanethidine, hydralazine, methyldopa, metoprolol, spironolactone, verapamil, nadolol, oxprenolol, pindolol, propranolol, timolol)	Possible increased effect of hypertensive medication.

POSSIBLE INTERACTION WITH OTHER SUBSTANCES

INTERACTS WITH	COMBINED EFFECT
Alcohol:	Unknown. Best to avoid.
Beverages: Coffee, tea or other caffeine-containing beverages.	May decrease effectiveness of pentoxifylline.
Cocaine:	Reduces pentoxifylline effect.
Foods:	None expected.
Marijuana:	Decreased effect of pentoxifylline.
Tobacco:	Decreased effect of pentoxifylline.

*See Glossary

PERPHENAZINE

BRAND NAMES

Apo-Perphenazine
Etrafon
PMS Levazine

Phenazine
Triavil
Trilafon

BASIC INFORMATION

Habit forming? No
Prescription needed? Yes
Available as generic? No
Drug class: Tranquilizer, antiemetic
(phenothiazine)

USES

- Stops nausea, vomiting, hiccups.
- Reduces anxiety, agitation.

DOSAGE & USAGE INFORMATION

How to take:
- Sustained-released tablet—Swallow with liquid or food to lessen stomach irritation.
- Drops or liquid—Dilute dose in beverage.

When to take:
- Nervous and mental disorders—Take at the same times each day.
- Nausea and vomiting—Take as needed, no more often than every 4 hours.

If you forget a dose:
- Nervous and mental disorders—Take up to 2 hours late. If more than 2 hours, wait for next scheduled dose (don't double this dose).
- Nausea and vomiting—Take as soon as you remember. Wait 4 hours for next dose.

What drug does:
- Suppresses brain's vomiting center.
- Suppresses brain centers that control abnormal emotions and behavior.

Continued next column

OVERDOSE

SYMPTOMS:
Stupor, convulsions, coma.
WHAT TO DO:
- Dial 0 (operator) or 911 (emergency) for an ambulance or medical help. Then give first aid immediately.
- See emergency information on inside covers.

Time lapse before drug works:
- Nausea and vomiting—1 hour or less.
- Nervous and mental disorders—4-6 weeks.

Don't take with:
- Antacid or medicine for diarrhea.
- Non-prescription drug for cough, cold or allergy.
- See Interaction column and consult doctor.

POSSIBLE ADVERSE REACTIONS OR SIDE EFFECTS

SYMPTOMS	WHAT TO DO
Life-threatening:	
Uncontrolled muscle movements of tongue, face and other muscles (neuroleptic malignant syndrome, rare).	Discontinue. Seek emergency treatment.
Common:	
• Muscle spasms of face and neck, unsteady gait.	Discontinue. Seek emergency treatment.
• Restlessness, tremor, drowsiness.	Discontinue. Call doctor right away.
• Decreased sweating, dry mouth, runny nose, constipation.	Continue. Call doctor when convenient.
Infrequent:	
• Fainting.	Discontinue. Seek emergency treatment.
• Rash.	Discontinue. Call doctor right away.
• Difficult urination, diminished sex drive, swollen breasts, menstrual irregularities.	Continue. Call doctor when convenient.
Rare:	
Change in vision, jaundice, sore throat, fever, abdominal pain.	Discontinue. Call doctor right away.

WARNINGS & PRECAUTIONS

Don't take if:
- You are allergic to any phenothiazine.
- You have a blood or bone-marrow disease.

Before you start, consult your doctor:
- If you will have surgery within 2 months, including dental surgery, requiring general or spinal anesthesia.
- If you have asthma, emphysema or other lung disorder, glaucoma, prostate trouble.
- If you take non-prescription ulcer medicine, asthma medicine or amphetamines.

Over age 60:
Adverse reactions and side effects may be more frequent and severe than in younger persons. More likely to develop involuntary movement of jaws, lips, tongue, chewing. Report this to your doctor immediately. Early treatment can help.

Pregnancy:
Risk to unborn child outweighs drug benefits. Don't use.

Breast-feeding:
Drug passes into milk. Avoid drug or discontinue nursing until you finish medicine. Consult doctor for advice on maintaining milk supply.

Infants & children:
Don't give to children younger than 2.

Prolonged use:
May lead to tardive dyskinesia (involuntary movement of jaws, lips, tongue, chewing).

Skin & sunlight:
May cause rash or intensify sunburn in areas exposed to sun or sunlamp. Skin may remain sensitive for 3 months after discontinuing.

Driving, piloting or hazardous work:
Don't drive or pilot aircraft until you learn how medicine affects you. Don't work around dangerous machinery. Don't climb ladders or work in high places. Danger increases if you drink alcohol or take medicine affecting alertness and reflexes.

Discontinuing:
- Nervous and mental disorders—Don't discontinue without doctor's advice until you complete prescribed dose, even though symptoms diminish or disappear.
- Nausea and vomiting—May be unnecessary to finish medicine. Follow doctor's instructions.

Others:
No problems expected.

POSSIBLE INTERACTION WITH OTHER DRUGS

GENERIC NAME OR DRUG CLASS	COMBINED EFFECT
Anticholinergics*	Increased anti-cholinergic effect.
Antidepressants, tricyclic (TCA)*	Increased perphenazine effect.
Antihistamines*	Increased antihistamine effect.
Appetite suppressants*	Decreased suppressant effect.
Dronabinol	Increased effects of both drugs. Avoid.
Guanethidine	Decreased guanethidine effect.
Levodopa	Decreased levodopa effect.
Mind-altering drugs*	Increased effect of mind-altering drugs.
Molindone	Increased tranquilizer effect.
Nabilone	Greater depression of central nervous system.
Narcotics*	Increased narcotic effect.
Phenytoin	Increased phenytoin effect.
Procarbazine	Increased sedation.
Quinidine	Impaired heart function. Dangerous mixture.
Sedatives*	Increased sedation.
Tranquilizers, other*	Increased tranquilizer effect.

POSSIBLE INTERACTION WITH OTHER SUBSTANCES

INTERACTS WITH	COMBINED EFFECT
Alcohol:	Dangerous oversedation.
Beverages:	None expected.
Cocaine:	Decreased perphenazine effect. Avoid.
Foods:	None expected.
Marijuana:	Drowsiness. May increase antinausea effect.
Tobacco:	None expected.

*See Glossary

BRAND NAMES

Etrafon   Triavil
PMS Levazine

BASIC INFORMATION

Habit forming? No
Prescription needed? Yes
Available as generic? Yes
Drug class: Tranquilizer (phenothiazine),
   antidepressant

 ## USES

* Decreases nausea, vomiting, hiccups.
* Gradually relieves, but doesn't cure,
  symptoms of depression, anxiety, agitation.
* Pain relief (sometimes).

 ## DOSAGE & USAGE
INFORMATION

How to take:
Tablet or liquid—Swallow with liquid.

When to take:
At the same time each day.

If you forget a dose:
Bedtime dose—If you forget your once-a-day
bedtime dose, don't take it more than 3 hours
late. If more than 3 hours, wait for next
scheduled dose (don't double this dose).

What drug does:
* Suppresses brain's vomiting center.
* Suppresses brain centers that control
  abnormal emotions and behavior.
* Probably affects part of brain that controls
  messages between nerve cells.

Continued next column

 ## OVERDOSE

SYMPTOMS:
Stupor, convulsions, hallucinations, coma.
WHAT TO DO:
* Dial 0 (operator) or 911 (emergency) for
  an ambulance or medical help. Then give
  first aid immediately.
* If patient is unconscious and not
  breathing, give mouth-to-mouth
  breathing. If there is no heartbeat, use
  cardiac massage and mouth-to-mouth
  breathing (CPR). Don't try to make patient
  vomit. If you can't get help quickly, take
  patient to nearest emergency facility,
* See emergency information on inside
  covers.

Time lapse before drug works:
* Nausea and vomiting—1 hour or less.
* Nervous and mental disorders—4-6 weeks.
* Begins in 1 to 2 weeks. May require 4 to 6
  weeks for maximum benefit.

Don't take with:
* Antacid or medicine for diarrhea.
* Non-prescription drug for cough, cold or
  allergy.
* Non-prescription drugs without consulting
  doctor.
* See Interaction column and consult doctor.

 ## POSSIBLE
ADVERSE REACTIONS
OR SIDE EFFECTS

SYMPTOMS	WHAT TO DO
Life-threatening:	
Seizures; irregular heartbeat; weak pulse; fainting; muscle spasms; uncontrolled muscle movements of tongue, face and other muscles (neuroleptic malignant syndrome, rare).	Discontinue. Seek emergency treatment.
Common:	
• Headache, constipation, nausea, vomiting, irregular heartbeat, drowsiness.	Discontinue. Call doctor right away.
• Insomnia, dry mouth, "sweet tooth," decreased sweating, runny nose, constipation.	Continue. Call doctor when convenient.
Infrequent:	
• Hallucinations, dizziness, tremor, blurred vision, eye pain, vomiting, inflamed tongue, joint pain, back pain, hiccups.	Discontinue. Call doctor right away.
• Frequent urination, diminished sex drive, breast swelling, menstrual irregularities, nasal congestion.	Continue. Call doctor when convenient.
Rare:	
• Rash; itchy skin; jaundice; change in vision; sore throat, fever, mouth sores; abdominal pain; constipation.	Discontinue. Call doctor right away.
• Fatigue, weakness.	Continue. Call doctor when convenient.

WARNINGS & PRECAUTIONS

Don't take if:
- You are allergic to any phenothiazine, tricyclic antidepressant.
- You have a blood or bone-marrow disease, glaucoma, prostate trouble.
- You drink alcohol.
- You have had a heart attack within 6 weeks.
- You have taken MAO inhibitors within 2 weeks.
- Patient is younger than 12.

Before you start, consult your doctor:
- If you have asthma, emphysema or other lung disorder.
- If you have an enlarged prostate, heart disease, high blood pressure, stomach or intestinal problems, overactive thyroid, liver disease.
- If you take non-prescription ulcer medicine, asthma medicine or amphetamines.
- If you will have surgery within 2 months, including dental surgery, requiring general or spinal anesthesia.

Over age 60:
Adverse reactions and side effects may be more frequent and severe than in younger persons. More likely to develop involuntary movement of jaws, lips, tongue, chewing, difficult urination. Report this to your doctor immediately. Early treatment can help.

Pregnancy:
Risk to unborn child outweighs drug benefits. Don't use.

Breast-feeding:
Drug passes into milk. Avoid drug or discontinue nursing until you finish medicine. Consult doctor for advice on maintaining milk supply.

Infants & children:
Don't give to children younger than 12.

Prolonged use:
May lead to tardive dyskinesia (involuntary movement of jaws, lips, tongue, chewing).

Skin & sunlight:
May cause rash or intensify sunburn in areas exposed to sun or sunlamp. Skin may remain sensitive for 3 months after discontinuing.

Driving, piloting or hazardous work:
Don't drive or pilot aircraft until you learn how medicine affects you. Don't work around dangerous machinery. Don't climb ladders or work in high places. Danger increases if you drink alcohol or take medicine affecting alertness and reflexes, such as antihistamines, tranquilizers, sedatives, pain medicine, narcotics and mind-altering drugs.

Discontinuing:
- Nervous and mental disorders—Don't discontinue without doctor's advice until you complete prescribed dose, even though symptoms diminish or disappear.

- Dose may require gradual reduction if you have taken drug for a long time. Doses of other drugs may also require adjustment.

Others:
No problems expected.

POSSIBLE INTERACTION WITH OTHER DRUGS

GENERIC NAME OR DRUG CLASS	COMBINED EFFECT
Anticholinergics*	Increased anticholinergic effect, increased sedation.
Anticoagulants, oral*	Increased anticoagulant effect.
Antihistamines*	Increased antihistamine effect.
Appetite suppressants*	Decreased suppressant effect.
Barbiturates*	Decreased antidepressant effect. Increased sedation.
Cimetidine	Possible increased effect and toxicity of perphenazine and amitriptyline.
Clonidine	Possible decreased clonidine effect.
Dronabinol	Increased effect of both drugs.
Ethchlorvynol	Delirium.

Continued page 1096

POSSIBLE INTERACTION WITH OTHER SUBSTANCES

INTERACTS WITH	COMBINED EFFECT
Alcohol: Beverages or medicines with alcohol.	Excessive intoxication. Avoid.
Beverages: Coffee.	Reduces effectiveness.
Cocaine:	Excessive intoxication. Avoid.
Foods:	None expected.
Marijuana:	Excessive drowsiness. Avoid.
Tobacco:	None expected.

*See Glossary

PHENACETIN

BRAND NAMES

A.P.C. Tablets
Aspirin Compound
  with Codeine
Emprazil
Florinal
P.A.C. Compound
Percodan

Propoxyphene
  Compound 65
Sinubid
SK-65 Compound
Soma Compound
Tabloid APC with
  Codeine

BASIC INFORMATION

Habit forming? No
Prescription needed? Yes
Available as generic? Yes
Drug class: Analgesic, fever reducer

USES

- Relieves pain.
- Reduces fever.

DOSAGE & USAGE INFORMATION

How to take:
- Tablet or capsule—Swallow with liquid or food to lessen stomach irritation. You may chew or crush tablets.
- Extended-release tablets or capsules— Swallow each dose whole with liquid.

When to take:
At the same times each day.

If you forget a dose:
Take as soon as you remember up to 2 hours late. If more than 2 hours, wait for next scheduled dose (don't double this dose).

What drug does:
Reduces level of prostaglandins, a chemical involved in producing inflammation, fever, pain.

Time lapse before drug works:
15 minutes.

Don't take with:
See Interaction column and consult doctor.

OVERDOSE

SYMPTOMS:
Sweating, bloody urine, convulsions, coma.
WHAT TO DO:
- Dial 0 (operator) or 911 (emergency) for an ambulance or medical help. Then give first aid immediately.
- See emergency information on inside covers.

POSSIBLE ADVERSE REACTIONS OR SIDE EFFECTS

SYMPTOMS	WHAT TO DO
Life-threatening: None expected.	
Common: None expected.	
Infrequent:	
• Rash; itchy skin; hives; sore throat, fever, mouth sores.	Discontinue. Call doctor right away.
• Confusion, drowsiness, nausea.	Continue. Call doctor when convenient.
Rare:	
• Black, bloody or tarry stools.	Discontinue. Seek emergency treatment.
• Easy bruising, swollen feet or legs, blood in urine, anemia, blue fingernails, fatigue, weakness.	Discontinue. Call doctor right away.

WARNINGS & PRECAUTIONS

Don't take if:
You are allergic to phenacetin, aspirin or any of the many mixtures which contain either.

Before you start, consult your doctor:
• If you have kidney or liver disease.
• If you have G6PD deficiency.

Over age 60:
Adverse reactions and side effects may be more frequent and severe than in younger persons.

Pregnancy:
May cause anemia in newborn. Avoid if possible.

Breast-feeding:
Drug passes into milk. Avoid drug or discontinue nursing until you finish medicine. Consult doctor for advice on maintaining milk supply.

Infants & children:
Not recommended.

Prolonged use:
Kidney damage. Don't take regularly without medical advice.

Skin & sunlight:
No problems expected.

Driving, piloting or hazardous work:
No problems expected.

Discontinuing:
May be unnecessary to finish medicine. Follow doctor's instructions.

Others:
No problems expected.

POSSIBLE INTERACTION WITH OTHER DRUGS

GENERIC NAME OR DRUG CLASS	COMBINED EFFECT
Phenobarbital	Decreased phenacetin effect.
Zidovudine (AZT)	Increased toxicity of zidovudine.

POSSIBLE INTERACTION WITH OTHER SUBSTANCES

INTERACTS WITH	COMBINED EFFECT
Alcohol:	None expected.
Beverages:	None expected.
Cocaine:	None expected.
Foods:	None expected.
Marijuana:	Increased pain relief.
Tobacco:	None expected.

PHENAZOPYRIDINE

BRAND NAMES

Azo-100
Azodine
Azo-Gantanol
Azo-Gantrisin
Azo-Mandelamine
Azo-Standard
Azotrex
Baridium
Di-Azo

Phen-Azo
Phenazodine
Pyridiate
Pyridium
Pyridium Plus
Pyrodine
Pyronium
Thiosulfil-A
Uroblotic

BASIC INFORMATION

Habit forming? No
Prescription needed? Yes
Available as generic? Yes
Drug class: Analgesic (urinary)

USES

Relieves pain of lower urinary-tract irritation, as in cystitis, urethritis or prostatitis. Relieves symptoms only. Phenazopyridine alone does not cure infections.

DOSAGE & USAGE INFORMATION

How to take:
Tablet—Swallow with liquid or food to lessen stomach irritation.

When to take:
At the same times each day.

If you forget a dose:
Take as soon as you remember up to 2 hours late. If more than 2 hours, wait for next scheduled dose (don't double this dose).

What drug does:
Anesthetizes lower urinary tract. Relieves pain, burning, pressure and urgency to urinate.

Time lapse before drug works:
1 to 2 hours.

Don't take with:
No restrictions.

OVERDOSE

SYMPTOMS:
Shortness of breath, weakness.
WHAT TO DO:
Overdose unlikely to threaten life. If person takes much larger amount than prescribed, call doctor, poison-control center or hospital emergency room for instructions.

POSSIBLE ADVERSE REACTIONS OR SIDE EFFECTS

SYMPTOMS	WHAT TO DO
Life-threatening: None expected.	
Common: Red-orange urine.	No action necessary.
Infrequent: Indigestion, fatigue, weakness.	Continue. Call doctor when convenient.
Rare:	
• Rash, jaundice.	Discontinue. Call doctor right away.
• Headache, anemia.	Continue. Call doctor when convenient.

PHENAZOPYRIDINE

WARNINGS & PRECAUTIONS

Don't take if:
- You have hepatitis.
- You are allergic to any urinary analgesic.

Before you start, consult your doctor:
If you have kidney or liver disease.

Over age 60:
Adverse reactions and side effects may be more frequent and severe than in younger persons.

Pregnancy:
No proven harm to unborn child. Avoid if possible.

Breast-feeding:
No problems expected.

Infants & children:
Not recommended.

Prolonged use:
- Orange or yellow skin.
- Anemia. Occasional blood studies recommended.

Skin & sunlight:
No problems expected.

Driving, piloting or hazardous work:
No problems expected.

Discontinuing:
May be unnecessary to finish medicine. Follow doctor's instructions.

Others:
No problems expected.

POSSIBLE INTERACTION WITH OTHER DRUGS

GENERIC NAME OR DRUG CLASS	COMBINED EFFECT
None expected.	

POSSIBLE INTERACTION WITH OTHER SUBSTANCES

INTERACTS WITH	COMBINED EFFECT
Alcohol:	None expected.
Beverages:	None expected.
Cocaine:	None expected.
Foods:	None expected.
Marijuana:	None expected.
Tobacco:	None expected.

PHENIRAMINE

BRAND NAMES

Citra Capsules
Citra Forte
Dri-Hist No. 2 Meta
  Caps
Dristan Nasal Spray
Flogesic
Inhistor
Poly-Histine D
Robitussin-AC
Ru-Tuss

S-T Forte
Symptrol
Triaminic
Triaminicin
Triaminicol
Tussagesic
Tussaminic
Tussirex Sugar-Free
Ursinus

BASIC INFORMATION

Habit forming? No
Prescription needed?
  High strength: Yes
  Low strength: No
Available as generic? Yes
Drug class: Antihistamine

USES

Reduces allergic symptoms such as hay fever, hives, rash or itching.

DOSAGE & USAGE INFORMATION

How to take:
- Tablet, syrup or capsule—Swallow with liquid or food to lessen stomach irritation.
- Extended-release tablets or capsules— Swallow each dose whole.

When to take:
Varies with form. Follow label directions.

If you forget a dose:
Take as soon as you remember up to 2 hours late. If more than 2 hours, wait for next scheduled dose (don't double this dose).

What drug does:
Blocks action of histamine after an allergic response triggers histamine release in sensitive cells.

Continued next column

OVERDOSE

SYMPTOMS:
Convulsions, red face, hallucinations, coma.
WHAT TO DO:
- **Dial 0 (operator) or 911 (emergency) for an ambulance or medical help. Then give first aid immediately.**
- **See emergency information on inside covers.**

Time lapse before drug works:
30 minutes.

Don't take with:
See Interaction column and consult doctor.

POSSIBLE ADVERSE REACTIONS OR SIDE EFFECTS

SYMPTOMS	WHAT TO DO
Life-threatening: None expected.	
Common: Drowsiness, dizziness, dry mouth, nose, throat, nausea.	Continue. Tell doctor at next visit.
Infrequent: • Change in vision.	Discontinue. Call doctor right away.
• Less tolerance for contact lenses, difficult urination.	Continue. Call doctor when convenient.
• Appetite loss.	Continue. Tell doctor at next visit.
Rare: Nightmares, agitation, irritability, sore throat, fever, rapid heartbeat, unusual bleeding or bruising, fatigue, weakness.	Discontinue. Call doctor right away.

WARNINGS & PRECAUTIONS

Don't take if:
You are allergic to any antihistamine.

Before you start, consult your doctor:
- If you have glaucoma.
- If you have enlarged prostate.
- If you have asthma.
- If you have kidney disease.
- If you have peptic ulcer.
- If you will have surgery within 2 months, including dental surgery, requiring general or spinal anesthesia.

Over age 60:
Don't exceed recommended dose. Adverse reactions and side effects may be more frequent and severe than in younger persons, especially urination difficulty, diminished alertness and other brain and nervous-system symptoms.

Pregnancy:
No proven harm to unborn child. Avoid if possible.

Breast-feeding:
Drug passes into milk. Avoid drug or discontinue nursing until you finish medicine. Consult doctor for advice on maintaining milk supply.

Infants & children:
Not recommended for premature or newborn infants. Otherwise, no problems expected.

Prolonged use:
Avoid. May damage bone-marrow and nerve cells.

Skin & sunlight:
May cause rash or intensify sunburn in areas exposed to sun or sunlamp.

Driving, piloting or hazardous work:
Don't drive or pilot aircraft until you learn how medicine affects you. Don't work around dangerous machinery. Don't climb ladders or work in high places. Danger increases if you drink alcohol or take medicine affecting alertness and reflexes, such as antihistamines, tranquilizers, sedatives, pain medicine, narcotics and mind-altering drugs.

Discontinuing:
No problems expected.

Others:
May mask symptoms of hearing damage from aspirin, other salicylates, cisplatin, paromomycin, vancomycin or anticonvulsants. Consult doctor if you use these.

POSSIBLE INTERACTION WITH OTHER DRUGS

GENERIC NAME OR DRUG CLASS	COMBINED EFFECT
Anticholinergics*	Increased anti-cholinergic effect.
Antidepressants, tricyclic (TCA)*	Increased pheniramine effect.
Antihistamines, other*	Excess sedation. Avoid.
Carteolol	Decreased antihistamine effect.
Dronabinol	Increased effects of both drugs. Avoid.
Hypnotics*	Excess sedation. Avoid.
MAO inhibitors*	Increased pheniramine effect.
Mind-altering drugs*	Excess sedation. Avoid.
Nabilone	Greater depression of central nervous system.
Narcotics*	Excess sedation. Avoid.
Sedatives*	Excess sedation. Avoid.
Sleep inducers*	Excess sedation. Avoid.
Sotalol	Increased antihistamine effect.
Tranquilizers*	Excess sedation. Avoid.

POSSIBLE INTERACTION WITH OTHER SUBSTANCES

INTERACTS WITH	COMBINED EFFECT
Alcohol:	Excess sedation. Avoid.
Beverages: Caffeine drinks.	Less pheniramine sedation.
Cocaine:	Decreased pheniramine effect. Avoid.
Foods:	None expected.
Marijuana:	Excess sedation. Avoid.
Tobacco:	None expected.

PHENOBARBITAL

BRAND NAMES

See complete list of brand names in the *Brand Name Directory,* page 1067.

BASIC INFORMATION

Habit forming? Yes
Prescription needed? Yes
Available as generic? Yes
Drug class: Sedative, hypnotic (barbiturate), anticonvulsant

 USES

- Relieves insomnia (higher bedtime dose).
- Prevents convulsions or seizures, such as epilepsy.

 DOSAGE & USAGE INFORMATION

How to take:
Tablet, liquid or capsule—Swallow with liquid or food to lessen stomach irritation. If you can't swallow whole, crumble tablet or open capsule and take with liquid or food.

When to take:
At the same times each day.

If you forget a dose:
Take as soon as you remember up to 2 hours late. If more than 2 hours, wait for next scheduled dose (don't double this dose).

What drug does:
May partially block nerve impulses at nerve-cell connections.

Time lapse before drug works:
60 minutes.

Don't take with:
- Non-prescription drugs without consulting doctor.
- See Interaction column and consult doctor.

 OVERDOSE

SYMPTOMS:
Deep sleep, weak pulse, coma.
WHAT TO DO:
- **Dial 0 (operator) or 911 (emergency) for an ambulance or medical help. Then give first aid immediately.**
- **See emergency information on inside covers.**

 POSSIBLE ADVERSE REACTIONS OR SIDE EFFECTS

SYMPTOMS	WHAT TO DO
Life-threatening:	
Hives, rash, intense itching, faintness soon after a dose (anaphylaxis).	Seek emergency treatment immediately.
Common:	
Dizziness, drowsiness, "hangover" effect.	Continue. Call doctor when convenient.
Infrequent:	
• Rash or hives, face or lip swelling, swollen eyelids, sore throat, fever.	Discontinue. Call doctor right away.
• Depression, confusion, slurred speech, diarrhea, nausea, vomiting, joint or muscle pain.	Continue. Call doctor when convenient.
Rare:	
• Agitation, slow heartbeat, difficult breathing, jaundice.	Discontinue. Call doctor right away.
• Unexplained bleeding or bruising.	Continue. Call doctor when convenient.

 WARNINGS & PRECAUTIONS

Don't take if:
- You are allergic to any barbiturate.
- You have porphyria.

Before you start, consult your doctor:
- If you have epilepsy, kidney or liver damage, asthma, anemia, chronic pain.
- If you will have surgery within 2 months, including dental surgery, requiring general or spinal anesthesia.

Over age 60:
Adverse reactions and side effects may be more frequent and severe than in younger persons. Use small doses.

Pregnancy:
Risk to unborn child outweighs drug benefits. Don't use.

Breast-feeding:
Drug passes into milk. Avoid drug or discontinue nursing until you finish medicine. Consult doctor for advice on maintaining milk supply.

Infants & children:
Use only under doctor's supervision.

Prolonged use:
- May cause addiction, anemia, chronic intoxication.
- May lower body temperature, making exposure to cold temperatures hazardous.

Skin & sunlight:
May cause rash or intensify sunburn in areas exposed to sun or sunlamp.

Driving, piloting or hazardous work:
Don't drive or pilot aircraft until you learn how medicine affects you. Don't work around dangerous machinery. Don't climb ladders or work in high places. Danger increases if you drink alcohol or take medicine affecting alertness and reflexes.

Discontinuing:
May be unnecessary to finish medicine. Follow doctor's instructions. If you develop withdrawal symptoms of hallucinations, agitation or sleeplessness after discontinuing, call doctor right away.

Others:
Great potential for abuse.

POSSIBLE INTERACTION WITH OTHER DRUGS

GENERIC NAME OR DRUG CLASS	COMBINED EFFECT
Anticoagulants, oral*	Decreased anti-coagulant effect.
Anticonvulsants*	Changed seizure patterns.
Antidepressants, tricyclics (TCA)*	Decreased anti-depressant effect. Possible dangerous oversedation.
Antidiabetics, oral*	Increased phenobarbital effect.
Antihistamines*	Dangerous sedation. Avoid.
Aspirin	Decreased aspirin effect.
Beta-adrenergic blockers*	Decreased effect of beta-adrenergic blocker.
Carteolol	Increased barbiturate effect. Dangerous sedation.
Contraceptives, oral*	Decreased contra-ceptive effect.
Cortisone drugs*	Decreased cortisone effect.
Cyclosporine	Decreased effect of cyclosporine.
Digitoxin	Decreased digitoxin effect.
Disulfiram	Possible increased phenobarbital effect.
Doxycycline	Decreased doxycycline effect.
Dronabinol	Increased effects of both drugs. Avoid.
Estrogens*	Decreased estrogen effect.
Griseofulvin	Decreased griseofulvin effect.
Indapamide	Increased indapamide effect.
Leucovorin (large doses)	May counteract anti-convulsant effect of barbiturate anticonvulsants.
Loxapine	Decreased anti-convulsant effect of all barbiturate anticonvulsants.
MAO inhibitors*	Increased phenobarbital effect.
Metronidazole	Possible decreased metronidazole effect.
Mind-altering drugs*	Dangerous sedation. Avoid.
Molindone	Increased sedative effect.

Continued page 1097

POSSIBLE INTERACTION WITH OTHER SUBSTANCES

INTERACTS WITH	COMBINED EFFECT
Alcohol:	Possible fatal oversedation. Avoid.
Beverages:	None expected.
Cocaine:	Decreased phenobarbital effect.
Foods:	None expected.
Marijuana:	Excessive sedation. Avoid.
Tobacco:	None expected.

PHENOLPHTHALEIN

BRAND NAMES

Agoral	Ex-Lax
Alophen	Ex-Lax Pills
Correctol	Feen-A-Mint Gum
Espotabs	Fructines-Vichy
Evac-Q-Kit	Modane
Evac-Q-Kwik	Phenolax
Evac-U-Gen	Prulet
Evac-U-Lax	Trilax

BASIC INFORMATION

Habit forming? No
Prescription needed? No
Available as generic? No
Drug class: Laxative (stimulant)

USES

Constipation relief.

DOSAGE & USAGE INFORMATION

How to take:
- Tablet or wafer—Swallow with liquid. If you can't swallow whole, chew or crumble and take with liquid or food.
- Liquid—Drink 6 to 8 glasses of water each day, in addition to one taken with each dose.
- Chewable tablets—Chew thoroughly before swallowing.

When to take:
Usually at bedtime with a snack, unless directed otherwise.

If you forget a dose:
Take as soon as you remember.

What drug does:
Acts on smooth muscles of intestine wall to cause vigorous bowel movement.

Time lapse before drug works:
6 to 10 hours.

Continued next column

OVERDOSE

SYMPTOMS:
Vomiting, electrolyte depletion.
WHAT TO DO:
Overdose unlikely to threaten life. If person takes much larger amount than prescribed, call doctor, poison-control center or hospital emergency room for instructions.

Don't take with:
- Don't take within 2 hours of taking another medicine. Laxative interferes with medicine absorption.
- See Interaction column and consult doctor.

POSSIBLE ADVERSE REACTIONS OR SIDE EFFECTS

SYMPTOMS	WHAT TO DO
Life-threatening:	
None expected.	
Common:	
• Rectal irritation.	Continue. Call doctor when convenient.
• Pink to orange urine.	No action necessary.
Infrequent:	
• Dangerous potassium loss.	Discontinue. Call doctor right away.
• Belching, cramps, nausea.	Continue. Call doctor when convenient.
Rare:	
Irritability, confusion, headache, rash, difficult breathing, irregular heartbeat, muscle cramps, unusual tiredness or weakness, burning on urination.	Discontinue. Call doctor right away.

WARNINGS & PRECAUTIONS

Don't take if:
- You have symptoms of appendicitis, inflamed bowel or intestinal blockage.
- You are allergic to a stimulant laxative.
- You have missed a bowel movement for only 1 or 2 days.

Before you start, consult your doctor:
- If you have a colostomy or ileostomy.
- If you have congestive heart disease.
- If you have diabetes.
- If you have high blood pressure.
- If you have a laxative habit.
- If you have rectal bleeding.
- If you take other laxatives.

Over age 60:
Adverse reactions and side effects may be more frequent and severe than in younger persons.

Pregnancy:
Risk to mother and unborn child outweighs drug benefits. Don't use.

Breast-feeding:
Drug passes into milk. Avoid drug or discontinue nursing until you finish medicine. Consult doctor for advice on maintaining milk supply.

Infants & children:
Use only under medical supervision.

Prolonged use:
Don't take for more than 1 week unless under a doctor's supervision. May cause laxative dependence.

Skin & sunlight:
No problems expected.

Driving, piloting or hazardous work:
No problems expected.

Discontinuing:
May be unnecessary to finish medicine. Follow doctor's instructions.

Others:
Don't take to "flush out" your system or as a "tonic."

POSSIBLE INTERACTION WITH OTHER DRUGS

GENERIC NAME OR DRUG CLASS	COMBINED EFFECT
Antacids*	Tablet coating may dissolve too rapidly, irritating stomach or bowel.
Antihypertensives*	May cause dangerous low potassium level.
Digitalis	Increased digitalis toxicity due to decreased serum potassium level.
Diuretics*	May cause dangerous low potassium level.

POSSIBLE INTERACTION WITH OTHER SUBSTANCES

INTERACTS WITH	COMBINED EFFECT
Alcohol:	None expected.
Beverages: Milk.	Tablet coating may dissolve too rapidly, irritating stomach or bowel.
Cocaine:	None expected.
Foods:	None expected.
Marijuana:	None expected.
Tobacco:	None expected.

PHENPROCOUMON

BRAND NAMES

Liquamar   Marcumar

BASIC INFORMATION

Habit forming? No
Prescription needed? Yes
Available as generic? Yes
Drug class: Anticoagulant

 ## USES

Reduces blood clots. Used for abnormal clotting inside blood vessels.

 ## DOSAGE & USAGE INFORMATION

How to take:
Tablet—Swallow with liquid. If you can't swallow whole, crumble tablet and take with liquid or food.

When to take:
At the same time each day, usually afternoon.

If you forget a dose:
Take as soon as you remember up to 12 hours late. If more than 12 hours, wait for next scheduled dose (don't double this dose). Inform your doctor of any missed doses.

What drug does:
Blocks action of vitamin K necessary for blood clotting.

Time lapse before drug works:
36 to 48 hours.

Don't take with:
See Interaction column and consult doctor.

 ## OVERDOSE

SYMPTOMS:
Bloody vomit and bloody or black stools, red urine.
WHAT TO DO:
- **Dial 0 (operator) or 911 (emergency) for an ambulance or medical help. Then give first aid immediately.**
- **See emergency information on inside covers.**

 ## POSSIBLE ADVERSE REACTIONS OR SIDE EFFECTS

SYMPTOMS	WHAT TO DO
Life-threatening: None expected.	
Common: Bloating, gaseousness.	Continue. Tell doctor at next visit.
Infrequent:	
• Black stools or bloody vomit, coughing up blood, necrosis of breast and buttocks.	Discontinue. Seek emergency treatment.
• Rash, hives, itchy skin, blurred vision, sore throat, easy bruising or bleeding, cloudy or red urine, back pain, jaundice, fever, chills, fatigue, weakness.	Discontinue. Call doctor right away.
• Diarrhea, cramps, nausea, vomiting, swollen feet or legs, hair loss.	Continue. Call doctor when convenient.
Rare: Dizziness, headache, mouth sores, change in color of toe.	Discontinue. Call doctor right away.

 ## WARNINGS & PRECAUTIONS

Don't take if:
- You have been allergic to any oral anticoagulant.
- You have a bleeding disorder.
- You have an active peptic ulcer.
- You have ulcerative colitis.

Before you start, consult your doctor:
- If you take any other drugs, including non-prescription drugs.
- If you have high blood pressure.
- If you have heavy or prolonged menstrual periods.
- If you have diabetes.
- If you have a bladder catheter.
- If you have serious liver or kidney disease.
- If you will have surgery within 2 months, including dental surgery, requiring general or spinal anesthesia.

Over age 60:
Adverse reactions and side effects may be more frequent and severe than in younger persons.

Pregnancy:
Risk to unborn child outweighs drug benefits. Don't use.

Breast-feeding:
Drug filters into milk. May harm child. Avoid.

Infants & children:
Use only under doctor's supervision.

Prolonged use:
No problems expected.

Skin & sunlight:
No problems expected.

Driving, piloting or hazardous work:
- Avoid hazardous activities that could cause injury.
- Don't drive if you feel dizzy or have blurred vision.

Discontinuing:
Don't discontinue without consulting doctor. Dose may require gradual reduction if you have taken drug for a long time. Doses of other drugs may also require adjustment.

Others:
- Carry identification to state you take anticoagulants.
- Before taking any new medication or stopping medication, consult your doctor or pharmacist.

POSSIBLE INTERACTION WITH OTHER DRUGS

GENERIC NAME OR DRUG CLASS	COMBINED EFFECT
Acetaminophen	Increased phenprocoumon effect.
Allopurinol	Increased phenprocoumon effect.
Amiodarone	Increased phenprocoumon effect.
Androgens*	Increased phenprocoumon effect.
Antacids* (large doses)	Decreased phenprocoumon effect.
Antibiotics*	Increased phenprocoumon effect.
Anticonvulsants, hydantoin*	Increased effect of both drugs.
Antidepressants, tricyclic (TCA)*	Possible increased phenprocoumon effect.
Antidiabetics, oral*	Increased phenprocoumon effect.
Antihistamines*	Unpredictable increased or decreased anticoagulant effect.

Barbiturates*	Decreased phenprocoumon effect.
Bismuth subsalicylate	Increased risk of bleeding.
Carbamazepine	Decreased phenprocoumon effect.
Chloral hydrate	Increased anticoagulant effect.
Chloramphenicol	Increased phenprocoumon effect.
Chlorpromazine	Decreased phenprocoumon effect.
Cholestyramine	May decrease phenprocoumon effect.
Cimetidine	Increased phenprocoumon effect.
Ciprofloxacin	Possible increased anticoagulant effect.
Clofibrate	Increased phenprocoumon effect.
Contraceptives, oral*	Decreased phenprocoumon effect.
Cortisone drugs*	Unpredictable increased or decreased phenprocoumon effect.
Co-trimoxazole (sulfa/trimethoprim)	Increased anticoagulant effect.
Danazol	Increased phenprocoumon effect.
Diclofenac	Increased risk of bleeding.
Dicloxacillin	Possible decreased phenprocoumon effect.

Continued page 1097

POSSIBLE INTERACTION WITH OTHER SUBSTANCES

INTERACTS WITH	COMBINED EFFECT
Alcohol:	Can increase or decrease effect of anticoagulant. Use with caution.
Beverages:	None expected.
Cocaine:	None expected.
Foods: High in vitamin K such as fish, liver, spinach, cabbage.	May decrease anticoagulant effect.
Marijuana:	None expected.
Tobacco:	None expected.

*See Glossary

PHENSUXIMIDE

BRAND NAMES

Milontin

BASIC INFORMATION

Habit forming? No
Prescription needed? Yes
Available as generic? No
Drug class: Anticonvulsant (succinimide)

 ## USES

Controls seizures in treatment of epilepsy.

 ## DOSAGE & USAGE INFORMATION

How to take:
Capsule—Swallow with liquid or food to lessen stomach irritation.

When to take:
Every day in regularly-spaced doses, according to prescription.

If you forget a dose:
Take as soon as you remember up to 2 hours late. If more than 2 hours, wait for next scheduled dose (don't double this dose).

What drug does:
Depresses nerve transmissions in part of brain that controls muscles.

Time lapse before drug works:
3 hours.

Don't take with:
See Interaction column and consult doctor.

 ## OVERDOSE

SYMPTOMS:
Coma
WHAT TO DO:
- **Dial 0 (operator) or 911 (emergency) for an ambulance or medical help. Then give first aid immediately.**
- **If patient is unconscious and not breathing, give mouth-to-mouth breathing. If there is no heartbeat, use cardiac massage and mouth-to-mouth breathing (CPR). Don't try to make patient vomit. If you can't get help quickly, take patient to nearest emergency facility.**
- **See emergency information on inside covers.**

 ## POSSIBLE ADVERSE REACTIONS OR SIDE EFFECTS

SYMPTOMS	WHAT TO DO
Life-threatening: None expected.	
Common: Nausea, vomiting, stomach cramps, appetite loss, dizziness, drowsiness.	Continue. Call doctor when convenient.
Infrequent: Headache, irritability, mood change, blurred vision.	Continue. Call doctor when convenient.
Rare: • Rash, sore throat, fever, unusual bleeding or bruising, depression, confusion, eye swelling, blood in urine, vaginal bleeding, gum swelling.	Discontinue. Call doctor right away.
• Swollen lymph glands.	Continue. Call doctor when convenient.

WARNINGS & PRECAUTIONS

Don't take if:
You are allergic to any succinimide anticonvulsant.

Before you start, consult your doctor:
- If you plan to become pregnant within medication period.
- If you take other anticonvulsants.
- If you have blood disease.
- If you have kidney or liver disease.

Over age 60:
Adverse reactions and side effects may be more frequent and severe than in younger persons.

Pregnancy:
Risk to unborn child outweighs drug benefits. Don't use.

Breast-feeding:
Drug passes into milk. Avoid drug or discontinue nursing.

Infants & children:
Use only under medical supervision.

Prolonged use:
No problems expected.

Skin & sunlight:
No problems expected.

Driving, piloting or hazardous work:
Don't drive or pilot aircraft until you learn how medicine affects you. Don't work around dangerous machinery. Don't climb ladders or work in high places. Danger increases if you drink alcohol or take medicine affecting alertness and reflexes, such as antihistamines, tranquilizers, sedatives, pain medicine, narcotics and mind-altering drugs.

Discontinuing:
Don't discontinue without doctor's advice until you complete prescribed dose, even though symptoms diminish or disappear.

Others:
- Your response to medicine should be checked regularly by your doctor. Dose and schedule may have to be altered frequently to fit individual needs.
- Periodic blood-cell counts, kidney- and liver-function studies recommended.
- May discolor urine pink to red-brown. No action needed.

POSSIBLE INTERACTION WITH OTHER DRUGS

GENERIC NAME OR DRUG CLASS	COMBINED EFFECT
Anticonvulsants, other*	Increased effect of both drugs.
Antidepressants, tricyclic (TCA)*	May provoke seizures.
Antipsychotics*	May provoke seizures.

POSSIBLE INTERACTION WITH OTHER SUBSTANCES

INTERACTS WITH	COMBINED EFFECT
Alcohol:	May provoke seizures.
Beverages:	None expected.
Cocaine:	May provoke seizures.
Foods:	None expected.
Marijuana:	May provoke seizures.
Tobacco:	None expected.

*See Glossary

PHENYLBUTAZONE

BRAND NAMES

Algoverine
Alka-Butazolidin
Alkabutazone
Alka-phenylbutazone
Apo-Phenylbutazone
Azolid
Buffazone
Butagesic
Butazolidin

Intrabutazone
Malgesic
Nadozone
Neo-Zoline
Novobutazone
Phenbuff
Phenbutazone
Sterazolidin

BASIC INFORMATION

Habit forming? No
Available as generic? Yes
Prescription needed? Yes
Drug class: Anti-inflammatory (non-steroid)

 USES

- Treatment for joint pain, stiffness, inflammation and swelling of arthritis and gout.
- Pain reliever.
- Treatment for dysmenorrhea (painful or difficult menstruation).

 DOSAGE & USAGE INFORMATION

How to take:
Tablet or capsule—Swallow with liquid or food to lessen stomach irritation. If you can't swallow whole, crumble tablet or open capsule and take with liquid or food.

When to take:
At the same times each day.

If you forget a dose:
Take as soon as you remember up to 2 hours late. If more than 2 hours, wait for next scheduled dose (don't double this dose).

Continued next column

 OVERDOSE

SYMPTOMS:
Confusion, agitation, incoherence, convulsions, possible hemorrhage from stomach or intestine, upper abdominal pain, nausea, vomiting, coma.
WHAT TO DO:
- **Dial 0 (operator) or 911 (emergency) for an ambulance or medical help. Then give first aid immediately.**
- **See emergency information on inside covers.**

What drug does:
Reduces tissue concentration of prostaglandins (hormones which produce inflammation and pain).

Time lapse before drug works:
Begins in 4 to 24 hours. May require 3 weeks regular use for maximum benefit.

Don't take with:
See Interaction column and consult doctor.

 POSSIBLE ADVERSE REACTIONS OR SIDE EFFECTS

SYMPTOMS	WHAT TO DO
Life-threatening:	
Hives, rash, intense itching, faintness soon after a dose (anaphylaxis).	Seek emergency treatment immediately.
Common:	
• Dizziness, stomach upset.	Continue. Call doctor when convenient.
• Headache, swollen feet or legs.	Continue. Tell doctor at next visit.
Infrequent:	
Depression, drowsiness, ringing in ears, constipation or diarrhea, vomiting.	Continue. Call doctor when convenient.
Rare:	
• Convulsions; stomach pain; confusion; rash, hives or itchy skin; blurred vision; sore throat, fever, mouth ulcers; black stools; vomiting blood; difficult breathing; tightness in chest; unusual bleeding or bruising; blood in urine, heartburn.	Discontinue. Call doctor right away.
• Frequent, painful or difficult urination; fatigue; weakness; weight gain.	Continue. Call doctor when convenient.

WARNINGS & PRECAUTIONS

Don't take if:
- You are allergic to aspirin or any non-steroid, anti-inflammatory drug.
- You have gastritis, peptic ulcer, enteritis, ileitis, ulcerative colitis.
- Patient is younger than 15.

Before you start, consult your doctor:
- If you have epilepsy.
- If you have Parkinson's disease.
- If you have been mentally ill.
- If you have had kidney disease or impaired kidney function, asthma, high blood pressure, heart failure, temporal arthritis, or polymyalgia rheumatica.

Over age 60:
Adverse reactions and side effects may be more frequent and severe than in younger persons.

Pregnancy:
Studies inconclusive on harm to unborn child. Animal studies show fetal abnormalities. Decide with your doctor whether drug benefits justify risk to unborn child.

Breast-feeding:
Drug filters into milk. May harm child. Avoid.

Infants & children:
Not recommended for those younger than 15. Use only under medical supervision.

Prolonged use:
- Eye damage.
- May cause rare bone-marrow damage, jaundice (yellow skin and eyes), reduced hearing.
- Periodic blood counts recommended if you use a long time.

Skin & sunlight:
No problems expected.

Driving, piloting or hazardous work:
Don't drive or pilot aircraft until you learn how medicine affects you. Don't work around dangerous machinery. Don't climb ladders or work in high places. Danger increases if you drink alcohol or take medicine affecting alertness and reflexes, such as antihistamines, tranquilizers, sedatives, pain medicine, narcotics and mind-altering drugs.

Discontinuing:
Don't discontinue without consulting doctor. Dose may require gradual reduction if you have taken drug for a long time. Doses of other drugs may also require adjustment.

Others:
No problems expected.

POSSIBLE INTERACTION WITH OTHER DRUGS

GENERIC NAME OR DRUG CLASS	COMBINED EFFECT
Acebutolol	Decreased acebutolol effect.
Anticoagulants, oral*	Increased anti-coagulant effect.
Aspirin	Possible stomach ulcer.
Antidiabetics, oral*	Increased antidiabetic effect.
Antihypertensives*	May decrease anti-hypertensive effect.
Barbiturates*	Decreased phenyl-butazone effect.
Beta-adrenergic blockers*	Decreased antihyper-tensive effect.
Carteolol	Decreased anti-hypertensive effect of carteolol.
Cholestyramine	Possible decreased phenylbutazone absorption.
Chloroquine	Possible skin toxicity.
Colestipol	Possible decreased phenylbutazone absorption.
Cortisone	Decreased cortisone effect.

Continued page 1099

POSSIBLE INTERACTION WITH OTHER SUBSTANCES

INTERACTS WITH	COMBINED EFFECT
Alcohol:	Possible stomach ulcer or bleeding. May increase sedation.
Beverages:	None expected.
Cocaine:	None expected.
Foods:	None expected.
Marijuana:	Increased pain relief from phenylbutazone.
Tobacco:	None expected.

PHENYLEPHRINE

BRAND NAMES

See complete list of brand names in the *Brand Name Directory,* page 1067.

BASIC INFORMATION

Habit forming? No
Prescription needed? No
Available as generic? Yes
Drug class: Sympathomimetic

USES

Temporary relief of congestion of nose, sinuses and throat caused by allergies, colds or sinusitis.

DOSAGE & USAGE INFORMATION

How to take:
- Capsule—Swallow with liquid or food to lessen stomach irritation.
- Nasal solution, nasal spray, nasal jelly—Take as directed on package.

When to take:
As needed, no more often than every 4 hours.

If you forget a dose:
Take when you remember. Wait 4 hours for next dose. Never double a dose.

What drug does:
Contracts blood-vessel walls of nose, sinus and throat tissues, enlarging airways.

Time lapse before drug works:
5 to 30 minutes.

Don't take with:
- Non-prescription drugs for asthma, cough, cold, allergy, appetite suppressants, sleeping pills or drugs containing caffeine without consulting doctor.
- See Interaction column and consult doctor.

OVERDOSE

SYMPTOMS:
Headache, heart palpitations, vomiting, blood-pressure rise, slow and forceful pulse.
WHAT TO DO:
- **Dial 0 (operator) or 911 (emergency) for an ambulance or medical help. Then give first aid immediately.**
- **See emergency information on inside covers.**

POSSIBLE ADVERSE REACTIONS OR SIDE EFFECTS

SYMPTOMS	WHAT TO DO
Life-threatening: None expected.	
Common:	
• Fast or pounding heartbeat.	Discontinue. Call doctor right away.
• Headache or dizziness; shakiness; insomnia; burning, dryness, stinging inside nose.	Continue. Call doctor when convenient.
Infrequent: Paleness.	Continue. Call doctor when convenient.
Rare: Unusual sweating.	Discontinue. Call doctor right away.

PHENYLEPHRINE

WARNINGS & PRECAUTIONS

Don't take if:
You are allergic to any sympathomimetic.

Before you start, consult your doctor:
- If you have high blood pressure.
- If you have heart disease.
- If you have diabetes.
- If you have overactive thyroid.
- If you have taken MAO inhibitors in past 2 weeks.

Over age 60:
Adverse reactions and side effects may be more frequent and severe than in younger persons.

Pregnancy:
Risk to unborn child outweighs drug benefits. Don't use.

Breast-feeding:
Drug passes into milk. Avoid drug or discontinue nursing until you finish medicine. Consult doctor for advice on maintaining milk supply.

Infants & children:
Use only under close supervision.

Prolonged use:
- Rebound* congestion and chemical irritation of nasal membranes.
- May cause functional dependence.

Skin & sunlight:
No problems expected.

Driving, piloting or hazardous work:
No problems expected.

Discontinuing:
May be unnecessary to finish medicine. Follow doctor's instructions.

Others:
No problems expected.

POSSIBLE INTERACTION WITH OTHER DRUGS

GENERIC NAME OR DRUG CLASS	COMBINED EFFECT
Amphetamines*	Increased nervousness.
Antiasthmatics*	Nervous stimulation.
Antidepressants, tricyclic (TCA)*	Increased phenylephrine effect.
Antihypertensives*	Decreased antihypertensive effect.
Beta-adrenergic blockers*	Decreased effects of both drugs.
Digitalis	Decreased digitalis effect.
Guanadrel	Decreased effect of both drugs.
MAO inhibitors*	Dangerous blood-pressure rise.
Methyldopa	Possible increased blood pressure.
Nitrates*	Possible decreased effects of both drugs.
Oxprenolol	Decreased effects of both drugs.
Phenothiazines*	Possible increased phenylephrine toxicity. Possible decreased phenylephrine effect.
Rauwolfia	Decreased rauwolfia effect.
Sedatives*	Decreased sedative effect.
Sympathomimetics, other*	Increased stimulant effect.
Tranquilizers*	Decreased tranquilizer effect.

POSSIBLE INTERACTION WITH OTHER SUBSTANCES

INTERACTS WITH	COMBINED EFFECT
Alcohol:	None expected.
Beverages: Caffeine drinks.	Excess brain stimulation.
Cocaine:	Excess brain stimulation.
Foods:	None expected.
Marijuana:	None expected.
Tobacco:	None expected.

PHENYLEPHRINE (Ophthalmic)

BRAND NAMES

Ak-Dilate   Mydfrin
Ak-Nefrin   Neo-Synephrine
Isopto Frin   Prefrin Liquifilm

BASIC INFORMATION

Habit forming? No
Prescription needed? Yes, some strengths
Available as generic? No
Drug class: Mydriatic (dilates pupils),
   decongestant

USES

- High concentration drops—Dilates pupils.
- Low concentration drops (available without prescription)—Relieves minor eye irritations caused by colds, hay fever, dust, wind, swimming, sun, smog, hard contact lenses, eye strain, smoke.

DOSAGE & USAGE INFORMATION

How to use:
Eye drops
- Wash hands.
- Apply pressure to inside corner of eye with middle finger.
- Continue pressure for 1 minute after placing medicine in eye.
- Tilt head backward. Pull lower lid away from eye with index finger of the same hand.
- Drop eye drops into pouch and close eye. Don't blink.
- Keep eyes closed for 1 to 2 minutes.
- Don't touch applicator tip to any surface (including the eye). If you accidentally touch tip, clean with warm soap and water.
- Keep container tightly closed.
- Keep cool, but don't freeze.
- Wash hands immediately after using.

When to use:
As directed on label.

Continued next column

OVERDOSE

SYMPTOMS:
None expected.
WHAT TO DO:
Not intended for internal use. If child accidentally swallows, call poison-control center.

If you forget a dose:
Use as soon as you remember.

What drug does:
Acts on small blood vessels to make them constrict.

Time lapse before drug works:
15 to 90 minutes.

Don't use with:
- Other eye drops or ointment without consulting your eye doctor.
- Antidepressants, guanadrel, guanethidine, maprotiline, pargyline, any MAO inhibitor.

POSSIBLE ADVERSE REACTIONS OR SIDE EFFECTS

SYMPTOMS	WHAT TO DO
Life-threatening None expected, unless you use much more than directed.	Discontinue. Call doctor right away.
Common None expected.	
Infrequent None expected, unless you use much more than directed. If too much is used—Burning or stinging eyes, headache, watery eyes, eye irritation not present before.	Continue. Call doctor when convenient.
Rare None expected, unless you use much more than directed. If too much gets absorbed—Paleness, dizziness, tremor, increased sweating, irregular or fast heartbeat.	Discontinue. Call doctor right away.

792

PHENYLEPHRINE (Ophthalmic)

WARNINGS & PRECAUTIONS

Don't use if:
- You are allergic to phenylephrine.
- You have glaucoma.

Before you start, consult your doctor:
- If you have heart disease with irregular heartbeat, high blood pressure, diabetes.
- If you take antidepressants, guanadrel, guanethidine, maprotiline, pargyline, any MAO inhibitor.

Over age 60:
Adverse reactions and side effects may be more frequent and severe than in younger persons. Ask doctor about smaller doses.

Pregnancy:
Safety to unborn child unestablished. Avoid if possible.

Breast-feeding:
Safety not established.

Infants & children:
Use only under close medical supervision.

Prolonged use:
Avoid if possible.

Skin & sunlight:
Sometimes causes increased sensitivity to sunlight.

Driving, piloting or hazardous work:
No problems expected.

Discontinuing:
No problems expected.

Others:
- Keep cool, but don't freeze.
- Consult doctor if condition doesn't improve in 3 to 4 days.

POSSIBLE INTERACTION WITH OTHER DRUGS

GENERIC NAME OR DRUG CLASS	COMBINED EFFECT
Clinically significant interactions with oral or injected medicines unlikely.	

POSSIBLE INTERACTION WITH OTHER SUBSTANCES

INTERACTS WITH	COMBINED EFFECT
Alcohol:	None expected.
Beverages:	None expected.
Cocaine:	None expected.
Foods:	None expected.
Marijuana:	None expected.
Tobacco:	None expected.

PHENYLPROPANOLAMINE

BRAND NAMES

See complete list of brand names in the *Brand Name Directory*, page 1068.

BASIC INFORMATION

Habit forming? No
Prescription needed?
  High strength: Yes
  Low strength: No
Available as generic? Yes
Drug class: Sympathomimetic

USES

- Relieves bronchial asthma.
- Decreases congestion of breathing passages.
- Suppresses allergic reactions.
- Decreases appetite.

DOSAGE & USAGE INFORMATION

How to take:
- Tablet—Swallow with liquid. You may chew or crush tablet.
- Extended-release capsules—Swallow each dose whole.

When to take:
As needed, no more often than every 4 hours.

If you forget a dose:
Take up to 2 hours late. If more than 2 hours, wait for next dose (don't double this dose).

What drug does:
- Prevents cells from releasing allergy-causing chemicals (histamines).
- Relaxes muscles of bronchial tubes.
- Decreases blood-vessel size and blood flow, thus causing decongestion.

Time lapse before drug works:
30 to 60 minutes.

Continued next column

OVERDOSE

SYMPTOMS:
Severe anxiety, confusion, delirium, muscle tremors, rapid and irregular pulse.
WHAT TO DO:
- **Dial 0 (operator) or 911 (emergency) for an ambulance or medical help. Then give first aid immediately.**
- **See emergency information on inside covers.**

Don't take with:
- Non-prescription drugs for cough, cold, allergy or asthma without consulting doctor.
- See Interaction column and consult doctor.

POSSIBLE ADVERSE REACTIONS OR SIDE EFFECTS

SYMPTOMS	WHAT TO DO
Life-threatening:	
None expected.	
Common:	
Rapid heartbeat.	Discontinue. Call doctor right away.
Nervousness, headache, paleness.	Continue. Call doctor when convenient.
Insomnia.	Continue. Tell doctor at next visit.
Infrequent:	
Irregular heartbeat.	Discontinue. Call doctor right away.
Dizziness, appetite loss, nausea, vomiting, difficult urination.	Continue. Call doctor when convenient.
Rare:	
Tightness in chest.	Discontinue. Call doctor right away.

WARNINGS & PRECAUTIONS

Don't take if:
You are allergic to any sympathomimetic drug.

Before you start, consult your doctor:
- If you have high blood pressure, diabetes, overactive thyroid gland, difficulty urinating.
- If you have taken any MAO inhibitors in past 2 weeks.
- If you have taken digitalis preparations in the last 7 days.
- If you will have surgery within 2 months, including dental surgery, requiring general or spinal anesthesia.

Over age 60:
More likely to develop high blood pressure, heart-rhythm disturbances, angina and to feel drug's stimulant effects.

Pregnancy:
No proven harm to unborn child. Avoid if possible.

Breast-feeding:
Drug passes into milk. Avoid drug or discontinue nursing until you finish medicine. Consult doctor for advice on maintaining milk supply.

Infants & children:
No special problems expected.

Prolonged use:
- Excessive doses—Rare toxic psychosis.
- Men with enlarged prostate gland may have more urination difficulty.

Skin & sunlight:
No known problems.

Driving, piloting or hazardous work:
No restrictions unless you feel dizzy.

Discontinuing:
May be unnecessary to finish medicine. Follow doctor's instructions.

Others:
No problems expected.

POSSIBLE INTERACTION WITH OTHER DRUGS

GENERIC NAME OR DRUG CLASS	COMBINED EFFECT
Anesthetics, general*	Increased phenylpropanolamine effect.
Antidepressants, tricyclic (TCA)*	Increased effect of phenylpropanolamine. Excessive stimulation of heart and blood pressure.
Antihypertensives*	Decreased antihypertensive effect.
Beta-adrenergic blockers*	Decreased effects of both drugs.
Digitalis preparations*	Serious heart-rhythm disturbances.
Epinephrine	Increased epinephrine effect.
Ergot preparations*	Serious blood-pressure rise.
Guanethidine	Decreased effect of both drugs.
Guanadrel	Decreased effect of both drugs.
MAO inhibitors*	Increased phenylpropanolamine effect. Dangerous blood-pressure rise.
Methyldopa	Possible increased blood pressure.
Nitrates*	Possible decreased effects of both drugs.
Phenothiazines*	Possible increased phenylpropanolamine toxicity. Possible decreased phenylpropanolamine effect.
Rauwolfia	Decreased rauwolfia effect.
Sympathomimetics*	Increased phenylpropanolamine effect.
Terazosin	Decreases effectiveness of terazosin.

POSSIBLE INTERACTION WITH OTHER SUBSTANCES

INTERACTS WITH	COMBINED EFFECT
Alcohol:	None expected.
Beverages: Caffeine drinks.	Nervousness or insomnia.
Cocaine:	High risk of heartbeat irregularities and high blood pressure.
Foods:	None expected.
Marijuana:	Rapid heartbeat, possible heart-rhythm disturbance. Avoid.
Tobacco:	None expected.

PHENYLTOLOXAMINE

BRAND NAMES

See complete list of brand names in the *Brand Name Directory*, page 1068.

BASIC INFORMATION

Habit forming? No
Prescription needed? Yes
Available as generic? No
Drug class: Antihistamine

 USES

Relieves symptoms of hay fever, allergic reactions and infections of nose and throat.

 DOSAGE & USAGE INFORMATION

How to take:
- Extended-release tablets or capsules— Swallow each dose whole with liquid.
- Syrup—Take as directed on label.
- Pediatric drops—Dilute dose in beverage before swallowing.

When to take:
As needed, no more often than every 3 hours.

If you forget a dose:
Take as soon as you remember. Wait 3 hours for next dose (don't double this dose).

What drug does:
Blocks histamine action in sensitized tissues.

Time lapse before drug works:
30 minutes.

Don't take with:
- Non-prescription drugs containing alcohol without consulting doctor.
- See Interaction column and consult doctor.

 OVERDOSE

SYMPTOMS:
- **Adults—Drowsiness, confusion, incoordination, unsteadiness, muscle tremors, stupor, coma.**
- **Children—Excitement, hallucinations, overactivity, convulsions.**

WHAT TO DO:
- **Dial 0 (operator) or 911 (emergency) for an ambulance or medical help. Then give first aid immediately.**
- **See emergency information on inside covers.**

 POSSIBLE ADVERSE REACTIONS OR SIDE EFFECTS

SYMPTOMS	WHAT TO DO
Life-threatening: None expected.	
Common: Drowsiness, thick bronchial secretions.	Continue. Tell doctor at next visit.
Infrequent:	
• Stomach upset or pain, rapid heartbeat.	Discontinue. Call doctor right away.
• Confusion; dry mouth, nose, throat; ringing or buzzing in ears; painful or difficult urination, appetite loss.	Continue. Call doctor when convenient.
Rare:	
• Nightmares, agitation, irritability, (especially children), change in vision, sore throat, fever, unusual bleeding or bruising, fatigue, weakness.	Discontinue. Call doctor right away.
• Unusual sweating.	Continue. Call doctor when convenient.

WARNINGS & PRECAUTIONS

Don't take if:
- You are allergic to any antihistamine.
- You have asthma attacks.
- You have glaucoma.
- You have urination difficulty.

Before you start, consult your doctor:
- If you have reacted badly to any antihistamine.
- If you have had peptic ulcer disease.
- If you will have surgery within 2 months, including dental surgery, requiring general or spinal anesthesia.

Over age 60:
Likely to be drowsy, dizzy or lethargic and have impaired thinking, judgment and memory. Increases urination problems from enlarged prostate gland.

Pregnancy:
No proven problems. Consult doctor.

Breast-feeding:
Drug passes into milk. Avoid drug or discontinue nursing until you finish medicine. Consult doctor for advice on maintaining milk supply.

Infants & children:
Use only under medical supervision.

Prolonged use:
No problems expected.

Skin & sunlight:
May cause rash or intensify sunburn in areas exposed to sun or sunlamp.

Driving, piloting or hazardous work:
Don't drive or pilot aircraft until you learn how medicine affects you. Don't work around dangerous machinery. Don't climb ladders or work in high places. Danger increases if you drink alcohol or take medicine affecting alertness and reflexes.

Discontinuing:
May be unnecessary to finish medicine. Follow doctor's instructions.

Others:
No problems expected.

POSSIBLE INTERACTION WITH OTHER DRUGS

GENERIC NAME OR DRUG CLASS	COMBINED EFFECT
Amphetamines*	Decreased effect of phenyltoloxamine, especially drowsiness.
Anticholinergics*	Increased anticholinergic effect.
Anticonvulsants, hydantoin*	Changed pattern of epileptic seizures.
Antidepressants, tricyclic (TCA)*	Increased phenyltoloxamine effect.
Carteolol	Decreased antihistamine effect.
Dronabinol	Increased effects of both drugs. Avoid.
Nabilone	Greater depression of central nervous system.
Narcotics*	Increased sedation.
Pain relievers*	Increased sedation.
Sedatives*	Increased sedation.
Sleep inducers*	Increased sedation.
Sotalol	Increased antihistamine effect.
Tranquilizers*	Increased sedation.

POSSIBLE INTERACTION WITH OTHER SUBSTANCES

INTERACTS WITH	COMBINED EFFECT
Alcohol:	Rapid, excessive sedation. Use caution.
Beverages:	None expected.
Cocaine:	Decreased phenyltoloxamine effect.
Foods:	None expected.
Marijuana:	Excessive sedation.
Tobacco:	None expected.

*See Glossary

PHENYTOIN

BRAND NAMES

Dantoin
Dilantin
Dilantin Infatabs
Dilantin Kapseals
Dilantin-125

Dilantin-30-Pediatric
Di-Phen
Diphenylan
Diphenylhydantoin
Novophenytoin

BASIC INFORMATION

Habit forming? No
Prescription needed? Yes
Available as generic? Yes
Drug class: Anticonvulsant (hydantoin)

USES

- Prevents epileptic seizures.
- Stabilizes irregular heartbeat.

DOSAGE & USAGE INFORMATION

How to take:
- Capsule—Swallow with liquid.
- Chewable tablets—Chew carefully before swallowing.
- Suspension—Shake well before taking with liquid.

When to take:
At the same time each day.

If you forget a dose:
- If drug taken 1 time per day—Take as soon as you remember up to 12 hours late. If more than 12 hours, wait for next scheduled dose (don't double this dose).
- If taken several times per day—Take as soon as possible, then return to regular schedule.

What drug does:
Promotes sodium loss from nerve fibers. This lessens excitability and inhibits spread of nerve impulses.

Continued next column

OVERDOSE

SYMPTOMS:
Jerky eye movements; stagger; slurred speech; imbalance; drowsiness; blood-pressure drop; slow, shallow breathing; coma.
WHAT TO DO:
- Dial 0 (operator) or 911 (emergency) for an ambulance or medical help. Then give first aid immediately.
- See emergency information on inside covers.

Time lapse before drug works:
7 to 10 days continual use.

Don't take with:
See Interaction column and consult doctor.

POSSIBLE ADVERSE REACTIONS OR SIDE EFFECTS

SYMPTOMS	WHAT TO DO
Life-threatening: None expected.	
Common: Enlarged, tender, receding gums with increased likelihood of bleeding; nausea; vomiting; constipation; mild dizziness; sleeplessness.	Continue. Call doctor when convenient.
Infrequent: • Hallucinations, confusion, slurred speech, stagger, rash, change in vision.	Discontinue. Call doctor right away.
• Headache, diarrhea, drowsiness, muscle twitching.	Continue. Call doctor when convenient.
• Increased body and facial hair.	Continue. Tell doctor at next visit.
Rare: Sore throat, fever, stomach pain, unusual bleeding or bruising, swollen lymph glands, jaundice.	Discontinue. Call doctor right away.

WARNINGS & PRECAUTIONS

Don't take if:
You are allergic to any hydantoin anticonvulsant.

Before you start, consult your doctor:
- If you have had impaired liver function or disease.
- If you will have surgery within 2 months, including dental surgery, requiring general or spinal anesthesia.

Over age 60:
Adverse reactions and side effects may be more frequent and severe than in younger persons.

Pregnancy:
Risk to unborn child outweighs drug benefits. Don't use.

Breast-feeding:
Drug passes into milk. Avoid drug or discontinue nursing until you finish medicine. Consult doctor for advice on maintaining milk supply.

Infants & children:
Use only under medical supervision.

Prolonged use:
- Weakened bones.
- Lymph gland enlargement.
- Possible liver damage.
- Numbness and tingling of hands and feet.
- Continual back-and-forth eye movements.
- Bleeding, swollen or tender gums.

Skin & sunlight:
May cause rash or intensify sunburn in areas exposed to sun or sunlamp.

Driving, piloting or hazardous work:
Don't drive or pilot aircraft until you learn how medicine affects you. Don't work around dangerous machinery. Don't climb ladders or work in high places. Danger increases if you drink alcohol or take medicine affecting alertness and reflexes.

Discontinuing:
Don't discontinue without consulting doctor. Dose may require gradual reduction if you have taken drug for a long time. Doses of other drugs may also require adjustment.

Others:
No problems expected.

POSSIBLE INTERACTION WITH OTHER DRUGS

GENERIC NAME OR DRUG CLASS	COMBINED EFFECT
Anticoagulants*	Increased effect of anticoagulant.
Antidepressants, tricyclic (TCA)*	Decreased phenytoin effect. Phenytoin dose requires adjustment.
Barbiturates*	Changed seizure pattern.
Carbamazepine	Possible increased phenytoin metabolism.
Carbonic anhydrase inhibitors*	Increased chance of bone disease.
Carteolol	Decreased carteolol effect.
Chloramphenicol	Increased phenytoin effect.
Cimetidine	Increased phenytoin toxicity.
Contraceptives, oral*	Increased seizures. Menstrual irregularities.
Cortisone drugs*	Decreased cortisone effect.
Cyclosporine	May decrease cyclosporine effect.
Digitalis preparations*	Decreased digitalis effect.
Disopyramide	Decreased disopyramide effect.
Disulfiram	Increased phenytoin effect.

Continued page 1099

POSSIBLE INTERACTION WITH OTHER SUBSTANCES

INTERACTS WITH	COMBINED EFFECT
Alcohol:	Possible decreased anticonvulsant effect. Use with caution.
Beverages:	None expected.
Cocaine:	Possible seizures.
Foods:	None expected.
Marijuana:	Drowsiness, unsteadiness, decreased anticonvulsant effect.
Tobacco:	None expected.

PILOCARPINE

BRAND NAMES

Adsorbocarpine
Akarpine
Almocarpine
I-Pilopine
Isopto Carpine
Minims
Minims Pilocarpine
Miocarpine
Nova-Carpine
Ocusert Pilo

Pilocar
Pilocel
Pilokair
Pilomiotin
Pilopine HS
Piloptic
P.V. Carpine
P.V. Carpine
  Liquifilm

BASIC INFORMATION

Habit forming? No
Prescription needed?
  U.S.: Yes
  Canada: No
Available as generic? Yes
Drug class: Antiglaucoma

USES

Treatment for glaucoma.

DOSAGE & USAGE INFORMATION

How to take:
- Drops—Apply to eyes. Close eyes for 1 or 2 minutes to absorb medicine.
- Eye system—Follow label directions.
- Gel—Follow label directions.

When to take:
As directed on label.

Continued next column

OVERDOSE

SYMPTOMS:
If swallowed—Nausea, vomiting, diarrhea, forceful urination, profuse sweating, rapid pulse, breathing difficulty, loss of consciousness.
WHAT TO DO:
- Dial 0 (operator) or 911 (emergency) for an ambulance or medical help. Then give first aid immediately.
- If patient is unconscious and not breathing, give mouth-to-mouth breathing. If there is no heartbeat, use cardiac massage and mouth-to-mouth breathing (CPR). Don't try to make patient vomit. If you can't get help quickly, take patient to nearest emergency facility.
- See emergency information on inside covers.

If you forget a dose:
Apply as soon as possible and return to prescribed schedule. Don't double dose.

What drug does:
Reduces internal-eye pressure.

Time lapse before drug works:
15 to 30 minutes.

Don't take with:
See Interaction column and consult doctor.

POSSIBLE ADVERSE REACTIONS OR SIDE EFFECTS

SYMPTOMS	WHAT TO DO
Life-threatening: None expected.	
Common: Pain, blurred or altered vision.	Continue. Call doctor when convenient.
Infrequent: • Headache, eye irritation or twitching, nausea, vomiting, diarrhea, difficult breathing, muscle tremors.	Discontinue. Call doctor right away.
• Profuse sweating, unusual saliva flow.	Continue. Call doctor when convenient.
Rare: None expected.	

WARNINGS & PRECAUTIONS

Don't take if:
You are allergic to pilocarpine.

Before you start, consult your doctor:
- If you take sedatives, sleeping pills, tranquilizers, antidepressants, antihistamines, narcotics or mind-altering drugs.
- If you have asthma.
- If you have conjunctivitis (pink eye).

Over age 60:
Adverse reactions and side effects may be more frequent and severe than in younger persons.

Pregnancy:
No proven harm to unborn child. Avoid if possible.

Breast-feeding:
No proven problems. Consult doctor.

Infants & children:
Not recommended.

Prolonged use:
You may develop tolerance for drug, making it ineffective.

Skin & sunlight:
No problems expected.

Driving, piloting or hazardous work:
Don't drive or pilot aircraft until you learn how medicine affects you. Don't work around dangerous machinery. Don't climb ladders or work in high places. Danger increases if you drink alcohol or take medicine affecting alertness and reflexes, such as antihistamines, tranquilizers, sedatives, pain medicine, narcotics and mind-altering drugs.

Discontinuing:
Doctor may discontinue and substitute another drug to keep treatment effective.

Others:
- Can provoke asthma attack in susceptible individuals.
- Drops may impair vision for 2 to 3 hours.

POSSIBLE INTERACTION WITH OTHER DRUGS

GENERIC NAME OR DRUG CLASS	COMBINED EFFECT
Amphetamines*	Decreased pilocarpine effect.
Anticholinergics*	Decreased pilocarpine effect.
Appetite suppressants*	Decreased pilocarpine effect.
Beta-adrenergic blockers*	Increased pilocarpine effect.
Carbonic anhydrase inhibitors, oral*	Increased pilocarpine effect.
Cortisone drugs*	Decreased pilocarpine effect.
Epinephrine, topical	Increased pilocarpine effect.
Glycopyrrolate	Increased glycopyrrolate effect.
Phenothiazines*	Decreased pilocarpine effect.

POSSIBLE INTERACTION WITH OTHER SUBSTANCES

INTERACTS WITH	COMBINED EFFECT
Alcohol:	May prolong alcohol's effect on brain.
Beverages:	None expected.
Cocaine:	Decreased pilocarpine effect. Avoid.
Foods:	None expected.
Marijuana:	Used once or twice weekly—May help lower internal eye pressure.
Tobacco:	None expected.

PINDOLOL

BRAND NAMES

Pindolol Visken

BASIC INFORMATION

Habit forming? No
Prescription needed? Yes
Available as generic? No
Drug class: Beta-adrenergic blocker

 USES

- Lowers blood pressure.
- Other uses prescribed by your doctor.

 DOSAGE & USAGE INFORMATION

How to take:
Tablet—Swallow with liquid. If you can't swallow whole, crumble tablet and take with liquid or food.

When to take:
With meals or immediately after.

If you forget a dose:
Take as soon as you remember. Return to regular schedule, but allow 3 hours between doses.

What drug does:
- Blocks certain actions of sympathetic nervous system.
- Lowers heart's oxygen requirements.
- Slows nerve impulses through heart.
- Reduces blood vessel contraction in heart, scalp and other body parts.

Time lapse before drug works:
1 to 4 hours.

Don't take with:
Non-prescription drugs or drugs in Interaction column without consulting doctor.

 OVERDOSE

SYMPTOMS:
Weakness, slow or weak pulse, blood-pressure drop, fainting, difficulty breathing, convulsions, cold and sweaty skin.
WHAT TO DO:
- **Dial 0 (operator) or 911 (emergency) for an ambulance or medical help. Then give first aid immediately.**
- **See emergency information on inside covers.**

 POSSIBLE ADVERSE REACTIONS OR SIDE EFFECTS

SYMPTOMS	WHAT TO DO
Life-threatening:	
Congestive heart failure.	Discontinue. Seek emergency treatment.
Common:	
• Pulse slower than 50 beats per minute.	Discontinue. Call doctor right away.
• Drowsiness, fatigue, numbness or tingling of fingers or toes, dizziness, diarrhea, nausea, weakness.	Continue. Call doctor when convenient.
• Cold hands, feet; dry mouth, eyes, skin.	Continue. Tell doctor at next visit.
Infrequent:	
• Hallucinations, nightmares, insomnia, headache, difficult breathing, joint pain.	Discontinue. Call doctor right away.
• Confusion, reduced alertness, depression.	Continue. Call doctor when convenient.
• Constipation.	Continue. Tell doctor at next visit.
Rare:	
• Rash, sore throat, fever, breathing difficulty.	Discontinue. Call doctor right away.
• Unusual bleeding and bruising; dry, burning eyes; impotence.	Continue. Call doctor when convenient.

 WARNINGS & PRECAUTIONS

Don't take if:
- You are allergic to any beta-adrenergic blocker.
- You have asthma or hay fever symptoms.
- You have taken MAO inhibitors in past 2 weeks.

Before you start, consult your doctor:
- If you have heart disease or poor circulation to the extremities.
- If you have hay fever, asthma, chronic bronchitis, emphysema.
- If you have overactive thyroid function, diabetes, hypoglycemia, impaired liver or kidney function.
- If you will have surgery within 2 months, including dental surgery, requiring general or spinal anesthesia.

Over age 60:
Adverse reactions and side effects may be more frequent and severe than in younger persons.

Pregnancy:
Risk to unborn child outweighs drug benefits.
Don't use.

Breast-feeding:
Drug passes into milk. Avoid drug or discontinue
nursing until you finish medicine. Consult doctor
for advice on maintaining milk supply.

Infants & children:
Not recommended.

Prolonged use:
Weakens heart muscle contractions.

Skin & sunlight:
No problems expected.

Driving, piloting or hazardous work:
Don't drive or pilot aircraft until you learn how
medicine affects you. Don't work around
dangerous machinery. Don't climb ladders or
work in high places. Danger increases if you
drink alcohol or take medicine affecting alertness
and reflexes.

Discontinuing:
Don't discontinue without consulting doctor.
Dose may require gradual reduction if you have
taken drug for a long time. Doses of other drugs
may also require adjustment.

Others:
May mask hypoglycemia.

POSSIBLE INTERACTION WITH OTHER DRUGS

GENERIC NAME OR DRUG CLASS	COMBINED EFFECT
ACE inhibitors: captopril, enalapril, lisinopril*	Increased antihypertensive effects of both drugs. Dosages may require adjustment.
Antidiabetics*	Increased antidiabetic effect.
Antihistamines*	Decreased antihistamine effect.
Antihypertensives*	Increased antihypertensive effect.
Barbiturates*	Increased barbiturate effect. Dangerous sedation.
Beta-agonists*	Decreased beta-agonist effect.
Betaxolol eyedrops	Possible increased pindolol effect.
Digitalis preparations*	Can either increase or decrease heart rate. Improves irregular heartbeat.
Indomethacin	Decreased pindolol effect.
Insulin	Hypoglycemic effects may be prolonged.
Levobunolol eyedrops	Possible increased pindolol effect.
Narcotics*	Increased narcotic effect. Dangerous sedation.
Nicardipine	Possible irregular heartbeat and congestive heart failure.
Nitrates*	Possible decreased blood pressure.
Non-steroidal anti-inflammatory drugs (NSAIDs)*	Decreased antihypertensive effect of pindolol.
Phenytoin	Decreased pindolol effect.
Quinidine	Slows heart excessively.
Reserpine	Increased reserpine effect. Excessive sedation and depression.
Rifampin	Decreased pindolol effect.
Timolol eyedrops	Possible increased pindolol effect.
Tocainide	May worsen congestive heart failure.
Verapamil	Increased effect of both drugs.

POSSIBLE INTERACTION WITH OTHER SUBSTANCES

INTERACTS WITH	COMBINED EFFECT
Alcohol:	Excessive blood-pressure drop. Avoid.
Beverages:	None expected.
Cocaine:	Irregular heartbeat. Avoid.
Foods:	None expected.
Marijuana:	Daily use—Impaired circulation to hands and feet.
Tobacco:	Possible irregular heartbeat.

*See Glossary

PIROXICAM

BRAND NAMES

Apo-Piroxicam   Novopirocam
Feldene

BASIC INFORMATION

Habit forming? No
Prescription needed? Yes
Available as generic? No
Drug class: Anti-inflammatory (non-steroid)

USES

- Relieves symptoms of rheumatoid arthritis, osteoarthritis and gout.
- Relieves symptoms of ankylosing spondylitis.
- Treats juvenile rheumatoid arthritis.

DOSAGE & USAGE INFORMATION

How to take:
Capsule—Swallow with liquid or food to lessen stomach irritation. If you can't swallow whole, open capsule and take with liquid or food.

When to take:
At the same times each day.

If you forget a dose:
Take as soon as you remember up to 2 hours late. If more than 2 hours, wait for next scheduled dose (don't double this dose).

What drug does:
Reduces tissue concentration of prostaglandins (hormones that produce inflammation and pain).

Time lapse before drug works:
Begins in 4 to 24 hours. May require 3 weeks regular use for maximum benefit.

Don't take with:
See Interaction column and consult doctor.

OVERDOSE

SYMPTOMS:
Confusion, agitation, incoherence, convulsions, possible hemorrhage from stomach or intestine, coma.
WHAT TO DO:
- **Dial 0 (operator) or 911 (emergency) for an ambulance or medical help. Then give first aid immediately.**
- **See emergency information on inside covers.**

POSSIBLE ADVERSE REACTIONS OR SIDE EFFECTS

SYMPTOMS	WHAT TO DO
Life-threatening: Hives, rash, intense itching, faintness soon after a dose (anaphylaxis in aspirin-sensitive persons).	Seek emergency treatment immediately.
Common: • Dizziness, nausea, pain. • Headache.	Continue. Call doctor when convenient. Continue. Tell doctor at next visit.
Infrequent: Depression, drowsiness, ringing in ears, swollen feet or legs, constipation or diarrhea, vomiting.	Continue. Call doctor when convenient.
Rare: • Convulsions; confusion; rash, hives or itchy skin; blurred vision; black, bloody or tarry stool; difficult breathing; tightness in chest; rapid heartbeat; unusual bleeding or bruising; blood in urine; jaundice; severe abdominal pain, psychosis. • Painful, difficult or frequent urination; fatigue; weakness; swollen breasts in males; impotence; menstrual irregularities.	Discontinue. Call doctor right away. Continue. Call doctor when convenient.

WARNINGS & PRECAUTIONS

Don't take if:
- You are allergic to aspirin or any non-steroid, anti-inflammatory drug.
- You have gastritis, peptic ulcer, enteritis, ileitis, ulcerative colitis, asthma, heart failure, high blood pressure or bleeding problems.
- Patient is younger than 15.

Before you start, consult your doctor:
- If you have epilepsy.
- If you have Parkinson's disease.
- If you have been mentally ill.
- If you have had kidney disease or impaired kidney function.
- If you will have surgery within 2 months, including dental surgery, requiring general or spinal anesthesia.

Over age 60:
Adverse reactions and side effects may be more frequent and severe than in younger persons. Smaller than average doses may reduce unpleasant side effects.

Pregnancy:
Studies inconclusive on harm to unborn child. Animal studies show fetal abnormalities. Decide with your doctor whether drug benefits justify risk to unborn child.

Breast-feeding:
May harm child. Avoid.

Infants & children:
Not recommended for anyone younger than 15. Use only under medical supervision.

Prolonged use:
- Eye damage, reduced hearing, sore throat, fever.
- Weight gain.
- Request liver-function and bleeding time studies.

Skin & sunlight:
Increased sensitivity to sunlight.

Driving, piloting or hazardous work:
Don't drive or pilot aircraft until you learn how medicine affects you. Don't work around dangerous machinery. Don't climb ladders or work in high places. Danger increases if you drink alcohol or take medicine affecting alertness and reflexes.

Discontinuing:
Don't discontinue without consulting doctor. Dose may require gradual reduction if you have taken drug for a long time. Doses of other drugs may also require adjustment.

Others:
No problems expected.

POSSIBLE INTERACTION WITH OTHER DRUGS

GENERIC NAME OR DRUG CLASS	COMBINED EFFECT
ACE inhibitors: captopril, enalapril, lisinopril*	May decrease ACE inhibitor effect.
Anticoagulants, oral*	Increased risk of bleeding.
Aspirin	Increased risk of stomach ulcer.
Beta-adrenergic blockers*	Decreased antihypertensive effect.
Carteolol	Decreased anti-hypertensive effect of carteolol.
Cortisone drugs*	Increased risk of stomach ulcer.
Diuretics*	May decrease diuretic effect.
Lithium	Possible increased lithium effect and toxicity.
Methotrexate	May increase toxicity.
Minoxidil	Decreased minoxidil effect.
Oxyphenbutazone	Possible stomach ulcer.
Phenylbutazone	Possible stomach ulcer.
Probenecid	Increased piroxicam effect.

Continued page 1100

POSSIBLE INTERACTION WITH OTHER SUBSTANCES

INTERACTS WITH	COMBINED EFFECT
Alcohol:	Possible stomach ulcer or bleeding.
Beverages:	None expected.
Cocaine:	Depression following cocaine use. Avoid.
Foods:	None expected.
Marijuana:	Increased pain relief from piroxicam, but may be depressing.
Tobacco:	Decreased absorption of piroxicam. Avoid tobacco.

*See Glossary

POLOXAMER 188

BRAND NAMES

Alaxin   Poloxalkol

BASIC INFORMATION

Habit forming? No
Prescription needed? No
Available as generic? No
Drug class: Laxative (emollient)

 USES

Constipation relief.

DOSAGE & USAGE INFORMATION

How to take:
Capsule—Swallow with liquid. Don't open capsules.

When to take:
At the same time each day, preferably bedtime.

If you forget a dose:
Take as soon as you remember. Wait 12 hours for next dose. Return to regular schedule.

What drug does:
Makes stool hold fluid so it is easier to pass.

Time lapse before drug works:
2 to 3 days of continual use.

Don't take with:
- Other medicines at same time. Wait 2 hours.
- See Interaction column and consult doctor.

 OVERDOSE

SYMPTOMS:
Appetite loss, nausea, vomiting, diarrhea.
WHAT TO DO:
Overdose unlikely to threaten life. If person takes much larger amount than prescribed, call doctor, poison-control center or hospital emergency room for instructions.

POSSIBLE ADVERSE REACTIONS OR SIDE EFFECTS

SYMPTOMS	WHAT TO DO
Life-threatening: None expected.	
Common: None expected.	
Infrequent: Throat irritation (liquid only), intestinal and stomach cramps.	Continue. Call doctor when convenient.
Rare: Rash.	Discontinue. Call doctor right away.

WARNINGS & PRECAUTIONS

Don't take if:
- You are allergic to any emollient laxative.
- You have abdominal pain and fever that might be appendicitis.

Before you start, consult your doctor:
- If you are taking other laxatives.
- To be sure constipation isn't a sign of a serious disorder.

Over age 60:
You must drink 6 to 8 glasses of fluid every 24 hours for drug to work.

Pregnancy:
No problems expected. Consult doctor.

Breast-feeding:
No problems expected.

Infants & children:
No problems expected.

Prolonged use:
Avoid. Overuse of laxatives may damage intestine lining.

Skin & sunlight:
No problems expected.

Driving, piloting or hazardous work:
No problems expected.

Discontinuing:
May be unnecessary to finish medicine. Follow doctor's instructions.

Others:
No problems expected.

POSSIBLE INTERACTION WITH OTHER DRUGS

GENERIC NAME OR DRUG CLASS	COMBINED EFFECT
Danthron	Possible liver damage.
Digitalis preparations*	Toxic absorption of digitalis.
Mineral oil	Increased mineral oil absorption into bloodstream. Avoid.
Phenolphthalein	Increased phenolphthalein absorption. Possible toxicity.

POSSIBLE INTERACTION WITH OTHER SUBSTANCES

INTERACTS WITH	COMBINED EFFECT
Alcohol:	None expected.
Beverages:	None expected.
Cocaine:	None expected.
Foods:	None expected.
Marijuana:	None expected.
Tobacco:	None expected.

*See Glossary

POLYCARBOPHIL CALCIUM

BRAND NAMES

FiberCon   **Mitrolan**

BASIC INFORMATION

Habit forming? No
Prescription needed? No
Available as generic? No
Drug class: Laxative (bulk-forming),
   antidiarrheal

USES

- Relieves constipation and prevents straining for bowel movement.
- Stops diarrhea.

DOSAGE & USAGE INFORMATION

How to take:
- Tablets (laxative)—Swallow with 8 oz. cold liquid. Drink 6 to 8 glasses of water each day in addition to the one with each dose.
- Tablets (diarrhea)—Take without water at half-hour intervals.
- Chewable tablets—Chew well before swallowing.

When to take:
At the same times each day.

If you forget a dose:
Take as soon as you remember. Resume regular schedule.

What drug does:
Absorbs water, stimulating the bowel to form a soft, bulky stool and decreasing watery diarrhea.

Time lapse before drug works:
May require 2 or 3 days to begin, then works in 12 to 24 hours.

Don't take with:
- See Interaction column and consult doctor.
- Don't take within 2 hours of taking another medicine.

OVERDOSE

SYMPTOMS:
None expected.
WHAT TO DO:
Overdose unlikely to threaten life. If person takes much larger amount than prescribed, call doctor, poison-control center or hospital emergency room for instructions.

POSSIBLE ADVERSE REACTIONS OR SIDE EFFECTS

SYMPTOMS	WHAT TO DO
Life-threatening: None expected.	
Common: None expected.	
Infrequent: Swallowing difficulty, "lump in throat" sensation, nausea, vomiting, diarrhea.	Continue. Call doctor when convenient.
Rare: Itchy skin, rash, intestinal blockage, asthma.	Discontinue. Call doctor right away.

WARNINGS & PRECAUTIONS

Don't take if:
- You are allergic to any bulk-forming laxative.
- You have symptoms of appendicitis, inflamed bowel or intestinal blockage.
- You have missed a bowel movement for only 1 or 2 days.

Before you start, consult your doctor:
- If you have diabetes.
- If you have a laxative habit.
- If you have rectal bleeding.
- If you have difficulty swallowing.
- If you take other laxatives.

Over age 60:
Adverse reactions and side effects may be more frequent and severe than in younger persons.

Pregnancy:
Most bulk-forming laxatives contain sodium or sugars which may cause fluid retention. Avoid if possible.

Breast-feeding:
No problems expected.

Infants & children:
Use only under medical supervision.

Prolonged use:
Don't take for more than 1 week unless under a doctor's supervision. May cause laxative dependence.

Skin & sunlight:
No problems expected.

Driving, piloting or hazardous work:
No problems expected.

Discontinuing:
May be unnecessary to finish medicine. Follow doctor's instructions.

Others:
Don't take to "flush out" your system or as a "tonic."

POSSIBLE INTERACTION WITH OTHER DRUGS

GENERIC NAME OR DRUG CLASS	COMBINED EFFECT
Digitalis preparations*	Decreased digitalis effect.
Salicylates* (including aspirin)	Decreased salicylate effect.
Tetracyclines*	Decreased tetracycline effect.

POSSIBLE INTERACTION WITH OTHER SUBSTANCES

INTERACTS WITH	COMBINED EFFECT
Alcohol:	None expected.
Beverages:	None expected.
Cocaine:	None expected.
Foods:	None expected.
Marijuana:	None expected.
Tobacco:	None expected.

POLYTHIAZIDE

BRAND NAMES

Renese

BASIC INFORMATION

Habit forming? No
Prescription needed? Yes
Available as generic? No
Drug class: Antihypertensive, diuretic
(thiazide)

 USES

- Controls, but doesn't cure, high blood pressure.
- Reduces fluid retention (edema) caused by conditions such as heart disorders and liver disease.

 DOSAGE & USAGE INFORMATION

How to take:
Tablet—Swallow with 8 oz. of liquid. If you can't swallow whole, crumble tablet and take with liquid or food. Don't exceed dose.

When to take:
At the same time each day.

If you forget a dose:
Take as soon as you remember up to 2 hours late. If more than 2 hours, wait for next scheduled dose (don't double this dose).

What drug does:
- Forces sodium and water excretion, reducing body fluid.
- Relaxes muscle cells of small arteries.
- Reduced body fluid and relaxed arteries lower blood pressure.

Time lapse before drug works:
4 to 6 hours. May require several weeks to lower blood pressure.

Continued next column

 OVERDOSE

SYMPTOMS:
Cramps, weakness, drowsiness, weak pulse, coma.
WHAT TO DO:
- **Dial 0 (operator) or 911 (emergency) for an ambulance or medical help. Then give first aid immediately.**
- **See emergency information on inside covers.**

Don't take with:
- See Interaction column and consult doctor.
- Non-prescription drugs without consulting doctor.

 POSSIBLE ADVERSE REACTIONS OR SIDE EFFECTS

SYMPTOMS	WHAT TO DO
Life-threatening: None expected.	
Common: None expected.	
Infrequent:	
• Blurred vision, severe abdominal pain, nausea, vomiting, irregular heartbeat, weak pulse.	Discontinue. Call doctor right away.
• Dizziness, mood change, headache, weakness, tiredness, weight changes.	Continue. Call doctor when convenient.
• Dry mouth, thirst.	Continue. Tell doctor at next visit.
Rare:	
• Rash or hives.	Discontinue. Seek emergency treatment.
• Jaundice, sore throat, fever.	Discontinue. Call doctor right away.

 WARNINGS & PRECAUTIONS

Don't take if:
You are allergic to any thiazide diuretic drug.

Before you start, consult your doctor:
- If you are allergic to any sulfa drug.
- If you have gout.
- If you have liver, pancreas or kidney disorder.

Over age 60:
Adverse reactions and side effects may be more frequent and severe than in younger persons, especially dizziness and excessive potassium loss.

Pregnancy:
Risk to unborn child outweighs drug benefits. Don't use.

Breast-feeding:
Drug passes into milk. Avoid drug or discontinue nursing.

Infants & children:
No problems expected.

Prolonged use:
You may need medicine to treat high blood pressure for the rest of your life.

POLYTHIAZIDE

Skin & sunlight:
May cause rash or intensify sunburn in areas exposed to sun or sunlamp.

Driving, piloting or hazardous work:
Don't drive or pilot aircraft until you learn how medicine affects you. Don't work around dangerous machinery. Don't climb ladders or work in high places. Danger increases if you drink alcohol or take medicine affecting alertness and reflexes, such as antihistamines, tranquilizers, sedatives, pain medicine, narcotics and mind-altering drugs.

Discontinuing:
Don't discontinue without medical advice.

Others:
- Hot weather and fever may cause dehydration and drop in blood pressure. Dose may require temporary adjustment. Weigh daily and report any unexpected weight decreases to your doctor.
- May cause rise in uric acid, leading to gout.
- May cause blood-sugar rise in diabetics.

POSSIBLE INTERACTION WITH OTHER DRUGS

GENERIC NAME OR DRUG CLASS	COMBINED EFFECT
ACE inhibitors: captopril, enalapril, lisinopril*	Decreased blood pressure. Possible excessive potassium in blood.
Allopurinol	Decreased allopurinol effect.
Amiodarone	Increased risk of heartbeat irregularity due to low potassium.
Amphotericin B	Increased potassium.
Antidepressants, tricyclic (TCA)*	Dangerous drop in blood pressure. Avoid combination unless under medical supervision.
Antidiabetic agents, oral*	Increased blood sugar.
Antihypertensives*	Increased hypertensive effect.
Beta-adrenergic blockers*	Increased antihypertensive effect. Dosages of both drugs may require adjustment.
Barbiturates*	Increased polythiazide effect.

Calcium supplements*	Increased calcium in blood.
Carteolol	Increased antihypertensive effect.
Colestipol	Decreased polythiazide effect.
Cholestyramine	Decreased polythiazide effect.
Cortisone drugs*	Excessive potassium loss that causes dangerous heart rhythms.
Digitalis preparations*	Excessive potassium loss that causes dangerous heart rhythms.
Diuretics, thiazide*	Increased effect of other thiazide diuretics.
Indapamide	Increased diuretic effect.
Indomethacin	Decreased polythiazide effect.
Lithium	Increased effect of lithium.
MAO inhibitors*	Increased polythiazide effect.
Nicardipine	Blood-pressure drop. Dosages may require adjustment.
Nitrates*	Excessive blood-pressure drop.
Opiates*	Weakness and faintness when arising from bed or chair.

Continued page 1100

POSSIBLE INTERACTION WITH OTHER SUBSTANCES

INTERACTS WITH	COMBINED EFFECT
Alcohol:	Dangerous blood-pressure drop.
Beverages:	None expected.
Cocaine:	Increased risk of heart block and high blood pressure.
Foods: Licorice.	Excessive potassium loss that causes dangerous heart rhythms.
Marijuana:	May increase blood pressure.
Tobacco:	None expected.

*See Glossary

811

POTASSIUM PHOSPHATES

BRAND NAMES

K-Phos Original   Neutra-Phos K

BASIC INFORMATION

Habit forming? No
Prescription needed? Yes
Available as generic? No
Drug class: Electrolyte replenisher

USES

- Provides supplement of phosphorous for people with diseases which decrease phosphorous absorption from food.
- Treatment of hypercalcemia due to cancer.

DOSAGE & USAGE INFORMATION

How to take:
Tablets—Dissolve tablets in 3/4 to 1 glass of water. Let tablets soak 2 to 5 minutes, then stir to completely dissolve.

When to take:
After meals or with food to prevent or lessen stomach irritation or loose stools.

If you forget a dose:
Take within 1 hour then return to original schedule. If later than 1 hour, skip dose. Don't double-dose.

What drug does:
- Provides supplemental phosphates.
- Makes uric acid.

Time lapse before drug works:
30-60 minutes.

Don't take with:
See Interaction column and consult doctor.

OVERDOSE

SYMPTOMS:
Irregular heartbeat, blood-pressure drop with weakness, coma, cardiac arrest.
WHAT TO DO:
- Dial 0 (operator) or 911 (emergency) for an ambulance or medical help. Then give first aid immediately.
- See emergency information on inside covers.

POSSIBLE ADVERSE REACTIONS OR SIDE EFFECTS

SYMPTOMS	WHAT TO DO
Life-threatening: Irregular heartbeat, shortness of breath.	Discontinue. Seek emergency treatment.
Common: Muscle cramps.	Discontinue. Call doctor right away.
Infrequent: Bone and joint pain, numbness or tingling in hands or feet, unusual tiredness, weakness, diarrhea, nausea, abdominal pain, vomiting.	Discontinue. Call doctor right away.
Rare: None expected.	

POTASSIUM PHOSPHATES

WARNINGS & PRECAUTIONS

Don't take if:
You have had allergic reaction to potassium, sodium or phosphates; severe kidney disease; severe burns.

Before you start, consult your doctor:
If you have heart problems, adrenal insufficiency, liver disease, high blood pressure, pregnancy, hypoparathyroidism, chronic kidney disease, osteomalacia, pancreatitis, rickets.

Over age 60:
Adverse reactions and side effects may be more frequent and severe than in younger persons. Ask doctor about smaller doses.

Pregnancy:
Risk to unborn child outweighs drug benefits. Don't use.

Breast-feeding:
No data available in humans.

Infants & children:
Use only under medical supervision.

Prolonged use:
Monitor ECG, serum calcium, phosphorous and potassium levels.

Skin & sunlight:
No problems expected.

Driving, piloting or hazardous work:
Avoid if medicine causes dizziness or confusion.

Discontinuing:
Don't discontinue without consulting doctor. Dose may require gradual reduction if you have taken drug for a long time. Doses of other drugs may also require adjustment.

Others:
Protect liquid medicine from freezing.

POSSIBLE INTERACTION WITH OTHER DRUGS

GENERIC NAME OR DRUG CLASS	COMBINED EFFECT
ACE inhibitors: captopril, enalapril, lisinopril*	Level of potassium in blood too high.
Antacids*	May decrease potassium absorption.
Calcium	Decreased potassium effect.
Cortisone drugs*	Increased fluid retention.
Digitalis preparations*	Level of potassium in blood too high.
Diuretics* (amiloride, spironolactone, triamterene)	Level of potassium in blood too high.
Male hormones*	Fluid retention.
Potassium supplements*	Level of potassium in blood too high.
Vitamin D (calcifidiol and calcitriol)	Level of phosphorous in blood too high.

POSSIBLE INTERACTION WITH OTHER SUBSTANCES

INTERACTS WITH	COMBINED EFFECT
Alcohol:	None expected.
Beverages: Salty drinks such as tomato juice, commercial thirst quenchers, salt substitutes.	Increased fluid retention.
Cocaine:	May cause irregular heartbeat.
Foods: Salty foods such as canned soups, potato chips, TV dinners, hot dogs, pickles.	Increased fluid retention.
Marijuana:	May cause irregular heartbeat.
Tobacco:	May aggravate irregular heartbeat.

POTASSIUM & SODIUM PHOSPHATES

BRAND AND GENERIC NAMES

DIBASIC POTASSIUM
  & SODIUM
  PHOSPHATES
K-Phos M.F.
K-Phos Neutral
K-Phos 2
MONOBASIC
  POTASSIUM &
  SODIUM
  PHOSPHATES

Neutra-Phos
Neutra-Phos-K
POTASSIUM &
  SODIUM
  PHOSPHATES
Uro-KP-Neutral

BASIC INFORMATION

Habit forming? No
Prescription needed? Yes
Available as generic? Yes
Drug class: Electrolyte replenisher

USES

- Provides supplement of phosphorous for people with diseases which decrease phosphorous absorption from food.
- Treatment of hypercalcemia due to cancer.

DOSAGE & USAGE INFORMATION

How to take:
- Tablets or capsules—Dissolve tablets or open capsules in 3/4 to 1 glass of water. Let tablets soak 2 to 5 minutes, then stir to completely dissolve.
- Oral solution—Take after meals with liquid to decrease stomach irritation.

When to take:
After meals or with food to prevent or lessen stomach irritation or loose stools.

If you forget a dose:
Take within 1 hour then return to original schedule. If later than 1 hour, skip dose. Don't double-dose.

Continued next column

OVERDOSE

SYMPTOMS:
Irregular heartbeat, blood-pressure drop with weakness, coma, cardiac arrest.
WHAT TO DO:
- Dial 0 (operator) or 911 (emergency) for an ambulance or medical help. Then give first aid immediately.
- See emergency information on inside covers.

What drug does:
- Provides supplemental phosphates.
- Makes uric acid.

Time lapse before drug works:
30-60 minutes.

Don't take with:
See Interaction column and consult doctor.

POSSIBLE ADVERSE REACTIONS OR SIDE EFFECTS

SYMPTOMS	WHAT TO DO
Life-threatening: Irregular heartbeat, difficult breathing, anxiety, weak legs.	Discontinue. Seek emergency treatment.
Common: None expected.	
Infrequent: Numbness or tingling in hands or feet, diarrhea, nausea, abdominal pain, vomiting, headache, dizziness, muscle cramps, swollen feet and ankles, thirst, weakness.	Discontinue. Call doctor right away.
Rare: Confusion.	Discontinue. Call doctor right away.

WARNINGS & PRECAUTIONS

Don't take if:
You have had allergic reaction to potassium, sodium or phosphates; severe kidney disease; severe burns.

Before you start, consult your doctor:
If you have heart problems, adrenal insufficiency, liver disease, high blood pressure, pregnancy, hypoparathyroidism, chronic kidney disease, osteomalacia, pancreatitis, rickets.

Over age 60:
Adverse reactions and side effects may be more frequent and severe than in younger persons. Ask doctor about smaller doses.

Pregnancy:
Risk to unborn child outweighs drug benefits. Don't use.

Breast-feeding:
No data available in humans.

Infants & children:
Use only under medical supervision.

Prolonged use:
Monitor ECG, serum calcium, phosphorous and potassium levels.

Skin & sunlight:
No problems expected.

Driving, piloting or hazardous work:
Avoid if medicine causes dizziness or confusion.

Discontinuing:
Don't discontinue without consulting doctor. Dose may require gradual reduction if you have taken drug for a long time. Doses of other drugs may also require adjustment.

Others:
Protect liquid medicine from freezing.

POSSIBLE INTERACTION WITH OTHER DRUGS

GENERIC NAME OR DRUG CLASS	COMBINED EFFECT
ACE inhibitors: captopril, enalapril, lisinopril*	Level of potassium in blood too high.
Antacids*	May decrease potassium absorption.
Calcium	Decreased potassium effect.
Cortisone drugs*	Increased fluid retention.
Digitalis preparations*	Level of potassium in blood too high.
Diuretics* (amiloride, spironolactone, triamterene)	Level of potassium in blood too high.
Male hormones*	Fluid retention.
Potassium supplements*	Level of potassium in blood too high.
Vitamin D (calcifidiol and calcitriol)	Level of phosphorous in blood too high.

POSSIBLE INTERACTION WITH OTHER SUBSTANCES

INTERACTS WITH	COMBINED EFFECT
Alcohol:	None expected.
Beverages: Salty drinks such as tomato juice, commercial thirst quenchers, salt substitutes.	Increased fluid retention.
Cocaine:	May cause irregular heartbeat.
Foods: Salty foods such as canned soups, potato chips, TV dinners, hot dogs, pickles.	Increased fluid retention.
Marijuana:	May cause irregular heartbeat.
Tobacco:	May aggravate irregular heartbeat.

*See Glossary

POTASSIUM SUPPLEMENTS

BRAND NAMES

See complete list of brand names in the *Brand Name Directory*, page 1069.

BASIC INFORMATION

Habit forming? No
Prescription needed? Yes
Available as generic? Yes
Drug class: Mineral supplement (potassium)

USES

- Treatment for potassium deficiency from diuretics, cortisone or digitalis medicines.
- Treatment for low potassium associated with some illnesses.

DOSAGE & USAGE INFORMATION

How to take:
- Tablet or capsule—Swallow with liquid or food to lessen stomach irritation. You may chew or crush tablet.
- Extended-release tablets or capsules— Swallow each dose whole with liquid.
- Effervescent tablets, granules, powder or liquid—Dilute dose in water.

When to take:
At the same time each day, preferably with food or immediately after meals.

If you forget a dose:
Take as soon as you remember. Don't double next dose.

What drug does:
Preserves or restores normal function of nerve cells, heart and skeletal-muscle cells, kidneys, and stomach-juice secretions.

Continued next column

OVERDOSE

SYMPTOMS:
Paralysis of arms and legs, irregular heartbeat, blood-pressure drop, convulsions, coma, cardiac arrest.
WHAT TO DO:
- **Dial 0 (operator) or 911 (emergency) for an ambulance or medical help. Then give first aid immediately.**
- **See emergency information on inside covers.**

Time lapse before drug works:
1 to 2 hours. Full benefit may require 12 to 24 hours.

Don't take with:
See Interaction column and consult doctor.

POSSIBLE ADVERSE REACTIONS OR SIDE EFFECTS

SYMPTOMS	WHAT TO DO
Life-threatening: None expected.	
Common: None expected.	
Infrequent: Diarrhea, nausea, vomiting, stomach discomfort, skin rash.	Continue. Call doctor when convenient.
Rare:	
• Confusion; irregular heartbeat; difficult breathing; unusual fatigue; weakness; heaviness of legs; small bowel ulcers, hemorrhage, perforation with enteric-coated tablets (rarely with wax matrix tablets); esophageal ulceration with tablets.	Discontinue. Call doctor right away.
• Numbness or tingling in hands or feet.	Continue. Call doctor when convenient.

WARNINGS & PRECAUTIONS

Don't take if:
- You are allergic to any potassium supplement.
- You have acute or chronic kidney disease.

Before you start, consult your doctor:
- If you have Addison's disease or familial periodic paralysis.
- If you have heart disease.
- If you have intestinal blockage.
- If you have a stomach ulcer.
- If you use diuretics.
- If you use heart medicine.
- If you use laxatives or have chronic diarrhea.
- If you use salt substitutes or low-salt milk.

Over age 60:
Observe dose schedule strictly. Potassium balance is critical. Deviation above or below normal can have serious results.

Pregnancy:
No problems expected if you adhere strictly to prescribed dose.

Breast-feeding:
Studies inconclusive on harm to infant. Consult doctor.

Infants & children:
Use only under doctor's supervision.

Prolonged use:
- Slows absorption of vitamin B-12. May cause anemia.
- Request frequent lab tests to monitor potassium levels in blood, especially if you take digitalis preparations.

Skin & sunlight:
No problems expected.

Driving, piloting or hazardous work:
No problems expected.

Discontinuing:
Don't discontinue without consulting doctor. Dose may require gradual reduction if you have taken drug for a long time. Doses of other drugs may also require adjustment.

Others:
- Overdose or underdose serious. Frequent EKGs and laboratory blood studies to measure serum electrolytes and kidney function recommended.
- Prolonged diarrhea may call for increased dosage of potassium.
- Serious injury may necessitate temporary *decrease* in potassium.
- Some products contain tartrazine dye. Avoid, especially if you are allergic to aspirin.

POSSIBLE INTERACTION WITH OTHER DRUGS

GENERIC NAME OR DRUG CLASS	COMBINED EFFECT
ACE inhibitors: captopril, enalapril, lisinopril*	Possible increased potassium effect.
Amiloride	Dangerous rise in blood potassium.
Anticholinergics, other*	Increased possibility of intestinal ulcers, which sometimes occur with oral potassium tablets.
Atropine	Increased possibility of intestinal ulcers, which sometimes occur with oral potassium tablets.
Belladonna	Increased possibility of intestinal ulcers, which sometimes occur with oral potassium tablets.
Cortisone medicines*	Decreased effect of potassium.
Digitalis preparations*	Possible irregular heartbeat.
Diuretics, thiazide or loop*	Decreased potassium effect.
Laxatives*	Possible decreased potassium effect.
Spironolactone	Dangerous rise in blood potassium.
Triamterene	Dangerous rise in blood potassium.
Vitamin B-12	Extended-release tablets may decrease vitamin B-12 absorption and increase vitamin B-12 requirements.

POSSIBLE INTERACTION WITH OTHER SUBSTANCES

INTERACTS WITH	COMBINED EFFECT
Alcohol:	None expected.
Beverages: Salty drinks such as tomato juice, commercial thirst quenchers.	Increased fluid retention.
Cocaine:	May cause irregular heartbeat.
Foods: Salty foods.	Increased fluid retention.
Marijuana:	May cause irregular heartbeat.
Tobacco:	None expected.

PRAZEPAM

BRAND NAMES

Centrax

BASIC INFORMATION

Habit forming? Yes
Prescription needed? Yes
Available as generic? No
Drug class: Tranquilizer (benzodiazepine)

 ## USES

Treatment for nervousness or tension.

 ## DOSAGE & USAGE INFORMATION

How to take:
Tablet or capsule—Swallow with liquid. If you can't swallow whole, crumble tablet or open capsule and take with liquid or food.

When to take:
At the same time each day, according to instructions on prescription label.

If you forget a dose:
Take as soon as you remember up to 2 hours late. If more than 2 hours, wait for next scheduled dose (don't double this dose).

What drug does:
Affects limbic system, the part of the brain that controls emotions.

Time lapse before drug works:
2 hours. May take 6 weeks for full benefit.

Don't take with:
See Interaction column and consult doctor.

 ## OVERDOSE

SYMPTOMS:
Drowsiness, weakness, tremor, stupor, coma.
WHAT TO DO:
- **Dial 0 (operator) or 911 (emergency) for an ambulance or medical help. Then give first aid immediately.**
- **If patient is unconscious and not breathing, give mouth-to-mouth breathing. If there is no heartbeat, use cardiac massage and mouth-to-mouth breathing (CPR). Don't try to make patient vomit. If you can't get help quickly, take patient to nearest emergency facility.**
- **See emergency information on inside covers.**

 ## POSSIBLE ADVERSE REACTIONS OR SIDE EFFECTS

SYMPTOMS	WHAT TO DO
Life-threatening: None expected.	
Common: Clumsiness, dizziness, drowsiness.	Continue. Call doctor when convenient.
Infrequent:	
• Hallucinations, confusion, irritability, depression, rash, itchy skin, change in vision.	Discontinue. Call doctor right away.
• Constipation or diarrhea, nausea, vomiting, difficult urination, vivid dreams.	Continue. Call doctor when convenient.
Rare:	
• Slow heartbeat, difficult breathing.	Discontinue. Seek emergency treatment.
• Mouth and throat ulcers, jaundice.	Discontinue. Call doctor right away.
• Decreased libido.	Continue. Call doctor when convenient.

WARNINGS & PRECAUTIONS

Don't take if:
- You are allergic to any benzodiazepine.
- You have myasthenia gravis.
- You have glaucoma.
- You are active or recovering alcoholic.
- Patient is younger than 6 months.

Before you start, consult your doctor:
- If you have liver, kidney or lung disease.
- If you have diabetes, epilepsy or porphyria.

Over age 60:
Adverse reactions and side effects may be more frequent and severe than in younger persons. You need smaller doses for shorter periods of time. May develop agitation, rage or "hangover" effect.

Pregnancy:
Risk to unborn child outweighs drug benefits. Don't use.

Breast-feeding:
Drug passes into milk. Avoid drug or discontinue nursing until you finish medicine. Consult doctor for advice on maintaining milk supply.

Infants & children:
Use only under medical supervision for children older than 6 months.

Prolonged use:
May impair liver function.

Skin & sunlight:
No problems expected.

Driving, piloting or hazardous work:
Don't drive or pilot aircraft until you learn how medicine affects you. Don't work around dangerous machinery. Don't climb ladders or work in high places. Danger increases if you drink alcohol or take medicine affecting alertness and reflexes.

Discontinuing:
Don't discontinue without consulting doctor. Dose may require gradual reduction if you have taken drug for a long time. Doses of other drugs may also require adjustment.

Others:
• Hot weather, heavy exercise and profuse sweat may reduce excretion and cause overdose.
• Blood sugar may rise in diabetics, requiring insulin adjustment.

POSSIBLE INTERACTION WITH OTHER DRUGS

GENERIC NAME OR DRUG CLASS	COMBINED EFFECT
Anticonvulsants*	Change in seizure frequency or severity.
Antidepressants*	Increased sedative effect of both drugs.
Antihistamines*	Increased sedative effect of both drugs.
Antihypertensives*	Excessively low blood pressure.
Contraceptives, oral*	Increased prazepam effect.
Disulfiram	Increased prazepam effect.
Dronabinol	Increased effects of both drugs. Avoid.
Levodopa	Possible decreased levodopa effect.
MAO inhibitors*	Convulsions, deep sedation, rage.
Molindone	Increased tranquilizer effect.
Nabilone	Greater depression of central nervous system.
Narcotics*	Increased sedative effect of both drugs.
Probenecid	Increased prazepam effect.
Sedatives*	Increased sedative effect of both drugs.
Sleep inducers*	Increased sedative effect of both drugs.
Tranquilizers*	Increased sedative effect of both drugs.

POSSIBLE INTERACTION WITH OTHER SUBSTANCES

INTERACTS WITH	COMBINED EFFECT
Alcohol:	Heavy sedation. Avoid.
Beverages:	None expected.
Cocaine:	Decreased prazepam effect.
Foods:	None expected.
Marijuana:	Heavy sedation. Avoid.
Tobacco:	Decreased prazepam effect.

PRAZOSIN

BRAND NAMES

Minipress

BASIC INFORMATION

Habit forming? No
Prescription needed? Yes
Available as generic? No
Drug class: Antihypertensive

 USES

- Treatment for high blood pressure.
- May improve congestive heart failure.
- Treatment for Raynaud's disease.

 DOSAGE & USAGE INFORMATION

How to take:
Tablet or capsule—Swallow with liquid. If you can't swallow whole, crumble tablet or open capsule and take with liquid or food.

When to take:
At the same times each day.

If you forget a dose:
Take as soon as you remember up to 2 hours late. If more than 2 hours, wait for next scheduled dose (don't double this dose).

What drug does:
Expands and relaxes blood-vessel walls to lower blood pressure.

Time lapse before drug works:
30 minutes.

Don't take with:
See Interaction column and consult doctor.

 OVERDOSE

SYMPTOMS:
Extreme weakness; loss of consciousness; cold, sweaty skin; weak, rapid pulse; coma.
WHAT TO DO:
- Dial 0 (operator) or 911 (emergency) for an ambulance or medical help. Then give first aid immediately.
- If patient is unconscious and not breathing, give mouth-to-mouth breathing. If there is no heartbeat, use cardiac massage and mouth-to-mouth breathing (CPR). Don't try to make patient vomit. If you can't get help quickly, take patient to nearest emergency facility.
- See emergency information on inside covers.

 POSSIBLE ADVERSE REACTIONS OR SIDE EFFECTS

SYMPTOMS	WHAT TO DO
Life-threatening: None expected.	
Common:	
● Rapid heartbeat.	Discontinue. Call doctor right away.
● Vivid dreams, drowsiness, dizziness.	Continue. Call doctor when convenient.
Infrequent:	
● Rash or itchy skin, blurred vision, shortness of breath, difficult breathing, chest pain.	Discontinue. Call doctor right away.
● Appetite loss, constipation or diarrhea, stomach pain, nausea, vomiting, fluid retention, joint or muscle aches, weakness and faintness when arising from bed or chair.	Continue. Call doctor when convenient.
● Headache, irritability, depression, dry mouth, stuffy nose, increased urination.	Continue. Tell doctor at next visit.
Rare:	
Decreased sexual function.	Continue. Call doctor when convenient.

 WARNINGS & PRECAUTIONS

Don't take if:
- You are allergic to prazosin.
- You are depressed.
- You will have surgery within 2 months, including dental surgery, requiring general or spinal anesthesia.

Before you start, consult your doctor:
- If you experience lightheadedness or fainting with other antihypertensive drugs.
- If you are easily depressed.
- If you have impaired brain circulation or have had a stroke.
- If you have coronary heart disease (with or without angina).
- If you have kidney disease or impaired liver function.

Over age 60:
Begin with no more than 1 mg. per day for first 3 days. Increases should be gradual and supervised by your doctor. Don't stand while taking. Sudden changes in position may cause falls. Sit or lie down promptly if you feel dizzy. If you have impaired brain circulation or coronary heart disease, excessive lowering of blood pressure should be avoided. Report problems to your doctor immediately.

Pregnancy:
Studies inconclusive on harm to unborn child. Animal studies show fetal abnormalities. Decide with your doctor whether drug benefits justify risk to child.

Breast-feeding:
No proven problems. Consult doctor.

Infants & children:
Not recommended.

Prolonged use:
No problems expected.

Skin & sunlight:
No problems expected.

Driving, piloting or hazardous work:
Don't drive or pilot aircraft until you learn how medicine affects you. Don't work around dangerous machinery. Don't climb ladders or work in high places.

Discontinuing:
Don't discontinue without doctor's advice until you complete prescribed dose, even though symptoms diminish or disappear.

Others:
First dose likely to cause fainting. Take it at night and get out of bed slowly next morning.

POSSIBLE INTERACTION WITH OTHER DRUGS

GENERIC NAME OR DRUG CLASS	COMBINED EFFECT
Amphetamines*	Decreased prazosin effect.
Antihypertensives, other*	Increased antihypertensive effect. Dosages may require adjustments.
Carteolol	Increased antihypertensive effect.
Estrogen	Decreased effect of prazosin.
Guanfacine	Increased effect of both medicines.

Lisinopril	Increased antihypertensive effect. Dosage of each may require adjustment.
MAO inhibitors*	Blood-pressure drop.
Nicardipine	Blood-pressure drop. Dosages may require adjustment.
Nifedipine	Weakness and faintness when arising from bed or chair.
Nitrates*	Possible excessive blood-pressure drop.
Non-steroidal anti-inflammatory drugs (NSAIDs)*	Decreased effect of prazosin.
Sotalol	Increased antihypertensive effect.
Sympathomimetics*	Decreased effect of prazosin.
Terazosin	Decreases effectiveness of terazosin.
Verapamil	Weakness and faintness when arising from bed or chair.

POSSIBLE INTERACTION WITH OTHER SUBSTANCES

INTERACTS WITH	COMBINED EFFECT
Alcohol:	Excessive blood-pressure drop.
Beverages:	None expected.
Cocaine:	Increased risk of heart block and high blood pressure.
Foods:	None expected.
Marijuana:	Possible fainting. Avoid.
Tobacco:	Possible spasm of coronary arteries. Avoid.

PRAZOSIN & POLYTHIAZIDE

BRAND NAMES

Minizide

BASIC INFORMATION

Habit forming? No
Prescription needed? Yes
Available as generic? No
Drug class: Antihypertensive, thiazide diuretic

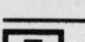

USES

- Controls, but doesn't cure, high blood pressure.
- Reduces fluid retention (edema) caused by conditions such as heart disorders and liver disease.
- Treatment for Raynaud's disease.

DOSAGE & USAGE INFORMATION

How to take:
Tablet or capsule—Swallow with 8 oz. of liquid. If you can't swallow whole, crumble tablet or open capsule and take with liquid or food. Don't exceed dose.

When to take:
At the same times each day.

If you forget a dose:
Take as soon as you remember up to 2 hours late. If more than 2 hours, wait for next scheduled dose (don't double this dose).

Continued next column

OVERDOSE

SYMPTOMS:
Extreme weakness; loss of consciousness; cold, sweaty skin; weak, rapid pulse; cramps; weakness; drowsiness; coma.
WHAT TO DO:
- **Dial 0 (operator) or 911 (emergency) for an ambulance or medical help. Then give first aid immediately.**
- **If patient is unconscious and not breathing, give mouth-to-mouth breathing. If there is no heartbeat, use cardiac massage and mouth-to-mouth breathing (CPR). Don't try to make patient vomit. If you can't get help quickly, take patient to nearest emergency facility.**
- **See emergency information on inside covers.**

What drug does:
- Expands and relaxes blood-vessel walls to lower blood pressure.
- Forces sodium and water excretion, reducing body fluid.
- Relaxes muscle cells of small arteries.
- Reduced body fluid and relaxed arteries lower blood pressure.

Time lapse before drug works:
4 to 6 hours. May require several weeks to lower blood pressure.

Don't take with:
- Non-prescription drugs without consulting doctor.
- See Interaction column and consult doctor.

POSSIBLE ADVERSE REACTIONS OR SIDE EFFECTS

SYMPTOMS	WHAT TO DO
Life-threatening: Irregular heartbeat, weak pulse, fast heartbeat, difficult breathing, chest pain.	Discontinue. Seek emergency treatment.
Common: Nightmares, vivid dreams, drowsiness, dizziness, dry mouth, stuffy nose.	Continue. Call doctor when convenient.
Infrequent: • Blurred vision, abdominal pain, nausea, vomiting, difficult breathing.	Discontinue. Call doctor right away.
• Dizziness, mood change, headache, dry mouth, muscle pain, urgent urination, weakness, tiredness, weight gain or loss, runny nose, joint or muscle pain, agitation, depression, rash, appetite loss, weakness and faintness when arising from bed or chair, constipation.	Continue. Call doctor when convenient.
Rare: • Sore throat, fever, mouth sores; jaundice.	Discontinue. Call doctor right away.
• Diminished sex drive.	Continue. Call doctor when convenient.

WARNINGS & PRECAUTIONS

Don't take if:
- You are allergic to any thiazide diuretic drug or prazosin.
- You are depressed.
- You will have surgery within 2 months, including dental surgery, requiring general or spinal anesthesia.

Before you start, consult your doctor:
- If you are allergic to any sulfa drug.
- If you have gout, impaired brain circulation or have had a stroke, coronary heart disease (with or without angina), kidney disease or impaired liver function.
- If you experience lightheadedness or fainting with other antihypertensive drugs.
- If you are easily depressed.

Over age 60:
- Adverse reactions and side effects may be more frequent and severe than in younger persons, especially dizziness and excessive potassium loss.
- Don't stand while taking. Sudden changes in position may cause falls. Sit or lie down promptly if you feel dizzy. If you have impaired brain circulation or coronary heart disease, excessive lowering of blood pressure should be avoided. Report problems to your doctor immediately.

Pregnancy:
Risk to unborn child outweighs drug benefits. Don't use.

Breast-feeding:
Drug passes into milk. Avoid drug or discontinue nursing until you finish medicine. Consult doctor for advice on maintaining milk supply.

Infants & children:
Not recommended.

Prolonged use:
You may need medicine to treat high blood pressure for the rest of your life.

Skin & sunlight:
May cause rash or intensify sunburn in areas exposed to sun or sunlamp.

Driving, piloting or hazardous work:
Don't drive or pilot aircraft until you learn how medicine affects you. Don't work around dangerous machinery. Don't climb ladders or work in high places. Danger increases if you drink alcohol or take medicine affecting alertness and reflexes, such as antihistamines, tranquilizers, sedatives, pain medicine, narcotics and mind-altering drugs.

Discontinuing:
Don't discontinue without consulting doctor.

Others:
- First dose likely to cause fainting. Take it at night and get out of bed slowly next morning.
- Hot weather and fever may cause dehydration and drop in blood pressure. Dose may require temporary adjustment. Weigh daily and report any unexpected weight decreases to your doctor.
- May cause rise in uric acid, leading to gout.
- May cause blood-sugar rise in diabetics.

POSSIBLE INTERACTION WITH OTHER DRUGS

GENERIC NAME OR DRUG CLASS	COMBINED EFFECT
Acebutolol	Increased antihypertensive effect. Dosages may require adjustments.
ACE inhibitors: captopril, enalapril lisinopril*	Decreased blood pressure.
Allopurinol	Decreased allopurinol effect.
Amphetamines*	Decreased prazosin effect.
Amphotericin B	Increased potassium.
Antidepressants, tricyclic (TCA)*	Dangerous drop in blood pressure. Avoid combination unless under medical supervision.

Continued page 1100

POSSIBLE INTERACTION WITH OTHER SUBSTANCES

INTERACTS WITH	COMBINED EFFECT
Alcohol:	Dangerous blood-pressure drop. Avoid.
Beverages:	None expected.
Cocaine:	Increased risk of heart block and high blood pressure.
Foods: Licorice.	Excessive potassium loss that causes dangerous heart rhythms.
Marijuana:	Possible fainting, may increase blood pressure. Avoid.
Tobacco:	Possible spasm of coronary arteries. Avoid.

PREDNISOLONE

BRAND NAMES

See complete list of brand names in the *Brand Name Directory,* page 1069.

BASIC INFORMATION

Habit forming? No
Prescription needed? Yes
Available as generic? Yes
Drug class: Cortisone drug (adrenal corticosteroid)

 USES

- Reduces inflammation caused by many different medical problems.
- Treatment for some allergic diseases, blood disorders, kidney diseases, asthma and emphysema.
- Replaces corticosteroid deficiencies.

 DOSAGE & USAGE INFORMATION

How to take:
Tablet or liquid—Swallow with liquid or food to lessen stomach irritation. If you can't swallow whole, crumble tablet and take with liquid or food.

When to take:
At the same times each day. Take once-a-day or once-every-other-day doses in mornings.

If you forget a dose:
- Several-doses-per-day prescription—Take as soon as you remember up to 2 hours late. If more than 2 hours, wait for next scheduled dose (don't double this dose).
- Once-a-day dose or less—Wait for next dose. Double this dose.

What drug does:
Decreases inflammatory responses.

Time lapse before drug works:
2 to 4 days.

Don't take with:
See Interaction column and consult doctor.

 OVERDOSE

SYMPTOMS:
Headache, convulsions, heart failure.
WHAT TO DO:
- Dial 0 (operator) or 911 (emergency) for an ambulance or medical help. Then give first aid immediately.
- See emergency information on inside covers.

 POSSIBLE ADVERSE REACTIONS OR SIDE EFFECTS

SYMPTOMS	WHAT TO DO
Life-threatening: Hives, rash, intense itching, faintness soon after a dose (anaphylaxis).	Seek emergency treatment immediately.
Common: Acne, poor wound healing, thirst, indigestion, nausea, vomiting, decreased growth in children.	Continue. Call doctor when convenient.
Infrequent: • Black, bloody or tarry stool.	Discontinue. Seek emergency treatment.
• Blurred vision, halos around lights, sore throat, fever, muscle cramps, swollen legs or feet.	Discontinue. Call doctor right away.
• Mood change, fatigue, insomnia, weakness, restlessness, frequent urination, weight gain, round face, TB recurrence, irregular menstrual periods.	Continue. Call doctor when convenient.
Rare: • Irregular heartbeat.	Discontinue. Seek emergency treatment.
• Rash, numbness or tingling of hands or feet, pancreatitis, hallucinations, thrombophlebitis, convulsions.	Discontinue. Call doctor right away.

 WARNINGS & PRECAUTIONS

Don't take if:
- You are allergic to any cortisone drug.
- You have tuberculosis or fungus infection.
- You have herpes infection of eyes, lips or genitals.

Before you start, consult your doctor:
- If you have had tuberculosis.
- If you have congestive heart failure, diabetes, peptic ulcer, glaucoma, underactive thyroid, high blood pressure, myasthenia gravis, blood clots in legs or lungs.

Over age 60:
Adverse reactions and side effects may be more frequent and severe than in younger persons. Likely to aggravate edema, diabetes or ulcers. Likely to cause cataracts and osteoporosis (softening of the bones).

Pregnancy:
Risk to unborn child outweighs drug benefits. Don't use.

Breast-feeding:
Drug passes into milk. Avoid drug or discontinue nursing until you finish medicine. Consult doctor for advice on maintaining milk supply.

Infants & children:
Use only under medical supervision.

Prolonged use:
- Retards growth in children.
- Possible glaucoma, cataracts, diabetes, fragile bones and thin skin.
- Functional dependence.

Skin & sunlight:
No problems expected.

Driving, piloting or hazardous work:
No problems expected.

Discontinuing:
- Don't discontinue without doctor's advice until you complete prescribed dose, even though symptoms diminish or disappear.
- Drug affects your response to surgery, illness, injury or stress for 2 years after discontinuing. Tell anyone who takes medical care of you within 2 years about drug.

Others:
Avoid immunizations if possible.

POSSIBLE INTERACTION WITH OTHER DRUGS

GENERIC NAME OR DRUG CLASS	COMBINED EFFECT
Amphotericin B	Potassium depletion.
Anticholinergics*	Possible glaucoma.
Anticoagulants, oral*	Decreased anticoagulant effect.
Anticonvulsants, hydantoin*	Decreased prednisolone effect.
Antidiabetics, oral*	Decreased antidiabetic effect.
Antihistamines*	Decreased prednisolone effect.
Aspirin	Increased prednisolone effect.

Attenuated virus vaccines*	Possible viral infection.
Barbiturates*	Decreased prednisolone effect. Oversedation.
Beta-adrenergic blockers*	Decreased prednisolone effect.
Chloral hydrate	Decreased prednisolone effect.
Chlorthalidone	Potassium depletion.
Cholestyramine	Decreased prednisolone absorption effect.
Cholinergics*	Decreased cholinergic effect.
Colestipol	Decreased prednisolone absorption effect.
Contraceptives, oral*	Increased prednisolone effect.
Digitalis preparations*	Dangerous potassium depletion. Possible digitalis toxicity.
Diuretics, thiazide*	Potassium depletion.
Ephedrine	Decreased prednisolone effect.
Estrogens*	Increased prednisolone effect.
Ethacrynic acid	Potassium depletion.
Furosemide	Potassium depletion.
Glutethimide	Decreased prednisolone effect.
Indapamide	Possible excessive potassium loss, causing dangerous heartbeat irregularity.

Continued page 1101

POSSIBLE INTERACTION WITH OTHER SUBSTANCES

INTERACTS WITH	COMBINED EFFECT
Alcohol:	Risk of stomach ulcers.
Beverages:	No proven problems.
Cocaine:	Overstimulation. Avoid.
Foods:	No proven problems.
Marijuana:	Decreased immunity.
Tobacco:	Increased prednisolone effect. Possible toxicity.

*See Glossary

PREDNISONE

BRAND NAMES

Apo-Prednisone	Panasol
Colisone	Paracort
Cortan	Prednicen-M
Deltasone	SK-Prednisone
Liquid-Pred	Sterapred
Meticorten	Sterazolidin
Novoprednisone	Winpred
Orasone	

BASIC INFORMATION

Habit forming? No
Prescription needed? Yes
Available as generic? Yes
Drug class: Cortisone drug (adrenal corticosteroid)

 ## USES

- Reduces inflammation caused by many different medical problems.
- Treatment for some allergic diseases, blood disorders, kidney diseases, asthma and emphysema.
- Replaces corticosteroid deficiencies.

 ## DOSAGE & USAGE INFORMATION

How to take:
Tablet or liquid—Swallow with liquid or food to lessen stomach irritation. If you can't swallow whole, crumble tablet.

When to take:
At the same times each day. Take once-a-day or once-every-other-day doses in mornings.

If you forget a dose:
- Several-doses-per-day prescription—Take as soon as you remember up to 2 hours late. If more than 2 hours, wait for next scheduled dose (don't double this dose).
- Once-a-day dose or less—Wait for next dose. Double this dose.

Continued next column

 ## OVERDOSE

SYMPTOMS:
Headache, convulsions, heart failure.
WHAT TO DO:
- Dial 0 (operator) or 911 (emergency) for an ambulance or medical help. Then give first aid immediately.
- See emergency information on inside covers.

What drug does:
Decreases inflammatory responses.

Time lapse before drug works:
2 to 4 days.

Don't take with:
See Interaction column and consult doctor.

 ## POSSIBLE ADVERSE REACTIONS OR SIDE EFFECTS

SYMPTOMS	WHAT TO DO
Life-threatening: Hives, rash, intense itching, faintness soon after a dose (anaphylaxis).	Seek emergency treatment immediately.
Common: Acne, poor wound healing, thirst, indigestion, nausea, vomiting, decreased growth in children.	Continue. Call doctor when convenient.
Infrequent: • Black, bloody or tarry stool.	Discontinue. Seek emergency treatment.
• Blurred vision, halos around lights, sore throat, fever, muscle cramps, swollen legs or feet.	Discontinue. Call doctor right away.
• Mood change, fatigue, insomnia, weakness, restlessness, frequent urination, weight gain, round face, TB recurrence, irregular menstrual periods.	Continue. Call doctor when convenient.
Rare: • Irregular heartbeat.	Discontinue. Seek emergency treatment.
• Skin rash, fever, joint pain, acute psychosis, hair loss, pancreatitis, numbness or tingling in hands or feet, convulsions, thrombophlebitis, hallucinations.	Discontinue. Call doctor right away.

WARNINGS & PRECAUTIONS

Don't take if:
- You are allergic to any cortisone drug.
- You have tuberculosis or fungus infection.
- You have herpes infection of eyes, lips or genitals.

Before you start, consult your doctor:
- If you have had tuberculosis.
- If you have congestive heart failure.
- If you have diabetes.
- If you have peptic ulcer.
- If you have glaucoma.
- If you have underactive thyroid.
- If you have high blood pressure.
- If you have myasthenia gravis.
- If you have blood clots in legs or lungs.

Over age 60:
Adverse reactions and side effects may be more frequent and severe than in younger persons. Likely to aggravate edema, diabetes or ulcers. Likely to cause cataracts and osteoporosis (softening of the bones).

Pregnancy:
Risk to unborn child outweighs drug benefits. Don't use.

Breast-feeding:
Drug passes into milk. Avoid drug or discontinue nursing until you finish medicine. Consult doctor for advice on maintaining milk supply.

Infants & children:
Use only under medical supervision.

Prolonged use:
- Retards growth in children.
- Possible glaucoma, cataracts, diabetes, fragile bones and thin skin.
- Functional dependence.

Skin & sunlight:
No problems expected.

Driving, piloting or hazardous work:
No problems expected.

Discontinuing:
- Don't discontinue without doctor's advice until you complete prescribed dose, even though symptoms diminish or disappear.
- Drug affects your response to surgery, illness, injury or stress for 2 years after discontinuing. Tell anyone who takes medical care of you within 2 years about drug.

Others:
Avoid immunizations if possible.

POSSIBLE INTERACTION WITH OTHER DRUGS

GENERIC NAME OR DRUG CLASS	COMBINED EFFECT
Amphotericin B	Potassium depletion.
Anticholinergics*	Possible glaucoma.
Anticoagulants, oral*	Decreased anti-coagulant effect.
Anticonvulsants, hydantoin*	Decreased prednisone effect.
Antidiabetics, oral*	Decreased anti-diabetic effect.
Antihistamines*	Decreased prednisone effect.
Aspirin	Increased prednisone effect.
Attenuated virus vaccines*	Possible viral infection.
Barbiturates*	Decreased prednisone effect. Oversedation.
Chloral hydrate	Decreased prednisone effect.
Chlorthalidone	Potassium depletion.
Cholestyramine	Decreased prednisone absorption.
Cholinergics*	Decreased cholinergic effect.
Colestipol	Decreased prednisone absorption.

Continued page 1101

POSSIBLE INTERACTION WITH OTHER SUBSTANCES

INTERACTS WITH	COMBINED EFFECT
Alcohol:	Risk of stomach ulcers.
Beverages:	No proven problems.
Cocaine:	Overstimulation. Avoid.
Foods:	No proven problems.
Marijuana:	Decreased immunity.
Tobacco:	Increased prednisone effect. Possible toxicity.

*See Glossary

PRIMIDONE

BRAND NAMES

Apo-Primidone   Mysoline
Myidone   Sertan

BASIC INFORMATION

Habit forming? No
Prescription needed? Yes
Available as generic? Yes
Drug class: Anticonvulsant

 ## USES

Prevents epileptic seizures.

 ## DOSAGE & USAGE INFORMATION

How to take:
- Tablet—Swallow with liquid. If you can't swallow whole, crumble tablet and take with liquid or food.
- Liquid—If desired, dilute dose in beverage before swallowing.

When to take:
Daily in regularly spaced doses, according to doctor's prescription.

If you forget a dose:
Take as soon as you remember up to 2 hours late. If more than 2 hours, wait for next scheduled dose (don't double this dose).

What drug does:
Probably inhibits repetitious spread of impulses along nerve pathways.

Continued next column

 ## OVERDOSE

SYMPTOMS:
Slow, shallow breathing; weak, rapid pulse; confusion, deep sleep, coma.
WHAT TO DO:
- Dial 0 (operator) or 911 (emergency) for an ambulance or medical help. Then give first aid immediately.
- If patient is unconscious and not breathing, give mouth-to-mouth breathing. If there is no heartbeat, use cardiac massage and mouth-to-mouth breathing (CPR). Don't try to make patient vomit. If you can't get help quickly, take patient to nearest emergency facility.
- See emergency information on inside covers.

Time lapse before drug works:
2 to 3 weeks.

Don't take with:
See Interaction column and consult doctor.

 ## POSSIBLE ADVERSE REACTIONS OR SIDE EFFECTS

SYMPTOMS	WHAT TO DO
Life-threatening: None expected.	
Common:	
• Difficult breathing.	Discontinue. Call doctor right away.
• Confusion, change in vision.	Continue. Call doctor when convenient.
• Clumsiness, dizziness, drowsiness.	Continue. Tell doctor at next visit.
Infrequent:	
• Unusual excitement, particularly in children; nausea; vomiting.	Discontinue. Call doctor right away.
• Headache, fatigue, weakness.	Continue. Call doctor when convenient.
Rare:	
• Rash or hives, appetite loss, acute psychosis, hair loss, fever, joint pain.	Discontinue. Call doctor right away.
• Swollen eyelids or legs.	Continue. Call doctor when convenient.
• Decreased sexual ability.	Continue. Tell doctor at next visit.

 ## WARNINGS & PRECAUTIONS

Don't take if:
- You are allergic to any barbiturate.
- You have had porphyria.

Before you start, consult your doctor:
- If you have had liver, kidney or lung disease or asthma.
- If you have lupus.

Over age 60:
Adverse reactions and side effects may be more frequent and severe than in younger persons.

Pregnancy:
Studies inconclusive on harm to unborn child. Animal studies show fetal abnormalities. Decide with your doctor whether drug benefits justify risk to unborn child.

Breast-feeding:
Drug filters into milk. May harm child. Avoid.

Infants & children:
Use only under medical supervision.

Prolonged use:
- Enlarged lymph and thyroid glands.
- Anemia.
- Rickets in children and osteomalacia (insufficient calcium to bones) in adults.

Skin & sunlight:
None expected.

Driving, piloting or hazardous work:
Don't drive or pilot aircraft until you learn how medicine affects you. Don't work around dangerous machinery. Don't climb ladders or work in high places. Danger increases if you drink alcohol or take medicine affecting alertness and reflexes.

Discontinuing:
Don't discontinue abruptly or without doctor's advice until you complete prescribed dose, even though symptoms diminish or disappear.

Others:
- Tell doctor if you become ill or injured and must interrupt dose schedule.
- Periodic laboratory blood tests of drug level recommended.

POSSIBLE INTERACTION WITH OTHER DRUGS

GENERIC NAME OR DRUG CLASS	COMBINED EFFECT
Anticoagulants, oral*	Decreased primidone effect.
Anticonvulsants, other*	Changed seizure pattern.
Antidepressants*	Increased anti-depressant effect.
Antidiabetics*	Increased effect of primidone sedation.
Antihistamines*	Increased effect of primidone sedation.
Aspirin	Decreased aspirin effect.
Carbamazepine	Unpredictable increase or decrease of primidone effect.
Carbonic anhydrase inhibitors*	Possible decreased primidone effect.
Contraceptives, oral*	Decreased contraceptive effect.
Cortisone drugs*	Decreased cortisone effect.
Cyclosporine	Decreased effect of cyclosporine.
Digitalis preparations*	Decreased digitalis effect.
Disulfiram	Possible increased primidone effect.
Estrogens*	Decreased estrogen effect.
Griseofulvin	Possible decreased griseofulvin effect.
Isoniazid	Decreased primidone effect.
Leucovorin (large dose)	May counteract anti-convulsant effect of primidone.
Loxapine	Decreased anti-convulsant effect of primidone.
MAO inhibitors*	Increased effect of primidone sedation.
Metronidazole	Possible decreased metronidazole effect.
Mind-altering drugs*	Increased effect of mind-altering drugs.
Nabilone	Greater depression of central nervous system.
Narcotics*	Increased narcotic effect.
Oxyphenbutazone	Decreased oxyphen-butazone effect.
Phenylbutazone	Decreased phenyl-butazone effect.
Phenytoin	Possible increased primidone toxicity.
Rifampin	Possible decreased primidone effect.

Continued page 1102

POSSIBLE INTERACTION WITH OTHER SUBSTANCES

INTERACTS WITH	COMBINED EFFECT
Alcohol:	Dangerous sedative effect. Avoid.
Beverages:	None expected.
Cocaine:	Decreased primidone effect.
Foods:	Possible need for more vitamin D.
Marijuana:	Decreased anticon-vulsant effect of primidone. Drowsiness, unsteadiness.
Tobacco:	None expected.

*See Glossary

829

PROBENECID

BRAND NAMES

Benacen
Benemid
Benuryl
ColBENEMID

Col-Probenecid
Polycillin-PRB
Probalan
SK-Probenecid

BASIC INFORMATION

Habit forming? No
Prescription needed? Yes
Available as generic? Yes
Drug class: Antigout (uricosuric)

USES

- Treatment for chronic gout.
- Increases blood levels of penicillins and cephalosporins.

DOSAGE & USAGE INFORMATION

How to take:
Tablet—Swallow with liquid or food to lessen stomach irritation. If you can't swallow whole, crumble tablet and take with liquid or food.

When to take:
At the same time each day.

If you forget a dose:
Take as soon as you remember up to 12 hours late. If more than 12 hours, wait for next scheduled dose (don't double this dose).

What drug does:
- Forces kidneys to excrete uric acid.
- Reduces amount of penicillin excreted in urine.

Time lapse before drug works:
May require several months of regular use to prevent acute gout.

Continued next column

OVERDOSE

SYMPTOMS:
Breathing difficulty, severe nervous agitation, vomiting, seizures, convulsions, delirium, coma.
WHAT TO DO:
- Dial 0 (operator) or 911 (emergency) for an ambulance or medical help. Then give first aid immediately.
- See emergency information on inside covers.

Don't take with:
- Non-prescription drugs containing aspirin or caffeine.
- See Interaction column and consult doctor.

POSSIBLE ADVERSE REACTIONS OR SIDE EFFECTS

SYMPTOMS	WHAT TO DO
Life-threatening: None expected.	
Common: Headache, appetite loss, nausea, vomiting.	Continue. Call doctor when convenient.
Infrequent: • Blood in urine, low back pain. worsening gout.	Discontinue. Call doctor right away.
• Dizziness, flushed face, itchy skin.	Continue. Call doctor when convenient.
• Painful or frequent urination.	Continue. Tell doctor at next visit.
Rare: Sore throat; difficult breathing; unusual bleeding or bruising; red, painful joint; jaundice; fever.	Discontinue. Call doctor right away.

WARNINGS & PRECAUTIONS

Don't take if:
- You are allergic to any uricosuric.
- You have acute gout.
- Patient is younger than 2.

Before you start, consult your doctor:
- If you have had kidney stones or kidney disease.
- If you have a peptic ulcer.
- If you have bone-marrow or blood-cell disease.

Over age 60:
Adverse reactions and side effects may be more frequent and severe than in younger persons.

Pregnancy:
Studies inconclusive on harm to unborn child. Animal studies show fetal abnormalities. Decide with your doctor whether drug benefits justify risk to unborn child.

Breast-feeding:
No proven problems.

Infants & children:
Not recommended.

Prolonged use:
Possible kidney damage.

Skin & sunlight:
No problems expected.

Driving, piloting or hazardous work:
Avoid if you feel dizzy. Otherwise, no problems expected.

Discontinuing:
Don't discontinue without consulting doctor. Dose may require gradual reduction if you have taken drug for a long time. Doses of other drugs may also require adjustment.

Others:
If signs of gout attack develop while taking medicine, consult doctor.

POSSIBLE INTERACTION WITH OTHER DRUGS

GENERIC NAME OR DRUG CLASS	COMBINED EFFECT
Allopurinol	Increased effect of each drug.
Anticoagulants, oral*	Increased anti-coagulant effect.
Aspirin	Decreased probenecid effect.
Bismuth subsalicylate	Decreased effect of probenecid.
Cephalosporins*	Increased cephalosporin effect.
Ciprofloxacin	May cause kidney dysfunction.
Dapsone	Increased dapsone effect. Increased toxicity.
Diclofenac	Increased diclofenac effect.
Diuretics, thiazide*	Decreased probenecid effect.
Hypoglycemics, oral*	Increased hypo-glycemic effect.
Indomethacin	Increased adverse effects of indomethacin.
Methotrexate	Increased methotrexate toxicity.
Nitrofurantoin	Incresed effect of nitrofurantoin.
Para-aminosalicylic acid (PAS)	Increased effect of para-aminosalicylic acid.
Penicillins*	Enhanced penicillin effect.
Pyrazinamide	Decreased probenecid effect.
Salicylates*	Decreased probenecid effect.
Sulfa drugs*	Slows elimination. May cause harmful accumulation of sulfa.

POSSIBLE INTERACTION WITH OTHER SUBSTANCES

INTERACTS WITH	COMBINED EFFECT
Alcohol:	Decreased probenecid effect.
Beverages: Caffeine drinks.	Loss of probenecid effectiveness.
Cocaine:	None expected.
Foods:	None expected.
Marijuana:	Daily use— Decreased probenecid effect.
Tobacco:	None expected.

*See Glossary

PROBENECID & COLCHICINE

BRAND NAMES

Colabid
Col Benemid
Col-Probencid
Proben-C

BASIC INFORMATION

Habit forming? No
Prescription needed? Yes
Available as generic? Yes
Drug class: Antigout (uricosuric)

USES

- Increases blood levels of penicillins and cephalosporins.
- Relieves joint pain, inflammation, swelling from gout.
- Also used for familial Mediterranean fever, dermatitis herpetiformis.

DOSAGE & USAGE INFORMATION

How to take:
Tablet—Swallow with liquid or food to lessen stomach irritation. If you can't swallow whole, crumble tablet and take with liquid or food.

When to take:
At the same time each day.

If you forget a dose:
Take as soon as you remember up to 12 hours late. If more than 12 hours, wait for next scheduled dose (don't double this dose).

What drug does:
- Forces kidneys to excrete uric acid.
- Reduces amount of penicillin excreted in urine.
- Decreases acidity of joint tissues and prevents deposits of uric-acid crystals.

Continued next column

OVERDOSE

SYMPTOMS:
Breathing difficulty, severe nervous agitation, convulsions, bloody urine, diarrhea, vomiting, muscle weakness, fever, stupor, seizures, delirium, coma.
WHAT TO DO:
- **Dial 0 (operator) or 911 (emergency) for an ambulance or medical help. Then give first aid immediately.**
- **See emergency information on inside covers.**

Time lapse before drug works:
12 to 48 hours.

Don't take with:
- Non-prescription drugs containing aspirin or caffeine.
- See Interaction column and consult doctor.

POSSIBLE ADVERSE REACTIONS OR SIDE EFFECTS

SYMPTOMS	WHAT TO DO
Life-threatening: Blood in urine; convulsions; severe muscle weakness; difficult breathing; burning feeling of stomach, throat or skin; worsening gout.	Discontinue. Seek emergency treatment.
Common: Diarrhea, headache, abdominal pain.	Discontinue. Call doctor right away.
Infrequent: • Back pain; painful, difficult urination.	Discontinue. Call doctor right away.
• Dizziness, red or flushed face, urgent urination, sore gums, hair loss.	Continue. Call doctor when convenient.
Rare: Sudden decrease in urine output; nausea; vomiting; mood change; fever; diarrhea; jaundice; numbness or tingling in hands or feet; rash; sore throat, fever, mouth sores; swollen feet and ankles; unexplained bleeding or bruising; weight gain or loss; low white or red blood cells.	Discontinue. Call doctor right away.

WARNINGS & PRECAUTIONS

Don't take if:
You are allergic to any uricosuric or colchicine.

Before you start, consult your doctor:
- If you have had kidney stones, kidney disease, heart or liver disease, peptic ulcers or ulcerative colitis.
- If you have bone-marrow or blood-cell disease.
- If you will have surgery within 2 months, including dental surgery, requiring general or spinal anesthesia.

Over age 60:
Adverse reactions and side effects may be more frequent and severe than in younger persons. Colchicine has a narrow margin of safety for people in this age group.

Pregnancy:
Risk to unborn child outweighs drug benefits. Don't use.

Breast-feeding:
No problems expected, but consult doctor.

Infants & children:
Not recommended.

Prolonged use:
- Possible kidney damage.
- Permanent hair loss.
- Anemia. Request blood counts.
- Numbness or tingling in hands and feet.

Skin & sunlight:
No problems expected.

Driving, piloting or hazardous work:
Don't drive or pilot aircraft until you learn how medicine affects you. Don't work around dangerous machinery. Don't climb ladders or work in high places. Danger increases if you drink alcohol or take medicine affecting alertness and reflexes, such as antihistamines, tranquilizers, sedatives, pain medicine, narcotics and mind-altering drugs.

Discontinuing:
- May be unnecessary to finish medicine. Follow doctor's instructions.
- Stop taking if severe digestive upsets occur before symptoms are relieved.

Others:
- If signs of gout attack develop while taking medicine, consult doctor.
- Limit each course of treatment to 8 mg. Don't exceed 3 mg. per 24 hours.
- Possible sperm damage. May cause birth defects if child conceived while father taking colchicine.

POSSIBLE INTERACTION WITH OTHER DRUGS

GENERIC NAME OR DRUG CLASS	COMBINED EFFECT
Acetohexamide	Increased acetohexamide effect.
Allopurinol	Increased effect of each drug.
Anticoagulants*	Irregular effect on anticoagulation, sometimes increased, sometimes decreased. Follow prothrombin times.
Antidepressants*	Oversedation.
Antihistamines*	Oversedation.
Antihypertensives*	Decreased antihypertensive effect.
Appetite suppressants*	Increased suppressant effect.
Bismuth subsalicylate	Decreased effect of probenecid.
Cephalosporins*	Increased cephalosporin effect.
Dapsone	Increased dapsone effect. Increased toxicity.
Diclofenac	Increased diclofenac effect.

Continued page 1102

POSSIBLE INTERACTION WITH OTHER SUBSTANCES

INTERACTS WITH	COMBINED EFFECT
Alcohol:	Decreased probenecid effect.
Beverages: Caffeine drinks.	Loss of probenecid effectiveness.
Herbal teas.	Increased colchicine effect. Avoid.
Cocaine:	Overstimulation. Avoid.
Foods:	No proven problems.
Marijuana:	Decreased colchicine and probenecid effect.
Tobacco:	No proven problems.

*See Glossary

PROBUCOL

BRAND NAMES

Lorelco

BASIC INFORMATION

Habit forming? No
Prescription needed? Yes
Available as generic? No
Drug class: Antihyperlipidemic

 USES

Lowers cholesterol level in blood in persons with type IIa hyperlipoproteinemia.

 DOSAGE & USAGE INFORMATION

How to take:
Tablet—Swallow with liquid. If you can't swallow whole, crumble tablet and take with liquid or food.

When to take:
With morning and evening meals.

If you forget a dose:
Take as soon as you remember up to 2 hours late. If more than 2 hours, wait for next scheduled dose (don't double this dose).

What drug does:
Reduces serum cholesterol without reducing liver cholesterol.

Time lapse before drug works:
3 to 4 months.

Don't take with:
Other medicines or vitamins. Separate by 1 to 2 hours.

 OVERDOSE

SYMPTOMS:
None reported.
WHAT TO DO:
Overdose unlikely to threaten life. If person takes much larger amount than prescribed, call doctor, poison-control center or hospital emergency room for instructions.

 POSSIBLE ADVERSE REACTIONS OR SIDE EFFECTS

SYMPTOMS	WHAT TO DO
Life-threatening: None expected.	
Common: Bloating, diarrhea, nausea, vomiting, stomach pain, flatus.	Continue. Call doctor when convenient.
Infrequent: • Dizziness, headache.	Discontinue. Call doctor right away.
• Numbness or tingling in feet, toes, fingers, face.	Continue. Call doctor when convenient.
Rare: • Swelling of hands, face, feet, mouth; difficult breathing.	Discontinue. Seek emergency treatment.
• Rash, gastrointestinal bleeding.	Discontinue. Call doctor right away.
• Insomnia, blurred vision, diminished taste, appetite loss, spots under skin, easy bruising, impotence.	Continue. Call doctor when convenient.

WARNINGS & PRECAUTIONS

Don't take if:
You are allergic to probucol.

Before you start, consult your doctor:
- If you have liver disease such as cirrhosis.
- If you have heartbeat irregularity.
- If you have congestive heart failure that is not under control.
- If you have gallstones.

Over age 60:
Adverse reactions and side effects may be more frequent and severe than in younger persons.

Pregnancy:
No proven problems. Avoid if possible. Continue using birth-control methods for 6 months after discontinuing medicine.

Breast-feeding:
Not recommended. Animal studies show drug passes into milk. Studies not available for human beings.

Infants & children:
Not recommended. Safety and dosage have not been established.

Prolonged use:
Request serum cholesterol and serum triglyceride laboratory studies every 2 to 4 months.

Skin & sunlight:
No problems expected.

Driving, piloting or hazardous work:
If medicine does not cause dizziness, no problems expected.

Discontinuing:
Don't discontinue without consulting doctor. Dose may require gradual reduction if you have taken drug for a long time. Doses of other drugs may also require adjustment.

Others:
Medicine works best in conjunction with low-fat, low-cholesterol diet and an active, regular exercise program.

POSSIBLE INTERACTION WITH OTHER DRUGS

GENERIC NAME OR DRUG CLASS	COMBINED EFFECT
Clofibrate	Combination no more effective than one drug only, so don't take both.

POSSIBLE INTERACTION WITH OTHER SUBSTANCES

INTERACTS WITH	COMBINED EFFECT
Alcohol:	May aggravate liver problems. Avoid.
Beverages:	None expected.
Cocaine:	None expected.
Foods:	None expected.
Marijuana:	None expected.
Tobacco:	None expected.

PROCAINAMIDE

BRAND NAMES

Procan
Procan SR
Procamide
Procapan
Promine

Pronestyl
Pronestyl SR
Rhythmin
Sub-Quin

BASIC INFORMATION

Habit forming? No
Prescription needed? Yes
Available as generic? Yes
Drug class: Antiarrhythmic

USES

Stabilizes irregular heartbeat.

DOSAGE & USAGE INFORMATION

How to take:
* Tablet or capsule—Swallow with liquid.
* Extended-release tablets—Swallow each dose whole. Do not crush them.

When to take:
Best taken on empty stomach, 1 hour before or 2 hours after meals. If necessary, may be taken with food or milk to lessen stomach upset.

If you forget a dose:
Take as soon as you remember up to 2 hours late. If more than 2 hours, wait for next scheduled dose (don't double this dose).

What drug does:
Slows activity of pacemaker (rhythm-control center of heart) and delays transmission of electrical impulses.

Time lapse before drug works:
30 to 60 minutes.

Don't take with:
See Interaction column and consult doctor.

OVERDOSE

SYMPTOMS:
Fast and irregular heartbeat, confusion, stupor, decreased blood pressure, fainting, cardiac arrest.
WHAT TO DO:
* Dial 0 (operator) or 911 (emergency) for an ambulance or medical help. Then give first aid immediately.
* See emergency information on inside covers.

POSSIBLE ADVERSE REACTIONS OR SIDE EFFECTS

SYMPTOMS	WHAT TO DO
Life-threatening: Hives, rash, intense itching, faintness soon after dose (anaphylaxis).	seek emergency treatment immediately.
Common: Diarrhea, appetite loss, nausea, vomiting, bitter taste.	Continue. Call doctor when convenient.
Infrequent:	
• Joint pain, painful breathing.	Discontinue. Call doctor right away.
• Dizziness.	Continue. Call doctor when convenient.
Rare:	
• Hallucinations, depression, confusion, psychosis, itchy skin, rash, sore throat, fever, jaundice, convulsions.	Discontinue. Call doctor right away.
• Headache, fatigue	Continue. Call doctor when convenient.

WARNINGS & PRECAUTIONS

Don't take if:
- You are allergic to procainamide.
- You have myasthenia gravis.

Before you start, consult your doctor:
- If you are allergic to local anesthetics that end in "caine."
- If you have had liver or kidney disease or impaired kidney function.
- If you have had lupus.
- If you take digitalis preparations.
- If you will have surgery within 2 months, including dental surgery, requiring general or spinal anesthesia.

Over age 60:
Adverse reactions and side effects may be more frequent and severe than in younger persons.

Pregnancy:
No proven harm to unborn child. Avoid if possible.

Breast-feeding:
No proven problems. Consult doctor.

Infants & children:
Not recommended.

Prolonged use:
May cause lupus-like illness.

Skin & sunlight:
No problems expected.

Driving, piloting or hazardous work:
Use caution if you feel dizzy or weak. Otherwise, no problems expected.

Discontinuing:
Don't discontinue without doctor's advice until you complete prescribed dose, even though symptoms diminish or disappear.

Others:
Some products contain tartrazine dye. Avoid, especially if you are allergic to aspirin.

POSSIBLE INTERACTION WITH OTHER DRUGS

GENERIC NAME OR DRUG CLASS	COMBINED EFFECT
Acetazolamide	Increased procainamide effect.
Ambenonium	Decreased ambenonium effect.
Aminoglycosides*	Possible severe muscle weakness, impaired breathing.
Antiarrhythmics, other*	Increased likelihood of adverse reactions with either drug. Possible increased effect of both drugs.
Antihypertensives*	Increased antihypertensive effect.
Antimyasthenics*	Decreased antimyasthenic effect.
Anticholinergics*	Increased anticholinergic effect.
Cimetidine	Increased procainamide effect.
Encainide	Increased effect of toxicity on heart muscle.
Guanfacine	Increased effect of both medicines.
Kanamycin	Possible severe muscle weakness, impaired breathing.
Neomycin	Possible severe muscle weakness, impaired breathing.
Nicardipine	Possible increased effect and toxicity of each drug.
Nizatidine	Increased effect and toxicity of procainamide.

POSSIBLE INTERACTION WITH OTHER SUBSTANCES

INTERACTS WITH	COMBINED EFFECT
Alcohol:	None expected.
Beverages: Caffeine drinks, iced drinks.	Irregular heartbeat.
Cocaine:	Decreased procainamide effect.
Foods:	None expected.
Marijuana:	None expected.
Tobacco:	Decreased procainamide effect.

*See Glossary

PROCARBAZINE

BRAND NAMES

Matulane   Natulan

BASIC INFORMATION

Habit forming? No
Prescription needed? Yes
Available as generic? No
Drug class: Antineoplastic

 ## USES

Treatment for some kinds of cancer.

 ## DOSAGE & USAGE INFORMATION

How to take:
Capsule—Swallow with liquid after light meal.
Don't drink fluids with meals. Drink extra fluids
between meals. Avoid sweet or fatty foods.

When to take:
At the same time each day.

If you forget a dose:
Take as soon as you remember. Don't double
dose ever.

What drug does:
Inhibits abnormal cell reproduction. Procarbazine
is an alkylating agent and a MAO inhibitor.

Time lapse before drug works:
Up to 6 weeks for full effect.

Don't take with:
See Interaction column and consult doctor.

 ## OVERDOSE

SYMPTOMS:
**Restlessness, agitation, fever, convulsions,
bleeding.**
WHAT TO DO:
- **Dial 0 (operator) or 911 (emergency) for
  an ambulance or medical help. Then give
  first aid immediately.**
- **If patient is unconscious and not
  breathing, give mouth-to-mouth
  breathing. If there is no heartbeat, use
  cardiac massage and mouth-to-mouth
  breathing (CPR). Don't try to make patient
  vomit. If you can't get help quickly, take
  patient to nearest emergency facility.**
- **See emergency information on inside
  covers.**

 ## POSSIBLE ADVERSE REACTIONS OR SIDE EFFECTS

SYMPTOMS	WHAT TO DO
Life-threatening: None expected.	
Common:	
• Nausea, vomiting, decreased urination, numbness or tingling in hands or feet, hair loss.	Discontinue. Call doctor right away.
• Fatigue, weakness.	Continue. Call doctor when convenient.
• Dizziness when changing position, dry mouth, inflamed tongue, constipation, difficult urination.	Continue. Tell doctor at next visit.
Infrequent:	
• Fainting.	Discontinue. Seek emergency treatment.
• Severe headache; abnormal bleeding or bruising; muscle, joint or chest pain.	Discontinue. Call doctor right away.
• Hallucinations, insomnia, nightmares, diarrhea, rapid or pounding heartbeat, swollen feet or legs, nervousness.	Continue. Call doctor when convenient.
• Diminished sex drive.	Continue. Tell doctor at next visit.
Rare: Rash, stiff neck, jaundice, fever, sore throat.	Discontinue. Call doctor right away.

 ## WARNINGS & PRECAUTIONS

Don't take if:
- You are allergic to any MAO inhibitor.
- You have heart disease, congestive heart
  failure, heart-rhythm irregularities or high
  blood pressure.
- You have liver or kidney disease.

Before you start, consult your doctor:
- If you are alcoholic.
- If you have asthma.
- If you have had a stroke.
- If you have diabetes or epilepsy.
- If you have overactive thyroid.
- If you have schizophrenia.
- If you have Parkinson's disease.
- If you have adrenal-gland tumor.
- If you will have surgery within 2 months,
  including dental surgery, requiring general or
  spinal anesthesia.

Over age 60:
Not recommended.

Pregnancy:
Avoid if possible.

Breast-feeding:
Safety not established. Consult doctor.

Infants & children:
Not recommended.

Prolonged use:
May be toxic to liver.

Skin & sunlight:
May cause rash or intensify sunburn in areas exposed to sun or sunlamp.

Driving, piloting or hazardous work:
Don't drive or pilot aircraft until you learn how medicine affects you. Don't work around dangerous machinery. Don't climb ladders or work in high places. Danger increases if you drink alcohol or take medicine affecting alertness and reflexes.

Discontinuing:
- Don't discontinue without doctor's advice until you complete prescribed dose, even though symptoms diminish or disappear.
- Follow precautions regarding foods, drinks and other medicines for 2 weeks after discontinuing.

Others:
- May affect blood-sugar levels in patients with diabetes.
- Fever may indicate that MAO inhibitor dose requires adjustment.

POSSIBLE INTERACTION WITH OTHER DRUGS

GENERIC NAME OR DRUG CLASS	COMBINED EFFECT
Amphetamines*	Blood-pressure rise to life-threatening level.
Anticonvulsants*	Changed seizure pattern.
Antidepressants, tricyclic (TCA)*	Blood-pressure rise to life-threatening level.
Antidiabetics, oral and insulin*	Excessively low blood sugar.
Antihistamines*	Increased sedation.
Barbiturates*	Increased sedation.
Caffeine	Irregular heartbeat or high blood pressure.
Carbamazepine	Fever, seizures. Avoid.
Cyclobenzaprine	Fever, seizures. Avoid.

Diuretics*	Excessively low blood pressure.
Ethinamate	Dangerous increased effects of ethinamate. Avoid combining.
Fluoxetine	Increased depressant effects of both drugs.
Guanethidine	Blood-pressure rise to life-threatening level.
Guanfacine	May increase depressant effects of either medicine.
Levodopa	Sudden, severe blood-pressure rise.
Leucovorin	High alcohol content of leucovorin may cause adverse effects.
MAO inhibitors, other*	High fever, convulsions, death.
Methyprylon	May increase sedative effect to dangerous level. Avoid.
Nabilone	Greater depression of central nervous system.
Narcotics*	Increased sedation.
Phenothiazines*	Increased sedation.
Reserpine	Increased blood pressure, excitation.

POSSIBLE INTERACTION WITH OTHER SUBSTANCES

INTERACTS WITH	COMBINED EFFECT
Alcohol:	Increased sedation to dangerous level. Disulfiram-like reaction.
Beverages: Caffeine drinks.	Irregular heartbeat or high blood pressure.
Drinks containing tyramine*	Blood-pressure rise to life-threatening level.
Cocaine:	Overstimulation. Possibly fatal.
Foods: Foods containing tyramine*	Blood-pressure rise to life-threatening level.
Marijuana:	Overstimulation. Avoid.
Tobacco:	No proven problems.

PROCHLORPERAZINE

BRAND NAMES

Chlorazine
Combid
Compazine
Eskatrol

Prochlor-Iso
Pro-Iso
Stemetil

BASIC INFORMATION

Habit forming? No
Prescription needed? Yes
Available as generic? Yes
Drug class: Tranquilizer, antiemetic
(phenothiazine)

 USES

- Stops nausea, vomiting, hiccups.
- Reduces anxiety, agitation.

 DOSAGE & USAGE INFORMATION

How to take:
- Tablet, sustained-release capsule or syrup—Swallow with liquid or food to lessen stomach irritation.
- Suppositories—Remove wrapper and moisten suppository with water. Gently insert into rectum, large end first.
- Drops or liquid—Dilute dose in beverage.

When to take:
- Nervous and mental disorders—Take at the same times each day.
- Nausea and vomiting—Take as needed, no more often than every 4 hours.

If you forget a dose:
- Nervous and mental disorders—Take up to 2 hours late. If more than 2 hours, wait for next scheduled dose (don't double this dose).
- Nausea and vomiting—Take as soon as you remember. Wait 4 hours for next dose.

Continued next column

 OVERDOSE

SYMPTOMS:
Stupor, convulsions, coma.
WHAT TO DO:
- Dial 0 (operator) or 911 (emergency) for an ambulance or medical help. Then give first aid immediately.
- See emergency information on inside covers.

What drug does:
- Suppresses brain's vomiting center.
- Suppresses brain centers that control abnormal emotions and behavior.

Time lapse before drug works:
- Nausea and vomiting—1 hour or less.
- Nervous and mental disorders—4-6 weeks.

Don't take with:
- Antacid or medicine for diarrhea.
- Non-prescription drug for cough, cold or allergy.
- See Interaction column and consult doctor.

 POSSIBLE ADVERSE REACTIONS OR SIDE EFFECTS

SYMPTOMS	WHAT TO DO
Life-threatening:	
Uncontrolled muscle movements of tongue, face and other muscles (neuroleptic malignant syndrome, rare).	Discontinue. Seek emergency treatment.
Common:	
Muscle spasms of face and neck, unsteady gait.	Discontinue. Seek emergency treatment.
Restlessness, tremor, drowsiness.	Discontinue. Call doctor right away.
Decreased sweating, dry mouth, runny nose, constipation.	Continue. Call doctor when convenient.
Infrequent:	
Fainting.	Discontinue. Seek emergency treatment.
Rash.	Discontinue. Call doctor right away.
Difficult urination, diminished sex drive, swollen breasts, menstrual irregularities.	Continue. Call doctor when convenient.
Rare:	
Change in vision, sore throat, fever, jaundice, abdominal pain.	Discontinue. Call doctor right away.

WARNINGS & PRECAUTIONS

Don't take if:
- You are allergic to any phenothiazine.
- You have a blood or bone-marrow disease.

Before you start, consult your doctor:
- If you will have surgery within 2 months, including dental surgery, requiring general or spinal anesthesia.
- If you have asthma, emphysema or other lung disorder, glaucoma, prostate trouble.
- If you take non-prescription ulcer medicine, asthma medicine or amphetamines.

Over age 60:
Adverse reactions and side effects may be more frequent and severe than in younger persons. More likely to develop involuntary movement of jaws, lips, tongue, chewing. Report this to your doctor immediately. Early treatment can help.

Pregnancy:
Risk to unborn child outweighs drug benefits. Don't use.

Breast-feeding:
Drug passes into milk. Avoid drug or discontinue nursing until you finish medicine. Consult doctor for advice on maintaining milk supply.

Infants & children:
Don't give to children younger than 2.

Prolonged use:
May lead to tardive dyskinesia (involuntary movement of jaws, lips, tongue, chewing).

Skin & sunlight:
May cause rash or intensify sunburn in areas exposed to sun or sunlamp. Skin may remain sensitive for 3 months after discontinuing.

Driving, piloting or hazardous work:
Don't drive or pilot aircraft until you learn how medicine affects you. Don't work around dangerous machinery. Don't climb ladders or work in high places. Danger increases if you drink alcohol or take medicine affecting alertness and reflexes.

Discontinuing:
- Nervous and mental disorders—Don't discontinue without doctor's advice until you complete prescribed dose, even though symptoms diminish or disappear.
- Nausea and vomiting—May be unnecessary to finish medicine. Follow doctor's instructions.

Others:
No problems expected.

POSSIBLE INTERACTION WITH OTHER DRUGS

GENERIC NAME OR DRUG CLASS	COMBINED EFFECT
Anticholinergics*	Increased anticholinergic effect.
Antidepressants, tricyclic (TCA)*	Increased prochlorperazine effect.
Antihistamines*	Increased antihistamine effect.
Appetite suppressants*	Decreased suppressant effect.
Dronabinol	Increased effects of both drugs. Avoid.
Guanethidine	Decreased guanethidine effect.
Levodopa	Decreased levodopa effect.
Mind-altering drugs*	Increased effect of mind-altering drugs.
Molindone	Increased tranquilizer effect.
Nabilone	Greater depression of central nervous system.
Narcotics*	Increased narcotic effect.
Phenytoin	Increased phenytoin effect.
Procarbazine	Increased sedation.
Quinidine	Impaired heart function. Dangerous mixture.
Sedatives*	Increased sedation.
Tranquilizers, other*	Increased tranquilizer effect.

POSSIBLE INTERACTION WITH OTHER SUBSTANCES

INTERACTS WITH	COMBINED EFFECT
Alcohol:	Dangerous oversedation.
Beverages:	None expected.
Cocaine:	Decreased prochlorperazine effect. Avoid.
Foods:	None expected.
Marijuana:	Drowsiness. May increase antinausea effect.
Tobacco:	None expected.

*See Glossary

PROCHLORPERAZINE & ISOPROPAMIDE

BRAND NAMES

Combid Spansules

BASIC INFORMATION

Habit forming? No
Prescription needed? Yes
Available as generic? No
Drug class: Antispasmodic, antiemetic,
**   tranquilizer (phenothiazine)**

 ## USES

- Stops nausea, vomiting, hiccups.
- Reduces anxiety, agitation.
- Reduces spasms of digestive system.

 ## DOSAGE & USAGE INFORMATION

How to take:
- Tablet or capsule—Swallow with liquid or food to lessen stomach irritation.
- Extended-release tablets or capsules— Swallow each dose whole. If you take regular tablets, you may chew or crush them.

When to take:
30 minutes before meals (unless directed otherwise by doctor).

If you forget a dose:
Take as soon as you remember up to 2 hours late. If more than 2 hours, wait for next scheduled dose (don't double this dose).

What drug does:
- Suppresses brain's vomiting center.
- Suppresses brain centers that control abnormal emotions and behavior.
- Blocks nerve impulses at parasympathetic nerve endings, preventing muscle contractions and gland secretions of organs involved.

Continued next column

 ## OVERDOSE

SYMPTOMS:
Dilated pupils, rapid pulse and breathing, dizziness, fever, hallucinations, confusion, slurred speech, agitation, flushed face, convulsions, stupor, coma.
WHAT TO DO:
- **Dial 0 (operator) or 911 (emergency) for an ambulance or medical help. Then give first aid immediately.**
- **See emergency information on inside covers.**

Time lapse before drug works:
15 to 30 minutes.

Don't take with:
- Antacid or medicine for diarrhea.
- Non-prescription drugs for cough, cold or allergy.
- See Interaction column and consult doctor.

 ## POSSIBLE ADVERSE REACTIONS OR SIDE EFFECTS

SYMPTOMS	WHAT TO DO
Life-threatening:	
Fainting; dilated pupils; rapid pulse; muscle spasms; hallucinations; unsteady gait; uncontrolled muscle movements of tongue, face and other muscles (neuroleptic malignant syndrome, rare).	Discontinue. Seek emergency treatment.
Common:	
• Restlessness, tremor, confusion, drowsiness, rash.	Discontinue. Call doctor right away.
• Decreased sweating, dry mouth, runny nose, constipation, nausea.	Continue. Call doctor when convenient.
Infrequent:	
• Painful, difficult urination; vomiting.	Discontinue. Call doctor right away.
• Headache, diminished sex drive, swollen breasts, menstrual irregularities.	Continue. Call doctor when convenient.
Rare:	
Hives; change in vision; eye pain; sore throat, fever, mouth sores.	Discontinue. Call doctor right away.

 ## WARNINGS & PRECAUTIONS

Don't take if:
- You are allergic to any anticholinergic or phenothiazine.
- You have trouble with stomach bloating, difficulty emptying your bladder completely, narrow-angle glaucoma, severe ulcerative colitis, a blood or bone-marrow diease.

PROCHLORPERAZINE & ISOPROPAMIDE

Before you start, consult your doctor:
- If you have open-angle glaucoma, angina, chronic bronchitis or asthma, hiatal hernia, liver disease, enlarged prostate, myasthenia gravis, peptic ulcer, emphysema or other lung disorder.
- If you take non-prescription ulcer medicine, asthma medicine or amphetamines.
- If you will have surgery within 2 months, including dental surgery, requiring general or spinal anesthesia.

Over age 60:
Adverse reactions and side effects may be more frequent and severe than in younger persons. More likely to develop involuntary movement of jaws, lips, tongue, chewing. Report this to your doctor immediately. Early treatment can help.

Pregnancy:
Risk to unborn child outweighs drug benefits. Don't use.

Breast-feeding:
Drug passes into milk. Avoid drug or discontinue nursing until you finish medicine. Consult doctor for advice on maintaining milk supply.

Infants & children:
Use only under medical supervision.

Prolonged use:
- Chronic constipation, possible fecal impaction.
- May lead to tardive dyskinesia (involuntary movement of jaws, lips, tongue, chewing).

Skin & sunlight:
May cause rash or intensify sunburn in areas exposed to sun or sunlamp. Skin may remain sensitive for 3 months after discontinuing.

Driving, piloting or hazardous work:
Don't drive or pilot aircraft until you learn how medicine affects you. Don't work around dangerous machinery. Don't climb ladders or work in high places. Danger increases if you drink alcohol or take medicine affecting alertness and reflexes, such as antihistamines, tranquilizers, sedatives, pain medicine, narcotics and mind-altering drugs.

Discontinuing:
- May be unnecessary to finish medicine. Follow doctor's instructions.
- If you develop withdrawal symptoms of hallucinations, agitation or sleeplessness after discontinuing, call doctor right away.

Others:
No problems expected.

POSSIBLE INTERACTION WITH OTHER DRUGS

GENERIC NAME OR DRUG CLASS	COMBINED EFFECT
Amantadine	Increased isopropamide effect.
Anticholinergics*	Increased anticholingeric effect.
Antidepressants, tricyclic (TCA)*	Increased atropine effect. Increased sedation.
Antihistamines*	Increased isopropamide effect.
Appetite suppressants*	Decreased suppressant effect.
Cortisone drugs*	Increased internal-eye pressure.
Dronabinol	Increased effect of both drugs. Avoid.
Guanethidine	Decreased guanethidine effect.
Haloperidol	Increased internal-eye pressure.
Levodopa	Decreased levodopa effect.
MAO inhibitors*	Increased isopropamide effect.
Meperidine	Increased isopropamide effect.
Methylphenidate	Increased isopropamide effect.

Continued page 1102

POSSIBLE INTERACTION WITH OTHER SUBSTANCES

INTERACTS WITH	COMBINED EFFECT
Alcohol:	Dangerous oversedation.
Beverages:	None expected.
Cocaine:	Excessively rapid heartbeat. Avoid.
Foods:	None expected.
Marijuana:	Drowsiness and dry mouth. May increase antinausea effect.
Tobacco:	None expected.

*See Glossary

PROCYCLIDINE

BRAND NAMES

Kemadrin   Procyclid
PMS Procyclidine

BASIC INFORMATION

Habit forming? No
Prescription needed? Yes
Available as generic? No
Drug class: Antidyskinetic, antiparkinsonism

 ## USES

- Treatment of Parkinson's disease.
- Treatment of adverse effects of phenothiazines.

 ## DOSAGE & USAGE INFORMATION

How to take:
Tablets or elixer—Take with food to lessen stomach irritation.

When to take:
At the same times each day.

If you forget a dose:
Take as soon as you remember up to 2 hours late. If more than 2 hours, wait for next scheduled dose (don't double this dose).

What drug does:
- Balances chemical reactions necessary to send nerve impulses within base of brain.
- Improves muscle control and reduces stiffness.

Continued next column

 ## OVERDOSE

SYMPTOMS:
Agitation, dilated pupils, hallucinations, dry mouth, rapid heartbeat, sleepiness.
WHAT TO DO:
- Dial 0 (operator) or 911 (emergency) for an ambulance or medical help. Then give first aid immediately.
- If patient is unconscious and not breathing, give mouth-to-mouth breathing. If there is no heartbeat, use cardiac massage and mouth-to-mouth breathing (CPR). Don't try to make patient vomit. If you can't get help quickly, take patient to nearest emergency facility.
- See emergency information on inside covers.

Time lapse before drug works:
1 to 2 hours.

Don't take with:
- Non-prescription drugs for colds, cough or allergy.
- See Interaction column and consult doctor.

 ## POSSIBLE ADVERSE REACTIONS OR SIDE EFFECTS

SYMPTOMS	WHAT TO DO
Life-threatening: None expected.	
Common: • Blurred vision, light sensitivity, constipation, nausea, vomiting.	Continue. Call doctor when convenient.
• Frequent, painful or difficult urination, dry mouth.	Continue. Tell doctor at next visit.
Infrequent: None expected.	
Rare: • Rash, hives, fever, eye pain, amnesia, delusions, paranoia, hallucinations, swollen neck glands, weakness and faintness when arising from bed or chair.	Discontinue. Call doctor right away.
• Confusion, dizziness, sore mouth or tongue, muscle cramps, numbness or weakness in hands or feet.	Continue. Call doctor when convenient.

844

WARNINGS & PRECAUTIONS

Don't take if:
You are allergic to any antidyskinetic.

Before you start, consult your doctor:
- If you have had glaucoma.
- If you have had high blood pressure or heart disease.
- If you have had impaired liver function.
- If you have had kidney disease or urination difficulty.

Over age 60:
More sensitive to drug. Aggravates symptoms of enlarged prostate. Causes impaired thinking, hallucinations, nightmares. Consult doctor about any of these.

Pregnancy:
Studies inconclusive on harm to unborn child. Animal studies show fetal abnormalities. Decide with your doctor whether drug benefits justify risk to unborn child.

Breast-feeding:
No problems expected.

Infants & children:
Not recommended for children 3 and younger. Use for older children only under doctor's supervision.

Prolonged use:
Possible glaucoma.

Skin & sunlight:
No problems expected.

Driving, piloting or hazardous work:
Don't drive or pilot aircraft until you learn how medicine affects you. Don't work around dangerous machinery. Don't climb ladders or work in high places. Danger increases if you drink alcohol or take medicine affecting alertness and reflexes, such as antihistamines, tranquilizers, sedatives, pain medicine, narcotics and mind-altering drugs.

Discontinuing:
Don't discontinue without consulting doctor. Dose may require gradual reduction if you have taken drug for a long time. Doses of other drugs may also require adjustment.

Others:
- Internal eye pressure should be measured regularly.
- Avoid becoming overheated.

POSSIBLE INTERACTION WITH OTHER DRUGS

GENERIC NAME OR DRUG CLASS	COMBINED EFFECT
Amantadine	Increased amantadine effect.
Antacids*	Possible decreased absorption.
Anticholinergics*	Increased anticholinergic effect.
Antidepressants, tricyclic (TCA)*	Increased procyclidine effect. May cause glaucoma.
Antihistamines*	Increased procyclidine effect.
Digoxin	Possible increased toxicity of digoxin.
Disopyramide	Increased anticholinergic effect.
Haloperidol	Behavior changes possible.
Levodopa	Possible increased levodopa effect.
Meperidine	Increased procyclidine effect.
MAO inhibitors*	Increased procyclidine effect.
Nabilone	Greater depression of central nervous system.
Phenothiazines*	Behavior changes.
Primidone	Excessive sedation.
Quinidine	Increased procyclidine effect.
Slow-k (extended-release potassium)	Increased risk of gastric irritation.
Tranquilizers*	Excessive sedation.

POSSIBLE INTERACTION WITH OTHER SUBSTANCES

INTERACTS WITH	COMBINED EFFECT
Alcohol:	None expected.
Beverages:	None expected.
Cocaine:	Decreased procyclidine effect. Avoid.
Foods:	None expected.
Marijuana:	None expected.
Tobacco:	None expected.

*See Glossary

PROMAZINE

BRAND NAMES

Norzine	Prozine
Promanyl	Sparine

BASIC INFORMATION

Habit forming? No
Prescription needed? Yes
Available as generic? Yes
Drug class: Tranquilizer, antiemetic
(phenothiazine)

USES

- Stops nausea, vomiting, hiccups.
- Reduces anxiety, agitation.

DOSAGE & USAGE INFORMATION

How to take:
Tablet—Swallow with liquid or food to lessen stomach irritation.

When to take:
- Nervous and mental disorders—Take at the same times each day.
- Nausea and vomiting—Take as needed, no more often than every 4 hours.

If you forget a dose:
- Nervous and mental disorders—Take up to 2 hours late. If more than 2 hours, wait for next scheduled dose (don't double this dose).
- Nausea and vomiting—Take as soon as you remember. Wait 4 hours for next dose.

What drug does:
- Suppresses brain's vomiting center.
- Suppresses brain centers that control abnormal emotions and behavior.

Time lapse before drug works:
- Nausea and vomiting—1 hour or less.
- Nervous and mental disorders—4-6 weeks.

Don't take with:
- Antacid or medicine for diarrhea.
- Non-prescription drug for cough, cold or allergy.
- See Interaction column and consult doctor.

OVERDOSE

SYMPTOMS:
Stupor, convulsions, coma.
WHAT TO DO:
- Dial 0 (operator) or 911 (emergency) for an ambulance or medical help. Then give first aid immediately.
- See emergency information on inside covers.

POSSIBLE ADVERSE REACTIONS OR SIDE EFFECTS

SYMPTOMS	WHAT TO DO
Life-threatening:	
Uncontrolled muscle movements of tongue, face and other muscles (neuroleptic malignant syndrome, rare).	Discontinue. Seek emergency treatment.
Common:	
• Muscle spasms of face and neck, unsteady gait.	Discontinue. Seek emergency treatment.
• Restlessness, tremor, drowsiness.	Discontinue. Call doctor right away.
• Decreased sweating, dry mouth, runny nose, constipation.	Continue. Call doctor when convenient.
Infrequent:	
• Fainting.	Discontinue. Seek emergency treatment.
• Rash.	Discontinue. Call doctor right away.
• Difficult urination, diminished sex drive, swollen breasts, menstrual irregularities.	Continue. Call doctor when convenient.
Rare:	
Change in vision, sore throat, fever, jaundice, abdominal pain.	Discontinue. Call doctor right away.

WARNINGS & PRECAUTIONS

Don't take if:
- You are allergic to any phenothiazine.
- You have a blood or bone-marrow disease.

Before you start, consult your doctor:
- If you will have surgery within 2 months, including dental surgery, requiring general or spinal anesthesia.
- If you have asthma, emphysema or other lung disorder, glaucoma, prostate trouble.
- If you take non-prescription ulcer medicine, asthma medicine or amphetamines.

Over age 60:
Adverse reactions and side effects may be more frequent and severe than in younger persons. More likely to develop involuntary movement of jaws, lips, tongue, chewing. Report this to your doctor immediately. Early treatment can help.

Pregnancy:
Risk to unborn child outweighs drug benefits. Don't use.

Breast-feeding:
Drug passes into milk. Avoid drug or discontinue nursing until you finish medicine. Consult doctor for advice on maintaining milk supply.

Infants & children:
Don't give to children younger than 2.

Prolonged use:
May lead to tardive dyskinesia (involuntary movement of jaws, lips, tongue, chewing).

Skin & sunlight:
May cause rash or intensify sunburn in areas exposed to sun or sunlamp. Skin may remain sensitive for 3 months after discontinuing.

Driving, piloting or hazardous work:
Don't drive or pilot aircraft until you learn how medicine affects you. Don't work around dangerous machinery. Don't climb ladders or work in high places. Danger increases if you drink alcohol or take medicine affecting alertness and reflexes.

Discontinuing:
- Nervous and mental disorders—Don't discontinue without doctor's advice until you complete prescribed dose, even though symptoms diminish or disappear.
- Nausea and vomiting—May be unnecessary to finish medicine. Follow doctor's instructions.

Others:
No problems expected.

POSSIBLE INTERACTION WITH OTHER DRUGS

GENERIC NAME OR DRUG CLASS	COMBINED EFFECT
Anticholinergics*	Increased anticholinergic effect.
Antidepressants, tricyclic (TCA)*	Increased promazine effect.
Antihistamines*	Increased antihistamine effect.
Appetite suppressants*	Decreased suppressant effect.
Dronabinol	Increased effects of both drugs. Avoid.
Guanethidine	Decreased guanethidine effect.
Levodopa	Decreased levodopa effect.
Mind-altering drugs*	Increased effect of mind-altering drugs.
Molindone	Increased tranquilizer effect.
Nabilone	Greater depression of central nervous system.
Narcotics*	Increased narcotic effect.
Phenytoin	Increased phenytoin effect.
Procarbazine	Increased sedation.
Quinidine	Impaired heart function. Dangerous mixture.
Sedatives*	Increased sedation.
Tranquilizers, other*	Increased tranquilizer effect.

POSSIBLE INTERACTION WITH OTHER SUBSTANCES

INTERACTS WITH	COMBINED EFFECT
Alcohol:	Dangerous oversedation.
Beverages:	None expected.
Cocaine:	Decreased promazine effect. Avoid.
Foods:	None expected.
Marijuana:	Drowsiness. May increase antinausea effect.
Tobacco:	None expected.

*See Glossary

PROMETHAZINE

BRAND NAMES

See complete list of brand names in the *Brand Name Directory*, page 1069.

BASIC INFORMATION

Habit forming? No
Prescription needed? Yes
Available as generic? Yes
Drug class: Antihistamine, tranquilizer (phenothiazine)

 USES

- Stops nausea, vomiting and dizziness of motion sickness.
- Produces mild sedation and light sleep.
- Reduces allergic symptoms of hay fever and hives.

 DOSAGE & USAGE INFORMATION

How to take:
- Tablets, sustained-release capsules or liquid—Swallow with water.
- Suppositories—Remove wrapper and moisten suppository with water. Gently insert larger end into rectum. Push well into rectum with finger.

When to take:
Take as needed, no more often than every 12 hours.

If you forget a dose:
Take as soon as you remember. Wait 12 hours for next dose.

What drug does:
- Blocks stimulation of brain's vomiting center.
- Suppresses brain centers that control abnormal emotions and behavior.
- Blocks histamine action in sensitized cells.

Time lapse before drug works:
1 to 2 hours.

Continued next column

 OVERDOSE

SYMPTOMS:
Stupor, convulsions, coma.
WHAT TO DO:
- Dial 0 (operator) or 911 (emergency) for an ambulance or medical help. Then give first aid immediately.
- See emergency information on inside covers.

Don't take with:
- Antacid or medicine for diarrhea.
- Non-prescription drug for cough, cold or allergy.
- See Interaction column and consult doctor.

 POSSIBLE ADVERSE REACTIONS OR SIDE EFFECTS

SYMPTOMS	WHAT TO DO
Life-threatening:	
Uncontrolled muscle movements of tongue, face and other muscles (neuroleptic malignant syndrome, rare).	Discontinue. Seek emergency treatment.
Common:	
• Restlessness, tremor, drowsiness.	Discontinue. Call doctor right away.
• Decreased sweating, dry mouth, runny nose, constipation.	Continue. Call doctor when convenient.
Infrequent:	
• Fainting.	Discontinue. Seek emergency treatment.
• Rash, muscle spasms of face and neck, unsteady gait.	Discontinue. Call doctor right away.
• Difficult urination, diminished sex drive, swollen breasts, menstrual irregularities.	Continue. Call doctor when convenient.
Rare:	
Change in vision, sore throat, fever, jaundice, abdominal pain.	Discontinue. Call doctor right away.

 WARNINGS & PRECAUTIONS

Don't take if:
- You are allergic to any phenothiazine.
- You have a blood or bone-marrow disease.

Before you start, consult your doctor:
- If you will have surgery within 2 months, including dental surgery, requiring general or spinal anesthesia.
- If you have asthma, emphysema or other lung disorder, glaucoma, prostate trouble.
- If you take non-prescription ulcer medicine, asthma medicine or amphetamines.

Over age 60:
Adverse reactions and side effects may be more frequent and severe than in younger persons. More likely to develop tardive dyskinesia (involuntary movement of jaws, lips, tongue, chewing). Report this to your doctor immediately. Early treatment can help.

Pregnancy:
Risk to unborn child outweighs drug benefits. Don't use.

Breast-feeding:
Drug passes into milk. Avoid drug or discontinue nursing until you finish medicine. Consult doctor for advice on maintaining milk supply.

Infants & children:
Don't give to children younger than 2.

Prolonged use:
May lead to tardive dyskinesia (involuntary movement of jaws, lips, tongue, chewing).

Skin & sunlight:
May cause rash or intensify sunburn in areas exposed to sun or sunlamp. Skin may remain sensitive for 3 months after discontinuing.

Driving, piloting or hazardous work:
Don't drive or pilot aircraft until you learn how medicine affects you. Don't work around dangerous machinery. Don't climb ladders or work in high places. Danger increases if you drink alcohol or take medicine affecting alertness and reflexes.

Discontinuing:
- Nervous and mental disorders—Don't discontinue without doctor's advice until you complete prescribed dose, even though symptoms diminish or disappear.
- Nausea, vomiting or allergy—May be unnecessary to finish medicine. Follow doctor's instructions.

Others:
No problems expected.

 POSSIBLE INTERACTION WITH OTHER DRUGS

GENERIC NAME OR DRUG CLASS	COMBINED EFFECT
Antacids*	Decreased promethazine effect.
Anticholinergics*	Increased anticholinergic effect.
Anticonvulsants, hydantoin*	Increased anticonvulsant effect.
Antidepressants, tricyclic (TCA)*	Increased promethazine effect.
Antihistamines, other*	Increased antihistamine effect.
Appetite suppressants*	Decreased suppressant effect.
Barbiturates*	Oversedation.
Carteolol	Decreased antihistamine effect.

Dronabinol	Increased effects of both drugs. Avoid.
Ethinamate	Dangerous increased effects of ethinamate. Avoid combining.
Fluoxetine	Increased depressant effects of both drugs.
Glycopyrrolate	Possible increased glycopyrrolate effect.
Guanethidine	Decreased guanethidine effect.
Guanfacine	May increase depressant effects of either medicine.
Levodopa	Decreased levodopa effect.
Leucovorin	High alcohol content of leucovorin may cause adverse effects.
MAO inhibitors*	Increased promethazine effect.
Methyprylon	May increase sedative effect to dangerous level. Avoid.
Mind-altering drugs*	Increased effect of mind-altering drugs.
Molindone	Increased sedative and antihistamine effect.
Nabilone	Greater depression of central nervous system.
Narcotics*	Increased narcotic effect.
Procarbazine	Increased sedation.
Sedatives*	Increased sedative effect.

Continued page 1102

 POSSIBLE INTERACTION WITH OTHER SUBSTANCES

INTERACTS WITH	COMBINED EFFECT
Alcohol:	Dangerous sedation.
Beverages:	None expected.
Cocaine:	Decreased effect of promethazine. Avoid.
Foods:	None expected.
Marijuana:	Drowsiness. May increase antinausea effect.
Tobacco:	None expected.

*See Glossary

PROPANTHELINE

BRAND NAMES

Banlin
Norpanth
Novopropanthil
Pro-Banthine

Pro-Banthine with
  Phenobarbital
Propanthel
Ropanth
SK-Propantheline

BASIC INFORMATION

Habit forming? No
Prescription needed?
  High strength: Yes
  Low strength: No
Available as generic? No
Drug class: Antispasmodic, anticholinergic

USES

Reduces spasms of digestive system, bladder and urethra.

DOSAGE & USAGE INFORMATION

How to take:
Tablet—Swallow with liquid or food to lessen stomach irritation.

When to take:
30 minutes before meals (unless directed otherwise by doctor).

If you forget a dose:
Take as soon as you remember up to 2 hours late. If more than 2 hours, wait for next scheduled dose (don't double this dose).

What drug does:
Blocks nerve impulses at parasympathetic nerve endings, preventing muscle contractions and gland secretions of organs involved.

Time lapse before drug works:
15 to 30 minutes.

Don't take with:
See Interaction column and consult doctor.

OVERDOSE

SYMPTOMS:
Dilated pupils, blurred vision, rapid pulse and breathing, dizziness, fever, hallucinations, confusion, slurred speech, agitation, flushed face, convulsions, coma.
WHAT TO DO:
- **Dial 0 (operator) or 911 (emergency) for an ambulance or medical help. Then give first aid immediately.**
- **See emergency information on inside covers.**

POSSIBLE ADVERSE REACTIONS OR SIDE EFFECTS

SYMPTOMS	WHAT TO DO
Life-threatening: Hives, rash, intense itching, faintness soon after a dose (anaphylaxis).	Seek emergency treatment immediately.
Common:	
• Confusion, delirium, rapid heartbeat.	Discontinue. Call doctor right away.
• Nausea, vomiting, decreased sweating.	Continue. Call doctor when convenient.
• Constipation, loss of taste.	Continue. Tell doctor at next visit.
• Dry ears, nose, throat.	No action necessary.
Infrequent: Headache, difficult urination.	Continue. Call doctor when convenient.
Rare: Rash or hives, pain, blurred vision.	Discontinue. Call doctor right away.

WARNINGS & PRECAUTIONS

Don't take if:
- You are allergic to any anticholinergic.
- You have trouble with stomach bloating.
- You have difficulty emptying your bladder completely.
- You have narrow-angle glaucoma.
- You have severe ulcerative colitis.

Before you start, consult your doctor:
- If you have open-angle glaucoma.
- If you have angina.
- If you have chronic bronchitis or asthma.
- If you have hiatal hernia.
- If you have liver disease.
- If you have enlarged prostate.
- If you have myasthenia gravis.
- If you have peptic ulcer.
- If you will have surgery within 2 months, including dental surgery, requiring general or spinal anesthesia.

Over age 60:
Adverse reactions and side effects may be more frequent and severe than in younger persons.

Pregnancy:
Studies inconclusive on harm to unborn child. Animal studies show fetal abnormalities. Decide with your doctor whether drug benefits justify risk to unborn child.

Breast-feeding:
Drug passes into milk and decreases milk flow. Avoid drug or discontinue nursing until you finish medicine. Consult doctor for advice on maintaining milk supply.

Infants & children:
Use only under medical supervision.

Prolonged use:
Chronic constipation, possible fecal impaction. Consult doctor immediately.

Skin & sunlight:
No problems expected.

Driving, piloting or hazardous work:
Use disqualifies you for piloting aircraft. Otherwise, no problems expected.

Discontinuing:
May be unnecessary to finish medicine. Follow doctor's instructions.

Others:
No problems expected.

POSSIBLE INTERACTION WITH OTHER DRUGS

GENERIC NAME OR DRUG CLASS	COMBINED EFFECT
Amantadine	Increased propantheline effect.
Antacids*	Decreased propantheline effect.
Anticholinergics, other*	Increased propantheline effect.
Antidepressants, tricyclic (TCA)*	Increased propantheline effect. Increased sedation.
Antihistamines*	Increased propantheline effect.
Buclizine	Increased propantheline effect.
Cortisone drugs*	Increased internal eye pressure.
Digitalis	Possible decreased absorption of digitalis.
Haloperidol	Increased internal eye pressure.
MAO inhibitors*	Increased propantheline effect.
Meperidine	Increased propantheline effect.
Methylphenidate	Increased propantheline effect.
Molindone	Increased anticholinergic effect.
Nitrates*	Increased internal-eye pressure.
Nizatidine	Increased nizatidine effect.
Orphenadrine	Increased propantheline effect.
Phenothiazines*	Increased propantheline effect.
Pilocarpine	Loss of pilocarpine effect in glaucoma treatment.
Potassium supplements*	Increased possibility of intestinal ulcers with oral potassium tablets.
Quinidine	Increased propantheline effect.
Terfenadine	Possible increased propantheline effect.
Vitamin C	Decreased propantheline effect. Avoid large doses of vitamin C.

POSSIBLE INTERACTION WITH OTHER SUBSTANCES

INTERACTS WITH	COMBINED EFFECT
Alcohol:	None expected.
Beverages:	None expected.
Cocaine:	Excessively rapid heartbeat. Avoid.
Foods:	None expected.
Marijuana:	Drowsiness and dry mouth.
Tobacco:	None expected.

*See Glossary

PROPRANOLOL

BRAND NAMES

Apo-Propranolol	Inderide
Detensol	Novopranol
Inderal	Panolol
Inderal LA	pms-Propranolol

BASIC INFORMATION

Habit forming? No
Prescription needed? Yes
Available as generic? Yes
Drug class: Beta-adrenergic blocker

USES

- Reduces angina attacks.
- Stabilizes irregular heartbeat.
- Lowers blood pressure.
- Reduces frequency of migraine headaches. (Does not relieve headache pain.)
- Other uses prescribed by your doctor.

DOSAGE & USAGE INFORMATION

How to take:
Tablet, liquid or extended-release capsule—Swallow with liquid. If you can't swallow whole, crumble tablet or open capsule and take with liquid or food. Don't crush capsule.

When to take:
With meals or immediately after.

If you forget a dose:
Take as soon as you remember. Return to regular schedule, but allow 3 hours between doses.

What drug does:
- Blocks certain actions of sympathetic nervous system.
- Lowers heart's oxygen requirements.
- Slows nerve impulses through heart.
- Reduces blood vessel contraction in heart, scalp and other body parts.

Continued next column

OVERDOSE

SYMPTOMS:
Weakness, slow or weak pulse, blood-pressure drop, fainting, difficulty breathing, convulsions, cold and sweaty skin.
WHAT TO DO:
- Dial 0 (operator) or 911 (emergency) for an ambulance or medical help. Then give first aid immediately.
- See emergency information on inside covers.

Time lapse before drug works:
1 to 4 hours.

Don't take with:
Non-prescription drugs or drugs in Interaction column without consulting doctor.

POSSIBLE ADVERSE REACTIONS OR SIDE EFFECTS

SYMPTOMS	WHAT TO DO
Life-threatening:	
Congestive heart failure.	Discontinue. Seek emergency treatment.
Common:	
• Pulse slower than 50 beats per minute.	Discontinue. Call doctor right away.
• Drowsiness, fatigue, numbness or tingling of fingers or toes, dizziness, diarrhea, nausea, weakness.	Continue. Call doctor when convenient.
• Cold hands or feet; dry mouth, eyes and skin.	Continue. Tell doctor at next visit.
Infrequent:	
• Hallucinations, nightmares, insomnia, headache, difficult breathing, joint pain, anxiety.	Discontinue. Call doctor right away.
• Confusion, reduced alertness, depression, impotence.	Continue. Call doctor when convenient.
• Constipation.	Continue. Tell doctor at next visit.
Rare:	
• Rash, sore throat, fever.	Discontinue. Call doctor right away.
• Unusual bleeding and bruising; dry, burning eyes; impotence.	Continue. Call doctor when convenient.

WARNINGS & PRECAUTIONS

Don't take if:
- You are allergic to any beta-adrenergic blocker.
- You have asthma.
- You have hay fever symptoms.
- You have taken MAO inhibitors in past 2 weeks.

Before you start, consult your doctor:
- If you have heart disease or poor circulation to the extremities.
- If you have hay fever, asthma, chronic bronchitis, emphysema.
- If you have overactive thyroid function.
- If you have impaired liver or kidney function.
- If you will have surgery within 2 months, including dental surgery, requiring general or spinal anesthesia.
- If you have diabetes or hypoglycemia.

Over age 60:
Adverse reactions and side effects may be more frequent and severe than in younger persons.

Pregnancy:
Risk to unborn child outweighs drug benefits. Don't use.

Breast-feeding:
Drug passes into milk. Avoid drug or discontinue nursing until you finish medicine. Consult doctor for advice on maintaining milk supply.

Infants & children:
Not recommended.

Prolonged use:
Weakens heart muscle contractions.

Skin & sunlight:
No problems expected.

Driving, piloting or hazardous work:
Don't drive or pilot aircraft until you learn how medicine affects you. Don't work around dangerous machinery. Don't climb ladders or work in high places. Danger increases if you drink alcohol or take medicine affecting alertness and reflexes.

Discontinuing:
Don't discontinue without consulting doctor. Dose may require gradual reduction if you have taken drug for a long time. Doses of other drugs may also require adjustment.

Others:
May mask hypoglycemia.

POSSIBLE INTERACTION WITH OTHER DRUGS

GENERIC NAME OR DRUG CLASS	COMBINED EFFECT
ACE inhibitors: captopril, enalapril, lisinopril*	Increased antihypertensive effects of both drugs. Dosages may require adjustment.
Antidiabetics*	Increased antidiabetic effect.
Antihistamines*	Decreased antihistamine effect.
Antihypertensives*	Increased antihypertensive effect.
Barbiturates*	Increased barbiturate effect. Dangerous sedation.
Beta-agonists*	Decreased beta-agonist effect.
Betaxolol eyedrops	Possible increased propranolol effect.
Digitalis preparations*	Can either increase or decrease heart rate. Improves irregular heartbeat.
Encainide	Increased effect of toxicity on heart muscle.
Indomethacin	Decreased effect of propranolol.
Insulin	Hypoglycemic effects may be prolonged.

Continued page 1103

POSSIBLE INTERACTION WITH OTHER SUBSTANCES

INTERACTS WITH	COMBINED EFFECT
Alcohol:	Excessive blood-pressure drop. Avoid.
Beverages:	None expected.
Cocaine:	Irregular heartbeat. Avoid.
Foods:	None expected.
Marijuana:	Daily use—Impaired circulation to hands and feet.
Tobacco:	Possible irregular heartbeat.

***See Glossary**

PROTECTANT (Ophthalmic)

BRAND AND GENERIC NAMES

Gonak
Goniosol
HYDROXYPROPYL
   CELLULOSE
HYDROXYPROPYL
   METHYL-CELLULOSE
Isopto Alkaline
Isopto Plain

Isopto Tears
Lacril (ophthalmic)
Lacrisert
Muro tears
Tearisol
Tears Naturale
Ultra Tears

BASIC INFORMATION

Habit forming? No
Prescription needed? Yes
Available as generic? No
Drug class: Protectant (ophthalmic),
   artificial tears

 ## USES

- Relieves eye dryness and irritation caused by inadequate flow of tears.
- Moistens contact lenses and artificial eyes.

 ## DOSAGE & USAGE INFORMATION

How to use:
Eye drops
- Wash hands.
- Apply pressure to inside corner of eye with middle finger.
- Continue pressure for 1 minute after placing medicine in eye.
- Tilt head backward. Pull lower lid away from eye with index finger of the same hand.
- Drop eye drops into pouch and close eye. Don't blink.
- Keep eyes closed for 1 to 2 minutes.
- Don't touch applicator tip to any surface (including the eye). If you accidentally touch tip, clean with warm soap and water.
- Keep container tightly closed.
- Keep cool, but don't freeze.
- Wash hands immediately after using.

Continued next column

 ## OVERDOSE

SYMPTOMS:
None expected.
WHAT TO DO:
Not intended for internal use. If child accidentally swallows, call poison-control center.

When to use:
As directed. Usually every 3 or 4 hours.

If you forget a dose:
Use as soon as you remember.

What drug does:
- Stabilizes and thickens tear film.
- Lubricates and protects eye.

Time lapse before drug works:
2 to 10 minutes.

Don't use with:
Other eye drops without consulting your doctor.

 ## POSSIBLE ADVERSE REACTIONS OR SIDE EFFECTS

SYMPTOMS	WHAT TO DO
Life-threatening None expected.	
Common None expected.	
Infrequent Eye irritation not present before using artificial tears.	Discontinue. Call doctor right away.
Rare None expected.	

PROTECTANT (Ophthalmic)

 ## WARNINGS & PRECAUTIONS

Don't use if:
You are allergic to any artificial tears.

Before you start, consult your doctor:
If you use any other eye drops.

Over age 60:
No problems expected.

Pregnancy:
No problems expected, but check with doctor.

Breast-feeding:
No problems expected, but check with doctor.

Infants & children:
Don't use.

Prolonged use:
Don't use for more than 3 or 4 days.

Skin & sunlight:
No problems expected.

Driving, piloting or hazardous work:
No problems expected.

Discontinuing:
May not need all the medicine in container. If symptoms disappear, stop using.

Others:
- Keep cool, but don't freeze.
- Check with your doctor if eye irritation continues or becomes worse.

 ## POSSIBLE INTERACTION WITH OTHER DRUGS

GENERIC NAME OR DRUG CLASS	COMBINED EFFECT
Clinically significant interactions with oral or injected medicines unlikely.	

 ## POSSIBLE INTERACTION WITH OTHER SUBSTANCES

INTERACTS WITH	COMBINED EFFECT
Alcohol:	None expected.
Beverages:	None expected.
Cocaine:	None expected.
Foods:	None expected.
Marijuana:	None expected.
Tobacco:	None expected.

PSEUDOEPHEDRINE

BRAND NAMES

See complete list of brand names in the *Brand Name Directory*, page 1069.

BASIC INFORMATION

Habit forming? No
Prescription needed?
  U.S.: High strength—Yes
       Low strength—No
  Canada: No
Available as generic? Yes
Drug class: Sympathomimetic

USES

Reduces congestion of nose, sinuses and throat from allergies and infections.

DOSAGE & USAGE INFORMATION

How to take:
- Tablet—Swallow with liquid. You may chew or crush tablet.
- Extended-release capsules—Swallow each dose whole.
- Syrup—Take as directed on label.
- Drops—Place directly on tongue and swallow.

When to take:
- At the same times each day.
- To prevent insomnia, take last dose of day a few hours before bedtime.

If you forget a dose:
Take up to 2 hours late. If more than 2 hours, wait for next dose (don't double this dose).

What drug does:
Decreases blood volume in nasal tissues, shrinking tissues and enlarging airways.

Continued next column

OVERDOSE

SYMPTOMS:
Nervousness, restlessness, headache, rapid or irregular heartbeat, sweating, nausea, vomiting, anxiety, confusion, delirium, muscle tremors.
WHAT TO DO:
- **Dial 0 (operator) or 911 (emergency) for an ambulance or medical help. Then give first aid immediately.**
- **See emergency information on inside covers.**

Time lapse before drug works:
15 to 20 minutes.

Don't take with:
- Non-prescription drugs with caffeine without consulting doctor.
- See Interaction column and consult doctor.

POSSIBLE ADVERSE REACTIONS OR SIDE EFFECTS

SYMPTOMS	WHAT TO DO
Life-threatening: None expected.	
Common: Agitation, insomnia.	Continue. Tell doctor at next visit.
Infrequent:	
• Nausea or vomiting, irregular or slow heartbeat, difficult breathing, unusually fast or pounding heartbeat, painful or difficult urination, increased sweating.	Discontinue. Call doctor right away.
• Dizziness, headache, shakiness, weakness.	Continue. Call doctor when convenient.
• Paleness.	Continue. Tell doctor at next visit.
Rare: Hallucinations, seizures.	Discontinue. Seek emergency treatment.

PSEUDOEPHEDRINE

WARNINGS & PRECAUTIONS

Don't take if:
You are allergic to any sympathomimetic drug.

Before you start, consult your doctor:
- If you have overactive thyroid or diabetes.
- If you have taken any MAO inhibitors in past 2 weeks.
- If you take digitalis preparations or have high blood pressure or heart disease.
- If you will have surgery within 2 months, including dental surgery, requiring general or spinal anesthesia.
- If you have urination difficulty.

Over age 60:
Adverse reactions and side effects may be more frequent and severe than in younger persons.

Pregnancy:
No proven harm to unborn child. Avoid if possible.

Breast-feeding:
Drug passes into milk. Avoid drug or discontinue nursing until you finish medicine. Consult doctor for advice on maintaining milk supply.

Infants & children:
Keep dose low or avoid.

Prolonged use:
No proven problems.

Skin & sunlight:
No problems expected.

Driving, piloting or hazardous work:
Avoid if you feel dizzy. Otherwise, no problems expected..

Discontinuing:
May be unnecessary to finish medicine. Follow doctor's instructions.

Others:
No problems expected.

POSSIBLE INTERACTION WITH OTHER DRUGS

GENERIC NAME OR DRUG CLASS	COMBINED EFFECT
Antidepressants, tricyclic (TCA)*	Increased pseudo-ephedrine effect.
Antihypertensives*	Decreased antihypertensive effect.
Beta-adrenergic blockers*	Decreased effect of both drugs.
Calcium supplements*	Increased pseudo-ephedrine effect.
Digitalis preparations*	Irregular heartbeat.
Epinephrine	Increased epinephrine effect. Excessive heart stimulation and blood-pressure increase.
Ergot preparations*	Serious blood-pressure rise.
Guanadrel	Decreased effect of both drugs.
Guanethidine	Decreased effect of both drugs.
MAO inhibitors*	Increased pseudo-ephedrine effect.
Methyldopa	Possible increased blood pressure.
Nitrates*	Possible decreased effects of both drugs.
Phenothiazines*	Possible increased pseudoephedrine toxicity. Possible decreased pseudo-ephedrine effect.
Rauwolfia	Decreased rauwolfia effect.
Sympathomimetics*	Increased pseudo-ephedrine effect.
Terazosin	Decreases effectiveness of terazosin.

POSSIBLE INTERACTION WITH OTHER SUBSTANCES

INTERACTS WITH	COMBINED EFFECT
Alcohol:	None expected.
Beverages: Caffeine drinks.	Nervousness or insomnia.
Cocaine:	High risk of heartbeat irregularities and high blood pressure.
Foods:	None expected.
Marijuana:	Rapid heartbeat.
Tobacco:	None expected.

*See Glossary

PSORALENS

BRAND AND GENERIC NAMES

METHOXSALEN
Methoxsalen Lotion
   (Topical)
Oxsoralen
Oxsoralen-Ultra

Oxsoralen (Topical)
TRIOXSALEN
Trisoralen
UltraMOP

BASIC INFORMATION

Habit forming? No
Prescription needed? Yes
Available as generic? No
Drug class: Repigmenting agent (psoralen)

USES

- Repigmenting skin affected with vitiligo (absence of skin pigment).
- Treatment for psoriasis, when other treatments haven't helped.
- Treatment for mycosis fungoides.

DOSAGE & USAGE INFORMATION

How to take or apply:
- Tablet or capsule—Swallow with liquid or food to lessen stomach irritation.
- Topical—As directed by doctor.

When to take or apply:
2 to 4 hours before exposure to sunlight or sunlamp.

If you forget a dose:
Take as soon as you remember. Delay sun exposure for at least 2 hours after taking.

What drug does:
Helps pigment cells when used in conjunction with ultraviolet light.

Time lapse before drug works:
- For vitiligo, 6 to 9 months.
- For psoriasis, 10 weeks or longer.
- For tanning, 3 to 4 days.

Don't take with:
Any other medicine which causes skin sensitivity to sun. Ask pharmacist.

OVERDOSE

SYMPTOMS:
Blistering skin, swelling feet and legs.
WHAT TO DO:
Overdose unlikely to threaten life. If person takes much larger amount than prescribed, call doctor, poison-control center or hospital emergency room for instructions.

POSSIBLE ADVERSE REACTIONS OR SIDE EFFECTS

SYMPTOMS	WHAT TO DO
Life-threatening: None expected.	
Always: • Increased skin sensitivity to sun. • Increased eye sensitivity to sunlight.	Always protect from overexposure. Always protect with wrap-around sunglasses.
Infrequent: None expected.	
Rare: Hepatitis with jaundice, blistering and peeling.	Discontinue. Call doctor right away.

WARNINGS & PRECAUTIONS

Don't take if:
- You are allergic to any other psoralen.
- You are unwilling or unable to remain under close medical supervision.

Before you start, consult your doctor:
- If you have heart or liver disease.
- If you have allergy to sunlight.
- If you have cataracts.
- If you have albinism.
- If you have lupus erythematosis, porphyria, chronic infection, skin cancer or peptic ulcer.
- If you will have surgery within 2 months, including dental surgery, requiring general or spinal anesthesia.

Over age 60:
Adverse reactions and side effects may be more frequent and severe than in younger persons.

Pregnancy:
Risk to unborn child outweighs drug benefits. Don't use.

Breast-feeding:
Drug passes into milk. Avoid drug or discontinue nursing until you finish medicine. Consult doctor for advice on maintaining milk supply.

Infants & children:
Not recommended.

Prolonged use:
Increased chance of toxic effects.

Skin & sunlight:
Too much can burn skin. Cover skin for 24 hours before and 8 hours following treatments.

Driving, piloting or hazardous work:
No problems expected. Protect eyes and skin from bright light.

Discontinuing:
Skin may remain sensitive for some time after treatment stops. Use extra protection from sun.

Others:
- Use sunblock on lips.
- Don't use just to make skin tan.

POSSIBLE INTERACTION WITH OTHER DRUGS

GENERIC NAME OR DRUG CLASS	COMBINED EFFECT
Any medicine causing sensitization to sunlight, such as: acetohexamide, amitriptyline, anthralin, barbiturates, bendroflumethiazide, carbamazepine, chlordiazepoxide, chloroquine, chlorothiazide, chloropromazine, chloropropamide, chlortetracycline, chlorthalidone, clindamycin, coal tar derivatives, cyproheptadine, demeclocycline, desipramine, diethylstilbestrol, diphenhydramine, doxepin, doxycycline, estrogen, fluphenazine, gold preparations, glyburide, griseofulvin, hydrochlorothiazide, hydroflumethiazide, imipramine, lincomycin, mesoridazine, methacycline, nalidixic acid, nortriptyline, oral contraceptives, oxyphenbutazone, oxytetracycline,	Greatly increased likelihood of extreme sensitivity to sunlight.

perphenazine, phenobarbital, phenylbutazone, phenytoin, prochlorperazine, promazine, promethazine, protriptyline, pyrazinamide, sulfonamides, tetracycline, thioridazine, thiazide diuretics, tolazamide, tolbutamide, tranylcypromine, triamterene, trifluoperazine, trimeprazine, trimipramine, triprolidine.

POSSIBLE INTERACTION WITH OTHER SUBSTANCES

INTERACTS WITH	COMBINED EFFECT
Alcohol:	May increase chance of liver toxicity.
Beverages: Lime drinks.	Avoid—toxic.
Cocaine:	Increased chance of toxicity. Avoid.
Foods: Those containing furocoumarin (limes, parsley, figs, parsnips, carrots, celery, mustard).	May cause toxic effects to psoralens.
Marijuana:	Increased chance of toxicity. Avoid.
Tobacco:	May cause uneven absorption of medicine. Avoid.

PSYLLIUM

BRAND NAMES

See complete list of brand names in the *Brand Name Directory*, page 1070.

BASIC INFORMATION

Habit forming? No
Prescription needed? No
Available as generic? No
Drug class: Laxative (bulk-forming)

 ## USES

Relieves constipation and prevents straining for bowel movement.

 ## DOSAGE & USAGE INFORMATION

How to take:
* Powder or granules—Dilute dose in 8 oz. cold water or fruit juice.
* Wafers or chewable pieces—Chew and swallow with liquid.

When to take:
At the same time each day, preferably morning.

If you forget a dose:
Take as soon as you remember. Resume regular schedule.

What drug does:
Absorbs water, stimulating the bowel to form a soft, bulky stool.

Time lapse before drug works:
May require 2 or 3 days to begin, then works in 12 to 24 hours.

Don't take with:
* See Interaction column and consult doctor.
* Don't take within 2 hours of taking another medicine.

 ## OVERDOSE

SYMPTOMS:
None expected.
WHAT TO DO:
Overdose unlikely to threaten life. If person takes much larger amount than prescribed, call doctor, poison-control center or hospital emergency room for instructions.

 ## POSSIBLE ADVERSE REACTIONS OR SIDE EFFECTS

SYMPTOMS	WHAT TO DO
Life-threatening None expected.	
Common: None expected.	
Infrequent: Swallowing difficulty, "lump in throat" sensation.	Continue. Call doctor when convenient.
Rare: Rash, itchy skin, intestinal blockage, asthma.	Discontinue. Call doctor right away.

WARNINGS & PRECAUTIONS

Don't take if:
- You are allergic to any bulk-forming laxative.
- You have symptoms of appendicitis, inflamed bowel or intestinal blockage.
- You have missed a bowel movement for only 1 or 2 days.

Before you start, consult your doctor:
- If you have diabetes.
- If you have kidney disease.
- If you have a laxative habit.
- If you have rectal bleeding.
- If you have difficulty swallowing.
- If you take other laxatives.

Over age 60:
Adverse reactions and side effects may be more frequent and severe than in younger persons.

Pregnancy:
Most bulk-forming laxatives contain sodium or sugars which may cause fluid retention. Avoid if possible.

Breast-feeding:
No problems expected.

Infants & children:
Use only under medical supervision.

Prolonged use:
Don't take for more than 1 week unless under a doctor's supervision. May cause laxative dependence.

Skin & sunlight:
No problems expected.

Driving, piloting or hazardous work:
No problems expected.

Discontinuing:
May be unnecessary to finish medicine. Follow doctor's instructions.

Others:
Don't take to "flush out" your system, or as a "tonic."

POSSIBLE INTERACTION WITH OTHER DRUGS

GENERIC NAME OR DRUG CLASS	COMBINED EFFECT
Digitalis preparations*	Decreased digitalis effect.
Salicylates* (including aspirin)	Decreased salicylate effect.

POSSIBLE INTERACTION WITH OTHER SUBSTANCES

INTERACTS WITH	COMBINED EFFECT
Alcohol:	None expected.
Beverages:	None expected.
Cocaine:	None expected.
Foods:	None expected.
Marijuana:	None expected.
Tobacco:	None expected.

*See Glossary

PYRIDOSTIGMINE

BRAND NAMES

Mestinon   Regonol
Mestinon Timespans

BASIC INFORMATION

Habit forming? No
Prescription needed? Yes
Available as generic? No
Drug class: Cholinergic (anticholinesterase)

 ## USES

- Treatment of myasthenia gravis.
- Treatment of urinary retention and abdominal distention.
- Antidote to adverse effects of muscle relaxants used in surgery.

 ## DOSAGE & USAGE INFORMATION

How to take:
- Tablet or syrup—Swallow with liquid or food to lessen stomach irritation.
- Extended-release tablets—Swallow each dose whole. If you take regular tablets, you may chew or crush them.

When to take:
As directed, usually 3 or 4 times a day.

If you forget a dose:
Take as soon as you remember up to 2 hours late. If more than 2 hours, wait for next scheduled dose (don't double this dose).

What drug does:
Inhibits the chemical activity of an enzyme (cholinesterase) so nerve impulses can cross the junction of nerves and muscles.

Continued next column

 ## OVERDOSE

SYMPTOMS:
Muscle weakness, cramps, twitching or clumsiness; severe diarrhea, nausea, vomiting, stomach cramps or pain; breathing difficulty; confusion, irritability, nervousness, restlessness, fear; unusually slow heartbeat; seizures.

WHAT TO DO:
- Dial 0 (operator) or 911 (emergency) for an ambulance or medical help. Then give first aid immediately.
- See emergency information on inside covers.

Time lapse before drug works:
3 hours.

Don't take with:
See Interaction column and consult doctor.

 ## POSSIBLE ADVERSE REACTIONS OR SIDE EFFECTS

SYMPTOMS	WHAT TO DO
Life-threatening: None expected.	
Common:	
• Mild diarrhea, nausea, vomiting, stomach cramps or pain.	Discontinue. Call doctor right away.
• Excess saliva, unusual sweating.	Continue. Call doctor when convenient.
Infrequent:	
• Confusion, irritability.	Discontinue. Seek emergency treatment.
• Constricted pupils, watery eyes, lung congestion, frequent urge to urinate.	Continue. Call doctor when convenient.
Rare:	
Bronchospasm, slow heartbeat, weakness.	Discontinue. Call doctor right away.

WARNINGS & PRECAUTIONS

Don't take if:
- You are allergic to any cholinergic or bromide.
- You take mecamylamine.

Before you start, consult your doctor:
- If you plan to become pregnant within medication period.
- If you have bronchial asthma.
- If you have heartbeat irregularities.
- If you have urinary obstruction or urinary-tract infection.

Over age 60:
Adverse reactions and side effects may be more frequent and severe than in younger persons.

Pregnancy:
No proven harm to unborn child. Avoid if possible. May increase uterus contractions close to delivery.

Breast-feeding:
No problems expected, but consult doctor.

Infants & children:
Not recommended.

Prolonged use:
Medication may lose effectiveness. Discontinuing for a few days may restore effect.

Skin & sunlight:
No problems expected.

Driving, piloting or hazardous work:
Don't drive or pilot aircraft until you learn how medicine affects you. Don't work around dangerous machinery. Don't climb ladders or work in high places. Danger increases if you drink alcohol or take medicine affecting alertness and reflexes, such as antihistamines, tranquilizers, sedatives, pain medicine, narcotics and mind-altering drugs.

Discontinuing:
Don't discontinue without doctor's advice until you complete prescribed dose, even though symptoms diminish or disappear.

Others:
No problems expected.

POSSIBLE INTERACTION WITH OTHER DRUGS

GENERIC NAME OR DRUG CLASS	COMBINED EFFECT
Anesthetics, local or general*	Decreased pyridostigmine effect.
Antiarrhythmics*	Decreased pyridostigmine effect.
Anticholinergics*	Decreased pyridostigmine effect. May mask severe side effects.
Cholinergics, other*	Reduced intestinal-tract function. Possible brain and nervous-system toxicity.
Mecamylamine	Decreased pyridostigmine effect.
Nitrates*	Decreased pyridostigmine effect.
Quinidine	Decreased pyridostigmine effect.

POSSIBLE INTERACTION WITH OTHER SUBSTANCES

INTERACTS WITH	COMBINED EFFECT
Alcohol:	No proven problems with small doses.
Beverages:	None expected.
Cocaine:	Decreased pyridostigmine effect. Avoid.
Foods:	None expected.
Marijuana:	No proven problems.
Tobacco:	No proven problems.

*See Glossary

PYRIDOXINE (Vitamin B-6)

BRAND NAMES

Alba-Lybe	Hexa-Betalin
Al-Vite	Hexacrest
Beelith	Hexavibex
Beesix	Mega-B
Bendectin	Nu-Iron-V
Eldertonic	Pyroxine
Glutofac	Rodex
Hemo-vite	Tex Six T.R.
Herpecin-L	Vicon

BASIC INFORMATION

Habit forming? No
Prescription needed?
  High strength: Yes
  Low strength: No
Available as generic? Yes
Drug class: Vitamin supplement

USES

- Prevention and treatment of pyridoxine deficiency.
- Treatment of some forms of anemia.
- Treatment of INH (isonicotinic acid hydrozide), cycloserine poisoning.

DOSAGE & USAGE INFORMATION

How to take:
- Tablets—Swallow with liquid.
- Extended-release capsules—Swallow each dose whole with liquid.

When to take:
At the same times each day.

If you forget a dose:
Take as soon as you remember, then resume regular schedule.

What drug does:
Acts as co-enzyme in carbohydrate, protein and fat metabolism.

Time lapse before drug works:
15 to 20 minutes.

Continued next column

OVERDOSE

SYMPTOMS:
None expected.
WHAT TO DO:
Overdose unlikely to threaten life.

Don't take with:
- Levodopa—Small amounts of pyridoxine will nullify levodopa effect. Carbidopa-levodopa combination not affected by this interaction.
- See Interaction column and consult doctor.

POSSIBLE ADVERSE REACTIONS OR SIDE EFFECTS

SYMPTOMS	WHAT TO DO
Life-threatening: None expected.	
Common: None expected.	
Infrequent: Nausea, headache.	Discontinue. Call doctor right away.
Rare: Numbness or tingling in hands or feet (large doses).	Discontinue. Call doctor right away.

WARNINGS & PRECAUTIONS

Don't take if:
You are allergic to pyridoxine.

Before you start, consult your doctor:
If you are pregnant or breast-feeding.

Over age 60:
No problems expected.

Pregnancy:
Don't exceed recommended dose.

Breast-feeding:
Don't exceed recommended dose.

Infants & children:
Don't exceed recommended dose.

Prolonged use:
Large doses for more than 1 month may cause toxicity.

Skin & sunlight:
No problems expected.

Driving, piloting or hazardous work:
No problems expected.

Discontinuing:
No problems expected.

Others:
Regular pyridoxine supplements recommended if you take chloramphenicol, cycloserine, ethionamide, hydralazine, immunosuppressants, isoniazid or penicillamine. These decrease pyridoxine absorption and can cause anemia or tingling and numbness in hands and feet.

POSSIBLE INTERACTION WITH OTHER DRUGS

GENERIC NAME OR DRUG CLASS	COMBINED EFFECT
Contraceptives, oral*	Decreased pyridoxine effect.
Cycloserine	Decreased pyridoxine effect.
Hydralazine	Decreased pyridoxine effect.
Hypnotics, barbiturates*	Decreased hypnotic effect.
Immunosuppressants*	Decreased pyridoxine effect.
Isoniazid	Decreased pyridoxine effect.
Levodopa	Decreased levodopa effect.
Penicillamine	Decreased pyridoxine effect.
Phenobarbital	Possible decreased phenobarbital effect.
Phenytoin	Decreased phenytoin effect.

POSSIBLE INTERACTION WITH OTHER SUBSTANCES

INTERACTS WITH	COMBINED EFFECT
Alcohol:	None expected.
Beverages:	None expected.
Cocaine:	None expected.
Foods:	None expected.
Marijuana:	None expected.
Tobacco:	May decrease pyridoxine absorption. Decreased pyridoxine effect.

PYRILAMINE

BRAND NAMES

See complete list of brand names in the *Brand Name Directory*, page 1070.

BASIC INFORMATION

Habit forming? No
Prescription needed? No
Available as generic? Yes
Drug class: Antihistamine

 ## USES

- Reduces allergic symptoms such as hay fever, hives, rash or itching.
- Prevents motion sickness, nausea, vomiting.
- Induces sleep.

 ## DOSAGE & USAGE INFORMATION

How to take:
Tablet—Swallow with liquid or food to lessen stomach irritation.

When to take:
Varies with form. Follow label directions.

If you forget a dose:
Take as soon as you remember up to 2 hours late. If more than 2 hours, wait for next scheduled dose (don't double this dose).

What drug does:
Blocks action of histamine after an allergic response triggers histamine release in sensitive cells.

Time lapse before drug works:
30 minutes.

Don't take with:
See Interaction column and consult doctor.

 ## OVERDOSE

SYMPTOMS:
Convulsions, red face, hallucinations, coma.
WHAT TO DO:
- Dial 0 (operator) or 911 (emergency) for an ambulance or medical help. Then give first aid immediately.
- If patient is unconscious and not breathing, give mouth-to-mouth breathing. If there is no heartbeat, use cardiac massage and mouth-to-mouth breathing (CPR). Don't try to make patient vomit. If you can't get help quickly, take patient to nearest emergency facility.
- See emergency information on inside covers.

 ## POSSIBLE ADVERSE REACTIONS OR SIDE EFFECTS

SYMPTOMS	WHAT TO DO
Life-threatening: None expected.	
Common: Drowsiness; dizziness; dry mouth, nose and throat; nausea.	Continue. Tell doctor at next visit.
Infrequent: • Change in vision.	Discontinue. Call doctor right away.
• Less tolerance for contact lenses, urination difficulty.	Continue. Call doctor when convenient.
• Appetite loss.	Continue. Tell doctor at next visit.
Rare: Nightmares, agitation, irritability, sore throat, fever, rapid heartbeat, unusual bleeding or bruising, fatigue, weakness.	Discontinue. Call doctor right away.

WARNINGS & PRECAUTIONS

Don't take if:
You are allergic to any antihistamine.

Before you start, consult your doctor:
- If you have glaucoma.
- If you have enlarged prostate.
- If you have asthma.
- If you have kidney disease.
- If you have peptic ulcer.
- If you will have surgery within 2 months, including dental surgery, requiring general or spinal anesthesia.

Over age 60:
Don't exceed recommended dose. Adverse reactions and side effects may be more frequent and severe than in younger persons, especially urination difficulty, diminished alertness and other brain and nervous-system symptoms.

Pregnancy:
No proven harm to unborn child. Avoid if possible.

Breast-feeding:
Drug passes into milk. Avoid drug or discontinue nursing until you finish medicine. Consult doctor for advice on maintaining milk supply.

Infants & children:
Not recommended for premature or newborn infants. Otherwise, no problems expected.

Prolonged use:
Avoid. May damage bone marrow and nerve cells.

Skin & sunlight:
May cause rash or intensify sunburn in areas exposed to sun or sunlamp.

Driving, piloting or hazardous work:
Don't drive or pilot aircraft until you learn how medicine affects you. Don't work around dangerous machinery. Don't climb ladders or work in high places. Danger increases if you drink alcohol or take medicine affecting alertness and reflexes, such as antihistamines, tranquilizers, sedatives, pain medicine, narcotics and mind-altering drugs.

Discontinuing:
No problems expected.

Others:
May mask symptoms of hearing damage from aspirin, other salicylates, cisplatin, paromomycin, vancomycin or anticonvulsants. Consult doctor if you use these.

POSSIBLE INTERACTION WITH OTHER DRUGS

GENERIC NAME OR DRUG CLASS	COMBINED EFFECT
Anticholinergics*	Increased anticholinergic effect.
Antidepressants, tricyclic (TCA)*	Increased pyrilamine effect. Excess sedation.
Antihistamines, other*	Excess sedation. Avoid.
Carteolol	Decreased antihistamine effect.
Dronabinol	Increased effects of both drugs. Avoid.
Hypnotics*	Excess sedation. Avoid.
MAO inhibitors*	Increased pyrilamine effect.
Mind-altering drugs*	Excess sedation. Avoid.
Molindone	Increased sedative and antihistamine effect.
Nabilone	Greater depression of central nervous system.
Narcotics*	Excess sedation. Avoid.
Sedatives*	Excess sedation. Avoid.
Sleep inducers*	Excess sedation. Avoid.
Sotalol	Increased antihistamine effect.
Tranquilizers*	Excess sedation. Avoid.

POSSIBLE INTERACTION WITH OTHER SUBSTANCES

INTERACTS WITH	COMBINED EFFECT
Alcohol:	Excess sedation. Avoid.
Beverages: Caffeine drinks.	Less pyrilamine sedation.
Cocaine:	Decreased pyrilamine effect. Avoid.
Foods:	None expected.
Marijuana:	Excess sedation. Avoid.
Tobacco:	None expected.

PYRILAMINE & PENTOBARBITAL

BRAND NAMES

Wans

BASIC INFORMATION

Habit forming? Yes
Prescription needed? Yes
Available as generic? No
Drug class: Antihistamine, sedative
(barbiturate)

USES

- Prevents and relieves motion sickness, nausea, vomiting.
- Induces sleep.

DOSAGE & USAGE INFORMATION

How to take:
Suppositories—Remove wrapper and moisten suppository with water. Gently insert larger end into rectum. Push well into rectum with finger.

When to take:
As directed when needed.

If you forget a dose:
Take as soon as you remember up to 2 hours late. If more than 2 hours, wait for next scheduled dose (don't double this dose).

What drug does:
- May partially block nerve impulses at nerve-cell connections in nausea center of brain.
- Blocks action of histamine after an allergic response triggers histamine release in sensitive cells.

Continued next column

OVERDOSE

SYMPTOMS:
Deep sleep, weak pulse, convulsions, red face, hallucinations, coma.
WHAT TO DO:
- **Dial 0 (operator) or 911 (emergency) for an ambulance or medical help. Then give first aid immediately.**
- **If patient is unconscious and not breathing, give mouth-to-mouth breathing. If there is no heartbeat, use cardiac massage and mouth-to-mouth breathing (CPR). Don't try to make patient vomit. If you can't get help quickly, take patient to nearest emergency facility.**
- **See emergency information on inside covers.**

Time lapse before drug works:
30 minutes.

Don't take with:
- Non-prescription drugs without consulting doctor.
- See Interaction column and consult doctor.

POSSIBLE ADVERSE REACTIONS OR SIDE EFFECTS

SYMPTOMS	WHAT TO DO
Life-threatening: Slow or fast heartbeat, difficult breathing.	Discontinue. Seek emergency treatment.
Common: • Drowsiness, agitation.	Discontinue. Call doctor right away.
• Dizziness, "hangover" effect, dry mouth.	Continue. Call doctor when convenient.
Infrequent: • Rash; swelling of face, lip or eyelid; change in vision; nausea; vomiting; diarrhea; appetite loss.	Discontinue. Call doctor right away.
• Less tolerance for contact lens, joint or muscle pain, frequent urination.	Continue. Call doctor when convenient.
Rare: Sore throat, fever, mouth sores; urgent urination; jaundice.	Discontinue. Call doctor right away.

WARNINGS & PRECAUTIONS

Don't take if:
- You are allergic to any antihistamine or barbiturate.
- You have porphyria.

Before you start, consult your doctor:
- If you have glaucoma, enlarged prostate, peptic ulcer, epilepsy, kidney or liver damage, asthma, anemia, chronic pain.
- If you will have surgery within 2 months, including dental surgery, requiring general or spinal anesthesia.

PYRILAMINE & PENTOBARBITAL

Over age 60:
Don't exceed recommended dose. Adverse reactions and side effects may be more frequent and severe than in younger persons, especially urination difficulty, diminished alertness and other brain and nervous-system symptoms.

Pregnancy:
Risk to unborn child outweighs drug benefits. Don't use.

Breast-feeding:
Drug passes into milk. Avoid drug or discontinue nursing until you finish medicine. Consult doctor for advice on maintaining milk supply.

Infants & children:
Not recommended for premature or newborn infants. Use only under doctor's supervision.

Prolonged use:
- May damage bone marrow and nerve cells. Avoid.
- May cause addiction, anemia, chronic intoxication.
- May lower body temperature, making exposure to cold temperatures hazardous.

Skin & sunlight:
May cause rash or intensify sunburn in areas exposed to sun or sunlamp.

Driving, piloting or hazardous work:
Don't drive or pilot aircraft until you learn how medicine affects you. Don't work around dangerous machinery. Don't climb ladders or work in high places. Danger increases if you drink alcohol or take medicine affecting alertness and reflexes, such as antihistamines, tranquilizers, sedatives, pain medicine, narcotics and mind-altering drugs.

Discontinuing:
- May be unnecessary to finish medicine. Follow doctor's instructions.
- If you develop withdrawal symptoms of hallucinations, agitation or sleeplessness after discontinuing, call doctor right away.

Others:
- May mask symptoms of hearing damage from aspirin, other salicylates, cisplatin, paromomycin, vancomycin or anticonvulsants. Consult your doctor if you use these.
- Great potential for abuse.

 POSSIBLE INTERACTION WITH OTHER DRUGS

GENERIC NAME OR DRUG CLASS	COMBINED EFFECT
Anticholinergics*	Increased anticholinergics effect.
Anticoagulants*	Decreased anticoagulant effect.
Anticonvulsants*	Changed seizure patterns.
Antidepressants, tricyclics (TCA)*	Possible dangerous oversedation. Increased pyrilamine effect.
Antidiabetics*	Increased pentobarbital effect.
Antihistamines*	Dangerous sedation. Avoid.
Aspirin	Decreased aspirin effect.
Beta-adrenergic blockers*	Decreased effect of beta-adrenergic blocker.
Carteolol	Decreased antihistamine effect.
Contraceptives, oral*	Decreased contraceptive effect.
Cortisone drugs*	Decreased cortisone effect.
Digitoxin	Decreased digitoxin effect.
Doxycycline	Decreased doxycycline effect.

Continued page 1103

 POSSIBLE INTERACTION WITH OTHER SUBSTANCES

INTERACTS WITH	COMBINED EFFECT
Alcohol:	Possible fatal oversedation. Avoid.
Beverages: Caffeine drinks.	Less pyrilamine sedation.
Cocaine:	Decreased Wans effect. Avoid.
Foods:	None expected.
Marijuana:	Excessive sedation. Avoid.
Tobacco:	None expected.

*See Glossary

PYRVINIUM

BRAND NAMES

Pamovin   Vanquin
Povan   Viprynium
Pyr-pam

BASIC INFORMATION

Habit forming? No
Prescription needed? Yes
Available as generic? No
Drug class: Antihelminthic (antiworm
   medication)

 ## USES

Treatment for pinworm infestation.

 ## DOSAGE & USAGE
INFORMATION

How to take:
Tablet—Swallow whole with food or liquid. Don't
crush or chew tablet.

When to take:
According to label instructions. Usually a single
dose, which may be repeated in 2 or 3 weeks.

If you forget a dose:
Take when remembered.

What drug does:
Interferes with a metabolic process in the
infecting parasite and kills it.

Time lapse before drug works:
12 hours.

Don't take with:
Non-prescription drugs for pinworms.

 ## OVERDOSE

SYMPTOMS:
Increased severity of adverse reactions and
side effects.
WHAT TO DO:
Overdose unlikely to threaten life. If person
takes much larger amount than prescribed,
call doctor, poison-control center or hospital
emergency room for instructions.

 ## POSSIBLE
ADVERSE REACTIONS
OR SIDE EFFECTS

SYMPTOMS	WHAT TO DO
Life-threatening: None expected.	
Common: None expected.	
Infrequent: None expected.	
Rare: ● Rash.	Discontinue. Call doctor right away.
● Dizziness, stomach cramps, nausea, vomiting.	Continue. Call doctor when convenient.

WARNINGS & PRECAUTIONS

Don't take if:
You are allergic to any antihelminthic drug.

Before you start, consult your doctor:
- If you have kidney or liver disease.
- If you have a bowel disease or inflammation.

Over age 60:
Adverse reactions and side effects may be more frequent and severe than in younger persons.

Pregnancy:
No proven harm to unborn child. Avoid if possible.

Breast-feeding:
No problems expected, but consult doctor.

Infants & children:
No problems expected.

Prolonged use:
Not recommended.

Skin & sunlight:
May cause rash or intensify sunburn in areas exposed to sun or sunlamp.

Driving, piloting or hazardous work:
Avoid if you feel dizzy. Otherwise, no problems expected.

Discontinuing:
Don't discontinue without doctor's advice until you complete prescribed dose, even though symptoms diminish or disappear.

Others:
- This medicine is a dye that permanently stains most materials. Teeth will be stained a few days. Stool and vomit may be red.
- Pinworm infestations are highly contagious. All family members should be treated at the same time.

POSSIBLE INTERACTION WITH OTHER DRUGS

GENERIC NAME OR DRUG CLASS	COMBINED EFFECT
None expected.	

POSSIBLE INTERACTION WITH OTHER SUBSTANCES

INTERACTS WITH	COMBINED EFFECT
Alcohol:	None expected.
Beverages:	None expected.
Cocaine:	None expected.
Foods:	None expected.
Marijuana:	None expected.
Tobacco:	None expected.

QUINACRINE

BRAND NAMES

Atabrine

BASIC INFORMATION

Habit forming? No
Prescription needed? Yes
Available as generic? Yes
Drug class: Antiprotozoal (destroys microscopic-sized, one-celled animals)

USES

Treats disease caused by the intestinal parasite *Giardia lamblia*.

DOSAGE & USAGE INFORMATION

How to take:
Tablets—Swallow with full glass of water, tea or fruit juice.

When to take:
After meals.

If you forget a dose:
Take as soon as you remember up to 2 hours late. If more than 2 hours, wait for next scheduled dose (don't double this dose).

What drug does:
Destroys *Gardia lamblia* parasites in the gastrointestinal system.

Time lapse before drug works:
1 day.

Don't take with:
See Interaction column and consult doctor.

OVERDOSE

SYMPTOMS:
Severe abdominal cramps, convulsions, severe diarrhea, fainting, irregular heartbeat, restlessness.
WHAT TO DO:
- Dial 0 (operator) or 911 (emergency) for an ambulance or medical help. Then give first aid immediately.
- If patient is unconscious and not breathing, give mouth-to-mouth breathing. If there is no heartbeat, use cardiac massage and mouth-to-mouth breathing (CPR). Don't try to make patient vomit. If you can't get help quickly, take patient to nearest emergency facility.
- See emergency information on inside covers.

POSSIBLE ADVERSE REACTIONS OR SIDE EFFECTS

SYMPTOMS	WHAT TO DO
Life-threatening: None expected.	
Common:	
• Dizziness, nausea, headache.	Discontinue. Call doctor right away.
• Yellow eyes, skin, urine (due to dye-like characteristics of quinacrine).	Report to doctor, but no action necessary.
Infrequent: Mild abdominal cramps; mild diarrhea; appetite loss; skin rash, itching or peeling.	Discontinue. Call doctor right away.
Rare: Hallucinations, nightmares.	Discontinue. Call doctor right away.

WARNINGS & PRECAUTIONS

Don't take if:
You are allergic to quinacrine.

Before you start, consult your doctor:
- If you have porphyria.
- If you have had psoriasis.
- If you have a history of severe mental disorders.
- If you are on a low-salt, low-sugar or other special diet.

Over age 60:
No special problems.

Pregnancy:
Studies inconclusive on harm to unborn child. Decide with your doctor whether drug benefits justify risk to unborn child. Treatment best begun after child has been delivered.

Breast-feeding:
No problems documented.

Infants & children:
Children tolerate quinacrine poorly. Quinacrine may cause vomiting due to bitter taste. Try crushing tablets in jam, honey or chocolate syrup.

Prolonged use:
Can cause eye problems, liver disease, aplastic anemia. Don't use for more than 5 days.

Skin & sunlight:
No problems expected.

Driving, piloting or hazardous work:
Don't drive or pilot aircraft until you learn how medicine affects you. Don't work around dangerous machinery. Don't climb ladders or work in high places. Danger increases if you drink alcohol or take medicine affecting alertness and reflexes, such as antihistamines, tranquilizers, sedatives, pain medicine, narcotics and mind-altering drugs.

Discontinuing:
Don't discontinue before 5 days without consulting doctor.

Others:
Request 3 stool exams several days apart.

POSSIBLE INTERACTION WITH OTHER DRUGS

GENERIC NAME OR DRUG CLASS	COMBINED EFFECT
Primaquine	Decreased effect of primaquine.

POSSIBLE INTERACTION WITH OTHER SUBSTANCES

INTERACTS WITH	COMBINED EFFECT
Alcohol:	Increase adverse effects of both. Avoid.
Beverages:	Increase adverse effects of both. Avoid.
Cocaine:	Increase adverse effects of both. Avoid.
Foods:	Increase adverse effects of both. Avoid.
Marijuana:	Increase adverse effects of both. Avoid.
Tobacco:	Increase adverse effects of both. Avoid.

QUINESTROL

BRAND NAMES

Estrovis

BASIC INFORMATION

Habit forming? No
Prescription needed? Yes
Available as generic? No
Drug class: Female sex hormone (estrogen)

USES

- Treatment for symptoms of menopause and menstrual-cycle irregularity.
- Replacement for female hormone deficiency.

DOSAGE & USAGE INFORMATION

How to take:
Tablet—Swallow with liquid. If you can't swallow whole, crumble tablet and take with liquid or food.

When to take:
At the same time each day.

If you forget a dose:
Take as soon as you remember up to 12 hours late. If more than 12 hours, wait for next scheduled dose (don't double this dose).

What drug does:
Restores normal estrogen level in tissues.

Time lapse before drug works:
10 to 20 days.

Don't take with:
See Interaction column and consult doctor.

OVERDOSE

SYMPTOMS:
Nausea, vomiting, fluid retention, breast enlargement and discomfort, abnormal vaginal bleeding.
WHAT TO DO:
Overdose unlikely to threaten life. If person takes much larger amount than prescribed, call doctor, poison-control center or hospital emergency room for instructions.

POSSIBLE ADVERSE REACTIONS OR SIDE EFFECTS

SYMPTOMS	WHAT TO DO
Life-threatening: None expected.	
Common:	
• Stomach cramps.	Discontinue. Call doctor right away.
• Appetite loss.	Continue. Call doctor when convenient.
• Nausea; diarrhea; swollen ankles, feet; swollen, tender breasts.	Continue. Tell doctor at next visit.
Infrequent:	
• Rash, stomach or side pain.	Discontinue. Call doctor right away.
• Dizziness, vomiting, irritability, headache, depression, breast lumps.	Continue. Call doctor when convenient.
• Brown blotches, hair loss, vaginal discharge or bleeding, changes in sex drive.	Continue. Tell doctor at next visit.
Rare: Jaundice, hypercalcemia in breast cancer, intolerance of contact lenses.	Discontinue. Call doctor right away.

WARNINGS & PRECAUTIONS

Don't take if:
- You are allergic to any estrogen-containing drugs.
- You have impaired liver function.
- You have had blood clots, stroke or heart attack.
- You have unexplained vaginal bleeding.

Before you start, consult your doctor:
- If you have had cancer of breast or reproductive organs, fibrocystic breast disease, fibroid tumors of the uterus or endometriosis.
- If you have had migraine headaches, epilepsy or porphyria.
- If you have diabetes, high blood pressure, asthma, congestive heart failure, kidney disease or gallstones.
- If you plan to become pregnant within 3 months.

Over age 60:
Controversial. You and your doctor must decide if drug risks outweigh benefits.

Pregnancy:
Risk to unborn child outweighs drug benefits. Don't use.

Breast-feeding:
Drug filters into milk. May harm child. Avoid.

Infants & children:
Not recommended.

Prolonged use:
Increased growth of fibroid tumors of uterus. Possible association with cancer of uterus.

Skin & sunlight:
May cause rash or intensify sunburn in areas exposed to sun or sunlamp.

Driving, piloting or hazardous work:
No problems expected.

Discontinuing:
You may need to discontinue quinestrol periodically. Consult your doctor.

Others:
In rare instances, may cause blood clot in lung, brain or leg. Symptoms are *sudden* severe headache, coordination loss, vision change, chest pain, breathing difficulty, slurred speech, pain in legs or groin. Seek emergency treatment immediately.

POSSIBLE INTERACTION WITH OTHER DRUGS

GENERIC NAME OR DRUG CLASS	COMBINED EFFECT
Anticoagulants, oral*	Decreased anti-coagulant effect.
Anticonvulsants, hydantoin*	Decreased estrogen effect.
Antidepressants, tricyclic (TCA)*	Increased toxicity of TCAs.
Antidiabetics, oral*	Unpredictable increase or decrease in blood sugar.
Antifibrinolytic agents*	Increased possibility of blood clotting.
Carbamazepine	Decreased estrogen effect.

Clofibrate	Decreased clofibrate effect.
Insulin	Possible decreased insulin effect. Dosages may require adjustment.
Meprobamate	Increased quinestrol effect.
Phenobarbital	Decreased quinestrol effect.
Primidone	Decreased quinestrol effect.
Rifampin	Decreased quinestrol effect.
Terazosin	Decreases effectiveness of terazosin.
Thyroid hormones*	Decreased thyroid effect.
Ursodiol	Decreased effect of ursodiol.
Vitamin C	Possible increased estrogen effect.

POSSIBLE INTERACTION WITH OTHER SUBSTANCES

INTERACTS WITH	COMBINED EFFECT
Alcohol:	None expected.
Beverages:	None expected.
Cocaine:	No proven problems.
Foods:	None expected.
Marijuana:	Possible menstrual irregularities and bleeding between periods.
Tobacco:	Increased risk of blood clots leading to stroke or heart attack.

QUINETHAZONE

BRAND NAMES

Aquamox   Hydromox

BASIC INFORMATION

Habit forming? No
Prescription needed? Yes
Available as generic? No
Drug class: Antihypertensive, diuretic
(thiazide)

USES

- Controls, but doesn't cure, high blood pressure.
- Reduces fluid retention (edema) caused by conditions such as heart disorders and liver disease.

DOSAGE & USAGE INFORMATION

How to take:
Tablet—Swallow with liquid. If you can't swallow whole, crumble tablet and take with liquid or food. Don't exceed dose.

When to take:
At the same time each day.

If you forget a dose:
Take as soon as you remember up to 2 hours late. If more than 2 hours, wait for next scheduled dose (don't double this dose).

What drug does:
- Forces sodium and water excretion, reducing body fluid.
- Relaxes muscle cells of small arteries.
- Reduced body fluid and relaxed arteries lower blood pressure.

Time lapse before drug works:
4 to 6 hours. May require several weeks to lower blood pressure.

Continued next column

OVERDOSE

SYMPTOMS:
Cramps, weakness, drowsiness, weak pulse, coma.
WHAT TO DO:
- **Dial 0 (operator) or 911 (emergency) for an ambulance or medical help. Then give first aid immediately.**
- **See emergency information on inside covers.**

Don't take with:
- Non-prescription drugs without consulting doctor.
- See Interaction column and consult doctor.

POSSIBLE ADVERSE REACTIONS OR SIDE EFFECTS

SYMPTOMS	WHAT TO DO
Life-threatening: None expected.	
Common: None expected.	
Infrequent:	
• Blurred vision, severe abdominal pain, nausea, vomiting, irregular heartbeat, weak pulse.	Discontinue. Call doctor right away.
• Dizziness, mood change, headache, weakness, tiredness, weight changes.	Continue. Call doctor when convenient.
• Dry mouth, thirst.	Continue. Tell doctor at next visit.
Rare:	
• Rash or hives.	Discontinue. Seek emergency treatment.
• Sore throat, fever, jaundice.	Discontinue. Call doctor right away.

WARNINGS & PRECAUTIONS

Don't take if:
You are allergic to any thiazide diuretic drug.

Before you start, consult your doctor:
- If you are allergic to any sulfa drug.
- If you have gout.
- If you have liver, pancreas or liver disorder.

Over age 60:
Adverse reactions and side effects may be more frequent and severe than in younger persons, especially dizziness and excessive potassium loss.

Pregnancy:
Risk to unborn child outweighs drug benefits. Don't use.

Breast-feeding:
Drug passes into milk. Avoid drug or discontinue nursing.

Infants & children:
No problems expected.

Prolonged use:
You may need medicine to treat high blood pressure for the rest of your life.

Skin & sunlight:
May cause rash or intensify sunburn in areas exposed to sun or sunlamp.

Driving, piloting or hazardous work:
Don't drive or pilot aircraft until you learn how medicine affects you. Don't work around dangerous machinery. Don't climb ladders or work in high places. Danger increases if you drink alcohol or take medicine affecting alertness and reflexes, such as antihistamines, tranquilizers, sedatives, pain medicine, narcotics and mind-altering drugs.

Discontinuing:
Don't discontinue without medical advice.

Others:
- Hot weather and fever may cause dehydration and drop in blood pressure. Dose may require temporary adjustment. Weigh daily and report any unexpected weight decreases to your doctor.
- May cause rise in uric acid, leading to gout.
- May cause blood-sugar rise in diabetics.

POSSIBLE INTERACTION WITH OTHER DRUGS

GENERIC NAME OR DRUG CLASS	COMBINED EFFECT
ACE inhibitors: captopril, enalapril, lisinopril*	Decreased blood pressure. Possible excessive potassium in blood.
Allopurinol	Decreased allopurinol effect.
Amiodarone	Increased risk of heartbeat irregularity due to low potassium.
Amphotericin B	Increased potassium.
Antidepressants, tricyclic (TCA)*	Dangerous drop in blood pressure. Avoid combination unless under medical supervision.
Antidiabetic agents, oral*	Increased blood sugar.
Antihypertensives, other*	Increased hypertensive effect of both drugs.
Barbiturates*	Increased quinethazone effect.
Beta-adrenergic blockers*	Increased antihypertensive effect. Dosages of both drugs may require adjustments.

Calcium supplements*	Increased calcium in blood.
Carteolol	Increased antihypertensive effect.
Cholestyramine	Decreased quinethazone effect.
Colestipol	Decreased quinethazone effect.
Cortisone drugs*	Excessive potassium loss that causes dangerous heart rhythms.
Digitalis preparations*	Excessive potassium loss that causes dangerous heart rhythms.
Diuretics, thiazide*	Increased effect of other thiazide diuretics.
Indapamide	Increased diuretic effect.
Indomethacin	Decreased quinethazone effect.
Labetalol	Increased antihypertensive effects.
Lithium	Increased effect of lithium.
MAO inhibitors*	Increased quinethazone effect.
Nicardipine	Blood-pressure drop. Dosages may require adjustment.

Continued page 1103

POSSIBLE INTERACTION WITH OTHER SUBSTANCES

INTERACTS WITH	COMBINED EFFECT
Alcohol:	Dangerous blood-pressure drop.
Beverages:	None expected.
Cocaine:	Increased risk of heart block and high blood pressure.
Foods: Licorice.	Excessive potassium loss that causes dangerous heart rhythms.
Marijuana:	May increase blood pressure.
Tobacco:	None expected.

QUINIDINE

BRAND NAMES

Apo-Quinidine
Biquin Durules
Cardioquin
Cin-Quin
Duraquin
Novoquinidin
Quinaglute Dura-Tabs

Quinalan
Quinate
Quinidex Extentabs
Quinobarb
Quinora
SK-Quinidine
 Sulfate

BASIC INFORMATION

Habit forming? No
Prescription needed?
 U.S.: Yes
 Canada: No
Available as generic? Yes
Drug class: Antiarrhythmic

USES

Corrects heart-rhythm disorders.

DOSAGE & USAGE INFORMATION

How to take:
* Tablet or capsule—Swallow with liquid or food to lessen stomach irritation.
* Extended-release tablets—Swallow each dose whole. Don't crush them.

When to take:
At the same times each day.

If you forget a dose:
Take as soon as you remember up to 2 hours late. If more than 2 hours, wait for next scheduled dose (don't double this dose).

Continued next column

OVERDOSE

SYMPTOMS:
Confusion, severe blood-pressure drop, lethargy, breathing difficulty, fainting, seizures, coma.
WHAT TO DO:
* Dial 0 (operator) or 911 (emergency) for an ambulance or medical help. Then give first aid immediately.
* If patient is unconscious and not breathing, give mouth-to-mouth breathing. If there is no heartbeat, use cardiac massage and mouth-to-mouth breathing (CPR). Don't try to make patient vomit. If you can't get help quickly, take patient to nearest emergency facility.
* See emergency information on inside covers.

What drug does:
Delays nerve impulses to the heart to regulate heartbeat.

Time lapse before drug works:
2 to 4 hours.

Don't take with:
See Interaction column and consult doctor.

POSSIBLE ADVERSE REACTIONS OR SIDE EFFECTS

SYMPTOMS	WHAT TO DO
Life-threatening:	
Hives, rash, intense itching, faintness soon after a dose (anaphylaxis).	Seek emergency treatment immediately.
Common:	
Bitter taste, diarrhea, nausea, vomiting.	Discontinue. Call doctor right away.
Infrequent:	
• Dizziness, lightheadedness, fainting, headache, confusion, rash, change in vision, difficult breathing, rapid heartbeat.	Discontinue. Call doctor right away.
• Ringing in ears.	Continue. Call doctor when convenient.
Rare:	
• Unusual bleeding or bruising, difficulty or pain on swallowing, fever, joint pain, jaundice, hepatitis.	Discontinue. Call doctor right away.
• Weakness.	Continue. Call doctor when convenient.

WARNINGS & PRECAUTIONS

Don't take if:
- You are allergic to quinidine.
- You have an active infection.

Before you start, consult your doctor:
About any drug you take, including non-prescription drugs.

Over age 60:
Adverse reactions and side effects may be more frequent and severe than in younger persons.

Pregnancy:
Risk to unborn child outweighs drug benefits. Don't use.

Breast-feeding:
Drug filters into milk. May harm child. Avoid.

Infants & children:
No problems expected.

Prolonged use:
No problems expected.

Skin & sunlight:
No problems expected.

Driving, piloting or hazardous work:
Don't drive or pilot aircraft until you learn how medicine affects you. Don't work around dangerous machinery. Don't climb ladders or work in high places. Danger increases if you drink alcohol or take medicine affecting alertness and reflexes, such as antihistamines, tranquilizers, sedatives, pain medicine, narcotics and mind-altering drugs.

Discontinuing:
Don't discontinue without doctor's advice until you complete prescribed dose, even though symptoms diminish or disappear.

Others:
No problems expected.

POSSIBLE INTERACTION WITH OTHER DRUGS

GENERIC NAME OR DRUG CLASS	COMBINED EFFECT
Alkaline urine	Slows quinidine elimination, increases effect and toxicity.
Antiarrhythmics*	May increase or decrease effect or toxicity of quinidine.
Anticholinergics*	Increased anti-cholinergic effect.
Anticoagulants, oral*	Possible increased anticoagulant effect.

	COMBINED EFFECT
Antihypertensives*	Increased antihypertensive effect.
Beta-adrenergic blockers*	May slow heartbeat excessively.
Cholinergics*	Decreased cholinergic effect.
Cimetidine	Increased quinidine effect.
Digitalis preparations*	May slow heartbeat excessively. Dose adjustments may be needed.
Encainide	Increased effect of toxicity on heart muscle.
Flecainide	Possible irregular heartbeat.
Guanfacine	Increased effect of both medicines.
Nicardipine	Possible increased effect and toxicity of each drug.
Nifedipine	Possible decreased quinidine effect.
Phenobarbital	Decreased quinidine effect.
Phenothiazines*	Possible increased quinidine effect.
Phenytoin	Decreased quinidine effect.
Rauwolfia alkaloids*	Possibly disturbs heart rhythms.
Tocainide	Increased possibility of adverse reactions from either drug.
Rifampin	Decreased quinidine effect.
Verapamil	Hypotension.

POSSIBLE INTERACTION WITH OTHER SUBSTANCES

INTERACTS WITH	COMBINED EFFECT
Alcohol:	None expected.
Beverages: Caffeine drinks.	Causes rapid heartbeat. Use sparingly.
Cocaine:	Irregular heartbeat. Avoid.
Foods:	None expected.
Marijuana:	Can cause fainting.
Tobacco:	Irregular heartbeat. Avoid.

*See Glossary

QUININE

BRAND NAMES

Coco-Quinine	Quindan
Kinine	Quine
NovoQuinie	Quinite
Quinamm	Strema

BASIC INFORMATION

Habit forming? No
Prescription needed?
  High strength: Yes
  Low strength: No
Available as generic? Yes
Drug class: Antiprotozoal

USES

- Treatment or prevention of malaria.
- Relief of muscle cramps.

DOSAGE & USAGE INFORMATION

How to take:
Tablet or capsule—Swallow with liquid or food to lessen stomach irritation.

When to take:
- Prevention—At the same time each day, usually at bedtime.
- Treatment—At the same times each day in evenly spaced doses.

If you forget a dose:
- Prevention—Take as soon as you remember up to 12 hours late. If more than 12 hours, wait for next scheduled dose (don't double this dose).
- Treatment—Take as soon as you remember up to 2 hours late. If more than 2 hours, wait for next scheduled dose (don't double this dose).

Continued next column

OVERDOSE

SYMPTOMS:
Severe impairment of vision and hearing; severe nausea, vomiting, diarrhea; shallow breathing, fast heartbeat; apprehension, confusion, delirium.
WHAT TO DO:
Dial 0 (operator) or 911 (emergency) for an ambulance or medical help. Then give first aid immediately.

What drug does:
- Reduces contractions of skeletal muscles.
- Increases blood flow.
- Interferes with genes in malaria micro-organisms.

Time lapse before drug works:
May require several days or weeks for maximum effect.

Don't take with:
See Interaction column and consult doctor.

POSSIBLE ADVERSE REACTIONS OR SIDE EFFECTS

SYMPTOMS	WHAT TO DO
Life-threatening: None expected.	
Common:	
Blurred vision or change in vision.	Discontinue. Call doctor right away.
Dizziness, headache, stomach discomfort, mild nausea, vomiting, diarrhea.	Continue. Call doctor when convenient.
Ringing or buzzing in ears, impaired hearing.	Continue. Tell doctor at next visit.
Infrequent:	
Rash, hives, itchy skin, difficult breathing.	Discontinue. Call doctor right away.
Rare:	
Sore throat, fever, unusual bleeding or bruising, unusual tiredness or weakness, angina.	Discontinue. Call doctor right away.

WARNINGS & PRECAUTIONS

Don't take if:
You are allergic to quinine or quinidine.

Before you start, consult your doctor:
- If you plan to become pregnant within medication period.
- If you have asthma.
- If you have eye disease, hearing problems or ringing in the ears.
- If you have heart disease.
- If you have myasthenia gravis.

Over age 60:
Adverse reactions and side effects may be more frequent and severe than in younger persons.

Pregnancy:
Risk to unborn child outweighs drug benefits. Don't use.

Breast-feeding:
Drug filters into milk. May harm child. Avoid.

Infants & children:
Use only under medical supervision.

Prolonged use:
May develop headache, blurred vision, nausea, temporary hearing loss, but seldom need to discontinue because of these symptoms.

Skin & sunlight:
No problems expected.

Driving, piloting or hazardous work:
Avoid if you feel dizzy or have blurred vision. Otherwise, no problems expected.

Discontinuing:
Don't discontinue without doctor's advice until you complete prescribed dose, even though symptoms diminish or disappear.

Others:
Don't confuse with quinidine, a medicine for heart-rhythm problems.

POSSIBLE INTERACTION WITH OTHER DRUGS

GENERIC NAME OR DRUG CLASS	COMBINED EFFECT
Antacids* (with aluminum hydroxide)	Decreased quinine effect.
Anticoagulants, oral*	Increased anti-coagulant effect.
Digitalis	Possible increased digitalis effect.
Digoxin	Possible increased digoxin effect.
Quinidine	Possible toxic effects of quinine.
Sodium bicarbonate	Possible toxic effects of quinine.

POSSIBLE INTERACTION WITH OTHER SUBSTANCES

INTERACTS WITH	COMBINED EFFECT
Alcohol:	No proven problems.
Beverages:	None expected.
Cocaine:	No proven problems.
Foods:	None expected.
Marijuana:	No proven problems.
Tobacco:	None expected.

*See Glossary

RADIO-PHARMACEUTICALS

BRAND NAMES

See complete list of brand names in the *Brand Name Directory*, page 1070.

BASIC INFORMATION

Habit forming? No
Prescription needed? Yes
Available as generic? Yes
Drug class: Radio-pharmaceuticals

 ## USES

To help establish an accurate diagnosis for many medical problems, such as pernicious anemia, malabsorption, iron metabolism, cancer, abscess, infection, cerebrospinal fluid flow, blood volume, kidney diseases, lung diseases, pancreas diseases, red blood cell disorders, spleen diseases, thyroid diseases, thyroid cancer, brain diseases or tumor, bladder diseases, eye tumors, liver diseases, heart diseases, bone diseases, bone marrow diseases.

 ## DOSAGE & USAGE INFORMATION

How to take:
- As directed by nuclear medicine specialist. Most are given intravenously by the doctor, some are taken by mouth.
- Drink lots of liquids and urinate often after test to decrease possible radiation effect on the kidneys and urinary bladder.

When to take:
According to individual instructions.

If you forget a dose:
Take as soon as you remember.

What drug does:
Very small quantities of radioactive substances concentrate in various organs of the body and become measurable. Pictures or readings of the organ or system under study become possible.

Time lapse before drug works:
Varies between products.

Don't take with:
Any other medicine without consulting doctor.

 ## OVERDOSE

SYMPTOMS:
None expected.
WHAT TO DO:
None expected.

 ## POSSIBLE ADVERSE REACTIONS OR SIDE EFFECTS

SYMPTOMS	WHAT TO DO
Life-threatening:	
Hives, rash, intense itching, faintness soon after a dose (anaphylaxis).	Seek emergency treatment immediately.
Common:	
None expected.	
Infrequent:	
Drowsiness; fast heartbeat; swollen feet, ankles, hands or throat; abdominal pain; rash; hives; nausea; vomiting, headache; red or flushed face; fever; fainting.	Discontinue. Call doctor right away.
Rare:	
Constipation; coughing; bronchospasm; laryngeal edema; sneezing, rhinitis, lacrimation.	Discontinue. Call doctor right away.

WARNINGS & PRECAUTIONS

Don't take if:
You are allergic to the prescribed drug.

Before you start, consult your doctor:
- If you have had allergic reactions to human serum albumin.
- If you are allergic to anything.

Over age 60:
Adverse reactions and side effects may be more frequent and severe than in younger persons. Ask doctor about smaller doses.

Pregnancy:
Avoid during pregnancy if possible.

Breast-feeding:
Drug passes into milk. Avoid drug or discontinue nursing until you finish medicine. Consult doctor for advice on maintaining milk supply.

Infants & children:
No problems expected.

Prolonged use:
Not intended for prolonged use.

Skin & sunlight:
No problems expected.

Driving, piloting or hazardous work:
No problems expected.

Discontinuing:
No problems expected.

Others:
Some of these agents may accumulate in the urinary bladder. To decrease chance of excessive radiation, drink 8 oz. of fluid every 1 hour for 10 to 12 hours following the test, unless otherwise specified by your doctor.

POSSIBLE INTERACTION WITH OTHER DRUGS

GENERIC NAME OR DRUG CLASS	COMBINED EFFECT
None expected.	

POSSIBLE INTERACTION WITH OTHER SUBSTANCES

INTERACTS WITH	COMBINED EFFECT
Alcohol:	None expected.
Beverages:	None expected.
Cocaine:	None expected.
Foods:	None expected.
Marijuana:	None expected.
Tobacco:	None expected.

RANITIDINE

BRAND NAMES

Zantac

BASIC INFORMATION

Habit forming? No
Prescription needed? Yes
Available as generic? No
Drug class: Histamine H2 antagonist

 ## USES

- Treatment for duodenal ulcer.
- Decreases acid in stomach.

 ## DOSAGE & USAGE INFORMATION

How to take:
Tablets—Swallow with liquid.

When to take:
At same times each day.

If you forget a dose:
Take as soon as you remember up to 2 hours late. If more than 2 hours, wait for next scheduled dose (don't double this dose).

What drug does:
Decreases stomach-acid production.

Time lapse before drug works:
2 to 3 hours.

Don't take with:
- Alcohol.
- See Interaction column and consult doctor.

 ## OVERDOSE

SYMPTOMS:
Muscular tremors, vomiting, rapid breathing, coma.
WHAT TO DO:
- **Dial 0 (operator) or 911 (emergency) for an ambulance or medical help. Then give first aid immediately.**
- **If patient is unconscious and not breathing, give mouth-to-mouth breathing. If there is no heartbeat, use cardiac massage and mouth-to-mouth breathing (CPR). Don't try to make patient vomit. If you can't get help quickly, take patient to nearest emergency facility.**
- **See emergency information on inside covers.**

 ## POSSIBLE ADVERSE REACTIONS OR SIDE EFFECTS

SYMPTOMS	WHAT TO DO
Life-threatening: None expected.	
Common: None expected.	
Infrequent: • Rash, confusion, diarrhea.	Discontinue. Call doctor right away.
• Headache, dizziness, constipation, nausea, abdominal pain.	Continue. Call doctor when convenient.
Rare: Jaundice.	Discontinue. Call doctor right away.

WARNINGS & PRECAUTIONS

Don't take if:
You are allergic to any histamine H2 antagonist.

Before you start, consult your doctor:
If you have kidney disease.

Over age 60:
Adverse reactions and side effects may be more frequent and severe than in younger persons.

Pregnancy:
No proven harm to unborn child. Avoid if possible.

Breast-feeding:
Drug passes into milk. Avoid drug or discontinue nursing until you finish medicine. Consult doctor for advice on maintaining milk supply.

Infants & children:
Not recommended.

Prolonged use:
Not recommended. Use for short term only.

Skin & sunlight:
No problems expected.

Driving, piloting or hazardous work:
Avoid if you feel dizzy. Otherwise, no problems expected.

Discontinuing:
Don't discontinue without consulting doctor until you finish prescribed dose, even though symptoms diminish or disappear.

Others:
The drug interactions with ranitidine may occur in a small number of patients compared to cimetidine.

POSSIBLE INTERACTION WITH OTHER DRUGS

GENERIC NAME OR DRUG CLASS	COMBINED EFFECT
Antacids*	Decreased absorption of ranitidine if taken simultaneously.
Glipizide	Possible increased glipizide effect.
Ketoconazole	Decreased absorption of ranitidine.
Procainamide	Increased procainamide effect and toxicity.
Theophylline	Possible increased theophylline effect.
Warfarin	Increased warfarin effect.

POSSIBLE INTERACTION WITH OTHER SUBSTANCES

INTERACTS WITH	COMBINED EFFECT
Alcohol:	Decreased ranitidine effect.
Beverages:	None expected.
Cocaine:	No proven problems.
Foods:	None expected.
Marijuana:	No proven problems.
Tobacco:	Decreased ranitidine effect.

BRAND AND GENERIC NAMES

See complete list of brand and generic names in the *Brand Name Directory*, page 1070.

BASIC INFORMATION

Habit forming? No
Prescription needed? Yes
Available as generic? Yes
Drug class: Antihypertensive, tranquilizer (rauwolfia alkaloid)

 ## USES

- Treatment for high blood pressure.
- Tranquilizer for mental and emotional disturbances.

 ## DOSAGE & USAGE INFORMATION

How to take:
Tablet or timed-release capsule—Swallow with liquid or food to lessen stomach irritation. If you can't swallow whole, crumble tablet or open capsule and take with liquid or food.

When to take:
At the same times each day.

If you forget a dose:
Take as soon as you remember up to 2 hours late. If more than 2 hours, wait for next scheduled dose (don't double this dose).

What drug does:
- Interferes with nerve impulses and relaxes blood-vessel muscles, reducing blood pressure.
- Suppresses brain centers that control emotions.

Time lapse before drug works:
3 weeks continual use required to determine effectiveness.

Don't take with:
See Interaction column and consult doctor.

 ## OVERDOSE

SYMPTOMS:
Drowsiness; slow, weak pulse; slow, shallow breathing; diarrhea; coma; flush; low body temperature.
WHAT TO DO:
- Dial 0 (operator) or 911 (emergency) for an ambulance or medical help. Then give first aid immediately.
- See emergency information on inside covers.

 ## POSSIBLE ADVERSE REACTIONS OR SIDE EFFECTS

SYMPTOMS	WHAT TO DO
Life-threatening: None expected.	
Common:	
• Depression.	Continue. Call doctor when convenient.
• Headache, faintness, drowsiness, lethargy, red eyes, stuffy nose, impotence, diminished sex drive.	Continue. Tell doctor at next visit.
Infrequent:	
• Black stool; bloody vomit; chest pain; shortness of breath; irregular or slow heartbeat; stiffness in muscles, bones, joints.	Discontinue. Call doctor right away.
• Trembling hands.	Continue. Call doctor when convenient.
Rare:	
• Rash or itchy skin, sore throat, fever, stomach pain, nausea, vomiting, unusual bleeding or bruising, jaundice.	Discontinue. Call doctor right away.
• Painful urination.	Continue. Call doctor when convenient.

 ## WARNINGS & PRECAUTIONS

Don't take if:
- You are allergic to any rauwolfia alkaloid.
- You are depressed.
- You have active peptic ulcer.
- You have ulcerative colitis.

Before you start, consult your doctor:
- If you have been depressed.
- If you have had peptic ulcer, ulcerative colitis or gallstones.
- If you have epilepsy.
- If you will have surgery within 2 months, including dental surgery, requiring general or spinal anesthesia.

Over age 60:
Adverse reactions and side effects may be more frequent and severe than in younger persons.

Pregnancy:
Studies inconclusive on harm to unborn child. Animal studies show fetal abnormalities. Decide with your doctor whether drug benefits justify risk to unborn child.

Breast-feeding:
Drug passes into milk. Avoid drug or discontinue nursing until you finish medicine. Consult doctor for advice on maintaining milk supply.

Infants & children:
Not recommended.

Prolonged use:
Causes cancer in laboratory animals. Consult your doctor if you have family or personal history of cancer.

Skin & sunlight:
No problems expected.

Driving, piloting or hazardous work:
Avoid if you feel drowsy, dizzy or faint. Otherwise, no problems expected.

Discontinuing:
Don't discontinue without consulting doctor. Dose may require gradual reduction if you have taken drug for a long time. Doses of other drugs may also require adjustment.

Others:
Consult your doctor if you do isometric exercises. These raise blood pressure. Drug may intensify blood-pressure rise.

POSSIBLE INTERACTION WITH OTHER DRUGS

GENERIC NAME OR DRUG CLASS	COMBINED EFFECT
Anticoagulants, oral*	Unpredictable increased or decreased effect of anticoagulant.
Anticonvulsants*	Serious change in seizure pattern.
Antidepressants*	Increased antidepressant effect.
Antihistamines*	Increased antihistamine effect.
Antihypertensives, other*	Increased effect of rauwolfia.
Aspirin	Decreased aspirin effect.
Beta-adrenergic blockers*	Increased effect of rauwolfia alkaloids. Excessive sedation.
Carteolol	Increased antihypertensive effect.
Digitalis preparations*	Possible irregular heartbeat.
Dronabinol	Increased effects of both drugs. Avoid.
Ethinamate	Dangerous increased effects of ethinamate. Avoid combining.
Fluoxetine	Increased depressant effects of both drugs.
Guanfacine	May increase depressant effects of either medicine.
Leucovorin	High alcohol content of leucovorin may cause adverse effects.
Levodopa	Decreased levodopa effect.
Lisinopril	Increased antihypertensive effect. Dosage of each may require adjustment.
Loxapine	May increase toxic effects of both drugs.
MAO inhibitors*	Severe depression.
Methyprylon	May increase sedative effect to dangerous level. Avoid.
Mind-altering drugs*	Excessive sedation.
Nabilone	Greater depression of central nervous system.
Nicardipine	Blood-pressure drop. Dosages may require adjustment.
Sotalol	Increased antihypertensive effect.
Terazosin	Decreases effectiveness of terazosin.

POSSIBLE INTERACTION WITH OTHER SUBSTANCES

INTERACTS WITH	COMBINED EFFECT
Alcohol:	Increased intoxication. Use with extreme caution.
Beverages: Carbonated drinks.	Decreased rauwolfia alkaloids effect.
Cocaine:	Increased risk of heart block and high blood pressure.
Foods: Spicy foods.	Possible digestive upset.
Marijuana:	Occasional use—Mild drowsiness. Daily use—Moderate drowsiness, low blood pressure, depression.
Tobacco:	No problems expected.

RAUWOLFIA & THIAZIDE DIURETICS

BRAND NAMES

See complete list of brand names in the *Brand Name Directory*, page 1070.

BASIC INFORMATION

Habit forming? No
Prescription needed? Yes
Available as generic? Yes
Drug class: Antihypertensive, diuretic, tranquilizer

USES

- Controls, but doesn't cure, high blood pressure.
- Reduces fluid retention (edema).

DOSAGE & USAGE INFORMATION

How to take:
Tablet—Swallow with liquid. If you can't swallow whole, crumble tablet and take with liquid or food.

When to take:
At the same time each day.

If you forget a dose:
Take as soon as you remember up to 2 hours late. If more than 2 hours, wait for next scheduled dose (don't double this dose).

What drug does:
- Forces sodium and water excretion, reducing body fluid.
- Reduced body fluid and relaxed arteries lower blood pressure.
- Interferes with nerve impulses and relaxes blood-vessel muscles, reducing blood pressure.
- Suppresses brain centers that control emotion.

Continued next column

OVERDOSE

SYMPTOMS:
Cramps; weakness; drowsiness; slow, weak pulse; slow, shallow breathing; diarrhea; flush; low body temperature; coma.
WHAT TO DO:
- **Dial 0 (operator) or 911 (emergency) for an ambulance or medical help. Then give first aid immediately.**
- **See emergency information on inside covers.**

Time lapse before drug works:
3 weeks continual use required to determine effectiveness.

Don't take with:
- Non-prescription drugs without consulting doctor.
- See Interaction column and consult doctor.

POSSIBLE ADVERSE REACTIONS OR SIDE EFFECTS

SYMPTOMS	WHAT TO DO
Life-threatening:	
Irregular heartbeat, weak pulse, hives, black stool, bloody vomit.	Discontinue. Seek emergency treatment.
Common:	
Lethargy, drowsiness, tremor, depression, red eyes, runny nose.	Continue. Call doctor when convenient.
Infrequent:	
• Blurred vision, abdominal pain, nausea, vomiting, irregular heartbeat, joint pain.	Discontinue. Call doctor right away.
• Dizziness, mood change, headache, dry mouth, weakness, tiredness, weight gain or loss.	Continue. Call doctor when convenient.
Rare:	
• Sore throat, fever, mouth sores; jaundice; unexplained bleeding or bruising.	Discontinue. Call doctor right away.
• Rash, painful or difficult urination, tremor, impotence.	Continue. Call doctor when convenient.

WARNINGS & PRECAUTIONS

Don't take if:
- You are allergic to any thiazide diuretic drug or any rauwolfia alkaloid.
- You are depressed.
- You have active peptic ulcer or ulcerative colitis.

Before you start, consult your doctor:
- If you are allergic to any sulfa drug.
- If you have gout, liver, pancreas or kidney disorder, epilepsy.
- If you have had peptic ulcer, ulcerative colitis or gallstones.
- If you have been depressed.
- If you will have surgery within 2 months, including dental surgery, requiring general or spinal anesthesia.

Over age 60:
Adverse reactions and side effects may be more frequent and severe than in younger persons, especially dizziness and excessive potassium loss.

Pregnancy:
Risk to unborn child outweighs drug benefits. Don't use.

Breast-feeding:
Drug passes into milk. Avoid drug or discontinue nursing until you finish medicine. Consult doctor for advice on maintaining milk supply.

Infants & children:
Not recommended.

Prolonged use:
- You may need medicine to treat high blood pressure for the rest of your life.
- Causes cancer in laboratory animals. Consult your doctor if you have family or personal history of cancer.

Skin & sunlight:
May cause rash or intensify sunburn in areas exposed to sun or sunlamp.

Driving, piloting or hazardous work:
Don't drive or pilot aircraft until you learn how medicine affects you. Don't work around dangerous machinery. Don't climb ladders or work in high places. Danger increases if you drink alcohol or take medicine affecting alertness and reflexes, such as antihistamines, tranquilizers, sedatives, pain medicine, narcotics and mind-altering drugs.

Discontinuing:
Don't discontinue without consulting doctor. Dose may require gradual reduction if you have taken drug for a long time. Doses of other drugs may also require adjustment.

Others:
- Hot weather and fever may cause dehydration and drop in blood pressure. Dose may require temporary adjustment. Weigh daily and report any unexpected weight decreases to your doctor.
- May cause rise in uric acid, leading to gout.
- May cause blood-sugar rise in diabetics.
- Consult your doctor if you do isometric exercises. These raise blood pressure. Drug may intensify blood-pressure rise.

POSSIBLE INTERACTION WITH OTHER DRUGS

GENERIC NAME OR DRUG CLASS	COMBINED EFFECT
Anticoagulants, oral*	Unpredictable increased or decreased effect of anticoagulant.
Anticonvulsants*	Serious change in seizure pattern.
Antidepressants, tricyclic (TCA)*	Dangerous drop in blood pressure. Avoid combination unless under medical supervision.
Antihistamines*	Increased antihistamine effect.
Antihypertensives*	Increased effect of rauwolfia.
Aspirin	Decreased aspirin effect.
Barbiturates*	Increased hydro-chlorothiazide effect.
Beta-adrenergic blockers*	Increased effect of rauwolfia alkaloids. Excessive sedation.

Continued page 1104

POSSIBLE INTERACTION WITH OTHER SUBSTANCES

INTERACTS WITH	COMBINED EFFECT
Alcohol:	Increased intoxication. Dangerous blood-pressure drop. Avoid.
Beverages: Carbonated drinks.	Decreased rauwolfia effect.
Cocaine:	Increased risk of heart block and high blood pressure.
Foods: Spicy foods. Licorice.	Possible digestive upset. Excessive potassium loss that causes dangerous heart rhythms.
Marijuana:	Occasional use—Mild drowsiness. Daily use—Moderate drowsiness, low blood pressure, depression.
Tobacco:	No proven problems.

RESERPINE & HYDRALAZINE

BRAND NAMES

Serpasil-Apresoline

BASIC INFORMATION

Habit forming? No
Prescription needed? Yes
Available as generic? No
Drug class: Antihypertensive, tranquilizer (rauwolfia alkaloid)

 USES

Treatment for high blood pressure and congestive heart failure.

 DOSAGE & USAGE INFORMATION

How to take:
Tablet—Swallow with liquid or food to lessen stomach irritation. If you can't swallow whole, crumble tablet and take with liquid or food.

When to take:
At the same times each day.

If you forget a dose:
Take as soon as you remember up to 2 hours late. If more than 2 hours, wait for next scheduled dose (don't double this dose).

Continued next column

 OVERDOSE

SYMPTOMS:
Drowsiness, slow, shallow breathing; diarrhea; flush; low body temperature; rapid, weak heartbeat; fainting; extreme weakness; cold, sweaty skin; coma.
WHAT TO DO:
- **Dial 0 (operator) or 911 (emergency) for an ambulance or medical help. Then give first aid immediately.**
- **If patient is unconscious and not breathing, give mouth-to-mouth breathing. If there is no heartbeat, use cardiac massage and mouth-to-mouth breathing (CPR). Don't try to make patient vomit. If you can't get help quickly, take patient to nearest emergency facility.**
- **See emergency information on inside covers.**

What drug does:
- Interferes with nerve impulses and relaxes blood-vessel muscles, reducing blood pressure.
- Suppresses brain centers that control emotions.

Time lapse before drug works:
Regular use for several weeks may be necessary to determine drug's effectiveness.

Don't take with:
- Non-prescription drugs containing alcohol without consulting doctor.
- See Interaction column and consult doctor.

 POSSIBLE ADVERSE REACTIONS OR SIDE EFFECTS

SYMPTOMS	WHAT TO DO
Life-threatening: Fainting, black stool, black vomit, chest pain, rapid or irregular heartbeat.	Discontinue. Seek emergency treatment.
Common: • Nausea, vomiting.	Discontinue. Call doctor right away.
• Headache, diarrhea, drowsiness, runny nose, appetite loss.	Continue. Call doctor when convenient.
Infrequent: • Rash, hives, joint pain.	Discontinue. Call doctor right away.
• Confusion; dizziness; red or flushed face; irritated, red, watery eyes; constipation; joint stiffness; weakness; depression, chest pain.	Continue. Call doctor when convenient.
Rare: • Unexplained bleeding or bruising; sore throat; swollen lymph glands; abdominal pain; jaundice; swollen feet, ankles or abdomen; weakness and faintness when arising from bed or chair.	Discontinue. Call doctor right away.
• Numbness, tingling, burning feeling in feet and hands; nasal congestion; impotence.	Continue. Call doctor when convenient.

WARNINGS & PRECAUTIONS

Don't take if:
- If you are allergic to any rauwolfia alkaloid, hydralazine or tartrazine dye.
- You are depressed.
- You have active peptic ulcer, ulcerative colitis, or history of coronary-artery disease or rheumatic heart disease.

Before you start, consult your doctor:
- If you have been depressed.
- If you have had peptic ulcer, ulcerative colitis, gallstones, lupus, a stroke, kidney disease or impaired kidney function.
- If you have epilepsy.
- If you will have surgery within 2 months, including dental surgery, requiring general or spinal anesthesia.

Over age 60:
Adverse reactions and side effects may be more frequent and severe than in younger persons.

Pregnancy:
Risk to unborn child outweighs drug benefits. Don't use.

Breast-feeding:
Drug passes into milk. Avoid drug or discontinue nursing until you finish medicine. Consult doctor for advice on maintaining milk supply.

Infants & children:
Not recommended.

Prolonged use:
- Causes cancer in laboratory animals. Consult your doctor if you have family or personal history of cancer.
- May cause lupus (a connective tissue illness with arthritis, anemia and kidney malfunction).
- Possible psychosis.
- May cause numbness, tingling in hands or feet.

Skin & sunlight:
No problems expected.

Driving, piloting or hazardous work:
Don't drive or pilot aircraft until you learn how medicine affects you. Don't work around dangerous machinery. Don't climb ladders or work in high places. Danger increases if you drink alcohol or take medicine affecting alertness and reflexes, such as antihistamines, tranquilizers, sedatives, pain medicine, narcotics and mind-altering drugs.

Discontinuing:
Don't discontinue without consulting doctor. Dose may require gradual reduction if you have taken drug for a long time. Doses of other drugs may also require adjustment.

Others:
- Consult your doctor if you do isometric exercises. These raise blood pressure. Drug may intensify blood-pressure rise.
- Vitamin B-6 diet supplement may be advisable. Consult doctor.
- Some products contain tartrazine dye. Avoid, especially if you are allergic to aspirin.

POSSIBLE INTERACTION WITH OTHER DRUGS

GENERIC NAME OR DRUG CLASS	COMBINED EFFECT
Amphetamines*	Decreased hydralazine effect.
Anticoagulants, oral*	Unpredictable increased or decreased effect of anticoagulant.
Anticonvulsants*	Serious change in seizure pattern.
Antidepressants*	Increased antidepressant effect.
Antihistamines*	Increased antihistamine effect.
Antihypertensives, other*	Increased antihypertensive effect.

Continued page 1104

POSSIBLE INTERACTION WITH OTHER SUBSTANCES

INTERACTS WITH	COMBINED EFFECT
Alcohol:	Increased intoxication. Avoid.
Beverages: Carbonated drinks.	Decreased rauwolfia alkaloids effect.
Cocaine:	Dangerous blood-pressure rise. Avoid.
Foods: Spicy foods.	Possible digestive upset.
Marijuana:	Occasional use—Mild drowsiness. Daily use—Moderate drowsiness, low blood pressure, depression.
Tobacco:	Possible angina attacks.

*See Glossary

RESERPINE, HYDRALAZINE & HYDROCHLOROTHIAZIDE

BRAND NAMES

Hydrap-Es
Hyserp
R-HCTZ-H

Ser-Ap-Es
Tri-Hydroserpine
Unipres

BASIC INFORMATION

Habit forming? No
Prescription needed? Yes
Available as generic? Yes
Drug class: Antihypertensive

 USES

- Treatment for high blood pressure and congestive heart failure.
- Reduces fluid retention (edema).

 DOSAGE & USAGE INFORMATION

How to take:
Tablet—Swallow with liquid. If you can't swallow whole, crumble tablet and take with liquid or food.

When to take:
At the same times each day.

If you forget a dose:
Take as soon as you remember up to 2 hours late. If more than 2 hours, wait for next scheduled dose (don't double this dose).

What drug does:
- Interferes with nerve impulses and relaxes blood-vessel muscles, reducing blood pressure.
- Suppresses brain centers that control emotions.
- Forces sodium and water excretion, reducing body fluid. Reduced body fluid and relaxed arteries lower blood pressure.

Continued next column

 OVERDOSE

SYMPTOMS:
Drowsiness; slow, shallow breathing; diarrhea; flush; low body temperature; rapid, weak heartbeat; fainting; extreme weakness; cold, sweaty skin; cramps, coma.
WHAT TO DO:
- Dial 0 (operator) or 911 (emergency) for an ambulance or medical help. Then give first aid immediately.
- See emergency information on inside covers.

Time lapse before drug works:
Regular use for several weeks may be necessary to determine drug's effectiveness.

Don't take with:
- Non-prescription drugs containing alcohol without consulting doctor.
- See Interaction column and consult doctor.

 POSSIBLE ADVERSE REACTIONS OR SIDE EFFECTS

SYMPTOMS	WHAT TO DO
Life-threatening:	
Rapid or irregular heartbeat, weak pulse, fainting, black stool, black or bloody vomit, chest pain.	Discontinue. Seek emergency treatment.
Common:	
• Nausea, vomiting.	Discontinue. Call doctor right away.
• Headache, diarrhea, drowsiness, runny nose, appetite loss.	Continue. Call doctor when convenient.
Infrequent:	
• Blurred vision, abdominal pain, rash, hives, joint pain.	Discontinue. Call doctor right away.
• Dizziness; mood change; headache; dry mouth; weakness; tiredness; weight gain or loss; eyes red, watery, irritated; confusion; constipation; red or flushed face; joint stiffness; depression; anxiety; chest pain.	Continue. Call doctor when convenient.
Rare:	
• Jaundice; unexplained bleeding or bruising; sore throat, fever, mouth sores; swollen feet, ankles and abdomen; weakness and faintness when arising from bed or chair.	Discontinue. Call doctor right away.
• Numbness, tingling, burning feeling in feet and hands; nasal congestion; impotence.	Continue. Call doctor when convenient.

WARNINGS & PRECAUTIONS

Don't take if:
- You are allergic to any rauwolfia alkaloid, hydralazine, any thiazide diuretic drug, or tartrazine dye.
- You are depressed.
- You have active peptic ulcer, ulcerative colitis, history of coronary-artery disease or rheumatic heart disease.

Before you start, consult your doctor:
- If you have been depressed.
- If you have had peptic ulcer, ulcerative colitis, gallstones, kidney disease or impaired kidney function, lupus or a stroke.
- If you have epilepsy, gout, liver, pancreas or kidney disorder.
- If you feel pain in chest, neck or arms on physical exertion.
- If you are allergic to any sulfa drug.
- If you will have surgery within 2 months, including dental surgery, requiring general or spinal anesthesia.

Over age 60:
Adverse reactions and side effects may be more frequent and severe than in younger persons, especially dizziness and excessive potassium loss.

Pregnancy:
Risk to unborn child outweighs drug benefits. Don't use.

Breast-feeding:
Drug passes into milk. Avoid drug or discontinue nursing until you finish medicine.

Infants & children:
Not recommended.

Prolonged use:
- Causes cancer in laboratory animals. Consult your doctor if you have family or personal history of cancer.
- Possible psychosis.
- May cause lupus; numbness, tingling in hands or feet.

Skin & sunlight:
May cause rash or intensify sunburn in areas exposed to sun or sunlamp.

Driving, piloting or hazardous work:
Don't drive or pilot aircraft until you learn how medicine affects you. Don't work around dangerous machinery. Don't climb ladders or work in high places. Danger increases if you drink alcohol or take medicine affecting alertness and reflexes.

Discontinuing:
Don't discontinue without consulting doctor. Dose may require gradual reduction if you have taken drug for a long time. Doses of other drugs may also require adjustment.

Others:
- Consult your doctor if you do isometric exercises. These raise blood pressure. Drug may intensify blood-pressure rise.
- Vitamin B-6 supplement may be advisable. Consult doctor.
- Hot weather and fever may cause dehydration and drop in blood pressure. Dose may require temporary adjustment. Weigh daily and report any unexpected weight decreases to your doctor.
- May cause rise in uric acid, leading to gout.
- May cause blood-sugar rise in diabetics.
- Some products contain tartrazine dye. Avoid, especially if you are allergic to aspirin.

POSSIBLE INTERACTION WITH OTHER DRUGS

GENERIC NAME OR DRUG CLASS	COMBINED EFFECT
Acebutolol	Possible increased effects of drugs.

Continued page 1105

POSSIBLE INTERACTION WITH OTHER SUBSTANCES

INTERACTS WITH	COMBINED EFFECT
Alcohol:	Increased intoxication. Avoid.
Beverages: Carbonated drinks.	Decreased rauwolfia alkaloids effect.
Cocaine:	Dangerous blood-pressure rise. Avoid.
Foods: Spicy foods. Licorice.	Possible digestive upset. Excessive potassium loss that causes dangerous heart rhythms.
Marijuana:	Weakness on standing. May increase blood pressure. Occasional use—Mild drowsiness. Daily use—Moderate drowsiness, low blood pressure, depression.
Tobacco:	Possible angina attacks.

RIBAVIRIN

BRAND NAMES

Tribavirin
Vilona

Viramid
Virazole

BASIC INFORMATION

Habit forming? No
Prescription needed? Yes
Available as generic? No
Drug class: Antiviral

USES

- Treats severe viral pneumonia.
- Treats influenza A and B with some success.
- It does *not* treat other viruses such as the common cold.

DOSAGE & USAGE INFORMATION

How to take:
By inhalation of a fine mist through mouth. Requires a special sprayer attached to oxygen mask, face mask for infants or hood.

When to take:
As ordered by your doctor.

If you forget a dose:
Use as soon as you remember.

What drug does:
Kills virus or prevents its growth.

Time lapse before drug works:
Begins working in 1 hour. May require treatment for 12 to 18 hours per day for 3 to 7 days.

Don't take with:
See Interaction column and consult doctor.

OVERDOSE

SYMPTOMS:
None expected.
WHAT TO DO:
Overdose unlikely to threaten life. If person takes much larger amount than prescribed, call doctor, poison-control center or hospital emergency room for instructions.

POSSIBLE ADVERSE REACTIONS OR SIDE EFFECTS

SYMPTOMS	WHAT TO DO
Life-threatening: None expected.	
Common: None expected.	
Infrequent: Blurred vision; dizziness; fainting; eye irritation; eyes more sensitive to light; red, swollen or itchy eyes.	Discontinue. Call doctor right away.
Rare: Difficult breathing, low blood pressure.	Discontinue. Call doctor right away.

WARNINGS & PRECAUTIONS

Don't take if:
You are allergic to ribavirin.

Before you start, consult your doctor:
If you are now on low-salt, low-sugar or any special diet.

Over age 60:
Adverse reactions and side effects may be more frequent and severe than in younger persons. Ask doctor about smaller doses.

Pregnancy:
Risk to unborn child outweighs drug benefits. Don't use.

Breast-feeding:
Drug passes into milk. Avoid drug or discontinue nursing until you finish medicine. Consult doctor for advice on maintaining milk supply.

Infants & children:
Use only under close medical supervision.

Prolonged use:
No problems expected.

Skin & sunlight:
No problems expected.

Driving, piloting or hazardous work:
Don't drive or pilot aircraft until you learn how medicine affects you. Don't work around dangerous machinery. Don't climb ladders or work in high places. Danger increases if you drink alcohol or take medicine affecting alertness and reflexes, such as antihistamines, tranquilizers, sedatives, pain medicine, narcotics and mind-altering drugs.

Discontinuing:
Don't discontinue without consulting doctor. Dose may require gradual reduction if you have taken drug for a long time. Doses of other drugs may also require adjustment.

Others:
No problems expected.

POSSIBLE INTERACTION WITH OTHER DRUGS

GENERIC NAME OR DRUG CLASS	COMBINED EFFECT
None expected.	

POSSIBLE INTERACTION WITH OTHER SUBSTANCES

INTERACTS WITH	COMBINED EFFECT
Alcohol:	None expected.
Beverages:	None expected.
Cocaine:	None expected.
Foods:	None expected.
Marijuana:	None expected.
Tobacco:	None expected.

RIBOFLAVIN (Vitamin B-2)

BRAND NAMES

Riobin-50
Many multivitamin preparations

BASIC INFORMATION

Habit forming? No
Prescription needed? No
Available as generic? Yes
Drug class: Vitamin supplement

USES

- Dietary supplement to ensure normal growth and health.
- Dietary supplement to treat symptoms caused by deficiency of B-2: sores in mouth, eyes sensitive to light, itching and peeling skin.

DOSAGE & USAGE INFORMATION

How to take:
Tablet—Swallow with liquid or food to lessen stomach irritation. If you can't swallow whole, crumble tablet and take with liquid or food.

When to take:
At the same times each day.

If you forget a dose:
Take as soon as you remember. Resume regular schedule. Don't double dose.

What drug does:
Promotes normal growth and health.

Time lapse before drug works:
Requires continual intake.

Don't take with:
See Interaction column and consult doctor.

OVERDOSE

SYMPTOMS:
Dark urine, nausea, vomiting.
WHAT TO DO:
Overdose unlikely to threaten life. If person takes much larger amount than prescribed, call doctor, poison-control center or hospital emergency room for instructions.

POSSIBLE ADVERSE REACTIONS OR SIDE EFFECTS

SYMPTOMS	WHAT TO DO
Life-threatening: None expected.	
Common: Urine yellow in color.	No action necessary.
Infrequent: None expected.	
Rare: None expected.	

RIBOFLAVIN (Vitamin B-2)

WARNINGS & PRECAUTIONS

Don't take if:
- You are allergic to any B vitamin.
- You have chronic kidney failure.

Before you start, consult your doctor:
If you are pregnant or plan pregnancy.

Over age 60:
No problems expected.

Pregnancy:
Recommended. Consult doctor.

Breast-feeding:
Recommended. Consult doctor.

Infants & children:
Consult doctor.

Prolonged use:
No problems expected.

Skin & sunlight:
No problems expected.

Driving, piloting or hazardous work:
No problems expected.

Discontinuing:
No problems expected.

Others:
A balanced diet should provide all the vitamin B-2 a healthy person needs and make supplements unnecessary during periods of good health. Best sources are milk, meats and green leafy vegetables.

POSSIBLE INTERACTION WITH OTHER DRUGS

GENERIC NAME OR DRUG CLASS	COMBINED EFFECT
Anticholinergics*	Possible increased riboflavin absorption.
Antidepressants, tricyclic (TCA)*	Decreased riboflavin effect.
Phenothiazines*	Decreased riboflavin effect.
Probenecid	Decreased riboflavin effect.

POSSIBLE INTERACTION WITH OTHER SUBSTANCES

INTERACTS WITH	COMBINED EFFECT
Alcohol:	Prevents uptake and absorption of vitamin B-2.
Beverages:	No problems expected.
Cocaine:	No problems expected.
Foods:	No problems expected.
Marijuana:	No problems expected.
Tobacco:	Prevents absorption of vitamin B-2 and other vitamins and nutrients.

RIFAMPIN

BRAND NAMES

Rifadin
Rifamate
Rifampicin

Rifomycin
Rimactane
Rofact

BASIC INFORMATION

Habit forming? No
Prescription needed? Yes
Available as generic? No
Drug class: Antibiotic (rifamycin)

 USES

Treatment for tuberculosis and other infections. Requires daily use for 1 to 2 years.

 DOSAGE & USAGE INFORMATION

How to take:
Capsule—Swallow with liquid. If you can't swallow whole, open capsule and take with liquid or small amount of food. For child, mix with small amount of applesauce or jelly.

When to take:
1 hour before or 2 hours after a meal.

If you forget a dose:
Take as soon as you remember up to 2 hours late. If more than 2 hours, wait for next scheduled dose (don't double this dose).

What drug does:
Prevents multiplication of tuberculosis germs.

Continued next column

 OVERDOSE

SYMPTOMS:
Slow, shallow breathing; weak, rapid pulse; cold, sweaty skin; coma.
WHAT TO DO:
- **Dial 0 (operator) or 911 (emergency) for an ambulance or medical help. Then give first aid immediately.**
- **If patient is unconscious and not breathing, give mouth-to-mouth breathing. If there is no heartbeat, use cardiac massage and mouth-to-mouth breathing (CPR). Don't try to make patient vomit. If you can't get help quickly, take patient to nearest emergency facility.**
- **See emergency information on inside covers.**

Time lapse before drug works:
Usually 2 weeks. May require 1 to 2 years without missed doses for maximum benefit.

Don't take with:
See Interaction column and consult doctor.

 POSSIBLE ADVERSE REACTIONS OR SIDE EFFECTS

SYMPTOMS	WHAT TO DO
Life-threatening: None expected.	
Common: Diarrhea; reddish urine, stool, saliva, sweat and tears.	Continue. Call doctor when convenient.
Infrequent:	
• Rash; flushed, itchy skin of face and scalp; blurred vision; difficult breathing; nausea, vomiting; abdominal cramps.	Discontinue. Call doctor right away.
• Dizziness, unsteady gait, confusion, muscle or bone pain, heartburn, flatulence.	Continue. Call doctor when convenient.
• Headache.	Continue. Tell doctor at next visit.
Rare:	
• Sore throat, mouth or tongue; jaundice.	Discontinue. Call doctor right away.
• Appetite loss, vomiting, less urination.	Continue. Call doctor when convenient.

WARNINGS & PRECAUTIONS

Don't take if:
- You are allergic to rifampin.
- You wear soft contact lenses.

Before you start, consult your doctor:
If you are alcoholic or have liver disease.

Over age 60:
Adverse reactions and side effects may be more frequent and severe than in younger persons.

Pregnancy:
Studies inconclusive on harm to unborn child. Animal studies show fetal abnormalities. Decide with your doctor whether drug benefits justify risk to unborn child.

Breast-feeding:
No proven problems. Consult doctor.

Infants & children:
Use only under medical supervision.

Prolonged use:
You may become more susceptible to infections caused by germs not responsive to rifampin.

Skin & sunlight:
No problems expected.

Driving, piloting or hazardous work:
Don't drive or pilot aircraft until you learn how medicine affects you. Don't work around dangerous machinery. Don't climb ladders or work in high places. Danger increases if you drink alcohol or take medicine affecting alertness and reflexes, such as antihistamines, tranquilizers, sedatives, pain medicine, narcotics and mind-altering drugs.

Discontinuing:
Don't discontinue without doctor's advice until you complete prescribed dose, even though symptoms diminish or disappear.

Others:
No problems expected.

POSSIBLE INTERACTION WITH OTHER DRUGS

GENERIC NAME OR DRUG CLASS	COMBINED EFFECT
Anticoagulants, oral*	Decreased anticoagulant effect.
Barbiturates*	Decreased barbiturate effect.
Chloramphenicol	Decreased effect of both drugs.
Contraceptives, oral*	Decreased contraceptive effect.
Cortisone drugs*	Decreased effect of cortisone drugs.
Cyclosporine	Decreased effect of both drugs.
Dapsone	Decreased dapsone effect.
Digitoxin	Decreased digitoxin effect.
Estrogens*	Decreased effect of both drugs.
Flecainide	Possible decreased blood-cell production in bone marrow.
Isoniazid	Possible toxicity to liver.
Ketoconazole	Increased risk of liver toxicity.
Methadone	Decreased methadone effect.
Nicardipine	Decreased nicardipine effect.
Para-aminosalicylic acid (PAS)	Decreased rifampin effect.
Probenecid	Possible toxicity to liver.
Quinidine	Decreased effect of both drugs.
Tocainide	Possible decreased blood-cell production in bone marrow.
Tolbutamide and other oral antidiabetics*	Decreased tolbutamide effect.
Trimethoprim	Decreased trimethoprim effect.

POSSIBLE INTERACTION WITH OTHER SUBSTANCES

INTERACTS WITH	COMBINED EFFECT
Alcohol:	Possible toxicity to liver.
Beverages:	None expected.
Cocaine:	No proven problems.
Foods:	None expected.
Marijuana:	No proven problems.
Tobacco:	None expected.

*See Glossary

RITODRINE

BRAND NAMES

Yutopar

BASIC INFORMATION

Habit forming? No
Prescription needed? Yes
Available as generic? Yes
Drug class: Labor Inhibitor; beta-adrenergic
   stimulator

USES

Halts premature labor in pregnancies of 20 or
more weeks.

DOSAGE & USAGE INFORMATION

How to take:
Tablet—Swallow with liquid or food to lessen
stomach irritation. If you can't swallow whole,
crumble tablet and take with liquid or food.

When to take:
Every 4 to 6 hours until term.

If you forget a dose:
Take as soon as you remember up to 2 hours
late. If more than 2 hours, wait for next
scheduled dose (don't double this dose).

What drug does:
Inhibits contractions of uterus (womb).

Time lapse before drug works:
30 to 60 minutes (oral form). Faster
intravenously.

Don't take with:
See Interaction column and consult doctor.

OVERDOSE

SYMPTOMS:
Rapid, irregular heartbeat to 120 or more;
shortness of breath.
WHAT TO DO:
- Dial 0 (operator) or 911 (emergency) for
  an ambulance or medical help. Then give
  first aid immediately.
- If patient is unconscious and not
  breathing, give mouth-to-mouth
  breathing. If there is no heartbeat, use
  cardiac massage and mouth-to-mouth
  breathing (CPR). Don't try to make patient
  vomit. If you can't get help quickly, take
  patient to nearest emergency facility.
- See emergency information on inside
  covers.

POSSIBLE ADVERSE REACTIONS OR SIDE EFFECTS

SYMPTOMS	WHAT TO DO
Life-threatening:	
Hives, rash, intense itching, faintness soon after a dose (anaphylaxis).	See emergency treatment immediately.
Always:	
Increased heart rate.	Continue. Call doctor when convenient.
Common:	
● Irregular heartbeat.	Discontinue. Call doctor right away.
● Increased systolic blood pressure.	Continue. Tell doctor at next visit.
Infrequent:	
● Shortness of breath.	Discontinue. Call doctor right away.
● Nervousness, trembling, headache, nausea, vomiting.	Continue. Call doctor when convenient.
Rare:	
Rash, angina.	Discontinue. Call doctor right away.

WARNINGS & PRECAUTIONS

Don't take if:
- You have heart disease.
- You have eclampsia.
- You have lung congestion.
- You have infection in the uterus.
- You have an overactive thyroid.
- You have a bleeding disorder.

Before you start, consult your doctor:
- If you have asthma.
- If you have diabetes.
- If you have high blood pressure.
- If you have pre-eclampsia.

Over age 60:
Not used.

Pregnancy:
Ritodrine crosses placenta, but animal studies show that it causes no effects on fetuses. Benefits versus risks must be assessed by you and your doctor.

Breast-feeding:
Not applicable.

Infants & children:
Not used.

Prolonged use:
Request blood sugar and electrolytes measurements.

Skin & sunlight:
No problems expected.

Driving, piloting or hazardous work:
Don't drive or pilot aircraft until you learn how medicine affects you. Don't work around dangerous machinery. Don't climb ladders or work in high places. Danger increases if you drink alcohol or take medicine affecting alertness and reflexes, such as antihistamines, tranquilizers, sedatives, pain medicine, narcotics and mind-altering drugs.

Discontinuing:
Don't discontinue without consulting doctor. Dose may require gradual reduction if you have taken drug for a long time. Doses of other drugs may also require adjustment.

Others:
No problems expected.

POSSIBLE INTERACTION WITH OTHER DRUGS

GENERIC NAME OR DRUG CLASS	COMBINED EFFECT
Adrenal corticosteroids*	Increased chance of fluid in lungs of mother. Avoid.
Anesthetics, general*	Possible cardiac arrhythmias or hypotension.
Beta-adrenergic blockers*	Decreased effect of ritodrine.
Diazoxide	Possible cardiac arrhythmias or hypotension.
Magnesium sulfate	Possible cardiac arrhythmias or hypotension.
Meperidine	Possible cardiac arrhythmias or hypotension.
Sympathomimetics*	Increased side effects of both.

POSSIBLE INTERACTION WITH OTHER SUBSTANCES

INTERACTS WITH	COMBINED EFFECT
Alcohol:	Increased adverse effects. Avoid.
Beverages:	No problems expected.
Cocaine:	Injury to fetus. Avoid.
Foods:	No problems expected.
Marijuana:	Injury to fetus. Avoid.
Tobacco:	Injury to fetus. Avoid.

*See Glossary

SALICYLATES

BRAND AND GENERIC NAMES

See complete list of brand and generic names in the *Brand Name Directory*, page 1071.

BASIC INFORMATION

Habit forming? No
Prescription needed? For some
Available as generic? Yes
Drug class: Analgesic, anti-inflammatory (salicylate)

USES

- Reduces pain, fever, inflammation.
- Relieves swelling, stiffness, joint pain of arthritis or rheumatism.
- Decreases risk of myocardial infarction in unstable angina (aspirin only).

DOSAGE & USAGE INFORMATION

How to take:
- Tablet or capsule—Swallow with liquid.
- Extended-release tablets—Swallow each dose whole.
- Suppositories—Remove wrapper and moisten suppository with water. Gently insert into rectum, large end first.

When to take:
Pain, fever, inflammation—As needed, no more often than every 4 hours.

If you forget a dose:
- Pain, fever—Take as soon as you remember. Wait 4 hours for next dose.
- Arthritis—Take as soon as you remember up to 2 hours late. Return to regular schedule.

Continued next column

OVERDOSE

SYMPTOMS:
Ringing in ears; nausea; vomiting; dizziness; fever; deep, rapid breathing; hallucinations; convulsions; coma.
WHAT TO DO:
- **Dial 0 (operator) or 911 (emergency) for an ambulance or medical help. Then give first aid immediately.**
- **See emergency information on inside covers.**

What drug does:
- Affects hypothalamus, the part of the brain that regulates temperature by dilating small blood vessels in skin.
- Prevents clumping of platelets (small blood cells) so blood vessels remain open.
- Decreases prostaglandin effect.
- Suppresses body's pain messages.

Time lapse before drug works:
30 minutes for pain, fever, arthritis.

Don't take with:
- Tetracyclines. Space doses 1 hour apart.
- See Interaction column and consult doctor.

POSSIBLE ADVERSE REACTIONS OR SIDE EFFECTS

SYMPTOMS	WHAT TO DO
Life-threatening: Hives, rash, intense itching, faintness soon after a dose (anaphylaxis); black or bloody vomit; blood in urine.	Seek emergency treatment immediately.
Common:	
• Nausea, vomiting, abdominal pain.	Discontinue. Seek emergency treatment.
• Heartburn, indigestion.	Continue. Call doctor when convenient.
• Ringing in ears.	Continue. Tell doctor at next visit.
Infrequent: None expected.	
Rare:	
• Black stools, unexplained fever.	Discontinue. Seek emergency treatment.
• Rash, hives, itchy skin, diminished vision, shortness of breath, wheezing, jaundice.	Discontinue. Call doctor right away.
• Drowsiness.	Continue. Call doctor when convenient.

WARNINGS & PRECAUTIONS

Don't take if:
- You need to restrict sodium in your diet. Buffered effervescent tablets and sodium salicylate are high in sodium.
- Salicylates have a strong vinegar-like odor, which means it has decomposed.
- You have a peptic ulcer of stomach or duodenum.
- You have a bleeding disorder.

Before you start, consult your doctor:
- If you have had stomach or duodenal ulcers.
- If you have had gout.
- If you have asthma or nasal polyps.

Over age 60:
More likely to cause hidden bleeding in stomach or intestines. Watch for dark stools.

Pregnancy:
Risk to unborn child outweighs drug benefits. Don't use.

Breast-feeding:
Drug passes into milk. Avoid drug or discontinue nursing until you finish medicine. Consult doctor for advice on maintaining milk supply.

Infants & children:
Overdose frequent and severe. Keep bottles out of children's reach.

Prolonged use:
Kidney damage. Periodic kidney-function test recommended.

Skin & sunlight:
Aspirin combined with sunscreen may decrease sunburn.

Driving, piloting or hazardous work:
No restrictions unless you feel drowsy.

Discontinuing:
For chronic illness—Don't discontinue without doctor's advice until you complete prescribed dose, even though symptoms diminish or disappear.

Others:
- Salicylates can complicate surgery, pregnancy, labor and delivery, and illness.
- For arthritis—Don't change dose without consulting doctor.
- Urine tests for blood sugar may be inaccurate.

 ## POSSIBLE INTERACTION WITH OTHER DRUGS

GENERIC NAME OR DRUG CLASS	COMBINED EFFECT
ACE inhibitors: captopril, enalapril, lisinopril *	Decreased ACE inhibitor effect.
Allopurinol	Decreased allopurinol effect.
Antacids *	Decreased salicylate effect.
Anticoagulants *	Increased anticoagulant effect. Abnormal bleeding.
Antidiabetics, oral *	Low blood sugar.

Aspirin, other	Likely salicylate toxicity.
Beta-adrenergic blockers *	Decreased antihypertensive effect.
Bismuth subsalicylate	Increased risk of salicylate toxicity.
Bumetanide	Decreased diuretic effect.
Calcium supplements *	Increased salicylate effect.
Carteolol	Decreased antihypertensive effect of carteolol.
Cortisone drugs *	Increased cortisone effect. Risk of ulcers and stomach bleeding.
Ethacrynic acid	Decreased diuretic effect.
Furosemide	Possible salicylate toxicity.
Gold compounds *	Increased likelihood of kidney damage.
Indomethacin	Risk of stomach bleeding and ulcers.
Insulin	Decreased blood sugar.
Methotrexate	Increased methotrexate effect and toxicity.
Non-steroidal anti-inflammatory drugs (NSAIDs) *	Risk of stomach bleeding and ulcers.
Para-aminosalicylic acid (PAS)	Possible salicylate toxicity.

Continued page 1105

 ## POSSIBLE INTERACTION WITH OTHER SUBSTANCES

INTERACTS WITH	COMBINED EFFECT
Alcohol:	Possible stomach irritation and bleeding. Avoid.
Beverages:	None expected.
Cocaine:	None expected.
Foods:	None expected.
Marijuana:	Possible increased pain relief, but marijuana may slow body's recovery. Avoid.
Tobacco:	None expected.

*See Glossary

SCOPOLAMINE (Hyoscine)

BRAND NAMES

See complete list of brand names in the *Brand Name Directory*, page 1071.

BASIC INFORMATION

Habit forming? No
Prescription needed?
 High strength: Yes
 Low strength: No
Available as generic? Yes
Drug class: Antispasmodic, anticholinergic

 ## USES

- Reduces spasms of digestive system, bladder and urethra.
- Relieves painful menstruation.
- Prevents motion sickness.

 ## DOSAGE & USAGE INFORMATION

How to take:
- Capsules—Swallow with liquid or food to lessen stomach irritation.
- Drops—Dilute dose in beverage.
- Skin discs—Clean application site. Change application sites with each dose.

When to take:
- Motion sickness—Apply disc 30 minutes before departure.
- Other uses—Take 30 minutes before meals (unless directed otherwise by doctor).

If you forget a dose:
Take up to 2 hours late. If more than 2 hours, wait for next dose (don't double this dose).

What drug does:
Blocks nerve impulses at parasympathetic nerve endings, preventing muscle contractions and gland secretions of organs involved.

Continued next column

 ## OVERDOSE

SYMPTOMS:
Dilated pupils, blurred vision, rapid pulse and breathing, dizziness, fever, hallucinations, confusion, slurred speech, agitation, flushed face, convulsions, coma.
WHAT TO DO:
- **Dial 0 (operator) or 911 (emergency) for an ambulance or medical help. Then give first aid immediately.**
- **See emergency information on inside covers.**

Time lapse before drug works:
15 to 30 minutes.

Don't take with:
See Interaction column and consult doctor.

 ## POSSIBLE ADVERSE REACTIONS OR SIDE EFFECTS

SYMPTOMS	WHAT TO DO
Life-threatening:	
Hives, rash, intense itching, faintness soon after a dose (anaphylaxis).	Seek emergency treatment immediately.
Common:	
• Confusion, delirium, rapid heartbeat.	Discontinue. Call doctor right away.
• Nausea, vomiting, decreased sweating.	Continue. Call doctor when convenient.
• Constipation, loss of taste.	Continue. Tell doctor at next visit.
• Dryness in ears, nose, throat.	No action necessary.
Infrequent:	
Headache, difficult urination.	Continue. Call doctor when convenient.
Rare:	
Rash or hives, pain, blurred vision.	Discontinue. Call doctor right away.

 ## WARNINGS & PRECAUTIONS

Don't take if:
- You are allergic to any anticholinergic.
- You have trouble with stomach bloating.
- You have difficulty emptying your bladder completely.
- You have narrow-angle glaucoma.
- You have severe ulcerative colitis.

Before you start, consult your doctor:
- If you have open-angle glaucoma, angina, chronic bronchitis or asthma, hiatal hernia, liver disease, enlarged prostate, myasthenia gravis, peptic ulcer.
- If you will have surgery within 2 months, including dental surgery, requiring general or spinal anesthesia.

Over age 60:
Adverse reactions and side effects may be more frequent and severe than in younger persons.

Pregnancy:
Studies inconclusive on harm to unborn child. Animal studies show fetal abnormalities. Decide with your doctor whether drug benefits justify risk to unborn child.

SCOPOLAMINE (Hyoscine)

Breast-feeding:
Drug passes into milk and decreases milk flow. Avoid drug or discontinue nursing until you finish medicine. Consult doctor for advice on maintaining milk supply.

Infants & children:
Use only under medical supervision.

Prolonged use:
Chronic constipation, possible fecal impaction. Consult doctor immediately.

Skin & sunlight:
No problems expected.

Driving, piloting or hazardous work:
Use disqualifies you for piloting aircraft. Otherwise, no problems expected.

Discontinuing:
May be unnecessary to finish medicine. Follow doctor's instructions.

Others:
No problems expected.

 ## POSSIBLE INTERACTION WITH OTHER DRUGS

GENERIC NAME OR DRUG CLASS	COMBINED EFFECT
Amantadine	Increased scopolamine effect.
Antacids*	Decreased scopolamine effect.
Anticholinergics, other*	Increased scopolamine effect.
Antidepressants, tricyclic (TCA)*	Increased scopolamine effect. Increased sedation.
Antihistamines*	Increased scopolamine effect.
Buclizine	Increased scopolamine effect.
Cortisone drugs*	Increased internal-eye pressure.
Digitalis	Possible decreased absorption of scopolamine.
Encainide	Increased effect of toxicity on heart muscle.
Ethinamate	Dangerous increased effects of ethinamate. Avoid combining.
Fluoxetine	Increased depressant effects of both drugs.
Guanfacine	May increase depressant effects of either medicine.
Haloperidol	Increased internal-eye pressure.
Leucovorin	High alcohol content of leucovorin may cause adverse effects.
MAO inhibitors*	Increased scopolamine effect.
Meperidine	Increased scopolamine effect.
Methylphenidate	Increased scopolamine effect.
Methyprylon	May increase sedative effect to dangerous level. Avoid.
Molindone	Increased anti-cholinergic effect.
Nabilone	Greater depression of central nervous system.
Nitrates*	Increased internal-eye pressure.
Nizatidine	Increased nizatidine effect.
Orphenadrine	Increased scopolamine effect.
Phenothiazines*	Increased scopolamine effect.

Continued page 1106

 ## POSSIBLE INTERACTION WITH OTHER SUBSTANCES

INTERACTS WITH	COMBINED EFFECT
Alcohol:	None expected.
Beverages:	None expected.
Cocaine:	Excessively rapid heartbeat. Avoid.
Foods:	None expected.
Marijuana:	Drowsiness, dry mouth.
Tobacco:	None expected.

SECOBARBITAL

BRAND NAMES

Novo Secobarb   Seral
Secogen   Tuinal
Seconal

BASIC INFORMATION

Habit forming? Yes
Prescription needed? Yes
Available as generic? Yes
Drug class: Sedative, hypnotic (barbiturate)

 ## USES

Relieves insomnia (higher bedtime dose).

 ## DOSAGE & USAGE INFORMATION

How to take:
- Tablet, or capsule—Swallow with food or liquid to lessen stomach irritation. If you can't swallow whole, crumble tablet or open capsule and take with liquid or food.
- Suppositories—Remove wrapper and moisten suppository with water. Gently insert larger end into rectum. Push well into rectum with finger.
- Rectal solution—Follow package instructions.

When to take:
At the same times each day.

If you forget a dose:
Take as soon as you remember up to 2 hours late. If more than 2 hours, wait for next scheduled dose (don't double this dose).

What drug does:
May partially block nerve impulses at nerve-cell connections.

Time lapse before drug works:
60 minutes.

Don't take with:
- Non-prescription drugs without consulting doctor.
- See Interaction column and consult doctor.

 ## OVERDOSE

SYMPTOMS:
Deep sleep, weak pulse, coma.
WHAT TO DO:
- Dial 0 (operator) or 911 (emergency) for an ambulance or medical help. Then give first aid immediately.
- See emergency information on inside covers.

 ## POSSIBLE ADVERSE REACTIONS OR SIDE EFFECTS

SYMPTOMS	WHAT TO DO
Life-threatening:	
Hives, rash, intense itching, faintness soon after a dose (anaphylaxis).	Seek emergency treatment immediately.
Common:	
Dizziness, drowsiness, "hangover" effect.	Continue. Call doctor when convenient.
Infrequent:	
• Rash or hives; fever; swollen face, lip or eyelids; sore throat.	Discontinue. Call doctor right away.
• Depression, confusion, slurred speech, diarrhea, nausea, vomiting, joint or muscle pain.	Continue. Call doctor when convenient.
Rare:	
• Agitation, slow heartbeat, difficult breathing, jaundice.	Discontinue. Call doctor right away.
• Unexplained bleeding or bruising.	Continue. Call doctor when convenient.

 ## WARNINGS & PRECAUTIONS

Don't take if:
- You are allergic to any barbiturate.
- You have porphyria.

Before you start, consult your doctor:
- If you have epilepsy, kidney or liver damage, asthma, anemia, chronic pain.
- If you will have surgery within 2 months, including dental surgery, requiring general or spinal anesthesia.

Over age 60:
Adverse reactions and side effects may be more frequent and severe than in younger persons. Use small doses.

Pregnancy:
Risk to unborn child outweighs drug benefits. Don't use.

Breast-feeding:
Drug passes into milk. Avoid drug or discon°-tinue nursing until you finish medicine. Consult doctor for advice on maintaining milk supply.

Infants & children:
Use only under doctor's supervision.

Prolonged use:
- May cause addiction, anemia, chronic intoxication.
- May lower body temperature, making exposure to cold temperatures hazardous.

Skin & sunlight:
May cause rash or intensify sunburn in areas exposed to sun or sunlamp.

Driving, piloting or hazardous work:
Don't drive or pilot aircraft until you learn how medicine affects you. Don't work around dangerous machinery. Don't climb ladders or work in high places. Danger increases if you drink alcohol or take medicine affecting alertness and reflexes.

Discontinuing:
May be unnecessary to finish medicine. Follow doctor's instructions. If you develop withdrawal symptoms of hallucinations, agitation or sleeplessness after discontinuing, call doctor right away.

Others:
Great potential for abuse.

POSSIBLE INTERACTION WITH OTHER DRUGS

GENERIC NAME OR DRUG CLASS	COMBINED EFFECT
Anticoagulants, oral*	Decreased anti-coagulant effect.
Anticonvulsants*	Changed seizure patterns.
Antidepressants, tricyclics (TCA)*	Decreased anti-depressant effect. Increased sedation.
Antidiabetics, oral*	Increased secobarbital effect.
Antihistamines*	Dangerous sedation. Avoid.
Aspirin	Decreased aspirin effect.
Beta-adrenergic blockers*	Decreased effect of beta-adrenergic blocker.
Carteolol	Increased barbiturate effect. Dangerous sedation.
Contraceptives, oral*	Decreased contra-ceptive effect.
Cortisone drugs*	Decreased cortisone effect.
Digitoxin	Decreased digitoxin effect.
Disulfiram	Possible increased secobarbital effect.
Doxycycline	Decreased doxycycline effect.
Dronabinol	Increased effects of both drugs. Avoid.
Estrogens*	Decreased estrogen effect.
Griseofulvin	Decreased griseofulvin effect.
Indapamide	Increased indapamide effect.
MAO inhibitors*	Increased secobarbital effect.
Metronidazole	Possible decreased metronidazole effect.
Mind-altering drugs*	Dangerous sedation. Avoid.
Molindone	Increased sedative effect.
Nabilone	Greater depression of central nervous system.
Narcotics*	Dangerous sedation. Avoid.
Non-steroidal anti-inflammatory drugs (NSAIDs)*	Decreased anti-inflammatory effect.
Pain relievers*	Dangerous sedation. Avoid.
Rifampin	Possible decreased secobarbital effect.
Sedatives*	Dangerous sedation. Avoid.

Continued page 1106

POSSIBLE INTERACTION WITH OTHER SUBSTANCES

INTERACTS WITH	COMBINED EFFECT
Alcohol:	Possible fatal oversedation. Avoid.
Beverages:	None expected.
Cocaine:	Decreased secobarbital effect.
Foods:	None expected.
Marijuana:	Excessive sedation. Avoid.
Tobacco:	None expected.

*See Glossary

SENNA

BRAND NAMES

Black Draught	Fletcher's Castoria
Black-Draught	Senexon
Lax Senna	Senokot
Casa-Fru	Senolax
Dr. Caldwell's	Swiss Kriss
Senna Laxative	X-Prep Liquid

BASIC INFORMATION

Habit forming? No
Prescription needed? No
Available as generic? No
Drug class: Laxative (stimulant)

 ## USES

Constipation relief.

 ## DOSAGE & USAGE INFORMATION

How to take:
- Tablet—Swallow with liquid. If you can't swallow whole, chew or crumble tablet and take with liquid or food.
- Liquid, granules—Drink 6 to 8 glasses of water each day, in addition to one taken with each dose.
- Suppositories—Remove wrapper and moisten suppository with water. Gently insert larger end into rectum. Push well into rectum with finger.

When to take:
Usually at bedtime with a snack, unless directed otherwise.

If you forget a dose:
Take as soon as you remember.

What drug does:
Acts on smooth muscles of intestine wall to cause vigorous bowel movement.

Time lapse before drug works:
6 to 10 hours.

Continued next column

 ## OVERDOSE

SYMPTOMS:
Vomiting, electrolyte depletion.
WHAT TO DO:
Overdose unlikely to threaten life. If person takes much larger amount than prescribed, call doctor, poison-control center or hospital emergency room for instructions.

Don't take with:
- See Interaction column and consult doctor.
- Don't take within 2 hours of taking another medicine. Laxative interferes with medicine absorption.

 ## POSSIBLE ADVERSE REACTIONS OR SIDE EFFECTS

SYMPTOMS	WHAT TO DO
Life-threatening:	
None expected.	
Common:	
• Rectal irritation.	Continue. Call doctor when convenient.
• Yellow-brown or red-violet urine.	No action necessary.
Infrequent:	
• Dangerous potassium loss.	Discontinue. Call doctor right away.
• Belching, cramps, nausea.	Continue. Call doctor when convenient.
Rare:	
• Irritability, headache, confusion, rash, difficult breathing, irregular heartbeat, muscle cramps, unusual tiredness or weakness.	Discontinue. Call doctor right away.
• Burning on urination.	Continue. Call doctor when convenient.

908

WARNINGS & PRECAUTIONS

Don't take if:
- You have symptoms of appendicitis, inflamed bowel or intestinal blockage.
- You are allergic to a stimulant laxative.
- You have missed a bowel movement for only 1 or 2 days.

Before you start, consult your doctor:
- If you have a colostomy or ileostomy.
- If you have congestive heart disease.
- If you have diabetes.
- If you have high blood pressure.
- If you have a laxative habit.
- If you have rectal bleeding.
- If you take other laxatives.

Over age 60:
Adverse reactions and side effects may be more frequent and severe than in younger persons.

Pregnancy:
Risk to mother and unborn child outweighs drug benefits. Don't use.

Breast-feeding:
Drug passes into milk. Avoid drug or discontinue nursing until you finish medicine. Consult doctor for advice on maintaining milk supply.

Infants & children:
Use only under medical supervision.

Prolonged use:
Don't take for more than 1 week unless under a doctor's supervision. May cause laxative dependence.

Skin & sunlight:
No problems expected.

Driving, piloting or hazardous work:
No problems expected.

Discontinuing:
May be unnecessary to finish medicine. Follow doctor's instructions.

Others:
- Don't take to "flush out" your system or as a "tonic."
- May cause urine to get discolored. No action necessary.

POSSIBLE INTERACTION WITH OTHER DRUGS

GENERIC NAME OR DRUG CLASS	COMBINED EFFECT
Antihypertensives*	May cause dangerous low potassium level.
Digitalis	Increased digitalis toxicity.
Diuretics*	May cause dangerous low potassium level.

POSSIBLE INTERACTION WITH OTHER SUBSTANCES

INTERACTS WITH	COMBINED EFFECT
Alcohol:	None expected.
Beverages:	None expected.
Cocaine:	None expected.
Foods:	None expected.
Marijuana:	None expected.
Tobacco:	None expected.

SENNOSIDES A & B

BRAND NAMES

Glysennid	Senokot
Nytilax	X-Prep
Gentle Nature	

BASIC INFORMATION

Habit forming? No
Prescription needed? No
Available as generic? No
Drug class: Laxative (stimulant)

 ## USES

Constipation relief.

 ## DOSAGE & USAGE INFORMATION

How to take:
- Tablet—Swallow with liquid. If you can't swallow whole, chew or crumble tablet and take with liquid or food.
- Liquid, granules—Drink 6 to 8 glasses of water each day, in addition to one taken with each dose.

When to take:
Usually at bedtime with a snack, unless directed otherwise.

If you forget a dose:
Take as soon as you remember.

What drug does:
Acts on smooth muscles of intestine wall to cause vigorous bowel movement.

Time lapse before drug works:
6 to 10 hours.

Don't take with:
- See Interaction column and consult doctor.
- Don't take within 2 hours of taking another medicine. Laxative interferes with medicine absorption.

 ## OVERDOSE

SYMPTOMS:
Vomiting, electrolyte depletion.
WHAT TO DO:
Overdose unlikely to threaten life. If person takes much larger amount than prescribed, call doctor, poison-control center or hospital emergency room for instructions.

 ## POSSIBLE ADVERSE REACTIONS OR SIDE EFFECTS

SYMPTOMS	WHAT TO DO
Life-threatening: None expected.	
Common:	
• Rectal irritation.	Continue. Call doctor when convenient.
• Yellow-brown or red-violet urine.	No action necessary.
Infrequent:	
• Dangerous potassium loss.	Discontinue. Call doctor right away.
• Belching, cramps, nausea.	Continue. Call doctor when convenient.
Rare:	
• Irritability, headache, confusion, rash, difficult breathing, irregular heartbeat, muscle cramps, unusual tiredness or weakness.	Discontinue. Call doctor right away.
• Burning on urination.	Continue. Call doctor when convenient.

SENNOSIDES A & B

WARNINGS & PRECAUTIONS

Don't take if:
- You have symptoms of appendicitis, inflamed bowel or intestinal blockage.
- You are allergic to a stimulant laxative.
- You have missed a bowel movement for only 1 or 2 days.

Before you start, consult your doctor:
- If you have a colostomy or ileostomy.
- If you have congestive heart disease.
- If you have diabetes.
- If you have high blood pressure.
- If you have a laxative habit.
- If you have rectal bleeding.
- If you take other laxatives.

Over age 60:
Adverse reactions and side effects may be more frequent and severe than in younger persons.

Pregnancy:
Risk to mother and unborn child outweighs drug benefits. Don't use.

Breast-feeding:
Drug passes into milk. Avoid drug or discontinue nursing until you finish medicine. Consult doctor for advice on maintaining milk supply.

Infants & children:
Use only under medical supervision.

Prolonged use:
Don't take for more than 1 week unless under a doctor's supervision. May cause laxative dependence.

Skin & sunlight:
No problems expected.

Driving, piloting or hazardous work:
No problems expected.

Discontinuing:
May be unnecessary to finish medicine. Follow doctor's instructions.

Others:
- Don't take to "flush out" your system or as a "tonic."
- May cause urine to get discolored. No action necessary.

POSSIBLE INTERACTION WITH OTHER DRUGS

GENERIC NAME OR DRUG CLASS	COMBINED EFFECT
Antihypertensives*	May cause dangerous low potassium level.
Digitalis	Increased digitalis toxicity.
Diuretics*	May cause dangerous low potassium level.

POSSIBLE INTERACTION WITH OTHER SUBSTANCES

INTERACTS WITH	COMBINED EFFECT
Alcohol:	None expected.
Beverages:	None expected.
Cocaine:	None expected.
Foods:	None expected.
Marijuana:	None expected.
Tobacco:	None expected.

*See Glossary

SIMETHICONE

BRAND NAMES

Barriere
Celluzyme
Di-Gel
Gas-X
Gelusil
Mygel
Mylanta
Mylicon

Ovol
Phazyme
Phazyme 125
Riopan Plus
Simeco
Silain
Tri-Cone

BASIC INFORMATION

Habit forming? No
Prescription needed? No
Available as generic? No
Drug class: Antiflatulent

USES

- Treatment for retention of abdominal gas.
- Used prior to x-ray of abdomen to reduce gas shadows.

DOSAGE & USAGE INFORMATION

How to take:
- Tablet or capsule—Swallow with liquid.
- Liquid—Dissolve in water. Drink complete dose.
- Chewable tablets—Chew completely. Don't swallow whole.

When to take:
After meals and at bedtime.

If you forget a dose:
Take when remembered if needed.

What drug does:
Reduces surface tension of gas bubbles in stomach.

Time lapse before drug works:
10 minutes.

Don't take with:
No restrictions.

OVERDOSE

SYMPTOMS:
None expected.
WHAT TO DO:
Overdose unlikely to threaten life.

POSSIBLE ADVERSE REACTIONS OR SIDE EFFECTS

SYMPTOMS	WHAT TO DO
Life-threatening: None expected.	
Common: None expected.	
Infrequent: None expected.	
Rare: None expected.	

WARNINGS & PRECAUTIONS

Don't take if:
You are allergic to simethicone.

Before you start, consult your doctor:
No problems expected.

Over age 60:
No problems expected.

Pregnancy:
No proven harm to unborn child. Avoid if possible.

Breast-feeding:
No problems expected.

Infants & children:
Not recommended.

Prolonged use:
No problems expected.

Skin & sunlight:
No problems expected.

Driving, piloting or hazardous work:
No problems expected.

Discontinuing:
May be unnecessary to finish medicine. Discontinue when symptoms disappear.

Others:
No problems expected.

POSSIBLE INTERACTION WITH OTHER DRUGS

GENERIC NAME OR DRUG CLASS	COMBINED EFFECT
None expected.	

POSSIBLE INTERACTION WITH OTHER SUBSTANCES

INTERACTS WITH	COMBINED EFFECT
Alcohol:	None expected.
Beverages:	None expected.
Cocaine:	None expected.
Foods:	None expected.
Marijuana:	None expected.
Tobacco:	None expected.

SODIUM BICARBONATE

BRAND NAMES

Alka-Citrate
  Compound
Alka-Seltzer Antacid
Arm and Hammer
  Baking Soda
Bell/ans
Bisodol
Bisodol Powder
Brioschi
Bromo Seltzer

Ceo-Two
Chembicarb
Citrocarbonate
Eno
Fizrin
Infalyte
Neut
Seidlitz Powder
Soda Mint

BASIC INFORMATION

Habit forming? No
Prescription needed? No
Available as generic? Yes
Drug class: Antacid

USES

Treatment for hyperacidity in upper gastrointestinal tract, including stomach and esophagus. Symptoms may be heartburn or acid indigestion. Diseases include peptic ulcer, gastritis, esophagitis, hiatal hernia.

DOSAGE & USAGE INFORMATION

How to take:
- Tablet—Swallow with liquid.
- Powder—Dilute dose in beverage before swallowing.

When to take:
1 to 3 hours after meals unless directed otherwise by your doctor.

If you forget a dose:
Take as soon as you remember.

What drug does:
- Neutralizes some of the hydrochloric acid in the stomach.
- Reduces action of pepsin, a digestive enzyme.

Continued next column

OVERDOSE

SYMPTOMS:
Weakness, fatigue, dizziness.
WHAT TO DO:
Overdose unlikely to threaten life. If person takes much larger amount than prescribed, call doctor, poison-control center or hospital emergency room for instructions.

Time lapse before drug works:
15 minutes.

Don't take with:
Other medicines at the same time. Decreases absorption of other drugs.

POSSIBLE ADVERSE REACTIONS OR SIDE EFFECTS

SYMPTOMS	WHAT TO DO
Life-threatening: None expected.	
Common:	
• Constipation, appetite loss, weight gain.	Continue. Call doctor when convenient.
• Belching.	Continue. Tell doctor at next visit.
Infrequent:	
• Lower abdominal pain and swelling, bone pain, muscle weakness, swollen wrists or ankles.	Discontinue. Call doctor right away.
• Mood change, nausea, vomiting, weight loss.	Continue. Call doctor when convenient.
Rare: None expected.	

WARNINGS & PRECAUTIONS

Don't take if:
You are allergic to any antacid.

Before you start, consult your doctor:
- If you have kidney disease, liver disease, high blood pressure or congestive heart failure.
- If you have chronic constipation or diarrhea.
- If you have symptoms of appendicitis.
- If you have stomach or intestinal bleeding.

Over age 60:
Adverse reactions and side effects may be more frequent and severe than in younger persons. Diarrhea or constipation particularly likely.

Pregnancy:
Risk to unborn child outweighs drug benefits. Don't use.

Breast-feeding:
Drug passes into milk. Avoid drug or discontinue nursing until you finish medicine. Consult doctor for advice on maintaining milk supply.

Infants & children:
Use only under medical supervision.

Prolonged use:
Prolonged use with calcium supplements or milk leads to too much calcium in blood.

Skin & sunlight:
No problems expected.

Driving, piloting or hazardous work:
No problems expected.

Discontinuing:
May be unnecessary to finish medicine. Follow doctor's instructions.

Others:
Don't take longer than 2 weeks unless under medical supervision.

POSSIBLE INTERACTION WITH OTHER DRUGS

GENERIC NAME OR DRUG CLASS	COMBINED EFFECT
Amphetamine	Increased amphetamine effect.
Ciprofloxacin	May cause kidney dysfunction.
Flecainide	Increased flecainide effect.
Iron supplements*	Decreased iron effect.
Ketoconazole	Decreased ketoconazole effect.
Levodopa	Possible increased levodopa effect.
Lithium	Decreased lithium effect.
Meperidine	Increased meperidine effect.
Methenamine	Decreased methenamine effect.
Mexiletine	May slow elimination of mexiletine and cause need to adjust dosage.
Nalidixic acid	Decreased effect of nalidixic acid.
Nitrofurantoin	Possible decreased nitrofurantoin effect.
Nizatidine	Decreased nizatidine absorption.
Norfloxacin	Decreased effect of norfloxacin.
Oxyphenbutazone	Decreased oxyphen-butazone effect.

Para-aminosalicylic acid (PAS)	Decreased PAS effect.
Penicillins*	Decreased penicillin effect.
Pentobarbital	Decreased pentobarbital effect.
Phenylbutazone	Decreased phenyl-butazone effect.
Pseudoephedrine	Increased pseudo-ephedrine effect.
Quinidine	Increased quinidine effect.
Salicylates*	Decreased salicylate effect.
Sulfa drugs*	Decreased sulfa effect.
Tetracyclines*	Decreased tetracycline effect.

POSSIBLE INTERACTION WITH OTHER SUBSTANCES

INTERACTS WITH	COMBINED EFFECT
Alcohol:	Decreased antacid effect.
Beverages:	No proven problems.
Cocaine:	No proven problems.
Foods:	Decreased antacid effect. Wait 1 hour after eating.
Marijuana:	No proven problems.
Tobacco:	Decreased antacid effect.

*See Glossary

SODIUM CARBONATE

BRAND NAMES

Rolaids

BASIC INFORMATION

Habit forming? No
Prescription needed? No
Available as generic? No
Drug class: Antacid

 USES

Treatment for hyperacidity in upper gastrointestinal tract, including stomach and esophagus. Symptoms may be heartburn or acid indigestion. Diseases include peptic ulcer, gastritis, esophagitis, hiatal hernia.

 DOSAGE & USAGE INFORMATION

How to take:
Chewable tablets or wafers—Chew well before swallowing.

When to take:
1 to 3 hours after meals unless directed otherwise by your doctor.

If you forget a dose:
Take as soon as you remember.

What drug does:
- Neutralizes some of the hydrochloric acid in the stomach.
- Reduces action of pepsin, a digestive enzyme.

Time lapse before drug works:
15 minutes.

Don't take with:
Other medicines at the same time. Decreases absorption of other drugs.

 OVERDOSE

SYMPTOMS:
Weakness, fatigue, dizziness.
WHAT TO DO:
Overdose unlikely to threaten life. If person takes much larger amount than prescribed, call doctor, poison-control center or hospital emergency room for instructions.

 POSSIBLE ADVERSE REACTIONS OR SIDE EFFECTS

SYMPTOMS	WHAT TO DO
Life-threatening: None expected.	
Common: Constipation, appetite loss.	Continue. Call doctor when convenient.
Infrequent:	
• Lower abdominal pain and swelling, bone pain, muscle weakness, swollen wrists or ankles.	Discontinue. Call doctor right away.
• Mood change, nausea, vomiting, weight loss.	Continue. Call doctor when convenient.
Rare: None expected.	

SODIUM CARBONATE

WARNINGS & PRECAUTIONS

Don't take if:
You are allergic to any antacid.

Before you start, consult your doctor:
- If you have kidney disease, liver disease, high blood pressure or congestive heart failure.
- If you have chronic constipation or diarrhea.
- If you have symptoms of appendicitis.
- If you have stomach or intestinal bleeding.

Over age 60:
Adverse reactions and side effects may be more frequent and severe than in younger persons. Diarrhea or constipation particularly likely.

Pregnancy:
Risk to unborn child outweighs drug benefits. Don't use.

Breast-feeding:
Drug passes into milk. Avoid drug or discontinue nursing until you finish medicine. Consult doctor for advice on maintaining milk supply.

Infants & children:
Use only under medical supervision.

Prolonged use:
Fluid retention.

Skin & sunlight:
No problems expected.

Driving, piloting or hazardous work:
No problems expected.

Discontinuing:
May be unnecessary to finish medicine. Follow doctor's instructions.

Others:
Don't take longer than 2 weeks unless under medical supervision.

POSSIBLE INTERACTION WITH OTHER DRUGS

GENERIC NAME OR DRUG CLASS	COMBINED EFFECT
Chlorpromazine	Decreased chlorpromazine effect.
Ciprofloxacin	May cause kidney dysfunction.
Digitalis preparations*	Decreased digitalis effect.
Iron supplements*	Decreased iron effect.
Ketoconazole	Decreased ketoconazole effect.
Levodopa	Possible increased levodopa effect.
Lithium	Decreased lithium effect.
Meperidine	Increased meperidine effect.
Methenamine	Decreased methenamine effect.
Nalidixic acid	Decreased effect of nalidixic acid.
Nitrofurantoin	Possible decreased nitrofurantoin effect.
Nizatidine	Decreased nizatidine absorption.
Norfloxacin	Decreased norfloxacin effect.
Oxyphenbutazone	Decreased oxyphenbutazone effect.
Para-aminosalicylic acid (PAS)	Decreased PAS effect.
Penicillins*	Decreased penicillin effect.
Pentobarbital	Decreased pentobarbital effect.
Phenylbutazone	Decreased phenylbutazone effect.
Pseudoephedrine	Increased pseudoephedrine effect.
Sulfa drugs*	Decreased sulfa effect.
Tetracyclines*	Decreased tetracycline effect.
Vitamins A and C	Decreased vitamin effect.

POSSIBLE INTERACTION WITH OTHER SUBSTANCES

INTERACTS WITH	COMBINED EFFECT
Alcohol:	Decreased antacid effect.
Beverages:	No proven problems.
Cocaine:	No proven problems.
Foods:	Decreased antacid effect. Wait 1 hour after eating.
Marijuana:	No proven problems.
Tobacco:	Decreased antacid effect.

*See Glossary

917

SODIUM FLUORIDE

BRAND NAMES

Denta-Fl	Luride-SF
Flo-Tab	Nafeen
Fluor-A-Day	Pediaflor
Fluorident	Pedi-Dent
Fluoritab	Solu-Flur
Fluorodex	Stay-Flo
Flura	Studaflor
Karidium	Thera-Flur
Luride	

Numerous other multiple vitamin-mineral supplements.

BASIC INFORMATION

Habit forming? No
Prescription needed? Yes
Available as generic? No
Drug class: Mineral supplement (fluoride)

USES

- Reduces tooth cavities.
- Treatment for osteoporosis.

DOSAGE & USAGE INFORMATION

How to take:
- Tablet—Swallow with liquid or crumble tablet and take with liquid (*not* milk) or food.
- Liquid—Measure with dropper and take directly or with liquid.
- Chewable tablets—Chew slowly and thoroughly before swallowing.

When to take:
Usually at bedtime after teeth are thoroughly brushed.

Continued next column

OVERDOSE

SYMPTOMS:
Stomach cramps or pain, nausea, faintness, vomiting (possibly bloody), diarrhea, black stools, shallow breathing, muscle spasms, seizures, arrhythmias.
WHAT TO DO:
- Dial 0 (operator) or 911 (emergency) for an ambulance or medical help. Then give first aid immediately.
- See emergency information on inside covers.

If you forget a dose:
Take as soon as you remember. Don't double a forgotten dose. Return to schedule.

What drug does:
Provides supplemental fluoride to combat tooth decay.

Time lapse before drug works:
8 weeks to provide maximum effect.

Don't take with:
- Other medicine simultaneously.
- See Interaction column.

POSSIBLE ADVERSE REACTIONS OR SIDE EFFECTS

SYMPTOMS	WHAT TO DO
Life-threatening: None expected.	
Common: None expected.	
Infrequent: Rash.	Discontinue. Call doctor right away.
Rare: • Severe upsets (digestive) only with overdose.	Discontinue. Seek emergency treatment.
• Sores in mouth and lips.	Discontinue. Call doctor right away.

WARNINGS & PRECAUTIONS

Don't take if:
- Your water supply contains 0.7 parts fluoride per million. Too much fluoride stains teeth permanently.
- You are allergic to any fluoride-containing product.
- You have underactive thyroid.

Before you start, consult your doctor:
Not necessary.

Over age 60:
No problems expected.

Pregnancy:
No problems expected.

Breast-feeding:
No problems expected.

Infants & children:
No problems expected except accidental overdose. Keep vitamin-mineral supplements out of children's reach.

Prolonged use:
Excess may cause discolored teeth and decreased calcium in blood.

Skin & sunlight:
No problems expected.

Driving, piloting or hazardous work:
No problems expected.

Discontinuing:
No problems expected.

Others:
- Store in original plastic container. Fluoride decomposes glass.
- Some products contain tartrazine dye. Avoid, especially if you are allergic to aspirin.

POSSIBLE INTERACTION WITH OTHER DRUGS

GENERIC NAME OR DRUG CLASS	COMBINED EFFECT
None expected.	

POSSIBLE INTERACTION WITH OTHER SUBSTANCES

INTERACTS WITH	COMBINED EFFECT
Alcohol:	None expected.
Beverages: Milk.	Prevents absorption of fluoride. Space dose 2 hours before or after milk.
Cocaine:	None expected.
Foods:	None expected.
Marijuana:	None expected.
Tobacco:	None expected.

SODIUM PHOSPHATE

BRAND NAMES

Fleet Enema   Phospho-Soda
Fleet Phospho-Soda   Sal Hepatica

BASIC INFORMATION

Habit forming? No
Prescription needed? No
Available as generic? Yes
Drug class: Laxative (hyperosmotic)

 USES

Constipation relief.

 DOSAGE & USAGE INFORMATION

How to take:
Liquid, effervescent tablet or powder—Dilute dose in beverage before swallowing.

When to take:
Usually once a day, preferably in the morning.

If you forget a dose:
Take as soon as you remember up to 8 hours before bedtime. If later, wait for next scheduled dose (don't double this dose). Don't take at bedtime.

What drug does:
Draws water into bowel from other body tissues. Causes distention through fluid accumulation, which promotes soft stool and accelerates bowel motion.

Time lapse before drug works:
30 minutes to 3 hours.

Don't take with:
See Interaction column and consult doctor.

 OVERDOSE

SYMPTOMS:
Fluid depletion, weakness, vomiting, fainting.
WHAT TO DO:
Overdose unlikely to threaten life. If person takes much larger amount than prescribed, call doctor, poison-control center or hospital emergency room for instructions.

 POSSIBLE ADVERSE REACTIONS OR SIDE EFFECTS

SYMPTOMS	WHAT TO DO
Life-threatening:	
None expected.	
Common:	
None expected.	
Infrequent:	
• Irregular heartbeat.	Discontinue. Call doctor right away.
• Increased thirst, gaseousness, cramps, diarrhea, nausea.	Continue. Tell doctor at next visit.
Rare:	
Dizziness, confusion, tiredness or weakness.	Continue. Call doctor when convenient.

WARNINGS & PRECAUTIONS

Don't take if:
- You are allergic to any hyperosmotic laxative.
- You have symptoms of appendicitis, inflamed bowel or intestinal blockage.
- You have missed a bowel movement for only 1 or 2 days.

Before you start, consult your doctor:
- If you have congestive heart disease.
- If you have diabetes.
- If you have high blood pressure.
- If you have a colostomy or ileostomy.
- If you have kidney disease.
- If you have a laxative habit.
- If you have rectal bleeding.
- If you take another laxative.

Over age 60:
Adverse reactions and side effects may be more frequent and severe than in younger persons.

Pregnancy:
Salt content may cause fluid retention and swelling. Avoid if possible.

Breast-feeding:
No problems expected.

Infants & children:
Use only under medical supervision.

Prolonged use:
Don't take for more than 1 week unless under a doctor's supervision. May cause laxative dependence.

Skin & sunlight:
No problems expected.

Driving, piloting or hazardous work:
No problems expected.

Discontinuing:
May be unnecessary to finish medicine. Follow doctor's instructions.

Others:
- Don't take to "flush out" your system or as a "tonic."
- Don't take within 2 hours of taking another medicine.

POSSIBLE INTERACTION WITH OTHER DRUGS

GENERIC NAME OR DRUG CLASS	COMBINED EFFECT
Chlordiazepoxide	Decreased chlordiazepoxide effect.
Chlorpromazine	Decreased chlorpromazine effect.
Dicumarol	Decreased dicumarol effect.
Digoxin	Decreased digoxin effect.
Isoniazid	Decreased isoniazid effect.
Mexiletine	May decrease effectiveness of mexiletine.
Tetracyclines*	Possible intestinal blockage.

POSSIBLE INTERACTION WITH OTHER SUBSTANCES

INTERACTS WITH	COMBINED EFFECT
Alcohol:	None expected.
Beverages:	None expected.
Cocaine:	None expected.
Foods:	None expected.
Marijuana:	None expected.
Tobacco:	None expected.

SOTALOL

BRAND NAMES

Sotacor

BASIC INFORMATION

Habit forming? No
Prescription needed? Yes
Available as generic? Yes
Drug class: Beta-adrenergic blocker

 USES

- Aids in treatment of increased thyroid activity.
- Reduces anxiety, tremors, and angina attacks.
- Stabilizes irregular heartbeat.
- Lowers blood pressure.
- Reduces frequency of migraine headaches. (Does not relieve headache pain.)
- Treats glaucoma.

 DOSAGE & USAGE INFORMATION

How to take:
Tablet, liquid or extended-release capsule—Swallow with liquid. If you can't swallow whole, crumble tablet or open capsule and take with liquid or food. Don't crush capsule.

When to take:
With meals or immediately after.

If you forget a dose:
Take as soon as you remember. Return to regular schedule, but allow 3 hours between doses.

What drug does:
- Blocks certain actions of sympathetic nervous system.
- Lowers heart's oxygen requirements.
- Slows nerve impulses through heart.
- Reduces blood vessel contraction in heart, scalp and other body parts.

Continued next column

 OVERDOSE

SYMPTOMS:
Weakness, slow or weak pulse, blood-pressure drop, fainting, difficulty breathing, convulsions, cold and sweaty skin.
WHAT TO DO:
- Dial 0 (operator) or 911 (emergency) for an ambulance or medical help. Then give first aid immediately.
- See emergency information on inside covers.

Time lapse before drug works:
1 to 4 hours.

Don't take with:
Non-prescription drugs or drugs in Interaction column without consulting doctor.

 POSSIBLE ADVERSE REACTIONS OR SIDE EFFECTS

SYMPTOMS	WHAT TO DO
Life-threatening:	
Congestive heart failure.	Discontinue. Seek emergency treatment.
Common:	
• Pulse slower than 50 beats per minute.	Discontinue. Call doctor right away.
• Drowsiness, fatigue, numbness or tingling of fingers or toes, dizziness, diarrhea, nausea, weakness.	Continue. Call doctor when convenient.
• Cold hands or feet; dry mouth, eyes and skin.	Continue. Tell doctor at next visit.
Infrequent:	
• Nightmares, insomnia, headache, difficult breathing, anxiety.	Discontinue. Call doctor right away.
• Depression, reduced alertness, impotence.	Continue. Call doctor when convenient.
Rare:	
Rash, sore throat, fever.	Discontinue. Call doctor right away.

 WARNINGS & PRECAUTIONS

Don't take if:
- You are allergic to any beta-adrenergic blocker.
- You have asthma.
- You have hay fever symptoms.
- You have taken MAO inhibitors in past 2 weeks.

Before you start, consult your doctor:
- If you have heart disease or poor circulation to the extremities.
- If you have hay fever, asthma, chronic bronchitis, emphysema.
- If you have overactive thyroid function.
- If you have impaired liver or kidney function.
- If you will have surgery within 2 months, including dental surgery, requiring general or spinal anesthesia.
- If you have diabetes or hypoglycemia.

Over age 60:
Adverse reactions and side effects may be more frequent and severe than in younger persons.

Pregnancy:
Risk to unborn child outweighs drug benefits. Don't use.

Breast-feeding:
Drug passes into milk. Avoid drug or discontinue nursing until you finish medicine. Consult doctor for advice on maintaining milk supply.

Infants & children:
Not recommended.

Prolonged use:
Weakens heart muscle contractions.

Skin & sunlight:
No problems expected.

Driving, piloting or hazardous work:
Don't drive or pilot aircraft until you learn how medicine affects you. Don't work around dangerous machinery. Don't climb ladders or work in high places. Danger increases if you drink alcohol or take medicine affecting alertness and reflexes.

Discontinuing:
Don't discontinue without consulting doctor. Dose may require gradual reduction if you have taken drug for a long time. Doses of other drugs may also require adjustment.

Others:
May mask hypoglycemia.

POSSIBLE INTERACTION WITH OTHER DRUGS

GENERIC NAME OR DRUG CLASS	COMBINED EFFECT
ACE inhibitors: captopril, enalapril, lisinopril*	Increased antihypertensive effects of both drugs. Dosages may require adjustment.
Antidiabetics*	Increased antidiabetic effect.
Antihistamines*	Decreased antihistamine effect.
Antihypertensives*	Increased antihypertensive effect.
Barbiturates*	Increased barbiturate effect. Dangerous sedation.
Beta-agonists*	Decreased beta-agonist effect.
Betaxolol eyedrops	Possible increased sotatol effect.
Diclofenac	Decreased antihypertensive effect of sotalol.

Digitalis preparations*	Can either increase or decrease heart rate. Improves irregular heartbeat.
Encainide	Increased effect of toxicity on heart muscle.
Indomethacin	Decreased effect of sotalol.
Insulin	Hypoglycemic effects may be prolonged.
Levobunolol eyedrops	Possible increased sotalol effect.
Molindone	Increased tranquilizer effect.
Narcotics*	Increased narcotic effect. Dangerous sedation.
Nicardipine	Blood-pressure drop. Dosages may require adjustment.
Nitrates*	Possible excessive blood-pressure drop.
Non-steroidal anti-inflammatory drugs (NSAIDs)*	Decreased antihypertensive effect of sotalol.
Phenytoin	Decreased sotalol effect.

POSSIBLE INTERACTION WITH OTHER SUBSTANCES

INTERACTS WITH	COMBINED EFFECT
Alcohol:	Excessive blood-pressure drop. Avoid.
Beverages:	None expected.
Cocaine:	Irregular heartbeat. Avoid.
Foods:	None expected.
Marijuana:	Daily use—Impaired circulation to hands and feet.
Tobacco:	Possible irregular heartbeat.

SPIRONOLACTONE

BRAND NAMES

Aldactazide	Sincomen
Aldactone	Spironazide
Novospiroton	

BASIC INFORMATION

Habit forming? No
Prescription needed? Yes
Available as generic? Yes
Drug class: Antihypertensive, diuretic

USES

- Reduces high blood pressure.
- Prevents fluid retention.

DOSAGE & USAGE INFORMATION

How to take:
Tablet—Swallow with liquid or food to lessen stomach irritation. If you can't swallow whole, crumble tablet and take with liquid or food.

When to take:
- 1 dose a day—Take after breakfast.
- More than 1 dose a day—Take last dose no later than 6 p.m.

If you forget a dose:
- 1 dose a day—Take as soon as you remember up to 12 hours late. If more than 12 hours, wait for next scheduled dose (don't double this dose).
- More than 1 dose a day—Take as soon as you remember. Wait 6 hours for next dose.

What drug does:
- Increases sodium and water excretion through increased urine production, decreasing body fluid and blood pressure.
- Retains potassium.

Continued next column

OVERDOSE

SYMPTOMS:
Thirst, drowsiness, confusion, fatigue, weakness, nausea, vomiting, irregular heartbeat, excessive blood-pressure drop.
WHAT TO DO:
- **Dial 0 (operator) or 911 (emergency) for an ambulance or medical help. Then give first aid immediately.**
- **See emergency information on inside covers.**

Time lapse before drug works:
3 to 5 days.

Don't take with:
See Interaction column and consult doctor.

POSSIBLE ADVERSE REACTIONS OR SIDE EFFECTS

SYMPTOMS	WHAT TO DO
Life-threatening: None expected.	
Common: Drowsiness or headache, thirst, nausea, vomiting, diarrhea, cramping.	Continue. Call doctor when convenient.
Infrequent: • Confusion, irregular heartbeat, shortness of breath, unusual sweating.	Discontinue. Call doctor right away.
• Numbness, tingling in hands or feet; menstrual irregularities; tender breasts; change in sex drive.	Continue. Call doctor when convenient.
Rare: • Rash or itchy skin, fever.	Discontinue. Call doctor right away.
• Deep voice in women, excess hair growth, voice change, enlarged clitoris in women.	Continue. Tell doctor at next visit.

SPIRONOLACTONE

WARNINGS & PRECAUTIONS

Don't take if:
- You are allergic to spironolactone.
- You have impaired kidney function.
- Your serum potassium level is high.

Before you start, consult your doctor:
- If you have had kidney or liver disease.
- If you will have surgery within 2 months, including dental surgery, requiring general or spinal anesthesia.

Over age 60:
- Limit use to 2 to 3 weeks if possible.
- Adverse reactions and side effects may be more frequent and severe than in younger persons.
- Heat or fever can reduce blood pressure. May require dose adjustment.
- Overdose and extended use may cause blood clots.

Pregnancy:
No proven harm to unborn child. Avoid if possible.

Breast-feeding:
No proven problems. Consult doctor.

Infants & children:
Use only under medical supervision.

Prolonged use:
Potassium retention with irregular heartbeat, unusual weakness and confusion.

Skin & sunlight:
No problems expected.

Driving, piloting or hazardous work:
Avoid if you feel drowsy. Otherwise, no problems expected.

Discontinuing:
Consult doctor about adjusting doses of other drugs.

Others:
No problems expected.

POSSIBLE INTERACTION WITH OTHER DRUGS

GENERIC NAME OR DRUG CLASS	COMBINED EFFECT
ACE inhibitors: captopril, enalapril, lisinopril*	Possible excessive potassium in blood.
Amiloride	Dangerous potassium retention.
Anticoagulants, oral*	Possible decreased anticoagulant effect.
Antihypertensives, other*	Increased anti-hypertensive effect.
Aspirin	Decreased spironolactone effect.
Carteolol	Increased antihyper-tensive effect.
Digitalis preparations*	Decreased digitalis effect.
Diuretics, other*	Increased effect of both drugs. Beneficial if needed and dose is correct.
Laxatives*	Reduced potassium levels.
Lithium	Likely lithium toxicity.
Nicardipine	Blood-pressure drop. Dosages may require adjustment.
Nitrates*	Excessive blood-pressure drop.
Potassium supplements*	Dangerous potassium retention, causing possible heartbeat irregularity.
Salicylates*	May decrease spironolactone effect.
Sodium bicarbonate	Reduces high potassium levels.
Sotalol	Increased antihyper-tensive effect.
Terazosin	Decreases effective-ness of terazosin.
Triamterene	Dangerous potassium retention.

POSSIBLE INTERACTION WITH OTHER SUBSTANCES

INTERACTS WITH	COMBINED EFFECT
Alcohol:	None expected.
Beverages: Low-salt milk.	Possible potassium toxicity.
Cocaine:	Increased risk of heart block and high blood pressure.
Foods: Salt.	Don't restrict unless directed by doctor.
Salt substitutes.	Possible potassium toxicity.
Marijuana:	Increased thirst, fainting.
Tobacco:	None expected.

SPIRONOLACTONE & HYDROCHLOROTHIAZIDE

BRAND NAMES

Aldactazide   Novospirozine

BASIC INFORMATION

Habit forming? Yes
Prescription needed? Yes
Available as generic? Yes
Drug class: Antihypertensive, diuretic
(thiazide)

USES

- Controls, but doesn't cure, high blood pressure.
- Reduces fluid retention (edema).

DOSAGE & USAGE INFORMATION

How to take:
Tablet—Swallow with liquid. If you can't swallow whole, crumble tablet and take with liquid or food.

When to take:
- 1 dose a day—Take after breakfast.
- More than 1 dose a day—Take last dose no later than 6 p.m.

If you forget a dose:
- 1 dose a day—Take as soon as you remember up to 12 hours late. If more than 12 hours, wait for next scheduled dose (don't double this dose).
- More than 1 dose a day—Take as soon as you remember. Wait 6 hours for next dose.

Continued next column

OVERDOSE

SYMPTOMS:
Thirst, drowsiness, confusion, fatigue, weakness, nausea, vomiting, cramps, irregular heartbeat, weak pulse, excessive blood-pressure drop, coma.
WHAT TO DO:
- **Dial 0 (operator) or 911 (emergency) for an ambulance or medical help. Then give first aid immediately.**
- **See emergency information on inside covers.**

What drug does:
- Increases sodium and water excretion through increased urine production.
- Retains potassium.
- Relaxes muscle cells of small arteries.
- Reduced body fluid and relaxed arteries lower blood pressure.

Time lapse before drug works:
4 to 6 hours. May require several weeks to lower blood pressure.

Don't take with:
- Non-prescription drugs without consulting doctor.
- See Interaction column and consult doctor.

POSSIBLE ADVERSE REACTIONS OR SIDE EFFECTS

SYMPTOMS	WHAT TO DO
Life-threatening: Irregular heartbeat, weak pulse, shortness of breath.	Discontinue. Seek emergency treatment.
Common: Drowsiness, headache, thirst, cramping.	Continue. Call doctor when convenient.
Infrequent: • Blurred vision, abdominal pain, nausea, vomiting.	Discontinue. Call doctor right away.
• Dizziness, mood change, headache, dry mouth, menstrual irregularities, tender breasts, diminished sex drive, increased sweating, weakness, tiredness, weight gain or loss, confusion, numbness or tingling in hands or feet, diarrhea.	Continue. Call doctor when convenient.
Rare: • Sore throat, fever, rash, jaundice.	Discontinue. Call doctor right away.
• Excess growth of hair, deep voice in in women, enlarged clitoris in women.	Continue. Call doctor when convenient.

WARNINGS & PRECAUTIONS

Don't take if:
You are allergic to any thiazide diuretic drug.

Before you start, consult your doctor:
- If you are allergic to any sulfa drug.
- If you have gout, liver, pancreas or kidney disorder.
- If you have had kidney or liver disease.
- If you will have surgery within 2 months, including dental surgery, requiring general or spinal anesthesia.

Over age 60:
- Adverse reactions and side effects may be more frequent and severe than in younger persons, especially dizziness and excessive potassium loss.
- Limit use to 2 to 3 weeks if possible.
- Heat or fever can reduce blood pressure. May require dose adjustment.
- Overdose and extended use may cause blood clots.

Pregnancy:
Risk to unborn child outweighs drug benefits. Don't use.

Breast-feeding:
Drug passes into milk. Avoid drug or discontinue nursing until you finish medicine.

Infants & children:
Use only under medical supervision.

Prolonged use:
- You may need medicine to treat high blood pressure for the rest of your life.
- Potassium retention with irregular heartbeat, unusual weakness and confusion.

Skin & sunlight:
May cause rash or intensify sunburn in areas exposed to sun or sunlamp.

Driving, piloting or hazardous work:
Don't drive or pilot aircraft until you learn how medicine affects you. Don't work around dangerous machinery. Don't climb ladders or work in high places. Danger increases if you drink alcohol or take medicine affecting alertness and reflexes.

Discontinuing:
- Don't discontinue without medical advice.
- Consult doctor about adjusting doses of other drugs.

Others:
- Hot weather and fever may cause dehydration and drop in blood pressure. Dose may require temporary adjustment. Weigh daily and report any unexpected weight decreases to your doctor.
- May cause rise in uric acid, leading to gout.
- May cause blood-sugar rise in diabetics.

POSSIBLE INTERACTION WITH OTHER DRUGS

GENERIC NAME OR DRUG CLASS	COMBINED EFFECT
ACE inhibitors: captopril, enalapril, lisinopril *	Possible excessive potassium in blood.
Allopurinol	Decreased allopurinol effect.
Anticoagulants, oral	Decreased anticoagulant effect.
Antidepressants, tricyclic (TCA) *	Dangerous drop in blood pressure. Avoid combination unless under medical supervision.

Continued page 1106

POSSIBLE INTERACTION WITH OTHER SUBSTANCES

INTERACTS WITH	COMBINED EFFECT
Alcohol:	Dangerous blood-pressure drop.
Beverages: Low-salt milk.	Possible potassium toxicity.
Cocaine:	Decreased spironolactone effect.
Foods: Salt.	Don't restrict unless directed by doctor.
Salt substitutes.	Possible potassium toxicity.
Marijuana:	May increase blood pressure. Increased thirst, fainting.
Tobacco:	None expected.

*See Glossary

SUCRALFATE

BRAND NAMES

Carafate   Sulcrate

BASIC INFORMATION

Habit forming? No
Prescription needed? Yes
Available as generic? No
Drug class: Anti-ulcer

 ## USES

Treatment of duodenal ulcer.

 ## DOSAGE & USAGE INFORMATION

How to take:
Tablet—Take as directed on an empty stomach.

When to take:
1 hour before meals and at bedtime. Allow 2 hours to elapse before taking other prescription medicines.

If you forget a dose:
Take as soon as you remember up to 2 hours late. If more than 2 hours, wait for next scheduled dose (don't double this dose).

What drug does:
Covers ulcer site and protects from acid, enzymes and bile salts.

Time lapse before drug works:
Begins in 30 minutes. May require several days to relieve pain.

Don't take with:
See Interaction column and consult doctor.

 ## OVERDOSE

SYMPTOMS:
No data available yet for this new drug.
WHAT TO DO:
Overdose unlikely to threaten life. If person takes much larger amount than prescribed, call doctor, poison-control center or hospital emergency room for instructions.

 ## POSSIBLE ADVERSE REACTIONS OR SIDE EFFECTS

SYMPTOMS	WHAT TO DO
Life-threatening: None expected.	
Common: Constipation.	Continue. Call doctor when convenient.
Infrequent: • Diarrhea.	Discontinue. Call doctor right away.
• Dizziness, sleepiness, rash, itchy skin, abdominal pain, indigestion, vomiting, nausea, back pain.	Continue. Call doctor when convenient.
Rare: None expected.	

WARNINGS & PRECAUTIONS

Don't take if:
You are allergic to sucralfate.

Before you start, consult your doctor:
If you will have surgery within 2 months, including dental surgery, requiring general or spinal anesthesia.

Over age 60:
Adverse reactions and side effects may be more frequent and severe than in younger persons.

Pregnancy:
No proven harm to unborn child. Avoid if possible.

Breast-feeding:
Unknown effects.

Infants & children:
Safety not established.

Prolonged use:
Request blood counts if medicine needed longer than 8 weeks.

Skin & sunlight:
No problems expected.

Driving, piloting or hazardous work:
Don't drive or pilot aircraft until you learn how medicine affects you. Don't work around dangerous machinery. Don't climb ladders or work in high places. Danger increases if you drink alcohol or take medicine affecting alertness and reflexes, such as antihistamines, tranquilizers, sedatives, pain medicine, narcotics and mind-altering drugs.

Discontinuing:
Don't discontinue without consulting doctor. Dose may require gradual reduction if you have taken drug for a long time. Doses of other drugs may also require adjustment.

Others:
No problems expected.

POSSIBLE INTERACTION WITH OTHER DRUGS

GENERIC NAME OR DRUG CLASS	COMBINED EFFECT
Cimetidine	Possible decreased absorption of cimetidine if taken simultaneously.
Phenytoin	Possible decreased absorption of phenytoin if taken simultaneously.
Tetracyclines*	Possible decreased absorption of tetracycline if taken simultaneously.

POSSIBLE INTERACTION WITH OTHER SUBSTANCES

INTERACTS WITH	COMBINED EFFECT
Alcohol:	Irritates ulcer. Avoid.
Beverages: Caffeine.	Irritates ulcer. Avoid.
Cocaine:	May make ulcer worse. Avoid.
Foods:	No problems expected.
Marijuana:	May make ulcer worse. Avoid.
Tobacco:	May make ulcer worse. Avoid.

*See Glossary

SULFACYTINE

BRAND NAMES

Renoquid

BASIC INFORMATION

Habit forming? No
Prescription needed? Yes
Available as generic? No
Drug class: Sulfa (sulfonamide)

 USES

Treatment for urinary tract infections responsive to this drug.

 DOSAGE & USAGE INFORMATION

How to take:
Tablet—Swallow with liquid. Instructions to take on empty stomach mean 1 hour before or 2 hours after eating.

When to take:
At the same times each day, evenly spaced.

If you forget a dose:
Take as soon as you remember up to 2 hours late. If more than 2 hours, wait for next scheduled dose (don't double this dose).

What drug does:
Interferes with a nutrient (folic acid) necessary for growth and reproduction of bacteria. Will not attack viruses.

Time lapse before drug works:
2 to 5 days to affect infection.

Don't take with:
See Interaction column and consult doctor.

 OVERDOSE

SYMPTOMS:
Less urine, bloody urine, coma.
WHAT TO DO:
- **Dial 0 (operator) or 911 (emergency) for an ambulance or medical help. Then give first aid immediately.**
- **See emergency information on inside covers.**

 POSSIBLE ADVERSE REACTIONS OR SIDE EFFECTS

SYMPTOMS	WHAT TO DO
Life-threatening: None expected.	
Common:	
• Itchy skin, rash.	Discontinue. Call doctor right away.
• Headache, vomiting, nausea, diarrhea, appetite loss.	Continue. Call doctor when convenient.
Infrequent:	
• Red, peeling or blistering skin; sore throat; fever; swallowing difficulty; unusual bruising; aching joints or muscles; jaundice.	Discontinue. Call doctor right away.
• Dizziness.	Continue. Call doctor when convenient.
Rare:	
Painful urination, low back pain, numbness or tingling in hands or feet.	Discontinue. Call doctor right away.

WARNINGS & PRECAUTIONS

Don't take if:
You are allergic to any sulfa drug.

Before you start, consult your doctor:
- If you are allergic to carbonic anhydrase inhibitors, oral antidiabetics, thiazide or loop diuretics.
- If you are allergic by nature.
- If you have liver or kidney disease.
- If you have porphyria.
- If you have developed anemia from use of any drug.

Over age 60:
Adverse reactions and side effects may be more frequent and severe than in younger persons.

Pregnancy:
Risk to unborn child outweighs drug benefits. Don't use.

Breast-feeding:
Drug passes into milk. Avoid drug or discontinue nursing until you finish medicine. Consult doctor for advice on maintaining milk supply.

Infants & children:
Don't give to infants younger than 1 month.

Prolonged use:
- May enlarge thyroid gland.
- You may become more susceptible to infections caused by germs not responsive to this drug.
- Request frequent blood counts, liver- and kidney-function studies.

Skin & sunlight:
May cause rash or intensify sunburn in areas exposed to sun or sunlamp.

Driving, piloting or hazardous work:
Avoid if you feel dizzy. Otherwise, no problems expected.

Discontinuing:
Don't discontinue without doctor's advice until you complete prescribed dose, even though symptoms diminish or disappear.

Others:
- Drink 2 quarts of liquid each day to prevent adverse reactions.
- If you require surgery, tell anesthetist you take sulfa. Pentothal anesthesia should not be used.

POSSIBLE INTERACTION WITH OTHER DRUGS

GENERIC NAME OR DRUG CLASS	COMBINED EFFECT
Aminobenzoate potassium	Possible decreased sulfa effect.
Anticoagulants, oral*	Increased anticoagulant effect.
Anticonvulsants, hydantoin*	Toxic effect on brain.
Aspirin	Increased sulfa effect.
Calcium supplements*	Decreased sulfa effect.
Isoniazid	Possible anemia.
Methenamine	Possible kidney blockage.
Methotrexate	Increased methotrexate effect.
Oxyphenbutazone	Increased sulfa effect.
Para-aminosalicylic acid (PAS)	Decreased sulfa effect.
Penicillins*	Decreased penicillin effect.
Phenylbutazone	Increased sulfa effect.
Probenecid	Increased sulfa effect.
Sulfinpyrazone	Increased sulfa effect.
Sulfonureas*	May increase hypoglycemic action.
Trimethoprim	Increased sulfa effect.

POSSIBLE INTERACTION WITH OTHER SUBSTANCES

INTERACTS WITH	COMBINED EFFECT
Alcohol:	Increased alcohol effect.
Beverages: Less than 2 quarts of fluid daily.	Kidney damage.
Cocaine:	None expected.
Foods:	None expected.
Marijuana:	None expected.
Tobacco:	None expected.

*See Glossary

SULFAMETHOXAZOLE

BRAND NAMES

Apo-Sulfamethoxazole	Gantrisin
Apo-Sulfatrim	Methoxanol
Azo Gantanol	Novotrimel
Bactrim	Protrin
Cetamide	Roubac
Cotrim	Septra
Cotrim D.S.	SMZ-TMP
Co-trimoxazole	Sulfamethoprim
Gantanol	Sulmeprim

BASIC INFORMATION

Habit forming? No
Prescription needed? Yes
Available as generic? Yes
Drug class: Sulfa (sulfonamide)

 ## USES

Treatment for urinary tract infections responsive to this drug.

 ## DOSAGE & USAGE INFORMATION

How to take:
- Tablet—Swallow with liquid. Instructions to take on empty stomach mean 1 hour before or 2 hours after eating.
- Liquid—Shake carefully before measuring.

When to take:
At the same times each day, evenly spaced.

If you forget a dose:
Take as soon as you remember up to 2 hours late. If more than 2 hours, wait for next scheduled dose (don't double this dose).

What drug does:
Interferes with a nutrient (folic acid) necessary for growth and reproduction of bacteria. Will not attack viruses.

Time lapse before drug works:
2 to 5 days to affect infection.

Continued next column

 ## OVERDOSE

SYMPTOMS:
Less urine, bloody urine, coma.
WHAT TO DO:
- **Dial 0 (operator) or 911 (emergency) for an ambulance or medical help. Then give first aid immediately.**
- **See emergency information on inside covers.**

Don't take with:
See Interaction column and consult doctor.

 ## POSSIBLE ADVERSE REACTIONS OR SIDE EFFECTS

SYMPTOMS	WHAT TO DO
Life-threatening: None expected.	
Common:	
• Itchy skin, rash.	Discontinue. Call doctor right away.
• Headache, nausea, vomiting, diarrhea, appetite loss.	Continue. Call doctor when convenient.
Infrequent:	
• Red, peeling or blistering skin; sore throat; fever; swallowing difficulty; unusual bruising; aching joints or muscles; jaundice.	Discontinue. Call doctor right away.
• Dizziness.	Continue. Call doctor when convenient.
Rare:	
Painful urination; low back pain; numbness, tingling, burning feeling in feet and hands.	Discontinue. Call doctor right away.

WARNINGS & PRECAUTIONS

Don't take if:
You are allergic to any sulfa drug.

Before you start, consult your doctor:
- If you are allergic to carbonic anhydrase inhibitors, oral antidiabetics or thiazide or loop diuretics.
- If you are allergic by nature.
- If you have liver or kidney disease.
- If you have porphyria.
- If you have developed anemia from use of any drug.

Over age 60:
Adverse reactions and side effects may be more frequent and severe than in younger persons.

Pregnancy:
Risk to unborn child outweighs drug benefits. Don't use.

Breast-feeding:
Drug passes into milk. Avoid drug or discontinue nursing until you finish medicine. Consult doctor for advice on maintaining milk supply.

Infants & children:
Don't give to infants younger than 1 month.

Prolonged use:
- May enlarge thyroid gland.
- You may become more susceptible to infections caused by germs not responsive to this drug.
- Request frequent blood counts, liver- and kidney-function studies.

Skin & sunlight:
May cause rash or intensify sunburn in areas exposed to sun or sunlamp.

Driving, piloting or hazardous work:
Avoid if you feel dizzy. Otherwise, no problems expected.

Discontinuing:
Don't discontinue without doctor's advice until you complete prescribed dose, even though symptoms diminish or disappear.

Others:
- Drink 2 quarts of liquid each day to prevent adverse reactions.
- If you require surgery, tell anesthetist you take sulfa. Pentothal anesthesia should not be used.

POSSIBLE INTERACTION WITH OTHER DRUGS

GENERIC NAME OR DRUG CLASS	COMBINED EFFECT
Aminobenzoate potassium	Possible decreased sulfa effect.
Anticoagulants, oral*	Increased anticoagulant effect.
Anticonvulsants, hydantoin*	Toxic effect on brain.
Aspirin	Increased sulfa effect.
Calcium supplements*	Decreased sulfa effect.
Isoniazid	Possible anemia.
Methenamine	Possible kidney blockage.
Methotrexate	Increased methotrexate effect.
Oxyphenbutazone	Increased sulfa effect.
Para-aminosalicylic acid (PAS)	Decreased sulfa effect.
Penicillins*	Decreased penicillin effect.
Phenylbutazone	Increased sulfa effect.
Probenecid	Increased sulfa effect.
Sulfinpyrazone	Increased sulfa effect.
Sulfonureas*	May increase hypoglycemic action.
Trimethoprim	Increased sulfa effect.

POSSIBLE INTERACTION WITH OTHER SUBSTANCES

INTERACTS WITH	COMBINED EFFECT
Alcohol:	Increased alcohol effect.
Beverages: Less than 2 quarts of fluid daily.	Kidney damage.
Cocaine:	None expected.
Foods:	None expected.
Marijuana:	None expected.
Tobacco:	None expected.

*See Glossary

SULFASALAZINE

BRAND NAMES

Azulfidine
Azulfidine En-Tabs

Salazopyrin
SAS-500

BASIC INFORMATION

Habit forming? No
Prescription needed? Yes
Available as generic? Yes
Drug class: Sulfa (sulfonamide)

 USES

Treatment for ulceration and bleeding during active phase of ulcerative colitis.

 DOSAGE & USAGE INFORMATION

How to take:
- Tablet—Swallow with liquid. Instructions to take on empty stomach mean 1 hour before or 2 hours after eating.
- Liquid—Shake carefully before measuring.

When to take:
At the same times each day, evenly spaced.

If you forget a dose:
Take as soon as you remember up to 2 hours late. If more than 2 hours, wait for next scheduled dose (don't double this dose).

What drug does:
Anti-inflammatory action reduces tissue destruction in colon.

Time lapse before drug works:
2 to 5 days.

Don't take with:
See Interaction column and consult doctor.

 OVERDOSE

SYMPTOMS:
Less urine, bloody urine, coma.
WHAT TO DO:
- Dial 0 (operator) or 911 (emergency) for an ambulance or medical help. Then give first aid immediately.
- See emergency information on inside covers.

 POSSIBLE ADVERSE REACTIONS OR SIDE EFFECTS

SYMPTOMS	WHAT TO DO
Life-threatening: None expected.	
Common:	
• Itchy skin, rash.	Discontinue. Call doctor right away.
• Headache, nausea, vomiting, diarrhea, appetite loss.	Continue. Call doctor when convenient.
• Orange urine.	Continue. Tell doctor at next visit.
Infrequent:	
• Red, peeling or blistering skin; sore throat; fever; swallowing difficulty; unusual bruising; aching joints or muscles; jaundice.	Discontinue. Call doctor right away.
• Dizziness.	Continue. Call doctor when convenient.
Rare: Painful urination; low back pain; numbness, tingling, burning feeling in feet and hands.	Discontinue. Call doctor right away.

WARNINGS & PRECAUTIONS

Don't take if:
You are allergic to any sulfa drug.

Before you start, consult your doctor:
- If you are allergic to carbonic anhydrase inhibitors, oral antidiabetics or thiazide or loop diuretics.
- If you are allergic by nature.
- If you have liver or kidney disease.
- If you have porphyria.
- If you have developed anemia from use of any drug.

Over age 60:
Adverse reactions and side effects may be more frequent and severe than in younger persons.

Pregnancy:
Risk to unborn child outweighs drug benefits. Don't use.

Breast-feeding:
Drug passes into milk. Avoid drug or discontinue nursing until you finish medicine. Consult doctor for advice on maintaining milk supply.

Infants & children:
Don't give to infants younger than 1 month.

Prolonged use:
- May enlarge thyroid gland.
- You may become more susceptible to infections caused by germs not responsive to this drug.
- Request frequent blood counts, liver- and kidney-function studies.

Skin & sunlight:
May cause rash or intensify sunburn in areas exposed to sun or sunlamp.

Driving, piloting or hazardous work:
Avoid if you feel dizzy. Otherwise, no problems expected.

Discontinuing:
Don't discontinue without doctor's advice until you complete prescribed dose, even though symptoms diminish or disappear.

Others:
- Drink 2 quarts of liquid each day to prevent adverse reactions.
- If you require surgery, tell anesthetist you take sulfa. Pentothal anesthesia should not be used.

POSSIBLE INTERACTION WITH OTHER DRUGS

GENERIC NAME OR DRUG CLASS	COMBINED EFFECT
Aminobenzoate potassium	Possible decreased sulfa effect.
Antibiotics*	Decreased sulfa effect.
Anticoagulants, oral*	Increased anticoagulant effect.
Anticonvulsants, hydantoin*	Toxic effect on brain.
Aspirin	Increased sulfa effect.
Calcium supplements*	Decreased sulfa effect.
Digoxin	Decreased digoxin effect.
Iron supplements*	Decreased sulfa effect.
Isoniazid	Possible anemia.
Methenamine	Possible kidney blockage.
Methotrexate	Increased methotrexate effect.
Oxyphenbutazone	Increased sulfa effect.
Para-aminosalicylic acid (PAS)	Decreased sulfa effect.
Penicillins*	Decreased penicillin effect.
Phenylbutazone	Increased sulfa effect.
Probenecid	Increased sulfa effect.
Sulfinpyrazone	Increased sulfa effect.
Sulfonureas*	May increase hypoglycemic action.
Trimethoprim	Increased sulfa effect.
Vitamin C	Possible kidney damage. Avoid large doses of vitamin C.

POSSIBLE INTERACTION WITH OTHER SUBSTANCES

INTERACTS WITH	COMBINED EFFECT
Alcohol:	Increased alcohol effect.
Beverages: Less than 2 quarts of fluid daily.	Kidney damage.
Cocaine:	None expected.
Foods:	None expected.
Marijuana:	None expected.
Tobacco:	None expected.

SULFINPYRAZONE

BRAND NAMES

Antazone
Anturan
Anturane
Apo-Sulfinpyrazone

Aprazone
Novopyrazone
Zynol

BASIC INFORMATION

Habit forming? No
Prescription needed? Yes
Available as generic? Yes
Drug class: Antigout (uricosuric)

USES

- Treatment for chronic gout.
- Reduces severity of recurrent heart attack. (This use is experimental and not yet approved by F.D.A.)

DOSAGE & USAGE INFORMATION

How to take:
Tablet or capsule—Swallow with liquid or food to lessen stomach irritation. If you can't swallow whole, crumble tablet or open capsule and take with liquid or food.

When to take:
At the same times each day.

If you forget a dose:
Take as soon as you remember up to 2 hours late. If more than 2 hours, wait for next scheduled dose (don't double this dose).

Continued next column

OVERDOSE

SYMPTOMS:
Breathing difficulty, vomiting, imbalance, seizures, convulsions, coma.
WHAT TO DO:
- Dial 0 (operator) or 911 (emergency) for an ambulance or medical help. Then give first aid immediately.
- If patient is unconscious and not breathing, give mouth-to-mouth breathing. If there is no heartbeat, use cardiac massage and mouth-to-mouth breathing (CPR). Don't try to make patient vomit. If you can't get help quickly, take patient to nearest emergency facility.
- See emergency information on inside covers.

What drug does:
Reduces uric-acid level in blood and tissues by increasing amount of uric acid secreted in urine by kidneys.

Time lapse before drug works:
May require 6 months to prevent gout attacks.

Don't take with:
See Interaction column and consult doctor.

POSSIBLE ADVERSE REACTIONS OR SIDE EFFECTS

SYMPTOMS	WHAT TO DO
Life-threatening: None expected.	
Common: None expected.	
Infrequent:	
• Painful or difficult urination, worsening gout.	Discontinue. Call doctor right away.
• Rash, nausea, vomiting, stomach pain, low back pain.	Continue. Call doctor when convenient.
Rare:	
• Black, bloody or tarry stools.	Discontinue. Seek emergency treatment.
• Sore throat; fever; unusual bleeding or bruising; red, painful joints; blood in urine; fatigue or weakness.	Discontinue. Call doctor right away.

WARNINGS & PRECAUTIONS

Don't take if:
- You are allergic to any uricosuric.
- You have acute gout.
- You have active ulcers (stomach or duodenal), enteritis or ulcerative colitis.
- You have blood-cell disorders.
- You are allergic to oxyphenbutazone or phenylbutazone.

Before you start, consult your doctor:
If you have kidney or blood disease.

Over age 60:
Adverse reactions and side effects may be more frequent and severe than in younger persons. You require lower dose because of decreased kidney function.

Pregnancy:
Studies inconclusive on harm to unborn child. Animal studies show fetal abnormalities. Decide with your doctor whether drug benefits justify risk to unborn child.

Breast-feeding:
No proven problems. Consult doctor.

Infants & children:
Not recommended.

Prolonged use:
Possible kidney damage.

Skin & sunlight:
No problems expected.

Driving, piloting or hazardous work:
No problems expected.

Discontinuing:
Don't discontinue without consulting doctor. Dose may require gradual reduction if you have taken drug for a long time. Doses of other drugs may also require adjustment.

Others:
- Drink 10 to 12 glasses of water each day you take this medicine.
- Periodic blood and urine laboratory tests recommended.

POSSIBLE INTERACTION WITH OTHER DRUGS

GENERIC NAME OR DRUG CLASS	COMBINED EFFECT
Allopurinol	Increased effect of each drug.
Anticoagulants, oral*	Increased anti-coagulant effect.
Antidiabetics, oral*	Increased antidiabetic effect.
Aspirin	Bleeding tendency. Decreased sulfin-pyrazone effect.
Bismuth subsalicylate	Decreased effect of sulfinpyrazone.
Cephalexin	Increased effect of cephalexin.
Cephradine	Increased effect of cephradine.
Cholestyramine	Decreased sulfin-pyrazone effect.
Contraceptives, oral*	Increased bleeding between menstrual periods.
Diuretics*	Decreased sulfin-pyrazone effect.
Penicillins*	Increased penicillin effect.
Salicylates*	Bleeding tendency. Decreased sulfin-pyrazone effect.
Sulfa drugs*	Increased effect of sulfa drugs.

POSSIBLE INTERACTION WITH OTHER SUBSTANCES

INTERACTS WITH	COMBINED EFFECT
Alcohol:	Decreased sulfin-pyrazone effect.
Beverages: Caffeine drinks.	Decreased sulfin-pyrazone effect.
Cocaine:	None expected.
Foods:	None expected.
Marijuana:	Occasional use—None expected. Daily use—May increase blood level of uric acid.
Tobacco:	None expected.

SULFISOXAZOLE

BRAND NAMES

See complete list of brand names in the *Brand Name Directory*, page 1071.

BASIC INFORMATION

Habit forming? No
Prescription needed? Yes
Available as generic? Yes
Drug class: Sulfa (sulfonamide)

 USES

Treatment for urinary tract infections responsive to this drug.

 DOSAGE & USAGE INFORMATION

How to take:
- Tablet—Swallow with liquid. Instructions to take on empty stomach mean 1 hour before or 2 hours after eating.
- Liquid—Shake carefully before measuring.

When to take:
At the same times each day, evenly spaced.

If you forget a dose:
Take as soon as you remember up to 2 hours late. If more than 2 hours, wait for next scheduled dose (don't double this dose).

What drug does:
Interferes with a nutrient (folic acid) necessary for growth and reproduction of bacteria. Will not attack viruses.

Time lapse before drug works:
2 to 5 days to affect infection.

Don't take with:
See Interaction column and consult doctor.

 OVERDOSE

SYMPTOMS:
Less urine, bloody urine, coma.
WHAT TO DO:
- Dial 0 (operator) or 911 (emergency) for an ambulance or medical help. Then give first aid immediately.
- See emergency information on inside covers.

 POSSIBLE ADVERSE REACTIONS OR SIDE EFFECTS

SYMPTOMS	WHAT TO DO
Life-threatening: None expected.	
Common:	
• Itchy skin, rash.	Discontinue. Call doctor right away.
• Headache, nausea, vomiting, diarrhea, appetite loss.	Continue. Call doctor when convenient.
Infrequent:	
• Red, peeling or blistering skin; sore throat; fever; swallowing difficulty; unusual bruising; aching joints or muscles; jaundice.	Discontinue. Call doctor right away.
• Dizziness.	Continue. Call doctor when convenient.
Rare:	
Painful urination; low back pain; numbness, tingling, burning feeling in feet and hands.	Discontinue. Call doctor right away.

WARNINGS & PRECAUTIONS

Don't take if:
You are allergic to any sulfa drug.

Before you start, consult your doctor:
- If you are allergic to carbonic anhydrase inhibitors, oral antidiabetics or thiazide or loop diuretics.
- If you are allergic by nature.
- If you have liver or kidney disease.
- If you have porphyria.
- If you have developed anemia from use of any drug.

Over age 60:
Adverse reactions and side effects may be more frequent and severe than in younger persons.

Pregnancy:
Risk to unborn child outweighs drug benefits. Don't use.

Breast-feeding:
Drug passes into milk. Avoid drug or discontinue nursing until you finish medicine. Consult doctor for advice on maintaining milk supply.

Infants & children:
Don't give to infants younger than 1 month.

Prolonged use:
- May enlarge thyroid gland.
- You may become more susceptible to infections caused by germs not responsive to this drug.
- Request frequent blood counts, liver- and kidney-function studies.

Skin & sunlight:
May cause rash or intensify sunburn in areas exposed to sun or sunlamp.

Driving, piloting or hazardous work:
Avoid if you feel dizzy. Otherwise, no problems expected.

Discontinuing:
Don't discontinue without doctor's advice until you complete prescribed dose, even though symptoms diminish or disappear.

Others:
- Drink 2 quarts of liquid each day to prevent adverse reactions.
- If you require surgery, tell anesthetist you take sulfa.

POSSIBLE INTERACTION WITH OTHER DRUGS

GENERIC NAME OR DRUG CLASS	COMBINED EFFECT
Aminobenzoate potassium	Possible decreased sulfisoxazole effect.
Anticoagulants, oral*	Increased anticoagulant effect.
Anticonvulsants, hydantoin*	Toxic effect on brain.
Aspirin	Increased sulfa effect.
Calcium supplements*	Decreased sulfa effect.
Flecainide	Possible decreased blood-cell production in bone marrow.
Isoniazid	Possible anemia.
Methenamine	Possible kidney blockage.
Methotrexate	Increased possibility of toxic side effects from methotrexate.
Oxyphenbutazone	Increased sulfa effect.
Para-aminosalicylic acid (PAS)	Decreased sulfa effect.
Penicillins*	Decreased penicillin effect.
Phenylbutazone	Increased sulfa effect.
Probenecid	Increased sulfa effect.
Sulfinpyrazone	Increased sulfa effect.
Sulfonureas*	May increase hypoglycemic action.
Tocainide	Possible decreased blood-cell production in bone marrow.
Trimethoprim	Increased sulfa effect.

POSSIBLE INTERACTION WITH OTHER SUBSTANCES

INTERACTS WITH	COMBINED EFFECT
Alcohol:	Increased alcohol effect.
Beverages: Less than 2 quarts of fluid daily.	Kidney damage.
Cocaine:	None expected.
Foods:	None expected.
Marijuana:	None expected.
Tobacco:	None expected.

*See Glossary

SULFONAMIDES & PHENAZOPYRIDINE

BRAND AND GENERIC NAMES

Azo Gantanol
Azo Gantrisin
Azo-Soxazole
Azo-Sulfamethoxazole
Azo-Sulfisoxazole
Suldiazo
Sulfafurazole &
  Phenazopyridine

SULFAMETHOXA-
  ZOLE & PHENAZO-
  PYRIDINE
SULFISOXAZOLE &
  PHENAZO-
  PYRIDINE
Uro-Gantanol

BASIC INFORMATION

Habit forming? No
Prescription needed? Yes
Available as generic? Yes
Drug class: Analgesic (urinary) sulfonamide

USES

- Treatment for infections responsive to this drug.
- Relieves pain of lower urinary-tract irritation, as in cystitis, urethritis or prostatitis.

DOSAGE & USAGE INFORMATION

How to take:
Tablet—Swallow with liquid. Instructions to take on empty stomach mean 1 hour before or 2 hours after eating.

When to take:
At the same times each day, after meals.

If you forget a dose:
Take as soon as you remember up to 2 hours late. If more than 2 hours, wait for next scheduled dose (don't double this dose).

Continued next column

OVERDOSE

SYMPTOMS:
Less urine, bloody urine, shortness of breath, weakness, coma.
WHAT TO DO:
- **Dial 0 (operator) or 911 (emergency) for an ambulance or medical help. Then give first aid immediately.**
- **See emergency information on inside covers.**

What drug does:
- Interferes with a nutrient (folic acid) necessary for growth and reproduction of bacteria. Will not attack viruses.
- Anesthetizes lower urinary tract. Relieves pain, burning, pressure and urgency to urinate.

Time lapse before drug works:
2 to 5 days to affect infection.

Don't take with:
See Interaction column and consult doctor.

POSSIBLE ADVERSE REACTIONS OR SIDE EFFECTS

SYMPTOMS	WHAT TO DO
Life-threatening: None expected.	
Common:	
Rash, itchy skin.	Discontinue. Call doctor right away.
Dizziness, diarrhea, headache, appetite loss, nausea, vomiting.	Continue. Call doctor when convenient.
Infrequent:	
Joint pain; swallowing difficulty; pale skin; blistering; peeling of skin; sore throat, fever, mouth sores; unexplained bleeding or bruising; weakness; jaundice; increased sun sensitivity.	Discontinue. Call doctor right away.
Abdominal pain, indigestion.	Continue. Call doctor when convenient.
Rare:	
Back pain; neck swelling; numbness, tingling, burning.	Discontinue. Call doctor right away. feeling in feet and hands.

SULFONAMIDES & PHENAZOPYRIDINE

WARNINGS & PRECAUTIONS

Don't take if:
- You are allergic to any sulfa drug or urinary analgesic.
- You have hepatitis.

Before you start, consult your doctor:
- If you are allergic to carbonic anhydrase inhibitors, oral antidiabetics or thiazide or loop diuretics.
- If you are allergic by nature.
- If you have liver or kidney disease, porphyria.
- If you have developed anemia from use of any drug.
- If you have G6PD deficiency.

Over age 60:
Adverse reactions and side effects may be more frequent and severe than in younger persons.

Pregnancy:
Risk to unborn child outweighs drug benefits. Don't use.

Breast-feeding:
Drug passes into milk. Avoid drug or discontinue nursing until you finish medicine. Consult doctor for advice on maintaining milk supply.

Infants & children:
Don't give to infants younger than 1 month.

Prolonged use:
- May enlarge thyroid gland.
- You may become more susceptible to infections caused by germs not responsive to this drug.
- Request frequent blood counts, liver- and kidney-function studies.
- Orange or yellow skin.
- Anemia. Occasional blood studies recommended.

Skin & sunlight:
May cause rash or intensify sunburn in areas exposed to sun or sunlamp.

Driving, piloting or hazardous work:
Avoid if you feel dizzy. Otherwise, no problems expected.

Discontinuing:
Don't discontinue without doctor's advice until you complete prescribed dose, even though symptoms diminish or disappear.

Others:
- Drink 2 quarts of liquid each day to prevent adverse reactions.
- If you require surgery, tell anesthetist you take sulfa.
- Will probably cause urine to be reddish orange. Requires no action.
- May stain fabrics.

POSSIBLE INTERACTION WITH OTHER DRUGS

GENERIC NAME OR DRUG CLASS	COMBINED EFFECT
Aminobenzoate potassium	Possible decreased sulfa effect.
Anticoagulants, oral*	Increased anti-coagulant effect.
Anticonvulsants, hydantoin*	Toxic effect on brain.
Aspirin	Increased sulfa effect.
Isoniazid	Possible anemia.
Methenamine	Possible kidney blockage.
Methotrexate	Increased methotrexate effect.
Oxyphenbutazone	Increased sulfa effect.
Para-aminosalicylic acid (PAS)	Decreased sulfa effect.
Penicillins*	Decreased penicillin effect.
Phenylbutazone	Increased sulfa effect.
Probenecid	Increased sulfa effect.
Sulfinpyrazone	Increased sulfa effect.
Sulfonureas*	May increase hypo-glycemic action.
Trimethoprim	Increased sulfa effect.

POSSIBLE INTERACTION WITH OTHER SUBSTANCES

INTERACTS WITH	COMBINED EFFECT
Alcohol:	Increased alcohol effect.
Beverages: Less than 2 quarts of fluid daily.	Kidney damage.
Cocaine:	None expected.
Foods:	None expected.
Marijuana:	None expected.
Tobacco:	None expected.

SULINDAC

BRAND NAMES

Clinoril

BASIC INFORMATION

Habit forming? No
Available as generic? No
Prescription needed? Yes
Drug class: Anti-inflammatory (non-steroid)

 USES

- Treatment for joint pain, stiffness, inflammation and swelling of arthritis and gout.
- Pain reliever.
- Treats juvenile rheumatoid arthritis.

 DOSAGE & USAGE INFORMATION

How to take:
Tablet—Swallow with liquid or food to lessen stomach irritation. If you can't swallow whole, crumble tablet and take with liquid or food.

When to take:
At the same times each day.

If you forget a dose:
Take as soon as you remember up to 2 hours late. If more than 2 hours, wait for next scheduled dose (don't double this dose).

What drug does:
Reduces tissue concentration of prostaglandins (hormones which produce inflammation and pain).

Time lapse before drug works:
Begins in 4 to 24 hours. May require 3 weeks regular use for maximum benefit.

Don't take with:
See Interaction column and consult doctor.

 OVERDOSE

SYMPTOMS:
Confusion, agitation, incoherence, convulsions, possible hemorrhage from stomach or intestine, coma.
WHAT TO DO:
- **Dial 0 (operator) or 911 (emergency) for an ambulance or medical help. Then give first aid immediately.**
- **See emergency information on inside covers.**

 POSSIBLE ADVERSE REACTIONS OR SIDE EFFECTS

SYMPTOMS	WHAT TO DO
Life-threatening:	
Hives, rash, intense itching, faintness soon after a dose (anaphylaxis in aspirin-sensitive persons).	Seek emergency treatment immediately.
Common:	
• Dizziness, nausea, pain.	Continue. Call doctor when convenient.
• Headache.	Continue. Tell doctor at next visit.
Infrequent:	
Depression, drowsiness, ringing in ears, constipation or diarrhea, vomiting, swollen feet or legs.	Continue. Call doctor when convenient.
Rare:	
• Convulsions; confusion; rash, hives or itchy skin; blurred vision; black, bloody or tarry stool; difficult breathing; tightness in chest; rapid heartbeat; unusual bleeding or bruising; blood in urine; jaundice; severe abdominal pain, psychosis.	Discontinue. Call doctor right away.
• Frequent, painful or difficult urination; fatigue; weakness; swollen breasts in males; impotence; menstrual irregularities.	Continue. Call doctor when convenient.

WARNINGS & PRECAUTIONS

Don't take if:
- You are allergic to aspirin or any non-steroid, anti-inflammatory drug.
- You have gastritis, peptic ulcer, enteritis, ileitis, ulcerative colitis, asthma, heart failure, high blood pressure or bleeding problems.
- You have had recent rectal bleeding and suppository form has been prescribed.
- Patient is younger than 15.

Before you start, consult your doctor:
- If you have epilepsy.
- If you have Parkinson's disease.
- If you have been mentally ill.
- If you have had kidney disease or impaired kidney function.

Over age 60:
Adverse reactions and side effects may be more frequent and severe than in younger persons.

Pregnancy:
Studies inconclusive on harm to unborn child. Decide with your doctor whether drug benefits justify risk to unborn child.

Breast-feeding:
May harm child. Avoid.

Infants & children:
Not recommended for those younger than 15. Use only under medical supervision.

Prolonged use:
- Eye damage.
- Reduced hearing.
- Sore throat, fever.
- Weight gain.

Skin & sunlight:
Increased sensitivity to sunlight.

Driving, piloting or hazardous work:
Don't drive or pilot aircraft until you learn how medicine affects you. Don't work around dangerous machinery. Don't climb ladders or work in high places. Danger increases if you drink alcohol or take medicine affecting alertness and reflexes, such as antihistamines, tranquilizers, sedatives, pain medicine, narcotics and mind-altering drugs.

Discontinuing:
Don't discontinue without consulting doctor. Dose may require gradual reduction if you have taken drug for a long time. Doses of other drugs may also require adjustment.

Others:
No problems expected.

POSSIBLE INTERACTION WITH OTHER DRUGS

GENERIC NAME OR DRUG CLASS	COMBINED EFFECT
ACE inhibitors: captopril, enalapril, lisinopril*	May decrease ACE inhibitor effect.
Anticoagulants, oral*	Increased risk of bleeding.
Aspirin	Increased risk of stomach ulcer.
Beta-adrenergic blockers*	Decreased antihypertensive effect.
Carteolol	Decreased antihypertensive effect of carteolol.
Cortisone drugs*	Increased risk of stomach ulcer.
Diuretics*	May decrease diuretic effect.
Lithium	Possible increased lithium effect and toxicity.
Methotrexate	May increase toxicity.
Minoxidil	Decreased minoxidil effect.
Oxyphenbutazone	Possible stomach ulcer.
Phenylbutazone	Possible stomach ulcer.
Probenecid	Increased sulindac effect.
Sotalol	Decreased antihypertensive effect of sotalol.

Continued page 1107

POSSIBLE INTERACTION WITH OTHER SUBSTANCES

INTERACTS WITH	COMBINED EFFECT
Alcohol:	Possible stomach ulcer or bleeding.
Beverages:	None expected.
Cocaine:	None expected.
Foods:	None expected.
Marijuana:	Increased pain relief from sulindac.
Tobacco:	None expected.

*See Glossary

TALBUTAL (Butalbital)

BRAND NAMES

Axotal	Lotusate
Buff-A-Comp	Marnal
Butal Compound	Plexonal
Fiorinal	Protensin
Isollyl	Sandoptal
Lanorinal	Tenstan

BASIC INFORMATION

Habit forming? Yes
Prescription needed? Yes
Available as generic? Yes
Drug class: Sedative, hypnotic (barbiturate)

USES

Relieves insomnia (higher bedtime dose).

DOSAGE & USAGE INFORMATION

How to take:
Tablet—Swallow with liquid or food to lessen stomach irritation. If you can't swallow whole, crumble tablet and take with liquid or food.

When to take:
At the same times each day.

If you forget a dose:
Take as soon as you remember up to 2 hours late. If more than 2 hours, wait for next scheduled dose (don't double this dose).

What drug does:
May partially block nerve impulses at nerve-cell connections.

Time lapse before drug works:
60 minutes.

Don't take with:
- Non-prescription drugs without consulting doctor.
- See Interaction column and consult doctor.

OVERDOSE

SYMPTOMS:
Deep sleep, weak pulse, coma.
WHAT TO DO:
- **Dial 0 (operator) or 911 (emergency) for an ambulance or medical help. Then give first aid immediately.**
- **See emergency information on inside covers.**

POSSIBLE ADVERSE REACTIONS OR SIDE EFFECTS

SYMPTOMS	WHAT TO DO
Life-threatening: Hives, rash, intense itching, faintness soon after a dose (anaphylaxis).	Seek emergency treatment immediately.
Common: Dizziness, drowsiness, "hangover" effect.	Continue. Call doctor when convenient.
Infrequent:	
• Rash or hives; fever; swollen face, lip, eyelids; sore throat.	Discontinue. Call doctor right away.
• Depression, confusion, slurred speech, diarrhea, nausea, vomiting, joint or muscle pain.	Continue. Call doctor when convenient.
Rare:	
• Agitation, slow heartbeat, difficult breathing, jaundice.	Discontinue. Call doctor right away.
• Unexplained bleeding or bruising.	Continue. Call doctor when convenient.

WARNINGS & PRECAUTIONS

Don't take if:
- You are allergic to any barbiturate.
- You have porphyria.

Before you start, consult your doctor:
- If you have epilepsy, kidney or liver damage, asthma, anemia, or chronic pain.
- If you will have surgery within 2 months, including dental surgery, requiring general or spinal anesthesia.

Over age 60:
Adverse reactions and side effects may be more frequent and severe than in younger persons. Use small doses.

Pregnancy:
Risk to unborn child outweighs drug benefits. Don't use.

Breast-feeding:
Drug passes into milk. Avoid drug or discontinue nursing until you finish medicine. Consult doctor for advice on maintaining milk supply.

Infants & children:
Use only under doctor's supervision.

TALBUTAL (Butalbital)

Prolonged use:
- May cause addiction, anemia, chronic intoxication.
- May lower body temperature, making exposure to cold temperatures hazardous.

Skin & sunlight:
May cause rash or intensify sunburn in areas exposed to sun or sunlamp.

Driving, piloting or hazardous work:
Don't drive or pilot aircraft until you learn how medicine affects you. Don't work around dangerous machinery. Don't climb ladders or work in high places. Danger increases if you drink alcohol or take medicine affecting alertness and reflexes.

Discontinuing:
May be unnecessary to finish medicine. Follow doctor's instructions. If you develop withdrawal symptoms of hallucinations, agitation or sleeplessness after discontinuing, call doctor right away.

Others:
No problems expected.

 POSSIBLE INTERACTION WITH OTHER DRUGS

GENERIC NAME OR DRUG CLASS	COMBINED EFFECT
Anticoagulants, oral*	Decreased anticoagulant effect.
Anticonvulsants*	Changed seizure patterns.
Antidepressants, tricyclics (TCA)*	Decreased antidepressant effect. Possible dangerous oversedation.
Antidiabetics, oral*	Increased talbutal (butalbital) effect.
Antihistamines*	Dangerous sedation. Avoid.
Aspirin	Decreased aspirin effect.
Beta-adrenergic blockers*	Decreased effect of beta-adrenergic blocker.
Carteolol	Increased barbiturate effect. Dangerous sedation.
Contraceptives, oral*	Decreased contraceptive effect.
Cortisone drugs*	Decreased cortisone effect.
Digitoxin	Decreased digitoxin effect.
Disulfiram	Possible increased talbutal effect.
Doxycycline	Decreased doxycycline effect.
Dronabinol	Increased effects of both drugs. Avoid.
Estrogens*	Decreased estrogen effect.
Griseofulvin	Possible decreased griseofulvin effect.
Indapamide	Increased indapamide effect.
MAO inhibitors*	Increased talbutal (butalbital) effect.
Metronidazole	Possible decreased metronidazole effect.
Mind-altering drugs*	Dangerous sedation. Avoid.
Molindone	Increased sedative effect.
Nabilone	Greater depression of central nervous system.
Narcotics*	Dangerous sedation. Avoid.
Non-steroidal anti-inflammatory drugs (NSAIDs)*	Decreased anti-inflammatory effect.
Pain relievers*	Dangerous sedation. Avoid.
Rifampin	Possible decreased talbutal effect.

Continued page 1107

 POSSIBLE INTERACTION WITH OTHER SUBSTANCES

INTERACTS WITH	COMBINED EFFECT
Alcohol:	Possible fatal oversedation. Avoid.
Beverages:	None expected.
Cocaine:	Decreased talbutal (butalbital) effect.
Foods:	None expected.
Marijuana:	Excessive sedation. Avoid.
Tobacco:	None expected.

TEMAZEPAM

BRAND NAMES

Razepam   Temaz
Restoril

BASIC INFORMATION

Habit forming? Yes
Prescription needed? Yes
Available as generic? Yes
Drug class: Tranquilizer (benzodiazepine)

 ## USES

Treatment for insomnia.

 ## DOSAGE & USAGE INFORMATION

How to take:
Capsule—Swallow with liquid. If you can't swallow whole, open capsule and take with liquid or food.

When to take:
At the same time each day, according to instructions on prescription label.

If you forget a dose:
Take as soon as you remember up to 2 hours late. If more than 2 hours, wait for next scheduled dose (don't double this dose).

What drug does:
Affects limbic system of brain—part that controls emotions. Induces near-normal sleep pattern.

Time lapse before drug works:
30 minutes.

Don't take with:
See Interaction column and consult doctor.

 ## OVERDOSE

SYMPTOMS:
Drowsiness, weakness, tremor, stupor, coma.
WHAT TO DO:
- **Dial 0 (operator) or 911 (emergency) for an ambulance or medical help. Then give first aid immediately.**
- **If patient is unconscious and not breathing, give mouth-to-mouth breathing. If there is no heartbeat, use cardiac massage and mouth-to-mouth breathing (CPR). Don't try to make patient vomit. If you can't get help quickly, take patient to nearest emergency facility.**
- **See emergency information on inside covers.**

 ## POSSIBLE ADVERSE REACTIONS OR SIDE EFFECTS

SYMPTOMS	WHAT TO DO
Life-threatening: None expected.	
Common: Clumsiness, dizziness, drowsiness.	Continue. Call doctor when convenient.
Infrequent:	
• Hallucinations, confusion, depression, irritability, rash, itchy skin, change in vision.	Discontinue. Call doctor right away.
• Constipation or diarrhea, nausea, vomiting, difficult urination.	Continue. Call doctor when convenient.
Rare:	
• Slow heartbeat, difficult breathing.	Discontinue. Seek emergency treatment.
• Mouth or throat ulcers, jaundice.	Discontinue. Call doctor right away.

TEMAZEPAM

 ## WARNINGS & PRECAUTIONS

Don't take if:
- You are allergic to any benzodiazepine.
- You have myasthenia gravis.
- You are active or recovering alcoholic.
- Patient is younger than 6 months.

Before you start, consult your doctor:
- If you have liver, kidney or lung disease.
- If you have diabetes, epilepsy or porphyria.

Over age 60:
Adverse reactions and side effects may be more frequent and severe than in younger persons. May develop agitation, rage or "hangover" effect.

Pregnancy:
Risk to unborn child outweighs drug benefits. Don't use.

Breast-feeding:
Drug passes into milk. Avoid drug or discontinue nursing until you finish medicine. Consult doctor for advice on maintaining milk supply.

Infants & children:
Use only under medical supervision for children older than 6 months.

Prolonged use:
May impair liver function.

Skin & sunlight:
No problems expected.

Driving, piloting or hazardous work:
Don't drive or pilot aircraft until you learn how medicine affects you. Don't work around dangerous machinery. Don't climb ladders or work in high places. Danger increases if you drink alcohol or take medicine affecting alertness and reflexes.

Discontinuing:
Don't discontinue without doctor's advice until you complete prescribed dose, even though symptoms diminish or disappear.

Others:
- Hot weather, heavy exercise and profuse sweat may reduce excretion and cause overdose.
- Blood sugar may rise in diabetics, requiring insulin adjustment.

 ## POSSIBLE INTERACTION WITH OTHER DRUGS

GENERIC NAME OR DRUG CLASS	COMBINED EFFECT
Anticonvulsants*	Change in seizure frequency or severity.
Antidepressants*	Increased sedative effect of both drugs.
Antihistamines	Increased sedative effect of both drugs.
Antihypertensives*	Excessively low blood pressure.
Cimetidine	Excess sedation.
Disulfiram	Increased temazepam effect.
Dronabinol	Increased effects of both drugs. Avoid.
MAO inhibitors*	Convulsions, deep sedation, rage.
Molindone	Increased sedative effect.
Nabilone	Greater depression of central nervous system.
Narcotics*	Increased sedative effect of both drugs.
Sedatives*	Increased sedative effect of both drugs.
Tranquilizers*	Increased sedative effect of both drugs.

 ## POSSIBLE INTERACTION WITH OTHER SUBSTANCES

INTERACTS WITH	COMBINED EFFECT
Alcohol:	Heavy sedation. Avoid.
Beverages:	None expected.
Cocaine:	Decreased temazepam effect.
Foods:	None expected.
Marijuana:	Heavy sedation. Avoid.
Tobacco:	Decreased temazepam effect.

*See Glossary

TERAZOSIN

BRAND NAMES

Hytrin

BASIC INFORMATION

Habit forming? No
Prescription needed? Yes
Available as generic? No
Drug class: Antihypertensive (alpha-adrenergic blocking agent)

 ## USES

Treats high blood pressure.

 ## DOSAGE & USAGE INFORMATION

How to take:
Tablet—Swallow with liquid or food to lessen stomach irritation. If you can't swallow whole, crumble tablet and take with liquid or food.

When to take:
Once a day (usually) at bedtime.

If you forget a dose:
Take as soon as you remember. Don't ever double the dose.

What drug does:
Relaxes smooth muscle in arteries, reducing blood pressure. Terazosin doesn't cure hypertension, but controls it. Persons with hypertension may need lifelong treatment.

Time lapse before drug works:
15 minutes.

Don't take with:
Any other drug (especially OTC medicines containing alcohol) without consulting your doctor.

 ## OVERDOSE

SYMPTOMS:
Difficult breathing, vomiting, fainting, slow heartbeat, coma, diminished reflexes.
WHAT TO DO:
- **Dial 0 (operator) or 911 (emergency) for an ambulance or medical help. Then give first aid immediately.**
- **If patient is unconscious and not breathing, give mouth-to-mouth breathing. If there is no heartbeat, use cardiac massage and mouth-to-mouth breathing (CPR). Don't try to make patient vomit. If you can't get help quickly, take patient to nearest emergency facility.**
- **See emergency information on inside covers.**

 ## POSSIBLE ADVERSE REACTIONS OR SIDE EFFECTS

SYMPTOMS	WHAT TO DO
Life-threatening: None expected.	
Common: Headache, dizziness, tiredness or weakness.	Continue. Call doctor right away.
Infrequent: • Chest pain; lightheadedness on arising from bed or chair (more likely to occur with first dose); increased or rapid heartbeat.	Discontinue. Call doctor right away.
• Fluid retention and weight gain.	Continue. Call doctor when convenient.
Rare: Back pain, joint pain, blurred vision, stuffy nose, drowsiness.	Continue. Call doctor when convenient.

WARNINGS & PRECAUTIONS

Don't take if:
- You are allergic to any alpha-adrenergic blocker.
- You are under age 12.

Before you start, consult your doctor:
- If you will have surgery within 2 months, including dental surgery, requiring general or spinal anesthesia.
- If you have heart disease or chronic kidney disease.
- If you have a peripheral circulation disorder (intermittent claudication, Buerger's disease).
- If you have history of depression.

Over age 60:
More sensitivity to drug causing weakness, fainting episodes, low temperature.

Pregnancy:
Studies inconclusive on harm to unborn child. Decide with your doctor whether drug benefits justify risk to unborn child.

Breast-feeding:
No proven problems.

Infants & children:
Not recommended for children. Adequate studies not complete.

Prolonged use:
No special problems expected.

Skin & sunlight:
No problems expected.

Driving, piloting or hazardous work:
Don't drive or pilot aircraft until you learn how medicine affects you. Don't work around dangerous machinery. Don't climb ladders or work in high places. Danger increases if you drink alcohol or take medicine affecting alertness and reflexes, such as antihistamines, tranquilizers, sedatives, pain medicine, narcotics and mind-altering drugs.

Discontinuing:
- Don't discontinue without consulting doctor. Dose may require gradual reduction if you have taken drug for a long time. Doses of other drugs may also require adjustment.
- Stopping abruptly may cause rebound high blood pressure, anxiety, chest pain, insomnia, headache, nausea, irregular heartbeat, flushed face, sweating.

Others:
- Avoid becoming overheated.
- Check blood pressure frequently.

POSSIBLE INTERACTION WITH OTHER DRUGS

GENERIC NAME OR DRUG CLASS	COMBINED EFFECT
Diclofenac	Decreases effectiveness of terazosin. Causes sodium and fluid retention.
Estrogens*	Decreases effectiveness of terazosin.
Lisinopril	Increased antihypertensive effect. Dosage of each may require adjustment.
Nicardipine	Blood-pressure drop. Dosages may require adjustment.
Non-steroidal anti-inflammatory drugs (NSAIDs)*	Decreases effectiveness of terazosin. Causes sodium and fluid retention.
Other medicines to treat high blood pressure (antihypertensives)*	Decreases effectiveness of terazosin.
Sympathomimetics*	Decreases effectiveness of terazosin.

POSSIBLE INTERACTION WITH OTHER SUBSTANCES

INTERACTS WITH	COMBINED EFFECT
Alcohol:	Increased sensitivity to sedative effect of alcohol and very low blood pressure. Avoid.
Beverages: Caffeine drinks.	Decreased terazosin effect.
Cocaine:	Blood pressure rise. Avoid.
Foods:	No problems expected.
Marijuana:	Weakness on standing.
Tobacco:	No problems expected.

TERBUTALINE

BRAND NAMES

Brethaire   Bricanyl
Brethine

BASIC INFORMATION

Habit forming? No
Prescription needed? Yes
Available as generic? No
Drug class: Sympathomimetic

 ## USES

Treatment of bronchial asthma, bronchitis and emphysema.

 ## DOSAGE & USAGE INFORMATION

How to take:
- Tablet—Swallow with liquid or food to lessen stomach irritation.
- Aerosol—Use according to package instructions.

When to take:
At the same times each day.

If you forget a dose:
Take as soon as you remember up to 2 hours late. If more than 2 hours, wait for next scheduled dose (don't double this dose).

What drug does:
Dilates constricted bronchial tubes.

Time lapse before drug works:
30 minutes.

Don't take with:
See Interaction column and consult doctor.

 ## OVERDOSE

SYMPTOMS:
Rapid heartbeat, chest pain, tremors.
WHAT TO DO:
- **Dial 0 (operator) or 911 (emergency) for an ambulance or medical help. Then give first aid immediately.**
- **If patient is unconscious and not breathing, give mouth-to-mouth breathing. If there is no heartbeat, use cardiac massage and mouth-to-mouth breathing (CPR). Don't try to make patient vomit. If you can't get help quickly, take patient to nearest emergency facility.**
- **See emergency information on inside covers.**

 ## POSSIBLE ADVERSE REACTIONS OR SIDE EFFECTS

SYMPTOMS	WHAT TO DO
Life-threatening: None expected.	
Common: Headache, trembling, restlessness, nervousness.	Continue. Call doctor when convenient.
Infrequent: • Drowsiness, nausea, vomiting, fast or pounding heartbeat, cramps, weakness.	Discontinue. Call doctor right away.
• Unusual sweating.	Continue. Call doctor when convenient.
Rare: None expected.	

WARNINGS & PRECAUTIONS

Don't take if:
You are allergic to any sympathomimetic.

Before you start, consult your doctor:
- If you have diabetes.
- If you have heart disease or high blood pressure.
- If you have overactive thyroid.
- If you have had seizures.
- If you take non-prescription amphetamines or other asthma medicines.

Over age 60:
Adverse reactions and side effects may be more frequent and severe than in younger persons.

Pregnancy:
No proven harm to unborn child. Avoid if possible. May prolong labor and delivery.

Breast-feeding:
No proven problems. Avoid if possible.

Infants & children:
Use only under medical supervision.

Prolonged use:
No problems expected.

Skin & sunlight:
No problems expected.

Driving, piloting or hazardous work:
Avoid if you feel drowsy. Otherwise, no problems expected.

Discontinuing:
May be unnecessary to finish medicine. Follow doctor's instructions.

Others:
If troubled breathing does not improve or worsens after using medicine, don't increase dose. Consult doctor.

POSSIBLE INTERACTION WITH OTHER DRUGS

GENERIC NAME OR DRUG CLASS	COMBINED EFFECT
Albuterol	Increased effect of both drugs, especially harmful side effects.
Antidepressants, tricyclics (TCA)*	Increased terbutaline effect.
Beta-adrenergic blockers*	Decreased effects of both drugs.
Carteolol	Decreased beta-agonist effect.
Ephedrine	Increased terbutaline effect. Excess heart stimulation.
Epinephrine	Increased terbutaline effect. Excess heart stimulation.
MAO inhibitors*	Increased terbutaline effect. Dangerous. Avoid.
Nitrates*	Possible decreased effects of both drugs.
Sotalol	Decreased beta-agonist effect.
Sympathomimetics*	Increased terbutaline effect.
Terazosin	Decreases effectiveness of terazosin.
Theophylline	Possible increased effect and toxicity of both drugs.

POSSIBLE INTERACTION WITH OTHER SUBSTANCES

INTERACTS WITH	COMBINED EFFECT
Alcohol:	None expected.
Beverages:	None expected.
Cocaine:	High risk of heartbeat irregularities and high blood pressure.
Foods:	None expected.
Marijuana:	Possible increased therapeutic effect of terbutaline. May cause lung disorders to worsen.
Tobacco:	No interactions expected, but smoking may slow body's recovery. Avoid.

TERFENADINE

BRAND NAMES

Seldane

BASIC INFORMATION

Habit forming? No
Prescription needed? Yes
Available as generic? No
Drug class: Antihistamine, hi-receptor
    antagonist

 ## USES

Reduces allergic symptoms such as hay fever, hives, rash or itching. Less likely to cause drowsiness than most other antihistamines.

 ## DOSAGE & USAGE INFORMATION

How to take:
Tablet—Swallow with water or food to lessen stomach irritation.

When to take:
Follow prescription instructions.

If you forget a dose:
Take as soon as you remember up to 2 hours late. If more than 2 hours, wait for next scheduled dose (don't double this dose).

What drug does:
Blocks effects of histamine, a chemical produced by the body as a result of contact with an allergen.

Time lapse before drug works:
1 to 2 hours; maximum effect at 3 to 4 hours.

Don't take with:
See Interaction column and consult doctor.

 ## OVERDOSE

SYMPTOMS:
Headache, nausea, confusion, heartbeat
rhythm disturbance.
WHAT TO DO:
* **Dial 0 (operator) or 911 (emergency) for**
  an ambulance or medical help. Then give
  first aid immediately.
* **See emergency information on inside**
  covers.

 ## POSSIBLE ADVERSE REACTIONS OR SIDE EFFECTS

SYMPTOMS	WHAT TO DO
Life-threatening: None expected.	
Common: None expected.	
Infrequent:	
• Nausea, vomiting sore throat, itching.	Discontinue. Call doctor right away.
• Drowsiness, fatigue, headache, dizziness, weakness.	Continue. Call doctor when convenient.
Rare:	
• Swollen lips. difficult breathing	Discontinue. Seek emergency treatment.
• Irregular heartbeat, nightmares, frequent urination.	Discontinue. Call doctor right away.
• Thinning hair.	Continue. Call doctor when convenient.

WARNINGS & PRECAUTIONS

Don't take if:
You are allergic to terfenadine.

Before you start, consult your doctor:
- If you are allergic to other antihistamines.
- If you have an enlarged prostrate or glaucoma.
- If you are under age 12.
- If you are allergic to any substance or any medicine.
- If you are pregnant or expect to become pregnant.
- If you have asthma.
- If you will have surgery within 2 months, including dental surgery, requiring general or spinal anesthesia.
- If you plan to have skin tests for allergies.

Over age 60:
Don't exceed recommended dose. Take only on advise of your doctor.

Pregnancy:
No proven harm to unborn child. Avoid if possible.

Breast-feeding:
Drug may pass into milk although this has not been proven. Consult doctor for advice on using while breast feeding.

Infants & children:
Safety and effectiveness in children under age 12 have not been established.

Prolonged use:
Take only on advice of your doctor.

Skin & sunlight:
No problems expected.

Driving, piloting or hazardous work:
Don't drive or pilot aircraft until you learn how medicine affects you. Sedation and dizziness are less likely to occur with terfenadine than with other antihistamines.

Discontinuing:
No problems expected.

Others:
No problems expected.

POSSIBLE INTERACTION WITH OTHER DRUGS

GENERIC NAME OR DRUG CLASS	COMBINED EFFECT
Carteolol	Decreased antihistamine effect.
Nabilone	Greater depression of central nervous system.
Sotalol	Increased antihistamine effect.

POSSIBLE INTERACTION WITH OTHER SUBSTANCES

INTERACTS WITH	COMBINED EFFECT
Alcohol:	Possible oversedation.
Beverages:	None expected.
Cocaine:	Decreased terfenadine effect.
Foods:	None expected.
Marijuana:	None expected.
Tobacco:	None expected.

TERPIN HYDRATE

BRAND NAMES

Cotussis
Prunicodeine
SK-Terpin Hydrate
  w/Codeine

Terpin Hydrate and
  Codeine Syrup
Terpin Hydrate
  Elixir

BASIC INFORMATION

Habit forming? Yes
Prescription needed? No
Available as generic? Yes
Drug class: Expectorant

 ## USES

Decreases cough due to simple bronchial
irritation.

 ## DOSAGE & USAGE INFORMATION

How to take:
Follow each dose with 8 oz. water or food to
decrease gastric distress. Works better in
combination with a cool-air vaporizer.

When to take:
3 to 4 times each day, spaced at least 4 hours
apart.

If you forget a dose:
Take as soon as you remember. Wait 4 hours for
next dose.

What drug does:
Loosens mucus in bronchial tubes to make
mucus easier to cough up.

Time lapse before drug works:
10 to 15 minutes.

Don't take with:
See Interaction column and consult doctor.

 ## OVERDOSE

SYMPTOMS:
Nausea, drowsiness.
WHAT TO DO:
Overdose unlikely to threaten life. If person
takes much larger amount than prescribed,
call doctor, poison-control center or hospital
emergency room for instructions.

 ## POSSIBLE ADVERSE REACTIONS OR SIDE EFFECTS

SYMPTOMS	WHAT TO DO
Life-threatening: None expected.	
Common: None expected.	
Infrequent: Nausea, vomiting, stomach pain.	Continue. Call doctor when convenient.
Rare: Symptoms of alcohol intoxication, especially in children.	Discontinue. Call doctor right away.

WARNINGS & PRECAUTIONS

Don't take if:
- You are allergic to terpin hydrate.
- You are a recovering or active alcoholic.

Before you start, consult your doctor:
If you plan to become pregnant within medication period.

Over age 60:
No problems expected.

Pregnancy:
Risk to unborn child outweighs drug benefits. Don't use.

Breast-feeding:
Drug filters into milk. May harm child. Avoid.

Infants & children:
Use only under medical supervision.

Prolonged use:
Habit forming.

Skin & sunlight:
No problems expected.

Driving, piloting or hazardous work:
Don't drive or pilot aircraft until you learn how medicine affects you. Don't work around dangerous machinery. Don't climb ladders or work in high places. Danger increases if you drink alcohol or take medicine affecting alertness and reflexes, such as antihistamines, tranquilizers, sedatives, pain medicine, narcotics and mind-altering drugs.

Discontinuing:
May be unnecessary to finish medicine. Follow doctor's instructions.

Others:
- Exceeding recommended doses may cause intoxication; drug is 42.5% alcohol.
- Frequently combined with codeine, which increases hazards.

POSSIBLE INTERACTION WITH OTHER DRUGS

GENERIC NAME OR DRUG CLASS	COMBINED EFFECT
Antidepressants*	Increased sedation.
Antihistamines*	Increased sedation.
Disulfiram	Possible disulfiram reaction.
Muscle relaxants*	Increased sedation.
Narcotics*	Increased sedation.
Sedatives*	Increased sedation.
Sleep inducers*	Increased sedation.
Tranquilizers*	Increased sedation.

POSSIBLE INTERACTION WITH OTHER SUBSTANCES

INTERACTS WITH	COMBINED EFFECT
Alcohol:	Contains alcohol. Increased sedative effect of both drugs. Avoid.
Beverages:	None expected.
Cocaine:	Unpredictable effect on nervous system. Avoid.
Foods:	None expected.
Marijuana:	Unpredictable effect on nervous system. Avoid.
Tobacco:	None expected.

*See Glossary

TESTOSTERONE & ESTRADIOL

BRAND NAMES

See complete list of brand names in the *Brand Name Directory,* page 1071.

BASIC INFORMATION

Habit forming? No
Prescription needed? Yes
Available as generic? Yes
Drug class: Androgens-estrogens

 ## USES

- Prevents breast fullness in new mothers after childbirth.
- Relieves menopause symptoms such as unnecessary sweating, hot flashes, chills, faintness and dizziness.

 ## DOSAGE & USAGE INFORMATION

How to take:
Given by injection, deeply intramuscular.

When to take:
When directed.

If you forget a dose:
Check with your doctor.

What drug does:
- Restores normal estrogen level in tissues.
- Stimulates cells that produce male sex characteristics.
- Replaces hormone deficiencies.
- Stimulates red-blood-cell production.
- Suppresses production of estrogen.

Time lapse before drug works:
10 to 20 days.

Don't take with:
See Interaction column and consult doctor.

 ## OVERDOSE

SYMPTOMS:
Nausea, vomiting, fluid retention, breast enlargement and discomfort, abnormal vaginal bleeding.
WHAT TO DO:
Overdose unlikely to threaten life. If person takes much larger amount than prescribed, call doctor, poison-control center or hospital emergency room for instructions.

 ## POSSIBLE ADVERSE REACTIONS OR SIDE EFFECTS

SYMPTOMS	WHAT TO DO
Life-threatening: Hives, black stool, black or bloody vomit, intense itching, weakness, loss of consciousness.	Discontinue. Seek emergency treatment.
Common: • Red or flushed face; rash; swollen, tender breasts.	Discontinue. Call doctor right away.
• Depression, irritability, dizziness, confusion, acne or oily skin (females), enlarged clitoris, deepened voice, appetite loss, increased sex drive.	Continue. Call doctor when convenient.
Infrequent: • Nausea, vomiting, diarrhea, unusual vaginal bleeding or discharge.	Discontinue. Call doctor right away.
• Swollen feet and ankles, increased libido in some women.	Continue. Call doctor when convenient.
Rare: • Jaundice, abdominal pain.	Discontinue. Call doctor right away.
• Brown blotches on skin; hair loss; sore throat, fever, mouth sores.	Continue. Call doctor when convenient.

 ## WARNINGS & PRECAUTIONS

Don't take if:
- You are allergic to any male hormone or any estrogen-containing drugs.
- You have impaired liver function.
- You have had blood clots, stroke or heart attack.
- You have unexplained vaginal bleeding.

Before you start, consult your doctor:
- If you might be pregnant or plan to become pregnant within 3 months.
- If you have heart disease, arteriosclerosis, diabetes, liver disease, high blood pressure, asthma, congestive heart failure, kidney disease or gallstones.
- If you have high level of blood calcium.
- If you have had migraine headaches, epilepsy or porphyria.
- If you have had cancer of breast or reproductive organs, fibrocystic breast disease, fibroid tumors of the uterus or endometriosis.

Over age 60:
- May stimulate sexual activity.
- Can make high blood pressure or heart disease worse.
- Controversial. You and your doctor must decide if drug risks outweigh benefits.

Pregnancy:
Risk to unborn child outweighs drug benefits. Don't use.

Breast-feeding:
Drug passes into milk. Avoid drug or discontinue nursing until you finish medicine. Consult doctor for advice on maintaining milk supply.

Infants & children:
Not recommended.

Prolonged use:
- Increased growth of fibroid tumors of uterus.
- Possible kidney stones.
- Unnatural hair growth and deep voice in women.

Skin & sunlight:
May cause rash or intensify sunburn in areas exposed to sun or sunlamp.

Driving, piloting or hazardous work:
No problems expected.

Discontinuing:
You may need to discontinue estrogens periodically. Consult your doctor.

Others:
- In rare instances, may cause blood clot in lung, brain or leg. Symptoms are *sudden* severe headache, coordination loss, vision change, chest pain, breathing difficulty, slurred speech, pain in legs or groin. Seek emergency treatment immediately.
- Will not increase strength in athletes.
- Carefully read the paper delivered with your prescription called "Information for the Patient."

POSSIBLE INTERACTION WITH OTHER DRUGS

GENERIC NAME OR DRUG CLASS	COMBINED EFFECT
Anticoagulants, oral*	Increased effect of of anticoagulant.
Anticonvulsants, hydantoin*	Increased seizures.
Antidiabetics, oral*	Unpredictable increase or decrease in blood sugar.
Antifibrinolytic agents*	Increased possibility of blood clotting.
Carbamazepine	Increased seizures.

Chlorzoxazone	Decreased androgen effect.
Cholestyramine	Decreased cholestyramine effect.
Clofibrate	Decreased clofibrate effect.
Colestipol	Decreased colestipol effect.
Insulin	Unpredictable increase or decrease in blood sugar.
Nicotinic acid	Decreased nicotinic acid.
Oxyphenbutazone	Decreased androgen and estrogen effect.
Phenobarbital	Decreased androgen and estrogen effect.
Phenylbutazone	Decreased androgen and testosterone effect.
Primidone	Decreased estrogen and testosterone effect.
Rifampin	Decreased estrogen and testosterone effect.
Terazosin	Decreases effectiveness of terazosin.
Thyroid hormones*	Decreased thyroid effect.
Ursodiol	Decreased effect of ursodiol.

POSSIBLE INTERACTION WITH OTHER SUBSTANCES

INTERACTS WITH	COMBINED EFFECT
Alcohol:	None expected.
Beverages:	None expected.
Cocaine:	No proven problems.
Foods: Salt.	Excessive fluid retention (edema). Decrease salt intake while taking male hormones.
Marijuana:	Decreased blood levels of androgens. Possible menstrual irregularities and bleeding between periods.
Tobacco:	Increased risk of blood clots leading to stroke or heart attack.

*See Glossary

TETRACYCLINES

BRAND NAMES

See complete list of brand and generic names in the *Brand Name Directory*, page 1071.

BASIC INFORMATION

Habit forming? No
Prescription needed? Yes
Available as generic? Yes
Drug class: Antibiotic (tetracycline)

USES

- Treatment for infections susceptible to any tetracycline. Will not cure virus infections such as colds or flu.
- Treatment for acne.

DOSAGE & USAGE INFORMATION

How to take:
- Tablet or capsule—Take on empty stomach 1 hour before or 2 hours after eating. If you can't swallow whole, crumble tablet or open capsule and take with liquid or food.
- Liquid—Shake well. Take with measuring spoon.

When to take:
At the same times each day, evenly spaced.

If you forget a dose:
Take as soon as you remember up to 2 hours late. If more than 2 hours, wait for next scheduled dose (don't double this dose).

What drug does:
Prevents germ growth and reproduction.

Time lapse before drug works:
- Infections—May require 5 days to affect infection.
- Acne—May require 4 weeks to affect acne.

Don't take with:
- Non-prescription drugs without consulting doctor.
- See Interaction column and consult doctor.

OVERDOSE

SYMPTOMS:
Severe nausea, vomiting, diarrhea.
WHAT TO DO:
Overdose unlikely to threaten life. If person takes much larger amount than prescribed, call doctor, poison-control center or hospital emergency room for instructions.

POSSIBLE ADVERSE REACTIONS OR SIDE EFFECTS

SYMPTOMS	WHAT TO DO
Life-threatening:	
Hives, rash, intense itching faintness soon after a dose (anaphylaxis).	Seek emergency treatment immediately.
Common:	
• Sore mouth or tongue, nausea, vomiting, diarrhea, abdominal burning.	Discontinue. Seek emergency treatment.
• Itching around rectum and genitals.	Discontinue. Call doctor right away.
• Vaginal discharge due to yeast.	Continue. Call doctor when convenient.
• Dark tongue.	Continue. Tell doctor at next visit.
Infrequent:	
• Headache, rash.	Discontinue. Call doctor right away.
• Excessive thirst, increased urination, dizziness (minocycline).	Continue. Call doctor when convenient.
Rare:	
Blurred vision, jaundice.	Discontinue. Call doctor right away.

WARNINGS & PRECAUTIONS

Don't take if:
You are allergic to any tetracycline antibiotic.

Before you start, consult your doctor:
• If you have kidney or liver disease.
• If you have lupus.
• If you have myasthenia gravis.

Over age 60:
Dosage usually less than in younger adults. More likely to cause itching around rectum. Ask your doctor how to prevent it.

Pregnancy:
Risk to unborn child outweighs drug benefits. Don't use.

Breast-feeding:
Drug passes into milk. Avoid drug or discontinue nursing until you finish medicine. Consult doctor for advice on maintaining milk supply.

Infants & children:
May cause permanent teeth malformation or discoloration in children less than 8 years old. Don't use.

Prolonged use:
• You may become more susceptible to infections caused by germs not responsive to tetracycline.
• May cause rare problems in liver, kidney or bone marrow. Periodic laboratory blood studies, liver- and kidney-function tests recommended if you use drug a long time.

Skin & sunlight:
May cause rash or intensify sunburn in areas exposed to sun or sunlamp.

Driving, piloting or hazardous work:
No problems expected.

Discontinuing:
Don't discontinue without doctor's advice until you complete prescribed dose, even though symptoms diminish or disappear.

Others:
Avoid using outdated drug.

POSSIBLE INTERACTION WITH OTHER DRUGS

GENERIC NAME OR DRUG CLASS	COMBINED EFFECT
Antacids*	Decreased tetracycline effect.
Anticoagulants, oral*	Increased anti-coagulant effect.
Bismuth subsalicylate	Decreased absorption of tetracycline.
Calcium supplements*	Decreased tetracycline effect.
Contraceptives, oral*	Decreased contra-ceptive effect.
Digitalis preparations*	Increased digitalis effect.
Etretinate	Increased chance of adverse reactions of etretinate.
Lithium	Increased lithium effect.
Mineral supplements* (iron, calcium, magnesium, zinc)	Decreased tetracycline absorption. Separate doses by 1 to 2 hours.
Penicillins*	Decreased penicillin effect.
Sodium bicarbonate	Decreased tetracycline effect.

POSSIBLE INTERACTION WITH OTHER SUBSTANCES

INTERACTS WITH	COMBINED EFFECT
Alcohol:	Possible liver damage. Avoid.
Beverages: Milk.	Decreased tetracycline absorption. Take dose 2 hours after or 1 hour before drinking.
Cocaine:	No proven problems.
Foods: Dairy products.	Decreased tetracycline absorption. Take dose 2 hours after or 1 hour before eating.
Marijuana:	No interactions ex-pected, but marijuana may slow body's recovery. Avoid.
Tobacco:	None expected.

*See Glossary

THEOPHYLLINE, EPHEDRINE & BARBITURATES

BRAND NAMES

Azma Aid	T.E.P.
Ephenyllin	Thalfed
Lardet	Theocord
Phedral	Theodrine
Primatene "P"	Theofed
Formula	Theofedral
Tedral	Theophenyllin
Tedral SA	Theoral
Tedrigen	

BASIC INFORMATION

Habit forming? Yes
Prescription needed? Some yes, others no
Available as generic? Some yes, others no
Drug class: Bronchodilator, barbiturate, sympathomimetic, sedative

USES

- Treatment for bronchial asthma symptoms.
- Decreases congestion of breathing passages.
- Suppresses allergic reactions.
- Reduces anxiety or nervous tension (low dose).

DOSAGE & USAGE INFORMATION

How to take:
- Tablet or elixir—Swallow with liquid.
- Extended-release tablets—Swallow each dose whole. If you take regular tablets, you may chew or crush them.

When to take:
Most effective taken on empty stomach 1 hour before or 2 hours after eating. However, may take with food to lessen stomach upset.

Continued next column

OVERDOSE

SYMPTOMS:
Restlessness, irritability, anxiety, confusion, delirium, muscle tremors, convulsions, rapid and irregular pulse, coma.
WHAT TO DO:
- Dial 0 (operator) or 911 (emergency) for an ambulance or medical help. Then give first aid immediately.
- See emergency information on inside covers.

If you forget a dose:
Take as soon as you remember up to 2 hours late. If more than 2 hours, wait for next scheduled dose (don't double this dose).

What drug does:
- Relaxes and expands bronchial tubes.
- Prevents cells from releasing allergy-causing chemicals (histamines).
- Decreases blood-vessel size and blood flow, thus causing decongestion.
- May partially block nerve impulses at nerve-cell connections.

Time lapse before drug works:
15 to 30 minutes.

Don't take with:
- Non-prescription drugs with ephedrine, pseudoephedrine or epinephrine.
- Non-prescription drugs for cough, cold, allergy or asthma without consulting doctor.
- See Interaction column and consult doctor.

POSSIBLE ADVERSE REACTIONS OR SIDE EFFECTS

SYMPTOMS	WHAT TO DO
Life-threatening:	
Difficult breathing, uncontrollable rapid heart rate, loss of consciousness.	Discontinue. Seek emergency treatment.
Common:	
• Headache, irritability, nervousness, restlessness, insomnia, nausea, vomiting, abdominal pain, "hangover" effect.	Discontinue. Call doctor right away.
• Dizziness, lightheadedness, paleness, irregular heartbeat.	Continue. Call doctor when convenient.
Infrequent:	
• Rash; hives; red or flushed face; appetite loss; diarrhea; cough; confusion; slurred speech; eyelid, face, lip swelling; joint pain.	Discontinue. Call doctor right away.
• Frequent urination.	Continue. Call doctor when convenient.
Rare:	
Agitation; sore throat, fever, mouth sores; jaundice.	Discontinue. Call doctor right away.

THEOPHYLLINE, EPHEDRINE & BARBITURATES

WARNINGS & PRECAUTIONS

Don't take if:
- You are allergic to any bronchodilator or barbiturate.
- You are allergic to ephedrine or any sympathomimetic drug.
- You have an active peptic ulcer or porphyria.

Before you start, consult your doctor:
- If you have gastritis, peptic ulcer, high blood pressure or heart disease, diabetes, overactive thyroid gland, difficulty urinating, epilepsy, kidney or liver damage, asthma, anemia, chronic pain, taken any MAO inhibitor in past 2 weeks, taken digitalis preparations in the last 7 days.
- If you have had impaired kidney or liver function.
- If you take medication for gout.
- If you will have surgery within 2 months, including dental surgery, requiring general or spinal anesthesia.

Over age 60:
- Adverse reactions and side effects may be more frequent and severe than in younger persons. Use small doses.
- More likely to develop high blood pressure, heart-rhythm disturbances, angina and to feel drug's stimulant effects.

Pregnancy:
Risk to unborn child outweighs drug benefits. Don't use.

Breast-feeding:
Drug passes into milk. Avoid drug or discontinue nursing until you finish medicine.

Infants & children:
Use only under medical supervision.

Prolonged use:
- Stomach irritation.
- Excessive doses—Rare toxic psychosis.
- Men with enlarged prostate gland may have more urination difficulty.
- May cause addiction, anemia, chronic intoxication.
- May lower body temperature, making exposure to cold temperatures hazardous.

Skin & sunlight:
May cause rash or intensify sunburn in areas exposed to sun or sunlamp.

Driving, piloting or hazardous work:
Don't drive or pilot aircraft until you learn how medicine affects you. Don't work around dangerous machinery. Don't climb ladders or work in high places. Danger increases if you drink alcohol or take medicine affecting alertness and reflexes.

Discontinuing:
- May be unnecessary to finish medicine. Follow doctor's instructions.
- If you develop withdrawal symptoms of hallucinations, agitation or sleeplessness after discontinuing, call doctor right away.

Others:
Potential for abuse.

POSSIBLE INTERACTION WITH OTHER DRUGS

GENERIC NAME OR DRUG CLASS	COMBINED EFFECT
Allopurinol	Decreased allopurinol effect.
Anticoagulants, oral*	Decreased anticoagulant effect.
Anticonvulsants*	Changed seizure patterns.
Antidepressants, tricyclics (TCA)*	Decreased antidepressant effect. Possible dangerous oversedation.
Antidiabetics, oral*	Increased phenobarbital effect.

Continued page 1107

POSSIBLE INTERACTION WITH OTHER SUBSTANCES

INTERACTS WITH	COMBINED EFFECT
Alcohol:	Possible fatal oversedation. Avoid.
Beverages: Caffeine drinks.	Nervousness or insomnia.
Cocaine:	High risk of heartbeat irregularities and high blood pressure.
Foods:	None expected.
Marijuana:	Rapid heartbeat, possible heart-rhythm disturbance.
Tobacco:	Decreased bronchodilator effect.

*See Glossary

THEOPHYLLINE, EPHEDRINE, GUAIFENESIN & BARBITURATES

BRAND NAMES

Bronkolixir
Bronkotabs
Guaiaphed

Lardet Expectorant
Mudrane GG
Quibron Plus

BASIC INFORMATION

Habit forming? Yes (barbiturates)
Prescription needed? Yes
Available as generic? Yes
Drug class: Bronchodilator (xanthine),
cough/cold preparation, sympathomimetic,
sedative

 ## USES

- Treatment for symptoms of bronchial asthma, emphysema, chronic bronchitis.
- Relieves wheezing, coughing and shortness of breath.

 ## DOSAGE & USAGE INFORMATION

How to take:
Tablet, capsule or elixir—Swallow with liquid.

When to take:
Most effective taken on empty stomach 1 hour before or 2 hours after eating. However, may take with food to lessen stomach upset.

If you forget a dose:
Take as soon as you remember up to 2 hours late. If more than 2 hours, wait for next scheduled dose (don't double this dose).

Continued next column

 ## OVERDOSE

SYMPTOMS:
Restlessness, irritability, confusion, muscle tremors, severe anxiety, rapid and irregular pulse, mild weakness, nausea, vomiting, delirium, coma.
WHAT TO DO:
- Overdose unlikely to threaten life. Depending on severity of symptoms and amount taken, call doctor, poison-control center or hospital emergency room for instructions.
- Dial 0 (operator) or 911 (emergency) for an ambulance or medical help. Then give first aid immediately.
- See emergency information on inside covers.

What drug does:
- Relaxes and expands bronchial tubes.
- Prevents cells from releasing allergy-causing chemicals (histamines).
- Relaxes muscles of bronchial tubes.
- Decreases blood-vessel size and blood flow, thus causing decongestion.
- Increases production of watery fluids to thin mucus so it can be coughed out or absorbed.
- May partially block nerve impulses at nerve-cell connections.

Time lapse before drug works:
30 to 60 minutes.

Don't take with:
- Non-prescription drugs with ephedrine, pseudoephedrine or epinephrine.
- Non-prescription drugs for cough, cold, allergy or asthma without consulting doctor.
- See Interaction column and consult doctor.

 ## POSSIBLE ADVERSE REACTIONS OR SIDE EFFECTS

SYMPTOMS	WHAT TO DO
Life-threatening:	
Difficult breathing, uncontrollable rapid heart rate, loss of consciousness.	Discontinue. Seek emergency treatment.
Common:	
• Headache, irritability, nervousness, restlessness, insomnia, nausea, vomiting, abdominal pain.	Discontinue. Call doctor right away.
• Dizziness, lightheadedness, paleness, irregular heartbeat.	Continue. Call doctor when convenient.
Infrequent:	
• Skin rash or hives, red or flushed face, appetite loss, diarrhea, abdominal pain.	Discontinue. Call doctor right away.
• Frequent urination.	Continue. Call doctor when convenient.
Rare:	
None expected.	

THEOPHYLLINE, EPHEDRINE, GUAIFENESIN & BARBITURATES

WARNINGS & PRECAUTIONS

Don't take if:
- You are allergic to any bronchodilator, ephedrine, any sympathomimetic drug, cough or cold preparation containing guaifenesin.
- You have an active peptic ulcer.

Before you start, consult your doctor:
- If you have had impaired kidney or liver function.
- If you have gastritis, peptic ulcer, high blood pressure, heart disease, diabetes, overactive thyroid gland, difficulty urinating, epilepsy, anemia, chronic pain, taken any MAO inhibitor in past 2 weeks, taken digitalis preparations in the last 7 days.
- If you take medication for gout.
- If you will have surgery within 2 months, including dental surgery, requiring general or spinal anesthesia.

Over age 60:
- Adverse reactions and side effects may be more frequent and severe than in younger persons. Use small doses. For drug to work, you must drink 8 to 10 glasses of fluid per day.
- More likely to develop high blood pressure, heart-rhythm disturbances, angina and to feel drug's stimulant effects.

Pregnancy:
Risk to unborn child outweighs drug benefits. Don't use.

Breast-feeding:
Drug passes into milk. Avoid drug or discontinue nursing until you finish medicine. Consult doctor for advice on maintaining milk supply.

Infants & children:
Use only under medical supervision.

Prolonged use:
- Stomach irritation.
- Excessive doses—Rare toxic psychosis.
- Men with enlarged prostate gland may have more urination difficulty.
- May cause addiction, anemia, chronic intoxication.
- May lower body temperature, making exposure to cold temperature hazardous.

Skin & sunlight:
May cause rash or intensify sunburn in areas exposed to sun or sunlamp.

Driving, piloting or hazardous work:
Don't drive or pilot aircraft until you learn how medicine affects you. Don't work around dangerous machinery. Don't climb ladders or work in high places. Danger increases if you drink alcohol or take medicine affecting alertness and reflexes, such as antihistamines, tranquilizers, sedatives, pain medicine, narcotics and mind-altering drugs.

Discontinuing:
- May be unnecessary to finish medicine. Follow doctor's instructions.
- If you develop withdrawal symptoms of hallucinations, agitation or sleeplessness after discontinuing, call doctor right away.

Others:
Great potential for abuse.

POSSIBLE INTERACTION WITH OTHER DRUGS

GENERIC NAME OR DRUG CLASS	COMBINED EFFECT
Allopurinol	Decreased allopurinol effect.
Anticonvulsants*	Changed seizure patterns.

Continued page 1108

POSSIBLE INTERACTION WITH OTHER SUBSTANCES

INTERACTS WITH	COMBINED EFFECT
Alcohol:	Possible fatal oversedation. Avoid.
Beverages:	You must drink 8 to 10 glasses of fluid per day for drug to work.
Caffeine drinks.	Nervousness and insomnia.
Cocaine:	High risk of heartbeat irregularities and high blood pressure.
Foods:	None expected.
Marijuana:	Excessive sedation, rapid heartbeat, possible heart-rhythm disturbance. Avoid.
Tobacco:	Decreased broncho-dilator effect. Smoking is damaging to all problems this medicine treats. Avoid.

THEOPHYLLINE, EPHEDRINE & HYDROXYZINE

BRAND NAMES

Brophed
Hydromax
Hydrophed
Hydrophed D.F.
Marax

Marax D.F.
Moxy Compound
T.E.H. Compound
Theozine

BASIC INFORMATION

Habit forming? No
Prescription needed? Yes
Available as generic? Yes
Drug class: Bronchodilator (xanthine),
sympathomimetic, antihistamine,
tranquilizer

USES

- Treatment for symptoms of bronchial asthma, emphysema, chronic bronchitis.
- Relieves wheezing, coughing and shortness of breath.

DOSAGE & USAGE INFORMATION

How to take:
Tablet, capsule or syrup—Swallow with liquid.

When to take:
Most effective taken on empty stomach 1 hour before or 2 hours after eating. However, may take with food to lessen stomach upset.

If you forget a dose:
Take as soon as you remember up to 2 hours late. If more than 2 hours, wait for next scheduled dose (don't double this dose).

Continued next column

OVERDOSE

SYMPTOMS:
Restlessness, irritability, confusion, severe anxiety, muscle tremors, rapid and irregular pulse, agitation, purposeless movements, delirium, convulsions, coma.
WHAT TO DO:
- **Dial 0 (operator) or 911 (emergency) for an ambulance or medical help. Then give first aid immediately.**
- **See emergency information on inside covers.**

What drug does:
- Relaxes and expands bronchial tubes.
- Prevents cells from releasing allergy-causing chemicals (histamines).
- Relaxes muscles of bronchial tubes.
- Decreases blood-vessel size and blood flow, thus causing decongestion.
- May reduce activity in areas of the brain that influence emotional stability.

Time lapse before drug works:
15 to 60 minutes.

Don't take with:
- Non-prescription drugs with ephedrine, pseudoephedrine or epinephrine.
- Non-prescription drugs for cough, cold, allergy or asthma without consulting doctor.
- See Interaction column and consult doctor.

POSSIBLE ADVERSE REACTIONS OR SIDE EFFECTS

SYMPTOMS	WHAT TO DO
Life-threatening: Difficult breathing, uncontrollable rapid heart rate, loss of consciousness.	Discontinue. Seek emergency treatment.
Common: • Headache, irritability, nervousness, restlessness, insomnia, nausea, vomiting, abdominal pain.	Discontinue. Call doctor right away.
• Dizziness, lightheadedness, paleness, irregular heartbeat.	Continue. Call doctor when convenient.
Infrequent: • Skin rash or hives, red or flushed face, appetite loss, diarrhea, abdominal pain.	Discontinue. Call doctor right away.
• Frequent urination.	Continue. Call doctor when convenient.
Rare: Tremor.	Discontinue. Call doctor right away.

THEOPHYLLINE, EPHEDRINE & HYDROXYZINE

WARNINGS & PRECAUTIONS

Don't take if:
- You are allergic to any bronchodilator, ephedrine, any sympathomimetic drug, or antihistamine.
- You have an active peptic ulcer.

Before you start, consult your doctor:
- If you have had impaired kidney or liver function.
- If you have gastritis, peptic ulcer, high blood pressure, heart disease, diabetes, overactive thyroid gland, difficulty urinating, epilepsy, taken any MAO inhibitor in past 2 weeks, taken digitalis preparations in the last 7 days.
- If you take medication for gout.
- If you will have surgery within 2 months, including dental surgery, requiring general or spinal anesthesia.

Over age 60:
- Adverse reactions and side effects may be more frequent and severe than in younger persons.
- More likely to develop increased urination difficulty, high blood pressure, heart-rhythm disturbances, angina and to feel drug's stimulant effects.

Pregnancy:
Risk to unborn child outweighs drug benefits. Don't use.

Breast-feeding:
Drug passes into milk. Avoid drug or discontinue nursing until you finish medicine. Consult doctor for advice on maintaining milk supply.

Infants & children:
Use only under medical supervision.

Prolonged use:
- Stomach irritation.
- Excessive doses—Rare toxic psychosis.
- Men with enlarged prostate gland may have more urination difficulty.
- Tolerance develops and reduces effectiveness.

Skin & sunlight:
No problems expected.

Driving, piloting or hazardous work:
Don't drive or pilot aircraft until you learn how medicine affects you. Don't work around dangerous machinery. Don't climb ladders or work in high places. Danger increases if you drink alcohol or take medicine affecting alertness and reflexes, such as antihistamines, tranquilizers, sedatives, pain medicine, narcotics and mind-altering drugs.

Discontinuing:
Don't discontinue without consulting doctor. Dose may require gradual reduction if you have taken drug for a long time. Doses of other drugs may also require adjustment.

Others:
No problems expected.

POSSIBLE INTERACTION WITH OTHER DRUGS

GENERIC NAME OR DRUG CLASS	COMBINED EFFECT
Allopurinol	Decreased allopurinol effect.
Antidepressants, tricyclics (TCA)*	Increased effect of ephedrine. Excess stimulation of heart and blood pressure.
Antihistamines*	Increased hydroxyzine effect.
Antihypertensives*	Decreased antihypertensive effect.
Beta-adrenergic blockers*	Decreased effect of drugs.
Carteolol	Decreased antihistamine effect.

Continued page 1109

POSSIBLE INTERACTION WITH OTHER SUBSTANCES

INTERACTS WITH	COMBINED EFFECT
Alcohol:	Increased sedation and intoxication. Avoid.
Beverages: Caffeine drinks.	Nervousness and insomnia.
Cocaine:	High risk of heartbeat irregularities and high blood pressure.
Foods:	None expected.
Marijuana:	Slightly increased anti-asthmatic effect of bronchodilator. Rapid heartbeat, possible heart-rhythm disturbance.
Tobacco:	Decreased bronchodilator effect. Smoking is damaging to all problems this medicine treats. Avoid.

*See Glossary

THEOPHYLLINE & GUAIFENESIN

BRAND NAMES

Asbron G
Asbron G Inlay
  Tablets
Bronchial
Elixophyllin-GG
Glycery T
Lanophyllin-GG

Quiagen
Quibron
Slo-Phyllin GG
Syncophylate-GG
Theocolate
Theolair-Plus
Theolate

BASIC INFORMATION

Habit forming? No
Prescription needed? Yes
Available as generic? Yes
Drug class: Bronchodilator, expectorant

 ## USES

- Treatment for bronchial asthma symptoms.
- Loosens mucus in respiratory passages.
- Relieves coughing, wheezing, shortness of breath.

 ## DOSAGE & USAGE INFORMATION

How to take:
Tablet, capsule, elixir or syrup—Swallow with liquid.

When to take:
Most effective taken on empty stomach 1 hour before or 2 hours after eating. However, may take with food to lessen stomach upset.

If you forget a dose:
Take as soon as you remember up to 2 hours late. If more than 2 hours, wait for next scheduled dose (don't double this dose).

Continued next column

 ## OVERDOSE

SYMPTOMS:
Restlessness, irritability, confusion, drowsiness, mild weakness, nausea, vomiting, delirium, convulsions, rapid pulse, coma.

WHAT TO DO:
- Dial 0 (operator) or 911 (emergency) for an ambulance or medical help. Then give first aid immediately.
- See emergency information on inside covers.

What drug does:
- Relaxes and expands bronchial tubes.
- Increases production of watery fluids to thin mucus so it can be coughed out or absorbed.

Time lapse before drug works:
15 to 30 minutes.

Don't take with:
See Interaction column and consult doctor.

 ## POSSIBLE ADVERSE REACTIONS OR SIDE EFFECTS

SYMPTOMS	WHAT TO DO
Life-threatening:	
Difficult breathing, uncontrollable heart rate, loss of consciousness.	Discontinue. Seek emergency treatment.
Common:	
• Headache, irritability, nervousness, restlessness, insomnia, drowsiness, nausea, vomiting, abdominal pain.	Discontinue. Call doctor right away.
• Dizziness, lightheadedness, diarrhea, abdominal pain.	Continue. Call doctor when convenient.
Infrequent:	
Skin rash or hives, red or flushed face, appetite loss, diarrhea.	Discontinue. Call doctor right away.
Rare:	
None expected.	

THEOPHYLLINE & GUAIFENESIN

WARNINGS & PRECAUTIONS

Don't take if:
- You are allergic to any bronchodilator or cough or cold preparation containing guaifenesin.
- You have an active peptic ulcer.

Before you start, consult your doctor:
- If you have had impaired kidney or liver function.
- If you have gastritis, peptic ulcer, high blood pressure or heart disease.
- If you take medication for gout.

Over age 60:
Adverse reactions and side effects may be more frequent and severe than in younger persons. For drug to work, you must drink 8 to 10 glasses of fluid per day.

Pregnancy:
Risk to unborn child outweighs drug benefits. Don't use.

Breast-feeding:
Drug passes into milk. Avoid drug or discontinue nursing until you finish medicine. Consult doctor for advice on maintaining milk supply.

Infants & children:
Use only under medical supervision.

Prolonged use:
Stomach irritation.

Skin & sunlight:
No problems expected.

Driving, piloting or hazardous work:
Avoid if lightheaded, drowsy or dizzy. Otherwise, no problems expected.

Discontinuing:
May be unnecessary to finish medicine. Follow doctor's instructions.

Others:
No problems expected.

POSSIBLE INTERACTION WITH OTHER DRUGS

GENERIC NAME OR DRUG CLASS	COMBINED EFFECT
Allopurinol	Decreased allopurinol effect.
Anticoagulants*	Possible risk of bleeding.
Ciprofloxacin	Increased possibility of central nervous system poisoning, such as nausea, vomiting, restlessness, palpitations.
Ephedrine	Increased effect of both drugs.
Epinephrine	Increased effect of both drugs.
Erythromycin	Increased bronchodilator effect.
Furosemide	Increased furosemide effect.
Lincomycins*	Increased bronchodilator effect.
Lithium	Decreased lithium effect.
Probenecid	Decreased effect of both drugs.
Propranolol	Decreased bronchodilator effect.
Rauwolfia alkaloids*	Rapid heartbeat.
Sulfinpyrazone	Decreased sulfinpyrazone effect.
Troleandomycin	Increased bronchodilator effect.

POSSIBLE INTERACTION WITH OTHER SUBSTANCES

INTERACTS WITH	COMBINED EFFECT
Alcohol:	No proven problems.
Beverages:	You must drink 8 to 10 glasses of fluid per day for drug to work.
Caffeine drinks.	Nervousness and insomnia.
Cocaine:	Excess stimulation. Avoid.
Foods:	None expected.
Marijuana:	Slightly increased antiasthmatic effect of bronchodilator.
Tobacco:	Decreased bronchodilator effect. Cigarette smoking makes worse all problems that this medicine treats. Avoid.

THIABENDAZOLE

BRAND NAMES

Foldan
Mintezol
Mintezol (Topical)

Minzolum
Triasox

BASIC INFORMATION

Habit forming? No
Prescription needed? Yes
Available as generic? No
Drug class: Antihelminthic (antiworm medication)

USES

Treatment of parasite infestations.

DOSAGE & USAGE INFORMATION

How to take or apply:
- Tablet—Swallow with liquid or food to lessen stomach irritation.
- Topical suspension—Apply to end of each tunnel or burrow made by worm.
- Chewable tablets—Chew thoroughly before swallowing.

When to take or apply:
- Tablet—According to instructions on prescription, after meals.
- Topical—2 to 4 times daily up to 14 days.

If you forget a dose:
Take as soon as you remember up to 2 hours late. If more than 2 hours, wait for next scheduled dose (don't double this dose).

What drug does:
Kills larvae and adult worms.

Continued next column

OVERDOSE

SYMPTOMS:
Aching, fever, blistered skin, seizures.
WHAT TO DO:
- Dial 0 (operator) or 911 (emergency) for an ambulance or medical help. Then give first aid immediately.
- If patient is unconscious and not breathing, give mouth-to-mouth breathing. If there is no heartbeat, use cardiac massage and mouth-to-mouth breathing (CPR). Don't try to make patient vomit. If you can't get help quickly, take patient to nearest emergency facility.
- See emergency information on inside covers.

Time lapse before drug works:
Varies according to degree of infestation.

Don't take with:
See Interaction column and consult doctor.

POSSIBLE ADVERSE REACTIONS OR SIDE EFFECTS

SYMPTOMS	WHAT TO DO
Life-threatening:	
None expected.	
Common:	
• Nausea, vomiting, abdominal pain.	Discontinue. Call doctor right away.
• Dizziness, headache, drowsiness, nausea, appetite loss, bedwetting.	Continue. Call doctor when convenient.
• Asparagus-like odor of urine.	Continue. Tell doctor at next visit.
Infrequent:	
• Redness, blistering with fever, rash with itchy skin, aching joints and muscles.	Discontinue. Call doctor right away.
• Ringing or buzzing in ears, numbness or tingling in hands and feet, swollen lymph nodes.	Continue. Call doctor when convenient.
Rare:	
Blurred or yellow vision, seizures.	Discontinue. Call doctor right away.

WARNINGS & PRECAUTIONS

Don't take if:
You are allergic to thiabendazole.

Before you start, consult your doctor:
- If you have kidney disease.
- If you have liver disease.

Over age 60:
Adverse reactions and side effects may be more frequent and severe than in younger persons.

Pregnancy:
Risk to unborn child outweighs drug benefits. Don't use.

Breast-feeding:
Unknown effect. Consult doctor.

Infants & children:
Use only under medical supervision.

Prolonged use:
Request follow-up stool exams 2 to 3 weeks following treatment.

Skin & sunlight:
No problems expected.

Driving, piloting or hazardous work:
Don't drive or pilot aircraft until you learn how medicine affects you. Don't work around dangerous machinery. Don't climb ladders or work in high places. Danger increases if you drink alcohol or take medicine affecting alertness and reflexes, such as antihistamines, tranquilizers, sedatives, pain medicine, narcotics and mind-altering drugs.

Discontinuing:
May be unnecessary to finish medicine. Follow doctor's instructions.

Others:
To prevent reinfection: Deworm household pets regularly. Cover sand boxes. Cook all pork until well done.

POSSIBLE INTERACTION WITH OTHER DRUGS

GENERIC NAME OR DRUG CLASS	COMBINED EFFECT
None expected.	

POSSIBLE INTERACTION WITH OTHER SUBSTANCES

INTERACTS WITH	COMBINED EFFECT
Alcohol:	Decreased thiabendazole effect.
Beverages:	No problems expected.
Cocaine:	Decreased thiabendazole effect.
Foods:	Take with foods to decrease nausea.
Marijuana:	Decreased thiabendazole effect.
Tobacco:	May decrease absorption of medicine.

THIAMINE (Vitamin B-1)

BRAND NAMES

Betalin S
Betaxin
Bewon
Numerous other multiple vitamin-mineral supplements.

Biamine
Pan-B-1

BASIC INFORMATION

Habit forming? No
Prescription needed? No
Available as generic? Yes
Drug class: Vitamin supplement

 ## USES

- Dietary supplement to promote normal growth, development and health.
- Treatment for beri-beri (a thiamine-deficiency disease).
- Dietary supplement for alcoholism, cirrhosis, overactive thyroid, infection, breast-feeding, absorption diseases, pregnancy, prolonged diarrhea, burns.

 ## DOSAGE & USAGE INFORMATION

How to take:
Tablet or liquid—Swallow with beverage or food to lessen stomach irritation.

When to take:
At the same time each day.

If you forget a dose:
Take when remembered. Return to regular schedule.

What drug does:
- Promotes normal growth and development.
- Combines with an enzyme to metabolize carbohydrates.

Time lapse before drug works:
15 minutes.

Don't take with:
See Interaction column and consult doctor.

 ## OVERDOSE

SYMPTOMS:
Increased severity of adverse reactions and side effects.
WHAT TO DO:
Overdose unlikely to threaten life. If person takes much larger amount than prescribed, call doctor, poison-control center or hospital emergency room for instructions.

 ## POSSIBLE ADVERSE REACTIONS OR SIDE EFFECTS

SYMPTOMS	WHAT TO DO
Life-threatening: Hives, rash, intense itching, faintness soon after a dose (anaphylaxis).	Seek emergency treatment immediately.
Common: None expected.	
Infrequent: None expected.	
Rare: • Wheezing.	Discontinue. Seek emergency treatment.
• Rash or itchy skin.	Discontinue. Call doctor right away.

THIAMINE (Vitamin B-1)

WARNINGS & PRECAUTIONS

Don't take if:
You are allergic to any B vitamin.

Before you start, consult your doctor:
If you have liver or kidney disease.

Over age 60:
No problems expected.

Pregnancy:
No problems expected.

Breast-feeding:
No problems expected.

Infants & children:
No problems expected.

Prolonged use:
No problems expected.

Skin & sunlight:
No problems expected.

Driving, piloting or hazardous work:
No problems expected.

Discontinuing:
No problems expected.

Others:
A balanced diet should provide enough thiamine for healthy people to make supplement unnecessary. Best dietary sources of thiamine are whole-grain cereals and meats.

POSSIBLE INTERACTION WITH OTHER DRUGS

GENERIC NAME OR DRUG CLASS	COMBINED EFFECT
Barbiturates*	Decreased thiamine effect.

POSSIBLE INTERACTION WITH OTHER SUBSTANCES

INTERACTS WITH	COMBINED EFFECT
Alcohol:	None expected.
Beverages: Carbonates, citrates (additives listed on many beverage labels).	Decreased thiamine effect.
Cocaine:	None expected.
Foods: Carbonates, citrates (additives listed on many food labels).	Decreased thiamine effect.
Marijuana:	None expected.
Tobacco:	None expected.

THIORIDAZINE

BRAND NAMES

Apo-Thioridazine
Mellaril
Mellaril S
Millazine
Novoridazine

PMS Thioridazine
SK-Thioridazine
Hydrochloride
Thioril

BASIC INFORMATION

Habit forming? No
Prescription needed? Yes
Available as generic? Yes
Drug class: Tranquilizer, antiemetic
(phenothiazine)

 USES

- Stops nausea, vomiting, hiccups.
- Reduces anxiety, agitation.

 DOSAGE & USAGE INFORMATION

How to take:
- Tablet—Swallow with liquid or food to lessen stomach irritation.
- Drops or liquid—Dilute dose in beverage.

When to take:
- Nervous and mental disorders—Take at the same times each day.
- Nausea and vomiting—Take as needed, no more often than every 4 hours.

If you forget a dose:
- Nervous and mental disorders—Take up to 2 hours late. If more than 2 hours, wait for next scheduled dose (don't double this dose).
- Nausea and vomiting—Take as soon as you remember. Wait 4 hours for next dose.

What drug does:
- Suppresses brain's vomiting center.
- Suppresses brain centers that control abnormal emotions and behavior.

Continued next column

 OVERDOSE

SYMPTOMS:
Stupor, convulsions, coma.
WHAT TO DO:
- Dial 0 (operator) or 911 (emergency) for an ambulance or medical help. Then give first aid immediately.
- See emergency information on inside covers.

Time lapse before drug works:
- Nausea and vomiting—1 hour or less.
- Nervous and mental disorders—4-6 weeks.

Don't take with:
- Antacid or medicine for diarrhea.
- Non-prescription drug for cough, cold or allergy.
- See Interaction column and consult doctor.

 POSSIBLE ADVERSE REACTIONS OR SIDE EFFECTS

SYMPTOMS	WHAT TO DO
Life-threatening:	
Uncontrolled muscle movements of tongue, face and other muscles (neuroleptic malignant syndrome, rare).	Discontinue. Seek emergency treatment.
Common:	
• Muscle spasms of face and neck, unsteady gait.	Discontinue. Seek emergency treatment.
• Restlessness, tremor, drowsiness.	Discontinue. Call doctor right away.
• Decreased sweating, dry mouth, nasal congestion, constipation.	Continue. Call doctor when convenient.
Infrequent:	
• Fainting.	Discontinue. Seek emergency treatment.
• Rash.	Discontinue. Call doctor right away.
• Difficult urination, less interest in sex, swollen breasts, menstrual irregularities.	Continue. Call doctor when convenient.
Rare:	
Change in vision, jaundice, sore throat, fever.	Discontinue. Call doctor right away.

WARNINGS & PRECAUTIONS

Don't take if:
- You are allergic to any phenothiazine.
- You have a blood or bone-marrow disease.

Before you start, consult your doctor:
- If you will have surgery within 2 months, including dental surgery, requiring general or spinal anesthesia.
- If you have asthma, emphysema or other lung disorder, glaucoma, prostate trouble.
- If you take non-prescription ulcer medicine, asthma medicine or amphetamines.

Over age 60:
Adverse reactions and side effects may be more frequent and severe than in younger persons. More likely to develop involuntary movement of jaws, lips, tongue, chewing. Report this to your doctor immediately. Early treatment can help.

Pregnancy:
Risk to unborn child outweighs drug benefits. Don't use.

Breast-feeding:
Drug passes into milk. Avoid drug or discontinue nursing until you finish medicine. Consult doctor for advice on maintaining milk supply.

Infants & children:
Don't give to children younger than 2.

Prolonged use:
May lead to tardive dyskinesia (involuntary movement of jaws, lips, tongue, chewing).

Skin & sunlight:
May cause rash or intensify sunburn in areas exposed to sun or sunlamp. Skin may remain sensitive for 3 months after discontinuing.

Driving, piloting or hazardous work:
Don't drive or pilot aircraft until you learn how medicine affects you. Don't work around dangerous machinery. Don't climb ladders or work in high places. Danger increases if you drink alcohol or take medicine affecting alertness and reflexes.

Discontinuing:
- Nervous and mental disorders—Don't discontinue without doctor's advice until you complete prescribed dose, even though symptoms diminish or disappear.
- Nausea and vomiting—May be unnecessary to finish medicine. Follow doctor's instructions.

Others:
No problems expected.

POSSIBLE INTERACTION WITH OTHER DRUGS

GENERIC NAME OR DRUG CLASS	COMBINED EFFECT
Anticholinergics*	Increased anticholinergic effect.
Antidepressants, tricyclic (TCA)*	Increased thioridazine effect.
Antihistamines*	Increased antihistamine effect.
Appetite suppressants*	Decreased suppressant effect.
Dronabinol	Increased effects of both drugs. Avoid.
Guanethidine	Decreased guanethidine effect.
Levodopa	Decreased levodopa effect.
Mind-altering drugs*	Increased effect of mind-altering drugs.
Molindone	Increased tranquilizer effect.
Nabilone	Greater depression of central nervous system.
Narcotics*	Increased narcotic effect.
Phenytoin	Increased phenytoin effect.
Procarbazine	Increased sedation.
Quinidine	Impaired heart function. Dangerous mixture.
Sedatives*	Increased sedation.
Tranquilizers, other*	Increased tranquilizer effect.

POSSIBLE INTERACTION WITH OTHER SUBSTANCES

INTERACTS WITH	COMBINED EFFECT
Alcohol:	Dangerous oversedation.
Beverages:	None expected.
Cocaine:	Decreased thioridazine effect. Avoid.
Foods:	None expected.
Marijuana:	Drowsiness. May increase antinausea effect.
Tobacco:	None expected.

THIOTHIXENE

BRAND NAMES

Navane

BASIC INFORMATION

Habit forming? No
Prescription needed? Yes
Available as generic? No
Drug class: Tranquilizer (thioxanthine), antiemetic

USES

- Reduces anxiety, agitation, psychosis.
- Stops vomiting, hiccups.

DOSAGE & USAGE INFORMATION

How to take:
- Capsule—Swallow with liquid. If you can't swallow whole, open capsule and take with liquid or food.
- Syrup—Dilute dose in beverage before swallowing.

When to take:
At the same time each day.

If you forget a dose:
Take as soon as you remember up to 2 hours late. If more than 2 hours, wait for next scheduled dose (don't double this dose).

What drug does:
Corrects imbalance of nerve impulses.

Continued next column

OVERDOSE

SYMPTOMS:
Drowsiness, dizziness, weakness, muscle rigidity, twitching, tremors, confusion, dry mouth, blurred vision, rapid pulse, shallow breathing, low blood pressure, convulsions, coma.
WHAT TO DO:
- **Dial 0 (operator) or 911 (emergency) for an ambulance or medical help. Then give first aid immediately.**
- **If patient is unconscious and not breathing, give mouth-to-mouth breathing. If there is no heartbeat, use cardiac massage and mouth-to-mouth breathing (CPR). Don't try to make patient vomit. If you can't get help quickly, take patient to nearest emergency facility.**
- **See emergency information on inside covers.**

Time lapse before drug works:
3 weeks.

Don't take with:
See Interaction column and consult doctor.

POSSIBLE ADVERSE REACTIONS OR SIDE EFFECTS

SYMPTOMS	WHAT TO DO
Life-threatening: Uncontrolled muscle movements of tongue, face and other muscles (neuroleptic malignant syndrome, rare).	Discontinue. Seek emergency treatment.
Common:	
• Fainting, jerky and involuntary movements, blurred vision, restlessness, rapid heartbeat.	Discontinue. Call doctor right away.
• Dizziness, drowsiness, constipation, muscle spasms, shuffling walk, decreased sweating.	Continue. Call doctor when convenient.
• Dry mouth, nasal congestion.	Continue. Tell doctor at next visit.
Infrequent:	
• Rash, abdominal pain.	Discontinue. Call doctor right away.
• Less sexual ability, difficult urination.	Continue. Call doctor when convenient.
• Menstrual irregularities, swollen breasts.	Continue. Tell doctor at next visit.
Rare: Sore throat, fever, jaundice.	Discontinue. Call doctor right away.

WARNINGS & PRECAUTIONS

Don't take if:
- You are allergic to any thioxanthine or phenothiazine tranquilizer.
- You have serious blood disorder.
- You have Parkinson's disease.
- Patient is younger than 12.

Before you start, consult your doctor:
- If you have had liver or kidney disease.
- If you have epilepsy, glaucoma, prostate trouble.
- If you have high blood pressure or heart disease (especially angina).
- If you use alcohol daily.
- If you will have surgery within 2 months, including dental surgery, requiring general or spinal anesthesia.

Over age 60:
Adverse reactions and side effects may be more frequent and severe than in younger persons.

Pregnancy:
No proven harm to unborn child. Avoid if possible.

Breast-feeding:
Studies inconclusive. Consult your doctor.

Infants & children:
Not recommended.

Prolonged use:
- Pigment deposits in lens and retina of eye.
- Involuntary movements of jaws, lips, tongue (tardive dyskinesia).

Skin & sunlight:
May cause rash or intensify sunburn in areas exposed to sun or sunlamp.

Driving, piloting or hazardous work:
Don't drive or pilot aircraft until you learn how medicine affects you. Don't work around dangerous machinery. Don't climb ladders or work in high places. Danger increases if you drink alcohol or take medicine affecting alertness and reflexes.

Discontinuing:
Don't discontinue without consulting doctor. Dose may require gradual reduction if you have taken drug for a long time. Doses of other drugs may also require adjustment.

Others:
Hot temperatures increase chance of heat stroke.

POSSIBLE INTERACTION WITH OTHER DRUGS

GENERIC NAME OR DRUG CLASS	COMBINED EFFECT
Anticholinergics*	Increased anticholinergic effect.
Anticonvulsants*	Change in seizure pattern.
Antidepressants, tricyclic (TCA)*	Increased thiothixene effect. Excessive sedation.
Antihistamines*	Increased thiothixene effect. Excessive sedation.
Antihypertensives*	Excessively low blood pressure.
Barbiturates*	Increased thiothixene effect. Excessive sedation.
Bethanechol	Decreased bethanechol effect.
Dronabinol	Increased effects of both drugs. Avoid.
Guanethidine	Decreased guanethidine effect.
Levodopa	Decreased levodopa effect.
MAO inhibitors*	Excessive sedation.
Mind-altering drugs*	Increased thiothixene effect. Excessive sedation.
Narcotics*	Increased thiothixene effect. Excessive sedation.
Procarbazine	Increased sedation.
Sedatives*	Increased thiothixene effect. Excessive sedation.
Sleep inducers*	Increased thiothixene effect. Excessive sedation.
Tranquilizers*	Increased thiothixene effect. Excessive sedation.

POSSIBLE INTERACTION WITH OTHER SUBSTANCES

INTERACTS WITH	COMBINED EFFECT
Alcohol:	Excessive brain depression. Avoid.
Beverages:	None expected.
Cocaine:	Decreased thiothixene effect. Avoid.
Foods:	None expected.
Marijuana:	Daily use—Fainting likely, possible psychosis.
Tobacco:	None expected.

*See Glossary

THYROGLOBULIN

BRAND NAMES

Proloid

BASIC INFORMATION

Habit forming? No
Prescription needed? Yes
Available as generic? No
Drug class: Thyroid hormone

 ## USES

Replacement for thyroid hormone deficiency.

 ## DOSAGE & USAGE INFORMATION

How to take:
Tablet—Swallow with liquid.

When to take:
At the same time each day before a meal or on awakening.

If you forget a dose:
Take as soon as you remember up to 12 hours late. If more than 12 hours, wait for next scheduled dose (don't double this dose).

What drug does:
Increases cell metabolism rate.

Time lapse before drug works:
48 hours.

Don't take with:
See Interaction column and consult doctor.

 ## OVERDOSE

SYMPTOMS:
"Hot" feeling, heart palpitations, nervousness, sweating, hand tremors, insomnia, rapid and irregular pulse, headache, irritability, diarrhea, weight loss, muscle cramps, angina, congestive heart failure possible.
WHAT TO DO:
Overdose unlikely to threaten life. If person takes much larger amount than prescribed, call doctor, poison-control center or hospital emergency room for instructions.

 ## POSSIBLE ADVERSE REACTIONS OR SIDE EFFECTS

SYMPTOMS	WHAT TO DO
Life-threatening: None expected.	
Common:	
• Tremor, headache, irritability, insomnia.	Discontinue. Call doctor right away.
• Appetite change, diarrhea, leg cramps, menstrual irregularities, fever, heat sensitivity, unusual sweating, weight loss.	Continue. Call doctor when convenient.
Infrequent: Hives, rash, vomiting, chest pain, rapid and irregular heartbeat, shortness of breath.	Discontinue. Call doctor right away.
Rare: None expected.	

WARNINGS & PRECAUTIONS

Don't take if:
- You have had a heart attack within 6 weeks.
- You have no thyroid deficiency, but use this to lose weight.

Before you start, consult your doctor:
- If you have heart disease or high blood pressure.
- If you have diabetes.
- If you have Addison's disease, have had adrenal gland deficiency or use epinephrine, ephedrine or isoproterenol for asthma.

Over age 60:
More sensitive to thyroid hormone. May need smaller doses.

Pregnancy:
Considered safe if for thyroid deficiency only.

Breast-feeding:
Present in milk. Considered safe if dose is correct.

Infants & children:
Use only under medical supervision.

Prolonged use:
No problems expected, if dose is correct.

Skin & sunlight:
No problems expected.

Driving, piloting or hazardous work:
No problems expected.

Discontinuing:
Don't discontinue without consulting doctor. Dose may require gradual reduction if you have taken drug for a long time. Doses of other drugs may also require adjustment.

Others:
- Digestive upsets, tremors, cramps, nervousness, insomnia or diarrhea may indicate need for dose adjustment.
- Different brands can cause different results. Do not change brands without consulting doctor.

POSSIBLE INTERACTION WITH OTHER DRUGS

GENERIC NAME OR DRUG CLASS	COMBINED EFFECT
Amphetamines*	Increased amphetamine effect.
Anticoagulants, oral*	Increased anticoagulant effect.
Antidepressants, tricyclic (TCA)*	Increased antidepressant effect. Irregular heartbeat.
Antidiabetics*	Antidiabetic may require adjustment.
Aspirin (large doses, continuous use)	Increased thyroglobulin effect.
Barbiturates*	Decreased barbiturate effect.
Beta-adrenergic blockers*	Possible decreased beta-blocker effect.
Cholestyramine	Decreased thyroglobulin effect.
Colestipol	Decreased thyroglobulin effect.
Contraceptives, oral*	Decreased thyroglobulin effect.
Cortisone drugs*	Requires dose adjustment to prevent cortisone deficiency.
Diclofenac	Rapid heartbeat, blood-pressure rise.
Digitalis preparations*	Decreased digitalis effect.
Estrogens*	Decreased thyroglobulin effect.
Ephedrine	Increased ephedrine effect.
Epinephrine	Increased epinephrine effect.
Methylphenidate	Increased methylphenidate effect.

POSSIBLE INTERACTION WITH OTHER SUBSTANCES

INTERACTS WITH	COMBINED EFFECT
Alcohol:	None expected.
Beverages:	None expected.
Cocaine:	Excess stimulation. Avoid.
Foods: Soybeans.	Heavy consumption interferes with thyroid function.
Marijuana:	None expected.
Tobacco:	None expected.

*See Glossary

THYROID

BRAND NAMES

Armour	Proloid
Cytomel	S-P-T
Eltroxin	Synthroid
Euthroid	Thyrar
Levothroid	Thyrocrine
Levoxine	Thyrolar

BASIC INFORMATION

Habit forming? No
Prescription needed? Yes
Available as generic? Yes
Drug class: Thyroid hormone

 USES

Replacement for thyroid hormone deficiency.

 DOSAGE & USAGE INFORMATION

How to take:
Tablet—Swallow with liquid.

When to take:
At the same time each day before a meal or on awakening.

If you forget a dose:
Take as soon as you remember up to 12 hours late. If more than 12 hours, wait for next scheduled dose (don't double this dose).

What drug does:
Increases cell metabolism rate.

Time lapse before drug works:
48 hours.

Don't take with:
See Interaction column and consult doctor.

 OVERDOSE

SYMPTOMS:
"Hot" feeling, heart palpitations, nervousness, sweating, hand tremors, insomnia, rapid and irregular pulse, headache, irritability, diarrhea, weight loss, muscle cramps, angina, congestive heart failure possible.
WHAT TO DO:
Overdose unlikely to threaten life. If person takes much larger amount than prescribed, call doctor, poison-control center or hospital emergency room for instructions.

 POSSIBLE ADVERSE REACTIONS OR SIDE EFFECTS

SYMPTOMS	WHAT TO DO
Life-threatening: None expected.	
Common: • Tremor, headache, irritability, insomnia.	Discontinue. Call doctor right away.
• Appetite change, diarrhea, leg cramps, menstrual irregularities, fever, heat sensitivity, unusual sweating, weight loss.	Continue. Call doctor when convenient.
Infrequent: Hives, rash, vomiting, chest pain, rapid and irregular heartbeat, shortness of breath.	Discontinue. Call doctor right away.
Rare: None expected.	

WARNINGS & PRECAUTIONS

Don't take if:
- You have had a heart attack within 6 weeks.
- You have no thyroid deficiency, but use this to lose weight.

Before you start, consult your doctor:
- If you have heart disease or high blood pressure.
- If you have diabetes.
- If you have Addison's disease, have had adrenal gland deficiency or use epinephrine, ephedrine or isoproterenol for asthma.

Over age 60:
More sensitive to thyroid hormone. May need smaller doses.

Pregnancy:
Considered safe if for thyroid deficiency only.

Breast-feeding:
Present in milk. Considered safe if dose is correct.

Infants & children:
Use only under medical supervision.

Prolonged use:
No problems expected, if dose is correct.

Skin & sunlight:
No problems expected.

Driving, piloting or hazardous work:
No problems expected.

Discontinuing:
Don't discontinue without consulting doctor. Dose may require gradual reduction if you have taken drug for a long time. Doses of other drugs may also require adjustment.

Others:
- Digestive upsets, tremors, cramps, nervousness, insomnia or diarrhea may indicate need for dose adjustment.
- Different brands can cause different results. Do not change brands without consulting doctor.

POSSIBLE INTERACTION WITH OTHER DRUGS

GENERIC NAME OR DRUG CLASS	COMBINED EFFECT
Amphetamines*	Increased amphetamine effect.
Anticoagulants, oral*	Increased anticoagulant effect.
Antidepressants, tricyclic (TCA)*	Increased antidepressant effect. Irregular heartbeat.
Antidiabetics*	Antidiabetic may require adjustment.
Aspirin (large doses, continuous use)	Increased thyroid effect.
Barbiturates*	Decreased barbiturate effect.
Beta-adrenergic blockers*	Possible decreased beta-blocker effect.
Cholestyramine	Decreased thyroid effect.
Colestipol	Decreased thyroid effect.
Contraceptives, oral*	Decreased thyroid effect.
Cortisone drugs*	Requires dose adjustment to prevent cortisone deficiency.
Diclofenac	Rapid heartbeat, blood-pressure rise.
Digitalis preparations*	Decreased digitalis effect.
Ephedrine	Increased ephedrine effect.
Epinephrine	Increased epinephrine effect.
Estrogens*	Decreased thyroid effect.
Methylphenidate	Increased methylphenidate effect.

POSSIBLE INTERACTION WITH OTHER SUBSTANCES

INTERACTS WITH	COMBINED EFFECT
Alcohol:	None expected.
Beverages:	None expected.
Cocaine:	Excess stimulation. Avoid.
Foods: Soybeans.	Heavy consumption interferes with thyroid function.
Marijuana:	None expected.
Tobacco:	None expected.

*See Glossary

THYROXINE (T-4, Levothyroxine)

BRAND NAMES

Choloxin	L-Thyroxine
Cytolen	L-T-S
Elthroxin	Noroxine
Euthroid	Ro-Thyroxine
Letter	Synthroid
Levoid	Thyrolar
Levothroid	

BASIC INFORMATION

Habit forming? No
Prescription needed? Yes
Available as generic? No
Drug class: Thyroid hormone

USES

Replacement for thyroid hormone deficiency.

DOSAGE & USAGE INFORMATION

How to take:
Tablet—Swallow with liquid.

When to take:
At the same time each day before a meal or on awakening.

If you forget a dose:
Take as soon as you remember up to 12 hours late. If more than 12 hours, wait for next scheduled dose (don't double this dose).

What drug does:
Increases cell metabolism rate.

Time lapse before drug works:
48 hours.

Don't take with:
See Interaction column and consult doctor.

OVERDOSE

SYMPTOMS:
"Hot" feeling, heart palpitations, nervousness, sweating, hand tremors, insomnia, rapid and irregular pulse, headache, irritability, diarrhea, weight loss, muscle cramps, angina, congestive heart failure possible.
WHAT TO DO:
Overdose unlikely to threaten life. If person takes much larger amount than prescribed, call doctor, poison-control center or hospital emergency room for instructions.

POSSIBLE ADVERSE REACTIONS OR SIDE EFFECTS

SYMPTOMS	WHAT TO DO
Life-threatening: None expected.	
Common:	
• Tremor, headache, irritability, insomnia.	Discontinue. Call doctor right away.
• Appetite change, diarrhea, leg cramps, menstrual irregularities, fever, heat sensitivity, unusual sweating, weight loss.	Continue. Call doctor when convenient.
Infrequent: Hives, rash, vomiting, chest pain, rapid and irregular heartbeat, shortness of breath.	Discontinue. Call doctor right away.
Rare: None expected.	

THYROXINE (T-4, Levothyroxine)

WARNINGS & PRECAUTIONS

Don't take if:
- You have had a heart attack within 6 weeks.
- You have no thyroid deficiency, but use this to lose weight.

Before you start, consult your doctor:
- If you have heart disease or high blood pressure.
- If you have diabetes.
- If you have Addison's disease, have had adrenal gland deficiency or use epinephrine, ephedrine or isoproterenol for asthma.

Over age 60:
More sensitive to thyroid hormone. May need smaller doses.

Pregnancy:
Considered safe if for thyroid deficiency only.

Breast-feeding:
Present in milk. Considered safe if dose is correct.

Infants & children:
Use only under medical supervision.

Prolonged use:
No problems expected, if dose is correct.

Skin & sunlight:
No problems expected.

Driving, piloting or hazardous work:
No problems expected.

Discontinuing:
Don't discontinue without consulting doctor. Dose may require gradual reduction if you have taken drug for a long time. Doses of other drugs may also require adjustment.

Others:
- Digestive upsets, tremors, cramps, nervousness, insomnia or diarrhea may indicate need for dose adjustment.
- Different brands can cause in different results. Do not change brands without consulting doctor.

POSSIBLE INTERACTION WITH OTHER DRUGS

GENERIC NAME OR DRUG CLASS	COMBINED EFFECT
Amphetamines*	Increased amphetamine effect.
Anticoagulants, oral*	Increased anticoagulant effect.
Antidepressants, tricyclic (TCA)*	Increased antidepressant effect. Irregular heartbeat.
Antidiabetics*	Antidiabetic may require adjustment.
Aspirin (large doses, continuous use)	Increased thyroxine effect.
Barbiturates*	Decreased barbiturate effect.
Beta-adrenergic blockers*	Possible decreased beta blockers effect.
Cholestyramine	Decreased thyroxine effect.
Colestipol	Decreased thyroxine effect.
Contraceptives, oral*	Decreased thyroxine effect.
Cortisone drugs*	Requires dose adjustment to prevent cortisone deficiency.
Digitalis preparations*	Decreased digitalis effect.
Ephedrine	Increased ephedrine effect.
Epinephrine	Increased epinephrine effect.
Estrogens*	Decreased thyroxine effect.
Methylphenidate	Increased methylphenidate effect.
Phenytoin	Possible decreased thyroxine effect.

POSSIBLE INTERACTION WITH OTHER SUBSTANCES

INTERACTS WITH	COMBINED EFFECT
Alcohol:	None expected.
Beverages:	None expected.
Cocaine:	Excess stimulation. Avoid.
Foods: Soybeans.	Heavy consumption interferes with thyroid function.
Marijuana:	None expected.
Tobacco:	None expected.

TICARCILLIN

BRAND NAMES

Ticar

BASIC INFORMATION

Habit forming? No
Prescription needed? Yes
Available as generic? No
Drug class: Antibiotic (penicillin)

 ## USES

Treatment of bacterial infections that are susceptible to ticarcillin.

 ## DOSAGE & USAGE INFORMATION

How to take:
By injection only.

When to take:
Follow doctor's instructions.

If you forget a dose:
Consult doctor.

What drug does:
Destroys susceptible bacteria. Does not kill viruses.

Time lapse before drug works:
May be several days before medicine affects infection.

Don't take with:
See Interaction column and consult doctor.

 ## OVERDOSE

SYMPTOMS:
Severe diarrhea, nausea, edema or vomiting.
WHAT TO DO:
Overdose unlikely to threaten life. If person takes much larger amount than prescribed, call doctor, poison-control center or hospital emergency room for instructions.

 ## POSSIBLE ADVERSE REACTIONS OR SIDE EFFECTS

SYMPTOMS	WHAT TO DO
Life-threatening: Hives, rash, intense itching, faintness soon after a dose (anaphylaxis).	Seek emergency treatment immediately.
Common: Dark or discolored tongue.	Continue. Tell doctor at next visit.
Infrequent: Mild nausea, vomiting, diarrhea.	Continue. Call doctor when convenient.
Rare: Unexplained bleeding; lowered blood potassium (as determined by a laboratory test). Symptoms may include weakness, hoarseness, heartbeat irregularities.	Discontinue. Call doctor right away.

WARNINGS & PRECAUTIONS

Don't take if:
You are allergic to ticarcillin, cephalosporin antibiotics, or other penicillins. Life-threatening reaction may occur.

Before you start, consult your doctor:
If you are allergic to any substance or drug.

Over age 60:
You may have skin reactions, particularly around genitals and anus.

Pregnancy:
Studies inconclusive on harm to unborn child. Animal studies show fetal abnormalities. Decide with your doctor whether drug benefits justify risk to unborn child.

Breast-feeding:
Drug passes into milk. Child may become sensitive to penicillins and have allergic reactions to penicillin drugs. Avoid ticarcillin or discontinue nursing until you finish medicine. Consult doctor for advice on maintaining milk supply.

Infants & children:
No problems expected.

Prolonged use:
You may become more susceptible to infections caused by germs not responsive to ticarcillin.

Skin & sunlight:
No problems expected.

Driving, piloting or hazardous work:
Usually not dangerous. Most hazardous reactions likely to occur a few minutes after taking ticarcillin.

Discontinuing:
Don't discontinue without doctor's advice until you complete prescribed dose, even though symptoms diminish or disappear.

Others:
No problems expected.

POSSIBLE INTERACTION WITH OTHER DRUGS

GENERIC NAME OR DRUG CLASS	COMBINED EFFECT
Beta-adrenergic blockers*	Increased chance of anaphylaxis (see emergency information on inside front cover).
Chloramphenicol	Decreased effect of both drugs.
Erythromycins*	Decreased effect of both drugs.
Loperamide	Decreased ticarcillin effect.
Paromomycin	Decreased effect of both drugs.
Tetracyclines*	Decreased effect of both drugs.
Troleandomycin	Decreased effect of both drugs.

POSSIBLE INTERACTION WITH OTHER SUBSTANCES

INTERACTS WITH	COMBINED EFFECT
Alcohol:	Occasional stomach irritation.
Beverages:	None expected.
Cocaine:	No proven problems.
Foods:	None expected.
Marijuana:	No proven problems.
Tobacco:	None expected.

TIMOLOL

BRAND NAMES

Blocadren   Timoptic
Timolide

BASIC INFORMATION

Habit forming? No
Prescription needed? Yes
Available as generic? No
Drug class: Beta-adrenergic blocker,
  antiglaucoma agent

 ## USES

- Reduces angina attacks.
- Stabilizes irregular heartbeat.
- Lowers blood pressure.
- Reduces frequency of migraine headaches.
  (Does not relieve headache pain.)
- Decreases internal-eye pressure of glaucoma
  (ophthalmic drops).
- After myocardial infarction, prevents another
  heart attack.

 ## DOSAGE & USAGE INFORMATION

How to take:
- Eye drops—Wash hands. Apply slight
  pressure with finger to inside corner of eye.
  Pull lower eyelid down. Put drop just above
  lowered eyelid. Close eye gently for 2
  minutes. Don't blink.
- Tablet—Swallow with liquid or crumble and
  take with food.

When to take:
- Tablet—With meals or immediately after.
- Eye drops—Follow prescription directions.

If you forget a dose:
Take as soon as you remember. Return to
regular schedule, but allow 3 hours between
doses.

Continued next column

 ## OVERDOSE

SYMPTOMS:
Weakness; slow or weak pulse; blood-
pressure drop; fainting; difficulty breathing,
convulsions; cold, sweaty skin.
WHAT TO DO:
- Dial 0 (operator) or 911 (emergency) for
  an ambulance or medical help. Then give
  first aid immediately.
- See emergency information on inside
  covers.

What drug does:
- Blocks certain actions of sympathetic nervous
  system.
- Lowers heart's oxygen requirements.
- Slows nerve impulses through heart.
- Reduces blood vessel contraction in heart,
  scalp and other body parts.
- Eye drops lower pressure inside eye.

Time lapse before drug works:
1 to 4 hours.

Don't take with:
Non-prescription drugs or drugs in Interaction
column without consulting doctor.

 ## POSSIBLE ADVERSE REACTIONS OR SIDE EFFECTS

SYMPTOMS	WHAT TO DO
Life-threatening:	
Congestive heart failure.	Discontinue. Seek emergency treatment.
Common:	
• Pulse slower than 50 beats per minute.	Discontinue. Call doctor right away.
• Drowsiness, fatigue, numbness or tingling of fingers or toes, dizziness, diarrhea, nausea, weakness.	Continue. Call doctor when convenient.
• Cold hands or feet; dry mouth, eyes and skin.	Continue. Tell doctor at next visit.
Infrequent:	
• Hallucinations, nightmares, insomnia, headache, difficult breathing.	Discontinue. Call doctor right away.
• Confusion, reduced alertness, depression. impotence.	Continue. Call doctor when convenient.
• Constipation.	Continue. Tell doctor at next visit.
Rare:	
• Rash, sore throat, fever.	Discontinue. Call doctor right away.
• Unusual bleeding and bruising; dry, burning eyes.	Continue. Call doctor when convenient.

WARNINGS & PRECAUTIONS

Don't take if:
- You are allergic to any beta-adrenergic blocker.
- You have asthma or hay fever symptoms.
- You have taken MAO inhibitors in past 2 weeks.

Before you start, consult your doctor:
- If you have heart disease or poor circulation to the extremities.
- If you have hay fever, asthma, chronic bronchitis, emphysema.
- If you have overactive thyroid function.
- If you have impaired liver or kidney function.
- If you will have surgery within 2 months, including dental surgery, requiring general or spinal anesthesia.
- If you have diabetes or hypoglycemia.

Over age 60:
Adverse reactions and side effects may be more frequent and severe than in younger persons.

Pregnancy:
Risk to unborn child outweighs drug benefits. Don't use.

Breast-feeding:
Drug passes into milk. Avoid drug or discontinue nursing until you finish medicine. Consult doctor about maintaining milk supply.

Infants & children:
Not recommended.

Prolonged use:
Weakens heart muscle contractions.

Skin & sunlight:
No problems expected.

Driving, piloting or hazardous work:
Don't drive or pilot aircraft until you learn how medicine affects you. Don't work around dangerous machinery. Don't climb ladders or work in high places. Danger increases if you drink alcohol or take medicine affecting alertness and reflexes.

Discontinuing:
Don't discontinue without consulting doctor. Dose may require gradual reduction if you have taken drug for a long time. Doses of other drugs may also require adjustment.

Others:
- May mask hypoglycemia.
- Side effects, such as burning or stinging of the eye, may also occur with timolol used as eye drops.

POSSIBLE INTERACTION WITH OTHER DRUGS

GENERIC NAME OR DRUG CLASS	COMBINED EFFECT
ACE inhibitors: captopril, enalapril, lisinopril*	Increased antihypertensive effects of both drugs. Dosages may require adjustment.
Antidiabetics*	Increased antidiabetic effect.
Antihistamines*	Decreased antihistamine effect.
Antihypertensives*	Increased antihypertensive effect.
Barbiturates*	Increased barbiturate effect. Dangerous sedation.
Beta-agonists*	Decreased beta-agonist effect.
Betaxolol eyedrops	Possible increased timolol effect.
Digitalis preparations*	Increased or decreased heart rate. Improves irregular heartbeat.
Encainide	Increased effect of toxicity on heart muscle.
Indomethacin	Decreased timolol effect.
Insulin	Hypoglycemic effects may be prolonged.
Levobunolol eyedrops	Possible increased timolol effect.

Continued page 1110

POSSIBLE INTERACTION WITH OTHER SUBSTANCES

INTERACTS WITH	COMBINED EFFECT
Alcohol:	Excessive blood-pressure drop. Avoid.
Beverages:	None expected.
Cocaine:	Irregular heartbeat. Avoid.
Foods:	None expected.
Marijuana:	Daily use—Impaired circulation to hands and feet.
Tobacco:	Possible irregular heartbeat.

*See Glossary

TOCAINIDE

BRAND NAMES

Tonocard

BASIC INFORMATION

Habit forming? No
Prescription needed? Yes
Available as generic? No
Drug class: Antiarrhythmic

 ## USES

Stabilizes irregular heartbeat, particularly irregular contractions of the ventricles of the heart or a too rapid heart rate.

 ## DOSAGE & USAGE INFORMATION

How to take:
Tablet—Swallow with food, water or milk. Dosage may need to be changed according to individual response.

When to take:
Take at regular times each day. For example, instructions to take 3 times a day means every 8 hours.

If you forget a dose:
Take as soon as you remember up to 4 hours late. If more than 4 hours, wait for next scheduled dose (don't double this dose).

What drug does:
Decreases excitability of cells of heart muscle.

Time lapse before drug works:
30 minutes to 2 hours.

Don't take with:
- See Interaction column and consult doctor.
- Wear identification information that states that you take this medicine so during an emergency a physician will know to avoid additional medicines that might be harmful or dangerous.

 ## OVERDOSE

SYMPTOMS:
Convulsions, depressed breathing, cardiac arrest.
WHAT TO DO:
- Dial 0 (operator) or 911 (emergency) for an ambulance or medical help. Then give first aid immediately.
- See emergency information on inside covers.

 ## POSSIBLE ADVERSE REACTIONS OR SIDE EFFECTS

SYMPTOMS	WHAT TO DO
Life-threatening: None expected.	
Common: Nausea, vomiting, lightheadedness, dizziness.	Discontinue. Call doctor right away.
Infrequent:	
• Trembling.	Discontinue. Call doctor right away.
• Numbness or tingling in hands or feet.	Continue. Call doctor when convenient.
Rare:	
• Sore throat, red tongue, mouth ulcers, unexplained bleeding or bruising, fever, chills, blurred vision, may accelerate heart rate or worsen irregular heartbeat, cough, difficult breathing, wheezing, may decrease white blood-cell count, double vision, disorientation, hallucinations, shakiness, seizures, jaundice, memory impairment, urinary retention, hiccups.	Discontinue. Call doctor right away.
• Rash, joint pain, swollen feet and ankles, unusual sweating, ringing in ears, joint pain, loss of taste.	Continue. Call doctor when convenient.

WARNINGS & PRECAUTIONS

Don't take if:
- You are allergic to tocainide or anesthetics whose names end in "caine."
- You have myasthenia gravis.

Before you start, consult your doctor:
- If you have congestive heart failure.
- If you are pregnant or plan to become pregnant.
- If you take anticancer drugs, trimethoprim, pyrimethamine, primaquine, phenylbutazone, penicillamine or oxyphenbutazone. These may affect blood-cell production in bone marrow.
- If you take any other heart medicine such as digitalis, flucystosine, colchicine, chloramphenicol, beta-adrenergic blockers or azathioprine. These can worsen heartbeat irregularity.
- If you will have surgery within 2 months, including dental surgery, requiring general, local or spinal anesthesia.
- If you have liver or kidney disease.

Over age 60:
Adverse reactions and side effects may be more frequent and severe than in younger persons.

Pregnancy:
No proven harm to unborn child. Nevertheless, avoid if possible.

Breast-feeding:
Avoid if possible.

Infants & children:
Not recommended. Safety and dosage have not been established.

Prolonged use:
Request periodic lab studies on blood, liver function, potassium levels.

Skin & sunlight:
No problems expected.

Driving, piloting or hazardous work:
Use caution if medicine causes you to feel dizzy or weak. Otherwise, no problems expected.

Discontinuing:
Don't discontinue without consulting doctor, even though symptoms diminish or disappear.

Others:
No problems expected.

POSSIBLE INTERACTION WITH OTHER DRUGS

GENERIC NAME OR DRUG CLASS	COMBINED EFFECT
Antiarrhythmics, others*	Increased possibility of adverse reactions from either drug.
Beta-adrenergic blockers*	Possible irregular heartbeat. May worsen congestive heart failure.
Bone-marrow depressants* (anticancer drugs, azathioprine, chloramphenicol, colchicine, flucytosine, oxyphenbutazone, penicillamine, phenylbutazone, primaquine, pyrimethamine, trimethoprim)	Possible decreased production of blood cells in bone marrow.
Cimetidine	May increase tocainide effect and toxicity.
Encainide	Increased effect of toxicity on heart muscle.
Guanfacine	Increased effect of both medicines.
Nicardipine	Possible increased effect and toxicity of each drug.

POSSIBLE INTERACTION WITH OTHER SUBSTANCES

INTERACTS WITH	COMBINED EFFECT
Alcohol:	Possible irregular heartbeat. Avoid.
Beverages: Caffeine drinks, iced drinks.	Possible irregular heartbeat.
Cocaine:	Possible light-headedness, dizziness, quivering, convulsions.
Foods:	None expected.
Marijuana:	None expected.
Tobacco:	Possible irregular heartbeat.

TOLAZAMIDE

BRAND NAMES

Ronase   Tolinase

BASIC INFORMATION

Habit forming? No
Prescription needed? Yes
Available as generic? Yes
Drug class: Antidiabetic (oral), sulfonurea

USES

- Treatment for diabetes in adults who can't control blood sugar by diet, weight loss and exercise.
- Treatment for diabetes insipidus.

DOSAGE & USAGE INFORMATION

How to take:
Tablet—Swallow with liquid or food to lessen stomach irritation. If you can't swallow whole, crumble tablet and take with liquid or food.

When to take:
At the same times each day.

If you forget a dose:
Take as soon as you remember up to 2 hours late. If more than 2 hours, wait for next scheduled dose (don't double this dose).

What drug does:
Stimulates pancreas to produce more insulin. Insulin in blood forces cells to use sugar in blood.

Time lapse before drug works:
3 to 4 hours. May require 2 weeks for maximum benefit.

Don't take with:
See Interaction column and consult doctor.

OVERDOSE

SYMPTOMS:
Excessive hunger, nausea, anxiety, cool skin, cold sweats, drowsiness, rapid heartbeat, weakness, unconsciousness, coma.
WHAT TO DO:
- **Dial 0 (operator) or 911 (emergency) for an ambulance or medical help. Then give first aid immediately.**
- **See emergency information on inside covers.**

POSSIBLE ADVERSE REACTIONS OR SIDE EFFECTS

SYMPTOMS	WHAT TO DO
Life-threatening: None expected.	
Common:	
• Dizziness.	Discontinue. Call doctor right away.
• Diarrhea, appetite loss, nausea, stomach pain, heartburn.	Continue. Call doctor when convenient.
Infrequent: Low blood sugar (hunger, anxiety, cold sweats, rapid pulse).	Discontinue. Seek emergency treatment.
Rare: Fatigue, itchy skin or rash, sore throat, fever, ringing in ears, unusual bleeding or bruising, jaundice, edema, weakness, confusion.	Discontinue. Call doctor right away.

WARNINGS & PRECAUTIONS

Don't take if:
- You are allergic to any sulfonurea.
- You have impaired kidney or liver function.

Before you start, consult your doctor:
- If you have a severe infection.
- If you have thyroid disease.
- If you take insulin.
- If you have heart disease.

Over age 60:
Dose usually smaller than for younger adults. Avoid "low-blood-sugar" episodes because repeated ones can damage brain permanently.

Pregnancy:
No proven harm to unborn child. Avoid if possible.

Breast-feeding:
Drug filters into milk. May lower baby's blood sugar. Avoid.

Infants & children:
Don't give to infants or children.

Prolonged use:
None expected.

Skin & sunlight:
May cause rash or intensify sunburn in areas exposed to sun or sunlamp.

Driving, piloting or hazardous work:
No problems expected unless you develop hypoglycemia (low blood sugar). If so, avoid driving or hazardous activity.

Discontinuing:
Don't discontinue without consulting doctor. Dose may require gradual reduction if you have taken drug for a long time. Doses of other drugs may also require adjustment.

Others:
Don't exceed recommended dose. Hypoglycemia (low blood sugar) may occur, even with proper dose schedule. You must balance medicine, diet and exercise.

POSSIBLE INTERACTION WITH OTHER DRUGS

GENERIC NAME OR DRUG CLASS	COMBINED EFFECT
Androgens*	Increased tolazamide effect.
Anticoagulants, oral*	Unpredictable prothrombin times.
Anticonvulsants, hydantoin*	Decreased tolazamide effect.
Aspirin	Increased tolazamide effect.
Beta-adrenergic blockers*	Increased tolazamide effect. Possible increased difficulty in regulating blood-sugar levels.
Bismuth subsalicylate	Increased insulin effect. May require dosage adjustment.
Chloramphenicol	Increased tolazamide effect.
Cimetidine	Possible increased tolazamide effect.
Clofibrate	Increased tolazamide effect.
Contraceptives, oral*	Decreased tolazamide effect.
Cortisone drugs*	Decreased tolazamide effect.
Digoxin	Possible decreased digoxin effect.
Diuretics* (loop, thiazide)	Decreased tolazamide effect.
Epinephrine	Decreased tolazamide effect.
Estrogens*	Decreased tolazamide effect.
Guanethidine	Unpredictable tolazamide effect.
Insulin	Increased tolazamide effect.
Isoniazid	Decreased tolazamide effect.
Labetalol	Increased antidiabetic effect, may mask hypoglycemia.
MAO inhibitors*	Increased tolazamide effect.
Nicotinic acid	Decreased tolazamide effect.
Non-steroidal anti-inflammatory drugs (NSAIDs)*	Increased tolazamide effect.
Oxyphenbutazone	Increased tolazamide effect.
Phenothiazines*	Decreased tolazamide effect.
Phenylbutazone	Increased tolazamide effect.
Phenyramidol	Increased tolazamide effect.
Phenytoin	Decreased tolazamide effect.
Probenecid	Increased tolazamide effect.
Pyrazinamide	Decreased tolazamide effect.
Ranitidine	Possible increased tolazamide effect.
Rifampin	Decreased tolazamide effect.
Sulfaphenazole	Increased tolazamide effect.
Sulfa drugs*	Increased tolazamide effect.
Thyroid hormones*	Decreased tolazamide effect.

POSSIBLE INTERACTION WITH OTHER SUBSTANCES

INTERACTS WITH	COMBINED EFFECT
Alcohol:	Disulfiram reaction.* Avoid.
Beverages:	None expected.
Cocaine:	No proven problems.
Foods:	None expected.
Marijuana:	Decreased tolazamide effect. Avoid.
Tobacco:	None expected.

*See Glossary

989

TOLBUTAMIDE

BRAND NAMES

Apo-Tolbutamide
Mobenol
Neo-Dibetic
Novobutamide
Oramide
Orinase
SK-Tolbutamide
Tolbutone

BASIC INFORMATION

Habit forming? No
Prescription needed? Yes
Available as generic? Yes
Drug class: Antidiabetic (oral), sulfonurea

 ## USES

- Treatment for diabetes in adults who can't control blood sugar by diet, weight loss and exercise.
- Treatment for diabetes insipidus.

 ## DOSAGE & USAGE INFORMATION

How to take:
Tablet—Swallow with liquid or food to lessen stomach irritation. If you can't swallow whole, crumble tablet and take with liquid or food.

When to take:
At the same times each day.

If you forget a dose:
Take as soon as you remember up to 2 hours late. If more than 2 hours, wait for next scheduled dose (don't double this dose).

What drug does:
Stimulates pancreas to produce more insulin. Insulin in blood forces cells to use sugar in blood.

Time lapse before drug works:
3 to 4 hours. May require 2 weeks for maximum benefit.

Don't take with:
See Interaction column and consult doctor.

 ## OVERDOSE

SYMPTOMS:
Excessive hunger, nausea, anxiety, cool skin, cold sweats, drowsiness, rapid heartbeat, weakness, unconsciousness, coma.
WHAT TO DO:
- Dial 0 (operator) or 911 (emergency) for an ambulance or medical help. Then give first aid immediately.
- See emergency information on inside covers.

 ## POSSIBLE ADVERSE REACTIONS OR SIDE EFFECTS

SYMPTOMS	WHAT TO DO
Life-threatening: None expected.	
Common: • Dizziness.	Discontinue. Call doctor right away.
• Diarrhea, appetite loss, nausea, stomach pain, heartburn.	Continue. Call doctor when convenient.
Infrequent: Low blood sugar (hunger, anxiety, cold sweats, rapid pulse).	Discontinue. Seek emergency treatment.
Rare: Fatigue, itchy skin or rash, sore throat, fever, ringing in ears, unusual bleeding or bruising, jaundice, edema, weakness, confusion.	Discontinue. Call doctor right away.

 ## WARNINGS & PRECAUTIONS

Don't take if:
- You are allergic to any sulfonurea.
- You have impaired kidney or liver function.

Before you start, consult your doctor:
- If you have a severe infection.
- If you have thyroid disease.
- If you take insulin.
- If you have heart disease.

Over age 60:
Dose usually smaller than for younger adults. Avoid "low-blood-sugar" episodes because repeated ones can damage brain permanently.

Pregnancy:
No proven harm to unborn child. Avoid if possible.

Breast-feeding:
Drug filters into milk. May lower baby's blood sugar. Avoid.

Infants & children:
Don't give to infants or children.

Prolonged use:
None expected.

Skin & sunlight:
May cause rash or intensify sunburn in areas exposed to sun or sunlamp.

Driving, piloting or hazardous work:
No problems expected unless you develop hypoglycemia (low blood sugar). If so, avoid driving or hazardous activity.

Discontinuing:
Don't discontinue without consulting doctor. Dose may require gradual reduction if you have taken drug for a long time. Doses of other drugs may also require adjustment.

Others:
Don't exceed recommended dose. Hypoglycemia (low blood sugar) may occur, even with proper dose schedule. You must balance medicine, diet and exercise.

 POSSIBLE INTERACTION WITH OTHER DRUGS

GENERIC NAME OR DRUG CLASS	COMBINED EFFECT
Androgens*	Increased tolbutamide effect.
Anticoagulants, oral*	Unpredictable prothrombin times.
Anticonvulsants, hydantoin*	Decreased tolbutamide effect.
Aspirin	Increased tolbutamide effect.
Beta-adrenergic blockers*	Increased tolbutamide effect. Possible increased difficulty in regulating blood-sugar levels.
Bismuth subsalicylate	Increased insulin effect. May require dosage adjustment.
Chloramphenicol	Increased tolbutamide effect.
Cimetidine	Possible increased tolbutamide effect.
Clofibrate	Increased tolbutamide effect.
Contraceptives, oral*	Decreased tolbutamide effect.
Cortisone drugs*	Decreased tolbutamide effect.
Digoxin	Possible decreased digoxin effect.
Diuretics* (loop, thiazide)	Decreased tolbutamide effect.
Epinephrine	Decreased tolbutamide effect.
Estrogens*	Increased tolbutamide effect.
Guanethidine	Unpredictable tolbutamide effect.
Insulin	Increased tolbutamide effect.
Isoniazid	Decreased tolbutamide effect.
Labetalol	Increased antidiabetic effect, may mask hypoglycemia.
MAO inhibitors*	Increased tolbutamide
Nicotinic acid	Decreased tolbutamide effect.
Non-steroidal anti-inflammatory drugs (NSAIDs)*	Increased tolbutamide effect.
Oxyphenbutazone	Increased tolbutamide effect.
Phenothiazines	Decreased tolbutamide effect.
Phenylbutazone	Increased tolbutamide effect.
Phenyramidol	Increased tolbutamide effect.
Phenytoin	Decreased tolbutamide effect.
Probenecid	Increased tolbutamide effect.
Pyrazinamide	Decreased tolbutamide effect.
Ranitidine	Possible increased tolbutamide effect.
Rifampin	Decreased tolbutamide effect.
Sulfa drugs*	Increased tolbutamide effect.
Sulfaphenazole	Increased tolbutamide effect.
Thyroid hormones*	Decreased tolbutamide effect.

 POSSIBLE INTERACTION WITH OTHER SUBSTANCES

INTERACTS WITH	COMBINED EFFECT
Alcohol:	Disulfiram reaction.* Avoid.
Beverages:	None expected.
Cocaine:	No proven problems.
Foods:	None expected.
Marijuana:	Decreased tolbutamide effect. Avoid.
Tobacco:	None expected.

TOLMETIN

BRAND NAMES

Tolectin   Tolectin DS

BASIC INFORMATION

Habit forming? No
Prescription needed? Yes
Available as generic? No
Drug class: Anti-inflammatory (non-steroid)

 USES

- Treatment for joint pain, stiffness, inflammation and swelling of arthritis and gout.
- Pain reliever.
- Treatment of juvenile rheumatoid arthritis.

 DOSAGE & USAGE INFORMATION

How to take:
Tablet or capsule—Swallow with liquid or food to lessen stomach irritation. If you can't swallow whole, crumble tablet or open capsule and take with liquid or food.

When to take:
At the same times each day.

If you forget a dose:
Take as soon as you remember up to 2 hours late. If more than 2 hours, wait for next scheduled dose (don't double this dose).

What drug does:
Reduces tissue concentration of prostaglandins (hormones which produce inflammation and pain).

Time lapse before drug works:
Begins in 4 to 24 hours. May require 3 weeks regular use for maximum benefit.

Don't take with:
See Interaction column and consult doctor.

 OVERDOSE

SYMPTOMS:
Confusion, agitation, incoherence, convulsions, possible hemorrhage from stomach or intestine, coma.
WHAT TO DO:
- **Dial 0 (operator) or 911 (emergency) for an ambulance or medical help. Then give first aid immediately.**
- **See emergency information on inside covers.**

 POSSIBLE ADVERSE REACTIONS OR SIDE EFFECTS

SYMPTOMS	WHAT TO DO
Life-threatening:	
Hives, rash, intense itching, faintness soon after a dose (anaphylaxis in aspirin-sensitive persons).	Seek emergency treatment immediately.
Common:	
• Dizziness, nausea, pain.	Continue. Call doctor when convenient.
• Headache.	Continue. Tell doctor at next visit.
Infrequent:	
Depression, drowsiness, ringing in ears, swollen feet or legs, constipation or diarrhea, vomiting.	Continue. Call doctor when convenient.
Rare:	
• Convulsions; confusion; rash, hives or itchy skin; blurred vision; black, bloody or tarry stools; difficult breathing; tightness in chest; rapid heartbeat; unusual bleeding or bruising; blood in urine; jaundice; severe abdominal pain, psychosis.	Discontinue. Call doctor right away.
• Painful, difficult or frequent urination; fatigue; weakness; swollen breasts in males; impotence; menstrual irregularities.	Continue. Call doctor when convenient.

 WARNINGS & PRECAUTIONS

Don't take if:
- You are allergic to aspirin or any non-steroid, anti-inflammatory drug.
- You have gastritis, peptic ulcer, enteritis, ileitis, ulcerative colitis, asthma, heart failure, high blood pressure or bleeding problems.
- Patient is younger than 15.

Before you start, consult your doctor:
- If you have epilepsy.
- If you have Parkinson's disease.
- If you have been mentally ill.
- If you have had kidney disease or impaired kidney function.

Over age 60:
Adverse reactions and side effects may be more frequent and severe than in younger persons.

Pregnancy:
Studies inconclusive on harm to unborn child. Decide with your doctor whether drug benefits justify risk to unborn child.

Breast-feeding:
May harm child. Avoid.

Infants & children:
Not recommended for anyone younger than 15. Use only under medical supervision.

Prolonged use:
- Eye damage.
- Reduced hearing.
- Sore throat, fever.
- Weight gain.

Skin & sunlight:
Increased sensitivity to sunlight.

Driving, piloting or hazardous work:
Don't drive or pilot aircraft until you learn how medicine affects you. Don't work around dangerous machinery. Don't climb ladders or work in high places. Danger increases if you drink alcohol or take medicine affecting alertness and reflexes, such as antihistamines, tranquilizers, sedatives, pain medicine, narcotics and mind-altering drugs.

Discontinuing:
Don't discontinue without consulting doctor. Dose may require gradual reduction if you have taken drug for a long time. Doses of other drugs may also require adjustment.

Others:
No problems expected.

POSSIBLE INTERACTION WITH OTHER DRUGS

GENERIC NAME OR DRUG CLASS	COMBINED EFFECT
ACE inhibitors: captopril, enalapril, lisinopril*	May decrease ACE inhibitor effect.
Anticoagulants, oral*	Increased risk of bleeding.
Aspirin	Increased risk of stomach ulcer.
Beta-adrenergic blockers*	Decreased antihypertensive effect.
Carteolol	Decreased antihypertensive effect of carteolol.

Cortisone drugs*	Increased risk of stomach ulcer.
Diuretics*	May decrease diuretic effect.
Lithium	Possible increased lithium effect and toxicity.
Methotrexate	May increase toxicity.
Minoxidil	Decreased minoxidil effect.
Oxyphenbutazone	Possible stomach ulcer.
Phenylbutazone	Possible stomach ulcer.
Probenecid	Increased tolmetin effect.
Sotalol	Decreased antihypertensive effect of sotalol.
Terazosin	Decreases effectiveness of terazosin. Causes sodium and fluid retention.
Thyroid hormones*	Rapid heartbeat, blood-pressure rise.

POSSIBLE INTERACTION WITH OTHER SUBSTANCES

INTERACTS WITH	COMBINED EFFECT
Alcohol:	Possible stomach ulcer or bleeding.
Beverages:	None expected.
Cocaine:	None expected.
Foods:	None expected.
Marijuana:	Increased pain relief from tolmetin.
Tobacco:	None expected.

TRAZODONE

BRAND NAMES

Desyrel   Trialodine
Desyrel Dividose

BASIC INFORMATION

Habit forming? No
Prescription needed? Yes
Available as generic? Yes
Drug class: Antidepressant (non-tricyclic)

USES

- Treats mental depression.
- Treats anxiety.

DOSAGE & USAGE INFORMATION

How to take:
Tablet—Swallow with liquid or food to lessen
stomach irritation. If you can't swallow whole,
crumble tablet and take with liquid or food.

When to take:
According to prescription directions. Bedtime
dose usually higher than other doses.

If you forget a dose:
Take as soon as you remember up to 2 hours
late. If more than 2 hours, wait for next
scheduled dose (don't double this dose).

What drug does:
Inhibits serotonin uptake in brain cells.

Time lapse before drug works:
2 to 4 weeks for full effect.

Don't take with:
See Interaction column and consult doctor.

OVERDOSE

SYMPTOMS:
Fainting, irregular heartbeat, respiratory
arrest, chest pain, seizures, coma.
WHAT TO DO:
- Dial 0 (operator) or 911 (emergency) for
  an ambulance or medical help. Then give
  first aid immediately.
- If patient is unconscious and not
  breathing, give mouth-to-mouth
  breathing. If there is no heartbeat, use
  cardiac massage and mouth-to-mouth
  breathing (CPR). Don't try to make patient
  vomit. If you can't get help quickly, take
  patient to nearest emergency facility.
- See emergency information on inside
  covers.

POSSIBLE ADVERSE REACTIONS OR SIDE EFFECTS

SYMPTOMS	WHAT TO DO
Life-threatening: None expected.	
Common: Drowsiness.	Continue. Call doctor when convenient.
Infrequent: • Prolonged penile erections.	Seek emergency treatment immediately.
• Tremor, fainting, incoordination, blood pressue rise or drop, rapid heartbeat, shortness of breath.	Discontinue. Call doctor right away.
• Disorientation, confusion, fatigue, dizziness on standing, excitement, headache, nervousness, rash, itchy skin, blurred vision, ringing in ears, dry mouth, bad taste, diarrhea, nausea, vomiting, constipation, aching, menstrual changes, diminished sex drive, nightmares, vivid dreams, seizures.	Continue. Call doctor when convenient.
Rare: None expected.	

WARNINGS & PRECAUTIONS

Don't take if:
- You are allergic to trazodone.
- You are thinking about suicide.

Before you start, consult your doctor:
- If you have heart rhythm problem.
- If you have any heart disease.
- If you will have surgery within 2 months, including dental surgery, requiring general or spinal anesthesia.

Over age 60:
Adverse reactions and side effects may be more frequent and severe than in younger persons.

Pregnancy:
Risk to unborn child outweighs drug benefits. Don't use.

Breast-feeding:
Drug passes into milk. Avoid drug or discontinue nursing until you finish medicine. Consult doctor for advice on maintaining milk supply.

Infants & children:
Not recommended.

Prolonged use:
Occasional blood counts, especially if you have fever and sore throat.

Skin & sunlight:
No problems expected.

Driving, piloting or hazardous work:
Don't drive or pilot aircraft until you learn how medicine affects you. Don't work around dangerous machinery. Don't climb ladders or work in high places. Danger increases if you drink alcohol or take medicine affecting alertness and reflexes, such as antihistamines, tranquilizers, sedatives, pain medicine, narcotics and mind-altering drugs.

Discontinuing:
Don't discontinue without consulting doctor. Dose may require gradual reduction if you have taken drug for a long time. Doses of other drugs may also require adjustment.

Others:
Electroshock therapy should be avoided.

POSSIBLE INTERACTION WITH OTHER DRUGS

GENERIC NAME OR DRUG CLASS	COMBINED EFFECT
Antidepressants, other*	Excess drowsiness.
Antihistamines*	Excess drowsiness.
Antihypertensives*	Possible too low blood pressure. Avoid.
Barbiturates*	Too low blood pressure. Avoid.
Digitalis preparations*	Possible increased digitalis level in blood.
Guanfacine	Increased effect of both medicines.
MAO inhibitors*	May add to toxic effect of each.
Nabilone	Greater depression of central nervous system.
Narcotics*	Excess drowsiness.
Phenytoin	Possible increased phenytoin level in blood.
Sedatives*	Excess drowsiness.
Tranquilizers*	Excess drowsiness.

POSSIBLE INTERACTION WITH OTHER SUBSTANCES

INTERACTS WITH	COMBINED EFFECT
Alcohol:	Excess sedation. Avoid.
Beverages: Caffeine.	May add to heartbeat irregularity. Avoid.
Cocaine:	May add to heartbeat irregularity. Avoid.
Foods:	No problems expected.
Marijuana:	May add to heartbeat irregularity. Avoid.
Tobacco:	May add to heartbeat irregularity. Avoid.

TRETINOIN (Topical)

BRAND NAMES

Retin-A StieVAA
Retinoic Acid Vitamin A Acid

BASIC INFORMATION

Habit forming? No
Prescription needed? Yes
Available as generic? Yes
Drug class: Antiacne (topical)

 USES

Treatment for acne, psoriasis, ichthyosis, keratosis, folliculitis, flat warts.

 DOSAGE & USAGE INFORMATION

How to use:
Wash skin with non-medicated soap, pat dry, wait 20 minutes before applying.
- Cream or gel—Apply to affected areas with fingertips and rub in gently.
- Solution—Apply to affected areas with gauze pad or cotton swab. Avoid getting too wet so medicine doesn't drip into eyes, mouth, lips or inside nose.
- Follow manufacturer's directions on container.

When to use:
At the same time each day.

If you forget an application:
Use as soon as you remember.

What drug does:
Increases skin-cell turnover so skin layer peels off more easily.

Time lapse before drug works:
2 to 3 weeks. May require 6 weeks for maximum improvement.

Don't use with:
- Benzoyl peroxide. Apply 12 hours apart.
- See Interaction column and consult doctor.

 OVERDOSE

SYMPTOMS:
None expected.
WHAT TO DO:
If person swallows drug, call doctor, poison-control center or hospital emergency room for instructions.

 POSSIBLE ADVERSE REACTIONS OR SIDE EFFECTS

SYMPTOMS	WHAT TO DO
Life-threatening: None expected.	
Common:	
• Pigment change in treated area, warmth or stinging, peeling.	Continue. Tell doctor at next visit.
• Sensitivity to wind or cold.	No action necessary.
Infrequent: Blistering, crusting, severe burning, swelling.	Discontinue. Call doctor right away.
Rare: None expected.	

WARNINGS & PRECAUTIONS

Don't take if:
- You are allergic to tretinoin.
- You are sunburned, windburned or have an open skin wound.

Before you start, consult your doctor:
If you have eczema.

Over age 60:
Not recommended.

Pregnancy:
No proven harm to unborn child. Avoid if possible.

Breast-feeding:
No problems expected.

Infants & children:
Not recommended.

Prolonged use:
No problems expected.

Skin & sunlight:
- May cause rash or intensify sunburn in areas exposed to sun or sunlamp.
- In some animal studies, tretinoin caused skin tumors to develop faster when treated area was exposed to ultraviolet light (sunlight or sunlamp). No proven similar effects in humans.

Driving, piloting or hazardous work:
No problems expected.

Discontinuing:
Don't discontinue without doctor's advice until you complete prescribed dose, even though symptoms diminish or disappear.

Others:
Acne may get worse before improvement starts in 2 or 3 weeks. Don't wash face more than 2 or 3 times daily.

POSSIBLE INTERACTION WITH OTHER DRUGS

GENERIC NAME OR DRUG CLASS	COMBINED EFFECT
Antiacne topical preparations, other*	Severe skin irritation.
Cosmetics (medicated)	Severe skin irritation.
Etretinate	Increased chance of toxicity of each drug.
Skin preparations with alcohol	Severe skin irritation.
Soaps or cleansers (abrasive)	Severe skin irritation.

POSSIBLE INTERACTION WITH OTHER SUBSTANCES

INTERACTS WITH	COMBINED EFFECT
Alcohol:	None expected.
Beverages:	None expected.
Cocaine:	None expected.
Foods:	None expected.
Marijuana:	None expected.
Tobacco:	None expected.

TRIAMCINOLONE

BRAND NAMES

See complete list of brand names in the *Brand Name Directory*, page 1072.

BASIC INFORMATION

Habit forming? No
Prescription needed? Yes
Available as generic? Yes
Drug class: Cortisone drug (adrenal corticosteroid)

 ## USES

- Reduces inflammation caused by many different medical problems.
- Treatment for some allergic diseases, blood disorders, kidney diseases, asthma and emphysema.
- Replaces corticosteroid deficiencies.

 ## DOSAGE & USAGE INFORMATION

How to take:
Tablet or syrup—Swallow with liquid or food to lessen stomach irritation. If you can't swallow whole, crumble tablet.

When to take:
At the same times each day. Take once-a-day or once-every-other-day doses in mornings.

If you forget a dose:
- Several-doses-per-day prescription—Take as soon as you remember up to 2 hours late. If more than 2 hours, wait for next scheduled dose (don't double this dose).
- Once-a-day dose or less—Wait for next dose. Double this dose.

What drug does:
Decreases inflammatory responses.

Time lapse before drug works:
2 to 4 days.

Don't take with:
See Interaction column and consult doctor.

 ## OVERDOSE

SYMPTOMS:
Headache, convulsions, heart failure.
WHAT TO DO:
- Dial 0 (operator) or 911 (emergency) for an ambulance or medical help. Then give first aid immediately.
- See emergency information on inside covers.

 ## POSSIBLE ADVERSE REACTIONS OR SIDE EFFECTS

SYMPTOMS	WHAT TO DO
Life-threatening: Hives, rash, intense itching, faintness soon after a dose (anaphylaxis).	Seek emergency treatment immediately.
Common: Acne, thirst, indigestion, nausea, vomiting, poor wound healing, decreased growth in children.	Continue. Call doctor when convenient.
Infrequent: • Black, bloody or tarry stool.	Discontinue. Seek emergency treatment.
• Blurred vision, halos around lights, muscle cramps, swollen legs and feet, sore throat, fever.	Discontinue. Call doctor right away.
• Mood change, fatigue, weakness, insomnia, restlessness, frequent urination, weight gain, round face, TB recurrence, menstrual irregularities.	Continue. Call doctor when convenient.
Rare: • Irregular heartbeat.	Discontinue. Seek emergency treatment.
• Rash, pancreatitis, numbness or tingling in hands or feet, thrombophlebitis, hallucinations, convulsions.	Discontinue. Call doctor right away.

 ## WARNINGS & PRECAUTIONS

Don't take if:
- You are allergic to any cortisone drug.
- You have tuberculosis or fungus infection.
- You have herpes infection of eyes, lips or genitals.

Before you start, consult your doctor:
- If you have had tuberculosis.
- If you have congestive heart failure, diabetes, peptic ulcer, glaucoma, underactive thyroid, high blood pressure, myasthenia gravis, blood clots in legs or lungs.

Over age 60:
Adverse reactions and side effects may be more frequent and severe than in younger persons. Likely to aggravate edema, diabetes or ulcers. Likely to cause cataracts and osteoporosis (softening of the bones).

Pregnancy:
Risk to unborn child outweighs drug benefits. Don't use.

Breast-feeding:
Drug passes into milk. Avoid drug or discontinue nursing until you finish medicine. Consult doctor for advice on maintaining milk supply.

Infants & children:
Use only under medical supervision.

Prolonged use:
- Retards growth in children.
- Possible glaucoma, cataracts, diabetes, fragile bones and thin skin.
- Functional dependence.

Skin & sunlight:
No problems expected.

Driving, piloting or hazardous work:
No problems expected.

Discontinuing:
- Don't discontinue without doctor's advice until you complete prescribed dose, even though symptoms diminish or disappear.
- Drug affects your response to surgery, illness, injury or stress for 2 years after discontinuing. Tell anyone who takes medical care of you within 2 years about drug.

Others:
Avoid immunizations if possible.

 ## POSSIBLE INTERACTION WITH OTHER DRUGS

GENERIC NAME OR DRUG CLASS	COMBINED EFFECT
Amphotericin B	Potassium depletion.
Anticholinergics*	Possible glaucoma.
Anticoagulants, oral*	Decreased anti-coagulant effect.
Anticonvulsants, hydantoin*	Decreased triamcinolone effect.
Antidiabetics, oral*	Decreased anti-diabetic effect.
Antihistamines*	Decreased triamcinolone effect.
Aspirin	Increased triamcinolone effect.
Attenuated virus vaccines*	Possible viral infection.

Barbiturates*	Decreased triamcinolone effect. Oversedation.
Chloral hydrate	Decreased triamcinolone effect.
Chlorthalidone	Potassium depletion.
Cholestyramine	Decreased triamcinolone absorption.
Cholinergics*	Decreased cholinergic effect.
Colestipol	Decreased triamcinolone absorption.
Contraceptives, oral*	Increased triamcinolone effect.
Digitalis preparations*	Dangerous potassium depletion. Possible digitalis toxicity.
Diuretics, thiazide*	Potassium depletion.
Ephedrine	Decreased triamcinolone effect.
Estrogens*	Increased triamcinolone effect.
Ethacrynic acid	Potassium depletion.
Furosemide	Potassium depletion.
Glutethimide	Decreased triamcinolone effect.
Indapamide	Possible excessive potassium loss, causing dangerous heartbeat irregularity.
Indomethacin	Increased triamcinolone effect.
Insulin	Decreased insulin effect.

Continued page 1110

 ## POSSIBLE INTERACTION WITH OTHER SUBSTANCES

INTERACTS WITH	COMBINED EFFECT
Alcohol:	Risk of stomach ulcers.
Beverages:	No proven problems.
Cocaine:	Overstimulation. Avoid.
Foods:	No proven problems.
Marijuana:	Decreased immunity.
Tobacco:	Increased triamcinolone effect. Possible toxicity.

*See Glossary

TRIAMTERENE

BRAND NAMES

Dyazide   **Maxzide**
Dyrenium

BASIC INFORMATION

Habit forming? No
Prescription needed? Yes
Available as generic? No
Drug class: Antihypertensive, diuretic

 ## USES

- Reduces fluid retention (edema).
- Reduces potassium loss.

 ## DOSAGE & USAGE INFORMATION

How to take:
Capsule—Swallow with liquid or food to lessen stomach irritation. If you can't swallow whole, open capsule and take with liquid or food.

When to take:
- 1 dose per day—Take after breakfast.
- More than 1 dose per day—Take last dose no later than 6 p.m.

If you forget a dose:
Take as soon as you remember up to 6 hours late. If more than 6 hours, wait for next scheduled dose (don't double this dose).

What drug does:
Increases urine production to eliminate sodium and water from body while conserving potassium.

Continued next column

 ## OVERDOSE

SYMPTOMS:
Lethargy, nausea, vomiting, hypotension, irregular heartbeat, coma.
WHAT TO DO:
- **Dial 0 (operator) or 911 (emergency) for an ambulance or medical help. Then give first aid immediately.**
- **If patient is unconscious and not breathing, give mouth-to-mouth breathing. If there is no heartbeat, use cardiac massage and mouth-to-mouth breathing (CPR). Don't try to make patient vomit. If you can't get help quickly, take patient to nearest emergency facility.**
- **See emergency information on inside covers.**

Time lapse before drug works:
2 hours. May require 2 to 3 days for maximum benefit.

Don't take with:
See Interaction column and consult doctor.

 ## POSSIBLE ADVERSE REACTIONS OR SIDE EFFECTS

SYMPTOMS	WHAT TO DO
Life-threatening:	
Hives, rash, intense itching, faintness soon after a dose (anaphylaxis).	Seek emergency treatment immediately.
Common:	
None expected.	
Infrequent:	
• Drowsiness, thirst, dry mouth, confusion, irregular heartbeat, shortness of breath, kidney stones, unusual tiredness, weakness.	Discontinue. Call doctor right away.
• Diarrhea.	Continue. Call doctor when convenient.
• Anxiety.	Continue. Tell doctor at next visit.
Rare:	
• Rash, sore throat, fever, red or inflamed tongue, unusual bleeding or bruising.	Discontinue. Call doctor right away.
• Headache.	Continue. Tell doctor at next visit.

WARNINGS & PRECAUTIONS

Don't take if:
- You are allergic to triamterene.
- You have had severe liver or kidney disease.

Before you start, consult your doctor:
- If you have gout, diabetes, kidney stones.
- If you will have surgery within 2 months, including dental surgery, requiring general or spinal anesthesia.

Over age 60:
- Warm weather or fever can decrease blood pressure. Dose may require adjustment.
- Extended use can increase blood clots.

Pregnancy:
No proven harm to unborn child. Avoid if possible.

Breast-feeding:
Present in milk. Avoid.

Infants & children:
Used infrequently. Use only under medical supervision.

Prolonged use:
Potassium retention which may lead to heart-rhythm problems.

Skin & sunlight:
May cause rash or intensify sunburn in areas exposed to sun or sunlamp.

Driving, piloting or hazardous work:
Avoid if you feel drowsy or confused. Otherwise, no problems expected.

Discontinuing:
Don't discontinue without consulting doctor. Dose may require gradual reduction if you have taken drug for a long time. Doses of other drugs may also require adjustment.

Others:
No problems expected.

POSSIBLE INTERACTION WITH OTHER DRUGS

GENERIC NAME OR DRUG CLASS	COMBINED EFFECT
ACE inhibitors: captopril, enalapril, lisinopril*	Possible excessive potassium in blood.
Amiloride	Dangerous retention of potassium.
Amiodarone	Increased risk of heartbeat irregularity due to low potassium.
Antihypertensives, other*	Increased effect of other antihypertensives.
Calcium supplements*	Increased calcium in blood.
Carteolol	Increased antihypertensive effect.
Digitalis preparations*	Possible decreased digitalis effect.
Indomethacin	Possible acute renal failure.
Lithium	Increased lithium effect.
Nicardipine	Blood-pressure drop. Dosages may require adjustment.
Nitrates*	Excessive blood-pressure drop.
Potassium supplements*	Possible excessive potassium retention.
Sotalol	Increased antihypertensive effect.
Spironolactone	Dangerous retention of potassium.
Terazosin	Decreases effectiveness of terazosin.

POSSIBLE INTERACTION WITH OTHER SUBSTANCES

INTERACTS WITH	COMBINED EFFECT
Alcohol:	None expected.
Beverages:	None expected.
Cocaine:	Increased risk of heart block and high blood pressure.
Foods: Salt.	Don't restrict unless directed by doctor.
Marijuana:	Daily use—Fainting likely.
Tobacco:	None expected.

TRIAMTERENE & HYDROCHLOROTHIAZIDE

BRAND NAMES

Apo-Triazide	Maxzide
Dyazide	Novotriamzide

BASIC INFORMATION

Habit forming? No
Prescription needed? Yes
Available as generic? Yes
Drug class: Diuretic

USES

- Reduces fluid retention (edema).
- Reduces potassium loss.
- Controls, but doesn't cure, high blood pressure.

DOSAGE & USAGE INFORMATION

How to take:
Tablet or capsule—Swallow with liquid. If you can't swallow whole, crumble tablet or open capsule and take with liquid or food.

When to take:
- 1 dose per day—Take after breakfast.
- More than 1 dose per day—Take last dose no later than 6 p.m.

If you forget a dose:
Take as soon as you remember up to 6 hours late. If more than 6 hours, wait for next scheduled dose (don't double this dose).

What drug does:
- Increases urine production to eliminate sodium and water from body while conserving potassium.
- Forces sodium and water excretion, reducing body fluid.
- Relaxes muscle cells of small arteries.
- Reduced body fluid and relaxed arteries lower blood pressure.

Continued next column

OVERDOSE

SYMPTOMS:
Lethargy, irregular heartbeat, cramps, nausea, vomiting, hypotension, weakness, drowsiness, weak pulse, coma.
WHAT TO DO:
- **Dial 0 (operator) or 911 (emergency) for an ambulance or medical help. Then give first aid immediately.**
- **See emergency information on inside covers.**

Time lapse before drug works:
4 to 6 hours. May require several weeks to lower blood pressure.

Don't take with:
- Non-prescription drugs without consulting doctor.
- See Interaction column and consult doctor.

POSSIBLE ADVERSE REACTIONS OR SIDE EFFECTS

SYMPTOMS	WHAT TO DO
Life-threatening: Irregular heartbeat, weak pulse, shortness of breath; hives, rash, intense itching, faintness soon after a dose (anaphylaxis).	Discontinue. Seek emergency treatment.
Common:	
• Mood change, muscle cramps.	Discontinue. Call doctor right away.
• Numbness or tingling in hands or feet.	Continue. Call doctor when convenient.
Infrequent:	
• Blurred vision, abdominal pain, nausea, vomiting, kidney stones.	Discontinue. Call doctor right away.
• Dizziness, mood change, headache, dry mouth, weakness, tiredness, weight gain or loss.	Continue. Call doctor when convenient.
Rare:	
• Sore throat, fever, mouth sores; jaundice; rash; joint or muscle pain; hives; unexplained bleeding or bruising.	Discontinue. Call doctor right away.
• Corners of mouth cracked, weakness.	Continue. Call doctor when convenient.

WARNINGS & PRECAUTIONS

Don't take if:
- If you are allergic to triamterene or any thiazide diuretic drug.
- If you have had severe liver or kidney disease.

Before you start, consult your doctor:
- If you have gout, diabetes, liver, pancreas or kidney disorder.
- You are allergic to any sulfa drug.
- If you will have surgery within 2 months, including dental surgery, requiring general or spinal anesthesia.

TRIAMTERENE & HYDROCHLOROTHIAZIDE

Over age 60:
- Adverse reactions and side effects may be more frequent and severe than in younger persons, especially dizziness and excessive potassium loss.
- Warm weather or fever can decrease blood pressure. Dose may require adjustment.
- Extended use can increase blood clots.

Pregnancy:
Risk to unborn child outweighs drug benefits. Don't use.

Breast-feeding:
Drug passes into milk. Avoid drug or discontinue nursing until you finish medicine. Consult doctor for advice on maintaining milk supply.

Infants & children:
Used infrequently. Use only under medical supervision.

Prolonged use:
Potassium retention which may lead to heart-rhythm problems.

Skin & sunlight:
May cause rash or intensify sunburn in areas exposed to sun or sunlamp.

Driving, piloting or hazardous work:
Don't drive or pilot aircraft until you learn how medicine affects you. Don't work around dangerous machinery. Don't climb ladders or work in high places. Danger increases if you drink alcohol or take medicine affecting alertness and reflexes, such as antihistamines, tranquilizers, sedatives, pain medicine, narcotics and mind-altering drugs.

Discontinuing:
Don't discontinue without consulting doctor. Dose may require gradual reduction if you have taken drug for a long time. Doses of other drugs may also require adjustment.

Others:
- Hot weather and fever may cause dehydration and drop in blood pressure. Dose may require temporary adjustment. Weigh daily and report any unexpected weight decreases to your doctor.
- May cause rise in uric acid, leading to gout.
- May cause blood-sugar rise in diabetics.

POSSIBLE INTERACTION WITH OTHER DRUGS

GENERIC NAME OR DRUG CLASS	COMBINED EFFECT
ACE inhibitors: captopril, enalapril, lisinopril*	Decreased blood pressure.
Allopurinol	Decreased allopurinol effect.
Amiloride	Dangerous retention of potassium.
Amphotericin B	Increased potassium.
Antidepressants*	Dangerous drop in blood pressure. Avoid combination unless under medical supervision.
Antihypertensives*	Increased hypertensive effect.
Barbiturates*	Increased hydro-chlorothiazide effect.
Beta-adrenergic blockers*	Increased antihyper-tensive effect. Dosages of both drugs may require adjustment.
Cholestyramine	Decreased hydro-chlorothiazide effect.
Cortisone drugs*	Excessive potassium loss that causes dangerous heart rhythms.
Digitalis preparations*	Excessive potassium loss that causes dangerous heart rhythms.
Diuretics, thiazide*	Increased effect of other thiazide diuretics.
Indapamide	Increased diuretic effect.

Continued page 1110

POSSIBLE INTERACTION WITH OTHER SUBSTANCES

INTERACTS WITH	COMBINED EFFECT
Alcohol:	Dangerous blood-pressure drop.
Beverages:	None expected.
Cocaine:	Decreased triamterene effect.
Foods: Salt.	Don't restrict unless directed by doctor.
Marijuana:	Daily use—Fainting likely.
Tobacco:	Decreases drug's effectiveness.

*See Glossary

TRIAZOLAM

BRAND NAMES

Halcion

BASIC INFORMATION

Habit forming? Yes
Prescription needed? Yes
Available as generic? No
Drug class: Tranquilizer (benzodiazepine)

 ## USES

Treatment of insomnia. Not recommended for more than 2 weeks maximum.

 ## DOSAGE & USAGE INFORMATION

How to take:
Tablet—Swallow with liquid. If you can't swallow whole, crumble tablet and take with liquid or food.

When to take:
At the same time each day, according to instructions on prescription label.

If you forget a dose:
Take as soon as you remember up to 2 hours late. If more than 2 hours, wait for next scheduled dose (don't double this dose).

What drug does:
Affects limbic system, the part of the brain that controls emotions.

Time lapse before drug works:
2 hours. May take 6 weeks for full benefit.

Don't take with:
See Interaction column and consult doctor.

 ## OVERDOSE

SYMPTOMS:
Drowsiness, weakness, tremor, stupor, coma.
WHAT TO DO:
- **Dial 0 (operator) or 911 (emergency) for an ambulance or medical help. Then give first aid immediately.**
- **If patient is unconscious and not breathing, give mouth-to-mouth breathing. If there is no heartbeat, use cardiac massage and mouth-to-mouth breathing (CPR). Don't try to make patient vomit. If you can't get help quickly, take patient to nearest emergency facility.**
- **See emergency information on inside covers.**

 ## POSSIBLE ADVERSE REACTIONS OR SIDE EFFECTS

SYMPTOMS	WHAT TO DO
Life-threatening: None expected.	
Common: Clumsiness, dizziness, drowsiness.	Continue. Call doctor when convenient.
Infrequent: • Hallucinations, confusion, irritability, depression, rash, itchy skin, change in vision.	Discontinue. Call doctor right away.
• Constipation or diarrhea, nausea, vomiting, difficult urination.	Continue. Call doctor when convenient.
Rare: • Slow heartbeat, difficult breathing.	Discontinue. Seek emergency treatment.
• Mouth or throat ulcers, jaundice.	Discontinue. Call doctor right away.

TRIAZOLAM

WARNINGS & PRECAUTIONS

Don't take if:
- You are allergic to any benzodiazepine.
- You have myasthenia gravis.
- You are active or recovering alcoholic.
- Patient is younger than 6 months.

Before you start, consult your doctor:
- If you have liver, kidney or lung disease.
- If you have diabetes, epilepsy or porphyria.
- If you will have surgery within 2 months, including dental surgery, requiring general or spinal anesthesia.

Over age 60:
Adverse reactions and side effects may be more frequent and severe than in younger persons. You need smaller doses for shorter periods of time. May develop agitation, rage or "hangover" effect.

Pregnancy:
Risk to unborn child outweighs drug benefits. Don't use.

Breast-feeding:
Drug passes into milk. Avoid drug or discontinue nursing until you finish medicine. Consult doctor for advice on maintaining milk supply.

Infants & children:
Use only under medical supervision for children older than 6 months.

Prolonged use:
May impair liver function.

Skin & sunlight:
No problems expected.

Driving, piloting or hazardous work:
Don't drive or pilot aircraft until you learn how medicine affects you. Don't work around dangerous machinery. Don't climb ladders or work in high places. Danger increases if you drink alcohol or take medicine affecting alertness and reflexes.

Discontinuing:
Don't discontinue without consulting doctor. Dose may require gradual reduction if you have taken drug for a long time. Doses of other drugs may also require adjustment.

Others:
- Hot weather, heavy exercise and profuse sweat may reduce excretion and cause overdose.
- Blood sugar may rise in diabetics, requiring insulin adjustment.

POSSIBLE INTERACTION WITH OTHER DRUGS

GENERIC NAME OR DRUG CLASS	COMBINED EFFECT
Anticonvulsants*	Change in seizure frequency or severity.
Antidepressants*	Increased sedative effect of both drugs.
Antihistamines*	Increased sedative effect of both drugs.
Antihypertensives*	Excessively low blood pressure.
Cimetidine	Excess sedation.
Disulfiram	Increased triazolam effect.
Dronabinol	Increased effects of both drugs. Avoid.
MAO inhibitors*	Convulsions, deep sedation, rage.
Molindone	Increased sedative effect.
Nabilone	Greater depression of central nervous system.
Narcotics*	Increased sedative effect of both drugs.
Sedatives*	Increased sedative effect of both drugs.
Sleep inducers*	Increased sedative effect of both drugs.
Tranquilizers*	Increased sedative effect of both drugs.

POSSIBLE INTERACTION WITH OTHER SUBSTANCES

INTERACTS WITH	COMBINED EFFECT
Alcohol:	Heavy sedation. Avoid.
Beverages:	None expected.
Cocaine:	Decreased triazolam effect.
Foods:	None expected.
Marijuana:	Heavy sedation. Avoid.
Tobacco:	Decreased triazolam effect.

*See Glossary

1005

TRICHLORMETHIAZIDE

BRAND NAMES

Metahydrin
Metatensin

Naqua
Naquival

BASIC INFORMATION

Habit forming? No
Prescription needed? Yes
Available as generic? Yes
Drug class: Antihypertensive, diuretic (thiazide)

 ## USES

- Controls, but doesn't cure, high blood pressure.
- Reduces fluid retention (edema) caused by conditions such as heart disorders and liver disease.

 ## DOSAGE & USAGE INFORMATION

How to take:
Tablet—Swallow with liquid. If you can't swallow whole, crumble tablet and take with liquid or food. Don't exceed dose.

When to take:
At the same time each day.

If you forget a dose:
Take as soon as you remember up to 2 hours late. If more than 2 hours, wait for next scheduled dose (don't double this dose).

What drug does:
- Forces sodium and water excretion, reducing body fluid.
- Relaxes muscle cells of small arteries.
- Reduced body fluid and relaxed arteries lower blood pressure.

Time lapse before drug works:
4 to 6 hours. May require several weeks to lower blood pressure.

Continued next column

 ## OVERDOSE

SYMPTOMS:
Cramps, weakness, drowsiness, weak pulse, coma.
WHAT TO DO:
- Dial 0 (operator) or 911 (emergency) for an ambulance or medical help. Then give first aid immediately.
- See emergency information on inside covers.

Don't take with:
- Non-prescription drugs without consulting doctor.
- See Interaction column and consult doctor.

 ## POSSIBLE ADVERSE REACTIONS OR SIDE EFFECTS

SYMPTOMS	WHAT TO DO
Life-threatening: None expected.	
Common: None expected.	
Infrequent:	
• Blurred vision, severe abdominal pain, nausea, vomiting, irregular heartbeat, weak pulse, sore throat, fever.	Discontinue. Call doctor right away.
• Dizziness, mood change, headache, weakness, tiredness, weight changes.	Continue. Call doctor when convenient.
• Dry mouth, thirst.	Continue. Tell doctor at next visit.
Rare:	
• Rash or hives.	Discontinue. Seek emergency treatment.
• Jaundice.	Discontinue. Call doctor right away.

 ## WARNINGS & PRECAUTIONS

Don't take if:
You are allergic to any thiazide diuretic drug.

Before you start, consult your doctor:
- If you are allergic to any sulfa drug.
- If you have gout.
- If you have liver, pancreas or kidney disorder.

Over age 60:
Adverse reactions and side effects may be more frequent and severe than in younger persons, especially dizziness and excessive potassium loss.

Pregnancy:
Risk to unborn child outweighs drug benefits. Don't use.

Breast-feeding:
Drug passes into milk. Avoid drug or discontinue nursing.

Infants & children:
No problems expected.

Prolonged use:
You may need medicine to treat high blood pressure for the rest of your life.

Skin & sunlight:
May cause rash or intensify sunburn in areas exposed to sun or sunlamp.

Driving, piloting or hazardous work:
Don't drive or pilot aircraft until you learn how medicine affects you. Don't work around dangerous machinery. Don't climb ladders or work in high places. Danger increases if you drink alcohol or take medicine affecting alertness and reflexes, such as antihistamines, tranquilizers, sedatives, pain medicine, narcotics and mind-altering drugs.

Discontinuing:
Don't discontinue without medical advice.

Others:
- Hot weather and fever may cause dehydration and drop in blood pressure. Dose may require temporary adjustment. Weigh daily and report any unexpected weight decreases to your doctor.
- May cause rise in uric acid, leading to gout.
- May cause blood-sugar rise in diabetics.

POSSIBLE INTERACTION WITH OTHER DRUGS

GENERIC NAME OR DRUG CLASS	COMBINED EFFECT
ACE inhibitors: captopril, enalapril, lisinopril*	Decreased blood pressure. Possible excessive potassium in blood.
Allopurinol	Decreased allopurinol effect.
Amiodarone	Increased risk of heartbeat irregularity due to low potassium.
Amphotericin B	Increased potassium.
Antidepressants, tricyclic (TCA)*	Dangerous drop in blood pressure. Avoid combination unless under medical supervision.
Antidiabetic agents, oral*	Increased blood sugar.
Antihypertensives*	Increased hypertensive effect.
Barbiturates*	Increased trichlormethiazide effect.
Beta-adrenergic blockers*	Increased antihypertensive effect. Dosages of both drugs may require adjustment.
Calcium supplements*	Increased calcium in blood.
Carteolol	Increased antihypertensive effect.
Cholestyramine	Decreased trichlormethiazide effect.
Colestipol	Decreased trichlormethiazide effect.
Cortisone drugs*	Excessive potassium loss that causes dangerous heart rhythms.
Digitalis preparations*	Excessive potassium loss that causes dangerous heart rhythms.
Diuretics, thiazide*	Increased effect of other thiazide diuretics.
Indapamide	Increased diuretic effect.
Indomethacin	Decreased trichlormethiazide effect.
Lithium	Increased effect of lithium.
MAO inhibitors*	Increased trichlormethiazide effect.
Nicardipine	Blood-pressure drop. Dosages may require adjustment.
Nitrates*	Excessive blood-pressure drop.
Opiates*	Weakness and faintness when arising from bed or chair.

Continued page 1110

POSSIBLE INTERACTION WITH OTHER SUBSTANCES

INTERACTS WITH	COMBINED EFFECT
Alcohol:	Dangerous blood-pressure drop.
Beverages:	None expected.
Cocaine:	Increased risk of heart block and high blood pressure.
Foods: Licorice.	Excessive potassium loss that causes dangerous heart rhythms.
Marijuana:	May increase blood pressure.
Tobacco:	None expected.

*See Glossary

1007

TRICYCLIC ANTIDEPRESSANTS

BRAND NAMES

See complete list of brand names in the *Brand Name Directory*, page 1072.

BASIC INFORMATION

Habit forming? No
Prescription needed? Yes
Available as generic? Yes
Drug class: Antidepressant (tricyclic)

 ## USES

- Gradually relieves, but doesn't cure, symptoms of depression.
- Imipramine is also used to decrease bedwetting.
- Pain relief (sometimes).

 ## DOSAGE & USAGE INFORMATION

How to take:
Tablet, capsule or syrup—Swallow with liquid.

When to take:
At the same time each day, usually at bedtime.

If you forget a dose:
Bedtime dose—If you forget your once-a-day bedtime dose, don't take it more than 3 hours late. If more than 3 hours, wait for next scheduled dose. Don't double this dose.

What drug does:
Probably affects part of brain that controls messages between nerve cells.

Time lapse before drug works:
Begins in 1 to 2 weeks. May require 4 to 6 weeks for maximum benefit.

Continued next column

 ## OVERDOSE

SYMPTOMS:
Hallucinations, respiratory failure, fever, cardiac arrhythmias, convulsions, coma.
WHAT TO DO:
- **Dial 0 (operator) or 911 (emergency) for an ambulance or medical help. Then give first aid immediately.**
- **If patient is unconscious and not breathing, give mouth-to-mouth breathing. If there is no heartbeat, use cardiac massage and mouth-to-mouth breathing (CPR). Don't try to make patient vomit. If you can't get help quickly, take patient to nearest emergency facility.**
- **See emergency information on inside covers.**

Don't take with:
- Non-prescription drugs without consulting doctor.
- See Interaction column and consult doctor.

 ## POSSIBLE ADVERSE REACTIONS OR SIDE EFFECTS

SYMPTOMS	WHAT TO DO
Life-threatening:	
Seizures.	Seek emergency treatment immediately.
Common:	
• Tremor.	Discontinue. Call doctor right away.
• Headache, dry mouth or unpleasant taste, constipation or diarrhea, nausea, indigestion, fatigue, weakness, drowsiness, nervousness, anxiety, excessive sweating.	Continue. Call doctor when convenient.
• Insomnia, "sweet tooth."	Continue. Tell doctor at next visit.
Infrequent:	
• Convulsions.	Discontinue. Seek emergency treatment.
• Hallucinations, shakiness, dizziness, fainting, blurred vision, eye pain, vomiting, irregular heartbeat or slow pulse, inflamed tongue, abdominal pain, jaundice, hair loss, rash, fever, chills, joint pain, palpitations, hiccups, visual changes.	Discontinue. Call doctor right away.
• Difficult or frequent urination; decreased, libido; muscle aches; abnormal dreams; nasal congestion; weakness and faintness when arising from bed or chair; back pain; absent, painful or heavy menstruation.	Continue. Call doctor when convenient.
Rare:	
Itchy skin; sore throat; involuntary movements of jaw, lips and tongue; nightmares; confusion; swollen breasts in males; decreased potassium by blood test.	Discontinue. Call doctor right away.

WARNINGS & PRECAUTIONS

Don't take if:
- You are allergic to any tricyclic antidepressant.
- You drink alcohol.
- You have had a heart attack within 6 weeks.
- You have glaucoma.
- You have taken MAO inhibitors within 2 weeks.
- Patient is younger than 12.

Before you start, consult your doctor:
- If you will have surgery within 2 months, including dental surgery, requiring general or spinal anesthesia.
- If you have an enlarged prostate.
- If you have heart disease or high blood pressure.
- If you have stomach or intestinal problems.
- If you have an overactive thyroid.
- If you have asthma.
- If you have liver disease.

Over age 60:
More likely to develop urination difficulty and side effects such as seizures, hallucinations, shaking, dizziness, fainting, headache, insomnia.

Pregnancy:
Studies inconclusive on harm to unborn child. Animal studies show fetal abnormalities. Decide with your doctor whether drug benefits justify risk to unborn child.

Breast-feeding:
Drug passes into milk. Avoid drug or discontinue nursing until you finish medicine. Consult doctor about maintaining milk supply.

Infants & children:
Don't give to children younger than 12.

Prolonged use:
No problems expected.

Skin & sunlight:
May cause rash or intensify sunburn in areas exposed to sun or sunlamp.

Driving, piloting or hazardous work:
Don't drive or pilot aircraft until you learn how medicine affects you. Don't work around dangerous machinery. Don't climb ladders or work in high places. Danger increases if you drink alcohol or take medicine affecting alertness and reflexes.

Discontinuing:
Don't discontinue without consulting doctor. Dose may require gradual reduction if you have taken drug for a long time. Doses of other drugs may also require adjustment.

Others:
No problems expected.

POSSIBLE INTERACTION WITH OTHER DRUGS

GENERIC NAME OR DRUG CLASS	COMBINED EFFECT
Anticoagulants, oral*	Possible increased anticoagulant effect.
Anticholinergics*	Increased anticholinergic effect.
Antihistamines*	Increased antihistamine effect.
Barbiturates*	Decreased antidepressant effect. Increased sedation.
Benzodiazepines*	Increased sedation.
Cimetidine	Possible increased tricyclic antidepressant effect and toxicity.
Clonidine	Possible decreased clonidine effect.
Disulfiram	Delirium.
Ethchlorvynol	Delirium.
Ethinamate	Dangerous increased effects of ethinamate. Avoid combining.
Fluoxetine	Increased depressant effects of both drugs.
Guanabenz	Decreased guanabenz effect.
Guanethidine	Decreased guanethidine effect.

Continued page 1111

POSSIBLE INTERACTION WITH OTHER SUBSTANCES

INTERACTS WITH	COMBINED EFFECT
Alcohol: Beverages or medicines with alcohol.	Excessive intoxication. Avoid.
Beverages:	None expected.
Cocaine:	Increased risk of heartbeat irregularity.
Foods:	None expected.
Marijuana:	Excessive drowsiness. Avoid.
Tobacco:	Possible decreased tricyclic antidepressant effect.

*See Glossary

TRIDIHEXETHYL

BRAND NAMES

Milpath   Pathilon
Pathibamate

BASIC INFORMATION

Habit forming? No
Prescription needed?
  Low strength: No
  High strength: Yes
Available as generic? No
Drug class: Antispasmodic, anticholinergic

USES

Reduces spasms of digestive system, bladder
and urethra.

DOSAGE & USAGE INFORMATION

How to take:
Tablet—Swallow with liquid or food to lessen
stomach irritation.

When to take:
30 minutes before meals (unless directed
otherwise by doctor).

If you forget a dose:
Take as soon as you remember up to 2 hours
late. If more than 2 hours, wait for next
scheduled dose (don't double this dose).

What drug does:
Blocks nerve impulses at parasympathetic nerve
endings, preventing muscle contractions and
gland secretions of organs involved.

Time lapse before drug works:
15 to 30 minutes.

Don't take with:
See Interaction column and consult doctor.

OVERDOSE

SYMPTOMS:
Dilated pupils, blurred vision, rapid pulse
and breathing, dizziness, fever,
hallucinations, confusion, slurred speech,
agitation, flushed face, convulsions, coma.
WHAT TO DO:
- Dial 0 (operator) or 911 (emergency) for
  an ambulance or medical help. Then give
  first aid immediately.
- See emergency information on inside
  covers.

POSSIBLE ADVERSE REACTIONS OR SIDE EFFECTS

SYMPTOMS	WHAT TO DO
Life-threatening:	
Hives, rash, intense itching, faintness soon after a dose (anaphylaxis).	Seek emergency treatment immediately.
Common:	
• Confusion, delirium, rapid heartbeat.	Discontinue. Call doctor right away.
• Nausea, vomiting, decreased sweating.	Continue. Call doctor when convenient.
• Constipation, loss of taste.	Continue. Tell doctor at next visit.
• Dryness in ears, nose, throat.	No action necessary.
Infrequent:	
Difficult urination, headache.	Continue. Call doctor when convenient.
Rare:	
Rash or hives, pain, blurred vision.	Discontinue. Call doctor right away.

WARNINGS & PRECAUTIONS

Don't take if:
- You are allergic to any anticholinergic.
- You have trouble with stomach bloating.
- You have difficulty emptying your bladder
  completely.
- You have narrow-angle glaucoma.
- You have severe ulcerative colitis.

Before you start, consult your doctor:
- If you have open-angle glaucoma.
- If you have angina.
- If you have chronic bronchitis or asthma.
- If you have hiatal hernia.
- If you have liver disease.
- If you have enlarged prostate.
- If you have myasthenia gravis.
- If you have peptic ulcer.
- If you will have surgery within 2 months,
  including dental surgery, requiring general or
  spinal anesthesia.

Over age 60:
Adverse reactions and side effects may be more
frequent and severe than in younger persons.

Pregnancy:
Studies inconclusive on harm to unborn child.
Animal studies show fetal abnormalities. Decide
with your doctor whether drug benefits justify
risk to unborn child.

Breast-feeding:
Drug passes into milk and decreases milk flow. Avoid drug or discontinue nursing until you finish medicine. Consult doctor for advice on maintaining milk supply.

Infants & children:
Use only under medical supervision.

Prolonged use:
Chronic constipation, possible fecal impaction. Consult doctor immediately.

Skin & sunlight:
No problems expected.

Driving, piloting or hazardous work:
Use disqualifies you for piloting aircraft. Otherwise, no problems expected.

Discontinuing:
May be unnecessary to finish medicine. Follow doctor's instructions.

Others:
No problems expected.

POSSIBLE INTERACTION WITH OTHER DRUGS

GENERIC NAME OR DRUG CLASS	COMBINED EFFECT
Amantadine	Increased tridihexethyl effect.
Antacids*	Decreased tridihexethyl effect.
Anticholinergics, other*	Increased tridihexethyl effect.
Antidepressants, tricyclic (TCA)*	Increased tridihexethyl effect. Increased sedation.
Antihistamines*	Increased tridihexethyl effect.
Buclizine	Increased tridihexethyl effect.
Cortisone drugs*	Increased internal-eye pressure.
Digitalis	Possible decreased absorption of digitalis.
Haloperidol	Increased internal-eye pressure.
MAO inhibitors*	Increased tridihexethyl effect.
Meperidine	Increased tridihexethyl effect.
Methylphenidate	Increased tridihexethyl effect.

Nitrates*	Increased internal-eye pressure.
Nizatidine	Increased nizatidine effect.
Orphenadrine	Increased tridihexethyl effect.
Phenothiazines*	Increased tridihexethyl effect.
Pilocarpine	Loss of pilocarpine effect in glaucoma treatment.
Potassium supplements*	Possible intestinal ulcers with oral potassium tablets.
Quinidine	Increased tridihexethyl effect.
Vitamin C	Decreased tridihexethyl effect. Avoid large doses of vitamin C.

POSSIBLE INTERACTION WITH OTHER SUBSTANCES

INTERACTS WITH	COMBINED EFFECT
Alcohol:	None expected.
Beverages:	None expected.
Cocaine:	Excessively rapid heartbeat. Avoid.
Foods:	None expected.
Marijuana:	Drowsiness and dry mouth.
Tobacco:	None expected.

*See Glossary

TRIFLUOPERAZINE

BRAND NAMES

Apo-Trifluoperazine	Stelazine
Clinazine	Suprazine
Novoflurazine	Terfluzine
Pentazine	Triflurin
Solazine	Tripazine

BASIC INFORMATION

Habit forming? No
Prescription needed? Yes
Available as generic? Yes
Drug class: Tranquilizer, antiemetic (phenothiazine)

USES

- Stops nausea, vomiting, hiccups.
- Reduces anxiety, agitation.

DOSAGE & USAGE INFORMATION

How to take:
- Tablet—Swallow with liquid or food to lessen stomach irritation.
- Drops or liquid—Dilute dose in beverage.

When to take:
- Nervous and mental disorders—Take at the same times each day.
- Nausea and vomiting—Take as needed, no more often than every 4 hours.

If you forget a dose:
- Nervous and mental disorders—Take up to 2 hours late. If more than 2 hours, wait for next scheduled dose (don't double this dose).
- Nausea and vomiting—Take as soon as you remember. Wait 4 hours for next dose.

What drug does:
- Suppresses brain's vomiting center.
- Suppresses brain centers that control abnormal emotions and behavior.

Continued next column

OVERDOSE

SYMPTOMS:
Stupor, convulsions, coma.
WHAT TO DO:
- Dial 0 (operator) or 911 (emergency) for an ambulance or medical help. Then give first aid immediately.
- See emergency information on inside covers.

Time lapse before drug works:
- Nausea and vomiting—1 hour or less.
- Nervous and mental disorders—4-6 weeks.

Don't take with:
- Antacid or medicine for diarrhea.
- Non-prescription drug for cough, cold or allergy.
- See Interaction column and consult doctor.

POSSIBLE ADVERSE REACTIONS OR SIDE EFFECTS

SYMPTOMS	WHAT TO DO
Life-threatening:	
Uncontrolled muscle movements of tongue, face and other muscles (neuroleptic malignant syndrome, rare).	Discontinue. Seek emergency treatment.
Common:	
• Muscle spasms of face and neck, unsteady gait.	Discontinue. Seek emergency treatment.
• Restlessness, tremor, drowsiness.	Discontinue. Call doctor right away.
• Decreased sweating, dry mouth, nasal congestion, constipation.	Continue. Call doctor when convenient.
Infrequent:	
• Fainting.	Discontinue. Seek emergency treatment.
• Rash.	Discontinue. Call doctor right away.
• Difficult urination, less interest in sex, swollen breasts, menstrual irregularities.	Continue. Call doctor when convenient.
Rare:	
Change in vision, sore throat, fever, jaundice, abdominal pain.	Discontinue. Call doctor right away.

WARNINGS & PRECAUTIONS

Don't take if:
- You are allergic to any phenothiazine.
- You have a blood or bone-marrow disease.

Before you start, consult your doctor:
- If you will have surgery within 2 months, including dental surgery, requiring general or spinal anesthesia.
- If you have asthma, emphysema or other lung disorder, glaucoma, prostate trouble.
- If you take non-prescription ulcer medicine, asthma medicine or amphetamines.

Over age 60:
Adverse reactions and side effects may be more frequent and severe than in younger persons. More likely to develop involuntary movement of jaws, lips, tongue, chewing. Report this to your doctor immediately. Early treatment can help.

Pregnancy:
Risk to unborn child outweighs drug benefits. Don't use.

Breast-feeding:
Drug passes into milk. Avoid drug or discontinue nursing until you finish medicine. Consult doctor for advice on maintaining milk supply.

Infants & children:
Don't give to children younger than 2.

Prolonged use:
May lead to tardive dyskinesia (involuntary movement of jaws, lips, tongue, chewing).

Skin & sunlight:
May cause rash or intensify sunburn in areas exposed to sun or sunlamp. Skin may remain sensitive for 3 months after discontinuing.

Driving, piloting or hazardous work:
Don't drive or pilot aircraft until you learn how medicine affects you. Don't work around dangerous machinery. Don't climb ladders or work in high places. Danger increases if you drink alcohol or take medicine affecting alertness and reflexes.

Discontinuing:
- Nervous and mental disorders—Don't discontinue without doctor's advice until you complete prescribed dose, even though symptoms diminish or disappear.
- Nausea and vomiting—May be unnecessary to finish medicine. Follow doctor's instructions.

Others:
No problems expected.

POSSIBLE INTERACTION WITH OTHER DRUGS

GENERIC NAME OR DRUG CLASS	COMBINED EFFECT
Anticholinergics*	Increased anticholinergic effect.
Antidepressants, tricyclic (TCA)*	Increased trifluoperazine effect.
Antihistamines*	Increased antihistamine effect.
Appetite suppressants*	Decreased suppressant effect.
Dronabinol	Increased effects of both drugs. Avoid.
Guanethidine	Decreased guanethidine effect.
Levodopa	Decreased levodopa effect.
Mind-altering drugs*	Increased effect of mind-altering drugs.
Molindone	Increased tranquilizer effect.
Nabilone	Greater depression of central nervous system.
Narcotics*	Increased narcotic effect.
Phenytoin	Increased phenytoin effect.
Procarbazine	Increased sedation.
Quinidine	Impaired heart function. Dangerous mixture.
Sedatives*	Increased sedation.
Tranquilizers, other*	Increased tranquilizer effect.

POSSIBLE INTERACTION WITH OTHER SUBSTANCES

INTERACTS WITH	COMBINED EFFECT
Alcohol:	Dangerous oversedation.
Beverages:	None expected.
Cocaine:	Decreased trifluoperazine effect. Avoid.
Foods:	None expected.
Marijuana:	Drowsiness. May increase antinausea effect.
Tobacco:	None expected.

TRIHEXYPHENIDYL

BRAND NAMES

Aparkane	T.H.P.
Apo-Trihex	Tremin
Artane	Trihexane
Artane Sequels	Trihexidyl
Novohexidyl	Trihexy

BASIC INFORMATION

Habit forming? No
Prescription needed? Yes
Available as generic? Yes
Drug class: Antidyskinetic, antiparkinsonism

USES

- Treatment of Parkinson's disease.
- Treatment of adverse effects of phenothiazines.

DOSAGE & USAGE INFORMATION

How to take:
Extended-release capsule or elixir—Take with food to lessen stomach irritation.

When to take:
At the same times each day.

If you forget a dose:
Take as soon as you remember up to 2 hours late. If more than 2 hours, wait for next scheduled dose (don't double this dose).

What drug does:
- Balances chemical reactions necessary to send nerve impulses within base of brain.
- Improves muscle control and reduces stiffness.

Continued next column

OVERDOSE

SYMPTOMS:
Agitation, dilated pupils, hallucinations, dry mouth, rapid heartbeat, sleepiness.
WHAT TO DO:
- Dial 0 (operator) or 911 (emergency) for an ambulance or medical help. Then give first aid immediately.
- If patient is unconscious and not breathing, give mouth-to-mouth breathing. If there is no heartbeat, use cardiac massage and mouth-to-mouth breathing (CPR). Don't try to make patient vomit. If you can't get help quickly, take patient to nearest emergency facility.
- See emergency information on inside covers.

Time lapse before drug works:
1 to 2 hours.

Don't take with:
- Non-prescription drugs for colds, cough or allergy.
- See Interaction column and consult doctor.

POSSIBLE ADVERSE REACTIONS OR SIDE EFFECTS

SYMPTOMS	WHAT TO DO
Life-threatening: None expected.	
Common:	
• Blurred vision, light sensitivity, constipation, nausea, vomiting.	Continue. Call doctor when convenient.
• Painful or difficult urination, dry mouth.	Continue. Tell doctor at next visit.
Infrequent: None expected.	
Rare:	
• Rash, eye pain, hives, delusions, hallucinations, amnesia, paranoia, fever, swollen neck glands, weakness and faintness when arising from bed or chair.	Discontinue. Call doctor right away.
• Confusion, dizziness, sore mouth or tongue, muscle cramps, numbness or tingling in hands or feet.	Continue. Call doctor when convenient.

WARNINGS & PRECAUTIONS

Don't take if:
You are allergic to any antidyskinetic.

Before you start, consult your doctor:
- If you have had glaucoma.
- If you have had high blood pressure or heart disease.
- If you have had impaired liver function.
- If you have had kidney disease or urination difficulty.

Over age 60:
More sensitive to drug. Aggravates symptoms of enlarged prostate. Causes impaired thinking, hallucinations, nightmares. Consult doctor about any of these.

Pregnancy:
Studies inconclusive on harm to unborn child. Animal studies show fetal abnormalities. Decide with your doctor whether drug benefits justify risk to unborn child.

Breast-feeding:
No problems expected.

Infants & children:
Not recommended for children 3 and younger. Use for older children only under doctor's supervision.

Prolonged use:
Possible glaucoma.

Skin & sunlight:
No problems expected.

Driving, piloting or hazardous work:
Don't drive or pilot aircraft until you learn how medicine affects you. Don't work around dangerous machinery. Don't climb ladders or work in high places. Danger increases if you drink alcohol or take medicine affecting alertness and reflexes, such as antihistamines, tranquilizers, sedatives, pain medicine, narcotics and mind-altering drugs.

Discontinuing:
Don't discontinue without consulting doctor. Dose may require gradual reduction if you have taken drug for a long time. Doses of other drugs may also require adjustment.

Others:
- Internal eye pressure should be measured regularly.
- Avoid becoming overheated.

POSSIBLE INTERACTION WITH OTHER DRUGS

GENERIC NAME OR DRUG CLASS	COMBINED EFFECT
Amantadine	Increased amantadine effect.
Antacids*	Possible decreased absorption.
Anticholinergics, others*	Increased anti-cholinergic effect.
Antidepressants, tricyclic (TCA)*	Increased trihexyphenidyl effect. May cause glaucoma.
Antihistamines	Increased trihexyphenidyl effect.
Digoxin	Possible increased toxicity of digoxin.
Disopyramide	Increased anti-cholinergic effect.
Haloperidol	Possible behavior changes.
Levodopa	Possible increased levodopa effect.
MAO inhibitors*	Increased trihexyphenidyl effect.
Meperidine	Increased trihexyphenidyl effect.
Nabilone	Greater depression of central nervous system.
Phenothiazines*	Behavior changes.
Primidone	Excessive sedation.
Quinidine	Increased trihexyphenidyl effect.
Slow-k (extended-release potassium)	Increased risk of gastric irritation.
Tranquilizers*	Excessive sedation.

POSSIBLE INTERACTION WITH OTHER SUBSTANCES

INTERACTS WITH	COMBINED EFFECT
Alcohol:	None expected.
Beverages:	None expected.
Cocaine:	Decreased trihexyphenidyl effect. Avoid.
Foods:	None expected.
Marijuana:	None expected.
Tobacco:	None expected.

*See Glossary

TRIMEPRAZINE

BRAND NAMES

Panectyl   Temaril

BASIC INFORMATION

Habit forming? No
Prescription needed? Yes
Available as generic? Yes
Drug class: Tranquilizer (phenothiazine),
   antihistamine

USES

Relieves itching of hives, skin allergies,
chickenpox.

DOSAGE & USAGE INFORMATION

How to take:
- Tablet or syrup—Swallow with liquid or food to
lessen stomach irritation.
- Extended-release capsules—Swallow each
dose whole. If you take regular tablets, you
may chew or crush them.

When to take:
At the same times each day.

If you forget a dose:
Take as soon as you remember up to 2 hours
late. If more than 2 hours, wait for next
scheduled dose (don't double this dose).

What drug does:
Blocks histamine action in skin.

Time lapse before drug works:
1 to 2 hours.

Don't take with:
- Antacid or medicine for diarrhea.
- Non-prescription drug for cough, cold or
allergy.
- See Interaction column and consult doctor.

OVERDOSE

SYMPTOMS:
Stupor, convulsions, coma.
WHAT TO DO:
- Dial 0 (operator) or 911 (emergency) for
an ambulance or medical help. Then give
first aid immediately.
- See emergency information on inside
covers.

POSSIBLE ADVERSE REACTIONS OR SIDE EFFECTS

SYMPTOMS	WHAT TO DO
Life-threatening: None expected.	
Common:	
• Restlessness, tremor, drowsiness.	Discontinue. Call doctor right away.
• Decreased sweating, dry mouth, nasal congestion, constipation.	Continue. Call doctor when convenient.
Infrequent:	
• Fainting.	Discontinue. Seek emergency treatment.
• Rash, muscle spasms of face and neck, unsteady gait.	Discontinue. Call doctor right away.
• Difficult urination, less interest in sex, swollen breasts, menstrual irregularities.	Continue. Call doctor when convenient.
Rare:	
Change in vision, sore throat, fever, jaundice.	Discontinue. Call doctor right away.

WARNINGS & PRECAUTIONS

Don't take if:
- You are allergic to any phenothiazine.
- You have a blood or bone-marrow disease.

Before you start, consult your doctor:
- If you will have surgery within 2 months,
including dental surgery, requiring general or
spinal anesthesia.
- If you have asthma, emphysema or other lung
disorder.
- If you take non-prescription ulcer medicine,
asthma medicine or amphetamines.

Over age 60:
Adverse reactions and side effects may be more
frequent and severe than in younger persons.
More likely to develop tardive dyskinesia
(involuntary movement of jaws, lips, tongue,
chewing). Report this to your doctor immediately.
Early treatment can help.

Pregnancy:
Risk to unborn child outweighs drug benefits.
Don't use.

Breast-feeding:
Drug passes into milk. Avoid drug or discontinue
nursing until you finish medicine. Consult doctor
for advice on maintaining milk supply.

Infants & children:
Don't give to children younger than 2.

Prolonged use:
May lead to tardive dyskinesia (involuntary movement of jaws, lips, tongue, chewing).

Skin & sunlight:
May cause rash or intensify sunburn in areas exposed to sun or sunlamp. Skin may remain sensitive for 3 months after discontinuing.

Driving, piloting or hazardous work:
Don't drive or pilot aircraft until you learn how medicine affects you. Don't work around dangerous machinery. Don't climb ladders or work in high places. Danger increases if you drink alcohol or take medicine affecting alertness and reflexes.

Discontinuing:
May be unnecessary to finish medicine. Follow doctor's instructions.

Others:
No problems expected.

 POSSIBLE INTERACTION WITH OTHER DRUGS

GENERIC NAME OR DRUG CLASS	COMBINED EFFECT
Antacids*	Decreased trimeprazine effect.
Anticholinergics*	Increased anticholinergic effect.
Anticonvulsants, hydantoin*	Increased anticonvulsant effect.
Antidepressants, tricyclic (TCA)*	Increased trimeprazine effect.
Antihistamines, other*	Increased antihistamine effect.
Appetite suppressants*	Decreased suppressant effect.
Barbiturates*	Oversedation.
Carteolol	Decreased antihistamine effect.
Dronabinol	Increased effects of both drugs. Avoid.
Ethinamate	Dangerous increased effects of ethinamate. Avoid combining.
Fluoxetine	Increased depressant effects of both drugs.
Guanfacine	May increase depressant effects of either medicine.
Guanethidine	Decreased guanethidine effect.
Leucovorin	High alcohol content of leucovorin may cause adverse effects.
Levodopa	Decreased levodopa effect.
MAO inhibitors*	Increased trimeprazine effect.
Methyprylon	May increase sedative effect to dangerous level. Avoid.
Mind-altering drugs*	Increased effect of mind-altering drugs.
Molindone	Increased sedative and antihistamine effect.
Nabilone	Greater depression of central nervous system.
Narcotics*	Increased narcotic effect.
Sedatives*	Increased sedative effect.
Sotalol	Increased antihistamine effect.
Tranquilizers*	Increased tranquilizer effect. Avoid.

 POSSIBLE INTERACTION WITH OTHER SUBSTANCES

INTERACTS WITH	COMBINED EFFECT
Alcohol:	Dangerous oversedation.
Beverages:	None expected.
Cocaine:	Decreased effect of trimeprazine. Avoid.
Foods:	None expected.
Marijuana:	Drowsiness.
Tobacco:	None expected.

TRIMETHOBENZAMIDE

BRAND NAMES

Stemetic	Tigan
Tegamide	Tiject-20
Ticon	

BASIC INFORMATION

Habit forming? No
Prescription needed? Yes
Available as generic? Yes
Drug class: Antiemetic

USES

Reduces nausea and vomiting.

DOSAGE & USAGE INFORMATION

How to take:
- Capsule—Swallow with liquid. If you can't swallow whole, open capsule and take with liquid or food.
- Suppositories—Remove wrapper and moisten suppository with water. Gently insert larger end into rectum. Push well into rectum with finger.

When to take:
When needed, no more often than label directs.

If you forget a dose:
Take when you remember. Wait as long as label directs for next dose.

What drug does:
Possibly blocks nerve impulses to brain's vomiting centers.

Time lapse before drug works:
20 to 40 minutes.

Continued next column

OVERDOSE

SYMPTOMS:
Confusion, convulsions, coma.
WHAT TO DO:
- Dial 0 (operator) or 911 (emergency) for an ambulance or medical help. Then give first aid immediately.
- If patient is unconscious and not breathing, give mouth-to-mouth breathing. If there is no heartbeat, use cardiac massage and mouth-to-mouth breathing (CPR). Don't try to make patient vomit. If you can't get help quickly, take patient to nearest emergency facility.
- See emergency information on inside covers.

Don't take with:
Non-prescription drugs or drugs in Interaction column without consulting doctor.

POSSIBLE ADVERSE REACTIONS OR SIDE EFFECTS

SYMPTOMS	WHAT TO DO
Life-threatening: None expected.	
Common: None expected.	
Infrequent:	
• Rash, blurred vision, low blood pressure.	Discontinue. Call doctor right away.
• Dizziness, headache, drowsiness, diarrhea, muscle cramps, unusual tiredness.	Continue. Call doctor when convenient.
Rare:	
• Convulsions.	Discontinue. Seek emergency treatment.
• Seizures, tremor, depression, sore throat, fever, repeated vomiting, back pain, jaundice, Parkinson symptoms, neck spasms.	Discontinue. Call doctor right away.

WARNINGS & PRECAUTIONS

Don't take if:
- You are allergic to trimethobenzamide.
- You are allergic to local anesthetics and have suppository form.

Before you start, consult your doctor:
If you have reacted badly to antihistamines.

Over age 60:
More susceptible to low blood pressure and sedative effects of this drug.

Pregnancy:
No proven harm to unborn child. Avoid if possible.

Breast-feeding:
No proven problems. Avoid if possible.

Infants & children:
- Injectable form not recommended.
- Avoid during viral infections. Drug may contribute to Reyes' syndrome.

Prolonged use:
- Damages blood-cell production of bone marrow.
- Causes Parkinson-like symptoms of tremors, rigidity.

Skin & sunlight:
Possible sun sensitivity. Use caution.

Driving, piloting or hazardous work:
- Use disqualifies you for piloting aircraft.
- Don't drive until you learn how medicine affects you. Don't work around dangerous machinery. Don't climb ladders or work in high places. Danger increases if you drink alcohol or take medicine affecting alertness and reflexes, such as antihistamines, tranquilizers, sedatives, pain medicine, narcotics and mind-altering drugs.

Discontinuing:
May be unnecessary to finish medicine. Follow doctor's instructions.

Others:
No problems expected.

POSSIBLE INTERACTION WITH OTHER DRUGS

GENERIC NAME OR DRUG CLASS	COMBINED EFFECT
Antidepressants*	Increased sedative effect.
Antihistamines*	Increased sedative effect.
Barbiturates*	Increased effect of both drugs.
Belladonna	Increased effect of both drugs.
Cholinergics*	Increased effect of both drugs.
Ethinamate	Dangerous increased effects of ethinamate. Avoid combining.
Fluoxetine	Increased depressant effects of both drugs.
Guanfacine	May increase depressant effects of either medicine.
Leucovorin	High alcohol content of leucovorin may cause adverse effects.
Methyprylon	May increase sedative effect to dangerous level. Avoid.
Mind-altering drugs*	Increased effect of mind-altering drug.
Nabilone	Greater depression of central nervous system.
Narcotics*	Increased sedative effect.
Phenothiazines*	Increased effect of both drugs.
Sedatives*	Increased sedative effect.
Sleep inducers*	Increased effect of sleep inducer.
Tranquilizers*	Increased sedative effect.

POSSIBLE INTERACTION WITH OTHER SUBSTANCES

INTERACTS WITH	COMBINED EFFECT
Alcohol:	Oversedation. Avoid.
Beverages:	None expected.
Cocaine:	None expected.
Foods:	None expected.
Marijuana:	Increased antinausea effect.
Tobacco:	None expected.

*See Glossary

TRIMETHOPRIM

BRAND NAMES

Apo-Sulfatrim	Rovbac
Bactrim	Septra
Cotrim	SMZ-TMP
Novotrimel	Syraprim
Proloprim	Trimpex
Protrin	

BASIC INFORMATION

Habit forming? No
Prescription needed? Yes
Available as generic? Yes
Drug class: Antimicrobial

USES

- Treatment for urinary-tract infections susceptible to trimethoprim.
- Helps prevent recurrent urinary-tract infections if taken once a day.

DOSAGE & USAGE INFORMATION

How to take:
Tablet—Swallow with liquid or food to lessen stomach irritation.

When to take:
Space doses evenly in 24 hours to keep constant amount in urine.

If you forget a dose:
Take as soon as possible. Wait 5 to 6 hours before next dose. Then return to regular schedule.

What drug does:
Stops harmful bacterial germs from multiplying. Will not kill viruses.

Time lapse before drug works:
2 to 5 days.

Don't take with:
See Interaction column and consult doctor.

OVERDOSE

SYMPTOMS:
Nausea, vomiting, diarrhea.
WHAT TO DO:
Overdose unlikely to threaten life. If person takes much larger amount than prescribed, call doctor, poison-control center or hospital emergency room for instructions.

POSSIBLE ADVERSE REACTIONS OR SIDE EFFECTS

SYMPTOMS	WHAT TO DO
Life-threatening: None expected.	
Common: Rash, itchy skin.	Discontinue. Seek emergency treatment.
Infrequent:	
• Diarrhea, nausea, vomiting, abdominal pain.	Discontinue. Call doctor right away.
• Headache.	Continue. Call doctor when convenient.
Rare:	
• Blue fingernails, lips and skin; difficult breathing.	Discontinue. Seek emergency treatment.
• Sore throat, fever, anemia, jaundice.	Discontinue. Call doctor right away.

WARNINGS & PRECAUTIONS

Don't take if:
- You are allergic to trimethoprim or any sulfa drug.
- You are anemic due to folic acid deficiency.

Before you start, consult your doctor:
If you have had liver or kidney disease.

Over age 60:
- Reduced liver and kidney function may require reduced dose.
- More likely to have severe anal and genital itch.
- Increased susceptibility to anemia.

Pregnancy:
Studies inconclusive on harm to unborn child. Animal studies show fetal abnormalities. Decide with your doctor whether drug benefits justify risk to unborn child.

Breast-feeding:
No proven harm to unborn child. Avoid if possible.

Infants & children:
Use under medical supervision only.

Prolonged use:
Anemia.

Skin & sunlight:
May cause rash or intensify sunburn in areas exposed to sun or sunlamp.

Driving, piloting or hazardous work:
No problems expected.

Discontinuing:
Don't discontinue without doctor's advice until you complete prescribed dose, even though symptoms diminish or disappear.

Others:
No problems expected.

POSSIBLE INTERACTION WITH OTHER DRUGS

GENERIC NAME OR DRUG CLASS	COMBINED EFFECT
Diuretics, thiazide*	Unusual bleeding or bruising.
Flecainide	Possible decreased blood-cell production in bone marrow.
Sulfamethoxazole	Beneficial increase of sulfamethoxazole effect.
Tocainide	Possible decreased blood-cell production in bone marrow.

POSSIBLE INTERACTION WITH OTHER SUBSTANCES

INTERACTS WITH	COMBINED EFFECT
Alcohol:	Increased alcohol effect with Bactrim or Septra.
Beverages:	None expected.
Cocaine:	No proven problems.
Foods:	None expected.
Marijuana:	None expected.
Tobacco:	None expected.

TRIPELENNAMINE

BRAND NAMES

PBZ   Pyribenzamine
PBZ-SR   Ro-Hist

BASIC INFORMATION

Habit forming? No
Prescription needed?
  High strength: Yes
  Low strength: No
Available as generic? Yes
Drug class: Antihistamine

 ## USES

- Reduces allergic symptoms such as hay fever, hives, rash or itching.
- Induces sleep.

 ## DOSAGE & USAGE INFORMATION

How to take:
- Tablet or liquid—Swallow with liquid or food to lessen stomach irritation.
- Extended-release tablets—Swallow each dose whole.

When to take:
Varies with form. Follow label directions.

If you forget a dose:
Take as soon as you remember up to 2 hours late. If more than 2 hours, wait for next scheduled dose (don't double this dose).

What drug does:
Blocks action of histamine after an allergic response triggers histamine release in sensitive cells.

Continued next column

 ## OVERDOSE

SYMPTOMS:
Convulsions, red face, hallucinations, coma.
WHAT TO DO:
- Dial 0 (operator) or 911 (emergency) for an ambulance or medical help. Then give first aid immediately.
- If patient is unconscious and not breathing, give mouth-to-mouth breathing. If there is no heartbeat, use cardiac massage and mouth-to-mouth breathing (CPR). Don't try to make patient vomit. If you can't get help quickly, take patient to nearest emergency facility.
- See emergency information on inside covers.

Time lapse before drug works:
30 minutes.

Don't take with:
See Interaction column and consult doctor.

 ## POSSIBLE ADVERSE REACTIONS OR SIDE EFFECTS

SYMPTOMS	WHAT TO DO
Life-threatening: None expected.	
Common: Drowsiness; dizziness; dry mouth, nose and throat; nausea.	Continue. Tell doctor at next visit.
Infrequent: • Change in vision.	Discontinue. Call doctor right away.
• Less tolerance for contact lenses, difficult urination.	Continue. Call doctor when convenient.
• Appetite loss.	Continue. Tell doctor at next visit.
Rare: Nightmares, agitation, irritability, sore throat, fever, rapid heartbeat, unusual bleeding or bruising, fatigue, weakness.	Discontinue. Call doctor right away.

WARNINGS & PRECAUTIONS

Don't take if:
You are allergic to any antihistamine.

Before you start, consult your doctor:
- If you have glaucoma.
- If you have enlarged prostate.
- If you have asthma.
- If you have kidney disease.
- If you have peptic ulcer.
- If you will have surgery within 2 months, including dental surgery, requiring general or spinal anesthesia.

Over age 60:
Don't exceed recommended dose. Adverse reactions and side effects may be more frequent and severe than in younger persons, especially urination difficulty, diminished alertness and other brain and nervous-system symptoms.

Pregnancy:
No proven harm to unborn child. Avoid if possible.

Breast-feeding:
Drug passes into milk. Avoid drug or discontinue nursing until you finish medicine. Consult doctor for advice on maintaining milk supply.

Infants & children:
Not recommended for premature or newborn infants. Otherwise, no problems expected.

Prolonged use:
Avoid. May damage bone marrow and nerve cells.

Skin & sunlight:
May cause rash or intensify sunburn in areas exposed to sun or sunlamp.

Driving, piloting or hazardous work:
Don't drive or pilot aircraft until you learn how medicine affects you. Don't work around dangerous machinery. Don't climb ladders or work in high places. Danger increases if you drink alcohol or take medicine affecting alertness and reflexes, such as antihistamines, tranquilizers, sedatives, pain medicine, narcotics and mind-altering drugs.

Discontinuing:
No problems expected.

Others:
May mask symptoms of hearing damage from aspirin, other salicylates, cisplatin, paromomycin, vancomycin or anticonvulsants. Consult doctor if you use these.

POSSIBLE INTERACTION WITH OTHER DRUGS

GENERIC NAME OR DRUG CLASS	COMBINED EFFECT
Anticholinergics*	Increased anti-cholinergic effect.
Anticoagulants, oral*	Decreased tripelennamine effect.
Antidepressants, tricyclic (TCA)*	Increased tripelennamine effect. Excess sedation.
Antihistamines, other*	Excess sedation. Avoid.
Carteolol	Decreased antihistamine effect.
Dronabinol	Increased effects of both drugs. Avoid.
Hypnotics*	Excess sedation. Avoid.
MAO inhibitors*	Increased tripelennamine effect.
Mind-altering drugs*	Excess sedation. Avoid.
Molindone	Increased antihistamine effect.
Nabilone	Greater depression of central nervous system.
Narcotics*	Excess sedation. Avoid.
Procarbazine	May increase sedation.
Sedatives*	Excess sedation. Avoid.
Sleep inducers*	Excess sedation. Avoid.
Sotalol	Increased antihistamine effect.
Tranquilizers*	Excess sedation. Avoid.

POSSIBLE INTERACTION WITH OTHER SUBSTANCES

INTERACTS WITH	COMBINED EFFECT
Alcohol:	Excess sedation. Avoid.
Beverages: Caffeine drinks.	Less tripelennamine sedation.
Cocaine:	Decreased tripelennamine effect. Avoid.
Foods:	None expected.
Marijuana:	Excess sedation. Avoid.
Tobacco:	None expected.

TRIPROLIDINE

BRAND NAMES

Actidil
Actifed
Bayidyl
Eldafed

Triafed-C
Trifed
Tripodrine

BASIC INFORMATION

Habit forming? No
Prescription needed?
  High Strength: Yes
  Low strength: No
Available as generic? Yes
Drug class: Antihistamine

USES

- Reduces allergic symptoms such as hay fever, hives, rash or itching.
- Induces sleep.

DOSAGE & USAGE INFORMATION

How to take:
Tablet or syrup—Swallow with liquid or food to lessen stomach irritation.

When to take:
Varies with form. Follow label directions.

If you forget a dose:
Take as soon as you remember up to 2 hours late. If more than 2 hours, wait for next scheduled dose (don't double this dose).

What drug does:
Blocks action of histamine after an allergic response triggers histamine release in sensitive cells.

Continued next column

OVERDOSE

SYMPTOMS:
Convulsions, red face, hallucinations, coma.
WHAT TO DO:
- Dial 0 (operator) or 911 (emergency) for an ambulance or medical help. Then give first aid immediately.
- If patient is unconscious and not breathing, give mouth-to-mouth breathing. If there is no heartbeat, use cardiac massage and mouth-to-mouth breathing (CPR). Don't try to make patient vomit. If you can't get help quickly, take patient to nearest emergency facility.
- See emergency information on inside covers.

Time lapse before drug works:
30 minutes.

Don't take with:
See Interaction column and consult doctor.

POSSIBLE ADVERSE REACTIONS OR SIDE EFFECTS

SYMPTOMS	WHAT TO DO
Life-threatening: None expected.	
Common: Drowsiness; dizziness; dry mouth, nose and throat; nausea.	Continue. Tell doctor at next visit.
Infrequent:	
• Change in vision.	Discontinue. Call doctor right away.
• Less tolerance for contact lenses, difficult urination.	Continue. Call doctor when convenient.
• Appetite loss.	Continue. Tell doctor at next visit.
Rare: Nightmares, agitation, irritability, sore throat, fever, rapid heartbeat, unusual bleeding or bruising, fatigue, weakness.	Discontinue. Call doctor right away.

WARNINGS & PRECAUTIONS

Don't take if:
You are allergic to any antihistamine.

Before you start, consult your doctor:
- If you have glaucoma.
- If you have enlarged prostate.
- If you have asthma.
- If you have kidney disease.
- If you have peptic ulcer.
- If you will have surgery within 2 months, including dental surgery, requiring general or spinal anesthesia.

Over age 60:
Don't exceed recommended dose. Adverse reactions and side effects may be more frequent and severe than in younger persons, especially urination difficulty, diminished alertness and other brain and nervous-system symptoms.

Pregnancy:
No proven harm to unborn child. Avoid if possible.

Breast-feeding:
Drug passes into milk. Avoid drug or discontinue nursing until you finish medicine. Consult doctor for advice on maintaining milk supply.

Infants & children:
Not recommended for premature or newborn infants. Otherwise, no problems expected.

Prolonged use:
Avoid. May damage bone marrow and nerve cells.

Skin & sunlight:
May cause rash or intensify sunburn in areas exposed to sun or sunlamp.

Driving, piloting or hazardous work:
Don't drive or pilot aircraft until you learn how medicine affects you. Don't work around dangerous machinery. Don't climb ladders or work in high places. Danger increases if you drink alcohol or take medicine affecting alertness and reflexes, such as antihistamines, tranquilizers, sedatives, pain medicine, narcotics and mind-altering drugs.

Discontinuing:
No problems expected.

Others:
May mask symptoms of hearing damage from aspirin, other salicylates, cisplatin, paromomycin, vancomycin or anticonvulsants. Consult doctor if you use these.

POSSIBLE INTERACTION WITH OTHER DRUGS

GENERIC NAME OR DRUG CLASS	COMBINED EFFECT
Anticholinergics*	Increased anticholinergic effect.
Anticoagulants, oral*	Decreased triprolidine effect.
Antidepressants, tricyclic (TCA)*	Increased triprolidine effect. Excess sedation.
Antihistamines, other*	Excess sedation. Avoid.
Carteolol	Decreased antihistamine effect.
Dronabinol	Increased effects of both drugs. Avoid.
Hypnotics*	Excess sedation. Avoid.
MAO inhibitors*	Increased triprolidine effect.
Mind-altering drugs*	Excess sedation. Avoid.
Molindone	Increased antihistamine effect.
Nabilone	Greater depression of central nervous system.
Narcotics*	Excess sedation. Avoid.
Procarbazine	May increase sedation.
Sedatives*	Excess sedation. Avoid.
Sleep inducers*	Excess sedation. Avoid.
Sotalol	Increased antihistamine effect.
Tranquilizers*	Excess sedation. Avoid.

POSSIBLE INTERACTION WITH OTHER SUBSTANCES

INTERACTS WITH	COMBINED EFFECT
Alcohol:	Excess sedation. Avoid.
Beverages: Caffeine drinks.	Less triprolidine sedation.
Cocaine:	Decreased triprolidine effect. Avoid.
Foods:	None expected.
Marijuana:	Excess sedation. Avoid.
Tobacco:	None expected.

URSODIOL

BRAND NAMES

Actigall

BASIC INFORMATION

Habit forming? No
Prescription needed? Yes
Available as generic? No
Drug class: Anticholethitic

USES

Dissolves cholesterol gallstones in selected patients who either can't tolerate surgery or don't require surgery for other reasons. Not used when surgery is clearly indicated.

DOSAGE & USAGE INFORMATION

How to take:
Tablets—Swallow with liquid or food to lessen stomach irritation. If you can't swallow whole, crumble tablet and take with liquid or food.

When to take:
With meals, 2 or 3 times a day according to your doctor's instructions.

If you forget a dose:
Take as soon as you remember up to 2 hours late. If more than 2 hours, wait for next scheduled time. Don't double this dose.

What drug does:
Decreases secretion of cholesterol into bile by suppressing production and secretion of cholesterol by the liver. Ursodiol will not help gallstone problems unless the gallstones are made of cholesterol. It works best when the stones are small.

Time lapse before drug works:
Unpredictable. Varies among patients.

Don't take with:
See Interaction column and consult doctor.

OVERDOSE

SYMPTOMS: Severe diarrhea.
WHAT TO DO:
Overdose not expected to threaten life. If person takes much larger amount than prescribed, call doctor, poison-control center or hospital emergency room for instructions.

POSSIBLE ADVERSE REACTIONS OR SIDE EFFECTS

SYMPTOMS	WHAT TO DO
Life-threatening: None expected.	
Common: None expected.	
Infrequent: None expected.	
Rare: Diarrhea.	Continue. Call doctor when convenient.

WARNINGS & PRECAUTIONS

Don't take if:
You can't tolerate other bile acids.

Before you start, consult your doctor:
- If you have complications of gallstones, such as infection or obstruction of the bile ducts.
- If you have had pancreatitis.
- If you have had chronically impaired liver function.
- If you take any other medicines for any reason.

Over age 60:
No special problems expected.

Pregnancy:
Studies have not been performed to determine effects on unborn child. Decide with your doctor whether drug benefits justify risk to unborn child.

Breast-feeding:
Unknown, but no documented problems.

Infants & children:
Not recommended. Adequate studies have not been performed.

Prolonged use:
No special problems expected.

Skin & sunlight:
No problems expected.

Driving, piloting or hazardous work:
Don't pilot aircraft until you learn how medicine affects you. Don't work around dangerous machinery. Don't climb ladders or work in high places. Danger increases if you drink alcohol or take medicine affecting alertness and reflexes, such as antihistamines, tranquilizers, sedatives, pain medicine, narcotics and mind-altering drugs.

Discontinuing:
Don't discontinue without consulting doctor.

Others:
Plan regular visits to your doctor while you take ursodiol. Have ultrasound and liver-function studies done at appropriate intervals. Liver damage is unlikely, but theoretically could happen.

POSSIBLE INTERACTION WITH OTHER DRUGS

GENERIC NAME OR DRUG CLASS	COMBINED EFFECT
Antacids* (aluminum-containing)	Decreased absorption of ursodiol.
Cholestyramine	Decreased absorption of ursodiol.
Clofibrate	Decreased effect of ursodiol.
Colestipol	Decreased absorption of ursodiol.
Estrogens*	Decreased effect of ursodiol.
Progesterone	Decreased effect of ursodiol.

POSSIBLE INTERACTION WITH OTHER SUBSTANCES

INTERACTS WITH	COMBINED EFFECT
Alcohol:	None expected, unless you have impaired liver function from alcohol abuse.
Beverages:	None expected.
Cocaine:	None expected.
Foods:	None expected.
Marijuana:	None expected.
Tobacco:	None reported. However, tobacco may possibly impair intestinal absorption from the intestinal tract. Better to avoid.

*See Glossary

VALPROIC ACID (Dipropylacetic Acid)

BRAND NAMES

Depakene
Depakote

Epival
Myproic Acid

BASIC INFORMATION

Habit forming? No
Prescription needed? Yes
Available as generic? Yes
Drug class: Anticonvulsant

USES

Controls petit mal (absence) seizures in treatment of epilepsy.

DOSAGE & USAGE INFORMATION

How to take:
Capsule or syrup—Swallow with liquid or food to lessen stomach irritation.

When to take:
Once a day.

If you forget a dose:
Take as soon as you remember. Don't ever double dose.

What drug does:
Increases concentration of gamma aminobutyric acid, which inhibits nerve transmission in parts of brain.

Time lapse before drug works:
1 to 4 hours.

Don't take with:
See Interaction column and consult doctor.

OVERDOSE

SYMPTOMS:
Coma
WHAT TO DO:
- Dial 0 (operator) or 911 (emergency) for an ambulance or medical help. Then give first aid immediately.
- If patient is unconscious and not breathing, give mouth-to-mouth breathing. If there is no heartbeat, use cardiac massage and mouth-to-mouth breathing (CPR). Don't try to make patient vomit. If you can't get help quickly, take patient to nearest emergency facility.
- See emergency information on inside covers.

POSSIBLE ADVERSE REACTIONS OR SIDE EFFECTS

SYMPTOMS	WHAT TO DO
Life-threatening: None expected.	
Common: Menstrual irregularities. nausea, vomiting, abdominal cramps.	Continue. Call doctor when convenient.
Infrequent: • Rash, blood spots under skin, hair loss, bleeding (heart and lungs), easy bruising.	Discontinue. Call doctor right away.
• Sleepiness, weakness, easily upset emotionally, depression, psychic changes, headache, incoordination, appetite change.	Continue. Call doctor when convenient.
Rare: • Double vision, unusual movements of eyes (nystagmus), severe abdominal pain; swelling of feet, ankles and abdomen; jaundice; increased bleeding tendency.	Discontinue. Call doctor right away.
• Anemia.	Continue. Call doctor when convenient.

VALPROIC ACID (Dipropylacetic Acid)

WARNINGS & PRECAUTIONS

Don't take if:
You are allergic to valproic acid.

Before you start, consult your doctor:
- If you have blood, kidney or liver disease.
- If you will have surgery within 2 months, including dental surgery, requiring general or spinal anesthesia.

Over age 60:
Adverse reactions and side effects may be more frequent and severe than in younger persons.

Pregnancy:
No proven harm to unborn child. Avoid if possible.

Breast-feeding:
Unknown effect.

Infants & children:
Under close medical supervision only.

Prolonged use:
Request periodic blood tests, liver- and kidney-function tests.

Skin & sunlight:
No problems expected.

Driving, piloting or hazardous work:
Don't drive or pilot aircraft until you learn how medicine affects you. Don't work around dangerous machinery. Don't climb ladders or work in high places. Danger increases if you drink alcohol or take medicine affecting alertness and reflexes, such as antihistamines, tranquilizers, sedatives, pain medicine, narcotics and mind-altering drugs.

Discontinuing:
Don't discontinue without consulting doctor. Dose may require gradual reduction if you have taken drug for a long time. Doses of other drugs may also require adjustment.

Others:
No problems expected.

POSSIBLE INTERACTION WITH OTHER DRUGS

GENERIC NAME OR DRUG CLASS	COMBINED EFFECT
Anticoagulants*	Increased chance of bleeding.
Aspirin	Increased chance of bleeding.
Central nervous system depressants*	Increased sedative effect.
Clonazepam	May prolong seizure.
Dypiradamole	Increased chance of bleeding.
Flecainide	Possible decreased blood-cell production in bone marrow.
Levocarnitine	Decreased levocarnitine. Patients taking valproic acid may need to take the supplement levocarnitine.
MAO inhibitors*	Increased sedative effect.
Nabilone	Greater depression of central nervous system.
Phenobarbital	Increases chance of toxicity.
Phenytoin	Unpredictable. Dose may require adjustment.
Primidone	Increased chance of toxicity.
Sulfinpyrazone	Increased chance of bleeding.
Tocainide	Possible decreased blood-cell production in bone marrow.

POSSIBLE INTERACTION WITH OTHER SUBSTANCES

INTERACTS WITH	COMBINED EFFECT
Alcohol:	Deep sedation. Avoid.
Beverages:	No problems expected.
Cocaine:	Increased brain sensitivity. Avoid.
Foods:	No problems expected.
Marijuana:	Increased brain sensitivity. Avoid.
Tobacco:	Decreased valproic acid effect.

*See Glossary

VERAPAMIL

BRAND NAMES

Calan	Isoptin
Calan SR	Isoptin SR

BASIC INFORMATION

Habit forming? No
Prescription needed? Yes
Available as generic? Yes
Drug class: Calcium-channel blocker, antiarrhythmic, antianginal

 ## USES

- Prevents angina attacks.
- Stabilizes irregular heartbeat.
- Treats high blood pressure.

 ## DOSAGE & USAGE INFORMATION

How to take:
Extended-release tablet—Swallow with liquid.

When to take:
At the same times each day 1 hour before or 2 hours after eating.

If you forget a dose:
Take as soon as you remember up to 2 hours late. If more than 2 hours, wait for next scheduled dose (don't double this dose).

What drug does:
- Reduces work that heart must perform.
- Reduces normal artery pressure.
- Increases oxygen to heart muscle.

Time lapse before drug works:
1 to 2 hours.

Don't take with:
See Interaction column and consult doctor.

 ## OVERDOSE

SYMPTOMS:
Unusually fast or unusually slow heartbeat, loss of consciousness, cardiac arrest.
WHAT TO DO:
- Dial 0 (operator) or 911 (emergency) for an ambulance or medical help. Then give first aid immediately.
- If patient is unconscious and not breathing, give mouth-to-mouth breathing. If there is no heartbeat, use cardiac massage and mouth-to-mouth breathing (CPR). Don't try to make patient vomit. If you can't get help quickly, take patient to nearest emergency facility.
- See emergency information on inside covers.

 ## POSSIBLE ADVERSE REACTIONS OR SIDE EFFECTS

SYMPTOMS	WHAT TO DO
Life-threatening: None expected.	
Common: Tiredness.	Continue. Tell doctor at next visit.
Infrequent:	
• Unusually fast or unusually slow heartbeat, wheezing, cough, shortness of breath.	Discontinue. Call doctor right away.
• Dizziness; numbness or tingling in hands and feet; swollen feet, ankles or legs; difficult urination.	Continue. Call doctor when convenient.
• Nausea, constipation.	Continue. Tell doctor at next visit.
Rare:	
• Fainting, depression, psychosis, rash, jaundice.	Discontinue. Call doctor right away.
• Headache, insomnia, vivid dreams, hair loss.	Continue. Tell doctor at next visit.

 ## WARNINGS & PRECAUTIONS

Don't take if:
- You are allergic to verapamil.
- You have very low blood pressure.

Before you start, consult your doctor:
- If you have kidney or liver disease.
- If you have high blood pressure.
- If you have heart disease other than coronary-artery disease.

Over age 60:
Adverse reactions and side effects may be more frequent and severe than in younger persons.

Pregnancy:
No proven harm to unborn child. Avoid if possible.

Breast-feeding:
Safety not established. Avoid if possible.

Infants & children:
Not recommended.

Prolonged use:
No problems expected.

Skin & sunlight:
No problems expected.

Driving, piloting or hazardous work:
Avoid if you feel dizzy. Otherwise, no problems expected.

Discontinuing:
Don't discontinue without doctor's advice until you complete prescribed dose, even though symptoms diminish or disappear.

Others:
Learn to check your own pulse rate. If it drops to 50 beats per minute or lower, don't take verapamil until your consult your doctor.

POSSIBLE INTERACTION WITH OTHER DRUGS

GENERIC NAME OR DRUG CLASS	COMBINED EFFECT
ACE Inhibitors: captopril, enalapril, lisinopril*	Possible excessive potassium in blood. Dosages may require adjustment.
Antiarrhythmics*	Possible increased effect and toxicity of each drug.
Anticoagulants, oral*	Possible increased anticoagulant effect.
Anticonvulsants, hydantoin*	Increased anticonvulsant effect.
Antihypertensives*	Blood-pressure drop. Dosages may require adjustment.
Beta-adrenergic blockers*	Possible irregular heartbeat and congestive heart failure.
Calcium (large doses)	Possible decreased verapamil effect.
Carbamazepine	May increase carbamazepine effect and toxicity.
Cimetidine	Possible increased verapamil effect and toxicity.
Digitalis preparations*	Increased digitalis effect. May need to reduce dose.
Disopyramide	May cause dangerously slow, fast or irregular heartbeat.
Diuretics*	Dangerous blood-pressure drop. Dosages may require adjustment.

Encainide	Increased effect of toxicity on heart muscle.
Lithium	Possible decreased lithium effect.
Nicardipine	Possible increased effect and toxicity of each drug.
Nitrates*	Reduced angina attacks.
Quinidine	Increased quinidine effect.
Rifampin	Decreased verapamil effect.
Theophylline	May increase theophylline effect and toxicity.
Phenytoin	Possible decreased verapamil effect.
Vitamin D (large doses)	Decreased verapamil effect.

POSSIBLE INTERACTION WITH OTHER SUBSTANCES

INTERACTS WITH	COMBINED EFFECT
Alcohol:	Dangerously low blood pressure. Avoid.
Beverages:	None expected.
Cocaine:	Possible irregular heartbeat. Avoid.
Foods:	None expected.
Marijuana:	Possible irregular heartbeat. Avoid.
Tobacco:	Possible rapid heartbeat. Avoid.

VITAMIN A

BRAND NAMES

Acon	Aquasol A
Afaxin	Dispatabs
Alphalin	Sust-A

Numerous multiple vitamin-mineral supplements.

BASIC INFORMATION

Habit forming? No
Prescription needed? No
Available as generic? Yes
Drug class: Vitamin supplement

 USES

- Dietary supplement to ensure normal growth and health, especially eyes and skin.
- Beta carotene form (Solatene) decreases severity of sun exposure in patients with porphyria.

 DOSAGE & USAGE INFORMATION

How to take:
- Drops or capsule—Swallow with liquid. If you can't swallow whole, open capsule and take with liquid or food.
- Oral solution—Swallow with liquid.

When to take:
At the same time each day.

If you forget a dose:
Take as soon as you remember. Resume regular schedule.

What drug does:
- Prevents night blindness.
- Promotes normal growth and health.

Time lapse before drug works:
Requires continual intake.

Don't take with:
See Interaction column and consult doctor.

 OVERDOSE

SYMPTOMS:
Increased adverse reactions and side effects. Jaundice (rare, but may occur with large doses), malaise, anorexia, vomiting, irritability.
WHAT TO DO:
Overdose unlikely to threaten life. If person takes much larger amount than prescribed, call doctor, poison-control center or hospital emergency room for instructions.

 POSSIBLE ADVERSE REACTIONS OR SIDE EFFECTS

SYMPTOMS	WHAT TO DO
Life-threatening: None expected.	
Common: None expected.	
Infrequent: Confusion; dizziness; drowsiness; headache; irritability; dry, cracked lips; peeling skin; hair loss.	Continue. Call doctor when convenient.
Rare:	
• Bulging soft spot on baby's head, double vision.	Discontinue. Call doctor right away.
• Diarrhea, appetite loss, nausea, vomiting.	Continue. Call doctor when convenient.

WARNINGS & PRECAUTIONS

Don't take if:
You have chronic kidney failure.

Before you start, consult your doctor:
If you have any kidney disorder.

Over age 60:
No problems expected.

Pregnancy:
Don't take more than 6,000 units daily.

Breast-feeding:
No problems expected.

Infants & children:
- Avoid large doses.
- Keep vitamin-mineral supplements out of children's reach.

Prolonged use:
No problems expected.

Skin & sunlight:
No problems expected.

Driving, piloting or hazardous work:
No problems expected.

Discontinuing:
Don't discontinue without doctor's advice until you complete prescribed dose, even though symptoms diminish or disappear.

Others:
- Don't exceed dose. Too much over a long time may be harmful.
- A balanced diet should provide all the vitamin A a healthy person needs and prevent need for supplements. Best sources are liver, yellow-orange fruits and vegetables, dark-green, leafy vegetables, milk, butter and margarine.

POSSIBLE INTERACTION WITH OTHER DRUGS

GENERIC NAME OR DRUG CLASS	COMBINED EFFECT
Anticoagulants*	Increased anticoagulant effect with large doses (over 10,000 I.U.) of vitamin A.
Calcium supplements*	Decreased vitamin effect.
Cholestyramine	Decreased vitamin A absorption.
Colestipol	Decreased vitamin absorption.
Contraceptives, oral*	Increased vitamin A levels.
Mineral oil (long term)	Decreased vitamin A absorption.
Neomycin	Decreased vitamin absorption.
Vitamin A derivatives, other	Increased toxicity risk.
Vitamin E (excess dose)	Vitamin A depletion.

POSSIBLE INTERACTION WITH OTHER SUBSTANCES

INTERACTS WITH	COMBINED EFFECT
Alcohol:	None expected.
Beverages:	None expected.
Cocaine:	None expected.
Foods:	None expected.
Marijuana:	None expected.
Tobacco:	None expected.

VITAMIN B-12 (Cyanocobalamin)

BRAND NAMES

See complete list of brand names in the *Brand Name Directory,* page 1072.

BASIC INFORMATION

Habit forming? No
Prescription needed? No
Available as generic? Yes
Drug class: Vitamin supplement

 ## USES

- Dietary supplement for normal growth, development and health.
- Treatment for nerve damage.
- Treatment for pernicious anemia.
- Treatment and prevention of vitamin B-12 deficiencies in people who have had stomach or intestines surgically removed.
- Prevention of vitamin B-12 deficiency in strict vegetarians and persons with absorption diseases.

 ## DOSAGE & USAGE INFORMATION

How to take:
- Tablets—Swallow with liquid.
- Injection—Follow doctor's directions.

When to take:
- Oral—At the same time each day.
- Injection—Follow doctor's directions.

If you forget a dose:
Take when remembered. Don't double next dose. Resume regular schedule.

What drug does:
Acts as enzyme to promote normal fat and carbohydrate metabolism and protein synthesis.

Time lapse before drug works:
15 minutes.

Don't take with:
See Interaction column and consult doctor.

 ## OVERDOSE

SYMPTOMS:
Increased adverse reactions and side effects.
WHAT TO DO:
Overdose unlikely to threaten life. If person takes much larger amount than prescribed, call doctor, poison-control center or hospital emergency room for instructions.

 ## POSSIBLE ADVERSE REACTIONS OR SIDE EFFECTS

SYMPTOMS	WHAT TO DO
Life-threatening: Hives, rash, intense itching, faintness soon after a dose (anaphylaxis).	Seek emergency treatment immediately.
Common: None expected.	
Infrequent: None expected.	
Rare:	
• Itchy skin, wheezing.	Discontinue. Call doctor right away.
• Diarrhea.	Continue. Call doctor when convenient.

VITAMIN B-12 (Cyanocobalamin)

WARNINGS & PRECAUTIONS

Don't take if:
You have Leber's disease (optic nerve atrophy).

Before you start, consult your doctor:
- If you have gout.
- If you have heart disease.

Over age 60:
Don't take more than 100 mg. per day unless prescribed by your doctor.

Pregnancy:
No problems expected.

Breast-feeding:
No problems expected.

Infants & children:
No problems expected.

Prolonged use:
No problems expected.

Skin & sunlight:
No problems expected.

Driving, piloting or hazardous work:
No problems expected.

Discontinuing:
Don't discontinue without doctor's advice until you complete prescribed dose, even though symptoms diminish or disappear.

Others:
- A balanced diet should provide all the vitamin B-12 a healthy person needs and make supplements unnecessary. Best sources are meat, fish, egg yolk and cheese.
- Tablets should be used only for diet supplements. All other uses of vitamin B-12 require injections.
- Don't take large doses of vitamin C (1,000 mg. or more per day) unless prescribed by your doctor.

POSSIBLE INTERACTION WITH OTHER DRUGS

GENERIC NAME OR DRUG CLASS	COMBINED EFFECT
Anticonvulsants*	Decreased absorption of vitamin B-12.
Chloramphenicol	Decreased vitamin B-12 effect.
Cimetidine	Decreased absorption of vitamin B-12.
Colchicine	Decreased absorption of vitamin B-12.
Famotidine	Decreased absorption of vitamin B-12.
H2 antagonists*	Decreased absorption of vitamin B-12.
Neomycin	Decreased absorption of vitamin B-12.
Para-aminosalicylic acid (PAS)	Decreased effects of PAS.
Potassium (extended-release forms)	Decreased absorption of vitamin B-12.
Ranitidine	Decreased absorption of vitamin B-12.
Vitamin C (ascorbic acid)	Destroys vitamin B-12 if taken at same time. Take 2 hours apart.

POSSIBLE INTERACTION WITH OTHER SUBSTANCES

INTERACTS WITH	COMBINED EFFECT
Alcohol:	Decreased absorption of vitamin B-12.
Beverages:	None expected.
Cocaine:	None expected.
Foods:	None expected.
Marijuana:	None expected.
Tobacco:	None expected.

VITAMIN C (Ascorbic Acid)

BRAND NAMES

See complete list of brand names in the *Brand Name Directory*, page 1072.

BASIC INFORMATION

Habit forming? No
Prescription needed? No
Available as generic? Yes
Drug class: Vitamin supplement

 ## USES

- Prevention and treatment of scurvy and other vitamin-C deficiencies.
- Treatment of anemia.
- Maintenance of acid urine.

 ## DOSAGE & USAGE INFORMATION

How to take:
- Tablets, capsules, liquid—Swallow with 8 oz. water.
- Extended-release tablets—Swallow whole.
- Drops—Squirt directly into mouth or mix with liquid or food.
- Chewable tablets—Chew well before swallowing.

When to take:
1, 2 or 3 times per day, as prescribed on label.

If you forget a dose:
Take as soon as you remember. Return to regular schedule.

What drug does:
- May help form collagen.
- Increases iron absorption from intestine.
- Contributes to hemoglobin and red-blood-cell production in bone marrow.

Time lapse before drug works:
1 week.

Don't take with:
See Interaction column and consult doctor.

 ## OVERDOSE

SYMPTOMS:
Diarrhea, vomiting, dizziness.
WHAT TO DO:
Overdose unlikely to threaten life. If person takes much larger amount than prescribed, call doctor, poison-control center or hospital emergency room for instructions.

 ## POSSIBLE ADVERSE REACTIONS OR SIDE EFFECTS

SYMPTOMS	WHAT TO DO
Life-threatening:	
None expected.	
Common:	
None expected.	
Infrequent:	
• Mild diarrhea, nausea, vomiting.	Discontinue. Call doctor right away.
• Flushed face.	Continue. Call doctor when convenient.
Rare:	
• Kidney stones with high doses, anemia.	Discontinue. Call doctor right away.
• Headache.	Continue. Tell doctor at next visit.

WARNINGS & PRECAUTIONS

Don't take if:
You are allergic to vitamin C.

Before you start, consult your doctor:
- If you have sickle-cell or other anemia.
- If you have had kidney stones.
- If you have gout.

Over age 60:
Don't take more than 100 mg. per day unless prescribed by your doctor.

Pregnancy:
No proven harm to unborn child. Avoid large doses.

Breast-feeding:
Avoid large doses.

Infants & children:
- Avoid large doses.
- Keep vitamin-mineral supplements out of children's reach.

Prolonged use:
Large doses for longer than 2 months may cause kidney stones.

Skin & sunlight:
No problems expected.

Driving, piloting or hazardous work:
No problems expected.

Discontinuing:
No problems expected.

Others:
- Store in cool, dry place.
- May cause inaccurate tests for sugar in urine or blood in stool.
- May cause crisis in patients with sickle-cell anemia.
- A balanced diet should provide all the vitamin C a healthy person needs and make supplements unnecessary. Best sources are citrus, strawberries, cantaloupe and raw peppers.
- Don't take large doses of vitamin C (1,000 mg. or more per day) unless prescribed by your doctor.
- Some products contain tartrazine dye. Avoid, if allergic (especially aspirin hypersensitivity).

POSSIBLE INTERACTION WITH OTHER DRUGS

GENERIC NAME OR DRUG CLASS	COMBINED EFFECT
Amphetamines*	Possible decreased amphetamine effect.
Anticholinergics*	Possible decreased anticholinergic effect.
Anticoagulants, oral*	Possible decreased anticoagulant effect.
Antidepressants, tricyclic (TCA)*	Possible decreased antidepressant effect.
Aspirin	Decreased vitamin C effect and salicylate excretion.
Barbiturates*	Decreased vitamin C effect. Increased barbiturate effect.
Contraceptives, oral*	Decreased vitamin C effect.
Estrogens*	Increased likelihood of adverse effects from estrogen with 1 gm or more of vitamin C per day.
Iron supplements*	Increased iron absorption.
Mexiletine	Possible decreased effectiveness of mexiletine.
Quinidine	Possible decreased quinidine effect.
Salicylates*	Decreased vitamin C effect and salicylate excretion. May lead to salicylate toxicity.
Tranquilizers* (phenothiazine)	May decrease phenothiazine effect if no vitamin C deficiency exists.

POSSIBLE INTERACTION WITH OTHER SUBSTANCES

INTERACTS WITH	COMBINED EFFECT
Alcohol:	None expected.
Beverages:	None expected.
Cocaine:	None expected.
Foods:	None expected.
Marijuana:	None expected.
Tobacco:	Increased requirement for vitamin C.

*See Glossary

VITAMIN D

BRAND NAMES

Calciferol	Dihydrotachysterol
Calcifidiol	Drisdol
Calcijex	Ergocalciferol
Calcitriol	Hytakerol
Calderol	Ostoforte
Deltalin	Radiostol
DHT	Radiostol Forte
DHT Intensol	Rocaltrol

Numerous other multiple vitamin-mineral supplements.

BASIC INFORMATION

Habit forming? No
Prescription needed?
  Low strength: No
  High strength: Yes
Available as generic? Yes
Drug class: Vitamin supplement

USES

- Dietary supplement.
- Prevention of rickets (bone disease).
- Treatment for hypocalcemia (low blood calcium) in kidney disease.
- Treatment for postoperative muscle contractions.

DOSAGE & USAGE INFORMATION

How to take:
- Tablet, capsule or liquid—Swallow with liquid.
- Drops—Dilute dose in beverage.
- Injection—Take under doctor's supervision.

When to take:
As directed, usually once a day at the same time each day.

Continued next column

OVERDOSE

SYMPTOMS:
Severe stomach pain, nausea, vomiting, weight loss; bone and muscle pain; increased urination, cloudy urine; mood or mental changes (possible psychosis); high blood pressure, irregular heartbeat; eye irritation or light sensitivity; itchy skin.
WHAT TO DO:
Overdose unlikely to threaten life. If person takes much larger amount than prescribed, call doctor, poison-control center or hospital emergency room for instructions.

If you forget a dose:
Take up to 12 hours late. If more than 12 hours, wait for next dose (don't double this dose).

What drug does:
- Maintains growth and health.
- Prevents rickets.
- Essential so body can use calcium and phosphate.

Time lapse before drug works:
2 hours. May require 2 to 3 weeks of continual use for maximum effect.

Don't take with:
Non-prescription drugs or drugs in Interaction column without consulting doctor.

POSSIBLE ADVERSE REACTIONS OR SIDE EFFECTS

SYMPTOMS	WHAT TO DO
Life-threatening: None expected.	
Common: None expected.	
Infrequent: Headache, metallic taste in mouth, thirst, dry mouth, constipation, appetite loss, nausea, vomiting, weakness.	Continue. Call doctor when convenient.
Rare:	
• Increased urination, increased thirst, pink eye, psychosis, severe abdominal pain, fever.	Discontinue. Call doctor right away.
• Muscle pain, bone pain.	Continue. Tell doctor when convenient.

WARNINGS & PRECAUTIONS

Don't take if:
You are allergic to medicine containing vitamin D.

Before you start, consult your doctor:
- If you plan to become pregnant while taking vitamin D.
- If you have epilepsy.
- If you have heart or blood-vessel disease.
- If you have kidney disease.

Over age 60:
Adverse reactions and side effects may be more frequent and severe than in younger persons.

Pregnancy:
Risk to unborn child outweighs drug benefits. Don't use.

Breast-feeding:
No problems expected, but consult doctor.

Infants & children:
- Avoid large doses.
- Keep vitamins out of children's reach.

Prolonged use:
No problems expected.

Skin & sunlight:
No problems expected.

Driving, piloting or hazardous work:
No problems expected.

Discontinuing:
Don't discontinue without doctor's advice until you complete prescribed dose, even though symptoms diminish or disappear.

Others:
- Don't exceed dose. Too much over a long time may be harmful.
- A balanced diet should provide all the vitamin D a healthy person needs and make supplements unnecessary. Best sources are fish and vitamin-D fortified milk and bread.
- Some products contain tartrazine dye. Avoid, if allergic (especially aspirin hypersensitivity).

POSSIBLE INTERACTION WITH OTHER DRUGS

GENERIC NAME OR DRUG CLASS	COMBINED EFFECT
Antacids* (magnesium-containing)	Possible excess magnesium.
Anticonvulsants, hydantoin*	Decreased vitamin D effect.
Calcium (high doses)	Excess calcium in blood.
Calcium-channel blockers*	Possible decreased effect of calcium-channel blockers.
Calcium supplements*	Excessive absorption of vitamin D.
Cholestyramine	Decreased vitamin D effect.
Colestipol	Decreased vitamin D absorption.
Cortisone	Decreased vitamin D effect.
Digitalis preparations*	Heartbeat irregularities.
Diuretics, thiazide*	Possible increased calcium.
Mineral oil	Decreased vitamin D effect.
Neomycin	Decreased vitamin D absorption.
Nicardipine	Decreased nicardipine effect.
Phenobarbital	Decreased vitamin D effect.
Phosphorous preparations*	Accumulation of excess phosphorous.
Rifampin	Possible decreased vitamin D effect.
Vitamin D, other	Possible toxicity.

POSSIBLE INTERACTION WITH OTHER SUBSTANCES

INTERACTS WITH	COMBINED EFFECT
Alcohol:	None expected.
Beverages:	None expected.
Cocaine:	None expected.
Foods:	None expected.
Marijuana:	None expected.
Tobacco:	None expected.

*See Glossary

VITAMIN E

BRAND NAMES

Aquasol E	Eprolin
Chew-E	Epsilan-M
Daltose	Pheryl-E
E-Ferol	Viterra E

Numerous other multiple vitamin-mineral supplements.

BASIC INFORMATION

Habit forming? No
Prescription needed? No
Available as generic? Yes
Drug class: Vitamin supplement

USES

- Dietary supplement to promote normal growth, development and health.
- Treatment and prevention of vitamin-E deficiency, especially in premature or low birth-weight infants.
- Treatment for fibrocystic disease of the breast.
- Treatment for circulatory problems to the lower extremities.
- Treatment for sickle-cell anemia.
- Treatment for lung toxicity from air pollution.

DOSAGE & USAGE INFORMATION

How to take:
- Tablet or capsule—Swallow with liquid or food to lessen stomach irritation.
- Drops—Dilute dose in beverage before swallowing or squirt directly into mouth.
- Injection—Take under doctor's supervision.

When to take:
At the same times each day.

If you forget a dose:
Take when you remember. Don't double next dose.

What drug does:
- Promotes normal growth and development.
- Prevents oxidation in body.

Continued next column

OVERDOSE

SYMPTOMS:
Nausea, vomiting, fatigue.
WHAT TO DO:
Overdose unlikely to threaten life. If person takes much larger amount than prescribed, call doctor, poison-control center or hospital emergency room for instructions.

Time lapse before drug works:
Not determined.

Don't take with:
See Interaction column and consult doctor.

POSSIBLE ADVERSE REACTIONS OR SIDE EFFECTS

SYMPTOMS	WHAT TO DO
Life-threatening:	
None expected.	
Common:	
None expected.	
Infrequent:	
Nausea, stomach pain, muscle aches, pain in lower legs, fever, tiredness, weakness.	Continue. Call doctor when convenient.
Rare:	
Blurred vision, diarrhea.	Discontinue. Call doctor right away.

WARNINGS & PRECAUTIONS

Don't take if:
You are allergic to vitamin E.

Before you start, consult your doctor:
- If you have had blood clots in leg veins (thrombophlebitis).
- If you have liver disease.

Over age 60:
No problems expected. Avoid excessive doses.

Pregnancy:
No problems expected with normal daily requirements. Don't exceed prescribed dose.

Breast-feeding:
No problems expected.

Infants & children:
Use only under medical supervision.

Prolonged use:
Toxic accumulation of vitamin E. Don't exceed recommended dose.

Skin & sunlight:
No problems expected.

Driving, piloting or hazardous work:
No problems expected.

Discontinuing:
No problems expected.

Others:
A balanced diet should provide all the vitamin E a healthy person needs and make supplements unnecessary. Best sources are vegetable oils, whole-grain cereals, liver.

POSSIBLE INTERACTION WITH OTHER DRUGS

GENERIC NAME OR DRUG CLASS	COMBINED EFFECT
Anticoagulants, oral*	Increased anti-coagulant effect.
Cholestyramine	Decreased vitamin E absorption.
Colestipol	Decreased vitamin E absorption.
Iron supplements*	Possible decreased effect of iron supplement in patients with iron-deficiency anemia. Decreased vitamin E effect in healthy persons.
Mineral oil	Decreased vitamin E effect.
Neomycin	Decreased vitamin E absorption.
Vitamin A	Recommended dose of vitamin E—Increased benefit and decreased toxicity of vitamin A. Excess dose of vitamin E—Vitamin A depletion.

POSSIBLE INTERACTION WITH OTHER SUBSTANCES

INTERACTS WITH	COMBINED EFFECT
Alcohol:	None expected.
Beverages:	None expected.
Cocaine:	None expected.
Foods:	None expected.
Marijuana:	None expected.
Tobacco:	None expected.

VITAMIN K

BRAND NAMES

AquaMEPHYTON	Mephyton
Konakion	Phytonadione
Menadione	Synkayvite
Menadiol	

BASIC INFORMATION

Habit forming? No
Prescription needed? No
Available as generic? No
Drug class: Vitamin supplement

 USES

- Dietary supplement.
- Treatment for bleeding disorders and malabsorption diseases due to vitamin K deficiency.
- Treatment for hemorrhagic disease of the newborn.
- Treatment for bleeding due to overdose of oral anticoagulants.

 DOSAGE & USAGE INFORMATION

How to take:
- Usually given by injection in hospital or doctor's office.
- Tablet—Swallow with liquid. If you can't swallow whole, crumble tablet and take with liquid or food.

When to take:
At the same time each day.

If you forget a dose:
Take as soon as you remember up to 12 hours late. If more than 12 hours, wait for next scheduled dose (don't double this dose).

What drug does:
- Promotes growth, development and good health.
- Supplies a necessary ingredient for blood clotting.

Continued next column

 OVERDOSE

SYMPTOMS:
Nausea, vomiting.
WHAT TO DO:
Overdose unlikely to threaten life. If person takes much larger amount than prescribed, call doctor, poison-control center or hospital emergency room for instructions.

Time lapse before drug works:
15 to 30 minutes to support blood clotting.

Don't take with:
See Interaction column and consult doctor.

 POSSIBLE ADVERSE REACTIONS OR SIDE EFFECTS

SYMPTOMS	WHAT TO DO
Life-threatening: None expected.	
Common: None expected.	
Infrequent: Unusual taste.	Continue. Call doctor when convenient.
Rare: Rash, hives.	Discontinue. Call doctor right away.

WARNINGS & PRECAUTIONS

Don't take if:
- You are allergic to vitamin K.
- You have G6PD deficiency.
- You have liver disease.

Before you start, consult your doctor:
If you are pregnant.

Over age 60:
No problems expected.

Pregnancy:
Don't exceed dose.

Breast-feeding:
No problems expected.

Infants & children:
Phytonadione is the preferred form for hemorrhagic disease of the newborn.

Prolonged use:
No problems expected.

Skin & sunlight:
No problems expected.

Driving, piloting or hazardous work:
No problems expected.

Discontinuing:
No problems expected.

Others:
- Tell all doctors and dentists you consult that you take this medicine.
- Don't exceed dose. Too much over a long time may be harmful.
- A balanced diet should provide all the vitamin K a healthy person needs and make supplements unnecessary. Best sources are green, leafy vegetables, meat or dairy products.

POSSIBLE INTERACTION WITH OTHER DRUGS

GENERIC NAME OR DRUG CLASS	COMBINED EFFECT
Anticoagulants, oral*	Decreased anti-coagulant effect.
Cholestyramine	Decreased vitamin K effect.
Colestipol	Decreased vitamin K absorption.
Mineral oil (long term)	Vitamin K deficiency.
Neomycin	Decreased vitamin K absorption.
Sulfa drugs*	Vitamin K deficiency.

POSSIBLE INTERACTION WITH OTHER SUBSTANCES

INTERACTS WITH	COMBINED EFFECT
Alcohol:	None expected.
Beverages:	None expected.
Cocaine:	None expected.
Foods:	None expected.
Marijuana:	None expected.
Tobacco:	None expected.

*See Glossary

VITAMINS & FLUORIDE

BRAND AND GENERIC NAMES

Adeflor
Carl-Tab
Mulvidren-F
Poly-Vi-Flor
MULTIPLE VITAMINS & FLUORIDE
VITAMINS A, D & C & FLUORIDE

Tri-Vi-Flor
Vi-Daylin/F
Vi-Penta F

BASIC INFORMATION

Habit forming? No
Prescription needed? Yes
Available as generic? No
Drug class: Vitamins, minerals

 USES

- Reduces incidence of tooth cavities (fluoride). Children who need supplements should take until age 16.
- Prevents deficiencies of vitamin included in formula (some contain multiple vitamins whose content varies among products, others contain only vitamins A, D and C).

 DOSAGE & USAGE INFORMATION

How to take:
- Chewable tablets—Chew or crush before swallowing.
- Oral liquid—Take by mouth measured with specially marked dropper. May mix with food, fruit juice, cereal.

When to take:
- Bedtime or with or just after meals.
- If at bedtime, brush teeth first.

If you forget a dose:
Take as soon as you remember up to 2 hours late. If more than 2 hours, wait for next scheduled dose (don't double this dose).

Continued next column

 OVERDOSE

SYMPTOMS:
Minor overdose—Black, brown or white spots on teeth.
Massive overdose—Shallow breathing, black or tarry stools, bloody vomit.
WHAT TO DO:
- **Dial 0 (operator) or 911 (emergency) for an ambulance or medical help. Then give first aid immediately.**
- **See emergency information on inside covers.**

What drug does:
Provides supplemental fluoride to combat tooth decay.

Time lapse before drug works:
8 weeks to provide maximum benefit.

Don't take with:
- Other medicine simultaneously.
- See Interaction column and consult doctor.

 POSSIBLE ADVERSE REACTIONS OR SIDE EFFECTS

SYMPTOMS	WHAT TO DO
Life-threatening: Fainting, bloody vomit, bloody or black stool.	Discontinue. Seek emergency treatment.
Common: White, black or brown spots on teeth; nausea; vomiting.	Discontinue. Call doctor right away.
Infrequent: • Drowsiness; abdominal pain; increased salivation; watery eyes; weight loss; sore throat, fever, mouth sores; constipation; bone pain; rash; muscle stiffness; weakness; tremor; agitation.	Discontinue. Call doctor right away.
• Diarrhea.	Continue. Call doctor when convenient.
Rare: None expected.	

WARNINGS & PRECAUTIONS

Don't take if:
- Your water supply contains 0.7 parts fluoride per million. Too much fluoride stains teeth permanently.
- You are allergic to any fluoride-containing product.
- You have underactive thyroid.

Before you start, consult your doctor or dentist:
For proper dosage.

Over age 60:
No problems expected.

Pregnancy:
No problems expected.

Breast-feeding:
No problems expected.

Infants & children:
No problems expected in children over 3 years of age except accidental overdose. Keep vitamin-mineral supplements out of children's reach.

Prolonged use:
Excess may cause discolored teeth and decreased calcium in blood.

Skin & sunlight:
No problems expected.

Driving, piloting or hazardous work:
No problems expected.

Discontinuing:
No problems expected.

Others:
- Store in original plastic container. Fluoride decomposes glass.
- Check with dentist once or twice a year to keep cavities at a minimum. Topical applications of fluoride may also be helpful.
- Fluoride probably not necessary if water contains about 1 part per million of fluoride or more. Check with health department.
- Don't freeze.
- Don't keep outdated medicine.

POSSIBLE INTERACTION WITH OTHER DRUGS

GENERIC NAME OR DRUG CLASS	COMBINED EFFECT
Iron supplements*	Decreased effect of any vitamin E if present in multivitamin product.
Vitamin A	May lead to vitamin A toxicity if vitamin A is in combination.
Vitamin D	May lead to vitamin D toxicity if vitamin D is in combination.

POSSIBLE INTERACTION WITH OTHER SUBSTANCES

INTERACTS WITH	COMBINED EFFECT
Alcohol:	None expected.
Beverages: Milk.	Prevents absorption of fluoride. Space dose 2 hours before or after milk.
Cocaine:	None expected.
Foods:	None expected.
Marijuana:	None expected.
Tobacco:	None expected.

XANTHINE BRONCHODILATORS

BRAND AND GENERIC NAMES

See complete list of brand names in the *Brand Name Directory*, page 1073.

BASIC INFORMATION

Habit forming? No
Prescription needed?
  Canada—No
  U.S.: High strength—Yes
         Low strength—No
Available as generic? Yes
Drug class: Bronchodilator (xanthine)

USES

Treatment for bronchial asthma symptoms.

DOSAGE & USAGE INFORMATION

How to take:
- Tablet or capsule—Swallow with liquid.
- Extended-release tablets or capsules—Swallow each dose whole. If you take regular tablets, you may chew or crush them.
- Suppositories—Remove wrapper and moisten suppository with water. Gently insert larger end into rectum. Push well into rectum with finger.
- Syrup—Take as directed on bottle.
- Enema—Use as directed on label.

When to take:
Most effective taken on empty stomach 1 hour before or 2 hours after eating. However, may take with food to lessen stomach upset.

If you forget a dose:
Take as soon as you remember up to 2 hours late. If more than 2 hours, wait for next scheduled dose (don't double this dose).

What drug does:
Relaxes and expands bronchial tubes.

Continued next column

OVERDOSE

SYMPTOMS:
Restlessness, irritability, confusion, delirium, convulsions, rapid pulse, coma.
WHAT TO DO:
- **Dial 0 (operator) or 911 (emergency) for an ambulance or medical help. Then give first aid immediately.**
- **See emergency information on inside covers.**

Time lapse before drug works:
15 to 30 minutes.

Don't take with:
See Interaction column and consult doctor.

POSSIBLE ADVERSE REACTIONS OR SIDE EFFECTS

SYMPTOMS	WHAT TO DO
Life-threatening: None expected.	
Common: Headache, irritability, nervousness, nausea, restlessness, insomnia, vomiting, stomach pain.	Continue. Call doctor when convenient.
Infrequent: • Rash or hives, flushed face, diarrhea, appetite loss, rapid breathing, irregular heartbeat.	Discontinue. Call doctor right away.
• Dizziness or lightheadedness.	Continue. Call doctor when convenient.
Rare: Frequent urination.	Continue. Call doctor when convenient.

XANTHINE BRONCHODILATORS

WARNINGS & PRECAUTIONS

Don't take if:
- You are allergic to any bronchodilator.
- You have an active peptic ulcer.

Before you start, consult your doctor:
- If you have had impaired kidney or liver function.
- If you have gastritis.
- If you have a peptic ulcer.
- If you have high blood pressure or heart disease.
- If you take medication for gout.

Over age 60:
Adverse reactions and side effects may be more frequent and severe than in younger persons.

Pregnancy:
Risk to unborn child outweighs drug benefits. Don't use.

Breast-feeding:
Drug passes into milk. Avoid drug or discontinue nursing until you finish medicine. Consult doctor for advice on maintaining milk supply.

Infants & children:
Use only under medical supervision.

Prolonged use:
Stomach irritation.

Skin & sunlight:
No problems expected.

Driving, piloting or hazardous work:
Avoid if lightheaded or dizzy. Otherwise, no problems expected.

Discontinuing:
May be unnecessary to finish medicine. Follow doctor's instructions.

Others:
No problems expected.

POSSIBLE INTERACTION WITH OTHER DRUGS

GENERIC NAME OR DRUG CLASS	COMBINED EFFECT
Allopurinol	Increased allopurinol effect.
Aminoglutethimide	Possible decreased bronchodilator effect.
Beta-agonists *	Increased effect of both drugs.
Beta-adrenergic blockers *	Decreased bronchodilator effect.
Cimetidine	Increased bronchodilator effect.
Clindamycin	May increase bronchodilator effect.
Corticosteroids *	Possible increased bronchodilator effect.
Erythromycin	Increased bronchodilator effect.
Furosemide	Increased furosemide effect.
Lincomycin	May increase bronchodilator effect.
Lithium	Decreased lithium effect.
Phenobarbital	Decreased bronchodilator effect.
Phenytoin	Decreased bronchodilator effect.
Probenecid	Increased effect of dyphylline.
Ranitidine	Possible increased bronchodilator effect and toxicity.
Rauwolfia alkaloids *	Rapid heartbeat.
Rifampin	Decreased bronchodilator effect.
Sulfinpyrazone	Increased effect of dyphylline.
Sympathomimetics *	Possible increased bronchodilator effect.
Troleandomycin	Increased bronchodilator effect.

POSSIBLE INTERACTION WITH OTHER SUBSTANCES

INTERACTS WITH	COMBINED EFFECT
Alcohol:	None expected.
Beverages: Caffeine drinks.	Nervousness and insomnia.
Cocaine:	Excess stimulation. Avoid.
Foods:	None expected.
Marijuana:	Slightly increased antiasthmatic effect of bronchodilator. Decreased effect with chronic use.
Tobacco:	Decreased bronchodilator effect.

XYLOMETAZOLINE

BRAND NAMES

See complete list of brand names in the *Brand Name Directory*, page 1073.

BASIC INFORMATION

Habit forming? No
Prescription needed? No
Available as generic? Yes
Drug class: Sympathomimetic

 USES

Relieves congestion of nose, sinuses and throat from allergies and infections.

 DOSAGE & USAGE INFORMATION

How to take:
Nasal solution, nasal spray—Use as directed on label. Avoid contamination. Don't use same container for more than 1 person.

When to take:
When needed, no more often than every 4 hours.

If you forget a dose:
Take as soon as you remember. Wait 4 hours for next dose.

What drug does:
Constricts walls of small arteries in nose, sinuses and eustachian tubes.

Time lapse before drug works:
5 to 30 minutes.

Continued next column

 OVERDOSE

SYMPTOMS:
Headache, sweating, anxiety, agitation, rapid and irregular heartbeat.
WHAT TO DO:
● **Dial 0 (operator) or 911 (emergency) for an ambulance or medical help. Then give first aid immediately.**
● **If patient is unconscious and not breathing, give mouth-to-mouth breathing. If there is no heartbeat, use cardiac massage and mouth-to-mouth breathing (CPR). If you can't get help quickly, take patient to nearest emergency facility.**
● **See emergency information on inside covers.**

Don't take with:
● Non-prescription drugs for allergy, cough or cold without consulting doctor.
● See Interaction column and consult doctor.

 POSSIBLE ADVERSE REACTIONS OR SIDE EFFECTS

SYMPTOMS	WHAT TO DO
Life-threatening: None expected.	
Common: Runny, stuffy, burning, dry or stinging nose; sneezing; fast, irregular or pounding heartbeat.	Continue. Call doctor when convenient.
Infrequent: Headache or lightheadedness, insomnia, nervousness.	Continue. Call doctor when convenient.
Rare: None expected.	

WARNINGS & PRECAUTIONS

Don't take if:
You are allergic to any sympathomimetic nasal spray.

Before you start, consult your doctor:
- If you have heart disease or high blood pressure.
- If you have diabetes.
- If you have overactive thyroid.
- If you have taken MAO inhibitors in past 2 weeks.

Over age 60:
Adverse reactions and side effects may be more frequent and severe than in younger persons.

Pregnancy:
No proven harm to unborn child. Avoid if possible.

Breast-feeding:
No proven problems. Consult doctor.

Infants & children:
Don't give to children younger than 2.

Prolonged use:
Drug may lose effectiveness, cause increased congestion (rebound effect*) and irritate nasal membranes.

Skin & sunlight:
No problems expected.

Driving, piloting or hazardous work:
No problems expected.

Discontinuing:
May be unnecessary to finish medicine. Follow doctor's instructions.

Others:
No problems expected.

POSSIBLE INTERACTION WITH OTHER DRUGS

GENERIC NAME OR DRUG CLASS	COMBINED EFFECT
Antidepressants, tricyclics (TCA)*	Increased xylometazoline effect.
Beta-adrenergic blockers*	Decreased effects of both drugs.
Guanadrel	Decreased effect of both drugs.
MAO inhibitors*	Dangerous blood-pressure rise.
Methyldopa	Possible increased blood pressure.
Minoxidil	Decreased minoxidil effect.
Nitrates*	Possible decreased effects of both drugs.
Phenothiazines*	Possible increased xylometazoline toxicity. Possible decreased xylometazoline effect.
Rauwolfia	Decreased rauwolfia effect.
Sympathomimetics*	Increased effect of both drugs, especially harmful side effects.
Terazosin	Decreases effectiveness of terazosin.

POSSIBLE INTERACTION WITH OTHER SUBSTANCES

INTERACTS WITH	COMBINED EFFECT
Alcohol:	None expected.
Beverages: Caffeine drinks.	Nervousness or insomnia.
Cocaine:	High risk of heartbeat irregularities and high blood pressure.
Foods:	None expected.
Marijuana:	Overstimulation. Avoid.
Tobacco:	None expected.

*See Glossary

ZIDOVUDINE (AZT, Azidothymidine)

BRAND NAMES

Retrovir

BASIC INFORMATION

Habit forming? No
Prescription needed? Yes
Available as generic? No
Drug class: Antiviral

 USES

Treatment of selected adult patients with AIDS (Acquired Immune Deficiency Syndrome) and advanced ARC (AIDS Related Complex) who have a history of pneumonia caused by *Pneumocystis carinii.*

 DOSAGE & USAGE INFORMATION

How to take:
Capsule—Swallow with liquid.

When to take:
Every 4 hours around the clock unless instructed otherwise.

If you forget a dose:
Take as soon as you remember.

What drug does:
Inhibits reproduction of some viruses, including HIV virus (the virus that causes AIDS).

Time lapse before drug works:
May require several weeks of treatment for full effect.

Don't take with:
See Interaction column and consult doctor.

 OVERDOSE

SYMPTOMS:
No cases reported. However, if overdose occurs, follow instructions below.
WHAT TO DO:
- Dial 0 (operator) or 911 (emergency) for an ambulance or medical help. Then give first aid immediately.
- See emergency information on inside covers.

 POSSIBLE ADVERSE REACTIONS OR SIDE EFFECTS

SYMPTOMS	WHAT TO DO
Life-threatening: None expected.	
Common:	
• Anemia, low white-blood-cell count.	Discontinue. Call doctor right away.
• Severe headache, nausea, insomnia.	Continue. Call doctor when convenient.
Infrequent: Severe headache, sweating, fever, appetite loss, abdominal pain, vomiting, aching muscles, dizziness, numbness in hands and feet, shortness of breath, skin rash, strange taste.	Continue. Call doctor when convenient.
Rare: Constipation, confusion.	Discontinue. Call doctor right away.

ZIDOVUDINE (AZT, Azidothymidine)

 ## WARNINGS & PRECAUTIONS

Don't take if:
You are allergic to any component of this capsule.

Before you start, consult your doctor:
- If you know you have a low white-blood-cell count or severe anemia.
- If you have severe kidney or liver disease.

Over age 60:
Adverse reactions and side effects may be more frequent and severe than in younger persons. Ask doctor about smaller doses.

Pregnancy:
Effect unknown at present.

Breast-feeding:
Drug passes into milk. If possible, avoid drug or discontinue until you finish medicine. Consult your doctor for advice on maintaining milk supply.

Infants & children:
Not recommended.

Prolonged use:
Not recommended.

Skin & sunlight:
No problems expected.

Driving, piloting, or hazardous work:
Don't drive or pilot aircraft until you learn how medicine affects you. Don't work around dangerous machinery. Don't climb ladders or work in high places. Danger increases if you drink alcohol or take medicine affecting alertness and reflexes, such as antihistamines, tranquilizers, sedatives, pain medicine, narcotics and mind-altering drugs.

Discontinuing:
Don't discontinue without consulting your doctor. Dose may require gradual reduction if you have taken drug for a long time. Doses of other drugs may also require adjustment.

Others:
- AZT does *not cure* HIV virus infections. Transfusions or dose modification may be necessary if toxicity develops.
- Have blood counts followed closely during treatment to detect anemia or lowered white-blood-cell count.
- AZT does not reduce risk of transmitting disease to others.

 ## POSSIBLE INTERACTION WITH OTHER DRUGS

GENERIC NAME OR DRUG CLASS	COMBINED EFFECT
Acetaminophen	May increase toxic effects of AZT. Avoid.
Acyclovir	Lethargy, convulsions.
Aspirin	May increase toxic effects of AZT.
Indomethacin	May increase toxic effects of AZT.
Probenecid	May increase toxic effects of AZT.

 ## POSSIBLE INTERACTION WITH OTHER SUBSTANCES

INTERACTS WITH	COMBINED EFFECT
Alcohol:	Unknown. Best avoid.
Beverages:	None expected.
Cocaine:	Unknown. Best avoid.
Foods:	None expected.
Marijuana:	Unknown. Best avoid.
Tobacco:	None expected.

Brand and Generic Name Directory

The following drugs are alphabetized by generic name or drug class, shown in large capital letters. The brand and generic names that follow each title in this list are the complete list referred to on the drug charts. Generic names are in all capital letters on the lists.

ACETAMINOPHEN

A'Cenol
Acephen
Aceta
Ace-Tabs
Aceta w/Codeine
Acetaco
Acetaminophen w/Codeine
Acetaminophen Uniserts
Actamin
Algisin
Amacodone
Amaphen
Amphenol
Anacin-3
Anapap
Anaphen
Anoquan
Anuphen
Apacet
Apamide Tablets
APAP
Apo-Acetaminophen
Arthralgen
Aspirin-Free Excedrin
Atasol
Axotal
Bancap w/Codeine
Banesin
Banesin Forte
Bayapap
Bromo-Seltzer
C2A
Cafadol
Campain
Capital
Capital w/Codeine
Chlorzone Forte
Co-Gesic
Co-Tylenol
Coastaldyne
Coastalgesic
Codalan
Codap
Colrex
Compal
Comtrex
Conacetol
Congespirin
Covangesic
D-Sinus
Dapa
Dapase
Darvocet-N
Datril
Dia-Gesic
Dialog
Dolacet
Dolanex
Dolene AP-65
Dolor
Dolprin
Dorcol
Dorcol Children's Fever and Pain Reducer

Dristan
Duadacin
Dularin
Duradyne DHC
Dynosal
Empracet w/Codeine
Endecon
Esgic
Excedrin
Exdol
Febrigesic
Febrinol
Febrogesic
Fendol
G-1
G-2
G-3
Gaysal
Genapap
Genebs
Genetabs
Gualamine
Halenol
Hasacode
Hi-Temp
Hyco-Pap
Hycomine Compound
Korigesic
Liquiprin
Liquix-C
Lorcet
Lyteca
Meda Cap
Meda Tab
Mejoral without aspirin
Mejoralito
Metrogesic
Midol PMS
Midrin
Migralam
Minotal
Myapap
Naldegesic
NAPAP
Nebs
Neopap
Oraphen-PD
Ornex
Ossonate-Plus
Pacaps
Pain Relief without aspirin
Panadol
Panasorb
Panex
Paracetamol
Parafon Forte
Paraphen
Pavadon
Pedric
Peedee Dose Aspirin
Percocet-5
Percogesic
Phenaphen
Phenaphen w/Codeine
Phendex

Phrenilin
Presalin
Prodolor
Protid
Proval
Repan
Rhinocaps
Robigesic
Ronuvex
Rounox
S-A-C
SK-65 APAP
SK-APAP
SK-Oxycodone w/Acetaminophen
Salatin
Saleto
Salimeph Forte
Salphenyl
Sedapap
Sinarest
Sine-Aid
Sine-Off
Singlet
Sinubid
Sinulin
Sinutab
St. Joseph Aspirin Free
Stopayne
Strascogesic
Sudoprin
Summit
Supac
Suppap
Sylapar
T.P.I.
Talacen
Tapanol
Tapar
Temlo
Tempra
Tenlap
Tenol
Triaminicin
Trigesic
Trind Sryup
Two-Dyne
Ty Caplets
Ty Pap
Ty-tabs
Tylenol
Tylenol w/Codeine
Tylox
Valadol
Valorin
Vanquish
Vicodin
Wygesic

ACETAMINOPHEN & SALICYLATES

445 Anti-Pain Compound
Accurate Forte
ACETAMINOPHEN & ASPIRIN

ACETAMINOPHEN, ASPIRIN &
  SALICYLAMIDE
ACETAMINOPHEN &
  SALICYLAMIDE
ACETAMINOPHEN & SODIUM
  SALICYLATE
APAP Fortified
Arthralgen
Banesin
Buffets II
Dinol
Doan's Pills
Double-A
Duoprin
Duoprin-S
Duradyne
Dynosal
Excedrin
Gaysal-S
Gemnisyn
Goody's Extra Strength Tablets
Goody's Headache Powders
Pain Reliever
Presalin
Rid-A-Pain Compound
S-A-C
Salatin
Saleto
Salimeph Forte
Salocol
Supac
Tisma
Trigesic
Tri-Pain
Vanquish

ADRENOCORTICOIDS
(Topical)
Acticort
Adcortyl
Adcortyl in Orabase
Aeroseb-Dex
Aeroseb-HC
Alphatrex
Aristocort
Aristocort A
Aristocort C
Aristocort D
Aristocort R
Bactine Hydrocortisone
Barriere-HC
Beben
Benisone
Beta-Val
Betacort
Betacort Scalp Lotion
Betaderm
Betaderm Scalp Lotion
Betatrex
Betnesol
Betnovate
CaldeCORT
Caldecort Anti-Itch
Carmol-HC
Celestoderm-V
Celestone
Cetacort
Clinicort
Cioderm
Cordran
Cordran SP
Cort-Dome

Cortaid
Cortate
Cortef
Corticaine
Corticosporin
Corticreme
Cortifoam
Cortiment
Cortisol
Cortizone
Cortoderm
Cortril
Cremocort
Cyclocort
Decaderm
Decadron
Decaspray
Delacort
Dermacort
DermiCort
Dermolate
Dermophyl
Dermovate
Dermovate Scalp Application
Dermtex HC
DesOwen
Dioderm
Diprolene
Diprosone
Drenison
EF cortelan
Ectosone
Ectosone Scalp Lotion
Eldecort
Emo-Cort
Epifoam
Florone
Fluocet
Fluoderm
Fluolar
Fluolean
Fluonid
Fluonide
Flurosyn
Flutex
Flutone
Gynecort
H2 Cort
HC-Jel
Halciderm
Halog
Halog E
Hexadrol
HI-Cor
HI-Cort
Hyderm
Hydro-Corilean
Hydro-Tex
Hydrocortone
Hytone
Kenalog
Kenalog-E
Kenalog-H
Kenalog in Orabase
Lacticare-HC
Lanacort
Lidemol
Lidex
Lidex-E
Locold
Locacorten
Lyderm
Maxiflor

Medrol
Metaderm
Meti-Derm
Metosyn
Metosyn FAPG
Neo-Cortef
Neo-Decadron
Novobetamet
Novohydrocort
Nutracort
Orabase HCA
Oxylone
Penecort
Pharma-Cort
Proctocort
Psorcon
Psorcon-E
Racet-SE
Rectocort
Rhulicort
Spencort
Stie-Cort
Synacort
Synalar
Synamol
Synandone
Synemol
Temovate
Texacort
Topicort
Topsyn
Triacet
Triaderm
Trianide
Triderm
Tridesilon
Trymex
Unicort
Uticort
Valisone
Valisone Scalp Lotion
Vioform
Westcort
Some of these brands are
  available as oral medicine.
  Look under specific generic
  name for each brand.

ALUMINUM HYDROXIDE
Alagel
Algenic Alka
Alka-mag
ALternaGEL
Alu-Cap
Alu-Tab
Aludrox
Alumid
Aluscop
Amphojel
Basaljel
Bisodol
Camalox
Chemgel
Creamalin
De Witts
Delcid
Di-Gel
Dialume
Dioval Ex
Ducon
Estomul-m
Gaviscon

Gelusil
Kolantyl
Kolantyl Wafers
Kudrox
Lowsium
Maalox
Magmalin
Magnagel
Magnatril
Maox
Marblen
Max-Ox 40
Maxamag
M.O.M.
Mucotin
Mygel
Mylanta
Neosorb Plus
Nephrox
Neutracomp
Neutralca-S
Par-mag
Pepsogel
Phillips Milk of Magnesia
Ratic
Riopan
Robalate
Rolaids
Rulox
Spastoced
Sterazolidin
Tralmag
Univol
Uro-Mag
Vanquish
Win Gel

ALUMINUM & MAGNESIUM ANTACIDS

Algenic Alka
Algenic Alka Improved
Alka-Med
Alma-Mag
Aludrox
Alumid
ALUMINA & MAGNESIA
ALUMINA & MAGENSIUM
   CARBONATE
ALUMINA, MAGNESIUM
   CARBONATE & MAGNESIUM
   OXIDE
ALUMINA & MAGNESIUM
   TRISILICATE
Aluscop
Amphojel 500
Creamalin
Delcid
DIHYDROXYALUMINUM
   AMINOACETATE & MAGNESIA
DIHYDROXYALUMINUM
   AMINOACETATE, MAGNESIA &
   ALUMINA
Diovol Ex
Estomul-M
Gaviscon
Gelamal
Gelusil
Gelusil Extra Strength
Kolantyl
Kudrox
Lowsium
Maalox

Maalox No. 1
Maalox No. 2
Maalox TC
Magmalin
Magnagel
Magnatril
MAGNESIUM TRISILICATE,
   ALUMINA & MAGNESIA
Mintox
Mylanta-2 Plain
Neosorb Plus
Neutracomp
Neutralca-S
Riopan
Rolox
Rulox
Rulox No. 1
Rulox No. 2
Tralmag
Univol
WinGel

ALUMINUM, MAGNESIUM, MAGALDRATE & SIMETHICONE ANTACIDS

Alma-Mag #4 Improved
Almacone
Almacone II
Alma-Mag Improved
Alumid Plus
ALUMINA, MAGNESIA &
   SIMETHICONE
Amphojel Plus
AntaGel
AntaGel-II
Di-Gel
Diovol
Gelusil
Gelusil-II
Gelusil-M
Maalox Plus
MAGALDRATE & SIMETHICONE
MI-Acid
Mygel
Mygel II
Mylanta
Mylanta-2
Mylanta-2 Extra Strength
Mylanta-II
Newtrogel II
Riopan Plus
Silain-Gel
Simaal Gel
Simaal 2 Gel
Simeco
SIMETHICONE, ALUMINA,
   MAGNESIUM CARBONATE &
   MAGNESIA

ANDROGENS

Anabolin
Anabolin LA 100
Anadrol-50
Anapolon 50
Anavar
Andro
Andro-Cyp
Andro-LA
Android
Android-F

Android-T
Androlone
Andron
Andronaq
Andronaq-LA
Andronate
Androyd
Andryl
Bay-Testone
Danabol
Deca-Durabolin
Delatestryl
Dep Andro
Depo-Testosterone
Depotest
Dianabol
Durabolin
Duratest
Durathate
ETHYLESTRENOL
Everone
FLUOXYMESTERONE
Halotestin
Histerone
Malogen
Malogex
Maxibolin
Metandren
Metandren Linguets
METHANDROSTENOLONE
METHYLTESTOSTERONE
NANDROLONE
Ora-Testryl
Oratestin
Oreton Methyl
OXANDROLONE
OXYMETHOLONE
STANOZOLOL
T-Cypionate
Teslonate
Testa-C
Testaqua
Testex
Testoject
Testoject-LA
Testolin
Testone L.A.
TESTOSTERONE
Testostroval P.A.
Testred
Testrin P.A.
T-Iontae
Virilon
Winstrol

ANESTHETICS (Topical)

Aero Caine
Aero Caine Aerosol
Aerotherm
Americaine
Americaine Aerosol
Americaine Anesthetic Lubricant
Americaine Ointment
Anbesol
Anestacon
Bactine
Benzocaine
Benzocaine Topical
Benzocal
BICozene
Burntame
BUTACAINE

BUTAMBEN
Butesin Picrate
Butyl aminobenzoate
Butyn
Butyn Sulfate
Caine Spray
Cal-Vi-Nol
Cetacaine
Cetacine
Chiggerex
Chiggertox
Clinicaine
Cyclaine
Cyclaine Solution
CYCLOMETHYCAINE
Derma-Medicone
Dermacoat
Dermo-Gen
Dermoplast
Dibucaine
Diothane
DIPERODON
Dyclone
DYCLONINE
Ethyl Aminobenzoate
Fleet Relief
Follie
Hexathricin Aerospra
HEXYLCAINE
Hurricaine
Isotraine
Ivy-Dry Cream
Lanacane
Lida-Mantle
Lidocaine
Lidocaine Ointment
Lignocaine
Medicone
Medicone Dressing
Mercurochrome II
Morusan
Nupercainal
Nupercainal Cream
Nupercainal Ointment
Nupercainal Spray
Orabase with Benzocaine
Orajel
Panthocal A & D
Perifoam
Pontocaine
Pontocaine Cream
Pontocaine Ointment
PRAMOXINE
Prax
Proctodon
Proctofoam
Proxine
Quotane
Rectal Medicone
Rid-A-Pain
Soft-N-Soothe
Solarcaine
Surfacaine
Tega-Caine
Tega-Dyne
TETRACAINE
Tronolane
Tronothane
Unguentine
Unguentine Plus
Unguentine Spray
Urolocaine
Velvacaine

Xylocaine
Xylocaine Ointment
Xylocaine Viscous

ANTI-ACNE (Topical)

Acne-Dome
Acno
Acnomel
Acnotex
Calicylic
Cuticura
Derma & Soft Creme
Domerine
Fomac
Fostex
Hydrisalic
Ionil
Keralyt
Klaron
Meted
Metid-2
Occlusal
OxyClean
P&S
Pernox
RESORCINOL
RESORCINOL AND SULFUR
Retin A
Retinoic Acid
Rezamid
SALICYLIC ACID
SALICYLIC ACID AND SULFUR
Saligel
Sastid
Sastid Plain
Sebex
Sebisol
Sebucare
Sebulex
Stie VAA
Sulforcin
Therac
TRETINOIN
Vanseb
Vitamin A Acid
Xseb

ANTIBACTERIALS (Ophthalmic)

Achromycin
Alcomicin
Aureomycin
Bleph-10
Cetamide
CHLORAMPHENICOL
CHLORTETRACYCLINE
Cortisporin
ERYTHROMYCIN
Gantrisin
Garamycin
Genoptic
Gentacidin
GENTAMYCIN
Ilotycin
Isopto Cetamide
Mycitracin
NEOMYCIN
NEOMYCIN, POLYMIXIN B AND
    BACITRACIN
NEOMYCIN, POLYMIXIN B AND
    CORTISOL

NEOMYCIN, POLYMIXIN B
    AND GRAMICIDIN
NEOMYCIN, POLYMIXIN B AND
    HYDROCORTISONE
Neosporin
Sulamyd
Sulf-10
Sulfafurazole
Sulfex
SULFONAMIDES
Sulten-10
TETRACYCLINE

ANTIBACTERIALS (Topical)

Baciguent
BACITRACIN
Bactroban
CHLORAMPHENICOL
CHLORTETRACYCLINE
CLINDAMYCIN
CLIOQUINOL
ERYTHROMYCIN
Flamazine
Flint SSD
Follie
FRAMYCETIN
FRAMYCETIN & GRAMICIDIN
FUSIDIC
FUSIDIC ACID
Garamycin
GENTAMICIN
MOMETASONE
MUPIROCIN
Myciguent
Mycitracin
NEOMYCIN
NEOMYCIN & POLYMYXIN B
NEOMYCIN, POLYMYXIN B AND
    BACITRACIN
Neo-Polycin
Neosporin
Silvadene
SILVER SULFADIAZINE
Thermazene

ANTIBACTERIALS, ANTIFUNGALS (Topical)

CLIOQUINOL AND CORTISOL
CLIOQUINOL CREAM
Dek-Quin
Flamazine
Flint SSD
HCV
Iodo
IODOCHLORHYDROXYQUIN
IODOCHLORHYDROXYQUIN AND
    CORTISOL
IODOCHLORHYDROXYQUIN AND
    HYDROCORTISONE
Mity-Quin
Myco Triacet
Mycolog
Mykacet
Mytrex
NAFTIDINE
Naftin
NYSTATIN, NEOMYCIN,
    GRAMICIDIN AND
    TRIAMCINOLONE

1055

Racet
Silvadene
SILVER SULFADIAZINE
Thermazene
Torofor
Vioform
Vioform-Hydrocortisone

ANTIFUNGALS (Topical)

Aftate
AMPHOTERACIN B
Candex
Canesten
CLOTRIMAZOLE
Cruex
Decylenes
Desenex
ECONAZOLE
Ecostatin
Fungizone
Haloprigin
Lotrimin
Micatin
MICONAZOLE
Monistat-Derm
Mycelex
Myclo
Mycostatin
Mykinac
Nadostine
NAFTIFINE
Naftine
Nilstat
Nyaderm
NYSTATIN
Nystex
Pevaryl
Pitrex
Quinsana Plus
Spectazole
Tinactin
Ting
TOLNAFTATE
UNDECYLENIC ACID
Undoquent

ANTIFUNGALS (Vaginal)

BUTOCAZOLE
Canesten
CLOTRIMAZOLE
ECONAZOLE
Ecostatin
Femstat
Genapax
Gentian Violet
Gyne-Lotrimin
Lotrimin
MICONAZOLE
Monistat
Monistat 3
Monistat 7
Mycelex
Mycelex-G
Myclo
Mycostatin
Nadostine
Nilstat
NYSTATIN
Terazol
TERCONAZOLE

ANTI-INFLAMMATORY, STEROIDAL (Ophthalmic)

Ak-Dex
Ak-Pred
Ak-Tate
BETAMETHASONE
Betnesol
Cortamed
Cortisol
Decadron
Dexair
DEXAMETHASONE
Econopred
Econopred Plus
FLUOROMETHOLONE
Fluor-Op
FML S.O.P.
FML Forte
FML Liquifilm
HMS Liquifilm
HYDROCORTISONE
Inflamase
Inflamase Forte
Maxidex
MEDRYSONE
Metroton
Ocu-Dex
Ocu-Pred
Ocu-Pred-A
Ocu-Pred Forte
Predair
Predair-A
Predair Forte
Pred Forte
Pred Mild
PREDNISOLONE
Predsol

APPETITE SUPPRESSANTS

Adipex-D
Adipex-P
Adipost
Adphen
Anorex
Bacarate
BENZPHETAMINE
B.O.F.
Bontril PDM
Bontril Slow Release
Chlor-Tripolon
Chlorophen
CHLORPHENTERMINE
CLORTERMINE
Dapex
Dapex-37.5
Delcozine
D.E.P.—75
Depletite
Dexatrim
DI-Ap-Trol
Didrex
Dietec
DIETHYLPROPION
Dyrexan-OD
Elephemet
Ex-Obese
Fastin
FENFLURAMINE
Hyrex

Hyrex-105
Inifast Unicelles
Ionamin
Limit
Limitite
MASINDOL
Mazanor
Melfiat
Menrium
Metra
Minus
Nobesine
Nobesine-75
Nu-Dispoz
Obalan
Obe-Nil TR
Obe-Nix
Obephen
Obermine
Obestin
Obestin-30
Obestrol
Obeval
Obezine
Oby-Trim
Parmine
Penderal Pacaps
Phenazine-35
Phendiet
PHENDIMETRAZINE
PHENMETRAZINE
Phentamine
PHENTERMINE
Phentrol
Phenzine
Plegine
Ponderal
Ponderal Pacaps
Pondimin
Pondimin Extentabs
Pre-Sate
Prelu-2
Preludin
Propion
P.S.P.R.X. 1,2 & 3
Reducto
Regibon
Ro-Diet
Sanorex
Slim-Tabs
Slynn-LL
Span-RD
Sprx-1
Sprx-105
Sprx-3
Statobex
Statobex-G
Symetra
Tenuate
Tenuate Dospan
Tepanil
Tepanil Ten-Tab
Teramine
Tora
Trimcaps
Trimstat
Trimtabs
Unicelles
Unifast
Voranil
Wehless

ASPIRIN

Weightrol
Wilpowr
X-Trozine
X-Trozine LA

4-Way Cold Tablets
8-Hour Bayer Timed Release
Acetophen
Acetylsalicylic Acid
Alka Seltzer
Alka-Seltzer
Alka-Seltzer Effervescent Pain
  Reliever & Antacid
Aluminum ASA
Amytal and Aspirin
Anacin
Anaphen
Ancasal
Anexsia w/Codeine
A.P.C.
A.P.C w/Codeine
Apo-Asen
Arthinol
Arthritis Bayer Timed-Release
Arthritis Pain Formula
A.S.A.
A.S.A. & Codeine Compound
A.S.A. Compound
A.S.A. Enseals
Ascodeen-30
Ascriptin
Ascriptin A/D
Ascriptin w/Codeine
Asperbuf
Aspergum
Aspir-10
Aspirin Compound w/Codeine
Aspirjen Jr.
Astrin
Axotal
Bancap w/Codeine
Bayer
Bayer Timed-Release Arthritic
  Pain Formula
Bexophene
Buff-A
Buff-A-Comp
Buffaprin
Buffered ASA
Bufferin
Buffex
Buffinol
Buf-Tabs
Calciphen
Cama Arthritis Reliever
Cama Inlay
Causalin
Cefinal
Cirin
Codalan
Codasa
Congespirin
Coralsone
Coricidin D
Coryphen
Cosprin
Darvon Compound
Dasicon
Decagesic
Dia-Gesic
Dihydrocodein Compound

Dolene Compound-65
Dolor
Dolprn #3
Dynosal
Easprin
Ecotrin
Elder 65 Compound
Emagrin
Empirin
Empirin Compound
Empirin Compound w/Codeine
Emprazil
Encaprin
Entrophen
Equagesic
Excedrin
Fiorinal
Fiorinal w/Codeine
Hiprin
Histadyl and ASA Compound
Hyco-Pap
ICN 65 Compound
Kengesin
Lanorinal
Lemidyne w/Codeine
Magnaprin
Maprin
Maprin I-B
Measurin
Mepro Compound
Metrogesic
Mobidin
Norgesic
Norwich Aspirin
Nova-Phase
Novasen
Pabirin Buffered
P-A-C Compound
P-A-C Compound w/Codeine
Pargesic Compound 65
Percodan
Persistin
Phenodyne w/Codeine
Poxy Compound-65
Presalin
Progesic Compound-65
Propoxychel Compound
Propoxyphene HCl Compound
Repro Compound 65
Rhinocaps
Riphen-10
Safety Coated APF Arthritis Pain
  Formula
St. Joseph
St. Joseph Aspirin for Children
Sal-Adult
Salatin
Salatin w/Codeine
Saleto
Salmeph Forte
Sal-Infant
Salocol
Salsprin
SK-65 Compound
Soma Compound
Soma Compound w/Codeine
Stero-Darvon
Supac
Supasa
Synalgos
Talwin Compound
Triaminic
Triaphen-10

Trigesic
Vanquish
Verin
Wesprin Buffered
Zorprin

ATROPINE

Almezyme
Amocine
Antrocol
Arco-Lase
Atrobarbital
Atromal
Atropine Bufopto
Atropisol
Atrosed
Barbella
Barbeloid
Barbidonna
Barbidonna-CR
Bar-Cy-Amine
Bar-Cy-A-Tab
Bar-Don
Bar-Tropin
Belbutal
Belkaloids
Belladenal
Bellergal-S
Bioxatphen
Briabell
Briaspaz
Brobella
Buren
Butibel
Cerebel
Chardonna
Comhist
Contac
Copin
Dallergy
Ditropan
Donnacin
Donnagel
Donnamine
Donnatal
Donnazyme
Drinus
Eldonal
G. B. S.
HASP
Haponal
Harvitrate
Hyatal
Hybephen
Hycodan
Hyonal
Hyonatol
Hytrona
Isopto Atropine
Kalmedic
Kinesed
Koryza
Levamine
Lyopine Vari-Dose
Magnased
Magnox
Maso-Donna
Neogel w/Sulfa
Nilspasm
Oxybutynin
P & A
Palbar No. 2

PAMA
Peece
Prydon
Renalgin
Ro Trim
Ru-Tuss
Sedamine
Sedapar
Sedatabs
Sedralex
Seds
SK-Diphenoxylate
SMP Atropine
Spabelin
Spasaid
Spasdel
Spasidon
Spasioids
Spasmate
Spasmolin
Spasquid
Spastolate
Spastosed
Stannitol
Thitrate
Trac
Unitral
Urised
Uriseptin
Urogesic
Zemarine

BELLADONNA

Amobel
Atrocap
Atrosed
Barbidonna
Bebetab
Belap
Belatol
Belbarb
Bellachar
Belladenal
Bellafedrol
Bellergal
Belikatal
Bello-phen
Belphen
B & O Supprettes
B-Sed
Butabar
Butabar Elixir
Butibel
Butibel Elixir
Butibel-Zyme
Chardonna
Comhist
Coryztime
Decobel
Donabarb
Donnafed Jr.
Donnatal
Donnazyme
Fitacol
Gastrolic
Gelcomul
Hycoff Cold Caps
Hynaldyne
Kamabel
Kinesed
Lanothal
Mallenzyme

Medi-Spas
Nilspasm
Phebe
Phen-o-bel
Rectacort
Sedapar
Sedatromine
Spabelin
Spasnil
Trac 2X
Ultabs
Urilief
Urised
U-Tract
Wigraine
Woltac
Wyanoids

BELLADONNA ALKALOIDS & BARBITURATES

Amobell
Anaspaz PB
Antrocol
ATROPINE, HYOSCYAMINE, SCOPOLAMINE & BUTABARBITAL
ATROPINE, HYOSCYAMINE, SCOPOLAMINE & PHENOBARBITAL
ATROPINE & PHENOBARBITAL
Barbidonna
Barophen
Bay-Ase
Belap
Belladenal
Belladenal-S
Belladenal Spacetabs
BELLADONNA & AMOBARBITAL
BELLADONNA & BUTABARBITAL
Bellalphen
Bellastal
Belikatal
Butibel
Chardonna-2
Donna-Sed
Donnapine
Donnatal
Donnatal Extentabs
Donphen
Hybephen
HYOSCYAMINE & PHENOBARBITAL
Hyosophen
Kinesed
Levsin-PB
Levsin with Phenobarbital
Levsinex with Phenobarbital Timecaps
Malatal
Palbar
Palbar No. 2
Pheno-Bella
Relaxadon
Seds
Spaslin
Spasmolin
Spasmophen
Spasquid
Susano
Vanatal
Vanodonnal

BENZOYL PEROXIDE

Acetoxyl
Acne-Aid
Allercreme Clear-Up
Alquam-X
Ben-Aqua
Ben-Aqua Mark
Benoxyl
Benzac
Benzac W
Benzagel
Buf-Oxal
Clear By Design
Clearasil
Clearasil BP(M)
Clearasil BP Plus
Cuticura Acne
Dermodex
Dermoxyl
Dermoxyl Aqua
Desquam-E
Desquam-X
Dry and Clean
Dry and Clear
Eloxyl
Epi-Clear
Fostex
Fostex BPO
H₂Oxyl
Intraderm-19
Loroxide
Neutrogena Acne Mask
Oxy
Oxyderm
Oxy-5
Oxy-10
PanOxyl
PanOxyl AQ
Persadox
Persadox HP
Persa-Gel
Persa-Gel W
PHisoAc BP
Porox 7
Propa P.H.
Propa P.H. Porox
Stri-Dex
Teen
Topex
Vanoxide
Vanoxide-HC
Xerac BP
Zeroxin

BETAMETHASONE

17-Valerate Celestone
17-Valerate Diprosone
Alphatrex
Beben
Benzoate
Beta-Val
Betacort
Betnelan
Betnesol
Betratrex
B-S-P
Celestoderm
Celestoject
Celestone
Celestone Phosphate
Celestone Soluspan
Cel-U-Sec

Dipropinate Metaderm
Diprosone
Disodium Phosphate Betnovate
Lotrisone
Prelestone
Selestoject
Uticort
Valerate Betaderm
Valerate Novobetamet
Valisone
Vancerace

BROMPHENIRAMINE

Brocon
Bromamine
Brombay
Bromepath
Bromfed
Bromphen
Chlorphed
Dehist
Dimetane
Dimetane Extentabs
Dimetane-Ten
Dimetapp
Disophrol Chronotabs
Drixoral
Dura Tap-PD
Eldatapp
E.N.T. Syrup
Histaject modified
Histatapp
Nasahist B
ND-Stat Revised
Oraminic II
Poly-Histine
Ralabromophen
Rynatapp
S-T Decongestant
Symptom 3
Taltapp
Tamine S.R.
Tapp
Tolabromophen
Veltane
Veltap

BUTABARBITAL

Barbased
Broncholate
Brondilate
Butabell HMB
Butalan
Butaserpazide
Butatran
Butibel
Buticaps
Butisol
Butizide
Cyclo-Bell
Cytospaz-SR
Day-Barb
Levamine
Neo-Barb
Numa-Dura-Tablets
Pyridium Plus
Quibron Plus
Sarisol No. 2
Scolate
Sidonna
Sinate-M
Tedral

CAFFEINE

Amaphen
Amaphen w/Codeine #3
Anacin
Anaphen
Anexsia w/Codeine
Anoquan
A.P.C.
A.S.A. Compound
Asphac-G
Aspirin Compound w/Codeine
Ban-Drow 2
Bexophene
Buff-A-Comp
Buffadyne
Butigetic
Cafacetin
Cafecon
Cafergot
Cafermine
Cafetrate
Caffedrine
Cefinal
Cenagesic
Citrated Caffeine
Coastalgesic
Codalan #3
Colrex
Compal
Coryban D
Coryzaid
Darvon Compound
Dasicon
Dexatrim
Dexitac
Dia-Gesic
Dihydrocodeine Compound
Dolor
Duadacin
Dularin
Dynosal
Elder 65 Compound
Emagrin
Empirin Compound
Emprazil
Esgic
Excedrin Extra Strength
Fendol
Fiorinal
G-1 Capsules
Hista-Derfule
Histadyl Compound
ICN 65 Compound
Kengesin
Kirkaffeine
Korigesic
Lanorinal
Lemidyne w/Codeine
Midol
Migralam
Nodaca
Nodoz
Pacaps
P-A-C Compound w/Codeine
Pargesic Compound 65
Percodan
Phenodyne
Phenodyne w/Codeine
Phensal
Phrenilin
Poxy Compound-65
Prodolor

Progesic Compound-65
Propoxychel Compound-65
Propoxyphene Compound
Pyrroxate
Quick Pep
Repro Compound 65
S-A-C
Salatin
Salatin w/Codeine
Saleto
Salocol
Sinarest
SK-65 Compound
Supac
Synalgos
Synalgos-DC
Tirend
Triaminic
Triaminicin
Trigesic
Two-Dyne
Vanquish
Vivarin
Wigraine

CALCIUM CARBONATE

Alka-mints
Alka-2
Alkets
Amitone
Bio Cal
Calcet
Calcilac
Calcitrate 600
Calglycine
Cal-Sup
Caltrate
Camalox
Chooz
Dicarbosil
Ducon
El-Da-Mint
Equilet
Fosfree
Gustalac
Iromin-G
Mallamint
Mission
Natacomp-FA
Natalins
Nu-Iron-V
Os-Cal
Os-Cal 500
Pama No. 1
Pramet FA
Pramilet FA
Prenate 90
Ratio
Suplical
Theracal
Titracid
Titralac
Trialka
Tums
Tums E-X
Zenate

CALCIUM SUPPLEMENTS

BioCal
CALCIUM CARBONATE (also
   used as an antacid)
CALCIUM CITRATE

CALCIUM GLUBIONATE
CALCIUM GLUCONATE
CALCIUM GLYCEROPHOSPHATE
   & CALCIUM LACTATE
CALCIUM LACTATE
Calphosan
Cal-Sup
Caltrate
Citracal
DIBASIC CALCIUM PHOSPHATE
Kalcinate
Neo-Calglucon
Os-Cal 500
Posture
Suplical
Theracal
TRIBASIC CALCIUM PHOSPHATE
Tums
Tums E-X

CHLORPHENIRAMINE

4-Way Cold Tablets
Acutuss
Acutuss Expectorant w/Codeine
Alermine
Alka-Seltzer Plus
Aller-chlor
Allerbid Tymcaps
Allerest
Allerform
Allergesic
Allerid - O.D.
AL-R
Alumadrine
Anafed
Anamine
Anatuss
Antagonate
Brexin
Bronkotuss
Cerose Compound
Children's Allerest
Chlo-Amine
Chlorafed
Chloramate Unicelles
Chlor-Histine
Chlor-MAL
Chlormine
Chlor-Niramine
Chlor-100
Chlorphen
Chlor-PRO
Chlor-Span
Chlortab
Chlor-Trimeton
Chlor-Trimeton w/Codeine
Chlor-Trimeton Repetabs
Chlor-Tripolon
Ciramine
Ciriforte
Citra Forte
Codimal
Coldene
Colrex
Comhist
Comtrex
Conex w/Codeine
Conex-DA
Cophene-X
Co-Pyronil 2
Coricidin
Coricidin "D"

Corilin
Coryban-D
Coryzaid
Cosea
Co-Tylenol
Covanamine
Covangesic
Dallergy
Deconamine
Dehist
Demazin
Dextromal
Dextro-Tussin
DM Plus
Donatussin
Dorcol
Drinus
Dristan
Drize M
Duadacin
Duphrene
Dura-Vent/A
E.N.T.
Expectrosed
Extendryl
Fedahist
Fernhist
Ginsopan
Guaiahist TT
Gualamine
Guistrey Fortis
Hal-Chlor
Histaiet
Histalon
Histamic
Histaspan
Hista-Vadrin
Histex
Histor-D Timecelles
Historal
Histrey
Hycoff
Hycomine Compound
Iophen-C
Isoclor
Korigesic
Koryza
Kronofed-A
Kronohist Kronocaps
Lanatuss
Marhist
Naldecon
Naldetuss
Napril Plateau
Narine Gyrocaps
Narspan
Nasahist
Neo-Codenyl-M
Neotep Granucaps
Nilcol
Nolamine
Novafed A
Novahistine
Novopheniram
Omni-Tuss
Ornade Spansule
P.R. Syrup
P-V-Tussin
Palohist
Partuss T.D.
Pediacof
Phenacol-DM
Phenate

Phenetron
Phenetron Lanacaps
Polaramine
Probahist
Protid Improved Formula
Pseudo-Hist
Pyma
Pyrroxate
Pyrroxate w/Codeine
Quadrahist
Quelidrine
Queltuss
Resaid T.D.
Rhinex
Rhinolar
Rhinolar-EX
Ru-Tuss
Rynatan
Rynatuss
Salphenyl
Scot-Tussin
Sinarest
Singlet
Sinovan
Sinulin
T.D. Alermine
Tedral Anti-H
Teldrin
Teldrin Spansules
T.P.I.
Triaminicin
Trymegen
Tusquelin
Tuss-Ornade
Tussar
Tussi-Organidin
U.R.I.
Wesmatic Forte

CONTRACEPTIVES (Oral)

Anoryol
Brevicon
Demulen
Enovid
Enovid-E
Genora 1/35
Genora 1/50
Levien
Loestrin
Lo-Ovral
Micronor
Minestrin
Min-Ovral
Modacon
Modicon
Nordette
Norinyl 1 + 35
Norinyl 1 + 50
Norinyl 1 + 80
Norinyl 2
Norlestrin
Norlinyl
Nor-Q.D.
Norquest
Ortho
Ortho-Novum
Ortho-Novum 0.5
Ortho-Novum 1/35
Ortho-Novum 1/50
Ortho-Novum 1/80
Ortho-Novum 2
Ortho-Novum 7/7/7

Ortho-Novum 10/11
Ovcon
Ovral
Ovrette
Ovulen
Program
Synphasic
Tri-Levlen
Tri-Norinyl
Triphasil

DEXAMETHASONE

Aeroseb-Dex
Ak-Dex
Congespirin
Cremacoat 1
Dalalone
Dalalone D.P.
Dalalone L.A.
Decaderm
Decadrol
Decadron
Decadron L.A.
Decadron Phosphate
Decadron Respihaler
Decadron Turbinaire
Decadron with Xylocaine
Decaject-L.A.
Decaject
Decameth
Decameth L.A.
Decaspray
Delsym
Demo-Cineol
Deronil
Dexacen
Dexacen L.A.
Dexasone
Dexasone L.A.
Dexon
Dexon LA
Dexone
Dexone LA
DM Cough
Extend-12
Hexadrol
Hexadrol Phosphate
Hexandrol
Hold
Maxidex
Mediquell
Oradexon
Pedia Care 1
Pertussin 8 Hour Cough Formula
SK-Dexamethasone
Solurex
Solurex LA
Sucrets

DEXTROMETHORPHAN

2/C-DM
216 DM
Anti-Tuss DM
Balminil DM
Benylin DM
Benylin DM Cough
Broncho-Grippol-DM
Cheracol
Congespirin
Contratuss
Cosanyl DM
Cremacoat 1

Delsym
Delsym Polistirex
Demo-Cineol
Dextro-Tussin GG
DM Cough
DM Syrup
Dormethan
Dristan
Dristan Cough Formula
Duad Koff Balls
Endotussin-NN
Extend-12
Formula 44-D
Glycotuss-dM
Gulatuss D-M
Hold
Hold Cough Suppressant
Koffex
Lixaminol AT
Mediquell
Neo-DM
Novahistine DMX
Nyquil
Ornacol
Pedia Care 1
Pertussin 8 Hour Cough Formula
Queltuss
Robidex
Robitussin
Robitussin-DM
Romilar
Romilar CF
Romilar Children's Cough
Sedatuss
Silence is Golden
Silexin
Sorbase
Sorbutuss
St. Joseph
St. Joseph Cough Syrup
St. Joseph for Children
Sucrets
Sucrets Cough Control
Trind DM
Trocal
Tussagesic
Tussaminic
Unproco
Vicks
Vicks Cough Syrup

DICYCLOMINE

Antispas
A-Spas
Baycyclomine
Bentyl
Bentylol
Byclomine
Cyclobec
Cyclocen
Dibent
Dicen
Di-Cyclonex
Dilomine
Di-Spaz
Dyspas
Formulex
Lomine
Menospasm
Neoquess
Nospaz
Or-Tyl

Protylol
Spasmoban
Spasmoject
Triactin
Viscerol

DIMENHYDRINATE

Apo-Dimenhydrinate
Calm X
Dimentabs
Dinate
Dommanate
Dramaban
Dramamine
Dramilin
Dramocen
Dramoject
Dymenate
Eldodram
Gravol
Hydrate
Marine
Marmine
Motion-Aid
Nauseatol
Novodimenate
PMS-Dimenhydrinate
Reidamine
Travamine
Trav-Arex
Vertiban
Wehamine

DIPHENHYDRAMINE

Allerdryl
Ambenyl Expectorant
Beldin
Bena-D
Benadryl
Benadryl Children's Allergy
Benadryl Complete Allergy
Benahist
Bendylate
Benoject-10
Benylin Cough Syrup
Caladryl
Compoz
Diahist
Dihydrex
Diphen
Diphenacen
Diphenadril
Eldadryl
Fenylhist
Fynex
Hydramine
Hydril
Hyrexin-50
Insomnal
Nervine Nighttime Sleep-Aid
Noradryl
Nordryl
Nytol
Nytol with DPH
Phen-Amin
Robalyn
SK-Diphenhydramine
Sleep-Eze
Sleep-Eze 3
Sominex
Sominex Formula 2
SominiFere

Tuestat
Twilite
Valdrene
Wehydryl

DOCUSATE SODIUM

Afko-Lube
Bilax
Bu-Lax
Colace
Colax
Coloctyl
Dialose
Dilax
Diocto
Dioctyl Sodium Sulfosuccinate
Dioeze
DioMedicone
Diosuccin
Dio-Sul
Disonate
Di-Sosul
Doctate
Doss
Doxidan
Doxinate
D-S-S
Duosol
Ferro-sequels
Geriplex-FS
Laxagel
Laxinate
Laxinate 100
Liqui-Doss
Modane Plus
Modane Soft
Molatoc
Neolax
Peri-Colase
Peritinic
Prenate 90
Pro-Sof
Pro-Sof 100
Pro-Sof Liquid Concentrate
Regulex
Regulex SS
Regutol
Senokot-S
Stulex
Therevac Plus
Therevac-SB
Trilax

EPHEDRINE

Acet-Am
Aladrine
Amesec
Amodrine
Asminyl
Benadryl w/Ephedrine
Broncholate
Brondilate
Bronkaid
Bronkolixir
Bronkotabs
Bronkotuss
Calcidrine
Coryza Brengle
Co-Xan Elixir
Dainite
Derma Medicone-HC
Duovent

Ectasule III
Ectasule Minus
Ephed II
Ephed-Organidin
Ephedrine and Amytal
Ephedrine and Nembutal-25
Ephedrine and Seconal
Ephedrol
Ephedrol w/Codeine
Epragen
Iso-Asminyl
Isuprel
Luasmin
Lufyllin-EPG
Marax
Mudrane
Numa-Dura-Tablets
Nyquil
Phyldrox
Primatene
Pyribenzamine w/Ephedrine
Quadrinal
Quelidrine
Quibron Plus
Slo-Fedrin A-60
Tedfern
Tedral
T.E.H.
T-E-P
Thalfed
Theofedral
Theotabs
Theozine
Wesmatic
Wyanoids

EPINEPHRINE

Adrenalin
Asmolin
Asthma Haler
Asthma Nefrin
Ayerst Epitrate
Bronitin
Bronkaid
Bronkaid Mist
Bronkaid Mistometer
Bronkaid Mist Suspension
Bronitin Mist
Dey-Dose Racepinephrine
Dysne-Inhal
Epifrin
Epi-Pen
EpiPen-Epinephrine Auto-Injector
Epi-Pen Jr.
Epitrate
Eppy
Glaucon
Marcaine Hydrochloride
  w/Epinephrine
Medihaler-Epi
microNEFRIN
Murocoll
Mytrate
Primatene
Primatene Mist
Primatene Mist Solution
Primatene Mist Suspension
S-2 Inhalent
Simplene
Sus-phrine
Vaponefrin

ERYTHROMYCINS

Apo-Erythro-S
A/T/S
Bristamycin
Dowmycin
E-Biotic
E.E.S.
E-Mycin
E-Mycin E
Eryc
Eryc Sprinkle
Ery-derm
EryPed
Erymax
Erypar
Ery-Tab
Erythrocin
Erythrocin Ethyl Succinate
Erythromid
ERYTHROMYCIN
ERYTHROMYCIN ESTOLATE
ERYTHROMYCIN
  ETHYLSUCCINATE
ERYTHROMYCIN GLUCEPTATE
ERYTHROMYCIN LACTOBIONATE
ERYTHROMYCIN STEARATE
Ethril
Ilosone
Ilosone Estolate
Ilotycin
Ilotycin Gluceptate
Kesso-mycin
Novorythro
PCE Dispersatabs
Pediazole
Pediamycin
Pendiamycin
Pfizer-E
Robimycin
RP-Mycin
SK-Erythromycin
Staticin
T-Star
Wyamycin
Wyamycin E
Wyamycin S

ESTROGEN

Amnestrogen
C.E.S.
Clinestrone
Conjugated Estrogens C.S.D.
Delestrogen
DES
DIENESTROL (vaginal)
DV (vaginal)
Estinyl
Estomed
Estrace
Estrace (vaginal)
ESTRADIOL (vaginal)
Estraguard (vaginal)
Estratab
Estrocon
ESTROGENS, CONJUGATED
  (vaginal)
ESTRONE (vaginal)
ESTROPIPATE (vaginal)
Estrovis
Evex
Feminone
Femogen

Formatrix
Hormonin
Menest
Menotrol
Menrium
Milprem
Oagen
Oestrilin
Oestrilin (vaginal)
Ogen
Ogen (vaginal)
Ortho Dienestrol (vaginal)
Piperazine Estrone Sulfate
   (vaginal)
PMB-200
PMB-400
Premarin
Premarin (vaginal)
Progens
Stilphostrol
Theogen

FERROUS FUMARATE

Cevi-Fer
Chromagen
Feco-T
Femiron
Feostat
Ferancee
Ferrofume
Ferro-sequels
Fersamal
Fetrin
Fumasorb
Fumerin
Hemocyte
Hemo-Vite
Ircon
Ircon-FA
Laud-Iron
Maniron
Natalins
Neo-Fer
Neo-Fer-50
Novofumar
Palafer
Palmiron
Poly-VI-Flor
Pramilet FA
Prenate 90
Span-FF
Stuartinic
Toleron
Tolfrinic
Tolifer
Trinsicon
Vitron C
Zenate

FERROUS SULFATE

Apo-Ferrous Sulfate
Feosol
Fer-In-Sol
Fer-Iron
Fero-folic-500
Fero-Grad
Fero-Grad-500
Fero-Gradumet
Ferospace
Ferralyn
Ferra-TD
Fesofor

Geritol Tablets
Hematinic
Iberet
Iberet-500
Iberet-Folic-500
Iromal
Mol-Iron
Novoferrosulfa
PMS Ferrous Sulfate
Slow-Fe

GUAIFENESIN

2/G
2/G-DM
Actol
Ambenyl
Anti-Tuss
Asbron
Asma
Balminil
Balminil Expectorant
Baytussin
Breonesin
Brexin
Bromphen
Broncholate
Brondecon
Bronkolizir
Bronkotabs
Bronkotuss
Caldrex Expectorant
Cetro Cirose
Cheracol
Cheracol Cough
Chlor-Trimeton
Codimal
Coditrate
Colrex Expectorant
Conar
Conex
Conex w/Codeine
Congess Jr. & Sr.
Corutol
Coryban-D
Co-Xan
Cremacoat
Cremacoat 2
Deproist w/Codeine
Detussin
Dilaudid
Dilor-G
Dimetane
Donatussin
Dorcol
Dristan
Dristan Cough
Duovent
Dura-Vent
Elixophyllin-GG
Emfaseen
Entex
Entuss-D
Expectorant
Fedahist
Formula
Formula 44-D
Gee-Gee
GG-CEN
Glyate
Glyceryl Guaiacolate
Glycotuss
Glytuss

Guaiahist
Guaifed
Guiamid
Guiatuss
Halotussin
Histalet X
Humibid L.A.
Hycotuss
Hytuss
Hytuss-2X
Luftodil
Lufyllin
Maiotuss
Mudrane GG
Naldecon
Neo-Spec
Neospect
Neothyllin-G
Nortussin
Novahistine
Nucofed
Pee Dee Dose Expectorant
Poly-Histine
P-V-Tussin
Queltuss
Quibron
Respaire-SR
Resyl
Robafen
Robitussin
Scot-Tussin Sugar-Free
Silexin
Sinufed Timecelles
Slo-Phyllin GG
Sorbase
Sorbutuss
S-T Expectorant
S-T Forte
Synophylate-GG
Syrup
Tedral
Theo-Guaia
Theolair-Plus
Triafed-C
Triaminic
Triaminic w/Codeine
Trind
Tussar
Tussend
Uproco
Vicks
Vicks Cough
Zephrex

HYDROCHLOROTHIAZIDE

Aldactazide
Aldoril
Apo-Hydro
Butaserpazide
Butizide
Diuchlor H
Diupres
Dyazide
Esidrix
Esimil
H-H-R
Hydrid
Hydro-Aquil
Hydrochlorothiazide Intensol
HydroDIURIL
Hydropres
Hydroserp

Hydroserpine
Hydrotensin
Hydrozide-Z-50
Hyperetic
Inderide
Mallopress
Maxzide
Mictrin
Moduretic
Naquival
Natrimax
Nefrol
Neo-Codema
Novohydrazide
Oretic
Oreticyl
Reserpazide
Ser-Ap-Es
Serpasil-Esidrix
Singoserp-Esidrix
SK-Hydrochlorothiazide
Spironazide
Thiuretic
Timolide
Timolol and Hydrochlorothiazide
Tri-Hydroserpine
Unipres
Urozide
Zide

HYDROCORTISONE
(Cortisol)

Aeroseb-HC
A-hydroCort
Barseb
Biosone
Colifoam
Cortald
Cortamed
Cortate
Cort-Dome
Cortef
Cortef Fluid
Cortenema
Corticreme
Cortifoam
Cortiment
Cortisol
Cortoderm
Cortril
Dermacort
Efcortelan Soluble
Efcortesol
Emo-Cort
Fernisone
Hycort
Hyderm
Hydro-Cortilean
Hydrocortistab
Hydrocortone
Hydrocortone Acetate
Hydrocortone Phosphate
Hytone
Lifocort
Microcort
Novohydrocort
Orabase HCA
Proctocort
Rectold
Restocort
Solu-Cortef

Texacort
Unicort
Westcort

HYDROXYZINE

Anxanil
Atarax
Ataraxoid
Atozine
Cartrax
Durrax
Enarax
E-Vista
Hydroxacen
Hy-Pam
Hyzine
Marax
Multipax
Neucalm 50
Orgatrax
Quiess
T.E.H. Tablets
Theozine
Vamate
Vistacon
Vistaject
Vistaquel
Vistaril
Vistazine
Vistrax

HYOSCYAMINE

Almezyme
Anaspa 3
Anaspaz
Anaspaz PB
Arco-Lase Plus
Barbella
Barbeloid
Barbidonna-CR
Bar-Cy-Amine
Bar-Cy-A-Tab
Bar-Don
Belbutal
Belkaloids
Bellafoline
Bellaspaz
Brobella-PB
Buren
Cytospaz
Cytospaz-M
De Tal
Donnacin
Donnagel
Donnamine
Donnatal
Donnazyme
Eldonal
Elixiril
Ergobel
Floramine
Gylanphen
Haponal
Hyatal
Hybephen
Hyonal
Hyonatol
Hytrona
Kinesed
Koryza
Kutrase

Levamine
Levsin
Levsinex
Levsinex Timecaps
Maso-Donna
Neoquess
Nevrotase
Nilspasm
Omnibel
Peece
Pyridium Plus
Renalgin
Restophen
Ru-Tuss
Sedajen
Sedamine
Sedapar
Sedatromine
Sedralex
Seds
Spabelin
Spasaid
Spasdel
Spasloids
Spasmolin
Spasquid
Spastolate
Trac 2X
Ultabs
Urised
Uriseptin
Urogesic
Zemarine

INSULIN

Actrapid
Globin Insulin
Humulin
Humulin BR
Humulin L
Humulin N
Humulin R
Insulatard
Insulatard NPH
Insulatard NPH Human
Lentard
Lente
Lente Iletin I
Lente Iletin II
Lente Insulin
Mixtard
Monotard
NPH
NPH Iletin I
NPH Iletin II
NPH Insulin
Novolin
Novolin L
Novolin N
Novolin R
Novolin 70/30
PZI
Protamine Zinc & Iletin
Protamine Zinc & Iletin I
Protamine Zinc & Iletin II
Protophane NPH
Regular
Regular (Concentrated) Iletin
Regular (Concentrated) Iletin II,
  U-500
Regular Iletin I

Regular Iletin II
Regular Insulin
Semilente
Semilente Iletin
Semilente Iletin I
Semitard
Ultralente
Ultratard
Utralente Iletin I
Velosulin
Velosulin Human

MAGNESIUM HYDROXIDE

Aludrox
Arthritis Pain Formula
Camalox
Creamalin
Delcid
Di-Gel
Dolprn #3
Ducon
Gelusil
Kolantyl
Maalox
Magnatril
Maxamag
Milk of Magnesia
M.O.M.
Mucotin
Mygel
Mylanta
Phillips' Milk of Magnesia
Silain-Gel
Simeco
Univol
Vanquish
Win-Gel

MEPROBAMATE

Apo-Meprobamate
Arcoban
Bamate
Bamo 400
Coprobate
Deprol
Equagesic
Equanil
Equanil Wyseals
Evenol
Kalmn
Lan-Dol
Medi-Tran
Mep-E
Mepriam
Mepro Compound
Meprocon
Meprospan
Meprotabs
Meribam
Miltown
Neo-Tran
Neuramate
Neurate
Novo-Mepro
Novomepro
Pathibamate
Pax 400
PMB
Protran
Quietal
Robam
Robamate

Sedabamate
SK-Bamate
Tranmep

METHYLPREDNISOLONE

A-methaPred
dep Medalone
Depoject
Depo-Medrol
Depo-medrone
Depopred
Depo-Pred-40
Depo-Pred-80
Depo-Predate
Duralone
Duralone-40
Duralone-80
Durameth
Medralone
Medralone-40
Medralone-80
Medrol
Medrol Enpak
Medrone
Medrone-80
Mepred-40
Methylone
m-Prednisol
Pre-Dep
Pro-Dep-40
Pro-Dep-80
Rep-Pred
Solu-Medrol
Solu-medrone

NARCOTIC & ACETAMINOPHEN

Acetaco
ACETAMINOPHEN & CODEINE
Aceta with Codeine
Amacodone
Anexsia
APAP with Codeine
Atasol with Codeine
Bancap-HC
Bayapap with Codeine
Capital with Codeine
Codap
Co-gesic
Compal
Cotabs
Damacet-P
Darvocet-N
Demerol-APAP
Dolacet
Dolene-AP
Dolo-Pap
Duradyne DHC
Empracet with Codeine
Emtec
Exdol with Codeine
Hycodaphen
Hydrocet
HYDROCODONE & ACETAMINOPHEN
Hydrocone with APAP
Hydrogesic
HY-PHEN
Lenoltec
Lorcet
Lorcet-HD

Lortab
Lortab 5
Lortab 7
MEPERIDINE & ACETAMINOPHEN
Norcet
Oxycocet
OXYCODONE & ACETAMINOPHEN
PENTAZOCINE & ACETAMINOPHEN
Percocet
Percocet-Demi
Phenaphen with Codeine
Propacet
Propain-HC
PROPOXYPHENE & ACETAMINOPHEN
Proval
Rounox with Codeine
Roxicet
SK-APAP with Codeine
SK-Oxycodone and Acetaminophen
SK-65 APAP
Stopayne
Talacen
T-Gesic Forte
Tylenol with Codeine
Tylox
Ty-Tabs
Vicodin
Wygesic

NARCOTIC ANALGESICS

642
Aceta w/Codeine
Acetaco
Acetaminophen w/Codeine
Actifed-C
Actifed-C Expectorant
Adatuss
Algodex
Ambenyl
Anaphen
A.P.C. w/Codeine Phosphate Tablets
A.P.C. w/Codeine Phosphate
Arthralgen
Ascriptin w/Codeine
Aspirin Compound w/Codeine
Astramorph
Astramorph-PF
Axotal
Bancap w/Codeine
Banesin Forte
BUTORPHANOL
Calcidrine
Calcidrine Syrup
Capital w/Codeine
Cetro Cirose
Cheracol
Coastaldyne
Coastalgesic
Codalan
Codalex
Codap
CODEINE
Codeine Sulfate
Codimal PH
Coditrate
Codone
Colrex Compound

Copavin
Corutol DH
Cotussis
Co-Xan
Dapase
Darvocet-N 100
Darvon
Darvon-N
Demer-idine
Demerol
Depronal-SA
Dialog
Dicodid
Dihydromorphinone
Dilaudid
Dilaudid-HP
Dimetane-DC
Dimetane Expectorant-DC
Dolene
Dolophine
Dolor
Doloxene
Doxaphene
Dromoran
Dularin
Duramorph PF
Dynosal
Empirin w/Codeine
Empracet w/Codeine
Emprazil-C
Ephedrol w/Codeine
Epimorph
Esgic
FL-Tussex
Florinal w/Codeine
Fortral
Gaysal
G-2
G-3
Hasacode
Hycodan
Hycotuss
HYDROCODONE
HYDROMORPHONE
Isoclor
Laudanum
Levo-Dromoran
Levorphan
LEVORPHANOL
Liquix-C
Lo-Tussin
Maxigesic
Mepergan Fortis
MEPERIDINE
METHADONE
Methadose
Metrogesic
Minotal
MORPHINE
Morphitec
M.O.S.
M.O.S. Syrup
MS Contin
MSIR
MST Continus
NALBUPHINE
Novahistine DH
Novahistine Expectorant
Novopropoxyn
Nubain
Numorphan
OPIUM
Ossonate-Plus

OXYCODONE
OXYMORPHONE
Pantapon
PAREGORIC
Pargesic
Pavadon
Paveral
Pediacof
PENTAZOCINE
Percodan
Pethadol
Pethidine
Phenaphen w/Codeine
Phenergan
Phrenilin
Physeptone
Poly-Histine w/Codeine
Presalin
Prodolor
Profene
Promethazine HCl w/Codeine
PROPOXYPHENE
Pro-65
Proxagesic
Proxene
Prunicodeine
RMS Uniserts
Robidone
Robitussin A-C
Roxanol
Roxanol SR
Roxicodone
S-A-C
Salatin
Saleto
Salimeph Forte
Sedapap
SK-65
SK-APAP w/Codeine
Soma Compound w/Codeine
Sorbase II
Stadol
Statex
Strascogesic
Supac
Supeudol
Sylapar
Synalgos-DC
Talwin
Talwin-NX
Terpin Hydrate w/Codeine
Triaminic w/Codeine
Trigesic
Tussar
Tussend
Tussi-Organidin
Tylenol w/Codeine
Tylox
Vicodin
Wygesic

NARCOTIC & ASPIRIN

222
282
292
293
692
A&C with Codeine
A.C.&C.
Anacin with Codeine
Ancasal
Anexsia with Codeine

Anexsia-D
A.S.A. and Codeine Compound
Ascriptin with Codeine
ASPIRIN & CODEINE
ASPIRIN, CODEINE & CAFFEINE
Bexophene
BUFFERED ASPIRIN & CODEINE
Codoxy
Coryphen with Codeine
C2 with Codeine
C2 Buffered with Codeine
Damason-P
Darvon Compound
Darvon-N Compound
Darvon with A.S.A.
Darvon-N with A.S.A.
Dolene Compound
Doxaphene Compound
Drocade and Aspirin
DROCODE, ASPIRIN & CAFFEINE
Emcodeine
Empirin with Codeine
HYDROCODONE, ASPIRIN &
   CAFFEINE
Instantine Plus
Novo AC&C
Oxycodan
OXYCODONE & ASPIRIN
PENTAZOCINE & ASPIRIN
Percodan
Percodan-Demi
PROPOXYPHENE & ASPIRIN
PROPOXYPHENE ASPIRIN &
   CAFFEINE
SK-65 Compound
SK-Oxycodone with Aspirin
Synalgos-DC
Talwin Compound
Talwin Compound-50

NIACIN (Nicotinic Acid)

Diacin
N-Caps
Niac
Niacin
Nicalex
Nico-400
Nico-Span
Nicobid
Nicocap
Nicolar
Nicotinex
Nicotinyl alcohol
Nicotym
Novoniacin
SK-Niacin
Span-Niacin
Tega-Span
Tri-B3
Vasotherm
Numerous other multiple vitamin-
   mineral supplements.

NITRATES

Ang-O-Span
Apo-ISDN
Cardilate
Coronex
Dilatrate-SR
Deponit
Duotrate

ERYTHRITYL TETRANITRATE
Glyceryl Trinitrate
Iso-Bid
Isochron
Isogard
Isonate
Isonate TR
Isordil
ISOSORBIDE DINITRATE
Isotrate
Kaytrate
Klavikordal
Naptrate
N-G-C
Niong
Nitro-Bid
Nitrobon
Nitrocap
Nitrocap T.D.
Nitrocardin
Nitrodisc
Nitro-Dur
Nitro-Dur II
Nitrogard-SR
NITROGLYCERIN (GLYCERYL TRINITRATE)
Nitroglyn
Nitrol
Nitrolin
Nitrolingual
Nitro-Long
Nitronet
Nitrong
Nitrong SR
Nitrospan
Nitrostablin
Nitrostat
Nitro-Time
Novosorbide
NTS
Onset
PENTAERYTHRITOL TETRANITRATE
Pentestan
Pentol
Pentol S.A.
Pentraspan
Pentraspan SR
Pentritol
Pentylan
Peritrate
Peritrate Forte
Peritrate SA
P.E.T.N.
Sorate
Sorbide
Sorbide T.D.
Sorbitrate
Sorbitrate SA
Susadrin
Transderm-Nitro
Trates
Tridil
Vaso-80
Vasoglyn

PAPAVERINE
Cerebid
Cerespan
Copavin
Dipav
Durapav

Dylate
Genabid
Hyobid
Kavrin
Lapav
Myobid
Octapav
Orapav
P-200
P-A-V
Pavabid
Pavabid HP
Pavacap
Pavacen
Pavadon
Pavadur
Pavagen
Pavakey
Pava-Par
Pavased
Pavasule
Pavatest
Pavatine
Pavatran
Pavatym
Paverolan
Payadur
Ro-Papan
Sustaverine
Therapav
Vasal
Vasospan

PHENOBARBITAL
Aminophylline-Phenobarbital
Anaspaz-PB
Antrocol
Asminyl
Banthine w/Phenobarbital
Barbidonna
Barbita
Bardase Filmseal
Bar-Tropin
Belap
Belbarb
Belladenal
Bellergal
Belkatal
Bentyl Phenobarbital
Bronkolixir
Bronkotabs
Cantil w/Phenobarbital
Chardonna
Cyclo-Bell
Dactil Phenobarbital
Dainite-KI
Daricon PB
Donna-Lix
Donnatal
Duovent
Eskabarb
Gardenal
Gastrolic
HASP
Hybephen
Hytrona
Iso-Asminyl
Isuprel Compound
Kinesed
Levsin PB
Levsin w/Phenobarbital
Luasmin

Luftodil
Lufyllin-EPG
Luminal
Matropinal
Mesopin PB
Mudrane
Neospect
Nova-Pheno
Oxoids
Pamine PB
Pathilon w/Phenobarbital
PBR/12
Phyldrox
Primatene, P Formula
Pro-Banthine w/Phenobarbital
Probital
Pyrdonnal Spansules
Quadrinal
Robinul-PH
Sedadrops
SK-Phenobarbital
Solfoton
Spasdel
Spasticol
Tedral
T-E-P
Thalfed
Theofedral
Theotabs
Tral w/Phenobarbital
Valpin-PB

PHENYLEPHRINE
4-Way Nasal Spray
4-Way Tablets
Albatussin
Alconefrin
Alka-Seltzer Plus
Allerest Nasal
Anamine T.D.
Bromepaph
Bromphen Compound
Callergy
Cenagesic
Children's Allerest
Chlor-Histine
Chlor-Trimeton
Citra
Clistin D
Codalex
Codimal
Colrex
Comhist
Conar
Congespirin
Contac
Coricidin
Coricidin Mist
Coricidin Nasal Mist
Coryban-D
Coryban-D Cough Syrup
Coryzaid
Cosea-D
Co-Tylenol
Covanamine
Covangesic
Dallergy
Dehist
Demazin
Dimetapp
doKtors Nose Drops
Donatussin DC

Dri-Hist No. Meta-Caps
Drinus Graduals
Dristan Advanced Formula
Dristan Nasal Spray
Drize M
Duadacin
Duo-Medihaler
Duphrene
Dura Tap-PD
Duration Mild
Dura-Vent/DA
Emagrin Forte
E.N.T.
Entex
Extendryl
Fendol
Fernhist
Ginospan
Gualahist
Hista-Vadrin
Histabid Duracaps
Histalet
Histaspan
Histatapp
Histor-D Timecelles
Historal No. 2
Hycomine Compound
Isophrin
Korigesic
Koryza
Marhist
Mydrin
Naldecon
Napril Plateau
Narine Cyrocaps
Narspan
Nasahist
Neo-Mist
Neo-Synephrine
NeoSynephrin Compound
Neotep Granucaps
Nostril
Novahistine
Palohist
Pediacof
Phenate
Phenergan VC
Phenergan VC w/Codeine
Prefrin
Protid Improved Formula
P-V-Tussin
Pyma Timed
Pyracort-D
Quelidrine
Rhinall
Rhinex
Rolabromophen
Rolahist
Ru-Tuss
Rynatan
Rynatapp
Salphenyl
Sinarest Nasal
Sinex
Singlet
Sinophen Intransal
Sinoran
S-T Forte
Super Anahist
Synasal
Taltapp
Tamine S.R.
Tapp

T.P.I.
Tussar DM
Tussirex
Tympagesic
U.R.I.
Vacon
Veltar

PHENYLPROPANOLAMINE

4-Way Cold Tablets
4-Way Nasal Spray
Acutrim
Acutrim Maximum Strength
Alka-Seltzer Plus
Allerest
Alumadrine
Asbron
Axon
Bayer Cold Tablets
Bayer Cough Syrup
Blu-Hist
Bromphen Compound
Caldecon
Children's Allerest
Cinsospan
Citra
Codimal
Coffee-Break
Colrex
Comtrex
Conex-DA
Congespirin
Conhist
Contac
Control
Coricidin "D" Decongestant
Cornex Plus
Coryban-D
Coryztime
CoTylenol Children's Liquid Cold
    Formula
Covanamine
Cremacoat
Dal-Sinus
Decongestant-P
Dehist
Dex-A-Diet
Dexatrim
Diadax
Dietac
Dieutrim
Dimetane
Dimetapp
Dri-Hist Meta-Kaps
Drinus Syrup
D-Sinus
Dura Tap-PD
Dura-Vent, /A
Efed II
Eldatapp
Endecon
E.N.T
Entex
Flogesic
Formula 44-D
Help
Histalet Forte
Histapp
Histatapp
Hycomine
Korigesic
Koryza

Kronohist Kronocaps
MSC Triaminic
Naldecon
Napril Plateau
Nasahist
Nolamine
Novahistine
Obestat
Ornacol
Ornade
Ornex
Partuss T.D.
Phenate
Phenylin
Poly-Histine-D
PPA
Prolamine
Prolamine, Maximum Strength
Propadrine
Propagest
Quadrahist
Resaid T.D.
Rescaps-D T.D.
Resolution I Maximum Strength
Resolution II Half-Strength
Rhindecon
Rhinex Ty-Med
Rhinidrin
Rhinocaps
Rhinolar
Robitussin-CF
Rolabromophen
Ru-Tuss
Rynatapp
Saleto-D
Sinarest
Sine-Off
Sinubid
Sinulin
Sinutab
S-T Decongestant
S-T Forte
Symtrol
Taltapp
Tapp
Tavist-D
T.P.I.
Triaminic
Triaminicin
Triaminicol
Tuss-Ade
Tussagesic
Tussaminic
Tuss-Ornade
Unitrol
U.R.I.
Ursinus
Veltap
Vernata Granucaps
Westrim
Westrim LA

PHENYLTOLOXAMINE

Amaril D
Amaril D Spantab
Comhist
Condecal
Decongestabs
Kutrase
Magsal
Naldecol
Naldecon

Naldelate
Percogesic
Poly-Histine-D
Quadra Hist
Sinocon
Sinubid
Sinutab
Trihista-Phen-25
Tri-Phen-Chlor
Tudecon
Tussionex

POTASSIUM SUPPLEMENTS

Apo-K
Bayon
BI-K
Cena-K
CHLORIDE
EM-K-10%
Infacyte
K-10
Kalium Durules
Kaochlor
Kaochlor S-F
Kaochlor-Eff
Kaon
Kaon-Cl
Kaon-Cl 10
Kaon-Cl 20
Kao-Nor
Kato
Kay Ciel
Kaylixir
KCL
K-Dur
KEFF
K-G Elixir
K-Long
K-Lor
Klor-10%
Klor-Con
Klor-Con/EF
Klor Con/25
Klorvess
Klotrix
K-Lyte
K-Lyte/CL Powder
K-Lyte DS
K-Lyte/Cl
K-Lyte/Cl 50
Kolyum
K-Tab
Micro-K
Micro-K 10
Neo-K
Novo-Lente-K
Pfiklor
Potachlor
Potage
Potasalan
Potassine
POTASSIUM ACETATE
POTASSIUM BICARBONATE
POTASSIUM BICARBONATE &
  POTASSIUM CHLORIDE
POTASSIUM BICARBONATE &
  POTASSIUM CITRATE
POTASSIUM CHLORIDE
POTASSIUM CHLORIDE,
  POTASSIUM BICARBONATE &
  POTASSIUM CITRATE

POTASSIUM GLUCONATE
POTASSIUM GLUCONATE &
  POTASSIUM CHLORIDE
POTASSIUM GLUCONATE &
  POTASSIUM CITRATE
POTASSIUM GLUCONATE,
  POTASSIUM CITRATE &
  AMMONIUM
Potassium Triplex
Potassium-Rougier
Potassium-Sandoz
Roychlor
Royonate
Rum-K
SK-Potassium Chloride
Slo-Pot
Slow-K
Ten K
Tri-K
TRIKATES
Twin-K
Twin-K-Cl

PREDNISOLONE

Ak-Pred
Ak-Tate
Articulose
Codesol
Cortalone
Delta-Cortef
Deltastab
Econopred
Fernisolone-P
Hydeltrasol
Hydeltra-TBA
Inflamase
Key-Pred
Key-Pred-SP
Metalone-TBA
Meticortelone
Meti-Derm
Metimyd
Metreton
Nor-Pred-TBA
Nova-Pred
Novaprednisolone
Pediapred
Predaject
Predate
Predate-S
Predate-TBA
Predcor
Pred Cor-TBA
Pred Forte
Pred Mild
Prednisol TBA
Predulose
Prelone
PSP-IV
Savacort 50 & 100
Sterane

PROMETHAZINE

Anergan
Baymethazine
Dihydrocodeine Compound
Fellozine
Ganphen
Histantil
Historest
K-Phen
Mallergan

Mepergan Fortis
Pentazine
Phenameth
Phenazine
Phencen-50
Phenergan
Phenergan Fortis
Phenergan Plain
Phenerhist
Phenoject-50
PMS Promethazine
Promet 50
Prometh
Prorex
Prosedin
Prothazine
Prothazine Plain
Provigan
Remsed
V-Gan
ZiPan

PSEUDOEPHEDRINE

Actifed
Afrinol
Afrinol Repetabs
Ambenyl-D
Anafed
Anamine
Brexin
Bromfed
Bronchobid
Cardec DM
Cenafed
Children's Sudafed Liquid
Chlorafed
Chlor-Trimeton
Codimal
Co-Pyronil 2
Cosanyl
Co-Tylenol
Cotrol-D
Decofed
Deconamine
D-Feda
Deproist w/Codeine
Detussin
Dimacol
Disobrom
Disophrol
Dorcol
Dorcol Pediatric Formula
Drixoral
Eltor
Emprazil
Entuss-D
Fedahist
Fedrazil
Gualfed
Halofed
Hista-Clopane
Histalet DM
Histamic
Historal
Isoclor
Kronofed-A Kronocaps
Naldegesic
Neo-Synephrinol Day Relief
Neobid
Neofed
Novafed
Novafed A

Novahistine DMX
Nucofed
PediaCare
Peedee Dose Decongestant
Phenergan
Phenergan-D
Poly-Histine-DX
Probahist
Pseudogest
Pseudo-Hist
Pseudofrin
Redahist Gyrocaps
Respaire-SR
Ro-Fedrin
Robidrine
Robitussin-DAC
Rondec
Sherafed
Sine-Aid Sinus Headache Tablets
Sinufed
Sinufed Timecelles
Sudafed
Sudafed S.A.
Sudagest
Sudahist
Suda-Prol
Sudolin
Sudrin
Triafed
Trifed
Trinalin Repetabs
Triphed
Tripodrine
Tussend
Tylenol Maximum Strength Sinus
   Medicine
Zephrex

PSYLLIUM

Cilium
Effersyllium
Fiberall
Hydrocil
Konsyl
Konsyl-D
Hydrocil Instant
L.A. Formula
Metamucil
Metamucil Instant Mix
Metamucil Instant Mix, Orange
   Flavor
Metamucil Orange Flavor
Metamucil Strawberry Flavor
Metamucil Sugar Free
Modane Bulk
Mucillium
Mucilose
Naturacil
Perdiem Plain
Piova
Prodiem
Pro-Lax
Prompt
Regacilium
Reguloid
Reguloid Natural
Reguloid Orange
Saraka
Senokot with Psyllium
Serutan
Serutan Toasted Granules
Siblin

Sof-Cil
Syllact
Versabran
V-Lax

PYRILAMINE

4-Way Nasal Spray
Albatussin
Allerstat
Allertoc
Citra Forte
Codimal DH, DM, PH
Covanamine
Dormarex
Duphrene
Excedrin P.M.
Flogesic
Histalet Forte
Kronohist Kronocaps
Midol PMS
Napril Plateau
Nervine Nighttime Sleep-Aid
Panadyl
Poly-Histine D
Primatene, M Formula
P-V-Tussin
Relemine
Ru-Tuss
Rynatan
Sominex
Somnicaps
Triaminic
Trihista-Phen-25
Tussanil

RADIO-
PHARMACEUTICALS

Cyanocobalamin Co 57
Cyanocobalamin Co 60
Ferrous Citrate Fe 59
Gallium Citrate Ga 67
Indium In 111 Pentetate
Iodinated I 131 Albumin
Iodohippurate Sodium I 123
Iodohippurate Sodium I 131
Iothalamate Sodium I 125
Krypton Kr 81m
Selenomethionine Se 75
Sodium Chromate Cr 51
Sodium Iodide I 123
Sodium Iodide I 131
Sodium Pertechnetate Tc 99m
Sodium Phosphate P 32
Technetium Tc 99m Albumin
   Aggregated
Technetium Tc 99m Disofenin
Technetium Tc 99m Gluceptate
Technetium Tc 99m Human
   Serum Albumin
Technetium Tc 99m Medronate
Technetium Tc 99m Oxidronate
Technetium Tc 99m Pentetate
Technetium Tc 99m
   Pyrophosphate
Technetium Tc 99m Succimer
Technetium Tc 99m Sulfur
   Colloid
Thallous Chloride Tl 201
Xenon Xe 127
Xenon Xe 133

RAUWOLFIA ALKALOIDS

Alkarau
ALSEROXYLON
Bonapene
Broserpine
Butiserpazide-50 Prestabs
Buytizide-25 Prestabs
Chloroserpine
Demi-Regroton
DESERPIDINE
Diupres
Diutensin-R
Draiserp
Enduronyl
Harmonyl
Harmonyl-D
H-H-R
Hydro-Fluserpine
Hydromox R
Hydropres
Hydroserp
Hydroserpine
Hydrotensin-50
Mallopress
Metatensin
Naquival
Novoreserpine
Oreticyl
Raudixin
Raulfia
Raunormine
Raupold
Rauraine
Rau-Sed
Rauserpa
Rautrax
Rauverid
Rauwiloid
Rauzide
RAUWOLFIA SERPENTINA
Regroton
Releserp-5
Renese-R
Reserfia
Reserpazide
RESERPINE
Reserpoid
Salutensin
Sandril
Ser-Ap-Es
Serpalan
Serpanray
Serpasil
Serpasil-Apresoline
Serpasil-Esidrix
SK-Reserpine
Serpate
Singoserp-Eisdrix
T-Serp
Unipres
Wolfina

RAUWOLFIA & THIAZIDE
DIURETICS

Demi-Regroton
DESERPIDINE &
   HYDROCHLOROTHIAZIDE
DESERPIDINE &
   METHYCLOTHIAZIDE
Diupres
Diutensen-R

Dureticyl
Enduronyl
Hydromox-R
Hydropres
Metatensin
Naquival
Oreticyl
Oreticyl Forte
RAUWOLFIA SERPENTINA &
  BENDROFLUMETHIAZIDE
Rauzide
Regroton
Renese-R
RESERPINE & CHLOROTHIAZIDE
RESERPINE &
  CHLORTHALIDONE
RESERPINE &
  HYDROCHLOROTHIAZIDE
RESERPINE &
  HYDROFLUMETHIAZIDE
RESERPINE &
  METHYCLOTHIAZIDE
RESERPINE & POLYTHIAZIDE
RESERPINE & QUINETHAZONE
RESERPINE &
  TRICHLORMETHIAZIDE
Salutensin
Salutensin-Demi
Serpasil-Esidrix

SALICYLATES

Arcylate
Artha-G
Arthropan
CHOLINE MAGNESIUM
  SALICYLATES
Choline Magnesium Trisalicylate
CHOLINE SALICYLATE
DIFLUNISAL
Disalcid
Doan's Pills
Durasil
Magan
MAGNESIUM SALICYLATE
Mobidin
Mono-Gesic
SALICYLAMIDE
SALSALATE
SODIUM SALICYLATE
S-60
Trilisate
Uracel
Uromide

SCOPOLAMINE
(Hyoscine)

Allerspan
Almezyme
Aluscop
Bar-Cy-Amine
Bar-Cy-A-Tab
Barbella
Barbeloid
Barbidonna
Barbidonna-CR
Bar-Don
Belbutal
Belkaloids
Bobid
Brobella-PB
Buren

Cenahist
Chlorpel
Conalsyn
Dallergy
Donnacin
Donnagel
Donnamine
Donnatal
Donnazyme
Drinus
Drize
Eldonal
Eulcin
Extendryl
Haponal
Histaspan-D
Historal
Hyatal
Hybephen
Hydrochol-Plus
Hyonal
Hyonatol
Hytrona
Kinesed
Kleer
Kleer-Tuss
Koryza
Levamine
Maso-Donna
Methnite
MSC Triaminic
Narine
Narspan
Nilspasm
Omnibel
Pamine
Pamine PB
Paraspan
Renalgin
Ru-Tuss
Sanhist
Scoline
Scoline-Amobarbital
Scopolamine Trans-Derm
Scotnord
Sedamine
Sedapar
Sedralex
Seds
Sinaprel
Sinodec
Sinoran
Sinunil
Spabelin
Spasdel
Spasloids
Spasmid
Spasmolin
Spasquid
Spastolate
Symptrol
Transderm
Transderm-Scop
Transderm-V
Triptone
Trisohist
Uriseptin
Urogesic
Vanodonnal
Zemarine

SULFISOXAZOLE

Apo-Sulfisoxazole
Azo-Gantrisin
Azo-Soxazole
Barazole
Chemovag
Gantrisin
G-Sox
Lipo Gantrisin
Koro-Sulf
Novosoxazole
Pediazole
Rosoxol
SK-Soxazole
Sosol
Soxa
Sulfafurazole
Sulfagen
Sulfizin
Sulfizole
Urisoxin

TESTOSTERONE &
ESTRADIOL

Andrest
Andro-Estro
Andro/Fem
Androgyn L.A.
De-Comberol
Deladumone
Deladumone OB
depAndrogyn
Depo-Testadiol
Depotestogen
Ditate
Ditate DS
Duo-Cyp
Duo-Gen L.A.
Duogex LA
Duoval PA
Duratestrin
Estrand
Estra-Testrin
Menoject-L.A.
Neo-Pause
Span-Est-Test
Teev
T.E.-Ionate P.A.
Testadiate-Depo
Test-Estra-C
Test-Estro Cypionates
TESTOSTERONE CYPIONATE &
  ESTRADIOL CYPIONATE
TESTOSTERONE ENANTHATE &
  ESTRADIOL VALERATE
Testradiol
Testradiol L.A.
Valertest

TETRACYCLINES

Achromycin
Achromycin V
Achrostatin V
Apo-Tetra
Bicycline
Bio-Tetra
Bristacycline
Cefracycline
Centet
Comycin
Cyclopar

1071

Declomycin
DEMECLOCYCLINE
Desamycin
Doryx
Doxy
Doxy-Caps
Doxychel
DOXYCYCLINE
Doxy-Lemmon
Doxy-Tabs
Fed-Mycin
G-Mycin
Kesso-Tetra
Lemtrex
Maytrex-BID
Medicycline
METHACYCLINE
Minocin
MINOCYCLINE
Muracine
Mysteclin F
Neo-Tetrine
Nor-Tet
Novotetra
Oxlopar
Oxy-Kesso-Tetra
OXYTETRACYCLINE
Paltet
Panmycin
Piracaps
PMS Tetracycline
Q'Dtet
Retet
Retet-S
Robitet
Ro-Cycline
Rondomycin
Sarocyclin
Scotrex
SK-Tetracycline
Sumycin
T-Caps
TETRACYCLINE
Terramycin
Tet-Cy
Tetet
Tetrachel
Tetra-Co
Tetracrine
Tetracyn
Tetracyrine
Tetralean
Tetram
Tetramax
Tetramine
Tetrastatin (M)
Tetrex
Tetrex-S
Topicycline
Trexin
Ultramycin
Uroblotic
Vibramycin
Vibratabs
Vivox

TRIAMCINOLONE

Acetospan
Amcort
Aristocort
Aristocort Forte
Aristocort Intralesional

Aristophan Intralesional
Aristospan
Articulose-L.A.
Azmacort
Cenocort
Cenocort A
Cenocort Forte
Cinalone 40
Cino-40
Cinonide
Cinonide 40
Cremocort
Intra-articular
Kenacort
Kenaject
Kenalog
Kenalog In Orabase
Kenalog-E
Kenalone
Ledercort
Lederspan
Mycolog
Myco-Triacet
Mytrex
Nust-Olone
Spencort
Tramacort
Triacet
Triacort
Triaderm
Trialean Acetonide
Triam
Triamcinair
Triam-Forte
Triamonide
Tri-Kort
Trilog
Trilone
Trim-A
Trimalone
Tristoject
Trymex
Some of these brands are
    available as topical medicines
    (ointments, creams or lotions).
See ADRENOCORTICOIDS
    (Topical) in this section.

TRICYCLIC ANTIDEPRESSANTS

Adapin
Amitid
Amitril
AMITRYPTILINE
AMOXAPINE
Anafranil
Anemtyl
Apo-Amitriptyline
Apo-Imipramine
Ascendin
Aventyl
CLOMIPRAMINE
DESIPRAMINE
Elavil
Emitrip
Endep
Enovil
Etrafon
IMIPRAMINE
Impril
Janimine
Levate

Meravil
Norpramin
NORTRIPTYLINE
Novopramine
Novotriptyn
Pamelor
Pertofrane
Presamine
PROTRIPTYLINE
Sinequan
SK-Amitriptyline
SK-Pramine
Surmontil
Tipramine
Tofranil
Tofranil-PM
Triadapin
Triavil
TRIMIPRAMINE
Triptil
Vivactil

VITAMIN B-12 (Cyanocobalamin)

Acti-B-12
Alphamin
Alpha Redisol
Anocobin
Bedoz
Berubigen
Betalin 12
Betalin 12 Crystalline
Codroxomin
Cyanabin
Droxomin
Kaybovite
Kaybovite-1000
Neo-Betalin
Neo-Rubex
Redisol
Rubion
Rubramin
Rubramin-PC
Sytobex
Numerous other multiple vitamin-
    mineral supplements.

VITAMIN C (Ascorbic Acid)

Adenex
Apo-C
Arco-Cee
Ascorbajen
Ascorbicap
Ascoril
Calscorbate
Cecon
Cemill
Cenolate
Ceri-Bid
Cetane
Cevalin
Cevi-Bid
Ce-Vi-Sol
Cevita
C-Ject
Flavorcee
Liqui-Cee
Megascorb
Redoxon
Numerous other multiple vitamin-
    mineral supplements.

XANTHINE BRONCHODILATORS

Accurbron
Aerolate
Aerophylline
Airet
Amesec
Aminodur
Aminodur Dura-tabs
Aminophyl
Aminophyllin
AMINOPHYLLINE
Aminophylline and Amytal
Aminophylline-Phenobarbital
Amodrine
Amoline
Amophylline
Apo-Oxtriphylline
Aquaphyllin
Asbron
Asma
Asmalix
Asminyl
Asthmophylline
Bronchobid Duracaps
Broncholate
Brondecon
Brondilate
Bronkodyl
Bronkodyl S-R
Bronkolixir
Bronkotabs
Brosema
Choledyl
Choledyl SA
Chophylline
Constant-T
Corophyllin
Corophylline
Co-Xan
Dilin
Dilor
Dilor-G
Droxine
Droxine L.A.
Droxine S.F.
Duovent
Duraphyl
Dyflex
Dyline
DYPHILLINE
Dy-Phyl-Lin
Elixicon
Elixomin
Elixophyllin
Elixophyllin SR
Emfaseem
G-Bron

Iso-Asminyl
Isuprel Compound
Kiophyllin
LABID
Lanophyllin
Liquophylline
Lixaminol
Lixaminol AT
Lixolin
Lodrane
Luasmin
Luftodil
Lufyllin
Marax
Marax DF
Mersalyl-Theophylline
Mini-Lix
Mudrane
Neospect
Neothylline
Neothylline-G
Novotriphyl
Numa-Dura-Tabs
Orthoxine & Aminophylline
OXTRIPHYLLINE
Oxystat
Palaron
Phenylin
Phyldrox
Phyllocontin
Physpan
PMS Theophylline
Primatene, M Formula
Primatene, P Formula
Protophylline
Pulmophylline
Quadrinal
Quibron
Quibron Plus
Quibron-T
Quibron-T Dividose
Quibron-T/SR Dividose
Respbid
Slo-Phyllin GG
Slo-Phyllin Gyrocaps
Slo-bid Gyrocaps
Slophyllin
Somophyllin
Somophyllin-12
Somophyllin-CRT
Somophyllin-DF
Somophyllin-T
Sudolin
Sustaire
Synophylate
Synophylate-GG
Tedfern
Tedral

T.E.H.
Thalfed
Theobid
Theobid Duracaps
Theobid Jr. Duracaps
Theochron
Theoclear
Theoclear L.A. Cenules
Theo-Dur
Theo-Dur Sprinkle
Theofedral
Theo-Guaia
Theolair
Theolair-Plus
Theolair-SR
Theolixir
Theon
Theo-Nar 100
Theo-Organidin
Theophyl
Theophyl-SR
THEOPHYLLINE
Theophylline Choline
Theospan
Theospan SR
Theostat
Theostate 80
Theotabs
Theo-Time
Theo-24
Theovent Long-acting
Theozine
Truphylline
Uniphyl

XYLOMETAZOLINE

4-Way Long-Acting Nasal
Afrin
Allerest 12-Hour Nasal
Bayfrin
Chlorohist
Corcidin Nasal Mist
Dristan Long Lasting
Duramist Plus
Duration
Nafrine
Neo-Spray Long-Acting
Neo-Synephrine II Long
Nostrilla
NTZ Long Acting Nasal
Ocuclear
Otrivin
Oxymeta-12 Nasal Spray
Sinarest 12-Hour
Sinex Long-Lasting
Sinutab
St. Joseph Decongestant for
Children

Additional Drug Interactions

The following lists of drugs and their interactions with other drugs are continuations of lists found in the alphabetized drug charts beginning on page 2. These lists are alphabetized by generic name or drug class name, shown in large capital letters. Only those lists too long for the drug charts are included in this section. For complete information about any generic drug, see the alphabetized chart.

GENERIC NAME OR DRUG CLASS	COMBINED EFFECT	GENERIC NAME OR DRUG CLASS	COMBINED EFFECT
ACEBUTOLOL			
Timolol eyedrops	Possible increased acebutolol effect.	Xanthine bronchodilators*	Decreased effects of both drugs.
Verapamil	Increased effect of both drugs.		
ACETAMINOPHEN & SALICYLATES			
Para-aminosalicylic acid (PAS)	Possible salicylate toxicity.	Spironolactone	Decreased spironolactone effect.
Phenobarbital	Decreased effect of acetaminophen and salicylates because of quicker elimination.	Sulfinpyrazone	Decreased sulfinpyrazone effect.
		Terazosin	Decreases effectiveness of terazosin. Causes sodium and fluid retention.
Phenytoin	Increased phenytoin effect.		
Probenecid	Decreased probenecid effect.	Tetracyclines* (effervescent granules or tablets)	May slow tetracycline absorption. Space doses 2 hours apart.
Propranolol	Decreased aspirin effect.	Vancomycin	Hearing loss.
Rauwolfia alkaloids*	Decreased aspirin effect.	Verapamil	Increased risk of toxicity.
Sotalol	Decreased antihypertensive effect of sotalol.	Vitamin C (large doses)	Possible aspirin toxicity.
AMILORIDE & HYDROCHLOROTHIAZIDE			
Digitalis preparations*	Excessive potassium loss that causes dangerous heart rhythms.	MAO inhibitors*	Increased hydrochlorothiazide effect.
		Nicardipine	Dangerous blood-pressure drop. Dosages may require djustment.
Diuretics, thiazide*	Increased diuretic effect.		
Diuretics, other*	Increased effect of both drugs.	Nitrates*	Excessive blood-pressure drop.
Indapamide	Increased diuretic effect.	Oxprenolol	Increased antihypertensive effect. Dosages may require adjustment.
Lisinopril	Increased antihypertensive effect. Dosage of each may require adjustment.		
		Probenecid	Decreased probenecid effect.
Lithium	Possible lithium toxicity.		

*See Glossary

GENERIC NAME OR DRUG CLASS	COMBINED EFFECT	GENERIC NAME OR DRUG CLASS	COMBINED EFFECT

AMILORIDE & HYDROCHLOROTHIAZIDE continued

GENERIC NAME OR DRUG CLASS	COMBINED EFFECT	GENERIC NAME OR DRUG CLASS	COMBINED EFFECT
Sodium bicarbonate	Decreased potassium levels.	Terazosin	Decreases effectiveness of terazosin.
Sotalol	Increased antihypertensive effect.		

AMOBARBITAL

GENERIC NAME OR DRUG CLASS	COMBINED EFFECT	GENERIC NAME OR DRUG CLASS	COMBINED EFFECT
Sleep inducers*	Dangerous sedation. Avoid.	Tranquilizers*	Dangerous sedation. Avoid.
Sotalol	Increased barbiturate effect. Dangerous sedation.	Valproic acid	Increased amobarbital effect.

ASPIRIN

GENERIC NAME OR DRUG CLASS	COMBINED EFFECT	GENERIC NAME OR DRUG CLASS	COMBINED EFFECT
Para-aminosalicylic acid (PAS)	Possible aspirin toxicity.	Spironolactone	Decreased spironolactone effect.
Penicillins*	Increased effect of both drugs.	Sulfinpyrazone	Decreased sulfinpyrazone effect.
Phenobarbital	Decreased aspirin effect.	Terazosin	Decreases effectiveness of terazosin. Causes sodium and fluid retention.
Phenytoin	Increased phenytoin effect.		
Probenecid	Decreased probenecid effect.	Terfenadine	May conceal symptoms of aspirin overdose, such as ringing in ears.
Propranolol	Decreased aspirin effect.		
Rauwolfia alkaloids*	Decreased aspirin effect.	Vitamin C (large doses)	Possible aspirin toxicity.
Salicylates, other*	Likely aspirin toxicity.	Valproic acid	May increase valproic acid effect.
Sotalol	Decreased antihypertensive effect of sotalol.		

ATROPINE, HYOSCYAMINE, METHENAMINE, METHYLENE BLUE, PHENYLSALICYLATE & BENZOIC ACID

GENERIC NAME OR DRUG CLASS	COMBINED EFFECT	GENERIC NAME OR DRUG CLASS	COMBINED EFFECT
Meperidine	Increased atropine and hyoscyamine effect.	Orphenadrine	Increased atropine and hyoscyamine effect.
Methylphenidate	Increased atropine and hyoscyamine effect.	Oxprenolol	Decreased antihypertensive effect of oxprenolol.
Minoxidil	Decreased minoxidil effect.	Para-aminosalicylic acid (PAS)	Possible salicylate toxicity.
Non-steroidal anti-inflammatory drugs (NSAIDs)*	Risk of stomach bleeding and ulcers.	Penicillins*	Increased effect of both drugs.
		Phenobarbital	Decreased salicylate effect.

*See Glossary

ADDITIONAL DRUG INTERACTIONS

GENERIC NAME OR DRUG CLASS	COMBINED EFFECT	GENERIC NAME OR DRUG CLASS	COMBINED EFFECT

ATROPINE, HYOSCYAMINE, METHENAMINE, METHYLENE BLUE, PHENYLSALICYLATE & BENZOIC ACID continued

GENERIC NAME OR DRUG CLASS	COMBINED EFFECT	GENERIC NAME OR DRUG CLASS	COMBINED EFFECT
Phenothiazines*	Increased atropine and hyoscyamine effect.	Sodium bicarbonate	Decreased methenamine effect.
Phenytoin	Increased phenytoin effect.	Spironolactone	Decreased spironolactone effect.
Pilocarpine	Loss of pilocarpine effect in glaucoma treatment.	Sulfa drugs*	Possible kidney damage.
		Sulfinpyrazone	Decreased sulfinpyrazone effect.
Potassium supplements*	Possible intestinal ulcers with oral potassium tablets.	Terfenadine	May conceal symptoms of salicylate overdose, such as ringing in ears.
Probenecid	Decreased probenecid effect.		
Propranolol	Decreased salicylate effect.	Vitamin C (1 to 4 grams per day)	Increased effect of methenamine, contributing to urine acidity; decreased atropine effect; possible salicylate toxicity.
Rauwolfia alkaloids*	Decreased salicylate effect.		
Salicylates, other*	Likely salicylate toxicity.		

BELLADONNA ALKALOIDS & BARBITURATES

GENERIC NAME OR DRUG CLASS	COMBINED EFFECT	GENERIC NAME OR DRUG CLASS	COMBINED EFFECT
Cortisone drugs*	Increased internal-eye pressure. Decreased cortisone effect.	Mind-altering drugs*	Dangerous sedation. Avoid.
Digitoxin	Decreased digitoxin effect.	Narcotics*	Dangerous sedation. Avoid.
Doxycycline	Decreased doxycycline effect.	Nitrates*	Increased internal-eye pressure.
Dronabinol	Increased effects of both drugs. Avoid.	Nizatidine	Increased nizatidine effect.
Furosemide	Possible orthostatic hypotension.	Non-steroidal anti-inflammatory drugs (NSAIDs)*	Decreased anti-inflammatory effect.
Griseofulvin	Decreased griseofulvin effect.	Orphenadrine	Increased belladonna effect.
Haloperidol	Increased internal-eye pressure.	Pain relievers*	Dangerous sedation. Avoid.
Indapamide	Increased indapamide effect.	Phenothiazines*	Increased belladonna effect. Danger of oversedation.
MAO inhibitors*	Increased belladonna and barbiturate effect.	Pilocarpine	Loss of pilocarpine effect in glaucoma treatment.
Meperidine	Increased belladonna effect.		
Methylphenidate	Increased belladonna effect.	Potassium supplements*	Possible intestinal ulcers with oral potassium tablets.
Metronidazole	Decreased metronidazole effect.	Quinidine	Increased belladonna effect.

*See Glossary

GENERIC NAME OR DRUG CLASS	COMBINED EFFECT	GENERIC NAME OR DRUG CLASS	COMBINED EFFECT
BELLADONNA ALKALOIDS & BARBITURATES continued			
Sedatives*	Dangerous sedation. Avoid.	Tranquilizers*	Dangerous sedation. Avoid.
Sleep inducers*	Dangerous sedation. Avoid.	Valproic acid	Increased barbiturate effect.
Sotalol	Increased barbiturate effect. Dangerous sedation.	Vitamin C	Decreased belladonna effect. Avoid large doses of vitamin C.

BENDROFLUMETHIAZIDE

Nicardipine	Dangerous blood-pressure drop. Dosages may require adjustment.	Potassium supplements*	Decreased potassium effect.
		Probenecid	Decreased probenecid effect.
Nitrates*	Excessive blood-pressure drop.	Sotalol	Increased antihypertensive effect.
Oxprenolol	Increased antihypertensive effect. Dosages of both drugs may require adjustments.	Terazosin	Decreases effectiveness of terazosin.
		Vitamin D	May increase calcium in blood.

BENZTHIAZIDE

Nicardipine	Blood-pressure drop. Dosages may require adjustment.	Potassium supplements*	Decreased potassium effect.
		Probenecid	Decreased probenecid effect.
Nitrates*	Excessive blood-pressure drop.	Sotalol	Increased antihypertensive effect.
Oxprenolol	Increased antihypertensive effect. Dosages of both drugs may require adjustments.	Terazosin	Decreases effectiveness of terazosin.
		Vitamin D	May increase calcium in blood.

BETA-ADRENERGIC BLOCKING AGENTS & THIAZIDE DIURETICS

Antihypertensives*	Increased antihypertensive effect.	Bumetanide	Increased diuretic effect.
Barbiturates*	Increased barbiturate effect. Dangerous sedation.	Cholestyramine	Decreased hydrochlorthiazide effect.
Beta-adrenergic blockers*	Increased antihypertensive effect. Dosages of both drugs may require adjustments.	Cortisone drugs*	Excessive potassium loss that causes dangerous heart rhythms.
		Diclofenac	Decreased antihypertensive effect.

*See Glossary

GENERIC NAME OR DRUG CLASS	COMBINED EFFECT	GENERIC NAME OR DRUG CLASS	COMBINED EFFECT

BETA-ADRENERGIC BLOCKING AGENTS & THIAZIDE DIURETICS continued

GENERIC NAME OR DRUG CLASS	COMBINED EFFECT	GENERIC NAME OR DRUG CLASS	COMBINED EFFECT
Digitalis preparations*	Excessive potassium loss that causes dangerous heart rhythms. Can either increase or decrease heart rate. Improves irregular heartbeat.	Metolazone	Increased diuretic effect.
		Narcotics*	Increased narcotic effect. Dangerous sedation.
Diuretics, thiazide*	Increased effect of other thiazide diuretics.	Nicardipine	Possible irregular heartbeat and congestive heart failure.
Ethacrynic acid	Increased diuretic effect.	Nitrates*	Excessive blood-pressure drop.
Furosemide	Increased diuretic effect.	Non-steroidal anti-inflammatory drugs (NSAIDs)*	Decreased anti-inflammatory effect.
Guanfacine	Increased effect of both drugs.	Phenytoin	Increased beta-adrenergic effect.
Hypoglycemics, oral*	Decreased ability to lower blood glucose.	Potassium supplements*	Decreased potassium effect.
Indapamide	Increased diuretic effect.	Probenecid	Decreased probenecid effect.
Insulin	Decreased ability to lower blood glucose.	Quinidine	Slows heart excessively.
Lisinopril	Increased antihypertensive effect. Dosage of each may require adjustment.	Reserpine	Increased reserpine effect. Excessive sedation and depression.
MAO inhibitors*	Increased hydrochlorothiazide effect.	Tocainide	May worsen congestive heart failure.

BETAMETHASONE

GENERIC NAME OR DRUG CLASS	COMBINED EFFECT	GENERIC NAME OR DRUG CLASS	COMBINED EFFECT
Potassium supplements	Decreased potassium effect.	Sympathomimetics*	Possible glaucoma.
Rifampin	Decreased betamethasone effect.		

BUTALBITAL & ASPIRIN (Also contains caffeine)

GENERIC NAME OR DRUG CLASS	COMBINED EFFECT	GENERIC NAME OR DRUG CLASS	COMBINED EFFECT
Aspirin, other	Likely aspirin toxicity.	Doxycycline	Decreased doxycycline effect.
Beta-adrenergic blockers*	Decreased effect of beta-adrenergic blocker.	Dronabinol	Increased effect of both drugs.
Contraceptives, oral*	Decreased contraceptive effect.	Furosemide	Possible aspirin toxicity.
Cortisone drugs*	Increased cortisone effect. Risk of ulcer and stomach bleeding.	Gold compounds*	Increased likelihood of kidney damage.
Digitoxin	Decreased digitoxin effect.	Griseofulvin	Decreased griseofulvin effect.

BUTALBITAL & ASPIRIN (Also contains caffeine) continued

GENERIC NAME OR DRUG CLASS	COMBINED EFFECT	GENERIC NAME OR DRUG CLASS	COMBINED EFFECT
Indapamide	Increased indapamide effect.	Salicylates, others*	Likely aspirin toxicity.
Indomethacin	Risk of stomach bleeding and ulcers.	Sedatives*	Dangerous sedation. Avoid.
MAO inhibitors*	Increased butalbital effect.	Sleep inducers*	Dangerous sedation. Avoid.
Methotrexate	Increased methotrexate effect.	Spironolactone	Decreased spironolactone effect.
Mind-altering drugs*	Dangerous sedation. Avoid.	Sulfinpyrazone	Decreased sulfin-pyrazone effect.
Minoxidil	Decreased minoxidil effect.	Terfenadine	May conceal symptoms of aspirin overdose, such as ringing in ears.
Narcotics*	Dangerous sedation. Avoid.		
Non-steroidal anti-inflammatory drugs (NSAIDs)*	Risk of stomach bleeding and ulcers.	Tranquilizers*	Dangerous sedation. Avoid.
Pain relievers*	Dangerous sedation. Avoid.	Valproic acid	Increased butalbital effect.
Rifampin	May decrease butalbital effect.	Vitamin C (large doses)	Possible aspirin toxicity.

BUTALBITAL, ASPIRIN & CODEINE (Also contains caffeine)

GENERIC NAME OR DRUG CLASS	COMBINED EFFECT	GENERIC NAME OR DRUG CLASS	COMBINED EFFECT
Antidepressants*	Decreased anti-depressant effect. Possible dangerous oversedation.	Doxycycline	Decreased doxycycline effect.
		Dronabinol	Increased effect of drugs.
Antidiabetics, oral*	Increased butalbital effect. Low blood sugar.	Furosemide	Possible aspirin toxicity.
Antihistamines*	Dangerous sedation. Avoid.	Gold compounds*	Increased likelihood of kidney damage.
Aspirin, other	Likely aspirin toxicity.	Griseofulvin	Decreased griseofulvin effect.
Beta-adrenergic blockers*	Decreased effect of beta-adrenergic blocker.	Indapamide	Increased indapamide effect.
Carteolol	Increased narcotic effect. Dangerous sedation.	Indomethacin	Risk of stomach bleeding and ulcers.
Contraceptives, oral*	Decreased contra-ceptive effect.	MAO inhibitors*	Increased butalbital effect.
Cortisone drugs*	Increased cortisone effect. Risk of ulcer and stomach bleeding.	Methotrexate	Increased methotrexate effect.
		Mind-altering drugs*	Dangerous sedation. Avoid.
Digitoxin	Decreased digitoxin effect.	Minoxidil	Decreased minoxidil effect.

*See Glossary

ADDITIONAL DRUG INTERACTIONS

BUTALBITAL, ASPIRIN & CODEINE (Also contains caffeine) continued

GENERIC NAME OR DRUG CLASS	COMBINED EFFECT	GENERIC NAME OR DRUG CLASS	COMBINED EFFECT
Narcotics*	Dangerous sedation. Avoid.	Rauwolfia alkaloids*	Decreased aspirin effect.
Nitrates*	Excessive blood-pressure drop.	Salicylates, others*	Likely aspirin toxicity.
Non-steroidal anti-inflammatory drugs (NSAIDs)*	Risk of stomach bleeding and ulcers.	Sedatives*	Dangerous sedation. Avoid.
Pain relievers*	Dangerous sedation. Avoid.	Sleep inducers*	Dangerous sedation. Avoid.
Para-aminosalicylic acid (PAS)	Possible aspirin toxicity.	Sotalol	Increased narcotic effect. Dangerous sedation.
Penicillins*	Increased effect of drugs.	Spironolactone	Decreased spironolactone effect.
Phenobarbital	Decreased aspirin effect.	Sulfinpyrazone	Decreased sulfin-pyrazone effect.
Phenothiazines*	Increased phenothiazine effect.	Terfenadine	May conceal symptoms of aspirin overdose, such as ringing in ears.
Phenytoin	Increased phenytoin effect.	Tranquilizers*	Dangerous sedation. Avoid.
Probenecid	Decreased probenecid effect.	Valproic acid	Increased phenobarbital effect.
Propranolol	Decreased aspirin effect.	Vitamin C (large doses)	Possible aspirin toxicity.

CAPTOPRIL & HYDROCHLOROTHIAZIDE

GENERIC NAME OR DRUG CLASS	COMBINED EFFECT	GENERIC NAME OR DRUG CLASS	COMBINED EFFECT
Lithium	Increased effect of lithium.	Potassium supplements*	Excessive potassium in blood.
MAO inhibitors*	Increased hydrochloro-thiazide effect.	Probenecid	Decreased probenecid effect.
Nicardipine	Blood-pressure drop. Dosages may require adjustment.	Sotalol	Increased antihyper-tensive effects of both drugs. Dosages may require adjustment.
Nitrates*	Excessive blood-pressure drop.	Spironolactone	Possible excessive potassium in blood.
Non-steroidal anti-inflammatory drugs (NSAIDs)*	Decreased captopril effect.	Triamterene	Possible excessive potassium in blood.

CARBAMAZEPINE

GENERIC NAME OR DRUG CLASS	COMBINED EFFECT	GENERIC NAME OR DRUG CLASS	COMBINED EFFECT
Leucovorin	High alcohol content of leucovorin may cause adverse effects.	Methyprylon	Increased sedative effect, perhaps to dangerous level. Avoid.
MAO inhibitors*	Dangerous over-stimulation. Avoid.	Nabilone	Greater depression of central nervous system.
Mebendazole	Decreased effect of mebendazole.	Nicardipine	May increase carbama-zepine effect and toxicity.

GENERIC NAME OR DRUG CLASS	COMBINED EFFECT	GENERIC NAME OR DRUG CLASS	COMBINED EFFECT

CARBAMAZEPINE continued

GENERIC NAME OR DRUG CLASS	COMBINED EFFECT	GENERIC NAME OR DRUG CLASS	COMBINED EFFECT
Nizatidine	Increased carbamazepine effect and toxicity.	Primidone	Decreased carbamazepine effect.
Phenytoin	Decreased carbamazepine effect.	Tranquilizers* (benzodiazepine)	Increased carbamazepine effect.
Phenobarbital	Decreased carbamazepine effect.	Verapamil	Possible increased carbamazepine effect.

CARTEOLOL

GENERIC NAME OR DRUG CLASS	COMBINED EFFECT	GENERIC NAME OR DRUG CLASS	COMBINED EFFECT
Insulin	Hypoglycemic effects may be prolonged.	Nitrates*	Possible excessive blood-pressure drop.
Levobunolol eyedrops	Possible increased carteolol effect.	Non-steroidal anti-inflammatory drugs (NSAIDs)*	Decreased antihypertensive effect of carteolol.
Molindone	Increased tranquilizer effect.	Phenytoin	Decreased carteolol effect.
Narcotics*	Increased narcotic effect. Dangerous sedation.		

CHLORDIAZEPOXIDE & AMITRIPTYLINE

GENERIC NAME OR DRUG CLASS	COMBINED EFFECT	GENERIC NAME OR DRUG CLASS	COMBINED EFFECT
Narcotics*	Dangerous oversedation.	Sleep inducers*	Increased sedative effect of both drugs.
Phenytoin	Decreased phenytoin effect.	Sympathomimetics*	Increased sympathomimetic effect.
Probenecid	Increased chlordiazepoxide effect.	Thyroid hormones*	Irregular heartbeat.
Quinidine	Irregular heartbeat.	Tranquilizers*	Increased sedative effect of both drugs.
Sedatives*	Dangerous oversedation.		

CHLORDIAZEPOXIDE & CLIDINIUM

GENERIC NAME OR DRUG CLASS	COMBINED EFFECT	GENERIC NAME OR DRUG CLASS	COMBINED EFFECT
Phenothiazines*	Increased clidinium effect.	Sleep inducers*	Increased sedative effect of both drugs.
Pilocarpine	Loss of pilocarpine effect in glaucoma treatment.	Tranquilizers*	Increased sedative effect of both drugs.
Potassium supplements*	Possible intestinal ulcers with oral potassium tablets.	Vitamin C	Decreased clidinium effect. Avoid large doses of vitamin C.
Sedatives*	Increased sedative effect of both drugs.		

CHLOROTHIAZIDE

GENERIC NAME OR DRUG CLASS	COMBINED EFFECT	GENERIC NAME OR DRUG CLASS	COMBINED EFFECT
Nicardipine	Blood-pressure drop. Dosages may require adjustment.	Nitrates*	Excessive blood-pressure drop.

*See Glossary

1081

GENERIC NAME OR DRUG CLASS	COMBINED EFFECT	GENERIC NAME OR DRUG CLASS	COMBINED EFFECT

CHLOROTHIAZIDE continued

GENERIC NAME OR DRUG CLASS	COMBINED EFFECT	GENERIC NAME OR DRUG CLASS	COMBINED EFFECT
Opiates*	Dizziness or weakness when standing up after sitting or lying down.	Probenecid	Decreased probenecid effect.
		Sotalol	Increased antihypertensive effect.
Pentoxifylline	Increased antihypertensive effect.	Terazosin	Decreases effectiveness of terazosin.
Potassium supplements*	Decreased potassium effect.		

CHLORTHALIDONE

GENERIC NAME OR DRUG CLASS	COMBINED EFFECT	GENERIC NAME OR DRUG CLASS	COMBINED EFFECT
Probenecid	Decreased probenecid effect.	Terazosin	Decreases effectiveness of terazosin.
Sotalol	Increased antihypertensive effect.		

CHLORZOXAZONE & ACETAMINOPHEN

GENERIC NAME OR DRUG CLASS	COMBINED EFFECT	GENERIC NAME OR DRUG CLASS	COMBINED EFFECT
Tetracyclines* (effervescent granules or tablets)	May slow tetracycline absorption. Space doses 2 hours apart.	Tranquilizers*	Increased sedation.
		Zidovudine	Increased toxicity of zidovudine.

CIMETIDINE

GENERIC NAME OR DRUG CLASS	COMBINED EFFECT	GENERIC NAME OR DRUG CLASS	COMBINED EFFECT
Ketoconazole	Decreased ketoconazole absorption.	Phenytoin	Increased effect and toxicity of phenytoin.
Labetalol	Increased antihypertensive effects.	Procainamide	Increased effect and toxicity of procainamide.
Methadone	Increased effect and toxicity of methadone.	Propranolol	May increase propranolol effect.
Metoclopramide	Decreased cimetidine absorption.	Quinidine	Increased quinidine effect.
Metoprolol	Increased effect and toxicity of metoprolol.	Theophylline	Increased theophylline effect.
Metronidazole	Increased effect and toxicity of metronidazole.	Triazolam	Increased effect and toxicity of triazolam.
Morphine	Increased effect and toxicity of morphine.	Verapamil	Increased effect and toxicity of verapamil.
Nicardipine	Possible increased nicardipine effect and toxicity.		

CLIDINIUM

GENERIC NAME OR DRUG CLASS	COMBINED EFFECT	GENERIC NAME OR DRUG CLASS	COMBINED EFFECT
Pilocarpine	Loss of pilocarpine effect in glaucoma treatment.	Tranquilizers*	Decreased clidinium effect.
Potassium supplements*	Possible intestinal ulcers with oral potassium tablets.	Vitamin C	Decreased clidinium effect. Avoid large doses of vitamin C.

*See Glossary

CLONIDINE & CHLORTHALIDONE

GENERIC NAME OR DRUG CLASS	COMBINED EFFECT	GENERIC NAME OR DRUG CLASS	COMBINED EFFECT
Cholestyramine	Decreased chlorthalidone effect.	MAO inhibitors*	Increased chlorthalidone effect.
Cortisone drugs*	Excessive potassium loss that causes dangerous heart rhythms.	Nabilone	Greater depression of central nervous system.
Digitalis preparations*	Excessive potassium loss that causes dangerous heart rhythms.	Nicardipine	Blood-pressure drop. Dosages may require adjustment.
Diuretics*	Excessive blood-pressure drop.	Nitrates*	Possible excessive blood-pressure drop.
Fenfluramine	Possible increased clonidine effect.	Potassium supplements*	Decreased potassium effect.
Guanfacine	Blood-pressure control impaired.	Probenecid	Decreased probenecid effect.
Indapamide	Increased diuretic effect.	Sotalol	Decreased antihypertensive effect.
Lithium	Increased effect of lithium.	Terazosin	Decreases effectiveness of terazosin.

CORTISONE

GENERIC NAME OR DRUG CLASS	COMBINED EFFECT	GENERIC NAME OR DRUG CLASS	COMBINED EFFECT
Indomethacin	Increased cortisone effect.	Oxyphenbutazone	Possible ulcers.
Insulin	Decreased insulin effect.	Phenobarbital	Decreased cortisone effect.
Isoniazid	Decreased isoniazid effect.	Phenylbutazone	Possible ulcers.
Ketoprofen	Increased risk of stomach ulcer and bleeding.	Potassium supplements*	Decreased potassium effect.
Mitotane	Decreased cortisone effect.	Rifampin	Decreased cortisone effect.
Non-steroidal anti-inflammatory drugs (NSAIDs)*	Increased risk of ulcers, increased cortisone effect.	Salicylates*	Decreased salicylate effect.
		Sympathomimetics*	Possible glaucoma.
		Theophylline	Possible increased theophylline effect.

CYCLOTHIAZIDE

GENERIC NAME OR DRUG CLASS	COMBINED EFFECT	GENERIC NAME OR DRUG CLASS	COMBINED EFFECT
Nicardipine	Blood-pressure drop. Dosages may require adjustment.	Pentoxifylline	Increased antihypertensive effect.
Nitrates*	Excessive blood-pressure drop.	Potassium supplements*	Decreased potassium effect.
Oplates*	Dizziness or weakness when standing up after sitting or lying down.	Probenecid	Decreased probenecid effect.
		Sotalol	Increased antihypertensive effect.

*See Glossary

ADDITIONAL DRUG INTERACTIONS

GENERIC NAME OR DRUG CLASS	COMBINED EFFECT	GENERIC NAME OR DRUG CLASS	COMBINED EFFECT

CYCLOTHIAZIDE continued

Terazosin	Decreases effectiveness of terazosin.	Vitamin D	May increase calcium in blood.

DEXAMETHASONE

Mitotane	Decreased dexamethasone effect.	Potassium supplements*	Decreased potassium effect.
Non-steroidal anti-inflammatory drugs (NSAIDs)*	Increased risk of ulcers and dexamethasone effect.	Rifampin	Decreased dexamethasone effect.
Oxyphenbutazone	Possible ulcers.	Salicylates*	Decreased salicylate effect.
Phenobarbital	Decreased dexamethasone effect.	Sympathomimetics*	Possible glaucoma.
Phenylbutazone	Possible ulcers.	Theophylline	Possible increased theophylline effect.

DIGITALIS PREPARATIONS

Quinidine	Increased digitalis effect.	Tetracycline	May increase digitalis absorption.
Rauwolfia alkaloids*	Increased digitalis effect.	Thyroid hormones*	Digitalis toxicity.
Rifampin	Possible decreased digitalis effect.	Trazodone	Possible increased digitalis toxicity.
Sulfasalazine	Decreased digitalis absorption.	Triamterene	Possible decreased digitalis effect.
Sotalol	Can either increase or decrease heart rate. Improves irregular heartbeat.	Verapamil	Increased digitalis effect.

ENALAPRIL

Sotalol	Increased antihypertensive effects of both drugs. Dosages may require adjustment.	Spironolactone	Possible excessive potassium in blood.
		Triamterene	Possible excessive potassium in blood.

ENALAPRIL & HYDROCHLOROTHIAZIDE

MAO Inhibitors*	Increased hydrochlorothiazide effect.	Potassium supplements*	Possible increased potassium in blood.
Nicardipine	Possible excessive potassium in blood. Dosages may require adjustment.	Probenecid	Decreased probenecid effect.
Nitrates*	Excessive blood-pressure drop.	Sotalol	Increased antihypertensive effect.
Non-steroidal anti-inflammatory drugs (NSAIDs)*	Decreased enalapril effect.	Spironolactone	Possible excessive potassium in blood.
		Triamterene	Possible excessive potassium in blood.

*See Glossary

ERGOTAMINE, BELLADONNA & PHENOBARBITAL

Generic Name or Drug Class	Combined Effect	Generic Name or Drug Class	Combined Effect
Digitoxin	Decreased digitoxin effect.	Nitrates*	Increased internal-eye pressure.
Doxycycline	Decreased doxycycline effect.	Orphenadrine	Increased belladonna effect.
Dronabinol	Increased effect of drugs.	Pain relievers*	Dangerous sedation. Avoid.
Ephedrine	Dangerous blood-pressure rise.	Phenothiazines*	Increased belladonna effect.
Epinephrine	Dangerous blood-pressure rise.	Pilocarpine	Loss of pilocarpine effect in glaucoma treatment.
Griseofulvin	Decreased griseofulvin effect.	Potassium supplements*	Possible intestinal ulcers with oral potassium tablets.
Guanethidine	Decreased belladonna effect.	Quinidine	Increased belladonna effect.
Haloperidol	Increased internal-eye pressure.	Reserpine	Decreased belladonna effect.
Indapamide	Increased indapamide effect.	Sedatives*	Dangerous sedation. Avoid.
MAO inhibitors*	Increased belladonna and phenobarbital effect.	Sleep inducers*	Dangerous sedation. Avoid.
Meperidine	Increased belladonna effect.	Tranquilizers*	Dangerous sedation. Avoid.
Methylphenidate	Increased belladonna effect.	Troleandomycin	Increased adverse reactions of ergotamine.
Metoclopramide	May decrease metoclopramide effect.	Valproic acid	Increased phenobarbital effect.
Mind-altering drugs*	Dangerous sedation. Avoid.	Vitamin C	Decreased belladonna effect. Avoid large doses of vitamin C.
Narcotics*	Dangerous sedation. Avoid.		

ERGOTAMINE, CAFFEINE, BELLADONNA & PENTOBARBITAL

Generic Name or Drug Class	Combined Effect	Generic Name or Drug Class	Combined Effect
Anticonvulsants*	Changed seizure patterns.	Beta-adrenergic blockers*	Decreased effect of beta-adrenergic blocker.
Antidepressants, tricyclics (TCA)*	Decreased anti-depressant effect. Possible dangerous oversedation.	Cimetidine	Increased caffeine effect.
Antidiabetics, oral*	Increased pento-barbital effect.	Contraceptives, oral*	Decreased contra-ceptive effect.
Antihistamines*	Dangerous sedation. Avoid.	Cortisone drugs*	Decreased cortisone effect. Increased internal-eye pressure.
Aspirin	Decreased aspirin effect.	Digitoxin	Decreased digitoxin effect.

*See Glossary

GENERIC NAME OR DRUG CLASS	COMBINED EFFECT	GENERIC NAME OR DRUG CLASS	COMBINED EFFECT

ERGOTAMINE, CAFFEINE, BELLADONNA & PENTOBARBITAL continued

GENERIC NAME OR DRUG CLASS	COMBINED EFFECT	GENERIC NAME OR DRUG CLASS	COMBINED EFFECT
Disulfiram	Possible increased pentobarbital effect.	Non-steroidal anti-inflammatory drugs (NSAIDs)*	Decreased anti-inflammatory effect.
Doxycycline	Decreased doxycycline effect.	Orphenadrine	Increased belladonna effect.
Dronabinol	Increased effect of drugs.	Pain relievers*	Dangerous sedation. Avoid.
Ephedrine	Dangerous blood-pressure rise.	Phenothiazines*	Increased belladonna effect.
Epinephrine	Dangerous blood-pressure rise.	Pilocarpine	Loss of pilocarpine effect in glaucoma treatment.
Estrogens*	Decreased estrogen effect.	Potassium supplements*	Possible intestinal ulcers with oral potassium tablets.
Griseofulvin	Possible decreased griseofulvin effect.		
Guanethidine	Decreased belladonna effect.	Quinidine	Increased belladonna effect.
Haloperidol	Increased internal-eye pressure.	Reserpine	Decreased belladonna effect.
Indapamide	Increased indapamide effect.	Rifampin	Possible decreased pentobarbital effect.
Isoniazid	Increased caffeine effect.	Sedatives*	Dangerous sedation. Avoid.
MAO inhibitors*	Increased belladonna effect, dangerous blood-pressure rise.	Sleep inducers*	Dangerous sedation. Avoid.
Meperidine	Increased belladonna effect.	Sympathomimetics*	Overstimulation, blood-pressure rise.
Methylphenidate	Increased belladonna effect.	Thyroid hormones*	Increased thyroid effect.
Metoclopramide	May decrease decrease metoclopramide effect.	Tranquilizers*	Dangerous sedation. Avoid.
Metronidazole	Possible decreased metronidazole effect.	Troleandomycin	Increased adverse reactions of ergotamine.
Mind-altering drugs*	Dangerous sedation. Avoid.	Valproic acid	Increased pentobarbital effect.
Narcotics*	Dangerous sedation. Avoid.	Vitamin C	Decreased belladonna effect. Avoid large doses of vitamin C.
Nitrates*	Increased internal-eye pressure.		

FLECAINIDE ACETATE

GENERIC NAME OR DRUG CLASS	COMBINED EFFECT	GENERIC NAME OR DRUG CLASS	COMBINED EFFECT
Sodium bicarbonate	Possible increased flecainide acetate effect.	Verapamil	Possible decreased efficiency of heart-muscle contraction, leading to congestive heart failure.

*See Glossary

FLUPREDNISOLONE

GENERIC NAME OR DRUG CLASS	COMBINED EFFECT	GENERIC NAME OR DRUG CLASS	COMBINED EFFECT
Non-steroidal anti-inflammatory drugs (NSAIDs)*	Increased risk of ulcers and fluprednisolone effect.	Rifampin	Decreased fluprednisolone effect.
Oxyphenbutazone	Possible ulcers.	Salicylates*	Decreased salicylate effect.
Phenobarbital	Decreased fluprednisolone effect.	Sympathomimetics*	Possible glaucoma.
Phenylbutazone	Possible ulcers.	Theophylline	Possible increased theophylline effect.
Potassium supplements*	Decreased potassium effect.		

GUANETHIDINE & HYDROCHLOROTHIAZIDE

GENERIC NAME OR DRUG CLASS	COMBINED EFFECT	GENERIC NAME OR DRUG CLASS	COMBINED EFFECT
Diuretics, thiazide,*	Increased thiazide and guanethidine effect.	Nicardipine	Blood-pressure drop. Dosages may require adjustment.
Haloperidol	Decreased guanethidine effect.	Nitrates*	Excessive blood-pressure drop.
Indapamide	Possible increased effects of both drugs. When monitored carefully, combination may be beneficial in controlling hypertension.	Oxprenolol	Increased antihypertensive effect. Dosages of both drugs may require adjustments.
Insulin	Increased insulin effect.	Phenothiazines*	Decreased guanethidine effect.
Lithium	Increased lithium effect.	Potassium supplements*	Decreased potassium effect.
MAO inhibitors*	Increased hydrochlorothiazide effect.	Probenecid	Decreased probenecid effect.
Minoxidil	Dosage adjustments may be necessary to keep blood pressure at proper level.	Sotalol	Increased antihypertensive effect.
		Terazosin	Decreases effectiveness of terazosin.

GUANFACINE

GENERIC NAME OR DRUG CLASS	COMBINED EFFECT	GENERIC NAME OR DRUG CLASS	COMBINED EFFECT
Non-steroidal anti-inflammatory drugs (NSAIDs)*	May decrease antihypertensive effects of guanfacine.	Sympathomimetics*	May decrease antihypertensive effects of guanfacine.
Sotalol	Increased antihypertensive effect.	Terazosin	Decreases effectiveness of terazosin.

HYDRALAZINE & HYDROCHLOROTHIAZIDE

GENERIC NAME OR DRUG CLASS	COMBINED EFFECT	GENERIC NAME OR DRUG CLASS	COMBINED EFFECT
Diazoxide	Increased antihypertensive effect.	Diuretics, oral*	Increased effect of both drugs. When monitored carefully, combination may be beneficial in controlling hypertension.
Digitalis preparations*	Excessive potassium loss that causes dangerous heart rhythms.		

ADDITIONAL DRUG INTERACTIONS

*See Glossary

GENERIC NAME OR DRUG CLASS	COMBINED EFFECT	GENERIC NAME OR DRUG CLASS	COMBINED EFFECT

HYDRALAZINE & HYDROCHLOROTHIAZIDE continued

GENERIC NAME OR DRUG CLASS	COMBINED EFFECT	GENERIC NAME OR DRUG CLASS	COMBINED EFFECT
Indapamide	Increased diuretic effect.	Nitrates*	Excessive blood-pressure drop.
Lithium	Increased effect of lithium.	Potassium supplements*	Decreased potassium effect.
MAO inhibitors*	Increased effect of drugs.	Probenecid	Decreased probenecid effect.

HYDROCHLOROTHIAZIDE

GENERIC NAME OR DRUG CLASS	COMBINED EFFECT	GENERIC NAME OR DRUG CLASS	COMBINED EFFECT
Opiates*	Dizziness or weakness when standing up after sitting or lying down.	Potassium supplements*	Decreased potassium effect.
		Probenecid	Decreased probenecid effect.
Oxprenolol	Increased antihypertensive effect. Dosages of both drugs may require adjustments.	Sotalol	Increased antihypertensive effect.
		Terazosin	Decreases effectiveness of terazosin.

HYDROCORTISONE (Cortisol)

GENERIC NAME OR DRUG CLASS	COMBINED EFFECT	GENERIC NAME OR DRUG CLASS	COMBINED EFFECT
Insulin	Decreased insulin effect.	Phenylbutazone	Possible ulcers.
Isoniazid	Decreased isoniazid effect.	Potassium supplements*	Decreased potassium effect.
Mitotane	Decreased hydrocortisone effect.	Rifampin	Decreased hydrocortisone effect.
Non-steroidal anti-inflammatory drugs (NSAIDs)*	Increased risk of ulcers and increased hydrocortisone effect.	Salicylates*	Decreased salicylate effect.
Oxyphenbutazone	Possible ulcers.	Sympathomimetics*	Possible glaucoma.
Phenobarbital	Decreased hydrocortisone effect.	Theophylline	Possible increased theophylline effect.

HYDROFLUMETHIAZIDE

GENERIC NAME OR DRUG CLASS	COMBINED EFFECT	GENERIC NAME OR DRUG CLASS	COMBINED EFFECT
Potassium supplements*	Decreased potassium effect.	Sotalol	Increased antihypertensive effect.
Probenecid	Decreased probenecid effect.	Terazosin	Decreases effectiveness of terazosin.

KAOLIN, PECTIN, BELLADONNA & OPIUM

GENERIC NAME OR DRUG CLASS	COMBINED EFFECT	GENERIC NAME OR DRUG CLASS	COMBINED EFFECT
Methylphenidate	Increased belladonna effect.	Orphenadrine	Increased belladonna effect.
Mind-altering drugs*	Increased sedative effect.	Phenothiazines*	Increased sedative effect of paregoric.
Narcotics, other*	Increased narcotic effect.	Pilocarpine	Loss of pilocarpine effect in glaucoma treatment.
Nitrates*	Increased internal-eye pressure.		

*See Glossary

GENERIC NAME OR DRUG CLASS	COMBINED EFFECT	GENERIC NAME OR DRUG CLASS	COMBINED EFFECT

KAOLIN, PECTIN, BELLADONNA & OPIUM continued

GENERIC NAME OR DRUG CLASS	COMBINED EFFECT	GENERIC NAME OR DRUG CLASS	COMBINED EFFECT
Potassium supplements*	Possible intestinal ulcers with oral potassium tablets.	Tranquilizers*	Increased tranquilizer effect.
Sedatives*	Excessive sedation.	Vitamin C	Decreased belladonna effect. Avoid large doses of vitamin C.
Sleep inducers*	Increased effect of sleep inducers.		
Sotalol	Increased narcotic effect. Dangerous sedation.	All other oral medicines	Decreases absorption of other medicines. Separate doses by at least 2 hours.

MAPROTILINE

GENERIC NAME OR DRUG CLASS	COMBINED EFFECT	GENERIC NAME OR DRUG CLASS	COMBINED EFFECT
Guanfacine	May increase depressant effects of either drug.	Methyprylon	Increased sedative effect, perhaps to dangerous level. Avoid.
Leucovorin	High alcohol content of leucovorin may cause adverse effects.	Molindone	Increased tranquilizer effect.
Levodopa	May increase blood pressure.	Narcotics*	Dangerous oversedation.
Lithium	Possible decreased seizure threshold.	Phenothiazine	Possible increased antidepressant effect and toxicity.
Nabilone	Greater depression of central nervous system.	Phenytoin	Decreased phenytoin effect.
MAO inhibitors*	Fever, delirium, convulsions.	Procainamide	Possible irregular heartbeat.
Methyldopa	Decreased methyldopa effect.	Quinidine	Irregular heartbeat.
		Sedatives*	Dangerous oversedation.
Methylphenidate	Possible increased antidepressant effect and toxicity.	Sympathomimetics*	Increased sympathomimetic effect.
		Thyroid hormones*	Irregular heartbeat.

MEPHENYTOIN

GENERIC NAME OR DRUG CLASS	COMBINED EFFECT	GENERIC NAME OR DRUG CLASS	COMBINED EFFECT
Sedatives*	Increased sedative effect.	Theophylline	Reduced anticonvulsant effect.
Sulfa drugs*	Increased mephenytoin effect.		

MEPROBAMATE & ASPIRIN

GENERIC NAME OR DRUG CLASS	COMBINED EFFECT	GENERIC NAME OR DRUG CLASS	COMBINED EFFECT
MAO inhibitors*	Increased meprobamate effect.	Narcotics*	Increased narcotic effect.
Methotrexate	Increased methotrexate effect.	Non-steroidal anti-inflammatory drugs (NSAIDs)*	Risk of stomach bleeding and ulcers.
Minoxidil	Decreased minoxidil effect.		

*See Glossary

GENERIC NAME OR DRUG CLASS	COMBINED EFFECT	GENERIC NAME OR DRUG CLASS	COMBINED EFFECT

MEPROBAMATE & ASPIRIN continued

GENERIC NAME OR DRUG CLASS	COMBINED EFFECT	GENERIC NAME OR DRUG CLASS	COMBINED EFFECT
Oxprenolol	Decreased antihypertensive effect of oxprenolol.	Salicylates, other*	Likely aspirin toxicity.
Para-aminosalicylic acid (PAS)	Possible aspirin toxicity.	Sedatives*	Increased sedative effect.
Penicillins*	Increased effect of both drugs.	Sleep inducers*	Increased effect of sleep inducer.
Phenobarbital	Decreased aspirin effect.	Spironolactone	Decreased spironolactone effect.
Phenytoin	Increased phenytoin effect.	Sulfinpyrazone	Decreased sulfinpyrazone effect.
Probenecid	Decreased probenecid effect.	Terfenadine	Possible excessive sedation. May conceal symptoms of aspirin overdose, such as ringing in ears.
Propranolol	Decreased aspirin effect.		
Rauwolfia alkaloids*	Decreased aspirin effect.	Tranquilizers*	Increased tranquilizer effect.
		Vitamin C (large doses)	Possible aspirin toxicity.

METHARBITAL

GENERIC NAME OR DRUG CLASS	COMBINED EFFECT	GENERIC NAME OR DRUG CLASS	COMBINED EFFECT
Sleep inducers*	Dangerous sedation. Avoid.	Tranquilizers*	Dangerous sedation. Avoid.
Sotalol	Increased barbiturate effect. Dangerous sedation.	Valproic acid	Increased metharbital effect.

METHYCLOTHIAZIDE

GENERIC NAME OR DRUG CLASS	COMBINED EFFECT	GENERIC NAME OR DRUG CLASS	COMBINED EFFECT
Potassium supplements*	Decreased potassium effect.	Sotalol	Increased antihypertensive effect.
Probenecid	Decreased probenecid effect.	Terazosin	Decreases effectiveness of terazosin.

METHYLDOPA & THIAZIDE DIURETICS

GENERIC NAME OR DRUG CLASS	COMBINED EFFECT	GENERIC NAME OR DRUG CLASS	COMBINED EFFECT
Cortisone drugs*	Excessive potassium loss that causes dangerous heart rhythms.	Lithium	Increased lithium effect.
Digitalis preparations*	Excessive potassium loss that causes dangerous heart rhythms.	MAO inhibitors*	Dangerous blood-pressure changes.
		Nabilone	Greater depression of central nervous system.
Diuretics, thiazide*	Increased effect of both drugs.	Nicardipine	Blood-pressure drop. Dosages may require adjustment.
Haloperidol	Increased sedation, possibly dementia.		
Indapamide	Increased diuretic effect.	Nitrates*	Excessive blood-pressure drop.
Levodopa	Increased effect of both drugs.	Phenoxybenzanine	Urinary retention.

*See Glossary

GENERIC NAME OR DRUG CLASS	COMBINED EFFECT	GENERIC NAME OR DRUG CLASS	COMBINED EFFECT

METHYLDOPA & THIAZIDE DIURETICS continued

GENERIC NAME OR DRUG CLASS	COMBINED EFFECT	GENERIC NAME OR DRUG CLASS	COMBINED EFFECT
Potassium supplements*	Decreased potassium effect.	Terazosin	Decreases effectiveness of terazosin.
Propranolol	Increased blood pressure (rarely).	Tolbutamide	Increased tolbutamide effect.
Sotalol	Increased antihypertensive effect.		

METHYLPREDNISOLONE

GENERIC NAME OR DRUG CLASS	COMBINED EFFECT	GENERIC NAME OR DRUG CLASS	COMBINED EFFECT
Indomethacin	Increased methylprednisolone effect.	Phenobarbital	Decreased methylprednisolone effect.
Insulin	Decreased insulin effect.	Phenylbutazone	Possible ulcers.
Isoniazid	Decreased isoniazid effect.	Potassium supplements*	Decreased potassium effect.
Mitotane	Decreased methylprednisolone effect.	Rifampin	Decreased methylprednisolone effect.
Non-steroidal anti-inflammatory drugs (NSAIDs)*	Increased risk of ulcers and methylprednisolone effect.	Salicylates*	Decreased salicylate effect.
		Sympathomimetics*	Possible glaucoma.
Oxyphenbutazone	Possible ulcers.	Theophylline	Possible increased theophylline effect.

METOLAZONE

GENERIC NAME OR DRUG CLASS	COMBINED EFFECT	GENERIC NAME OR DRUG CLASS	COMBINED EFFECT
Potassium supplements*	Decreased potassium effect.	Sotalol	Increased antihypertensive effect.
Probenecid	Decreased probenecid effect.	Terazosin	Decreases effectiveness of terazosin.

METOPROLOL

GENERIC NAME OR DRUG CLASS	COMBINED EFFECT	GENERIC NAME OR DRUG CLASS	COMBINED EFFECT
Phenytoin	Decreased metoprolol effect.	Rifampin	Decreased metoprolol effect.
Quinidine	Slows heart excessively.	Timolol eyedrops	Possible increased metoprolol effect.
Reserpine	Possible increased effects of both drugs. Slow heartbeat and low blood pressure may result.	Tocainide	May worsen congestive heart failure.
		Verapamil	Increased effect of both drugs.

MONAMINE OXIDASE (MAO) INHIBITORS

GENERIC NAME OR DRUG CLASS	COMBINED EFFECT	GENERIC NAME OR DRUG CLASS	COMBINED EFFECT
Leucovorin	High alcohol content of leucovorin may cause adverse effects.	MAO inhibitors* (others, when taken together)	High fever, convulsions, death.
Levodopa	Sudden, severe blood-pressure rise.	Methyldopa	Sudden, severe blood-pressure rise.

*See Glossary

ADDITIONAL DRUG INTERACTIONS

GENERIC NAME OR DRUG CLASS	COMBINED EFFECT	GENERIC NAME OR DRUG CLASS	COMBINED EFFECT

MONAMINE OXIDASE (MAO) INHIBITORS continued

GENERIC NAME OR DRUG CLASS	COMBINED EFFECT	GENERIC NAME OR DRUG CLASS	COMBINED EFFECT
Methylphenidate	Increased blood pressure.	Phenothiazines*	Possible increased phenothiazine toxicity.
Methyprylon	Increased sedative effect, perhaps to dangerous level. Avoid.	Phenylpropanolamine	Increased blood pressure.
		Pseudoephedrine	Increased blood pressure.
Nabilone	Greater depression of central nervous system.	Sympathomimetics*	Blood-pressure rise to life-threatening level.
		Tryptophan	Increased blood pressure.

NADOLOL

Timolol eyedrops	Possible increased nadolol effect.	Verapamil	Increased effects of both drugs.
Tocainide	May worsen congestive heart failure.		

NAPROXEN

Terazosin	Decreases effectiveness of terazosin. Causes sodium and fluid retention.	Thyroid hormones*	Rapid heartbeat, blood-pressure rise.

NARCOTIC ANALGESICS

Nitrates*	Excessive blood-pressure drop.	Rifampin	Possible decreased narcotic effect.
Non-steroidal anti-inflammatory drugs (NSAIDs)*	Increased narcotic effect.	Sedatives*	Increased sedative effect.
Pentazocine	Possibly precipitates withdrawal with chronic narcotic use.	Sleep inducers*	Increased sedative effect.
		Sotalol	Increased narcotic effect. Dangerous sedation.
Phenothiazines*	Increased sedative effect.	Tranquilizers*	Increased sedative effect.
Phenytoin	Possible decreased narcotic effect.		

NARCOTIC & ASPIRIN

Furosemide	Possible aspirin toxicity. May decrease furosemide effect.	Minoxidil	Decreased minoxidil effect.
		Narcotics, other*	Increased narcotic effect.
Gold compounds*	Increased likelihood of kidney damage.	Nitrates*	Excessive blood-pressure drop.
Indomethacin	Risk of stomach bleeding and ulcers.	Non-steroidal anti-inflammatory drugs (NSAIDs)*	Risk of stomach bleeding and ulcers.
Methotrexate	Increased methotrexate effect.		

*See Glossary

GENERIC NAME OR DRUG CLASS	COMBINED EFFECT	GENERIC NAME OR DRUG CLASS	COMBINED EFFECT
NARCOTIC & ASPIRIN continued			
Oxprenolol	Decreased antihypertensive effect of oxprenolol.	Sleep Inducers*	Increased sedative effect.
Para-aminosalicylic acid (PAS)	Possible aspirin toxicity.	Sotalol	Increased narcotic effect. Dangerous sedation.
Penicillins*	Increased effect of both drugs.	Spironolactone	Decreased spironolactone effect.
Phenobarbital	Decreased aspirin effect.	Sulfinpyrazone	Decreased sulfinpyrazone effect.
Phenytoin	Increased phenytoin effect.	Terfenadine	Possible excessive sedation. May conceal symptoms of aspirin overdose, such as ringing in ears.
Probenecid	Decreased probenecid effect.		
Propranolol	Decreased aspirin effect.	Tranquilizers*	Increased sedative effect.
Rauwolfia alkaloids*	Decreased aspirin effect.	Valproic acid	May increase valproic acid effect.
Salicylates, other*	Likely aspirin toxicity.	Vitamin C (large doses)	Possible aspirin toxicity.
Sedatives*	Increased sedative effect.		

ORPHENADRINE, ASPIRIN & CAFFEINE

GENERIC NAME OR DRUG CLASS	COMBINED EFFECT	GENERIC NAME OR DRUG CLASS	COMBINED EFFECT
Antidepressants, tricyclic (TCA)*	Increased sedation.	MAO inhibitors*	Dangerous blood-pressure rise.
Antidiabetics, oral*	Low blood sugar.	Methotrexate	Increased methotrexate effect.
Aspirin, other	Likely aspirin toxicity.		
Chlorpromazine	Hypoglycemia (low blood sugar).	Minoxidil	Decreased minoxidil effect.
Contraceptives, oral*	Increased caffeine effect.	Nitrates*	Increased internal-eye pressure.
Cortisone drugs*	Increased cortisone effect. Risk of ulcers and stomach bleeding.	Non-steroidal anti-inflammatory drugs (NSAIDs)*	Risk of stomach bleeding and ulcers.
Furosemide	Possible aspirin toxicity.	Para-aminosalicylic acid (PAS)	Possible aspirin toxicity.
Gold compounds*	Increased likelihood of kidney damage.	Penicillins*	Increased effect of drugs.
Griseofulvin	Decreased griseofulvin effect.	Phenobarbital	Decreased aspirin effect.
Indomethacin	Risk of stomach bleeding and ulcers.	Potassium supplements*	Increased possibility of intestinal ulcers with oral potassium tablets.
Isoniazid	Increased caffeine effect.	Probenecid	Decreased probenecid effect.
Levodopa	Increased effect of levodopa. (Improves effectiveness in treating Parkinson's disease.)	Propoxyphene	Possible confusion, nervousness, tremors.
		Propranolol	Decreased aspirin effect.

ADDITIONAL DRUG INTERACTIONS

GENERIC NAME OR DRUG CLASS	COMBINED EFFECT	GENERIC NAME OR DRUG CLASS	COMBINED EFFECT

ORPHENADRINE, ASPIRIN & CAFFEINE continued

GENERIC NAME OR DRUG CLASS	COMBINED EFFECT	GENERIC NAME OR DRUG CLASS	COMBINED EFFECT
Rauwolfia alkaloids*	Decreased aspirin effect.	Terfenadine	May conceal symptoms of aspirin overdose, such as ringing in ears.
Salicylates, other*	Likely aspirin toxicity.		
Sedatives*	Decreased sedative effect.	Thyroid hormones*	Increased thyroid effect.
Sleep inducers*	Decreased sedative effect.	Tranquilizers*	Decreased tranquilizer effect.
Spironolactone	Decreased spironolactone effect.	Valproic acid	May increase valproic acid effect.
Sulfinpyrazone	Decreased sulfin-pyrazone effect.	Vitamin C (large doses)	Possible aspirin toxicity.
Sympathomimetics*	Overstimulation.		

OXPRENOLOL

GENERIC NAME OR DRUG CLASS	COMBINED EFFECT	GENERIC NAME OR DRUG CLASS	COMBINED EFFECT
Reserpine	Possible excessively low blood pressure and slow heartbeat.	Sympathomimetics*	Decreased effects of both drugs.
		Timolol eyedrops	Possible increased oxprenolol effect.
Rifampin	Decreased oxprenolol effect.	Verapamil	Increased effect of both drugs.
Suprofen	Decreased antihyper-tensive effect of oxprenolol.	Xanthine bronchodilators*	Decreased effects of both drugs.

OXYPHENBUTAZONE

GENERIC NAME OR DRUG CLASS	COMBINED EFFECT	GENERIC NAME OR DRUG CLASS	COMBINED EFFECT
Non-steroidal anti-inflammatory drugs (NSAIDs)*	Increased possibility of ulcer.	Sotalol	Decreased antihyper-tensive effect of sotalol.
Penicillamine	Possible toxicity.	Terazosin	Decreases effective-ness of terazosin. Causes sodium and fluid retention.
Phenytoin	Possible toxic phenytoin effect.		
Rifampin	Decreased oxyphen-butazone effect.	Trimethoprim	Possible bone-marrow toxicity.

PANCREATIN, PEPSIN, BILE SALTS, HYOSCYAMINE, ATROPINE, SCOPOLAMINE & PHENOBARBITAL

GENERIC NAME OR DRUG CLASS	COMBINED EFFECT	GENERIC NAME OR DRUG CLASS	COMBINED EFFECT
Dronabinol	Increased phenobarbital effect.	Meperidine	Increased atropine effect.
Griseofulvin	Decreased griseofulvin effect.	Methylphenidate	Increased atropine effect.
Haloperidol	Increased internal-eye pressure.	Mind-altering drugs*	Dangerous sedation. Avoid.
Indapamide	Increased indapamide effect.	Narcotics*	Dangerous sedation. Avoid.
MAO inhibitors*	Increased atropine effect.	Nitrates*	Increased internal-eye pressure.

*See Glossary

GENERIC NAME OR DRUG CLASS	COMBINED EFFECT	GENERIC NAME OR DRUG CLASS	COMBINED EFFECT

PANCREATIN, PEPSIN, BILE SALTS, HYOSCYAMINE, ATROPINE, SCOPOLAMINE & PHENOBARBITAL continued

GENERIC NAME OR DRUG CLASS	COMBINED EFFECT	GENERIC NAME OR DRUG CLASS	COMBINED EFFECT
Nizatidine	Increased nizatidine effect.	Quinidine	Increased quinidine and scopolamine effect.
Non-steroidal anti-inflammatory drugs (NSAIDs)*	Decreased anti-inflammatory effects.	Sedatives*	Dangerous sedation. Avoid.
Orphenadrine	Increased atropine effect.	Sleep inducers*	Dangerous sedation. Avoid.
Phenothiazines*	Increased atropine effect.	Tranquilizers*	Dangerous sedation. Avoid.
Pilocarpine	Loss of pilocarpine effect in glaucoma treatment.	Valproic acid	Increased phenobarbital effect.
Potassium supplements*	Possible intestinal ulcers with oral potassium tablets.	Vitamin C	Decreased atropine effect. Avoid large doses of vitamin C.

PARAMETHASONE

GENERIC NAME OR DRUG CLASS	COMBINED EFFECT	GENERIC NAME OR DRUG CLASS	COMBINED EFFECT
Mitotane	Decreased paramethasone effect.	Potassium supplements*	Decreased potassium effect.
Non-steroidal anti-inflammatory drugs (NSAIDs)*	Increased risk of ulcers and para-methasone effect.	Rifampin	Decreased paramethasone effect.
Oxyphenbutazone	Possible ulcers.	Salicylates*	Decreased salicylate effect.
Phenobarbital	Decreased para-methasone effect.	Sympathomimetics*	Possible glaucoma.
Phenylbutazone	Possible ulcers.	Theophylline	Possible increased theophylline effect.

PARGYLINE & METHYCLOTHIAZIDE

GENERIC NAME OR DRUG CLASS	COMBINED EFFECT	GENERIC NAME OR DRUG CLASS	COMBINED EFFECT
Antihypertensives*	Excessively low blood pressure.	Cortisone drugs*	Excessive potassium loss that causes dangerous heart rhythms.
Barbiturates*	Increased methy-clothiazide effect.	Cyclobenzaprine	Fever, seizures. Avoid.
Beta-adrenergic blockers*	Increased anti-hypertensive effect. Dosages of both drugs may require adjustments.	Digitalis preparations*	Excessive potassium loss that causes dangerous heart rhythms.
Caffeine	Irregular heartbeat or high blood pressure.	Diuretics, other*	Excessively low blood pressure.
Carbamazepine	Fever, seizures. Avoid.	Ethinamate	Dangerous increased effects of ethinamate. Avoid combining.
Carteolol	Increased antihyper-tensive effect.	Fluoxetine	Increased depressant effects of both drugs.
Cholestyramine	Decreased methy-clothiazide effect.	Guanethidine	Blood-pressure rise to life-threatening level.

GENERIC NAME OR DRUG CLASS	COMBINED EFFECT	GENERIC NAME OR DRUG CLASS	COMBINED EFFECT

PARGYLINE & METHYCLOTHIAZIDE continued

GENERIC NAME OR DRUG CLASS	COMBINED EFFECT	GENERIC NAME OR DRUG CLASS	COMBINED EFFECT
Guanfacine	May increase depressant effects of either drug.	Nabilone	Greater depression of central nervous system.
Indapamide	Increased indapamide and diuretic effect.	Nitrates*	Excessive blood-pressure drop.
Leucovorin	High alcohol content of leucovorin may cause adverse effects.	Oxprenolol	Possible blood-pressure rise if MAO inhibitor is discontinued after simultaneous use with oxprenolol.
Levodopa	Sudden, severe blood-pressure rise.		
Lisinopril	Increased antihypertensive effect. Dosage of each may require adjustment.	Potassium supplements*	Decreased potassium effect.
		Probenecid	Decreased probenecid effect.
Lithium	Increased effect of lithium.	Sotalol	Increased antihypertensive effect.
MAO Inhibitors* (other, when taken together)	High fever, convulsions, death. Increased methyclothiazide effect.	Terazosin	Decreases effectiveness of terazosin.
		Terfenadine	Increased side effects of MAO inhibitors.
Methyprylon	Increased sedative effect, perhaps to dangerous level. Avoid.		

PENTOBARBITAL

GENERIC NAME OR DRUG CLASS	COMBINED EFFECT	GENERIC NAME OR DRUG CLASS	COMBINED EFFECT
Rifampin	Possible decreased pentobarbital effect.	Sotalol	Increased barbiturate effect. Dangerous sedation.
Sedatives*	Dangerous sedation. Avoid.	Tranquilizers*	Dangerous sedation. Avoid.
Sleep Inducers*	Dangerous sedation. Avoid.	Valproic acid	Increased pentobarbital effect.

PERPHENAZINE & AMITRIPTYLINE

GENERIC NAME OR DRUG CLASS	COMBINED EFFECT	GENERIC NAME OR DRUG CLASS	COMBINED EFFECT
Guanabenz	Possible decreased guanabenz effect.	Methylphenidate	Possible increased antidepressant effect.
Guanethidine	Decreased guanethidine effect.	Mind-altering drugs*	Increased effect of mind-altering drugs.
Guanfacine	Possible decreased guanfacine effect.	Nabilone	Greater depression of central nervous system.
Levodopa	Decreased levodopa effect.	Narcotics*	Increased narcotic effect and dangerous sedation.
Lithium	Possible decreased seizure threshold.		
MAO Inhibitors*	Fever, delirium, convulsions.	Phenothiazines*	Possible increased antidepressant effect.
		Procainamide	Possible irregular heartbeat.
Methyldopa	Possible decreased methyldopa effect.	Procarbazine	Increased sedation.

GENERIC NAME OR DRUG CLASS	COMBINED EFFECT	GENERIC NAME OR DRUG CLASS	COMBINED EFFECT

PERPHENAZINE & AMITRIPTYLINE continued

GENERIC NAME OR DRUG CLASS	COMBINED EFFECT	GENERIC NAME OR DRUG CLASS	COMBINED EFFECT
Quinidine	Impaired heart function. Dangerous mixture.	Sympathomimetics*	Increased sympathomimetics effect.
		Thyroid hormones*	Irregular heartbeat.
Sedatives*	Dangerous oversedation.	Tranquilizers, other*	Increased tranquilizer effect.

PHENOBARBITAL

GENERIC NAME OR DRUG CLASS	COMBINED EFFECT	GENERIC NAME OR DRUG CLASS	COMBINED EFFECT
Nabilone	Greater depression of central nervous system.	Sedatives*	Dangerous sedation. Avoid.
Narcotics*	Dangerous sedation. Avoid.	Sleep inducers*	Dangerous sedation. Avoid.
Non-steroidal anti-inflammatory drugs (NSAIDs)*	Decreased anti-inflammatory effect.	Sotalol	Increased barbiturate effect. Dangerous sedation.
Pain relievers*	Dangerous sedation. Avoid.	Tranquilizers*	Dangerous sedation. Avoid.
Quinidine	Decreased quinidine effect.	Valproic acid	Increased phenobarbital effect.
Rifampin	Possible decreased phenobarbital effect.		

PHENPROCOUMON

GENERIC NAME OR DRUG CLASS	COMBINED EFFECT	GENERIC NAME OR DRUG CLASS	COMBINED EFFECT
Chloramphenicol	Increased phenprocoumon effect.	Dicloxacillin	Possible decreased phenprocoumon effect.
Chlorpromazine	Decreased phenprocoumon effect.	Dipyridamole	Increased risk of bleeding with antiplatelet effect. Increased phenprocoumon effect.
Cholestyramine	Unpredictable increased or decreased phenprocoumon effect.		
Cimetidine	Increased phenprocoumon effect.	Disulfiram	Increased phenprocoumon effect.
Ciprofloxacin	Possible increased anticoagulant effect.	Erythromycin	Increased phenprocoumon effect.
Clofibrate	Increased phenprocoumon effect.	Estrogens*	Decreased phenprocoumon effect.
Contraceptives, oral*	Decreased phenprocoumon effect.	Ethacrynic acid	Increased phenprocoumon effect.
Cortisone drugs*	Unpredictable increased or decreased phenprocoumon effect.	Ethchlorvynol	Decreased phenprocoumon effect.
		Gemfibrozil	Increased phenprocoumon effect.
Co-trimoxazole (sulfa/trimethoprim)	Increased anticoagulant effect.	Glucagon	Increased phenprocoumon effect.
Danazol	Increased phenprocoumon effect.	Glutethimide	Decreased phenprocoumon effect.

GENERIC NAME OR DRUG CLASS	COMBINED EFFECT	GENERIC NAME OR DRUG CLASS	COMBINED EFFECT
PHENPROCOUMON continued			
Griseofulvin	Decreased phenprocoumon effect.	Para-aminosalicylic acid (PAS)	Increased phenprocoumon effect.
Guanethidine	Increased phenprocoumon effect.	Phenylbutazone	Unpredictable increased or decreased phenprocoumon effect.
Haloperidol	Decreased phenprocoumon effect.	Phenytoin	Decreased phenytoin levels.
Heparin	Increased risk of bleeding.	Probenecid	Increased phenprocoumon effect.
Hydroxyzine	Increased phenprocoumon effect.	Propoxyphene	Increased phenprocoumon effect.
Indomethacin	Increased phenprocoumon effect.	Propylthiouracil	Increased phenprocoumon effect.
Insulin	Increased insulin effect.	Quinidine	Increased phenprocoumon effect.
Isocarboxazid	Increased phenprocoumon effect.	Quinine	Increased phenprocoumon effect.
Isoniazid	Increased phenprocoumon effect.	Ranitidine	Possible decreased phenprocoumon effect.
Ketoconazole	Increased phenprocoumon effect.	Rauwolfia alkaloids*	Unpredictable increased or decreased phenprocoumon effect.
Meclofenamate	Increased phenprocoumon effect.	Rifampin	Decreased anticoagulant effect.
Mefenamic acid	Increased phenprocoumon effect.	Salicylates* (including aspirin)	Increased phenprocoumon effect.
Meprobamate	Decreased phenprocoumon effect.	Sulfa drugs*	Increased phenprocoumon effect.
Mercaptopurine	Decreased phenprocoumon effect.	Sulfinpyrazone	Increased phenprocoumon effect.
Methylphenidate	Increased phenprocoumon effect.	Tetracyclines*	Increased phenprocoumon effect.
Metronidazole	Increased phenprocoumon effect.	Thyroid hormones*	Increased phenprocoumon effect.
Nafcillin (IV)	Possible decreased phenprocoumon effect.	Trimethoprim	Increased phenprocoumon effect.
Nalidixic acid	Increased phenprocoumon effect.	Vaccine, influenza	May increase anticoagulant effect.
Neomycin (oral)	Increased phenprocoumon effect.	Vitamin C (large doses)	May decrease phenprocoumon effect.
Nicardipine	Possible increased anticoagulant effect.	Vitamin E (large doses)	Increased phenprocoumon effect.
Nizatidine	Increased anticoagulant effect.	Vitamin K	Decreased phenprocoumon effect.
Oxyphenbutazone	Increased phenprocoumon effect.		

*See Glossary

PHENYLBUTAZONE

GENERIC NAME OR DRUG CLASS	COMBINED EFFECT	GENERIC NAME OR DRUG CLASS	COMBINED EFFECT
Diclofenac	Possible stomach ulcer.	Non-steroidal anti-inflammatory drugs (NSAIDs)*	Increased possibility of ulcer.
Digitoxin	Decreased digitoxin effect.	Oxprenolol	Decreased antihypertensive effect of oxprenolol.
Flecainide	Possible decreased blood-cell production in bone marrow.	Penicillamine	Possible toxicity.
Gold compounds*	Possible increased likelihood of kidney damage.	Phenytoin	Possible toxic phenytoin effect.
Hydroxychloroquine	Possible skin toxicity.	Rifampin	Decreased phenylbutazone effect.
Insulin	Decreased insulin effect. Dosages may require adjustment.	Sotalol	Decreased antihypertensive effect of sotalol.
Ketoprofen	Increased possibility of internal bleeding.	Terazosin	Decreases effectiveness of terazosin. Causes sodium and fluid retention.
Lisinopril	Decreased lisinopril effect.		
Methotrexate	Increased toxicity of both drugs to bone marrow.	Tocainide	Possible decreased blood-cell production in bone marrow.
Minoxidil	Decreased minoxidil effect.	Trimethoprim	Possible bone-marrow toxicity.

PHENYTOIN

GENERIC NAME OR DRUG CLASS	COMBINED EFFECT	GENERIC NAME OR DRUG CLASS	COMBINED EFFECT
Encainide	Increased effect of toxicity on heart muscle.	MAO inhibitors*	Increased polythiazide effect.
Estrogens*	Increased estrogen effect.	Methadone	Decreased methadone effect.
Furosemide	Decreased furosemide effect.	Methylphenidate	Increased phenytoin effect.
Gold compounds*	Increased phenytoin blood levels. Phenytoin dose may require adjustment.	Molindone	Increased phenytoin effect.
		Nicardipine	Increased anticonvulsant effect.
Griseofulvin	Increased griseofulvin effect.	Nitrates*	Excessive bloodpressure drop.
Hypoglycemics, oral*	Possible decreased hypoglycemic effect.	Nizatidine	Increased effect and toxicity of phenytoin.
Isoniazid	Increased phenytoin effect.	Oxyphenbutazone	Increased phenytoin effect.
Leucovorin	May counteract the effect of phenytoin or any hydantoin anticonvulsant.	Para-aminosalicylic acid (PAS)	Increased phenytoin effect.
		Phenothiazines*	Increased phenytoin effect.
Loxapine	Decreased anticonvulsant effect of phenytoin or any hydantoin anticonvulsant.	Phenylbutazone	Increased phenytoin effect.

*See Glossary

ADDITIONAL DRUG INTERACTIONS

GENERIC NAME OR DRUG CLASS	COMBINED EFFECT	GENERIC NAME OR DRUG CLASS	COMBINED EFFECT

PHENYTOIN continued

GENERIC NAME OR DRUG CLASS	COMBINED EFFECT	GENERIC NAME OR DRUG CLASS	COMBINED EFFECT
Potassium supplements*	Decreased potassium effect.	Sotalol	Decreased sotalol effect.
Probenecid	Decreased probenecid effect.	Sulfa drugs*	Increased phenytoin effect.
Propranolol	Increased propranolol effect.	Theophylline	Reduced anticonvulsant effect.
Quinidine	Increased quinidine effect.	Trimethoprim	Increased phenytoin effect.
Sedatives*	Increased sedative effect.	Valproic acid	Unpredictable change in seizure control.

PIROXICAM

GENERIC NAME OR DRUG CLASS	COMBINED EFFECT	GENERIC NAME OR DRUG CLASS	COMBINED EFFECT
Sotalol	Decreased antihypertensive effect of sotalol.	Thyroid hormones*	Rapid heartbeat, blood-pressure rise.
Terazosin	Decreases effectiveness of terazosin. Causes sodium and fluid retention.		

POLYTHIAZIDE

GENERIC NAME OR DRUG CLASS	COMBINED EFFECT	GENERIC NAME OR DRUG CLASS	COMBINED EFFECT
Potassium supplements*	Decreased potassium effect.	Sotalol	Increased antihypertensive effect.
Probenecid	Decreased probenecid effect.	Terazosin	Decreases effectiveness of terazosin.

PRAZOSIN & POLYTHIAZIDE

GENERIC NAME OR DRUG CLASS	COMBINED EFFECT	GENERIC NAME OR DRUG CLASS	COMBINED EFFECT
Antidiabetics, other*	Increased blood sugar.	Estrogen	Decreased prazosin effect.
Antihypertensives*	Increased antihypertensive effect. Dosages may require adjustments.	Indapamide	Increased diuretic effect.
		Indomethacin	Decreased polythiazide effect.
Barbiturates*	Increased polythiazide effect.	Lithium	Increased effect of lithium.
Carteolol	Increased antihypertensive effect.	MAO inhibitors*	Blood-pressure drop. Increased polythiazide effect.
Cholestyramine	Decreased polythiazide effect.	Nicardipine	Blood-pressure drop. Dosages may require adjustment.
Chlorpromazine	Acute agitation.		
Cortisone drugs*	Excessive potassium loss that causes dangerous heart rhythms.	Nifedipine	Weakness and faintness when arising from bed or chair.
Digitalis preparations*	Excessive potassium loss that causes dangerous heart rhythms.	Nitrates	Possible excessive blood-pressure drop.
Diuretics, other*	Increased effect of other thiazide diuretics.	Non-steroidal anti-inflammatory drugs (NSAIDs)*	Decreased prazosin effect.

*See Glossary

GENERIC NAME OR DRUG CLASS	COMBINED EFFECT	GENERIC NAME OR DRUG CLASS	COMBINED EFFECT

PRAZOSIN & POLYTHIAZIDE continued

GENERIC NAME OR DRUG CLASS	COMBINED EFFECT	GENERIC NAME OR DRUG CLASS	COMBINED EFFECT
Opiates*	Weakness and faintness when arising from bed or chair.	Sympathomimetics*	Decreased prazosin effect.
Potassium	Decreased potassium effect.	Terazosin	Decreases effectiveness of terazosin.
Probenecid	Decreased probenecid effect.	Verapamil	Weakness and faintness when arising from bed or chair.
Sotalol	Decreased anti-hypertensive effect.		

PREDNISOLONE

GENERIC NAME OR DRUG CLASS	COMBINED EFFECT	GENERIC NAME OR DRUG CLASS	COMBINED EFFECT
Indomethacin	Increased prednisolone effect.	Phenobarbital	Decreased prednisolone effect.
Insulin	Decreased insulin effect.	Phenylbutazone	Possible ulcers.
Isoniazid	Decreased isoniazid effect.	Potassium supplements*	Decreased potassium effect.
Mitotane	Decreased prednisolone effect.	Rifampin	Decreased prednisolone effect.
Non-steroidal anti-inflammatory drugs (NSAIDs)*	Increased risk of ulcers, increased prednisolone effect.	Salicylates*	Decreased salicylate effect.
Oxyphenbutazone	Possible ulcers.	Sympathomimetics*	Possible glaucoma.
		Theophylline	Possible increased theophylline effect.

PREDNISONE

GENERIC NAME OR DRUG CLASS	COMBINED EFFECT	GENERIC NAME OR DRUG CLASS	COMBINED EFFECT
Contraceptives, oral*	Increased prednisone effect.	Insulin	Decreased insulin effect.
Digitalis preparations*	Dangerous potassium depletion. Possible digitalis toxicity.	Isoniazid	Decreased isoniazid effect.
Diuretics, thiazide*	Potassium depletion.	Mitotane	Decreased prednisone effect.
Ethacrynic acid	Potassium depletion.	Non-steroidal anti-inflammatory drugs (NSAIDs)*	Increased risk of ulcers and prednisone effect.
Ephedrine	Decreased prednisone effect.	Phenobarbital	Decreased prednisone effect.
Estrogens*	Increased prednisone effect.	Oxyphenbutazone	Possible ulcers.
Furosemide	Potassium depletion.	Phenylbutazone	Possible ulcers.
Glutethimide	Decreased prednisone effect.	Potassium supplements*	Decreased potassium effect.
Indapamide	Possible excessive potassium loss, causing dangerous heartbeat irregularity.	Rifampin	Decreased prednisone effect.
Indomethacin	Increased prednisone effect.	Salicylates*	Decreased salicylate effect.
		Sympathomimetics*	Possible glaucoma.
		Theophylline	Possible increased theophylline effect.

*See Glossary

ADDITIONAL DRUG INTERACTIONS

GENERIC NAME OR DRUG CLASS	COMBINED EFFECT	GENERIC NAME OR DRUG CLASS	COMBINED EFFECT

PRIMIDONE

GENERIC NAME OR DRUG CLASS	COMBINED EFFECT	GENERIC NAME OR DRUG CLASS	COMBINED EFFECT
Sedatives*	Increased sedative effect.	Tranquilizers*	Increased tranquilizer effect.
Sleep inducers*	Increased effect of sleep inducer.		

PROBENECID & COLCHICINE

GENERIC NAME OR DRUG CLASS	COMBINED EFFECT	GENERIC NAME OR DRUG CLASS	COMBINED EFFECT
Diuretics, thiazide*	Decreased probenecid effect.	Phenylbutazone	Decreased antigout effect of colchicine.
Indomethacin	Increased adverse effects of indomethacin.	Pyrazinamide	Decreased probenecid effect.
Methotrexate	Increased methotrexate effect.	Salicylates*	Decreased probenecid effect.
Mind-altering drugs	Oversedation.	Sedatives*	Oversedation.
Narcotics*	Oversedation.	Sleep inducers*	Oversedation.
Nitrofurantoin	Increased nitrofurantoin effect.	Sulfa drugs*	Slows elimination. May cause harmful accumulation of sulfa.
Para-aminosalicylic acid (PAS)	Increased effect of para-aminosalicylic acid.	Tranquilizers*	Oversedation.
Penicillins*	Enhanced penicillin effect.	Vitamin B-12	Decreased absorption of vitamin B-12.

PROCHLORPERAZINE & ISOPROPAMIDE

GENERIC NAME OR DRUG CLASS	COMBINED EFFECT	GENERIC NAME OR DRUG CLASS	COMBINED EFFECT
Mind-altering drugs*	Increased effect of mind-altering drugs.	Pilocarpine	Loss of pilocarpine effect in glaucoma treatment.
Nabilone	Greater depression of central nervous system.	Potassium supplements*	Possible intestinal ulcers with oral potassium tablets.
Narcotics*	Increased narcotic effect.	Quinidine	Impaired heart function. Dangerous mixture.
Nitrates*	Increased internal-eye pressure.	Sedatives*	Increased sedative effect.
Orphenadrine	Increased isopropamide effect.	Tranquilizers, other	Increased tranquilizer effect.
Phenothiazines*	Increased isopropamide effect.	Vitamin C	Decreased isopropamide effect. Avoid large doses of vitamin C.
Phenytoin	Increased phenytoin effect.		

PROMETHAZINE

GENERIC NAME OR DRUG CLASS	COMBINED EFFECT	GENERIC NAME OR DRUG CLASS	COMBINED EFFECT
Sotalol	Increased antihistamine effect.	Tranquilizers, other*	Increased tranquilizer effect.
Terfenadine	Possible oversedation.		

*See Glossary

GENERIC NAME OR DRUG CLASS	COMBINED EFFECT	GENERIC NAME OR DRUG CLASS	COMBINED EFFECT

PROPRANOLOL

GENERIC NAME OR DRUG CLASS	COMBINED EFFECT	GENERIC NAME OR DRUG CLASS	COMBINED EFFECT
Levobunolol eyedrops	Possible increased propranolol effect.	Phenytoin	Decreased propranolol effect.
Molindone	Increased tranquilizer effect.	Quinidine	Slows heart excessively.
Narcotics*	Increased narcotic effect. Dangerous sedation.	Reserpine	Increased reserpine effect. Excessive sedation and depression.
Nicardipine	Possible irregular heartbeat and congestive heart failure.	Rifampin	Decreased propranolol effect.
Nitrates*	Possible excessive blood-pressure drop.	Timolol eyedrops	Possible increased propranolol effect.
Non-steroidal anti-inflammatory drugs (NSAIDs)*	Decreased antihypertensive effect of propranolol.	Tocainide	May worsen congestive heart failure.
		Verapamil	Increased effects of both drugs.

PYRILAMINE & PENTOBARBITAL

GENERIC NAME OR DRUG CLASS	COMBINED EFFECT	GENERIC NAME OR DRUG CLASS	COMBINED EFFECT
Dronabinol	Increased effect of both drugs.	Narcotics*	Dangerous sedation. Avoid.
Griseofulvin	Decreased griseofulvin effect.	Non-steroidal anti-inflammatory drugs (NSAIDs)*	Decreased anti-inflammatory effect.
Hypnotics*	Excess sedation. Avoid.	Pain relievers*	Dangerous sedation. Avoid.
Indapamide	Increased indapamide effect.	Sedatives*	Dangerous sedation. Avoid.
MAO inhibitors*	Increased pentobarbital effect. Avoid mixture. May be toxic.	Sleep inducers*	Dangerous sedation. Avoid.
Mind-altering drugs*	Dangerous sedation. Avoid.	Sotalol	Decreased antihistamine effect.
Nabilone	Greater depression of central nervous system.	Tranquilizers*	Dangerous sedation. Avoid.
		Valproic acid	Dangerous sedation. Avoid.

QUINETHAZONE

GENERIC NAME OR DRUG CLASS	COMBINED EFFECT	GENERIC NAME OR DRUG CLASS	COMBINED EFFECT
Nitrates*	Excessive blood-pressure drop.	Potassium supplements*	Decreased potassium effect.
Opiates*	Weakness and faintness when arising from bed or chair.	Probenecid	Decreased probenecid effect.
Oxprenolol	Increased antihypertensive effect. Dosages of both drugs may require adjustments.	Sotalol	Increased antihypertensive effect.
		Terazosin	Decreases effectiveness of terazosin.

*See Glossary

GENERIC NAME OR DRUG CLASS	COMBINED EFFECT	GENERIC NAME OR DRUG CLASS	COMBINED EFFECT

RAUWOLFIA & THIAZIDE DIURETICS

GENERIC NAME OR DRUG CLASS	COMBINED EFFECT	GENERIC NAME OR DRUG CLASS	COMBINED EFFECT
Carteolol	Increased antihypertensive effect.	MAO inhibitors*	Increased hydrochlorothiazide effect. Severe depression.
Cholestyramine	Decreased hydrocholorothiazide effect.	Mind-altering drugs*	Excessive sedation.
Cortisone drugs*	Excessive potassium loss that causes dangerous heart rhythms.	Nicardipine	Blood-pressure drop. Dosages may require adjustment.
Digitalis preparations*	Excessive potassium loss that causes dangerous heart rhythms.	Nitrates*	Excessive blood-pressure drop.
Diuretics, thiazide*	Increased effect of other thiazide diuretics.	Oxprenolol	Increased antihypertensive effect. Dosages of both drugs may require adjustments.
Dronabinol	Increased effect of both drugs. Avoid.		
Indapamide	Increased diuretic effect.	Potassium supplements*	Decreased potassium effect.
Levodopa	Decreased levodopa effect.	Probenecid	Decreased probenecid effect.
Lisinopril	Increased antihypertensive effect. Dosage of each may require adjustment.	Sotalol	Decreased antihypertensive effect.
		Terazosin	Decreases effectiveness of terazosin.
Lithium	Increased effect of lithium.		

RESERPINE & HYDRALAZINE

GENERIC NAME OR DRUG CLASS	COMBINED EFFECT	GENERIC NAME OR DRUG CLASS	COMBINED EFFECT
Aspirin	Decreased aspirin effect.	Levodopa	Decreased levodopa effect.
Beta-adrenergic blockers*	Increased effect of rauwolfia alkaloids. Excessive sedation.	Lisinopril	Increased antihypertensive effect. Dosage of each may require adjustment.
Carteolol	Increased antihypertensive effect.	MAO inhibitors*	Severe depression.
Diazoxide	Increased antihypertensive effect.	Mind-altering drugs*	Excessive sedation.
Digitalis preparations*	Irregular heartbeat.	Nicardipine	Blood-pressure drop. Dosages may require adjustment.
Diuretics, oral*	Increased effect of both drugs. When monitored carefully, combination may be beneficial in controlling hypertension.	Non-steroidal anti-inflammatory drugs (NSAIDs)*	Decreased hydralazine effect.
		Sotalol	Decreased antihypertensive effect.
Dronabinol	Increased effect of both drugs. Avoid.	Terazosin	Decreases effectiveness of terazosin.

1104

*See Glossary

RESERPINE, HYDRALAZINE & HYDROCHLOROTHIAZIDE

GENERIC NAME OR DRUG CLASS	COMBINED EFFECT	GENERIC NAME OR DRUG CLASS	COMBINED EFFECT
Allopurinol	Decreased allopurinol effect.	Dronabinol	Increased effects of drugs.
Amphetamines*	Decreased hydralazine effect.	Indapamide	Increased diuretic effect.
Anticoagulants, oral*	Unpredictable increased or decreased effect of anticoagulant.	Levodopa	Decreased levodopa effect.
Anticonvulsants*	Serious change in seizure pattern.	Lisinopril	Increased antihypertensive effect. Dosage of each may require adjustment.
Antidepressants, tricyclic (TCA)*	Dangerous drop in blood pressure. Avoid combination unless under medical supervision.	Lithium	Increased lithium effect.
Antihistamines*	Increased antihistamine effect.	MAO inhibitors*	Increased effects of both drugs. Severe depression.
Antihypertensives, other*	Increased antihypertensive effect.	Mind-altering drugs*	Excessive sedation.
Aspirin	Decreased aspirin effect.	Nicardipine	Blood-pressure drop. Dosages may require adjustment.
Barbiturates*	Increased hydrochlorothiazide effect.	Nitrates*	Excessive blood-pressure drop.
Beta-adrenergic blockers*	Increased effect of rauwolfia alkaloids. Excessive sedation.	Non-steroidal anti-inflammatory drugs (NSAIDs)*	Decreased hydralazine effect.
Carteolol	Increased antihypertensive effect.	Oxprenolol	Increased antihypertensive effect. Dosages of drug may require adjustments.
Cholestyramine	Decreased hydrochlorothiazide effect.	Potassium supplements*	Decreased potassium effect.
Cortisone drugs*	Excessive potassium loss that causes dangerous heart rhythms.	Probenecid	Decreased probenecid effect.
Diazoxide	Increased antihypertensive effect.	Sotalol	Decreased antihypertensive effect.
Digitalis preparations*	Excessive potassium loss that causes dangerous heart rhythms.	Terazosin	Decreases effectiveness of terazosin.
Diuretics, oral*	Increased effects of drugs. When monitored carefully, combination may be beneficial in controlling hypertension.		

SALICYLATES

GENERIC NAME OR DRUG CLASS	COMBINED EFFECT	GENERIC NAME OR DRUG CLASS	COMBINED EFFECT
Penicillins*	Increased effect of both drugs.	Phenytoin	Increased phenytoin effect.
Phenobarbital	Decreased salicylate effect.	Probenecid	Decreased probenecid effect.

*See Glossary

ADDITIONAL DRUG INTERACTIONS

GENERIC NAME OR DRUG CLASS	COMBINED EFFECT	GENERIC NAME OR DRUG CLASS	COMBINED EFFECT

SALICYLATES continued

GENERIC NAME OR DRUG CLASS	COMBINED EFFECT	GENERIC NAME OR DRUG CLASS	COMBINED EFFECT
Rauwolfia alkaloids*	Decreased salicylate effect.	Terazosin	Decreases effectiveness of terazosin. Causes sodium and fluid retention.
Salicylates, other*	Likely salicylate toxicity.		
Sotalol	Decreased antihypertensive effect of sotalol.	Urinary acidifiers*	Decreased excretion, increased salicylate effect.
Spironolactone	Decreased spironolactone effect.	Urinary alkalizers*	Increased excretion, decreased salicylate effect.
Sulfinpyrazone	Decreased sulfinpyrazone effect.	Valproic acid	Possible increased valproic acid toxicity.
		Vitamin C (large doses)	Possible salicylate toxicity.

SCOPOLAMINE (Hyoscine)

GENERIC NAME OR DRUG CLASS	COMBINED EFFECT	GENERIC NAME OR DRUG CLASS	COMBINED EFFECT
Pilocarpine	Loss of pilocarpine effect in glaucoma treatment.	Quinidine	Increased scopolamine effect.
Potassium supplements*	Possible intestinal ulcers with oral potassium tablets.	Vitamin C	Decreased scopolamine effect. Avoid large doses of vitamin C.

SECOBARBITAL

GENERIC NAME OR DRUG CLASS	COMBINED EFFECT	GENERIC NAME OR DRUG CLASS	COMBINED EFFECT
Sleep inducers*	Dangerous sedation. Avoid.	Tranquilizers*	Dangerous sedation. Avoid.
Sotalol	Increased barbiturate effect. Dangerous sedation.	Valproic acid	Increased secobarbital effect.

SPIRONOLACTONE & HYDROCHLOROTHIAZIDE

GENERIC NAME OR DRUG CLASS	COMBINED EFFECT	GENERIC NAME OR DRUG CLASS	COMBINED EFFECT
Antidiabetics, oral*	Increased blood sugar.	Diuretics, other*	Increased effect of both drugs. Beneficial if needed and dose is correct.
Antihypertensives, other*	Increased antihypertensive effect.		
Aspirin	Decreased spironolactone effect.	Indapamide	Increased diuretic effect.
Barbiturates*	Increased hydrochlorothiazide effect.	Indomethacin	Decreased hydrochlorothiazide effect.
Carteolol	Increased antihypertensive effect.	Laxatives*	Reduced potassium levels.
Cholestyramine	Decreased hydrochlorothiazide effect.	Lithium	Increased effect of lithium. Likely lithium toxicity.
Cortisone drugs*	Excessive potassium loss that causes dangerous heart rhythms.	MAO inhibitors*	Increased hydrochlorothiazide effect.
		Nicardipine	Blood-pressure drop. Dosages may require adjustment.

*See Glossary

GENERIC NAME OR DRUG CLASS	COMBINED EFFECT	GENERIC NAME OR DRUG CLASS	COMBINED EFFECT

SPIRONOLACTONE & HYDROCHLOROTHIAZIDE continued

GENERIC NAME OR DRUG CLASS	COMBINED EFFECT	GENERIC NAME OR DRUG CLASS	COMBINED EFFECT
Nitrates*	Excessive blood-pressure drop.	Salicylates*	May decrease spironolactone effect.
Opiates*	Weakness and faintness when arising from bed or chair.	Sodium bicarbonate	Reduces high potassium levels.
		Sotalol	Decreased anti-hypertensive effect.
Potassium supplements*	Decreased potassium effect. Dangerous potassium retention, causing possible heartbeat irregularity.	Terazosin	Decreases effective-ness of terazosin.
		Triamterene	Dangerous potassium retention.
Probenecid	Decreased probenecid effect.		

SULINDAC

Terazosin	Decreases effective-ness of terazosin. Causes sodium and fluid retention.	Thyroid hormones*	Rapid heartbeat, blood-pressure rise.

TALBUTAL (Butalbital)

Sedatives*	Dangerous sedation. Avoid.	Tranquilizers*	Dangerous sedation. Avoid.
Sleep inducers*	Dangerous sedation. Avoid.	Valproic acid	Increased talbutal (butalbital) effect.
Sotalol	Increased barbiturate effect. Dangerous sedation.		

THEOPHYLLINE, EPHEDRINE & BARBITURATES

Antihistamines*	Dangerous sedation. Avoid.	Digitalis preparations*	Serious heart-rhythm disturbances.
Antihypertensives*	Decreased antihyper-tensive effect.	Doxycycline	Decreased doxycycline effect.
Aspirin	Decreased aspirin effect.	Dronabinol	Increased effect of drugs. Avoid.
Beta-adrenergic blockers*	Decreased effect of drugs.	Ephedrine	Increased effect of drugs.
Carteolol	Increased barbiturate effect. Dangerous sedation.	Epinephrine	Increased effect of drugs.
Ciprofloxacin	Increased possibility of central nervous system poisoning, such as nausea, vomiting, rest-lessness, palpitations.	Ergot preparations*	Serious blood-pressure rise.
		Erythromycin	Increased broncho-dilator effect.
Contraceptives, oral*	Decreased contra-ceptive effect.	Furosemide	Increased furosemide effect.
Cortisone drugs*	Decreased cortisone effect.	Griseofulvin	Decreased griseofulvin effect.

*See Glossary

GENERIC NAME OR DRUG CLASS	COMBINED EFFECT	GENERIC NAME OR DRUG CLASS	COMBINED EFFECT

THEOPHYLLINE, EPHEDRINE & BARBITURATES continued

GENERIC NAME OR DRUG CLASS	COMBINED EFFECT	GENERIC NAME OR DRUG CLASS	COMBINED EFFECT
Guanethidine	Decreased effect of drugs.	Non-steroidal anti-inflammatory drugs (NSAIDs)*	Decreased anti-inflammatory effect.
Indapamide	Increased indapamide effect.	Probenecid	Decreased effect of drugs.
Lincomycins*	Increased broncho-dilator effect.	Propranolol	Decreased broncho-dilator effect.
Lithium	Decreased lithium effect.	Pseudoephedrine	Increased pseudo-ephedrine effect.
MAO Inhibitors*	Increased ephedrine effect. Dangerous blood-pressure rise.	Rauwolfia alkaloids*	Rapid heartbeat.
Mind-altering drugs*	Dangerous sedation. Avoid.	Sotalol	Increased barbiturate effect. Dangerous sedation.
Narcotics*	Dangerous sedation. Avoid.	Sulfinpyrazone	Decreased sulfin-pyrazone effect.
Nicardipine	May increase theophylline effect and toxicity.	Terazosin	Decreased effect of terazosin.
Nitrates*	Possible decreased effect of drugs.	Troleandomycin	Increased broncho-dilator effect.
		Valproic acid	Increased barbiturate effect.

THEOPHYLLINE, EPHEDRINE, GUAIFENESIN & BARBITURATES

GENERIC NAME OR DRUG CLASS	COMBINED EFFECT	GENERIC NAME OR DRUG CLASS	COMBINED EFFECT
Antidepressants, tricyclics (TCA)*	Decreased anti-depressant effect.	Digitoxin	Decreased digitoxin effect.
Antidiabetics, oral*	Increased phenobarbital effect.	Doxycycline	Decreased doxycycline effect.
Antihistamines*	Dangerous sedation. Avoid.	Dronabinol	Increased effect of drugs.
Aspirin, other	Decreased aspirin effect.	Ephedrine	Increased effect of drugs.
Beta-adrenergic blockers*	Decreased effect of drugs.	Ergot preparations*	Serious blood-pressure rise.
Carteolol	Increased barbiturate effect. Dangerous sedation.	Erythromycin	Increased broncho-dilator effect.
Ciprofloxacin	Increased possibility of central nervous system poisoning, such as nausea, vomiting, restlessness, palpitations.	Furosemide	Increased furosemide effect.
		Griseofulvin	Decreased griseofulvin effect.
Contraceptives, oral*	Decreased contra-ceptive effect.	Guanethidine	Decreased effect of drugs.
Cortisone drugs*	Increased cortisone effect.	Indapamide	Increased indapamide effect.
Digitalis preparations*	Serious heart-rhythm disturbances.	Lincomycins*	Increased broncho-dilator effect.

*See Glossary

THEOPHYLLINE, EPHEDRINE, GUAIFENESIN & BARBITURATES continued

GENERIC NAME OR DRUG CLASS	COMBINED EFFECT	GENERIC NAME OR DRUG CLASS	COMBINED EFFECT
Lithium	Decreased lithium effect.	Propranolol	Decreased bronchodilator effect.
MAO inhibitors*	Increased phenobarbital effect.	Pseudoephedrine	Increased pseudoephedrine effect.
Mind-altering drugs*	Dangerous sedation. Avoid.	Rauwolfia alkaloids*	Rapid heartbeat.
Narcotics*	Dangerous sedation. Avoid.	Sedatives*	Dangerous sedation. Avoid.
Nicardipine	May increase theophylline effect and toxicity.	Sleep inducers*	Dangerous sedation. Avoid.
		Sulfinpyrazone	Decreased sulfinpyrazone effect.
Nitrates*	Possible decreased effect of drugs.	Terazosin	Decreased effect of terazosin.
Non-steroidal anti-inflammatory drugs (NSAIDs)*	Decreased anti-inflammatory effect.	Tranquilizers*	Dangerous sedation. Avoid.
Pain relievers*	Dangerous sedation. Avoid.	Troleandomycin	Increased bronchodilator effect.
Probenecid	Decreased effect of drugs.	Valproic acid	Increased phenobarbital effect.

THEOPHYLLINE, EPHEDRINE & HYDROXYZINE

GENERIC NAME OR DRUG CLASS	COMBINED EFFECT	GENERIC NAME OR DRUG CLASS	COMBINED EFFECT
Ciprofloxacin	May cause kidney dysfunction.	Nabilone	Greater depression of central nervous system.
Digitalis preparations*	Serious heart-rhythm disturbances.	Nicardipine	May increase theophylline effect and toxicity.
Dronabinol	Increased effect of drugs.	Nitrates*	Possible decreased effect of drugs.
Ephedrine	Increased effect of drugs.	Pain relievers	Increased effect of drugs.
Epinephrine	Increased effect of drugs.	Probenecid	Decreased effect of drugs.
Ergot preparations*	Serious blood-pressure rise.	Propranolol	Decreased bronchodilator effect.
Erythromycin	Increased bronchodilator effect.	Pseudoephedrine	Increased pseudoephedrine effect.
Furosemide	Increased furosemide effect.	Rauwolfia alkaloids*	Rapid heartbeat.
Guanethidine	Decreased effect of drugs.	Sotalol	Decreased antihistamine effect.
Lincomycins*	Increased bronchodilator effect.	Sulfinpyrazone	Decreased sulfinpyrazone effect.
Lithium	Decreased lithium effect.	Terazosin	Decreased effect of terazosin.
MAO inhibitors*	Increased ephedrine effect. Dangerous blood-pressure rise.	Tranquilizers*	Increased effect of drugs.
		Troleandomycin	Increased bronchodilator effect.

*See Glossary

ADDITIONAL DRUG INTERACTIONS

TIMOLOL

GENERIC NAME OR DRUG CLASS	COMBINED EFFECT	GENERIC NAME OR DRUG CLASS	COMBINED EFFECT
Narcotics*	Increased narcotic effect. Dangerous sedation.	Quinidine	Slows heart excessively.
Nicardipine	Possible irregular heartbeat and congestive heart failure.	Reserpine	Increased reserpine effect. Excessive sedation, depression.
Nitrates*	Possible decreased blood pressure.	Rifampin	Decreased timolol effect.
Non-steroidal anti-inflammatory drugs (NSAIDs)*	Decreased antihypertensive effect of timolol.	Timolol eyedrops	Possible increased timolol effect.
Phenytoin	Decreased timolol effect.	Tocainide	May worsen congestive heart failure.
		Verapamil	Increased effect of both drugs.

TRIAMCINOLONE

GENERIC NAME OR DRUG CLASS	COMBINED EFFECT	GENERIC NAME OR DRUG CLASS	COMBINED EFFECT
Isoniazid	Decreased isoniazid effect.	Phenylbutazone	Possible ulcers.
Mitotane	Decreased triamcinolone effect.	Potassium supplements*	Decreased potassium effect.
Non-steroidal anti-inflammatory drugs (NSAIDs)*	Increased risk of ulcers and triamcinolone effect.	Rifampin	Decreased triamcinolone effect.
Oxyphenbutazone	Possible ulcers.	Salicylates*	Decreased salicylate effect.
Phenobarbital	Decreased triamcinolone effect.	Sympathomimetics*	Possible glaucoma.
		Theophylline	Possible increased theophylline effect.

TRIAMTERINE & HYDROCHOLOROTHIAZIDE

GENERIC NAME OR DRUG CLASS	COMBINED EFFECT	GENERIC NAME OR DRUG CLASS	COMBINED EFFECT
Indomethacin	Possible acute renal failure.	Nitrates*	Excessive blood-pressure drop.
Lisinopril	Possible severe blood-pressure drop with first dose.	Opiates*	Weakness and faintness when arising from bed or chair.
Lithium	Increased lithium effect.	Potassium supplements*	Possible excessive potassium retention. Decreased potassium effect.
MAO inhibitors*	Increased hydrochlorothiazide effect.		
Nicardipine	Dangerous blood-pressure drop. Dosages may require adjustment.	Probenecid	Decreased probenecid effect.
		Spironolactone	Dangerous retention of potassium.

TRICHLORMETHIAZIDE

GENERIC NAME OR DRUG CLASS	COMBINED EFFECT	GENERIC NAME OR DRUG CLASS	COMBINED EFFECT
Potassium supplements*	Decreased potassium effect.	Sotalol	Increased antihypertensive effect.
Probenecid	Decreased probenecid effect.	Terazosin	Decreases effectiveness of terazosin.

*See Glossary

TRICYCLIC ANTIDEPRESSANTS

GENERIC NAME OR DRUG CLASS	COMBINED EFFECT	GENERIC NAME OR DRUG CLASS	COMBINED EFFECT
Leucovorin	High alcohol content of leucovorin may cause adverse effects.	**Nabilone**	Greater depression of central nervous system.
Levodopa	May increase blood pressure.	**Narcotics***	Oversedation.
Lithium	Possible decreased seizure threshold.	**Phenothiazines***	Possible increased tricyclic antidepressant effect and toxicity.
MAO Inhibitors*	Fever, delirium, convulsions.	**Phenytoin**	Decreased phenytoin effect.
Methyprylon	Increased sedative effect, perhaps to dangerous level. Avoid.	**Procainamide**	Possible irregular heartbeat.
Methyldopa	Possible decreased methyldopa effect.	**Quinidine**	Possible irregular heartbeat.
Methylphenidate	Possible increased tricyclic antidepressant effect and toxicity.	**Sedatives***	Dangerous oversedation.
		Sympathomimetics*	Increased sympathomimetic effect.
Molindone	Increased molindone effect.	**Thyroid hormones***	Irregular heartbeat.

ADDITIONAL DRUG INTERACTIONS

Glossary

The following medical terms are found in the drug charts. Where drug names are listed, the generic or drug class is first with brand names following in parentheses.

A

ACE Inhibitors—Angiotensin-Converting Enzyme (ACE)—A family of drugs used to treat hypertension and congestive heart failure. Inhibitors decrease the rate of conversion of Angiotensin I into Angiotensin II, which is the normal process for the angiotensin-converting enzyme. These drugs include: captopril (Capoten), enalapril (Vasotec), and lisinopril.

Acne Preparations—Creams, lotions and liquids applied to the skin to treat acne. These include: alcohol and acetone; alcohol and sulfur; benzoyl peroxide; clindamycin; erythromycin; erythromycin and benzoyl peroxide; isotretinoin; meclocycline; resorcinol; resorcinol and sulfur; salicylic acid gel USP; salicylic acid lotion; salicylic acid ointment; salicylic acid pads; salicylic acid soap; salicylic acid and sulfur bar soap; salicylic acid and sulfur cleansing lotion; salicylic acid and sulfur cleansing suspension; salicylic acid and sulfur lotion; sulfurated lime; sulfur bar soap; sulfur cream; sulfur lotion; tetracycline, oral; tetracycline hydrochloride for topical solution; tretinoin.

Acute—Having a short and relatively severe course.

Addiction—Psychological or physiological dependence upon a drug.

Addison's Disease—Changes in the body caused by a deficiency of hormones manufactured by the adrenal gland. Usually fatal if untreated.

Adrenal Cortex—Center of the adrenal gland.

Adrenal Gland—Gland next to the kidney that produces cortisone and epinephrine (adrenalin).

Alkalizers—These drugs neutralize acidic properties of the blood and urine by making them more alkaline (or basic). Systemic alkalizers include: potassium citrate and citric acid, sodium bicarbonate, sodium citrate and citric acid, and tricitrates. Urinary alkalizers include: potassium citrate, potassium citrate and citric acid, potassium citrate and sodium citrate, sodium citrate and citric acid.

Alkylating Agent—Chemical used to treat malignant diseases.

Allergy—Excessive sensitivity to a substance.

Amebiasis—Infection with amoeba, one-celled organisms. Causes diarrhea, fever and abdominal cramps.

Aminoglycosides—A family of antibiotics used for serious infections. Their usefulness is limited because of relative toxicity compared to some other antibiotics. These drugs include: amikacin, gentamicin, kanamycin, neomycin, netilmicin, streptomycin, tobramycin.

Amphetamines—A family of drugs that stimulates the central nervous system, prescribed to treat attention-deficit disorders in children and also for narcolepsy. They are habit-forming, controlled under U.S. law, and are no longer prescribed as appetite suppressants. These drugs include: amphetamine, dextroamphetamine, methamphetamine. They may be ingredients of several combination drugs.

Analgesic—Agent that reduces pain without reducing consciousness.

Anaphylaxis—Severe allergic response to a substance. Symptoms are wheezing, itching, hives, nasal congestion, intense burning of hands and feet, collapse, loss of consciousness and cardiac arrest. Symptoms appear within a few seconds or minutes after exposure. Anaphylaxis is a severe medical emergency. Without appropriate treatment, it can cause death. Instructions for home treatment for anaphylaxis are on the front inside cover.

Androgens—Male hormones, including: fluoxymesterone, methyltestosterone, testosterone.

Anemia—Not enough healthy red-blood cells in the bloodstream or too little hemoglobin in the red-blood cells. Anemia is caused by imbalance of blood loss and blood production.

Anemia, Hemolytic—Anemia caused by a shortened lifespan of red-blood cells. The body can't manufacture new cells fast enough to replace old cells.

Anemia, Iron-Deficiency—Anemia caused when iron necessary to manufacture red-blood cells is not available.

Anemia, Pernicious—Anemia caused by a vitamin B-12 deficiency. Symptoms include weakness, fatigue, numbness and tingling of the hands or feet, and degeneration of the central nervous system.

Anemia, Sickle-Cell—Anemia caused by defective hemoglobin that deprives red-blood cells of oxygen, making them sickle-shaped.

Anesthesias, General—Gases that are used in surgery to render patients unconscious and able to withstand the pain of surgical cutting and manipulation. They include: enflurane; etomidate; halothane; isoflurane; ketamine; methohexital; methoxyflurane; nitrous oxide; thiamylal; thiopental; alfentanil; amobarbital; butabarbital; butorphanol; chloral hydrate; etomidate; tentanyl; hydroxyzine; ketamine; levorphanol; meperidine; midazolam; morphine, parenteral; nalbuphine; oxymorphone; pentazocine; pentobarbital; phenobarbital; promethazine; propiomazine; scopolamine; secobarbital; sufentanil.

Anesthetic—Drug that eliminates the sensation of pain.

Angina (Angina Pectoris)—Chest pain with a sensation of suffocation and impending death. Caused by a temporary reduction in the amount of oxygen to the heart muscle through diseased coronary arteries.

Antacids—A large family of drugs prescribed to treat hyperacidity, peptic ulcer, esophageal reflux, and others. These drugs include: aluminum carbonate, basic (Basaljel); aluminum hydroxide (Alagel, ALternaGEL, Alu-Cap, Alu-Tab, Amphojel, Dialume, Nephrox); dihydroxyaluminum aminoacetate (Robalate); dihydroxyaluminum sodium carbonate (Rolaids); alumina, magnesia and calcium carbonate (Camalox); alumina, magnesium carbonate and calcium carbonate (Duracid); simethicone, alumina, calcium carbonate and magnesia (Tempo); alumina and magnesia (Algenic Alka Improved, Aludrox, Alumid, Amphojel 500, Creamalin, Delcid, Diovol Ex, Gelamal, Gelusil, Gelusil Extra Strength, Kolantyl, Kudrox, Maalox Maalox No. 1, Maalox No. 2, Maalox TC, Magmalin, Mintox, Mylanta 2 Plain, Neutralca-S, Rolox, Rulox, Rulox No. 1, Rulox No. 2, Univol, WinGel); alumina, magnesia and simethicone (Almacone, Almacone II, Alma-Mag Improved, Alma-Mag #4 Improved, Alumid Plus, Amphojel Plus, AntaGel, AntaGel-II, Di-Gel, Diovol, Gelusil, Gelusil-II, Gelusil-M, Maalox Plus, MiAcid, Mygel, Mygel II, Mylanta, Mylanta-II, Mylanta-2, Mylanta-2 Extra Strength, Newtrogel II, Silain-Gel, Simaal Gel, Simaal 2 Gel, Simeco); alumina and magnesium carbonate (Gaviscon, Liquimint, Magnagel, Remegel); alumina and magnesium trisilicate (Gaviscon, Gaviscon-2); dihydroxyaluminum aminoacetate, magnesia and alumina (Tralmag); magnesium trisilicate, alumina and magnesia (Magnatril); magnesium trisilicate, alumina and magnesium carbonate (Escot); simethicone, alumina, magnesium carbonate and magnesia (Amphojel Plus, Di-Gel); alumina, magnesium trisilicate and sodium bicarbonate (Gas-is-gon, Triconsil); calcium carbonate (Alka-Mints, Amitone, Chooz, Calcilac, Calglycine, Dicarbosil, Equilet, Gustalac, Pama No. 1, Titracin, Titralac, Tums, Tums E-X); calcium carbonate and magnesia (Bisodol, Calcitrel); calcium carbonate, magnesia and simethicone (Advanced Formula Di-Gel); calcium and magnesium carbonates (Marblen, Noralac, Spastosed); calcium and magnesium carbonates and magnesium oxide (Alkets); magaldrate (Lowsium, Riopan); magaldrate and simethicone (Riopan Plus, Lowsium); magnesium hydroxide (M.O.M., Phillips' Milk of Magnesia); magnesium oxide (Mag-Ox 400, Maox, Par-Mag, Uro-Mag); magnesium carbonate and sodium bicarbonate (Bisodol).

Antiacne Topical Preparations—See Acne Preparations.

Antianginals—A group of drugs used to treat *angina pectoris* (chest pain that comes and goes, caused by coronary artery disease). These drugs include: acebutolol, amyl nitrite, atenolol, diltiazem, erythrityl tetranitrate, isosorbide dinitrate, labetalol, metoprolol, nadolol, nifedipine, nitroglycerin, oxprenolol, pentaerythritol tetranitrate, pindolol, propranolol, sotalol, timolol, verapamil.

Antianxiety—A group of drugs prescribed to treat anxiety. These drugs include: alprazolam, bromazepam, buspirone, chlordiazepoxide, chlorpromazine, clomipramine, clorazepate, diazepam, halazepam, hydroxyzine, imipramine, ketazolam, lorazepam, meprobamate, mesoridazine, oxazepam, prazepam, prochlorperazine, thioridazine, trifluoperazine.

Antiarrhythimcs—A group of drugs used to treat heartbeat irregularities (arrhythmias). These drugs include: acebutolol, amiodarone, atenolol, atropine, bretylium, deslanoside, digitalis, digitoxin, disopyramide, edrophonium, encainide, esmolol, flecainide, glycopyrrolate, hyoscyamine, lidocaine, methoxamine, metoprolol, mexiletine, nadolol, oxprenolol, phenytoin, procainamide, propranolol, quinidine, scopolamine, sotalol, timolol, tocainide, verapamil.

Antiasthmatics—Medicines used to treat asthma, which may be tablets, liquids or aerosols (to be inhaled to get directly to the bronchial tubes rather than through the bloodstream). These medicines include: adrenocorticoids, glucocorticoid; albuterol; aminophylline; beclomethasone; bitolterol; corticotropin; cromolyn; dexamethasone; dyphylline; ephedrine; epinephrine; ethylnorepinephrine; fenoterol; flunisolide;

isoetharine; isoproterenol; isoproterenol and phenylephrine; metaproterenol; oxtriphylline; oxtriphylline and guaifenesin; pirbuterol; racepinephrine; terbutaline; theophylline; theophylline and guaifenesin; triamcinolone.

Antibacterials (Antibiotics)—A group of drugs prescribed to treat infections. These drugs include: aminocillin, amikacin, amoxicillin, amoxicillin and clavulanate, ampicillin, azlocillin, aztreonam, bacampicillin, carbenicillin, cefaclor, cefadroxil, cefamandole, cefazolin, cefonicid, cefoperazone, ceforanide, cefotaxime, cefotetan, cefoxitin, ceftazidime, ceftizoxime, ceftriaxone, cefuroxime, cephalexin, cephalothin, cephapirin, cephradine, chloramphenicol, cinoxacine, clindamycin, cloxacillin, cyclacillin, cycloserine, demeclocycline, dicloxacillin, doxycycline, erythromycin, erythromycin and sulfisoxazole, flucloxacillin, fusidic acid, gentamicin, imipenem and cilastatin, kanamycin, lincomycin, methacycline, methenamine, methicillin, metronidazole, mezlocillin, minocycline, moxalactam, nafcillin, nalidixic acid, netilmicin, nitrofurantoin, norfloxacin, oxacillin, oxytetracycline, penicillin G, penicillin V, piperacillin, pivampicillin, rifampin, spectinomycin, streptomycin, sulfacytine, sulfadiazine and trimethoprim, sulfamethoxazole, sulfamethoxazole and trimethoprim, sulfisoxazole, tetracycline, ticarcillin, ticarcillin and clavulanate, tobramycin, trimethoprim, vancomycin.

Antibiotics—Chemicals that inhibit the growth of or kill germs. See Antibacterials.

Anticholinergics—Drugs that chemically inhibit nerve impulses through the parasympathetic nervous system.

Anticoagulants—A family of drugs prescribed to slow the rate of blood-clotting. These drugs include: acenocoumarol, anisindione, dicumarol, heparin, warfarin, dihydroergotamine and heparin.

Anticonvulsants—A group of drugs prescribed to treat or prevent seizures (convulsions). These drugs include: amobarbital, carbamazepine, clonazepam, clorazepate, diazepam, divalproex, ethosuximide, ethotoin, lorazepam, magnesium sulfate, mephenytoin, mephobarbital, metharbital, methsuximide, nitrazepam, paraldehyde, paramethadione, pentobarbital, phenobarbital, phensuximide, phenytoin, primidone, secobarbital, trimethadione, valproic acid.

Antidepressants—A group of medicines prescribed to treat mental depression. These drugs include: amitriptyline, amoxapine, clomipramine, desipramine, doxepin,

imipramine, isocarboxazid, maprotiline, nortriptyline, phenelzine, protriptyline, tranylcypromine, trazodone, trimipramine.

Antidepressants, MAO (Monamine Oxidase Inhibitors)—A special group of drugs prescribed for mental depression. These are not as popular as in years past because of a relatively high incidence of adverse effects. These drugs include: isocarboxazid (Marplan), phenelzine (Nardil), tranylcypromine (Parnate).

Antidepressants, tricyclic (TCA)—A group of medicines with similar chemical structure and pharmacologic activity used to treat mental depression. These drugs include: amitriptyline (Amitril, Apo-Amitriptyline, Elavil, Emitrip, Endep, Levate, Meravil, Novotriptyn); amoxapine (Asendin); clomipramine (Anafranil); desipramine (Pertofrane, Norpramin); doxepin (Adapin, Sinequan, triadapin); imipramine (Apo-Imipramine, Impril, Janimine, Novopramine, Tipramine, Tofranil, Tofranil-PM); nortriptyline (Aventyl, Pamelor); protriptyline (Triptil, Vivactil); trimipramine (Surmontil).

Antidiabetics—A group of drugs used in the treatment of *diabetes mellitus*. These medicines all reduce blood sugar. These drugs include: acetohexamide, chlorpropamide, glipizide, glyburide, insulin, metformin, tolazamide, tolbutamide.

Antidiarrheal Preparations—Medicines that treat diarrhea symptoms. Most do not cure the cause. Oral medicines include: aluminum hydroxide; charcoal, activated; kaolin and pectin; loperamide; polycarbophil; psyllium hydrophilic mucilloid. Systemic medicines include: codeine; difenoxin and atropine; diphenoxylate and atropine; glucose and electrolytes; glycopyrrolate; kaolin, pectin, belladonna alkaloids and opium; kaolin, pectin and paregoric; opium tincture; paregoric.

Antidyskinetics—A group of drugs used for treatment of Parkinsonism (paralysis agitans) and drug-induced extrapyramidal reactions (see elsewhere in Glossary). These drugs include: amantadine, benztropine, biperiden, bromocriptine, carbidopa and levodopa, diphenhydramine, ethopropazine, levodopa, levodopa and benserazide.

Antiemetics—A group of drugs used to treat nausea and vomiting. These drugs include: buclizine, cyclizine, chlorpromazine, dimenhydrinate, diphenhydramine, diphenidol, domperidone, dronabinol, haloperidol, hydroxyzine, meclizine, metoclopramide, nabilone, perphenazine, prochlorperazine, promethazine, scopolamine, triflupromazine, trimethobenzamide.

Antifibronyltic Drugs—Drugs that are used to treat serious bleeding. These drugs include aminocaproic acid and tranexamic acid.

Antifungals—A group of drugs used to treat fungus infection. Those listed as systemic are taken orally or given by injection. Those listed as topical are applied directly to the skin and include liquids, powders, creams, ointments and liniments. Those listed as vaginal are used topically inside the vagina and sometimes on the vaginal lips. These drugs include: Systemic— amphotericin B, miconazole, flucytosine, griseofulvin, ketoconazole, potassium iodide. Topical—carbol-fuchsin; ciclopirox; clioquinol; clotrimazole; econazole; haloprogin; ketoconzaole; miconazole; nystatin; salicylic acid, sulfur and coal; tolnaftate. Vaginal— butoconazole, clotrimazole, gentian violet, miconazole, nystatin.

Antiglaucoma—Medicines used to treat glaucoma. Those listed as systemic are taken orally or given by injection. Those listed as ophthalmic are used as eye drops. These drugs include: Systemic—acetazolamide, dichlorphenamide, glycerin, mannitol, methazolamide, timolol, urea. Ophthalmic— betaxolol, carbachol ophthalmic solution, demecarium, dipivefrin, echothiophate, epinephrine, epinephrine bitartrate, epinephryl borate, isoflurophate, levobunolol, physostigmine, pilocarpine, timolol.

Antigout Drugs—Drugs to treat the metabolic disease called gout. Gout causes recurrent attacks of joint pain caused by deposits of uric acid in the joints. Antigout drugs include: allopurinol, carprofen, colchicine, fenoprofen, ibuprofen, indomethacin, ketoprofen, naproxen, phenylbutazone, piroxicam, probenecid, pro- benecid and colchicine, sulfinpyrazone, sulindac.

Antihelminthics—A family of drugs used to treat intestinal parasites. Names of these drugs include: niclosamide, piperazine, pyrantel, pyrvinium, quinacrine, mebendazole, metronidazole, oxamniquine, praziquantel, thiabendazole.

Antihistamines—A family of drugs used to treat allergic conditions, such as hay fever, allergic conjunctivitis, itching, sneezing, runny nose, motion sickness, dizziness, sedation, insomnia and others. These drugs include: azatadine (Optimine); brompheniramine (Bromamine, Brombay, Bromphen, Chlorphed, Dehist, Dimetane, Dimetane Extentabs, Dimetane-Ten, Histaject Modified, Nasahist B, ND-Stat Revised, Oraminic II, Veltane); carbinoxamine (Clistin); chlorpheniramine (Aller-Chlor, Allerid-

O.D., Chlo-Amine, Chlor-100, Chlor-Mal, Chlor-Niramine, Chlorphen, Chlor-Pro, Chlorspan, Chlortab, Chlor-Trimeton, Chlor-Trimeton Repetabs, Chlor-Tripolon, Hal-Chlor, Histrey, Novopheniram, Phenetron, Phenetron Lanacaps, T.D. Alermine, Teldrin, Trymegen); clemastine (Tavist); cyproheptadine (Periactin); dexchlorpheniramine (Polaramine, Polaramine Repetabs); dimenhydrinate (Apo-Dimenhydrinate, Calm X, Dimentabs, Dinate, Dommanate, Dramamine, Dramilin, Dramocen, Dramoject, Dymenate, Gravol, Hydrate, Marmine, Motion-Aid, Nauseatol, Novodimenate, PMS-Dimenhydrinate, Reidamine, Travamine, Wehamine); diphenhydramine (Beldin, Benadryl, Benadryl Children's Allergy, Benadryl Complete Allergy, Bendylate, Benylin, Compoz, Diahist, Diphen, Diphenadril, Fenylhist, Fynex, Hydramine, Hydril, Insomnal, Nervine Nighttime Sleep-Aid, Noradryl, Nordryl, Nytol with DPH, Robalyn, Sleep-Eze 3, Sominex Formula 2, Tusstate, Twilite, Valdrene); diphenylpyraline (Hispril); doxylamine (Unisom Nighttime Sleep-Aid); phenindamine (Nolahist); pyrilamine (Dormarex, Somnicaps, Sominex); terfenadine (Seldane); tripelennamine (PBZ, PBZ-SR); triprolidine (Actidil, Bayidyl).

Antihypertensives—Drugs used to treat high blood pressure. These medicines can be used singly or in combination with other drugs. They work best if accompanied by a low-salt, low-fat diet plus an active exercise program. These drugs include: acebutolol, alseroxylon, amiloride, amiloride and hydrochlorothiazide, atenolol, atenolol and chlorthalidone, bendroflumethiazide, benzthiazide, bumetanide, captopril, captopril and hydrochlorothiazide, chlorothiazide, chlorthalidone, clonidine, clonidine and chlorthalidone, cyclothiazide, debrisoquine, deserpidine, deserpidine and hydrochlorothiazide, deserpidine and methyclothiazide, diazoxide, diltiazem, enalapril, enalapril and hydrochlorothiazide, ethacrynic acid, furosemide, guanabenz, guanadrel, guanethidine, guanethidine and hydrochlorothiazide, guanfacine, hydralazine, hydralazine and hydrochlorothiazide, hydrochlorothiazide, hydroflumethiazide, indapamide, labetalol, labetalol and hydrochlorothiazide, mecamylamine, methyclothiazide, methyldopa, methyldopa and chlorothiazide, methyldopa and hydrochlorothiazide, metolazone, metoprolol, metoprolol and hydrochlorothiazide, minoxidil, nadolol, nadolol and bendroflumethiazide, nifedipine, nitroglycerin, nitroprusside, oxprenolol, pargyline, pargyline and methyclothiazide, pindolol, pindolol and hydrochlorothiazide, polythiazide, prazosin, prazosin and polythiazide, propranolol, propranolol and hydrochlorothiazide, quinethazone, rauwolfia serpentina, rauwolfia serpentina and bendroflumethazide, reserpine, reserpine and chlorothiazide, reserpine and chlorthalidone, reserpine and hydralazine, reserpine, hydralazine and hydrochlorothiazide, reserpine and hydrochlorothiazide, reserpine and hydroflumethiazide, reserpine and methyclothiazide, reserpine and polythiazide, reserpine and quinethazone, reserpine and trichlormethiazide, sotalol, spironolactone, spironolactone and hydrochlorothiazide, terazosin, timolol, timolol and hydrochlorothiazide, triamterene, triamterene and hydrochlorothiazide, trichlormethiazide, trimethaphan, verapamil.

Anti-inflammatory Analgesics, Non-steroidal (NSAIAs)—A family of drugs not related to cortisone or other steroids. NSAIAs help the body decrease inflammation and pain. These drugs include: fenoprofen, ibuprofen, indomethacin, meclofenamate, naproxen, oxyphenbutazone, phenylbutazone, salicylates, sulindac, tolmetin.

Anti-inflammatory, Non-steroidal (NSAIDs)— Drugs that decrease inflammation wherever it occurs in the body. Used for treatment of pain, fever, arthritis, gout, menstrual cramps and vascular headaches. These drugs include: aspirin; aspirin, alumina and magnesia tablets; buffered aspirin; bufexamac; choline salicylate; choline and magnesium salicylates; diflunisal; fenoprofen; ibuprofen; indomethacin; ketoprofen; magnesium salicylate; meclofenamate; naproxen; piroxicam; salsalate; sodium salicylate; sulindac; tolmetin.

Anti-inflammatory, steroidal—A family of drugs with similar pharmacologic characteristics of cortisone and cortisone-like drugs. They are used for many purposes to help the body deal with inflammation no matter what the cause. Steroidal drugs may be used orally or by injection (systemic), as local applications for the skin, eyes, ears, bronchial tubes (topical), and for others. These drugs include: Nasal— beclomethasone, dexamethasone, flunisolide. Ophthalmic (eyes)—betamethasone, dexamethasone, fluorometholone, hydrocortisone, medrysone, prednisolone. Otic (ears)— betamethasone, desonide and acetic acid, dexamethasone, hydrocortisone, hydrocortisone and acetic acid, prednisolone. Systemic— betamethasone, cortisone, dexamethasone, hydrocortisone, methylprednisolone,

paramethasone, prednisolone, prednisone, triamcinolone. Topical—alclometasone; amcinonide; beclomethasone; betamethasone; clobetasol; clobetasone; clocortolone; desonide; desoximetasone; dexamethasone; diflorasone; diflucortolone; flumethasone; fluocinolone; fluocinonide; fluocinonide, procinonide and ciprocinonide; flurandrenolid; halcinonide; hydrocortisone; methylprednisolone; mometasone; triamcinolone.

Antimalarials (also called antiprotozoals)—A group of drugs used to treat malaria. The choice depends on the precise type of malaria organism and its developmental state. These drugs include: amphotericin B, chloroquine, dapsone, demeclocycline, doxycycline, hydroxychloro- quine, iodoquinol, methacycline, metronidazole, minocycline, oxytetracycline, pentamidine, primaquine, pyrimethamine, quinacrine, quinine, sulfadoxine and pyrimethamine, sulfamethoxazole, sulfamethoxazole and trimethoprim, sulfisoxazole, tetracycline.

Antimuscarines—Drugs that block the muscarinic action of acetylcholine and therefore decrease spasm of smooth muscles. They are prescribed for peptic ulcers, dysmenorrhea, dizziness, seasickness, bedwetting, slow heart rate, treatment of toxicity from pesticides made from organophosphates, and other medical problems. These drugs include: anisotropine, atropine, belladonna, clidinium dicyclomine, glycopyrrolate, hexocyclium, homatropine, hyoscyamine, hyoscyamine and scopolamine, isopropamide, mepenzolate, methantheline, methscopolamine, oxyphencyclimine, oxyphenonium, pirenzepine, propantheline, scopolamine, tridihexethyl.

Antimyasthenics—Medicines to treat myasthenia gravis, a muscle disorder (especially of the face and head) with increasing fatigue and weakness as muscles tire from use. These medicines include: ambenonium, neostigmine, pyridostigmine.

Antineoplastic—Potent drugs used for malignant disease, they are listed here for completeness. Some of these are *not* described in this book. These drugs include: Systemic— aminoglutethimide, amsacrine, asparaginase, bleomycin, busulfan, carboplatin, carmustine, chlorambucil, chlorotrianisene, chromic phosphate, cisplatin, cyclophosphamide, cyproterone, cytarabine, dacarbazine, dactinomycin, daunorubicin, diethylstilbestrol, doxorubicin, dromostanolone, epirubicin, estradiol, estradiol valerate, estramustine, estrogens (conjugated and esterified), estrone, ethinyl estradiol, etoposide, floxuridine, fluorouracil, flutamide, fluoxymesterone, hexamethylmelamine, hydroxyprogesterone, hydroxyurea, interferon alfa-2a and alfa-2b (recombinant), ketoconazole, leuprolide, levothyroxine, liothyronine, liotrix, lomustine, mechlorethamine, medroxyprogesterone, megestrol, melphalan, methyltestosterone, mercaptopurine, methotrexate, mitomycin, mitotane, mitoxantrone, nandrolone phenpropionate, plicamycin, procarbazine, sodium iodide I 131, sodium phosphate P 32, streptozocin, tamoxifen, teniposide, testolactone, testosterone, thioguanine, thiotepa, thyroglobulin, thyroid, thyrotropin, uracil mustard, vinblastine, vincristine, vindesine. Topical—fluorouracil, mechlorethamine.

Antiparkisonism Drugs—Drugs used to treat Parkinson's Disease. A disease of the central nervous system in older adults, it's characterized by gradual progressive muscle rigidity, tremors and clumsiness. These drugs include: amantadine, benztropine, biperiden, bromocriptine, carbidopa and levodopa, diphenhydramine, ethopropazine, levodopa, levodopa and benserazide, procyclidine, trihexyphenidyl.

Antipsychotic—A group of drugs used to treat the mental disease of psychosis, such as schizophrenia, manic-depressive illness, anxiety states, severe behavior problems and others. These drugs include: acetophenazine, carbamazepine, chlorpromazine, chlorprothixene, fluphenazine, flupenthixol, fluspirilene, haloperidol, loxapine, mesoridazine, methotrimeprazine, molindone, pericyazine, perphenazine, pipotiazine, prochlorperazine, promazine, thioridazine, thiothixene, trifluoperazine, triflupromazine.

Antitussive—A group of drugs used to suppress cough. These drugs include: chlophedianol, codeine (oral), dextromethorphan, diphenhydramine syrup, hydrocodone, hydromorphone, methadone, morphine.

Antiulcer—A group of medicines used to treat peptic ulcer in the stomach, duodenum or the lower end of the esophagus. These drugs include: cimetidine, doxepin, famotidine, ranitidine, sucralfate, trimipramine.

Antiviral—A group of drugs to treat viral infection. These drugs include: Ophthalmic (eye)—idoxuridine, trifluridine, vidarabine. Systemic—acyclovir, amantadine, ribavirin, zidovudine. Topical—acyclovir.

Appendicitis—Inflammation or infection of the appendix. Symptoms include loss of appetite, nausea, low-grade fever and tenderness in the lower right of the abdomen.

Appetite Suppressants—A group of drugs used to decrease the appetite as part of an overall treatment for obesity. These drugs include: benzphetamine, cyproheptadine, diethylpropion, fenfluramine, mazindol, phendimetrazine, phenmetrazine, phentermine, phenylpropanolamine.

Artery—Blood vessel carrying blood away from the heart.

Asthma—Recurrent attacks of breathing difficulty due to spasms and contractions of the bronchial tubes.

Attentuated Virus Vaccines—Liquid products of killed germs used for injections to prevent certain diseases.

B

Bacteria—Microscopic organism. Some bacteria contribute to health; others (germs) cause disease.

Barbiturates—Powerful drugs used for sedation, to help induce sleep and sometimes to prevent seizures. Except for use in seizures (phenobarbital), barbiturates are being used less and less because there are better, less hazardous drugs that produce the same or better effects. These drugs include: amobarbital, aprobarbital, butabarbital, mephobarbital, metharbital, pentobarbital, phenobarbital, secobarbital, secobarbital and amobarbital, talbutal.

Basal Area of Brain—Part of the brain that regulates muscle control and tone.

Beta-agonists—A group of drugs that act directly on cells in the body (beta-adrenergic receptors) to relieve spasm of the bronchial tubes and other organs consisting of smooth muscles. These drugs include: albuterol, bitolerol, isoetharine, isoproterenol, methproterenol, terbutaline.

Beta-blockers (beta-adrenergic blocking agents)—A family of drugs with similar pharmacological actions with some variations. These drugs are prescribed for angina, heartbeat irregularities (arrhythmias), high blood pressure, hypertrophic subaortic stenosis, vascular headaches (as a preventative, not to treat once the pain begins), and others. Timolol is prescribed for treatment of open-angle glaucoma. These drugs include: acebutolol (Monitan, Sectral); atenolol (Esmolol); labetalol (Normodyne, Trandate); metoprolol (Apo-Metoprolol, Betaloc, Betaloc Durules, Lopresor, Lopresor SR, Lopressor, Novometoprol); nadolol (Corgard); oxprenolol (Trasicor, Slow-Trasicor); pindolol (Visken); propranolol (Apo-Propranolol, Detensol, Inderal, Inderal LA, Novopranol, pms-Propranolol); sotalol (Sotacor); timolol (Blocadren).

Benzodiazepines—A family of drugs prescribed to treat anxiety, alcohol withdrawal, and sometimes for sedation. These drugs include: alprazolam, bromazepam, chlordiazepoxide, clonazepam, clorazepate, diazepam, flurazepam, halazepam, ketazolam, lorazepam, midazolam, nitrazepam, oxazepam, prazepam, temazepam, triazolam.

Blood Count—Laboratory studies to count white-blood cells, red-blood cells, platelets and other elements of the blood.

Blood Pressure, Diastolic—Pressure (usually recorded in millimeters of mercury) in the large arteries of the body when the heart muscle is relaxed and filling for the next contraction.

Blood Pressure, Systolic—Pressure (usually recorded in millimeters of mercury) in the large arteries of the body at the instant the heart muscle contracts.

Blood Sugar (Blood Glucose)—Necessary element in the blood to sustain life.

Bone Marrow Depressants—Medicines that affect the bone marrow to depress the normal function of forming blood cells. These medicines include: anticancer drugs, antithyroid drugs, azathioprine, carbamazepine, chloramphenicol, flucytosine, penicillamine, phenylbutazone, primaquine, pyrimethamine, rifampin, sulfa drugs, tocainide, trimethoprim, valproic acid.

Brain Depressants—Any drug that depresses brain function, such as tranquilizers, narcotics, alcohol, barbiturates.

Bronchodilators—A group of drugs used to dilate the bronchial tubes to treat such problems as asthma, emphysema, bronchitis, bronchiectasis, allergies and others. These drugs include: albuterol, aminophylline, bitolterol, dyphylline, ephedrine, epinephrine, ethylnorepinephrine, fenoterol, ipratropium, isoetharine, isoproterenol, metaproterenol, oxtriphylline, oxtriphylline and guaifenesin, terbutaline, theophylline, theophylline and guaifenesin.

Bronchodilators, Xanthine Derivative—Drugs of similar chemical structure and pharmacological activity. They are prescribed to dilate bronchial tubes in disorders such as asthma, bronchitis, emphysema and other chronic lung diseases. These drugs include: aminophylline, dyphylline, oxtriphylline, theophylline.

C

Calcium-channel Blockers—A group of drugs used to treat angina and heartbeat irregularities. These drugs include diltiazem, nifedipine, verapamil.

Calcium Supplements—Supplements used to increase calcium concentration in the blood in hopes of making bones denser (as in osteoporosis). These supplements include: calcium citrate, calcium glubionate, calcium gluconate, calcium glycerophosphate and calcium lactate, calcium lactate, dibasic calcium phosphate, tribasic calcium phosphate.

Carbonic Anhydrase Inhibitors—Drugs used to treat glaucoma, seizures and prevent high altitude sickness. They include acetazolamide, dichlorphenamide, methazolamid.

Cataract—Loss of transparency in the lens of the eye.

Cell—Unit of protoplasm, the essential living matter of all plants and animals.

Central Nervous System (CNS) Depression-Producing Medications—These drugs cause sedation or otherwise diminish brain activity and other parts of the nervous system. These drugs include: alcohol, aminoglutethimide, anesthetics (general and injection-local), anticonvulsants, antidepressants (MAO inhibitors, TCA), antidyskinetics (except amantadine), antihistamines, apomorphine, baclofen, barbiturates, benzodiazepines, buclizine, carbamazepine, chloral hydrate, chlorzoxazone, clonidine, cyclizine, difenoxin and atropine, diphenoxylate and atropine, disulfiram, dronabinol, ethchlorvynol, ethinamate, etomidate, fenfluramine, flavoxate, glutethimide, guanabenz, guanfacine, haloperidol, hydroxyzine, interferon, loxapine, magnesium sulfate (injection), maprotiline, meclizine, meprobamate, methyldopa, methyprylon, metoclopramide, metyrosine, mitotane, molindone, opioid (narcotic) analgesics, oxybutynin, paraldehyde, paregoric, pargyline, phenothiazines, pimozide, procarbazine, promethazine, propiomazine, rauwolfia alkaloids, scopolamine, skeletal muscle relaxants (centrally acting), thioxanthenes, trazodone, trimeprazine, trimethobenzamide.

Central Nervous System (CNS) Stimulants—Drugs that cause excitation, anxiety, nervousness or otherwise stimulate the brain and other parts of the central nervous system. These drugs include: amantadine, amphetamines, anesthetics (local), appetite suppressants (except fenfluramine), bronchodilators (xanthine-derivative), caffeine, chlophedianol, cocaine, doxapram, methylphenidate, pemoline, sympathomimetics.

Cephalosporin—Antibiotic that kills many bacterial germs that penicillin and sulfa drugs can't destroy.

Cholinergic (Parasympathomimetic)— Chemical that facilitates passage of nerve impulses through the parasympathetic nervous system.

Chronic—Long-term, continuing. Chronic illnesses may not be curable, but they can often be prevented from becoming worse. Symptoms usually can be alleviated or controlled.

Cirrhosis—Disease that scars and destroys liver tissue.

Citrates—Medicines taken orally to make urine more acid. Citrates include: potassium citrate, potassium citrate and citric acid, potassium citrate and sodium citrate, sodium citrate and citric acid, tricitrates.

Coal Tar Preparations—Creams, ointments and lotions used on the skin for various skin ailments.

Cold Urticaria—Hives that appear in areas of the body exposed to the cold.

Colitis, Ulcerative—Chronic, recurring ulcers of the colon for unknown reasons.

Collagen—Support tissue of skin, tendon, bone, cartilage and connective tissue.

Colostomy—Surgical opening from the colon, the large intestine, to the outside of the body.

Congestive—Excess accumulation of blood. In congestive heart failure, congestion occurs in the lungs, liver, kidney and other parts of the body to cause shortness of breath, swelling of the ankles and feet, rapid heartbeat and other symptoms.

Constriction—Tightness or pressure.

Contraceptives (birth-control pills)—A group of hormones used to prevent ovulation, therefore preventing pregnancy. These hormones include: ethynodiol diacetate and ethinyl estradiol, ethynodiol diacetate and mestranol, levonorgestrel and ethinyl estradiol, medroxyprogesterone, norethindrone tablets, norethindrone acetate and ethinyl estradiol, norethindrone and ethinyl estradiol, norethindrone and mestranol, norethynodrel and mestranol, norgestrel, norgestrel and ethinyl estradiol.

Convulsions—Violent, uncontrollable contractions of the voluntary muscles.

Corticosteroid (Adrenocorticosteroid)—Steroid hormones produced by the body's adrenal cortex or their synthetic equivalents.

Cortisone (Adrenocorticoids, Glucocorticoids) and other Adrenal Steroids—Medicines that mimic the action of the steroid hormone cortisone, manufactured in the cortex of the adrenal gland. These drugs decrease the effects of inflammation within the body. They are available for injection, oral use, topical use

for the skin and nose and inhalation for the bronchial tubes. These drugs include: alclometasone; amcinonide; beclomethasone; benzyl benzoate; betamethasone; bismuth; clobetasol; clobetasone 17-butyrate; clocortolone; cortisone; desonide; desoximetasone; desoxycorticosterone; dexamethasone; diflorasone; diflucortolone; fludrocortisone; flumethasone; flunisolide; fluocinonide; fluocinonide, procinonide and ciprocinonide; fluorometholone; flurandrenolide; halcinonide; hydrocortisone; medrysone; methylprednisolone; mometasone; paramethasone; peruvian balsam; prednisolone; prednisone; triamcinolone; zinc oxide.

Cystitis—Inflammation of the urinary bladder.

D

Decongestants—Drugs used to open nasal passages by shrinking swollen lining membranes in the nose. These drugs include: Cough-suppressing—phenylephrine and dextromethorphan, phenylpropanolamine and caramiphen, phenylpropanolamine and dextromethorphan, phenylpropanolamine and hydrocodone, pseudoephedrine and codeine, pseudoephedrine and dextromethorphan, pseudoephedrine and hydrocodone. Cough-suppressing and pain-relieving—phenylpropanolamine, dextromethorphan and acetaminophen. Cough-suppressing and sputum-thinning—phenylephrine, dextromethorphan and guaifenesin; phenylephrine, hydrocodone and guaifenesin; phenylpropanolamine, codeine and guaifenesin; phenylpropanolamine, dextromethorphan and guaifenesin; pseudoephedrine, codeine and guaifenesin; pseudoephedrine, dextromethorphan and guaifenesin; pseudoephedrine, hydrocodone and guaifenesin; phenylephrine, dextromethorphan, guaifenesin and acetaminophen; pseudoephedrine, dextromethorphan, guaifenesin and acetaminophen. Sputum-thinning—ephedrine and guaifenesin; ephedrine and potassium iodide; phenylephrine, phenylpropanolamine and guaifenesin; phenylpropanolamine and guaifenesin; pseudoephedrine and guaifenesin. Nasal—ephedrine (oral), phenylpropanolamine, pseudoephedrine. Ophthalmic (eye)—naphazoline, oxymetazoline, phenylephrine. Topical—oxymetazoline, phenylephrine, xylometazoline.

Delirium—Temporary mental disturbance characterized by hallucinations, agitation and incoherence.

Diabetes—Metabolic disorder in which the body can't use carbohydrates efficiently. This leads to a dangerously high level of glucose (a carbohydrate) in the blood.

Dialysis—Procedure to filter waste products from the bloodstream of patients with kidney failure.

Digitalis Preparations (digitalis glycosides)—Important drugs to treat heart disease, such as congestive heart failure, heartbeat irregularities and cardiogenic shock. These drugs include: deslanoside (Cedilanid); powdered digitalis (Crystodigin); digoxin (Lanoxin, Lanoxicaps).

Digoxin—One of the digitalis drugs used to treat heart disease. All digitalis products were originally derived from the fox-glove plant.

Dilation—Enlargement.

Disulfiram Reaction—Disulfiram (Antabuse) is a drug to treat alcoholism. When alcohol in the bloodstream interacts with disulfiram, it causes a flushed face, severe headache, chest pains, shortness of breath, nausea, vomiting, sweating and weakness. Severe reactions may cause death. A disulfiram reaction is the interaction of any drug with alcohol or another drug to produce these symptoms.

Diuretics—Drugs that act on the kidneys to prevent reabsorption of electrolytes, especially chlorides. They are used to treat edema, high blood pressure, congestive heart failure, kidney and liver failure and others. These drugs include: amiloride, amiloride and hydrochlorothiazide, bendroflumethiazide, benzthiazide, bumetanide, chlorothiazide, chlorthalidone, cyclothiazide, ethacrynic acid, furosemide, glycerin, hydrochlorothiazide, hydroflumethiazide, indapamide, mannitol, methyclothiazide, metolazone, polythiazide, quinethazone, spironolactone, sprionolactone and hydrochlorothiazide, triamterene, triamterene and hydrochlorothiazide, trichlormethiazide, urea.

Diuretics, Loop—Drugs that act on the kidneys to prevent reabsorption of electrolytes, especially chlorides. They are used to treat edema, high blood pressure, congestive heart failure, kidney and liver failure and others. These drugs include: bumetanide, ethacrynic acid, furosemide.

Diuretics, Thiazide—Drugs that act on the kidneys to prevent reabsorption of electrolytes, especially chlorides. They are used to treat edema, high blood pressure, congestive heart failure, kidney and liver failure and others. These drugs include: bendroflumethiazide (Naturetin); benzthiazide (Aquatag, Exna, Hydrex); chlorothiazide (Diuril); chlorthalidone (Apo-Chlorthalidone, Hygroton, Novothalidone, Thalitone, Uridon); cyclothiazide (Anhydron,

Fluidil); hydrochlorothiazide (Apo-Hydro, Diuchlor H, Esidrix, Hydrochlorothiazide Intensol, HydroDIURIL, Mictrin, Natrimax, Neo-Codema, Novohydrazide, Oretic, Thiuretic, Urozide); hydroflumethiazide (Diucardin, Saluron); methyclothiazide (Aquatensen, Duretic, Enduron); metolazone (Diulo, Zaroxolyn); polythiazide (Renese); quinethazone (Aquamox, Hydromox); trichlormethiazide (Metahydrin, Naqua).

Diuretics, Potassium-Sparing—Drugs that act on the kidneys to prevent reabsorption of electrolytes, especially chlorides. They are used to treat edema, high blood pressure, congestive heart failure, kidney and liver failure and others. This particular group of diuretics does not allow the unwanted side effect of low potassium in the blood to occur. These drugs include: amiloride, spironolactone, triamterene.

Duodenum—The first 12 inches of the small intestine.

E

Eczema—Disorder of the skin with redness, itching, blisters, weeping and abnormal pigmentation.

Electrolyte—Substance that can transmit electrical impulses when dissolved in body fluids.

Embolism—Sudden blockage of an artery by a clot or foreign material in the blood.

Emphysema—Disease in which the lung's air sacs lose elasticity, and air accumulates in the lungs.

Endometriosis—Condition in which uterus tissue is found outside the uterus. Can cause pain, abnormal menstruation and infertility.

Enzyme—Protein chemical that can accelerate a chemical reaction in the body.

Epilepsy—Episodes of brain disturbance that cause convulsions and loss of consciousness.

Ergot Preparations—Medicines used to treat migraine and other types of throbbing headaches. Also used after delivery of babies to make the uterus clamp down and reduce excessive bleeding.

Erythromycins—A group of drugs with similar structure used to treat infections. These drugs include: erythromycin (Eryc, Eryc Sprinkle, Erythromid, Novorythro, E-Mycin, Ery-Tab, Ilotycin, PCE Dispersatabs, Robimycin, RP-Mycin); erythromycin estolate (Ilosone, Novorythro); erythromycin ethylsuccinate (E.E.S., E-Mycin E, Pediamycin, Wyamycin E, EryPed); erythromycin gluceptate (Ilotycin); erythromycin lactobionate (Erythrocin); erythromycin stearate (ApoErythro-S).

Esophagitis—Inflammation of the lower part of the esophagus, the tube connecting the throat and the stomach.

Estrogens—Female hormones used to replenish the body's stores after the ovaries have been removed or become non-functional after menopause. Also used with progesterone in some birth-control pills and for other purposes. These drugs include: Systemic—chlorotrianisene, diethylstilbestrol, estradiol, estrogens (conjugated and esterified), estrone, estropipate, ethinyl estradiol, quinestrol. Vaginal—dienestrol, estradiol, estrogens (conjugated), estrone, estropipate.

Eustachian Tube—Small passage from the middle ear to the sinuses and nasal passages.

Extrapyramidal Reactions—Drugs that may cause abnormal reactions in the power and coordination of posture and muscular movements. Movements are not under voluntary control. Some drugs associated with producing extrapyramidal reactions include: antidepressants (tricyclic), droperidol, haloperidol, loxapine, methyldopa, metoclopramide, metyrosine, molindone, pemoline, phenothiazines, pimozide, rauwolfia alkaloids, thioxanthenes.

Extremity—Arm, leg, hand or foot.

F

Fecal Impaction—Condition in which feces become firmly wedged in the rectum.

Fibrocystic Breast Disease—Overgrowth of fibrous tissue in the breast, producing non-malignant cysts.

Fibroid Tumors—Non-malignant tumors of the muscular layer of the uterus.

Flu (Influenza)—A virus infection of the respiratory tract that lasts three to ten days. Symptoms include headache, fever, runny nose, cough, tiredness and muscle aches.

Folliculitis—Inflammation of a follicle.

G

G6PD—Deficiency of glucose 6-phosphate, necessary for glucose metabolism.

Ganglionic Blockers—Medicines that block the passage of nerve impulses through a part of the nerve cell called a ganglion. Ganglionic blockers are used to treat urinary retention and other medical problems. Bethanechol is one of the best ganglionic blockers.

Gastritis—Inflammation of the stomach.

Gastrointestinal—Stomach and intestinal tract.

Gland—Cells that manufacture and excrete materials not required for their own metabolic needs.

Glaucoma—Eye disease in which increased pressure inside the eye damages the optic nerve, causes pain and changes vision.

Glucagon—Injectable drug that immediately elevates blood sugar by mobilizing glycogen from the liver.

Gold Compounds—Medicines which use gold as their base and are usually used to treat joint or arthritic disorders. These medicines include auranofin, aurothioglucose, gold sodium thiomalate.

H

Hangover Effect—The same feelings as a "hangover" after too much alcohol consumption. Symptoms include headache, irritability and nausea.

Hemochromatosis—Disorder of iron metabolism in which excessive iron is deposited in and damages body tissues, particularly liver and pancreas.

Hemoglobin—Pigment that carries oxygen in red-blood cells.

Hemorrhage—Heavy bleeding.

Hemorrheologic Agents—Medicines to help control bleeding.

Hemosiderosis—Increase of iron deposits in body tissues without tissue damage.

Hepatitis—Inflammation of liver cells, usually accompanied by jaundice.

Hepatotoxic—Medications that can possibly cause toxicity or decreased normal function of the liver. These drugs include: acetaminophen (with long-term, high-dose use or acute overdose), 4-aminoquinolines, amiodarone, anabolic steroids, androgens, antithyroid agents, asparaginase, azlocillin, carbamazepine, carmustine, contraceptives (estrogen-containing, oral), dantrolene, daunorubicin, disulfiram, divalproex, erythromycins, estrogens, etretinate, gold compounds, halothane, isoniazid, ketoconazole (oral), mercaptopurine, methotrexate, methyldopa, mezlocillin, naltrexone (with long-term, high-dose use), nitrofurans, phenothiazines, phenytoin, piperacillin, plicamycin, rifampin, sulfonamides (systemic), tetracycline (intravenous), valproic acid.

Hiatal Hernia—Section of stomach that protrudes into the chest cavity.

Histamine—Chemical in body tissues that dilates the smallest blood vessels, constricts the smooth muscle surrounding the bronchial tubes and stimulates stomach secretions.

History—Past medical events in a patient's life.

Hives—Elevated patches on the skin that are redder or paler than surrounding skin and often itch severely.

Hormone—Chemical substance produced in the body to regulate other body functions.

Hypertension—High blood pressure.

Hypnotics—Drugs used to induce a sleeping state. See Barbiturates.

Hypocalcemia—Abnormally low level of calcium in the blood.

Hypoglycemia—Low blood sugar (blood glucose). A critically low blood-sugar level will interfere with normal brain function and can damage the brain permanently.

Hypoglycemics, Oral—Drugs that reduce blood sugar. These include: insulin, acetohexamide, chlorpropamide, glipizide, glyburide, metformin, tolazamide, tolbutamide.

Hypotension—Blood pressure decreased below normal. Symptoms may include weakness, lightheadedness, dizziness. Some medications that might cause hypotension include: alcohol, alprostadil, amantadine, anesthetics (general), angiotensin-converting enzyme inhibitors (ACE inhibitors), antidepressants (MAO inhibitors, tricyclic), antihypertensives, benzodiazepines used as preanesthetics, beta-adrenergic blocking agents, bromocriptine, calcium channel-blocking agents, captopril, diuretics, edetate calcium disodium, edetate disodium, enalapril, encainide, haloperidol, hydralazine, levodopa, lidocaine (systemic), loxapine, maprotiline, molindone, nitrates, nitrites, opioid analgesics (including fentanil, fentanyl and sufentanil), pentamidine, phenothiazines, pimozide, prazosin, procainamide, quinidine, radiopaques (materials used in x-ray studies), thioxanthenes, tocainide, trazodone. If you take any of these medications, be sure to tell a dentist, anesthesiologist or anyone else who intends to give you an anesthetic to put you to sleep.

I

Ichthyosis—Skin disorder with dryness, scaling and roughness.

Ileitis—Inflammation of the ileum, the last section of the small intestine.

Ileostomy—Surgical opening from the ileum, the end of the small intestine, to the outside of the body.

Immunosuppressants—Powerful drugs that suppress the immune system. Immunosuppressants are used in patients who have had organ transplants or severe disease associated with the immune system. These drugs include: azathioprine, betamethasone, chlorambucil, corticotropin, cortisone, cyclophosphamide, cyclosporine, dexamethasone,

hydrocortisone, mercaptopurine, methylprednisolone, muromonab-CD3, paramethasone, prednisolone, prednisone, triamcinolone.

Impotence—Male's inability to achieve or sustain erection of the penis for sexual intercourse.

Insomnia—Sleeplessness.

Interaction—Change in the body's response to one drug when another is taken. Interaction may decrease the effect of one or both drugs, decrease the effect of one or both drugs, or cause toxicity.

Iron Supplements—Products that contain iron in a form that can be absorbed from the intestinal tract. Supplements include: ferrous fumarate, ferrous gluconate, ferrous sulfate, iron dextran, iron-polysaccharide.

J

Jaundice—Symptoms of liver damage, bile obstruction or red-blood-cell destruction. Symptoms include yellowed whites of the eyes, yellow skin, dark urine and light stool.

K

Keratosis—Growth that is an accumulation of cells from the outer skin layers.

Kidney Stones—Small, solid stones made from calcium, cholesterol, cysteine and other body chemicals.

L

Laxatives—Medicines prescribed to treat constipation. These medicines include: bisacodyl; bisacodyl and docusate; casanthranol; casanthranol and docusate; cascara sagrada; cascara sagrada and aloe; cascara sagrada and phenolphthalein; castor oil; danthron; danthron and docusate; danthron and poloxamer 188; dehydrocholic acid; dehydrocholic acid and docusate; docusate; docusate and phenolphthalein; docusate and mineral oil; docusate and phenolphthalein; docusate, carboxymethylcellulose and casanthranol glycerin; lactulose; magnesium citrate; magnesium hydroxide; magnesium hydroxide and mineral oil; magnesium oxide; magnesium sulfate; malt soup extract; malt soup extract and psyllium; methylcellulose; mineral oil; mineral oil and cascara sagrada; mineral oil and phenolphthalein; mineral oil, glycerin and phenolphthalein; phenolphthalein; poloxamer; polycarbophil; potassium bitartrate and sodium bicarbonate; psyllium; psyllium and senna; psyllium hydrophilic mucilloid; psyllium hydrophilic mucilloid and carboxymethyl-cellulose; psyllium hydrophilic mucilloid and sennosides; psyllium hydrophilic musilloid and senna; senna; senna and docusate; sennosides; sodium phosphate.

Lincomycins—A family of antibiotics used to treat certain infections. These antibiotics include: erythromycin, erythromycin estolate, erythromycin ethylsuccinate, erythromycin gluceptate, erythromycin lactobionate, erythromycin stearate.

Low-Purine Diet—A diet that avoids high-purine foods, such as liver, sweetbreads, kidneys, sardines, oysters and others. If you need a low-purine diet, request instructions from your doctor.

Lupus—Serious disorder of connective tissue that primarily affects women. Varies in severity with skin eruptions, joint inflammation, low white-blood cell count and damage to internal organs, especially the kidney.

Lymph Glands—Glands in the lymph vessels throughout the body that trap foreign and infectious matter and protect the bloodstream from infection.

M

MAO Inhibitors—Drugs that prevent the activity of the enzyme monoamine oxidase (MAO) in brain tissue, thus affecting mood. MAO inhibitors include antidepressants, the use of which is frequently restricted because of severe side effects. These side effects may be interactions with other drugs (such as ephedrine or amphetamine) or foods containing tyramine (such as cheese) and may produce a sudden increase in blood pressure. MAOs include isocarboxazid, pargyline, phenelzine, tranylcypromine.

Male Hormones—Chemical substances secreted by the testicles, ovaries and adrenal glands in humans. Some male hormones used by humans are derived synthetically. Male hormones include: testosterone cypionate and estradiol cypionate, testosterone enanthate and estradiol valerate.

Manic-Depressive Illness—Psychosis with alternating cycles of excessive enthusiasm and depression.

Mast Cell—Connective-tissue cell.

Menopause—The end of menstruation in the female, often accompanied by irritability, hot flushes, changes in the skin and bones and vaginal dryness.

Metabolism—Process of using nutrients and energy to build and break down wastes.

Migraine—Periodic headaches caused by constriction of arteries to the skull. Symptoms include severe pain, vision disturbances, nausea, vomiting and light sensitivity.

Mind-Altering Drugs—Any drug that decreases alertness, perception, concentration, contact with reality or muscular coordination.

Monoamine Oxidase (MAO) Inhibitors—See MAO Inhibitors.

Muscle Relaxants—Medicines to lessen painful contractions and spasms of muscles. These include: atracurium, carisoprodol, chlorphenesin, chlorzoxazone, cyclobenzaprine, metaxalone, methcarbamol, metocurine, orphenadrine citrate, pancuronium, succinylcholine, tubocurarine, vecuronium.

Myasthenia Gravis—Disease of the muscles characterized by fatigue and progressive paralysis. It is usually confined to muscles of the face, lips, tongue and neck.

N

Narcotics—A group of habit-forming, addicting drugs used for treatment of pain, diarrhea, cough, acute pulmonary edema and others. They are all dervied from opium, a milky exudate in capsules of *Papaver somniferum*. Law requires licensed physicians to dispense by prescription. These drugs include: alfentanil, buprenorphine, butorphanol, codeine, fentanyl, heroin, hydrocodone, hydromorphone, levorphanol, meperidine, methadone, morphine, nalbuphine, opium, oxycodone, oxymorphone, paregoric, pentazocine, propoxyphene, sufetanil.

Nephrotoxic Medications (Kidney-Poisoning)—Under some circumstances, these medicines can be toxic to the kidneys. These medicines include: acyclovir; aminoglycosides; amphotericin B (given internally); analgesic combinations containing acetaminophen and aspirin or other salicylates (with chronic high-dose use); anti-inflammatory analgesics (non-steroidal); bacitracin (given internally); capreomycin; captopril; carmustine; cisplatin; cyclosporine; demeclocycline (nephrogenic diabetes insipidus); edetate calcium disodium (with high doses); edetate disodium (with high dose); enalapril; gold compounds; lithium; methotrexate (with high dose therapy); methoxyflurane; neomycin (oral); penicillamine; pentamidine; plicamycin; polymyxins (given internally); radiopaques (materials used for special x-ray examinations); rifampin; streptozocin; sulfonamides; tetracyclines (other, except doxycycline and minocycline); vancomycin (given internally).

Neuromuscular Blocking Agents—A group of drugs prescribed to relax skeletal muscles. They are all given by injection and descriptions are not included in this book. These drugs include: atracurium, gallamine, metocurine, pancuronium, succinylcholine, tubocurarine, vecuronium.

Nitrates—Medicines made from a chemical with a nitrogen base. Nitrates include erythrityl tetranitrate, isosorbide dinitrate, nitroglycerin, pentaerythritol tetranitrate.

Non-steroidal Anti-inflammatory Drugs (NSAIDs)—See Anti-inflammatory, Non-steroidal.

Nutritional Supplements—Substances used to treat and prevent deficiencies when the body is unable to absorb them by eating a well-balanced, nutritional diet. These supplements include: Vitamins—ascorbic acid, ascorbic acid and sodium ascorbate, calcifediol, calcitriol, calcium pantothenate, cyanocobalamin, dihydrotachysterol, ergocalciferol, folate sodium, folic acid, hydroxocobalamin, niacin, niacinamide, pantothenic, pyridoxine, riboflavin, sodium ascorbate, thiamine, vitamin A, vitamin E. Minerals—calcium carbonate, calcium citrate, calcium glubionate, calcium gluconate, calcium lactate, calcium phosphate (dibasic and tribasic), sodium fluoride. Other—levocarnitine, omega-3 polyunsaturated fatty acids.

O

Opiates—Pain-killing medicines derived from opium that have a high index of addiction. Some of these include: butorphanol, codeine, hydrocodone, hydromorphone, levorphanol, meperidine, methadone, morphine, nalbuphine, opium, oxycodone, oxymorphone, paregoric, pentazocine, propoxyphene.

Osteoporosis—Softening of bones caused by a loss of chemicals usually found in bone.

Ototoxic Medications—These medicines may possibly cause hearing damage. They include: aminoglycosides, 4-aminoquinolines, anti-inflammatory analgesics (non-steroidal), bumetanide, capreomyucin, cisplatin, deferoxamine, erythromycins, ethacrynic acid, furosemide, minocycline, quinine, salicylates, vancomycin.

Ovary—Female sexual gland where eggs mature and ripen for fertilization.

P

Pain Relievers—Non-narcotic medicines to treat pain.

Palpitations—Rapid heartbeat noticeable to the patient.

Pancreatitis—Serious inflammation or infection of the pancreas that causes upper abdominal pain.

Parkinson's Disease—Disease of the central nervous system. Characteristics are a fixed, emotionless expression of the face, tremor, slower muscle movements, weakness, changed gait and a peculiar posture.

Pellagra—Disease caused by a deficiency of the water-soluble vitamin, thiamine (vitamin B-1). Symptoms include brain disturbance, diarrhea and skin inflammation.

Penicillin—Chemical substance (antibiotic) originally discovered as a product of mold, which can kill some bacterial germs.

Phenothiazines—Drugs used to treat mental, nervous and emotional conditions. These drugs include: acetophenazine, chlorpromazine, fluphenazine, mesoridazine, perphenazine, prochlorperazine, promazine, thioridazine, trifluoperazine, triflupromazine.

Phlegm—Thick mucus secreted by glands in the respiratory tract.

Photosensitizing Medications—Medicines that can cause abnormally-heightened skin reactions to the effects of sunlight. These medicines include: amiodarone, anthralin, antidiabetic agents (oral), antihistamines, benzocaine, coal tar, contraceptives (estrogen-containing, oral), diuretics, thiazide, estrogens, ethionamide, etretinate, fluorouracil, furosemide, griseofulvin, isotretinoin, ketoprofen, methotrexate, methoxsalen, nalidixic acid, naproxen, phenothiazines, phenylbutazone, piroxicam, pyrazinamide, sulfonamides, sulindac, tetracyclines, thioxanthenes, tretinoin, trioxsalen.

Pinworms—Common intestinal parasite that causes rectal itching and irritation.

Pituitary Gland—Gland at the base of the brain that secretes hormones to stimulate growth and other glands to produce hormones.

Platelet—Disc-shaped element of the blood, smaller than red- or white-blood cells, necessary for blood clotting.

Polyp—Growth on a mucous membrane.

Porphyria—Inherited metabolic disorder characterized by changes in the nervous system and kidney.

Post-partum—Following delivery of a baby.

Potassium—Important chemical found in body cells.

Potassium Foods—Foods high in potassium content, including dried apricots and peaches, lentils, raisins, citrus and whole-grain cereals.

Potassium Supplements—Medicines needed by people who don't have enough potassium in their diets or by those who develop a deficiency due to illness or taking diuretics and other medicines. These supplements include: chloride; potassium acetate; potassium bicarbonate; potassium bicarbonate and potassium chloride; potassium bicarbonate and potassium citrate; potassium chloride; potassium chloride, potassium bicarbonate and potassium citrate; potassium gluconate; potassium gluconate and potassium chloride; potassium gluconate and potassium citrate; potassium gluconate, potassium citrate and ammonium; trikates.

Prostate—Gland in the male that surrounds the neck of the bladder and the urethra.

Prothrombin—Blood substance essential in clotting.

Prothrombin Time—Laboratory study used to follow prothrombin activity and keep coagulation safe.

Psoriasis—Chronic, inherited skin disease. Symptoms are lesions with silvery scales on the edges.

Psychosis—Mental disorder characterized by deranged personality, loss of contact with reality and possible delusions, hallucinations or illusions.

Purine Foods—Foods that are metabolized into uric acid. Foods high in purines include anchovies, liver, brains, sweetbreads, sardines, kidney, oysters, gravy and meat extracts.

R

Rauwolfia Alkaloids—Drugs that belong to the family of antihypertensives (to lower blood pressure). Rauwolfia alkaloids are not used as extensively as in years past. They include: alseroxylon, deserpidine, rausolfia serpentina, reserpine.

RDA—Recommended daily allowance of a vitamin or mineral.

Rebound Effect—Return of a condition, often with increased severity, once the prescribed drug is withdrawn.

Renal—Pertaining to the kidney.

Retina—Innermost covering of the eyeball on which the image is formed.

Reye's Syndrome—Rare, sometimes fatal, disease of children that causes brain and liver damage.

Rickets—Bone disease caused by vitamin-D deficiency. Bones become bent and distorted during infancy or childhood.

S

Salicylates—Medicines to relieve pain and reduce fever. These include: aspirin, aspirin and caffeine, buffered aspirin, choline salicylate, choline and magnesium salicylates, magnesium salicylate, salicylamide, salsalate, sodium salicylate.

Sedative—Drug that reduces excitement or anxiety.

Seizure—Brain disorder causing changes of consciousness or convulsions.

Sick Sinus Syndrome—A complicated, serious heartbeat rhythm disturbance characterized by a slow heart rate alternating with a fast or slow heart rate with heart block.

Sinusitis—Inflammation or infection of the sinus cavities in the skull.

Skeletal Muscle Relaxants—A group of drugs prescribed to treat spasm of skeletal muscles. These drugs include: carisoprodol, chlorphenesin, chlorzoxazone, cyclobenzaprine, diazepam, lorazepam, metaxalone, methocarbamol, orphenadrine, phenytoin.

Sleep Inducers—Night-time sedatives to aid in falling asleep. See Benzodiazepines.

Stimulants, Central Nervous System (CNS)—Drugs that stimulate the brain and spinal cord nerves. These drugs include: amphetamine, caffeine, caffeine (citrated), caffeine and sodium benzoate, cocaine, dextroamphetamine, ephedrine (oral), methamphetamine, methylphenidate, pemoline.

Streptococcus—Bacteria that causes infections in the throat, respiratory system and skin. Improperly treated, can lead to disease in the heart, joints and kidneys.

Stroke—Sudden, severe attack. Usually sudden paralysis from injury to the brain or spinal cord caused by a blood clot or hemorrhage in the brain.

Stupor—Near unconsciousness.

Sublingual—Under the tongue. Some drugs are absorbed almost as quickly this way as by injection.

Sulfonamides—Sulfa drugs prescribed to treat infections. They include: sulfacytine, sulfamethoxazole, sulfamethoxazole and trimethoprin, sulfasalazine, sulfisoxazole.

Sympathomimetics—A large group of drugs that mimic the effects of stimulation of the *sympathetic* part of the autonomic nervous system. These drugs include: adrenalin (epinephrine); appetite suppressants (such as benzphetamine, diethylpropion, fenfluramine, mazindol, phendimetrazine, phenmetrazine, phentermine, phenylpropanolamine); aramine; dobutamine; ephedrine; mephentermine; methoxamine; phenylephrine; metaraminol; isoproterenol.

T

Tardive Dyskinesia—Involuntary movements of the jaw, lips and tongue caused by an unpredictable drug reaction.

Tartrazine Dye—A dye used in foods and medicine preparations that may cause an allergic reaction in some people.

Tetracyclines—A group of medicines with similar chemical structure used to treat infections. These drugs include: demeclocycline, doxycycline, methacycline, minocycline, oxytetracycline, tetracycline.

Thiazides—A group of chemicals that cause diuresis (loss of water through the kidney). Frequently used to treat high blood pressure and congestive heart failure. Thiazides include: bendroflumethiazide, benzthiazide, chlorothiazide, cyclothiazide, hydrochlorothiazide, hydroflumethiazide, methyclothiazide, polythiazide, trichlormethiazide.

Thiothixines—See Thioxanthenes.

Thioxanthenes—Drugs used to treat emotional, mental and nervous conditions. These drugs include chlorprothixene, fluphenthixol, thiothixene.

Thrombolytic Agents—Drugs that help to dissolve blood clots. They include alteplase, streptokinase, urokinase.

Thrombophlebitis—Inflammation of a vein caused by a blood clot in the vein.

Thyroid—Gland in the neck that manufactures and secretes several hormones.

Thyroid Hormones—Medications that mimic the action of the thyroid hormone made in the thyroid gland. They include: levothyroxine, liothyronine, liotrix, thyroglobulin, thyroid.

Tic-douloureaux—Painful condition caused by inflammation of a nerve in the face.

Toxicity—Poisonous reaction to a drug that impairs body functions or damages cells.

Transdermal Patches—There are more and more medications in a form known as transdermal (stick-on) patches. If you are using this form, follow these instructions: Choose an area of skin without cuts, scars or hair, such as the upper arm, chest or behind the ear. Thoroughly clean the area where patch is to be applied. If patch gets wet and loose, cover with an additional piece of plastic. Apply a fresh patch if the first one falls off. Apply each dose to a different area of skin if possible.

Tranquilizer—Drug that calms a person without clouding consciousness.

Tremor—Involuntary trembling.

Trichomoniasis—Infestation of the vagina by *trichomonas*, an infectious organism. The infection causes itching, vaginal discharge and irritation.

Triglyceride—Fatty chemical manufactured from carbohydrates for storage in fat cells.

Tyramine—Normal chemical component of the body that helps sustain blood pressure. Can rise to fatal levels in combination with some drugs.

Tyramine is found in many foods:

Beverages—Alcohol beverages, especially Chianti or robust red wines, vermouth, ale, beer.

Breads—Homemade bread with a lot of yeast and breads or crackers containing cheese.

Fats—Sour cream.

Fruits—Bananas, red plums, avocados, figs, raisins.

Meats and meat substitutes—Aged game, liver, canned meats, salami, sausage, cheese, salted dried fish, pickled herring.

Vegetables—Italian broad beans, green-bean pods, eggplant.

Miscellaneous—Yeast concentrates or extracts, marmite, soup cubes, commercial gravy, soy sauce, any protein food that has been stored improperly or is spoiled.

U

Ulcer, Peptic—Open sore on the mucous membrane of the esophagus, stomach or duodenum caused by stomach acid.

Urethra—Hollow tube through which urine (and semen in men) is discharged.

Urethritis—Inflammation or infection of the urethra.

Urinary Acidifiers—Medications that cause urine to become acid. These include: ascorbic acid, potassium phosphate, potassium and sodium phosphates.

Urinary Alkalizers—Medications that cause urine to become alkaline. These include: potassium citrate, potassium citrate and citric acid, potassium citrate and sodium citrate, sodium bicarbonate, sodium citrate and citric acid, tricitrate.

Uterus—Also called womb. A hollow muscular organ in the female in which the embryo develops into a fetus.

V

Vascular—Pertaining to blood vessels.

Vascular Headache (Preventative)—Medicines prescribed to prevent the occurrence of or reduce the frequency and severity of vascular headache such as migraine. These drugs include: atenolol; clonidine; ergotamine, belladonna alkaloids and phenobarbital; fenoprofen; ibuprofen; indomethacin; lithium; mefenamic acid; methysergide; metoprolol; nadolol; naproxen; pizotyline; propranolol; timolol.

Vascular Headache (Treatment)—Medicine prescribed to treat vascular headaches such as migraine. These drugs include: dihydroergotamine; ergotamine; ergotamine and caffeine; ergotamine, caffeine, belladonna alkaloids and pentobarbital; fenoprofen; ibuprofen; indomethacin (capsules, oral suspension, rectal); isometheptene, dichloralphenazone and acetaminophen; naproxen.

Virus—Infectious organism that reproduces in the cells of the infected host.

Y

Yeast—A single-cell organism that can cause infections of the mouth, vagina, skin and parts of the gastrointestinal system.

GUIDE TO INDEX

Alphabetical entries in the index include three categories—generic names, brand names and drug-class names.

1. Generic names appear in capital letters, following by their chart page number:
     ASPIRIN 112

2. Brand names appear in *italic*, followed by their generic ingredient and chart page number:
     Bayer - See ASPIRIN 112

   Some brand names contain two or more generic ingredients. These generic ingredients are listed in capital letters, following the brand name:
     Cefinal - See
       ASPIRIN 112
       CAFFEINE 172

3. Drug-class names appear in regular type, capital and lower-case letters. All generic drug names in this book that fall into a drug class are listed after the class name:
     Anticonvulsant - See
       CARBAMAZEPINE 184
       DIVALPOREX 374
       PHENOBARBITAL 780
       PRIMIDONE 828
       VALPROIC ACID (Dipropylacetic Acid) 1028

2/C-DM - See DEXTROMETHORPHAN 336
2/G - See GUAIFENESIN 480
2/G-DM - See GUAIFENESIN 480
4-Way Cold Tablets - See
  ASPIRIN 112
  CHLORPHENIRAMINE 236
  PHENYLPROPANOLAMINE 794
4-Way Long-Acting Nasal - See XYLOMETAZOLINE 1048
4-Way Nasal Spray - See
  PYRILAMINE 866
  PHENYLEPHRINE 790
  PHENYLPROPANOLAMINE 794
4-Way Tablets - See PHENYLEPHRINE 790
6-MP - See MERCAPTOPURINE 614
8-Hour Bayer Timed Release - See ASPIRIN 112
17-Valerate Celestone - See BETAMETHASONE 142
17-Valerate Diprosone - See BETAMETHASONE 142
216 DM - See DEXTROMETHORPHAN 336
222 - See NARCOTIC & ASPIRIN 692
282 - See NARCOTIC & ASPIRIN 692
292 - See NARCOTIC & ASPIRIN 692
293 - See NARCOTIC & ASPIRIN 692
445 Anti-Pain Compound - See ACETAMINOPHEN & SALICYLATES 6
642 - See NARCOTIC ANALGESICS 690
692 - See NARCOTIC & ASPIRIN 692

A

ABC Compound with Codeine - See BUTALBITAL, ASPIRIN & CODEINE (Also contains caffeine) 170
Abortifacient (a prostoglandin) - See DINOPROSTONE (Vaginal) 358
A&C with Codeine - See NARCOTIC & ASPIRIN 692
A.C.&C. - See NARCOTIC & ASPIRIN 692
Accurate Forte - See ACETAMINOPHEN & SALICYLATES 6

Accurbron - See XANTHINE BRONCHODILATORS 1046
Accutane - See ISOTRETINOIN 538
ACE inhibitor - See
  CAPTOPRIL 180
  CAPTOPRIL & HYDROCHLOROTHIAZIDE 182
  ENALAPRIL 386
  ENALAPRIL & HYDROCHLOROTHIAZIDE 388
  LISINOPRIL 568
ACEBUTOLOL 2
A'Cenol - See ACETAMINOPHEN 4
Acephen - See ACETAMINOPHEN 4
Ace-Tabs - See ACETAMINOPHEN 4
Aceta - See ACETAMINOPHEN 4
Aceta w/Codeine - See
  ACETAMINOPHEN 4
  NARCOTIC ANALGESICS 690
  NARCOTIC & ACETAMINOPHEN 688
Acetaco - See
  ACETAMINOPHEN 4
  NARCOTIC ANALGESICS 690
  NARCOTIC & ACETAMINOPHEN 688
Acet-Am - See EPHEDRINE 392
ACETAMINOPHEN 4
ACETAMINOPHEN & ASPIRIN - See ACETAMINOPHEN & SALICYLATES 6
ACETAMINOPHEN, ASPIRIN & SALICYLAMIDE - See ACETAMINOPHEN & SALICYLATES 6
ACETAMINOPHEN & CODEINE - See NARCOTIC & ACETAMINOPHEN 688
Acetaminophen w/Codeine - See
  ACETAMINOPHEN 4
  NARCOTIC ANALGESICS 690
ACETAMINOPHEN & SALICYLAMIDE - See ACETAMINOPHEN & SALICYLATES 6
ACETAMINOPHEN & SALICYLATES 6
ACETAMINOPHEN & SODIUM SALICYLATE - See ACETAMINOPHEN & SALICYLATES 6
Acetaminophen Uniserts - See ACETAMINOPHEN 4

INDEX

Acetazolam - See CARBONIC ANHYDRASE
   INHIBITORS 194
ACETOHEXAMIDE 8
ACETAZOLAMIDE - See CARBONIC ANHYDRASE
   INHIBITORS 194
ACETOHYDROXAMIC ACID (AHA) 10
Acetophen - See ASPIRIN 112
ACETOPHENAZINE 12
Acetospan - See TRIAMCINOLONE 998
Acetoxyl - See BENZOYL PEROXIDE 134
Acetylsaucylic Acid - See ASPIRIN 112
Achromycin (ophthalmic) - See ANTIBACTERIALS
   (Ophthalmic) 76
Achromycin (topical) - See ANTIBACTERIALS FOR
   ACNE (Topical) 84
Achrostatin V - See
   NYSTATIN 724
   TETRACYCLINES 958
Acne-Aid - See BENZOYL PEROXIDE 134
Acne Aid (topical) - See ANTI-ACNE, CLEANSING
   (Topical) 72
Acne-Dome (topical) - See ANTI-ACNE (Topical) 74
Acno (topical) - See ANTI-ACNE (Topical) 74
Acnomel (topical) - See ANTI-ACNE (Topical) 74
Acnotex (topical) - See ANTI-ACNE (Topical) 74
Acon - See VITAMIN A 1032
ACRISORCIN (Topical) 14
Acrisorcin Cream (topical) - See ACRISORCIN
   (Topical) 14
Acta-Char - See CHARCOAL, ACTIVATED 212
Acta-Char Liquid - See CHARCOAL, ACTIVATED
   212
Actamin - See ACETAMINOPHEN 4
Acti-B-12 - See VITAMIN B-12 (Cyanocobalamin)
   1034
Acticort - See ADRENOCORTICOIDS (Topical) 18
Actidil - See TRIPROLIDINE 1024
Actidose-Aqua - See CHARCOAL, ACTIVATED 212
Actifed - See
   PSEUDOEPHEDRINE 856
   TRIPROLIDINE 1024
Actifed-C - See NARCOTIC ANALGESICS 690
Actifed-C Expectorant - See NARCOTIC
   ANALGESICS 690
Actigall - See URSODIOL 1026
Actol - See GUAIFENESIN 480
Actrapid - See INSULIN 520
Acutrim - See PHENYLPROPANOLAMINE 794
Acutrim Maximum Strength - See
   PHENYLPROPANOLAMINE 794
Acutuss - See CHLORPHENIRAMINE 236
Acutuss Expectorant w/Codeine - See
   CHLORPHENIRAMINE 236
ACYCLOVIR (Oral & Topical) 16
Adalat - See NIFEDIPINE 706
Adapin - See TRICYCLIC ANTIDEPRESSANTS 1008
Adatuss - See NARCOTIC ANALGESICS 690
Adcortyl - See ADRENOCORTICOIDS (Topical) 18
Adcortyl in Orabase - See ADRENOCORTICOIDS
   (Topical) 18
Adeflor - See VITAMINS & FLUORIDE 1044
Adenex - See VITAMIN C (Ascorbic Acid) 1036
Adipex-D - See APPETITE SUPPRESSANTS 110
Adipex-P - See APPETITE SUPPRESSANTS 110
Adipost - See APPETITE SUPPRESSANTS 110
Adphen - See APPETITE SUPPRESSANTS 110
Adrenalin - See EPINEPHRINE 394

Adrenocorticoid (ophthalmic) - See ANTI-
   INFLAMMATORY, STEROIDAL (Ophthalmic)
   102
Adrenocorticoid (otic) - See ANTI-INFLAMMATORY
   (Otic) 100
Adrenocorticoid (topical) - See
   ADRENOCORTICOIDS (Topical) 18
ADRENOCORTICOIDS (Topical) 18
Adsorbocarpine - See PILOCARPINE 800
Advanced Formula Di-gel - See CALCIUM &
   MAGNESIUM ANTACIDS 176
Advil - See IBUPROFEN 514
Aero Caine - See ANESTHETICS (Topical) 62
Aero Caine Aerosol - See ANESTHETICS (Topical)
   62
Aerolate - See XANTHINE BRONCHODILATORS
   1046
Aerolone - See ISOPROTERENOL 534
Aerophylline - See XANTHINE
   BRONCHODILATORS 1046
Aeroseb-Dex - See
   ADRENOCORTICOIDS (Topical) 18
   DEXAMETHASONE 330
Aeroseb-HC - See
   ADRENOCORTICOIDS (Topical) 18
   HYDROCORTISONE (Cortisol) 502
Aerotherm - See ANESTHETICS (Topical) 62
Afaxin - See VITAMIN A 1032
Afko-Lube - See DOCUSATE SODIUM 380
Afrin - See XYLOMETAZOLINE 1048
Afrinol - See PSEUDOEPHEDRINE 856
Afrinol Repetabs - See PSEUDOEPHEDRINE 856
Aftate (topical) - See ANTIFUNGALS (Topical) 92
Agoral - See PHENOLPHTHALEIN 782
A-hydroCort - See HYDROCORTISONE (Cortisol)
   502
Airet - See XANTHINE BRONCHODILATORS 1046
Akarpine - See PILOCARPINE 800
Ak-Con (ophthalmic) - See DECONGESTANTS
   (Ophthalmic) 326
Ak-Dex - See DEXAMETHASONE 330
Ak-Dex (ophthalmic) - See ANTI-INFLAMMATORY,
   STEROIDAL (Ophthalmic) 102
Ak-Dilate (ophthalmic) - See PHENYLEPHRINE
   (Ophthalmic) 792
AK Homatropine (ophthalmic) - See CYCLOPEGIC,
   MYDRIATIC (Ophthalmic) 302
Akineton - See BIPERIDEN 146
Ak-Nefrin (ophthalmic) - See PHENYLEPHRINE
   (Ophthalmic) 792
Akne-mycin (topical) - See ANTIBACTERIALS FOR
   ACNE (Topical) 84
Ak-Pentolate (ophthalmic) - See CYCLOPENTOLATE
   (Ophthalmic) 304
Ak-Pred - See PREDNISOLONE 824
Ak-Pred (ophthalmic) - See ANTI-INFLAMMATORY,
   STEROIDAL (Ophthalmic) 102
AKshun - See DANTHRON 320
Ak-Taine (ophthalmic) - See ANESTHETICS, LOCAL
   (Ophthalmic) 68
Ak-Tate - See PREDNISOLONE 824
Ak-Tate (ophthalmic) - See ANTI-INFLAMMATORY,
   STEROIDAL (Ophthalmic) 102
Ak-Zol - See CARBONIC ANHYDRASE INHIBITORS
   194
Aladrine - See EPHEDRINE 392
Alagel - See ALUMINUM HYDROXIDE 28
Alaxin - See POLOXAMER 188 808

Aludrox - See
  ALUMINUM HYDROXIDE 28
  ALUMINUM & MAGNESIUM ANTACIDS 30
  MAGNESIUM HYDROXIDE 584
Aluline - See ALLOPURINOL 22
Alumadrine - See
  CHLORPHENIRAMINE 236
  PHENYLPROPANOLAMINE 794
Alumid - See
  ALUMINUM & MAGNESIUM ANTACIDS 30
  ALUMINUM HYDROXIDE 28
Alumid Plus - See ALUMINUM, MAGNESIUM,
  MAGALDRATE & SIMETHICONE ANTACIDS 32
ALUMINA & MAGNESIA - See ALUMINUM &
  MAGNESIUM ANTACIDS 30
ALUMINA, MAGNESIA & SIMETHICONE - See
  ALUMINUM, MAGNESIUM, MAGALDRATE &
  SIMETHICONE ANTACIDS 32
ALUMINA & MAGNESIUM CARBONATE - See
  ALUMINUM & MAGNESIUM ANTACIDS 30
ALUMINA, MAGNESIUM CARBONATE &
  MAGNESIUM OXIDE - See ALUMINUM &
  MAGNESIUM ANTACIDS 30
ALUMINA & MAGNESIUM TRISILICATE - See
  ALUMINUM & MAGNESIUM ANTACIDS 30
ALUMINUM & MAGNESIUM ANTACIDS 30
Aluminum ASA - See ASPIRIN 112
ALUMINUM, CALCIUM & MAGNESIUM ANTACIDS
  26
ALUMINUM HYDROXIDE 28
ALUMINUM, MAGNESIUM, MAGALDRATE &
  SIMETHICONE ANTACIDS 32
ALUMINUM, MAGNESIUM & SODIUM
  BICARBONATE ANTACIDS 34
Alupent - See METAPROTERENOL 620
Aluscop - See
  ALUMINUM HYDROXIDE 28
  ALUMINUM & MAGNESIUM ANTACIDS 30
  SCOPOLAMINE (Hyoscine) 904
Alu-Tab - See ALUMINUM HYDROXIDE 28
Al-Vite - See PYRIDOXINE (Vitamin B-6) 864
Alzapam - See LORAZEPAM 574
Amacodone - See
  ACETAMINOPHEN 4
  NARCOTIC & ACETAMINOPHEN 688
AMANTADINE 36
Amaphen - See
  ACETAMINOPHEN 4
  CAFFEINE 172
Amaphen w/Codeine #3 - See CAFFEINE 172
Amaril D - See PHENYLTOLOXAMINE 796
Amaril D Spantab - See PHENYLTOLOXAMINE 796
AMBENONIUM 38
Ambenyl - See
  GUAIFENESIN 480
  NARCOTIC ANALGESICS 690
Ambenyl-D - See PSEUDOEPHEDRINE 856
Ambenyl Expectorant - See
  BROMODIPHENHYDRAMINE 154
  DIPHENHYDRAMINE 360
Ambodryl - See BROMODIPHENHYDRAMINE 154
Amcill - See AMPICILLIN 54
Amcort - See TRIAMCINOLONE 998
Amen - See MEDROXYPROGESTERONE 600
Americaine - See ANESTHETICS (Topical) 62
Americaine (rectal) - See ANESTHETICS (Rectal) 60
Americaine (topical) - See ANESTHETICS, DENTAL
  (Topical) 66

Americaine Aerosol - See ANESTHETICS (Topical)
  62
Americaine Anesthetic Lubricant - See
  ANESTHETICS (Topical) 62
Americaine Ointment - See ANESTHETICS (Topical)
  62
Amersol - See IBUPROFEN 514
Amesec - See
  EPHEDRINE 392
  XANTHINE BRONCHODILATORS 1046
A-methaPred - See METHYLPREDNISOLONE 650
Amicar - See ANTIFIBRINOLYTIC AGENTS 90
Aminocaproic Acid - See ANTIFIBRINOLYTIC
  AGENTS 90
AMILORIDE 40
AMILORIDE & HYDROCHLOROTHIAZIDE 42
AMINOBENZOATE POTASSIUM 44
Aminodur - See XANTHINE BRONCHODILATORS
  1046
Aminodur Dura-tabs - See XANTHINE
  BRONCHODILATORS 1046
Aminophyl - See XANTHINE BRONCHODILATORS
  1046
Aminophyllin - See XANTHINE
  BRONCHODILATORS 1046
AMINOPHYLLINE - See XANTHINE
  BRONCHODILATORS 1046
Aminophylline and Amytal - See XANTHINE
  BRONCHODILATORS 1046
Aminophylline-Phenobarbital - See
  PHENOBARBITAL 780
  XANTHINE BRONCHODILATORS 1046
AMIODARONE 46
Amitid - See TRICYCLIC ANTIDEPRESSANTS 1008
Amitone - See CALCIUM CARBONATE 174
Amitril - See TRICYCLIC ANTIDEPRESSANTS 1008
AMITRYPTILINE - See TRICYCLIC
  ANTIDEPRESSANTS 1008
Amnestrogen - See
  ESTERIFIED ESTROGENS 412
  ESTROGEN 416
AMOBARBITAL 48
Amobel - See BELLADONNA 128
Amobell - See BELLADONNA ALKALOIDS &
  BARBITURATES 130
Amocine - See ATROPINE 116
Amodrine - See
  EPHEDRINE 392
  XANTHINE BRONCHODILATORS 1046
Amogel PG - See KAOLIN, PECTIN,
  BELLADONNA & OPIUM 544
Amoline - See XANTHINE BRONCHODILATORS
  1046
Amophylline - See XANTHINE
  BRONCHODILATORS 1046
AMOXAPINE - See TRICYCLIC
  ANTIDEPRESSANTS 1008
AMOXICILLIN 50
Amoxil - See AMOXICILLIN 50
Amphaplex - See DEXTROAMPHETAMINE 334
Amphenol - See ACETAMINOPHEN 4
AMPHETAMINE 52
Amphicol - See CHLORAMPHENICOL 220
Amphlaplex 10 & 20 - See AMPHETAMINE 52
Amphojel - See ALUMINUM HYDROXIDE 28
Amphojel 500 - See ALUMINUM & MAGNESIUM
  ANTACIDS 30

Apo-Allopurinol - See ALLOPURINOL 22
Apo-Amitriptyline - See TRICYCLIC
  ANTIDEPRESSANTS 1008
Apo-Amoxi - See AMOXICILLIN 50
Apo-Ampi - See AMPICILLIN 54
Apo-Asen - See ASPIRIN 112
Apo-Benztropine - See BENZTROPINE 138
Apo-Bisacodyl - See BISACODYL 148
Apo-C - See VITAMIN C (Ascorbic Acid) 1036
Apo-Carbamazepine - See CARBAMAZEPINE 184
Apo-Chlorax - See CHLORDIAZEPOXIDE &
  CLIDINIUM 226
Apo-Chlordiazepoxide - See CHLORDIAZEPOXIDE
  222
Apo-Chlorpromazine - See CHLORPROMAZINE
  238
Apo-Chlorpropamide - See CHLORPROPAMIDE
  240
Apo-Chlorthalide - See CHLORTHALIDONE 244
Apo-Chlorthalidone - See CHLORTHALIDONE 244
Apo-Cimetidine - See CIMETIDINE 252
Apo-Cloxi - See CLOXACILLIN 278
Apo-Diazepam - See DIAZEPAM 338
Apo-Dimenhydrinate - See DIMENHYDRINATE 356
Apo-Dipyridamole - See DIPYRIDAMOLE 368
Apo-Erythro-S - See ERYTHROMYCINS 408
Apo-Ferrous Gluconate - See FERROUS
  GLUCONATE 444
Apo-Ferrous Sulfate - See FERROUS SULFATE 446
Apo-Fluphenazine - See FLUPHENAZINE 456
Apo-Flurazepam - See FLURAZEPAM 460
Apo-Folic - See FOLIC ACID (Vitamin B-9) 462
Apo-Furosemide - See FUROSEMIDE 464
Apo-Guanethidine - See GUANETHIDINE 486
Apo-Haloperidol - See HALOPERIDOL 494
Apo-Hydro - See HYDROCHLOROTHIAZIDE 500
Apo-Ibuprofen - See IBUPROFEN 514
Apo-Imipramine - See TRICYCLIC
  ANTIDEPRESSANTS 1008
Apo-Indomethacin - See INDOMETHACIN 518
Apo-ISDN - See NITRATES 708
Apo-K - See POTASSIUM SUPPLEMENTS 816
Apo-Lorazepam - See LORAZEPAM 574
Apo-Meprobamate - See MEPROBAMATE 610
Apo-Methyldopa - See METHYLDOPA 642
Apo-metoprolol - See METOPROLOL 660
Apo-Metronidazole - See METRONIDAZOLE 662
Apo-Naproxen - See NAPROXEN 686
Apo-Nitrofurantoin - See NITROFURANTOIN 710
Apo-Oxazepam - See OXAZEPAM 732
Apo-Oxtriphylline - See XANTHINE
  BRONCHODILATORS 1046
Apo-Pen-VK - See PENICILLIN V 764
Apo-Perphenazine - See PERPHENAZINE 770
Apo-Phenylbutazone - See PHENYLBUTAZONE
  788
Apo-Piroxicam - See PIROXICAM 804
Apo-Prednisone - See PREDNISONE 826
Apo-Primidone - See PRIMIDONE 828
Apo-Propranolol - See PROPRANOLOL 852
Apo-Quinidine - See QUINIDINE 878
Apo-Sulfamethoxazole - See SULFAMETHOXAZOLE
  932
Apo-Sulfatrim - See
  SULFAMETHOXAZOLE 932
  TRIMETHOPRIM 1020
Apo-Sulfinpyrazone - See SULFINPYRAZONE 936
Apo-Sulfisoxazole - See SULFISOXAZOLE 938

Apo-Tetra - See TETRACYCLINES 958
Apo-Thioridazine - See THIORIDAZINE 972
Apo-Tolbutamide - See TOLBUTAMIDE 990
Apo-Triazide - See TRIAMTERENE &
  HYDROCHLOROTHIAZIDE 1002
Apo-Trifluoperazine - See TRIFLUOPERAZINE 1012
Apo-Trihex - See TRIHEXYPHENIDYL 1014
Appetite suppressant - See APPETITE
  SUPPRESSANTS 110
APPETITE SUPPRESSANTS 110
Aprazone - See SULFINPYRAZONE 936
Apresazide - See HYDRALAZINE &
  HYDROCHOLORTHIAZIDE 498
Apresodez - See HYDRALAZINE &
  HYDROCHOLORTHIAZIDE 498
Apresoline - See HYDRALAZINE 496
Apresoline-Esidrix - See HYDRALAZINE &
  HYDROCHOLORTHIAZIDE 498
Apsifen - See IBUPROFEN 514
Apsifen-F - See IBUPROFEN 514
Aquachloral - See CHLORAL HYDRATE 216
Aquachloral Supprettes - See CHLORAL HYDRATE
  216
AquaMEPHYTON - See VITAMIN K 1042
Aquamox - See QUINETHAZONE 876
Aquaphyllin - See XANTHINE BRONCHODILATORS
  1046
Aquasol A - See VITAMIN A 1032
Aquasol E - See VITAMIN E 1040
Aquastat - See BENZTHIAZIDE 136
Aquatag - See BENZTHIAZIDE 136
Aquatensen - See METHYCLOTHIAZIDE 638
Aqueous Charcodote - See CHARCOAL,
  ACTIVATED 212
Aralen - See CHLOROQUINE 228
Arcoban - See MEPROBAMATE 610
Arco-Cee - See VITAMIN C (Ascorbic Acid) 1036
Arco-Lase - See ATROPINE 116
Arco-Lase Plus - See HYOSCYAMINE 512
Arcylate - See SALICYLATES 902
Aristocort - See
  ADRENOCORTICOIDS (Topical) 18
  TRIAMCINOLONE 998
Aristocort A - See ADRENOCORTICOIDS (Topical)
  18
Aristocort C - See ADRENOCORTICOIDS (Topical)
  18
Aristocort D - See ADRENOCORTICOIDS (Topical)
  18
Aristocort Forte - See TRIAMCINOLONE 998
Aristocort Intralesional - See TRIAMCINOLONE 998
Aristocort R - See ADRENOCORTICOIDS (Topical)
  18
Aristophan Intralesional - See TRIAMCINOLONE
  998
Aristospan - See TRIAMCINOLONE 998
Arlidin - See NYLIDRIN 722
Arlidin Forte - See NYLIDRIN 722
Arm-a-Char - See CHARCOAL, ACTIVATED 212
Arm-a-Med Isoetharine - See ISOETHARINE 526
Arm and Hammer Baking Soda - See SODIUM
  BICARBONATE 914
Armour - See THYROID 978
Aromatic Cascara Fluidextract - See CASCARA 200
Artane - See TRIHEXYPHENIDYL 1014
Artane Sequels - See TRIHEXYPHENIDYL 1014
Artha-G - See SALICYLATES 902

Axid - See NIZATIDINE 712
Axon - See PHENYLPROPANOLAMINE 794
Axotal - See
  ACETAMINOPHEN 4
  ASPIRIN 112
  BUTALBITAL & ASPIRIN (Also contains caffeine)
    168
  NARCOTIC ANALGESICS 690
  TALBUTAL (Butalbital) 944
Ayercillin - See PENICILLIN G 762
Ayerst Epitrate - See EPINEPHRINE 394
Aygestin - See NORETHINDRONE ACETATE 716
Azapen - See METHICILLIN 630
AZATADINE 120
Azma Aid - See THEOPHYLLINE, EPHEDRINE &
    BARBITURATES 960
Azmacort - See TRIAMCINOLONE 998
Azo-100 - See PHENAZOPYRIDINE 776
Azodine - See PHENAZOPYRIDINE 776
Azo Gantanol - See
  PHENAZOPYRIDINE 776
  SULFAMETHOXAZOLE 932
  SULFONAMIDES & PHENAZOPYRIDINE 940
Azo-Gantrisin - See
  PHENAZOPYRIDINE 776
  SULFISOXAZOLE 938
  SULFONAMIDES & PHENAZOPYRIDINE 940
Azolid - See PHENYLBUTAZONE 788
Azolinic Acid - See CINOXACIN 254
Azo-Mandelamine - See
  METHENAMINE 628
  PHENAZOPYRIDINE 776
Azo-Soxazole - See
  SULFISOXAZOLE 938
  SULFONAMIDES & PHENAZOPYRIDINE 940
Azo-Standard - See PHENAZOPYRIDINE 776
Azo-Sulfamethoxazole - See SULFONAMIDES &
    PHENAZOPYRIDINE 940
Azo-Sulfisoxazole - See SULFONAMIDES &
    PHENAZOPYRIDINE 940
Azotrex - See PHENAZOPYRIDINE 776
Azulfidine - See SULFASALAZINE 934
Azulfidine En-Tabs - See SULFASALAZINE 934

B

B-A-C - See BUTALBITAL & ASPIRIN (Also contains
    caffeine) 168
B-A-C with Codeine - See BUTALBITAL, ASPIRIN &
    CODEINE (Also contains caffeine) 170
BACAMPICILLIN 122
Bacarate - See APPETITE SUPPRESSANTS 110
Baciguent (topical) - See ANTIBACTERIALS
    (Topical) 80
BACITRACIN (topical) - See ANTIBACTERIALS
    (Topical) 80
Back-Ese - See ORPHENADRINE, ASPIRIN &
    CAFFEINE 728
BACLOFEN 124
Bactine - See ANESTHETICS (Topical) 62
Bactine Hydrocortisone - See
    ADRENOCORTICOIDS (Topical) 18
Bactocill - See OXACILLIN 730
Bactopen - See CLOXACILLIN 278
Bactrim - See
  SULFAMETHOXAZOLE 932
  TRIMETHOPRIM 1020
Bactroban - See ANTIBACTERIALS (Topical) 80
Balminil - See GUAIFENESIN 480

Balminil DM - See DEXTROMETHORPHAN 336
Balminil Expectorant - See GUAIFENESIN 480
Bamate - See MEPROBAMATE 610
Bamo 400 - See MEPROBAMATE 610
Bancap w/Codeine - See
  ACETAMINOPHEN 4
  ASPIRIN 112
  NARCOTIC ANALGESICS 690
Bancap-HC - See NARCOTIC & ACETAMINOPHEN
    688
Ban-Drow 2 - See CAFFEINE 172
Banesin - See
  ACETAMINOPHEN 4
  ACETAMINOPHEN & SALICYLATES 6
Banesin Forte - See
  ACETAMINOPHEN 4
  NARCOTIC ANALGESICS 690
Banflex - See ORPHENADRINE 726
Banlin - See PROPANTHELINE 850
Banthine w/Phenobarbital - See PHENOBARBITAL
    780
Barazole - See SULFISOXAZOLE 938
Barbased - See BUTABARBITAL 166
Barbella - See
  ATROPINE 116
  HYOSCYAMINE 512
  SCOPOLAMINE (Hyoscine) 904
Barbeloid - See
  ATROPINE 116
  HYOSCYAMINE 512
  SCOPOLAMINE (Hyoscine) 904
Barbidonna - See
  ATROPINE 116
  BELLADONNA 128
  BELLADONNA ALKALOIDS & BARBITURATES
    130
  PHENOBARBITAL 780
  SCOPOLAMINE (Hyoscine) 904
Barbidonna-CR - See
  ATROPINE 116
  HYOSCYAMINE 512
  SCOPOLAMINE (Hyoscine) 904
Barbita - See PHENOBARBITAL 780
Barbiturate - See THEOPHYLLINE, EPHEDRINE &
    BARBITURATES 960
Barc (topical) - See PEDICULOSIDES (Topical) 756
Bar-Cy-Amine - See
  ATROPINE 116
  HYOSCYAMINE 512
  SCOPOLAMINE (Hyoscine) 904
Bar-Cy-A-Tab - See
  ATROPINE 116
  HYOSCYAMINE 512
  SCOPOLAMINE (Hyoscine) 904
Bardase Filmseal - See PHENOBARBITAL 780
Bar-Don - See
  ATROPINE 116
  HYOSCYAMINE 512
  SCOPOLAMINE (Hyoscine) 904
Baridium - See PHENAZOPYRIDINE 776
Barophen - See BELLADONNA ALKALOIDS &
    BARBITURATES 130
Barriere - See SIMETHICONE 912
Barriere-HC - See ADRENOCORTICOIDS (Topical)
    18
Barseb - See HYDROCORTISONE (Cortisol) 502

Bar-Tropin - See
   ATROPINE 116
   PHENOBARBITAL 780
Basaljel - See ALUMINUM HYDROXIDE 28
Bayapap - See ACETAMINOPHEN 4
Bayapap with Codeine - See NARCOTIC &
   ACETAMINOPHEN 688
Bay-Ase - See BELLADONNA ALKALOIDS &
   BARBITURATES 130
Baycyclomine - See DICYCLOMINE 344
Bayer - See ASPIRIN 112
Bayer Cold Tablets - See
   PHENYLPROPANOLAMINE 794
Bayer Cough Syrup - See
   PHENYLPROPANOLAMINE 794
Bayer Timed Release Arthritic Pain Formula - See
   ASPIRIN 112
Bayfrin - See XYLOMETAZOLINE 1048
Bayidyl - See TRIPROLIDINE 1024
Baymethazine - See PROMETHAZINE 848
Bayon - See POTASSIUM SUPPLEMENTS 816
Bay-Testone - See ANDROGENS 58
Baytussin - See GUAIFENESIN 480
Beben - See
   ADRENOCORTICOIDS (Topical) 18
   BETAMETHASONE 142
Bebetab - See BELLADONNA 128
BECLOMETHASONE 126
Beclovent - See BECLOMETHASONE 126
Beclovent Rotacaps - See BECLOMETHASONE 126
Beconase Inhaler - See BECLOMETHASONE 126
Becotide - See BECLOMETHASONE 126
Bedoz - See VITAMIN B-12 (Cyanocobalamin) 1034
Beelith - See PYRIDOXINE (Vitamin B-6) 864
Beepen-VK - See PENICILLIN V 764
Beesix - See PYRIDOXINE (Vitamin B-6) 864
Belap - See
   BELLADONNA 128
   BELLADONNA ALKALOIDS & BARBITURATES
      130
   PHENOBARBITAL 780
Belatol - See BELLADONNA 128
Belbarb - See
   BELLADONNA 128
   PHENOBARBITAL 780
Belbutal - See
   ATROPINE 116
   HYOSCYAMINE 512
   SCOPOLAMINE (Hyoscine) 904
Beldin - See DIPHENHYDRAMINE 360
Belkaloids - See
   ATROPINE 116
   HYOSCYAMINE 512
   SCOPOLAMINE (Hyoscine) 904
Bellachar - See BELLADONNA 128
Belladenal - See
   ATROPINE 116
   BELLADONNA 128
   BELLADONNA ALKALOIDS & BARBITURATES
      130
   PHENOBARBITAL 780
Belladenal-S - See BELLADONNA ALKALOIDS &
   BARBITURATES 130
Belladenal Spacetabs - See BELLADONNA
   ALKALOIDS & BARBITURATES 130
BELLADONNA 128
BELLADONNA ALKALOIDS & BARBITURATES 130

BELLADONNA & AMOBARBITAL - See
   BELLADONNA ALKALOIDS & BARBITURATES
      130
BELLADONNA & BUTABARBITAL - See
   BELLADONNA ALKALOIDS & BARBITURATES
      130
Bellafedrol - See BELLADONNA 128
Bellafoline - See HYOSCYAMINE 512
Bellalphen - See BELLADONNA ALKALOIDS &
   BARBITURATES 130
Bell/ans - See SODIUM BICARBONATE 914
Bellaspaz - See HYOSCYAMINE 512
Bellastal - See BELLADONNA ALKALOIDS &
   BARBITURATES 130
Bellergal - See
   BELLADONNA 128
   ERGOTAMINE, BELLADONNA &
      PHENOBARBITAL 402
   PHENOBARBITAL 780
Bellergal-S - See
   ATROPINE 116
   ERGOTAMINE, BELLADONNA &
      PHENOBARBITAL 402
Bellergal Spacetabs - See ERGOTAMINE,
   BELLADONNA & PHENOBARBITAL 402
Bellkatal - See
   BELLADONNA 128
   BELLADONNA ALKALOIDS & BARBITURATES
      130
   PHENOBARBITAL 780
Bello-phen - See BELLADONNA 128
Belphen - See BELLADONNA 128
Benacen - See PROBENECID 830
Bena-D - See DIPHENHYDRAMINE 360
Benadryl - See DIPHENHYDRAMINE 360
Benadryl Children's Allergy - See
   DIPHENHYDRAMINE 360
Benadryl Complete Allergy - See
   DIPHENHYDRAMINE 360
Benadryl w/Ephedrine - See EPHEDRINE 392
Benahist - See DIPHENHYDRAMINE 360
Ben-Aqua - See BENZOYL PEROXIDE 134
Ben-Aqua Mark - See BENZOYL PEROXIDE 134
Bendectin - See
   DOXYLAMINE 382
   PYRIDOXINE (Vitamin B-6) 864
Bendopa - See LEVODOPA 560
BENDROFLUMETHIAZIDE 132
Bendylate - See DIPHENHYDRAMINE 360
Benemid - See PROBENECID 830
Benisone - See ADRENOCORTICOIDS (Topical) 18
Benoject-10 - See DIPHENHYDRAMINE 360
Benoxyl - See BENZOYL PEROXIDE 134
Bensylate - See BENZTROPINE 138
Bentyl - See DICYCLOMINE 344
Bentyl Phenobarbital - See PHENOBARBITAL 780
Bentylol - See DICYCLOMINE 344
Benuryl - See PROBENECID 830
Benylin Cough Syrup - See DIPHENHYDRAMINE
   360
Benylin DM - See DEXTROMETHORPHAN 336
Benylin DM Cough - See DEXTROMETHORPHAN
   336
Benzac - See BENZOYL PEROXIDE 134
Benzac W - See BENZOYL PEROXIDE 134
Benzagel - See BENZOYL PEROXIDE 134
Benzedrine - See AMPHETAMINE 52
Benzoate - See BETAMETHASONE 142

Benzocaine - See ANESTHETICS (Topical) 62
BENZOCAINE (Rectal) - See ANESTHETICS
 (Rectal) 60
BENZOCAINE (Topical) - See ANESTHETICS,
 DENTAL (Topical) 66
Benzocaine Topical - See ANESTHETICS (Topical)
 62
Benzocal - See ANESTHETICS (Topical) 62
BENZOYL PEROXIDE 134
BENZPHETAMINE - See APPETITE
 SUPPRESSANTS 110
BENZTHIAZIDE 136
BENZTROPINE 138
Berubigen - See VITAMIN B-12 (Cyanocobalamin)
 1034
Besterone - See ESTRONE 418
Beta-2 - See ISOETHARINE 526
Beta-adrenergic blocker - See
 ACEBUTOLOL 2
 ATENOLOL 114
 BETA-ADRENERGIC BLOCKING AGENTS &
  THIAZIDE DIURETICS 140
 CARTEOLOL 198
 METOPROLOL 660
 NADOLOL 678
 OXPRENOLOL 734
 PINDOLOL 802
 PROPRANOLOL 852
 SOTALOL 922
 TIMOLOL 984
BETA-ADRENERGIC BLOCKING AGENTS &
 THIAZIDE DIURETICS 140
Beta-adrenergic stimulator - See RITODRINE 900
Betacort - See
 ADRENOCORTICOIDS (Topical) 18
 BETAMETHASONE 142
Betacort Scalp Lotion - See ADRENOCORTICOIDS
 (Topical) 18
Betaderm - See ADRENOCORTICOIDS (Topical) 18
Betaderm Scalp Lotion - See
 ADRENOCORTICOIDS (Topical) 18
Betalin 12 - See VITAMIN B-12 (Cyanocobalamin)
 1034
Betalin 12 Crystalline - See VITAMIN B-12
 (Cyanocobalamin) 1034
Betalin S - See THIAMINE (Vitamin B-1) 970
Betaloc - See METOPROLOL 660
Betaloc Durules - See METOPROLOL 660
BETAMETHASONE 142
BETAMETHASONE (Ophthalmic) - See ANTI-
 INFLAMMATORY, STEROIDAL (Ophthalmic)
 102
BETAMETHASONE (Otic) - See ANTI-
 INFLAMMATORY (Otic) 100
Betapen-VK - See PENICILLIN V 764
Betatrex - See ADRENOCORTICOIDS (Topical) 18
Beta-Val - See
 ADRENOCORTICOIDS (Topical) 18
 BETAMETHASONE 142
Betaxin - See THIAMINE (Vitamin B-1) 970
BETHANECHOL 144
Betnelan - See BETAMETHASONE 142
Betnesol - See
 ADRENOCORTICOIDS (Topical) 18
 BETAMETHASONE 142
Betnesol (ophthalmic) - See ANTI-INFLAMMATORY,
 STEROIDAL (Ophthalmic) 102

Betnesol (otic) - See ANTI-INFLAMMATORY (Otic)
 100
Betnovate - See ADRENOCORTICOIDS (Topical) 18
Betratrex - See BETAMETHASONE 142
Bewon - See THIAMINE (Vitamin B-1) 970
Bexedrine - See AMPHETAMINE 52
Bexophene - See
 ASPIRIN 112
 CAFFEINE 172
 NARCOTIC & ASPIRIN 692
Bicillin - See PENICILLIN G 762
Bicillin L.A. - See PENICILLIN G 762
Bicitra - See CITRATES 258
BiCozene - See ANESTHETICS (Topical) 62
Bicycline - See TETRACYCLINES 958
Bi-K - See POTASSIUM SUPPLEMENTS 816
Bilagog - See MAGNESIUM SULFATE 586
Bilax - See
 DEHYDROCHOLIC ACID 328
 DOCUSATE SODIUM 380
Bilivist - See GALLBLADDER X-RAY TEST DRUGS
 (Cholecystographic Agents) 466
Bilopaque - See GALLBLADDER X-RAY TEST
 DRUGS (Cholecystographic Agents) 466
BioCal - See
 CALCIUM CARBONATE 174
 CALCIUM SUPPLEMENTS 178
Biosone - See HYDROCORTISONE (Cortisol) 502
Bio-Tetra - See TETRACYCLINES 958
Bioxatphen - See ATROPINE 116
BIPERIDEN 146
Biphetamine - See
 AMPHETAMINE 52
 DEXTROAMPHETAMINE 334
Biquin-Durules - See QUINIDINE 878
BISACODYL 148
Bisco-Lax - See BISACODYL 148
BISMUTH SUBSALICYLATE 150
Bisodol - See
 ALUMINUM HYDROXIDE 28
 CALCIUM & MAGNESIUM ANTACIDS 176
 MAGNESIUM CARBONATE 580
 SODIUM BICARBONATE 914
Bisodol Powder - See SODIUM BICARBONATE 914
Bisorine - See ISOETHARINE 526
Black Draught - See SENNA 908
Black-Draught Lax Senna - See SENNA 908
Blamine - See THIAMINE (Vitamin B-1) 970
Blanex - See CHLORZOXAZONE &
 ACETAMINOPHEN 248
Bleph-10 (ophthalmic) - See ANTIBACTERIALS
 (Ophthalmic) 76
Blocadren - See TIMOLOL 984
Blue (topical) - See PEDICULOSIDES (Topical) 756
Blu-Hist - See PHENYLPROPANOLAMINE 794
B & O Supprettes - See BELLADONNA 128
Bobid - See SCOPOLAMINE (Hyoscine) 904
B.O.F. - See APPETITE SUPPRESSANTS 110
Bonamine - See MECLIZINE 596
Bonapene - See RAUWOLFIA ALKALOIDS 886
Bonine - See MECLIZINE 596
Bontril PDM - See APPETITE SUPPRESSANTS 110
Bontril Slow Release - See APPETITE
 SUPPRESSANTS 110
Breonesin - See GUAIFENESIN 480
Brethaire - See TERBUTALINE 950

BUFFERED ASPIRIN & CODEINE - See
    NARCOTIC & ASPIRIN 692
Bufferin - See ASPIRIN 112
Buffets II - See ACETAMINOPHEN & SALICYLATES
    6
Buffex - See ASPIRIN 112
Buffinol - See ASPIRIN 112
Buf-Oxal - See BENZOYL PEROXIDE 134
Buf-Tabs - See ASPIRIN 112
Bu-Lax - See DOCUSATE SODIUM 380
BUMETANIDE 160
Bumex - See BUMETANIDE 160
Buren - See
    ATROPINE 116
    HYOSCYAMINE 512
    SCOPOLAMINE (Hyoscine) 904
Burntame - See ANESTHETICS (Topical) 62
BuSpar - See BUSPIRONE 162
BUSPIRONE 162
BUSULFAN 164
Butabar - See BELLADONNA 128
Butabar Elixir - See BELLADONNA 128
BUTABARBITAL 166
Butabell HMB - See BUTABARBITAL 166
BUTACAINE - See ANESTHETICS (Topical) 62
BUTACAINE (Topical) - See ANESTHETICS,
    DENTAL (Topical) 66
Butagesic - See PHENYLBUTAZONE 788
Butal Compound - See
    BUTALBITAL & ASPIRIN (Also contains caffeine)
    168
    TALBUTAL (Butalbital) 944
Butalan - See BUTABARBITAL 166
Butalbital A-C - See BUTALBITAL & ASPIRIN (Also
    contains caffeine) 168
BUTALBITAL & ASPIRIN (Also contains caffeine)
    168
BUTALBITAL, ASPIRIN & CAFFEINE - See
    BUTALBITAL & ASPIRIN (Also contains
    caffeine) 168
BUTALBITAL, ASPIRIN & CODEINE (Also contains
    caffeine) 170
BUTAMBEN - See ANESTHETICS (Topical) 62
Butaserpazide - See
    BUTABARBITAL 166
    HYDROCHLOROTHIAZIDE 500
Butatran - See BUTABARBITAL 166
Butazolidin - See PHENYLBUTAZONE 788
Butesin Picrate - See ANESTHETICS (Topical) 62
Butibel - See
    ATROPINE 116
    BELLADONNA 128
    BELLADONNA ALKALOIDS & BARBITURATES
    130
    BUTABARBITAL 166
Butibel Elixir - See BELLADONNA 128
Butibel-Zyme - See BELLADONNA 128
Buticaps - See BUTABARBITAL 166
Butigetic - See CAFFEINE 172
Butiserpazide-50 Prestabs - See RAUWOLFIA
    ALKALOIDS 886
Butisol - See BUTABARBITAL 166
Butizide - See
    BUTABARBITAL 166
    HYDROCHLOROTHIAZIDE 500
BUTOCAZOLE - See ANTIFUNGALS (Vaginal) 94
BUTORPHANOL - See NARCOTIC ANALGESICS
    690

Butyl aminobenzoate - See ANESTHETICS (Topical)
    62
Butyn - See ANESTHETICS (Topical) 62
Butyn (topical) - See ANESTHETICS, DENTAL
    (Topical) 66
Butyn Sulfate - See ANESTHETICS (Topical) 62
Buytizide-25 Prestabs - See RAUWOLFIA
    ALKALOIDS 886
Byclomine - See DICYCLOMINE 344

C

C2 Buffered with Codeine - See NARCOTIC &
    ASPIRIN 692
C2 with Codeine - See NARCOTIC & ASPIRIN 692
C2A - See ACETAMINOPHEN 4
Cafacetin - See CAFFEINE 172
Cafadol - See ACETAMINOPHEN 4
Cafatine - See ERGOTAMINE & CAFFEINE 404
Cafatine PB - See ERGOTAMINE, CAFFEINE,
    BELLADONNA & PENTOBARBITAL 406
Cafecon - See CAFFEINE 172
Cafergot - See
    CAFFEINE 172
    ERGOTAMINE & CAFFEINE 404
Cafergot-PB - See ERGOTAMINE, CAFFEINE,
    BELLADONNA & PENTOBARBITAL 406
Cafermine - See CAFFEINE 172
Cafermine PB - See ERGOTAMINE, CAFFEINE,
    BELLADONNA & PENTOBARBITAL 406
Cafertabs - See ERGOTAMINE & CAFFEINE 404
Cafetrate -See
    CAFFEINE 172
    ERGOTAMINE & CAFFEINE 404
Cafetrate-PB - See
    ERGOTAMINE 400
    ERGOTAMINE, CAFFEINE, BELLADONNA &
    PENTOBARBITAL 406
Caffedrine - See CAFFEINE 172
CAFFEINE 172
Caine Spray - See ANESTHETICS (Topical) 62
Caladryl - See DIPHENHYDRAMINE 360
Calan - See VERAPAMIL 1030
Calan SR - See VERAPAMIL 1030
Calcet - See CALCIUM CARBONATE 174
Calcidrine - See
    EPHEDRINE 392
    NARCOTIC ANALGESICS 690
Calcidrine Syrup - See NARCOTIC ANALGESICS
    690
Calciferol—See VITAMIN D 1038
Calcifidiol - See VITAMIN D 1038
Calcijex - See VITAMIN D 1038
Calcilac - See CALCIUM CARBONATE 174
Calciphen - See ASPIRIN 112
Calcitrate 600 - See CALCIUM CARBONATE 174
Calcitrel - See
    CALCIUM & MAGNESIUM ANTACIDS 176
    MAGNESIUM CARBONATE 580
Calcitriol - See VITAMIN D 1038
CALCIUM CARBONATE 174
CALCIUM CARBONATE - See CALCIUM
    SUPPLEMENTS 178
CALCIUM CARBONATE & MAGNESIA - See
    CALCIUM & MAGNESIUM ANTACIDS 176
Calcium-channel blocker - See
    DILTIAZEM 354
    NICARDIPINE 702

Cenagesic - See
  CAFFEINE 172
  PHENYLEPHRINE 790
Cenahist - See SCOPOLAMINE (Hyoscine) 904
Cena-K - See POTASSIUM SUPPLEMENTS 816
Cenalax - See BISACODYL 148
Cenocort - See TRIAMCINOLONE 998
Cenocort A - See TRIAMCINOLONE 998
Cenocort Forte - See TRIAMCINOLONE 998
Cenolate - See VITAMIN C (Ascorbic Acid) 1036
Centet - See TETRACYCLINES 958
Central nervous system stimulant (amphetamine) -
    See
  AMPHETAMINE 52
  DEXTROAMPHETAMINE 334
  METHAMPHETAMINE 624
  PEMOLINE 758
Centrax - See PRAZEPAM 818
Ceo-Two - See SODIUM BICARBONATE 914
Cephalac - See LACTULOSE 554
CEPHALEXIN 208
CEPHRADINE 210
Ceporex - See CEPHALEXIN 208
Cerebel - See ATROPINE 116
Cerebid - See PAPAVERINE 746
Cerespan - See PAPAVERINE 746
Ceri-Bid - See VITAMIN C (Ascorbic Acid) 1036
Cerose Compound - See CHLORPHENIRAMINE
    236
C.E.S. - See
  CONJUGATED ESTROGENS 286
  ESTROGEN 416
Cesamet - See NABILONE 676
Cetacaine - See ANESTHETICS (Topical) 62
Cetacine - See ANESTHETICS (Topical) 62
Cetacort - See ADRENOCORTICOIDS (Topical) 18
Cetamide - See SULFAMETHOXAZOLE 932
Cetamide (ophthalmic) - See ANTIBACTERIALS
    (Ophthalmic) 76
Cetane - See VITAMIN C (Ascorbic Acid) 1036
Cetazol - See CARBONIC ANHYDRASE
    INHIBITORS 194
Cetro Cirose - See
  GUAIFENESIN 480
  NARCOTIC ANALGESICS 690
Cetroma - See MAGNESIUM CITRATE 582
Cetro-Nesia - See MAGNESIUM CITRATE 582
Cevalin - See VITAMIN C (Ascorbic Acid) 1036
Cevi-Bid - See VITAMIN C (Ascorbic Acid) 1036
Cevi-Fer - See FERROUS FUMARATE 442
Ce-Vi-Sol - See VITAMIN C (Ascorbic Acid) 1036
Cevita - See VITAMIN C (Ascorbic Acid) 1036
Charcoaid - See CHARCOAL, ACTIVATED 212
CHARCOAL, ACTIVATED 212
Charcoalanti Dote - See CHARCOAL, ACTIVATED
    212
Charcocaps - See CHARCOAL, ACTIVATED 212
Charcodote - See CHARCOAL, ACTIVATED 212
Chardonna - See
  ATROPINE 116
  BELLADONNA 128
  PHENOBARBITAL 780
Chardonna-2 - See BELLADONNA ALKALOIDS &
    BARBITURATES 130
Chelating agent - See PENICILLAMINE 760
Chembicarb - See SODIUM BICARBONATE 914
Chemgel - See ALUMINUM HYDROXIDE 28

Chemovag - See SULFISOXAZOLE 938
Cheracol - See
  DEXTROMETHORPHAN 336
  GUAIFENESIN 480
  NARCOTIC ANALGESICS 690
Cheracol Cough - See GUAIFENESIN 480
Chew-E - See VITAMIN E 1040
Chiggerex - See ANESTHETICS (Topical) 62
Chiggertox - See ANESTHETICS (Topical) 62
Children's Allerest - See
  CHLORPHENIRAMINE 236
  PHENYLEPHRINE 790
  PHENYLPROPANOLAMINE 794
Children's Sudafed Liquid - See
    PSEUDOEPHEDRINE 856
Chlor-100 - See CHLORPHENIRAMINE 236
Chlo-Amine - See CHLORPHENIRAMINE 236
CHLOPHEDIANOL 214
Chlor-Histine - See
  CHLORPHENIRAMINE 236
  PHENYLEPHRINE 790
Chlor-MAL - See CHLORPHENIRAMINE 236
Chlor-Niramine - See CHLORPHENIRAMINE 236
Chlor-PRO - See CHLORPHENIRAMINE 236
Chlor-Promanyl - See CHLORPROMAZINE 238
Chlor-Span - See CHLORPHENIRAMINE 236
Chlor-Trimeton - See
  CHLORPHENIRAMINE 236
  GUAIFENESIN 480
  PHENYLEPHRINE 790
  PSEUDOEPHEDRINE 856
Chlor-Trimeton w/Codeine - See
  CHLORPHENIRAMINE 236
Chlor-Trimeton Repetabs - See
  CHLORPHENIRAMINE 236
Chlor-Tripolon - See
  APPETITE SUPPRESSANTS 110
  CHLORPHENIRAMINE 236
Chlorafed - See
  CHLORPHENIRAMINE 236
  PSEUDOEPHEDRINE 856
CHLORAL HYDRATE 216
Chloramate Unicelles - See CHLORPHENIRAMINE
    236
CHLORAMBUCIL 218
Chloramead - See CHLORPROMAZINE 238
CHLORAMPHENICOL 220
CHLORAMPHENICOL (Ophthalmic) - See
    ANTIBACTERIALS (Ophthalmic) 76
CHLORAMPHENICOL (Otic) - See
    ANTIBACTERIALS (Otic) 78
CHLORAMPHENICOL (Topical) - See
    ANTIBACTERIALS (Topical) 80
Chlorazine - See PROCHLORPERAZINE 840
CHLORDIAZEPOXIDE 222
CHLORDIAZEPOXIDE & AMITRIPTYLINE 224
CHLORDIAZEPOXIDE & CLIDINIUM 226
CHLORIDE - See POTASSIUM SUPPLEMENTS 816
Chlormine - See CHLORPHENIRAMINE 236
Chlorofon-F - See CHLORZOXAZONE &
    ACETAMINOPHEN 248
Chlorohist - See XYLOMETAZOLINE 1048
Chloromide - See CHLORPROPAMIDE 240
Chloromycetin - See CHLORAMPHENICOL 220
Chloromycetin (otic) - See ANTIBACTERIALS (Otic)
    78
Chloronase - See CHLORPROPAMIDE 240

INDEX

Clipoxide - See
  CHLORDIAZEPOXIDE & CLIDINIUM 226
  CLIDINIUM 262
Clistin - See CARBINOXAMINE 190
Clistin D - See PHENYLEPHRINE 790
Clistin R-A - See CARBINOXAMINE 190
Cloderm - See ADRENOCORTICOIDS (Topical) 18
CLOFIBRATE 266
Clomid - See CLOMIPHENE 268
CLOMIPHENE 268
CLOMIPRAMINE - See TRICYCLIC
  ANTIDEPRESSANTS 1008
CLONIDINE 270
CLONIDINE & CHLORTHALIDONE 272
Clopa - See METOCLOPRAMIDE 656
CLORAZEPATE 274
Clorazine - See CHLORPROMAZINE 238
CLORTERMINE - See APPETITE SUPPRESSANTS
  110
CLOTRIMAZOLE (Oral-Local) 276
CLOTRIMAZOLE (Topical) - See ANTIFUNGALS
  (Topical) 92
CLOTRIMAZOLE (Vaginal) - See ANTIFUNGALS
  (Vaginal) 94
CLOXACILLIN 278
Cloxapen - See CLOXACILLIN 278
Cloxilean - See CLOXACILLIN 278
Clysodrast - See BISACODYL 148
CM with Paregoric - See PAREGORIC 752
Coastaldyne - See
  ACETAMINOPHEN 4
  NARCOTIC ANALGESICS 690
Coastalgesic - See
  ACETAMINOPHEN 4
  CAFFEINE 172
  NARCOTIC ANALGESICS 690
Co-Betaloc - See BETA-ADRENERGIC BLOCKING
  AGENTS & THIAZIDE DIURETICS 140
COCAINE 280
Cocaine - See COCAINE 280
Coco-Quinine - See QUININE 880
Codalan - See
  ACETAMINOPHEN 4
  ASPIRIN 112
  NARCOTIC ANALGESICS 690
Codalan –3 - See CAFFEINE 172
Codalex - See
  NARCOTIC ANALGESICS 690
  PHENYLEPHRINE 790
Codap - See
  ACETAMINOPHEN 4
  NARCOTIC ANALGESICS 690
  NARCOTIC & ACETAMINOPHEN 688
Codasa - See ASPIRIN 112
CODEINE - See NARCOTIC ANALGESICS 690
Codeine Sulfate - See NARCOTIC ANALGESICS
  690
Codesol - See PREDNISOLONE 824
Codimal - See
  CHLORPHENIRAMINE 236
  GUAIFENESIN 480
  PHENYLEPHRINE 790
  PHENYLPROPANOLAMINE 794
  PSEUDOEPHEDRINE 856
Codimal DH, DM, PH - See PYRILAMINE 866
Codimal PH - See NARCOTIC ANALGESICS 690

Coditrate - See
  GUAIFENESIN 480
  NARCOTIC ANALGESICS 690
Codone - See NARCOTIC ANALGESICS 690
Codoxy - See NARCOTIC & ASPIRIN 692
Codroxomin - See VITAMIN B-12 (Cyanocobalamin)
  1034
Codylax - See BISACODYL 148
Coffee-Break - See PHENYLPROPANOLAMINE 794
Cogentin - See BENZTROPINE 138
Co-Gesic - See
  ACETAMINOPHEN 4
  NARCOTIC & ACETAMINOPHEN 688
Colabid - See PROBENECID & COLCHICINE 832
Colace - See DOCUSATE SODIUM 380
Colax - See DOCUSATE SODIUM 380
ColBENEMID - See PROBENECID 830
ColBenemid - See
  COLCHICINE 282
  PROBENECID & COLCHICINE 832
COLCHICINE 282
Coldene - See CHLORPHENIRAMINE 236
Colestid - See COLESTIPOL 284
COLESTIPOL 284
Colidrate - See CHLORAL HYDRATE 216
Colifoam - See HYDROCORTISONE (Cortisol) 502
Colisone - See PREDNISONE 826
Colistin (otic) - See ANTIBACTERIALS (Otic) 78
Coloctyl - See DOCUSATE SODIUM 380
Cologel - See METHYLCELLULOSE 640
Colonil - See DIPHENOXYLATE & ATROPINE 364
Col-Probencid - See PROBENECID & COLCHICINE
  832
Col-Probenecid - See
  COLCHICINE 282
  PROBENECID 830
Colrex - See
  ACETAMINOPHEN 4
  CAFFEINE 172
  CHLORPHENIRAMINE 236
  PHENYLEPHRINE 790
  PHENYLPROPANOLAMINE 794
Colrex Compound - See NARCOTIC ANALGESICS
  690
Colrex Expectorant - See GUAIFENESIN 480
Coly-Mycin S (otic) - See ANTIBACTERIALS (Otic)
  78
Combid - See
  ISOPROPAMIDE 532
  PROCHLORPERAZINE 840
Combid Spansules - See PROCHLORPERAZINE &
  ISOPROPAMIDE 842
Combipres - See
  CHLORTHALIDONE 244
  CLONIDINE 270
  CLONIDINE & CHLORTHALIDONE 272
Comhist - See
  ATROPINE 116
  BELLADONNA 128
  CHLORPHENIRAMINE 236
  PHENYLEPHRINE 790
  PHENYLTOLOXAMINE 796
Compal - See
  ACETAMINOPHEN 4
  CAFFEINE 172
  NARCOTIC & ACETAMINOPHEN 688

CORTISONE 290
DEXAMETHASONE 330
FLUPREDNISOLONE 458
HYDROCORTISONE (Cortisol) 502
METHYLPREDNISOLONE 650
PARAMETHASONE 750
PREDNISOLONE 824
PREDNISONE 826
TRIAMCINOLONE 998

Cortisporin (ophthalmic) - See ANTIBACTERIALS
(Ophthalmic) 76
Cortisporin (otic) - See ANTIBACTERIALS (Otic) 78
Cortistab - See CORTISONE 290
Cortizone - See ADRENOCORTICOIDS (Topical) 18
Cortoderm - See
ADRENOCORTICOIDS (Topical) 18
HYDROCORTISONE (Cortisol) 502
Cortone Acetate - See CORTISONE 290
Cortril - See
ADRENOCORTICOIDS (Topical) 18
HYDROCORTISONE (Cortisol) 502
Corutol - See GUAIFENESIN 480
Corutol DH - See NARCOTIC ANALGESICS 690
Coryban D - See
CAFFEINE 172
CHLORPHENIRAMINE 236
GUAIFENESIN 480
PHENYLEPHRINE 790
PHENYLPROPANOLAMINE 794
Coryban-D Cough Syrup - See PHENYLEPHRINE
790
Coryphen - See ASPIRIN 112
Coryphen with Codeine - See NARCOTIC &
ASPIRIN 692
Coryza Brengle - See EPHEDRINE 392
Coryzaid - See
CAFFEINE 172
CHLORPHENIRAMINE 236
PHENYLEPHRINE 790
Coryztime - See
BELLADONNA 128
PHENYLPROPANOLAMINE 794
Corzide - See
BENDROFLUMETHIAZIDE 132
BETA-ADRENERGIC BLOCKING AGENTS &
THIAZIDE DIURETICS 140
NADOLOL 678
Cosanyl - See PSEUDOEPHEDRINE 856
Cosanyl DM - See DEXTROMETHORPHAN 336
Cosea - See CHLORPHENIRAMINE 236
Cosea-D - See PHENYLEPHRINE 790
Cosprin - See ASPIRIN 112
Cotabs - See NARCOTIC & ACETAMINOPHEN 688
Cotazym - See PANCRELIPASE 742
Cotazym E.C.S. - See PANCRELIPASE 742
Cotazym-S - See PANCRELIPASE 742
Cotrim - See
SULFAMETHOXAZOLE 932
TRIMETHOPRIM 1020
Cotrim D.S. - See SULFAMETHOXAZOLE 932
Co-trimoxazole - See SULFAMETHOXAZOLE 932
Cotrol-D - See PSEUDOEPHEDRINE 856
Cotussis - See
NARCOTIC ANALGESICS 690
TERPIN HYDRATE 954
Co-Tylenol - See
ACETAMINOPHEN 4
CHLORPHENIRAMINE 236

PHENYLEPHRINE 790
PSEUDOEPHEDRINE 856
Co-Tylenol Children's Liquid Cold Formula - See
PHENYLPROPANOLAMINE 794
Cough/cold preparation - See
GUAIFENESIN 480
OXTRIPHYLLINE & GUAIFENESIN 736
THEOPHYLLINE, EPHEDRINE, GUAIFENESIN &
BARBITURATES 962
Cough suppressant - See
CHLOPHEDIANOL 214
DEXTROMETHORPHAN 336
Coumadin - See ANTICOAGULANTS (Oral) 86
Covanamine - See
CHLORPHENIRAMINE 236
PHENYLEPHRINE 790
PHENYLPROPANOLAMINE 794
PYRILAMINE 866
Covangesic - See
ACETAMINOPHEN 4
CHLORPHENIRAMINE 236
PHENYLEPHRINE 790
Co-Xan - See
GUAIFENESIN 480
NARCOTIC ANALGESICS 690
XANTHINE BRONCHODILATORS 1046
Co-Xan Elixir - See EPHEDRINE 392
Creamalin - See
ALUMINUM & MAGNESIUM ANTACIDS 30
ALUMINUM HYDROXIDE 28
MAGNESIUM HYDROXIDE 584
Cremacoat - See
GUAIFENESIN 480
PHENYLPROPANOLAMINE 794
Cremacoat 1 - See
DEXAMETHASONE 330
DEXTROMETHORPHAN 336
Cremacoat 2 - See GUAIFENESIN 480
Cremacoat 4 - See DOXYLAMINE 382
Cremocort - See
ADRENOCORTICOIDS (Topical) 18
TRIAMCINOLONE 998
CROMOLYN 292
Cruex (topical) - See ANTIFUNGALS (Topical) 92
Crystapen - See PENICILLIN G 762
Crysticillin - See PENICILLIN G 762
Crystodigin - See DIGITALIS PREPARATIONS 352
Crystogin - See DIGITALIS PREPARATIONS 352
C.S.D. - See CONJUGATED ESTROGENS 286
Cuprimine - See PENICILLAMINE 760
Curretab - See MEDROXYPROGESTERONE 600
Cuticura (topical) - See ANTI-ACNE (Topical) 74
Cuticura Acne - See BENZOYL PEROXIDE 134
Cy clogyl (ophthalmic) - See CYCLOPENTOLATE
(Ophthalmic) 304
Cyanabin - See VITAMIN B-12 (Cyanocobalamin)
1034
Cyanocobalamin Co 57 - See RADIO-
PHARMACEUTICALS 882
Cyanocobalamin Co 60 - See RADIO-
PHARMACEUTICALS 882
Cyantin - See NITROFURANTOIN 710
CYCLACILLIN 294
Cyclaine - See ANESTHETICS (Topical) 62
Cyclaine Solution - See ANESTHETICS (Topical) 62
CYCLANDELATE 296
Cyclapen-W - See CYCLACILLIN 294
CYCLIZINE 298

Decapryn - See DOXYLAMINE 382
Decaspray - See
  ADRENOCORTICOIDS (Topical) 18
  DEXAMETHASONE 330
Decholin - See DEHYDROCHOLIC ACID 328
Declobese - See
  AMPHETAMINE 52
  DEXTROAMPHETAMINE 334
Declomycin - See TETRACYCLINES 958
Declostatin - See NYSTATIN 724
Decobel - See BELLADONNA 128
Decofed - See PSEUDOEPHEDRINE 856
De-Comberol - See TESTOSTERONE & ESTRADIOL
  956
Deconamine - See
  CHLORPHENIRAMINE 236
  PSEUDOEPHEDRINE 856
Decongestabs - See PHENYLTOLOXAMINE 796
Decongestant - See PHENYLEPHRINE
  (Ophthalmic) 792
Decongestant (ophthalmic) - See
  DECONGESTANTS (Ophthalmic) 326
Decongestant-P - See PHENYLPROPANOLAMINE
  794
DECONGESTANTS (Ophthalmic) 326
Decylenes (topical)—See ANTIFUNGALS (Topical)
  92
Deficol - See BISACODYL 148
Degest 2 (ophthalmic) - See DECONGESTANTS
  (Ophthalmic) 326
Dehist - See
  BROMPHENIRAMINE 156
  CHLORPHENIRAMINE 236
  PHENYLEPHRINE 790
  PHENYLPROPANOLAMINE 794
DEHYDROCHOLIC ACID 328
Dek-Quin (topical) - See ANTIBACTERIALS,
  ANTIFUNGALS (Topical) 82
Delacort - See ADRENOCORTICOIDS (Topical) 18
Deladumone - See TESTOSTERONE & ESTRADIOL
  956
Deladumone OB - See TESTOSTERONE &
  ESTRADIOL 956
Delatestryl - See ANDROGENS 58
Delaxin - See METHOCARBAMOL 632
Delcid - See
  ALUMINUM HYDROXIDE 28
  ALUMINUM & MAGNESIUM ANTACIDS 30
  MAGNESIUM HYDROXIDE 584
Delcozine - See APPETITE SUPPRESSANTS 110
Delestrogen - See
  ESTRODIOL 414
  ESTROGEN 416
Delsym - See
  DEXAMETHASONE 330
  DEXTROMETHORPHAN 336
Delsym Polistirex - See DEXTROMETHORPHAN
  336
Delta-Cortef - See PREDNISOLONE 824
Deltalin - See VITAMIN D 1038
Deltasone - See PREDNISONE 826
Deltastab - See PREDNISOLONE 824
Demazin - See
  CHLORPHENIRAMINE 236
  PHENYLEPHRINE 790
DEMECARIUM (Ophthalmic) - See
  ANTIGLAUCOMA, LONG-ACTING (Ophthalmic)
  96

DEMECLOCYCLINE - See TETRACYCLINES 958
Demer-Idine - See NARCOTIC ANALGESICS 690
Demerol - See NARCOTIC ANALGESICS 690
Demerol-APAP - See NARCOTIC &
  ACETAMINOPHEN 688
Demi-Regroton - See
  CHLORTHALIDONE 244
  RAUWOLFIA ALKALOIDS 886
  RAUWOLFIA & THIAZIDE DIURETICS 888
Demo-Cineol - See
  DEXAMETHASONE 330
  DEXTROMETHORPHAN 336
Demulen - See
  CONTRACEPTIVES (Oral) 288
  ETHINYL ESTRADIOL 428
Denta-Fl - See SODIUM FLUORIDE 918
D.E.P.-75 - See APPETITE SUPPRESSANTS 110
Depakene - See VALPROIC ACID (Dipropylacetic
  Acid) 1028
Depakote - See
  DIVALPOREX 374
  VALPROIC ACID (Dipropylacetic Acid) 1028
Dep Andro - See ANDROGENS 58
depAndrogyn - See TESTOSTERONE &
  ESTRADIOL 956
Depen - See PENICILLAMINE 760
Depletite - See APPETITE SUPPRESSANTS 110
dep Medalone - See METHYLPREDNISOLONE 650
Depoject - See METHYLPREDNISOLONE 650
Depo-Medrol - See METHYLPREDNISOLONE 650
Depo-medrone - See METHYLPREDNISOLONE
  650
Deponit - See NITRATES 708
Depopred - See METHYLPREDNISOLONE 650
Depo-Pred-40 - See METHYLPREDNISOLONE 650
Depo-Pred-80 - See METHYLPREDNISOLONE 650
Depo-Predate - See METHYLPREDNISOLONE 650
Depo-Provera - See MEDROXYPROGESTERONE
  600
Depotest - See ANDROGENS 58
Depo-Testadiol - See TESTOSTERONE &
  ESTRADIOL 956
Depotestogen - See TESTOSTERONE &
  ESTRADIOL 956
Depo-Testosterone - See ANDROGENS 58
Deproist w/Codeine - See
  GUAIFENESIN 480
  PSEUDOEPHEDRINE 856
Deprol - See MEPROBAMATE 610
Depronal-SA - See NARCOTIC ANALGESICS 690
Dermacoat - See ANESTHETICS (Topical) 62
Dermacort - See ADRENOCORTICOIDS (Topical) 18
Derma-Medicone - See ANESTHETICS (Topical) 62
Derma Medicone-HC - See EPHEDRINE 392
Derma & Soft Cream (topical) - See ANTI-ACNE
  (Topical) 74
DermiCort - See ADRENOCORTICOIDS (Topical) 18
Dermocort - See HYDROCORTISONE (Cortisol) 502
Dermodex - See BENZOYL PEROXIDE 134
Dermo-Gen - See ANESTHETICS (Topical) 62
Dermolate - See ADRENOCORTICOIDS (Topical) 18
Dermolate (rectal) - See HYDROCORTISONE
  (Rectal) 504
Dermophyl - See ADRENOCORTICOIDS (Topical)
  18
Dermoplast - See ANESTHETICS (Topical) 62

INDEX

Di-Sosul - See DOCUSATE SODIUM 380
Dispatabs - See VITAMIN A 1032
Di-Spaz - See DICYCLOMINE 344
Dispos-a Med Isoetharine - See ISOETHARINE 526
Dispose-a-Med Isoproterenol - See
   ISOPROTERENOL 534
Distamine - See PENICILLAMINE 760
DISULFIRAM 372
Ditate - See TESTOSTERONE & ESTRADIOL 956
Ditate DS - See TESTOSTERONE & ESTRADIOL
   956
Dithranol (topical) - See ANTHRALIN (Topical) 70
Ditropan - See ATROPINE 116
Diucardin - See HYDROFLUMETHIAZIDE 506
Diuchlor H - See HYDROCHLOROTHIAZIDE 500
Diulo - See METOLAZONE 658
Diupres - See
   CHLOROTHIAZIDE 230
   HYDROCHLOROTHIAZIDE 500
   RAUWOLFIA ALKALOIDS 886
   RAUWOLFIA & THIAZIDE DIURETICS 888
Diuretic - See
   AMILORIDE 40
   BUMETANIDE 160
   FUROSEMIDE 464
   INDAPAMIDE 516
   SPIRONOLACTONE 924
   TRIAMTERENE 1000
Diuretic (loop diuretic) - See ETHACRYNIC ACID
   422
Diuretic (thiazide) - See
   AMILORIDE & HYDROCHLOROTHIAZIDE 42
   BENDROFLUMETHIAZIDE 132
   BENZTHIAZIDE 136
   BETA-ADRENERGIC BLOCKING AGENTS &
     THIAZIDE DIURETICS 140
   CAPTOPRIL & HYDROCHLOROTHIAZIDE 182
   CHLOROTHIAZIDE 230
   CHLORTHALIDONE 244
   CYCLOTHIAZIDE 312
   ENALAPRIL & HYDROCHLOROTHIAZIDE 388
   HYDROCHLOROTHIAZIDE 500
   HYDROFLUMETHIAZIDE 506
   METHYCLOTHIAZIDE 638
   METHYLDOPA & THIAZIDE DIURETICS 644
   METOLAZONE 658
   POLYTHIAZIDE 810
   PRAZOSIN & POLYTHIAZIDE 822
   QUINETHAZONE 876
   RAUWOLFIA & THIAZIDE DIURETICS 888
   SPIRONOLACTONE & HYDROCHLOROTHIAZIDE
     926
   TRIAMTERENE & HYDROCHLOROTHIAZIDE
     1002
   TRICHLORMETHIAZIDE 1006
Diuril - See CHLOROTHIAZIDE 230
Diutensen - See METHYCLOTHIAZIDE 638
Diutensen-R - See
   RAUWOLFIA ALKALOIDS 886
   RAUWOLFIA & THIAZIDE DIURETICS 888
DIVALPOREX 374
Dixarit - See CLONIDINE 270
DM Cough - See
   DEXAMETHASONE 330
   DEXTROMETHORPHAN 336
DM Plus - See CHLORPHENIRAMINE 236
DM Syrup - See DEXTROMETHORPHAN 336

Doan's Pills - See
   ACETAMINOPHEN & SALICYLATES 6
   SALICYLATES 902
Doctate - See DOCUSATE SODIUM 380
DOCUSATE CALCIUM 376
DOCUSATE POTASSIUM 378
DOCUSATE SODIUM 380
doKtors Nose Drops - See PHENYLEPHRINE 790
Dolacet - See
   ACETAMINOPHEN 4
   NARCOTIC & ACETAMINOPHEN 688
Dolanex - See ACETAMINOPHEN 4
Dolene - See NARCOTIC ANALGESICS 690
Dolene-AP - See NARCOTIC & ACETAMINOPHEN
   688
Dolene AP-65 - See ACETAMINOPHEN 4
Dolene Compound - See NARCOTIC & ASPIRIN
   692
Dolene Compound-65 - See ASPIRIN 112
Dolobid - See DIFLUNISAL 350
Dolo-Pap - See NARCOTIC & ACETAMINOPHEN
   688
Dolophine - See NARCOTIC ANALGESICS 690
Dolor - See
   ACETAMINOPHEN 4
   ASPIRIN 112
   CAFFEINE 172
   NARCOTIC ANALGESICS 690
Doloxene - See NARCOTIC ANALGESICS 690
Dolprin - See ACETAMINOPHEN 4
Dolprn 3 - See
   ASPIRIN 112
   MAGNESIUM HYDROXIDE 584
Dolsed - See ATROPINE, HYOSCYAMINE,
     METHENAMINE, METHYLENE BLUE,
     PHENYLSALICYLATE & BENZOIC ACID 118
Domerine (topical) - See ANTI-ACNE (Topical) 74
Dommanate - See DIMENHYDRINATE 356
Donabarb - See BELLADONNA 128
Donatussin - See
   CHLORPHENIRAMINE 236
   GUAIFENESIN 480
Donatussin DC - See PHENYLEPHRINE 790
Donnacin - See
   ATROPINE 116
   HYOSCYAMINE 512
   SCOPOLAMINE (Hyoscine) 904
Donnafed Jr. - See BELLADONNA 128
Donnagel - See
   ATROPINE 116
   HYOSCYAMINE 512
   SCOPOLAMINE (Hyoscine) 904
Donnagel-MB - See KAOLIN & PECTIN 542
Donnagel-PG - See
   KAOLIN & PECTIN 542
   KAOLIN, PECTIN & PAREGORIC 546
   KAOLIN, PECTIN, BELLADONNA & OPIUM 544
   PAREGORIC 752
Donna-Lix - See PHENOBARBITAL 780
Donnamine - See
   ATROPINE 116
   HYOSCYAMINE 512
   SCOPOLAMINE (Hyoscine) 904
Donnapine - See BELLADONNA ALKALOIDS &
     BARBITURATES 130
Donna-Sed - See BELLADONNA ALKALOIDS &
     BARBITURATES 130

Donnatal - See
ATROPINE 116
BELLADONNA 128
BELLADONNA ALKALOIDS & BARBITURATES 130
HYOSCYAMINE 512
PHENOBARBITAL 780
SCOPOLAMINE (Hyoscine) 904
Donnatal Extentabs - See BELLADONNA ALKALOIDS & BARBITURATES 130
Donnazyme - See
ATROPINE 116
BELLADONNA 128
HYOSCYAMINE 512
PANCREATIN, PEPSIN, BILE SALTS, HYOSCYAMINE, ATROPINE, SCOPOLAMINE & PHENOBARBITAL 740
SCOPOLAMINE (Hyoscine) 904
Donphen - See BELLADONNA ALKALOIDS & BARBITURATES 130
Dopamet - See
METHYLDOPA 642
METHYLDOPA & THIAZIDE DIURETICS 644
Dopaminergic blocker - See METOCLOPRAMIDE 656
Dopar - See
CARBIDOPA & LEVODOPA 188
LEVODOPA 560
Dorbane - See DANTHRON 320
Dorbantyl L - See DANTHRON 320
Dorcol - See
ACETAMINOPHEN 4
CHLORPHENIRAMINE 236
GUAIFENESIN 480
PSEUDOEPHEDRINE 856
Dorcol Children's Fever and Pain Reducer - See ACETAMINOPHEN 4
Dorcol Pediatric Formula - See PSEUDOEPHEDRINE 856
Dormarex - See PYRILAMINE 866
Dormethan - See DEXTROMETHORPHAN 336
Doryx - See TETRACYCLINES 958
Doss - See DOCUSATE SODIUM 380
Double-A - See ACETAMINOPHEN & SALICYLATES 6
DOW-Isoniazid - See ISONIAZID 530
Dowmycin - See ERYTHROMYCINS 408
Doxaphene - See NARCOTIC ANALGESICS 690
Doxaphene Compound - See NARCOTIC & ASPIRIN 692
Doxidan - See
DANTHRON 320
DOCUSATE CALCIUM 376
DOCUSATE SODIUM 380
Doxinate - See DOCUSATE SODIUM 380
Doxy - See TETRACYCLINES 958
Doxy-Caps - See TETRACYCLINES 958
Doxychel - See TETRACYCLINES 958
DOXYCYCLINE - See TETRACYCLINES 958
DOXYLAMINE 382
Doxy-Lemmon - See TETRACYCLINES 958
Doxy-Tabs - See TETRACYCLINES 958
Dralserp - See RAUWOLFIA ALKALOIDS 886
Dralzine - See HYDRALAZINE 496
Dramaban - See DIMENHYDRINATE 356
Dramaject - See DIMENHYDRINATE 356
Dramamine - See DIMENHYDRINATE 356
Dramilin - See DIMENHYDRINATE 356

Dramocen - See DIMENHYDRINATE 356
Dr. Caldwell's Senna Laxative - See SENNA 908
Drenison - See ADRENOCORTICOIDS (Topical) 18
Dri-Hist Meta-Kaps - See PHENYLPROPANOLAMINE 794
Dri-Hist No. 2 Meta Caps - See
PHENIRAMINE 778
PHENYLEPHRINE 790
Drinus - See
ATROPINE 116
CHLORPHENIRAMINE 236
SCOPOLAMINE (Hyoscine) 904
Drinus Graduals - See PHENYLEPHRINE 790
Drinus Syrup - See PHENYLPROPANOLAMINE 794
Drisdol - See VITAMIN D 1038
Dristan - See
ACETAMINOPHEN 4
CHLORPHENIRAMINE 236
DEXTROMETHORPHAN 336
GUAIFENESIN 480
Dristan Advanced Formula - See PHENYLEPHRINE 790
Dristan Cough Formula - See
DEXTROMETHORPHAN 336
GUAIFENESIN 480
Dristan Long Lasting - See XYLOMETAZOLINE 1048
Dristan Nasal Spray - See
PHENIRAMINE 778
PHENYLEPHRINE 790
Drithocreme (topical) - See ANTHRALIN (Topical) 70
Drithocreme HP (topical) - See ANTHRALIN (Topical) 70
Drixoral - See
BROMPHENIRAMINE 156
PSEUDOEPHEDRINE 856
Drize - See SCOPOLAMINE (Hyoscine) 904
Drize M - See
CHLORPHENIRAMINE 236
PHENYLEPHRINE 790
Drocade and Aspirin - See NARCOTIC & ASPIRIN 692
DROCODE, ASPIRIN & CAFFEINE - See NARCOTIC & ASPIRIN 692
Dromoran - See NARCOTIC ANALGESICS 690
DRONABINOL 384
Droxine - See XANTHINE BRONCHODILATORS 1046
Droxine L.A. - See XANTHINE BRONCHODILATORS 1046
Droxine S.F. - See XANTHINE BRONCHODILATORS 1046
Droxomin - See VITAMIN B-12 (Cyanocobalamin) 1034
Dry and Clean - See BENZOYL PEROXIDE 134
Dry and Clear - See BENZOYL PEROXIDE 134
Drying agent - See CARBOL-FUCHSIN (Topical) 192
D-Sinus - See
ACETAMINOPHEN 4
PHENYLPROPANOLAMINE 794
D-S-S - See DOCUSATE SODIUM 380
D-Tran - See DIAZEPAM 338
Duadacin - See
ACETAMINOPHEN 4
CAFFEINE 172

Ectosone - See ADRENOCORTICOIDS (Topical) 18

Ectosone Scalp Lotion - See ADRENOCORTICOIDS (Topical) 18

Edecrin - See ETHACRYNIC ACID 422

E.E.S. - See ERYTHROMYCINS 408

EF cortelan - See ADRENOCORTICOIDS (Topical) 18

Efcortelan Soluble - See HYDROCORTISONE (Cortisol) 502

Efcortesol - See HYDROCORTISONE (Cortisol) 502

Efed II - See PHENYLPROPANOLAMINE 794

E-Ferol - See VITAMIN E 1040

Effersyllium - See PSYLLIUM 860

Efudex (topical) - See FLUOROURACIL (Topical) 452

Elavil - See TRICYCLIC ANTIDEPRESSANTS 1008

Eldadryl - See DIPHENHYDRAMINE 360

Eldafed - See TRIPROLIDINE 1024

El-Da-Mint - See CALCIUM CARBONATE 174

Eldatapp - See
BROMPHENIRAMINE 156
PHENYLPROPANOLAMINE 794

Eldecort - See ADRENOCORTICOIDS (Topical) 18

Elder 65 Compound - See
ASPIRIN 112   CAFFEINE 172

Eldercaps - See MAGNESIUM SULFATE 586

Eldertonic - See
MAGNESIUM SULFATE 586
PYRIDOXINE (Vitamin B-6) 864

Eldodram - See DIMENHYDRINATE 356

Eldonal - See
ATROPINE 116
HYOSCYAMINE 512
SCOPOLAMINE (Hyoscine) 904

Electrolyte replenisher - See
POTASSIUM & SODIUM PHOSPHATES 814
POTASSIUM PHOSPHATES 812

Elephemet - See APPETITE SUPPRESSANTS 110

Elixicon - See XANTHINE BRONCHODILATORS 1046

Elixiril - See HYOSCYAMINE 512

Elixomin - See XANTHINE BRONCHODILATORS 1046

Elixophyllin - See XANTHINE BRONCHODILATORS 1046

Elixophyllin-GG - See
GUAIFENESIN 480
THEOPHYLLINE & GUAIFENESIN 966

Elixophyllin SR - See XANTHINE BRONCHODILATORS 1046

Eloxyl - See BENZOYL PEROXIDE 134

Elthroxin - See THYROXINE (T-4, Levothyroxine) 980

Eltor - See PSEUDOEPHEDRINE 856

Eltroxin - See THYROID 978

Emagrin - See
ASPIRIN 112
CAFFEINE 172

Emagrin Forte - See PHENYLEPHRINE 790

Emcodeine - See NARCOTIC & ASPIRIN 692

Emex - See METOCLOPRAMIDE 656

Emfaseem - See XANTHINE BRONCHODILATORS 1046

Emfaseen - See GUAIFENESIN 480

Emitrip - See TRICYCLIC ANTIDEPRESSANTS 1008

EM-K-10% - See POTASSIUM SUPPLEMENTS 816

Emo-Cort - See
ADRENOCORTICOIDS (Topical) 18
HYDROCORTISONE (Cortisol) 502

Empirin - See ASPIRIN 112

Empirin w/Codeine - See
NARCOTIC ANALGESICS 690
NARCOTIC & ASPIRIN 688

Empirin Compound - See
ASPIRIN 112
CAFFEINE 172

Empirin Compound w/Codeine - See ASPIRIN 112

Empracet w/Codeine - See
ACETAMINOPHEN 4
NARCOTIC ANALGESICS 690
NARCOTIC & ACETAMINOPHEN 688

Emprazil - See
ASPIRIN 112
CAFFEINE 172
PHENACETIN 774
PSEUDOEPHEDRINE 856

Emprazil-C - See NARCOTIC ANALGESICS 690

Emtec - See NARCOTIC & ACETAMINOPHEN 688

Emulsoil - See CASTOR OIL 202

E-Mycin - See ERYTHROMYCINS 408

E-Mycin E - See ERYTHROMYCINS 408

ECONAZOLE - See ANTIFUNGALS (Vaginal) 94

Ecostatin - See ANTIFUNGALS (Vaginal) 94

ENALAPRIL 386

ENALAPRIL & HYDROCHLOROTHIAZIDE 388

Enarax - See HYDROXYZINE 510

ENCAINIDE 390

Encaprin - See ASPIRIN 112

Endecon - See
ACETAMINOPHEN 4
PHENYLPROPANOLAMINE 794

Endep - See TRICYCLIC ANTIDEPRESSANTS 1008

Endotussin-NN - See DEXTROMETHORPHAN 336

Enduron - See METHYCLOTHIAZIDE 638

Enduronyl - See
METHYCLOTHIAZIDE 638
RAUWOLFIA ALKALOIDS 886
RAUWOLFIA & THIAZIDE DIURETICS 888

Enkaid - See ENCAINIDE 390

Eno - See SODIUM BICARBONATE 914

Enovid - See CONTRACEPTIVES (Oral) 288

Enovid-E - See CONTRACEPTIVES (Oral) 288

Enovil - See TRICYCLIC ANTIDEPRESSANTS 1008

Enoxa - See DIPHENOXYLATE & ATROPINE 364

E.N.T. - See
CHLORPHENIRAMINE 236
PHENYLEPHRINE 790
PHENYLPROPANOLAMINE 794

E.N.T. Syrup - See BROMPHENIRAMINE 156

Entex - See
GUAIFENESIN 480
PHENYLEPHRINE 790
PHENYLPROPANOLAMINE 794

Entrophen - See ASPIRIN 112

Entuss-D - See
GUAIFENESIN 480
PSEUDOEPHEDRINE 856

Enzyme (pancreatic) - See PANCRELIPASE 742

E-Pam - See DIAZEPAM 338

Ephed II - See EPHEDRINE 392

Ephed-Organidin - See EPHEDRINE 392

EPHEDRINE 392

Ephedrine and Amytal - See EPHEDRINE 392

Ephedrine and Nembutal-25 - See EPHEDRINE 392

Estomul-M - See
   ALUMINUM & MAGNESIUM ANTACIDS 30
   MAGNESIUM CARBONATE 580
Estrace - See
   ESTRADIOL 414
   ESTROGEN 416
Estrace (vaginal) - See ESTROGEN 416
ESTRADIOL 414
ESTRADIOL (Vaginal) - See ESTROGEN 416
Estraguard (vaginal) - See ESTROGEN 416
Estrand - See TESTOSTERONE & ESTRADIOL 956
Estratab - See
   ESTERIFIED ESTROGENS 412
   ESTROGEN 416
Estratest - See ESTERIFIED ESTROGENS 412
Estra-Testrin - See TESTOSTERONE & ESTRADIOL
   956
Estrocon - See ESTROGEN 416
Estrofol - See ESTRONE 418
ESTROGEN 416
ESTROGENS, CONJUGATED (Vaginal) - See
   ESTROGEN 416
Estroject - See ESTRONE 418
Estromed - See ESTERIFIED ESTROGENS 412
ESTRONE 418
ESTRONE (Vaginal) - See ESTROGEN 416
Estrone-A - See ESTRONE 418
Estronol - See ESTRONE 418
ESTROPIPATE 420
ESTROPIPATE (Vaginal) - See ESTROGEN 416
Estrovis - See
   ESTROGEN 416
   QUINESTROL 874
ETHACRYNIC ACID 422
ETHCHLORVYNOL 424
ETHINAMATE 426
ETHINYL ESTRADIOL 428
Ethionamide - See ISONIAZID 530
ETHOPROPAZINE 430
ETHOSUXIMIDE 432
ETHOTOIN 434
Ethril - See ERYTHROMYCINS 408
Ethyl Aminobenzoate - See ANESTHETICS (Topical)
   62
Ethyl Aminobenzoate (rectal) - See ANESTHETICS
   (Rectal) 60
Ethyl Aminobenzoate (topical) - See ANESTHETICS,
   DENTAL (Topical) 66
ETHYLESTRENOL - See ANDROGENS 58
Etrafon - See
   PERPHENAZINE 770
   PERPHENAZINE & AMITRIPTYLINE 772
   TRICYCLIC ANTIDEPRESSANTS 1008
ETRETINATE 436
Euglucon - See GLYBURIDE 472
Eulcin - See SCOPOLAMINE (Hyoscine) 904
Euthroid - See
   LIOTRIX 566
   THYROID 978
   THYROXINE (T-4, Levothyroxine) 980
Eutonyl - See MONAMINE OXIDASE (MAO)
   INHIBITORS 674
Eutron - See PARGYLINE & METHYCLOTHIAZIDE
   754
Evac-Q-Kit - See
   MAGNESIUM CITRATE 582
   PHENOLPHTHALEIN 782

Evac-Q-Kwik - See
   BISACODYL 148
   MAGNESIUM CITRATE 582
   PHENOLPHTHALEIN 782
Evac-U-Gen - See PHENOLPHTHALEIN 782
Evac-U-Lax - See PHENOLPHTHALEIN 782
Evenol - See MEPROBAMATE 610
Everone - See ANDROGENS 58
Evex - See
   ESTERIFIED ESTROGENS 412
   ESTROGEN 416
E-Vista - See HYDROXYZINE 510
Excedrin - See
   ACETAMINOPHEN 4
   ACETAMINOPHEN & SALICYLATES 6
   ASPIRIN 112
Excedrin Extra Strength - See CAFFEINE 172
Excedrin P.M. - See PYRILAMINE 866
Excel (topical) - See ANTISEBORRHEIC (Topical)
   104
Exdol - See ACETAMINOPHEN 4
Exdol with Codeine - See NARCOTIC &
   ACETAMINOPHEN 688
Ex-Lax - See PHENOLPHTHALEIN 782
Ex-Lax Pills - See PHENOLPHTHALEIN 782
Exna - See BENZTHIAZIDE 136
Ex-Obese - See APPETITE SUPPRESSANTS 110
Expectorant - See
   TERPIN HYDRATE 954
   THEOPHYLLINE & GUAIFENESIN 966
Expectorant - See GUAIFENESIN 480
Expectrosed - See CHLORPHENIRAMINE 236
Extend-12 - See DEXAMETHASONE 330
Extendryl - See
   CHLORPHENIRAMINE 236
   PHENYLEPHRINE 790
   SCOPOLAMINE (Hyoscine) 904

F

FAMOTIDINE 438
Fastin - See APPETITE SUPPRESSANTS 110
Febrigesic - See ACETAMINOPHEN 4
Febrinol - See ACETAMINOPHEN 4
Febrogesic - See ACETAMINOPHEN 4
Feco-T - See FERROUS FUMARATE 442
Fedahist - See
   CHLORPHENIRAMINE 236
   GUAIFENESIN 480
   PSEUDOEPHEDRINE 856
Fedrazil - See PSEUDOEPHEDRINE 856
Fed-Mycin - See TETRACYCLINES 958
Feen-A-Mint Gum - See PHENOLPHTHALEIN 782
Feldene - See PIROXICAM 804
Fellozine - See PROMETHAZINE 848
Female sex hormone - See CONTRACEPTIVES
   (Oral) 288
Female sex hormone (estrogen) - See
   CHLOROTRIANISENE 232
   CONJUGATED ESTROGENS 286
   DIETHYLSTILBESTROL 346
   ESTERIFIED ESTROGENS 412
   ESTRADIOL 414
   ESTROGEN 416
   ESTRONE 418
   ESTROPIPATE 420
   ETHINYL ESTRADIOL 428
   QUINESTROL 874

Gelusil-II - See ALUMINUM, MAGNESIUM, MAGALDRATE & SIMETHICONE ANTACIDS 32

Gelusil Extra Strength - See ALUMINUM & MAGNESIUM ANTACIDS 30

Gelusil-M - See
  ALUMINUM, MAGNESIUM, MAGALDRATE & SIMETHICONE ANTACIDS 32
  MAGNESIUM TRISILICATE 588

GEMFIBROZIL 468

Gemnisyn - See ACETAMINOPHEN & SALICYLATES 6

Gemonil - See METHARBITAL 626

Genabid - See PAPAVERINE 746

Genapap - See ACETAMINOPHEN 4

Genapax (vaginal) - See ANTIFUNGALS (Vaginal) 94

Genebs - See ACETAMINOPHEN 4

Genetabs - See ACETAMINOPHEN 4

Genoptic (ophthalmic) - See ANTIBACTERIALS (Ophthalmic) 76

Genoptic (otic) - See ANTIBACTERIALS (Otic) 78

Genora 1/35 - See CONTRACEPTIVES (Oral) 288

Genora 1/50 - See CONTRACEPTIVES (Oral) 288

Gentacidin (ophthalmic) - See ANTIBACTERIALS (Ophthalmic) 76

GENTAMYCIN - See ANTIBACTERIALS (Topical) 80

GENTAMYCIN (ophthalmic) - See ANTIBACTERIALS (Ophthalmic) 76

GENTAMICIN (otic) - See ANTIBACTERIALS (Otic) 78

Gentian Violet (vaginal) - See ANTIFUNGALS (Vaginal) 94

Gentle Nature - See SENNOSIDES A & B 910

Geocillin - See CARBENICILLIN 186

Geopen - See CARBENICILLIN 186

Geopen Oral - See CARBENICILLIN 186

Geriplex-FS - See DOCUSATE SODIUM 380

Geritol Tablets - See FERROUS SULFATE 446

GG-CEN - See GUAIFENESIN 480

Ginsopan - See
  CHLORPHENIRAMINE 236
  PHENYLEPHRINE 790

Gitaligen - See DIGITALIS PREPARATIONS 352

GITALIN - See DIGITALIS PREPARATIONS 352

Glaucon - See EPINEPHRINE 394

Glaucon (ophthalmic) - See ANTIGLAUCOMA, SHORT-ACTING (Ophthalmic) 98

Glibenclamide - See GLYBURIDE 472

GLIPIZIDE 470

Globin Insulin - See INSULIN 520

Glucamide - See CHLORPROPAMIDE 240

Glucotrol - See GLIPIZIDE 470

Glutofac - See
  MAGNESIUM SULFATE 586
  PYRIDOXINE (Vitamin B-6) 864

Glyate - See GUAIFENESIN 480

GLYBURIDE 472

Glyceryl Guaiacolate - See GUAIFENESIN 480

Glyceryl Trinitrate - See NITRATES 708

Glycery T - See THEOPHYLLINE & GUAIFENESIN 966

GLYCOPYRROLATE 474

Glycotuss - See GUAIFENESIN 480

Glycotuss-dM - See DEXTROMETHORPHAN 336

Glysennid - See SENNOSIDES A & B 910

Glytinic - See FERROUS GLUCONATE 444

Glytuss - See GUAIFENESIN 480

G-Mycin - See TETRACYCLINES 958

GOLD COMPOUNDS 476

Gold compounds - See GOLD COMPOUNDS 476

Gold Sodium Thiomalate - See GOLD COMPOUNDS 476

Gonad stimulant - See CLOMIPHENE 268

Gonadotropin inhibitor - See DANAZOL 318

Gonak (ophthalmic) - See PROTECTANT (Ophthalmic) 854

Gonio-Gel - See METHYLCELLULOSE 640

Goniosol (ophthalmic) - See PROTECTANT (Ophthalmic) 854

Goody's Extra Strength Tablets - See ACETAMINOPHEN & SALICYLATES 6

Goody's Headache Powders - See ACETAMINOPHEN & SALICYLATES 6

Granulex - See CASTOR OIL 202

Gravol - See DIMENHYDRINATE 356

Grifulvin V - See GRISEOFULVIN 478

Grisactin - See GRISEOFULVIN 478

Grisactin Ultra - See GRISEOFULVIN 478

GRISEOFULVIN 478

Grisovin-FP - See GRISEOFULVIN 478

grisOwen - See GRISEOFULVIN 478

Gris-PEG - See GRISEOFULVIN 478

G-Sox - See SULFISOXAZOLE 938

Guaiahist - See
  GUAIFENESIN 480
  PHENYLEPHRINE 790

Guaiahist TT - See CHLORPHENIRAMINE 236

Guaiamine - See
  ACETAMINOPHEN 4
  CHLORPHENIRAMINE 236

Guaiaphed - See THEOPHYLLINE, EPHEDRINE, GUAIFENESIN & BARBITURATES 962

Guaifed - See
  GUAIFENESIN 480
  PSEUDOEPHEDRINE 856

GUAIFENESIN 480

GUANABENZ 482

GUANADREL 484

GUANETHIDINE 486

GUANETHIDINE & HYDROCHLOROTHIAZIDE 488

GUANFACINE 490

Guiamid - See GUAIFENESIN 480

Guiatuss - See GUAIFENESIN 480

Guiatuss D-M - See DEXTROMETHORPHAN 336

Guistrey Fortis - See CHLORPHENIRAMINE 236

Gustalac - See CALCIUM CARBONATE 174

G-well (topical) - See PEDICULOSIDES (Topical) 756

Gylanphen - See HYOSCYAMINE 512

Gynecort - See ADRENOCORTICOIDS (Topical) 18

Gynergen - See ERGOTAMINE 400

Gyne-Lotrimin - See ANTIFUNGALS (Vaginal) 94

Gynogen - See ESTRONE 418

H

H2 Cort - See ADRENOCORTICOIDS (Topical) 18

H_2Oxyl - See BENZOYL PEROXIDE 134

Hair growth stimulant - See
  ANTHRALIN (Topical) 70
  MINOXIDIL (Topical) 668

HALAZEPAM 492

Hal-Chlor - See CHLORPHENIRAMINE 236

Halciderm - See ADRENOCORTICOIDS (Topical) 18

Halcion - See TRIAZOLAM 1004

Haldol - See HALOPERIDOL 494

Haldol Decanoate - See HALOPERIDOL 494

Haldol LA - See HALOPERIDOL 494
Haldrone - See PARAMETHASONE 750
Halenol - See ACETAMINOPHEN 4
Halofed - See PSEUDOEPHEDRINE 856
Halog - See ADRENOCORTICOIDS (Topical) 18
Halog E - See ADRENOCORTICOIDS (Topical) 18
HALOPERIDOL 494
Haloprigin (topical) - See ANTIFUNGALS (Topical)
    92
Halotestin - See ANDROGENS 58
Halotex (topical) - See ANTIFUNGALS (Topical) 92
Halotussin - See GUAIFENESIN 480
Haltran - See IBUPROFEN 514
Haponal - See
    ATROPINE 116
    HYOSCYAMINE 512
    SCOPOLAMINE (Hyoscine) 904
Harmonyl - See RAUWOLFIA ALKALOIDS 886
Harmonyl-D - See RAUWOLFIA ALKALOIDS 886
Harvitrate - See ATROPINE 116
Hasacode - See
    ACETAMINOPHEN 4
    NARCOTIC ANALGESICS 690
HASP - See
    ATROPINE 116
    PHENOBARBITAL 780
HC-Jel - See ADRENOCORTICOIDS (Topical) 18
HCV (topical) - See ANTIBACTERIALS,
    ANTIFUNGALS (Topical) 82
Head and Shoulders (topical) - See
    ANTISEBORRHEIC (Topical) 104
Hedulin - See ANTICOAGULANTS (Oral) 86
Help - See PHENYLPROPANOLAMINE 794
Hemantinic - See FERROUS SULFATE 446
Hemocyte - See FERROUS FUMARATE 442
Hemorrheologic agent - See PENTOXIFYLLINE 768
Hemo-Vite - See
    FERROUS FUMARATE 442
    PYRIDOXINE (Vitamin B-6) 864
Hepahydrin - See DEHYDROCHOLIC ACID 328
Herpecin-L - See PYRIDOXINE (Vitamin B-6) 864
Herplex Eye Drops (ophthalmic) - See ANTIVIRALS
    (Ophthalmic) 108
Hexa-Betalin - See PYRIDOXINE (Vitamin B-6) 864
Hexacrest - See PYRIDOXINE (Vitamin B-6) 864
Hexadrol - See
    ADRENOCORTICOIDS (Topical) 18
    DEXAMETHASONE 330
Hexadrol Phosphate - See DEXAMETHASONE 330
Hexalol - See ATROPINE, HYOSCYAMINE,
    METHENAMINE, METHYLENE BLUE,
    PHENYLSALICYLATE & BENZOIC ACID 118
Hexamine - See METHENAMINE 628
Hexandrol - See DEXAMETHASONE 330
Hexathricin Aerospa - See ANESTHETICS (Topical)
    62
Hexavibex - See PYRIDOXINE (Vitamin B-6) 864
HEXYLCAINE - See ANESTHETICS (Topical) 62
H-H-R - See
    HYDRALAZINE 496
    HYDROCHLOROTHIAZIDE 500
    RAUWOLFIA ALKALOIDS 886
Hi-Cor - See ADRENOCORTICOIDS (Topical) 18
Hi-Cort - See ADRENOCORTICOIDS (Topical) 18
Hip-Rex - See METHENAMINE 628
Hiprex - See METHENAMINE 628
Hiprin - See ASPIRIN 112
Hi-receptor antagonist - See TERFENADINE 952

Hispril - See DIPHENYLPYRALINE 366
Histabid Duracaps - See PHENYLEPHRINE 790
Hista-Clopane - See PSEUDOEPHEDRINE 856
Hista-Derfule - See CAFFEINE 172
Histadyl and ASA Compound - See ASPIRIN 112
Histadyl Compound - See CAFFEINE 172
Histaject modified - See BROMPHENIRAMINE 156
Histalet - See
    CHLORPHENIRAMINE 236
    PHENYLEPHRINE 790
Histalet DM - See PSEUDOEPHEDRINE 856
Histalet Forte - See
    PHENYLPROPANOLAMINE 794
    PYRILAMINE 866
Histalet X - See GUAIFENESIN 480
Histalon - See CHLORPHENIRAMINE 236
Histamic - See
    CHLORPHENIRAMINE 236
    PSEUDOEPHEDRINE 856
Histamine H-2 antagonist - See
    CIMETIDINE 252
    NIZATIDINE 712
    RANITIDINE 884
Histantil - See PROMETHAZINE 848
Histapp - See PHENYLPROPANOLAMINE 794
Histaspan - See
    CHLORPHENIRAMINE 236
    PHENYLEPHRINE 790
Histaspan-D - See SCOPOLAMINE (Hyoscine) 904
Histatapp - See
    BROMPHENIRAMINE 156
    PHENYLEPHRINE 790
    PHENYLPROPANOLAMINE 794
Hista-Vadrin - See
    CHLORPHENIRAMINE 236
    PHENYLEPHRINE 790
Histerone - See ANDROGENS 58
Histex - See CHLORPHENIRAMINE 236
Historal - See
    CHLORPHENIRAMINE 236
    PSEUDOEPHEDRINE 856
    SCOPOLAMINE (Hyoscine) 904
Historal No. 2 - See PHENYLEPHRINE 790
Histor-D Timecelles - See
    CHLORPHENIRAMINE 236
    PHENYLEPHRINE 790
Historest - See PROMETHAZINE 848
Histrey - See CHLORPHENIRAMINE 236
Hi-Temp - See ACETAMINOPHEN 4
HMS Liquifilm (Ophthalmic) - See ANTI-
    INFLAMMATORY, STEROIDAL (Ophthalmic)
    102
Hold - See
    DEXAMETHASONE 330
    DEXTROMETHORPHAN 336
Hold Cough Suppressant - See
    DEXTROMETHORPHAN 336
HOMATROPINE (ophthalmic) - See CYCLOPEGIC,
    MYDRIATIC (Ophthalmic) 302
Honvol - See DIETHYLSTILBESTROL 346
Hormogen-A - See ESTRONE 418
Hormonin - See ESTROGEN 416
Humibid L.A. - See GUAIFENESIN 480
Humorsol (ophthalmic) - See ANTIGLAUCOMA,
    LONG-ACTING (Ophthalmic) 96
Humulin - See INSULIN 520
Humulin BR - See INSULIN 520
Humulin L - See INSULIN 520

INDEX

Kao-Con - See KAOLIN & PECTIN 542
Kaodene with Paregoric - See KAOLIN, PECTIN,
    BELLADONNA & OPIUM 544
Kaodonna-PG - See KAOLIN, PECTIN,
    BELLADONNA & OPIUM 544
KAOLIN & PECTIN 542
KAOLIN, PECTIN, BELLADONNA & OPIUM 544
KAOLIN, PECTIN & PAREGORIC 546
Kaon - See POTASSIUM SUPPLEMENTS 816
Kaon-Cl - See POTASSIUM SUPPLEMENTS 816
Kaon Cl 10 - See POTASSIUM SUPPLEMENTS 816
Kaon Cl 20 - See POTASSIUM SUPPLEMENTS 816
Kao-Nor - See POTASSIUM SUPPLEMENTS 816
Kaoparin - See PAREGORIC 752
Kaopectate - See KAOLIN & PECTIN 542
Kapectolin - See KAOLIN & PECTIN 542
Kapectolin with Paregoric and Parepectolin - See
    KAOLIN, PECTIN & PAREGORIC 546
Kapectolin PG - See KAOLIN, PECTIN,
    BELLADONNA & OPIUM 544
Karidium - See SODIUM FLUORIDE 918
Kasof - See DOCUSATE POTASSIUM 378
Kato - See POTASSIUM SUPPLEMENTS 816
Kavrin - See PAPAVERINE 746
Kaybovite - See VITAMIN B-12 (Cyanocobalamin)
    1034
Kaybovite-1000 - See VITAMIN B-12
    (Cyanocobalamin) 1034
Kay Ciel - See POTASSIUM SUPPLEMENTS 816
Kaylixir - See POTASSIUM SUPPLEMENTS 816
Kaypectol - See KAOLIN & PECTIN 542
Kaytrate - See NITRATES 708
K-C - See KAOLIN & PECTIN 542
KCL - See POTASSIUM SUPPLEMENTS 816
K-Dur - See POTASSIUM SUPPLEMENTS 816
KEFF - See POTASSIUM SUPPLEMENTS 816
Keflet - See CEPHALEXIN 208
Keflex - See CEPHALEXIN 208
Kellogg's Castor Oil - See CASTOR OIL 202
Kemadrin - See PROCYCLIDINE 844
Kenacort - See TRIAMCINOLONE 998
Kenaject - See TRIAMCINOLONE 998
Kenalog - See
    ADRENOCORTICOIDS (Topical) 18
    TRIAMCINOLONE 998
Kenalog in Orabase - See
    ADRENOCORTICOIDS (Topical) 18
    TRIAMCINOLONE 998
Kenalog-E - See ADRENOCORTICOIDS (Topical) 18
Kenalog-E - See TRIAMCINOLONE 998
Kenalog-H - See ADRENOCORTICOIDS (Topical) 18
Kenalone - See TRIAMCINOLONE 998
Kengesin - See
    ASPIRIN 112
    CAFFEINE 172
Keralyt (topical) - See ANTI-ACNE (Topical) 74
Kesso-mycin - See ERYTHROMYCINS 408
Kesso-Tetra - See TETRACYCLINES 958
Kestrin - See ESTRONE 418
Kestrin Aqueous - See ESTRONE 418
Kestrone - See ESTRONE 418
KETOCONAZOLE 548
KETOPROFEN 550
Key-Pred - See PREDNISOLONE 824
Key-Pred-SP - See PREDNISOLONE 824
K-Flex - See ORPHENADRINE 726
K-G Elixir - See POTASSIUM SUPPLEMENTS 816

Kinesed - See
    ATROPINE 116
    BELLADONNA 128
    BELLADONNA ALKALOIDS & BARBITURATES
    130
    HYOSCYAMINE 512
    PHENOBARBITAL 780
    SCOPOLAMINE (Hyoscine) 904
Kinine - See QUININE 880
Kirkaffeine - See CAFFEINE 172
Klaron (topical) - See ANTI-ACNE (Topical) 74
Klavikordal - See NITRATES 708
Kleer - See SCOPOLAMINE (Hyoscine) 904
Kleer-Tuss - See SCOPOLAMINE (Hyoscine) 904
K-Long - See POTASSIUM SUPPLEMENTS 816
Klophyllin - See XANTHINE BRONCHODILATORS
    1046
K-Lor - See POTASSIUM SUPPLEMENTS 816
Klor-10% - See POTASSIUM SUPPLEMENTS 816
Klor-Con - See POTASSIUM SUPPLEMENTS 816
Klor Con/25 - See POTASSIUM SUPPLEMENTS 816
Klor-Con/EF - See POTASSIUM SUPPLEMENTS 816
Klorvess - See POTASSIUM SUPPLEMENTS 816
Klotrix - See POTASSIUM SUPPLEMENTS 816
K-Lyte - See POTASSIUM SUPPLEMENTS 816
K-Lyte/Cl - See POTASSIUM SUPPLEMENTS 816
K-Lyte/Cl 50 - See POTASSIUM SUPPLEMENTS 816
K-Lyte/CL Powder - See POTASSIUM
    SUPPLEMENTS 816
K-Lyte DS - See POTASSIUM SUPPLEMENTS 816
Koffex - See DEXTROMETHORPHAN 336
Kolantyl - See
    ALUMINUM HYDROXIDE 28
    ALUMINUM & MAGNESIUM ANTACIDS 30
    MAGNESIUM HYDROXIDE 584
Kolantyl Wafers - See ALUMINUM HYDROXIDE 28
Kolyum - See POTASSIUM SUPPLEMENTS 816
Konakion - See VITAMIN K 1042
Konsyl - See PSYLLIUM 860
Konsyl-D - See PSYLLIUM 860
Korigesic - See
    ACETAMINOPHEN 4
    CAFFEINE 172
    CHLORPHENIRAMINE 236
    PHENYLEPHRINE 790
    PHENYLPROPANOLAMINE 794
Korostatin - See NYSTATIN 724
Koro-Sulf - See SULFISOXAZOLE 938
Koryza - See
    ATROPINE 116
    CHLORPHENIRAMINE 236
    HYOSCYAMINE 512
    PHENYLEPHRINE 790
    PHENYLPROPANOLAMINE 794
    SCOPOLAMINE (Hyoscine) 904
K-P - See KAOLIN & PECTIN 542
KPAB - See AMINOBENZOATE POTASSIUM 44
K-Pek - See KAOLIN & PECTIN 542
K-Phen - See PROMETHAZINE 848
K-Phos Original - See POTASSIUM PHOSPHATES
    812
K-Phos 2 - See POTASSIUM & SODIUM
    PHOSPHATES 814
K-Phos M.F. - See POTASSIUM & SODIUM
    PHOSPHATES 814
K-Phos Neutral - See POTASSIUM & SODIUM
    PHOSPHATES 814
Kronofed-A - See CHLORPHENIRAMINE 236

Kronofed-A Kronocaps - See PSEUDOEPHEDRINE
856
Kronohist Kronocaps - See
CHLORPHENIRAMINE 236
PHENYLPROPANOLAMINE 794
PYRILAMINE 866
Krypton Kr 81m - See RADIO-PHARMACEUTICALS
882
K-Tab - See POTASSIUM SUPPLEMENTS 816
Ku-Zyme HP - See PANCRELIPASE 742
Kudrox - See
ALUMINUM HYDROXIDE 28
ALUMINUM & MAGNESIUM ANTACIDS 30
Kutrase - See
HYOSCYAMINE 512
PHENYLTOLOXAMINE 796
Kwell (topical) - See PEDICULOSIDES (Topical) 756
Kwellada (topical) - See PEDICULOSIDES (Topical)
756
Kwildane (topical) - See PEDICULOSIDES (Topical)
756

L

LABETALOL 552
LABID - See XANTHINE BRONCHODILATORS
1046
Labor inhibitor - See RITODRINE 900
Lacril - See METHYLCELLULOSE 640
Lacril (ophthalmic) - See PROTECTANT
(Ophthalmic) 854
Lacrisert - See PROTECTANT (Ophthalmic) 854
Lacticare-HC - See ADRENOCORTICOIDS (Topical)
18
LACTULOSE 554
L.A. Formula - See PSYLLIUM 860
Lanacane - See ANESTHETICS (Topical) 62
Lanacort - See ADRENOCORTICOIDS (Topical) 18
Lanatuss - See CHLORPHENIRAMINE 236
Lan-Dol - See MEPROBAMATE 610
Laniazid - See ISONIAZID 530
Laniazid C.P. - See ISONIAZID 530
Lanophyllin - See XANTHINE BRONCHODILATORS
1046
Lanophyllin-GG - See THEOPHYLLINE &
GUAIFENESIN 966
Lanorinal - See
ASPIRIN 112
BUTALBITAL & ASPIRIN (Also contains caffeine)
168
CAFFEINE 172
TALBUTAL (Butalbital) 944
Lanothal - See BELLADONNA 128
Lanoxicaps - See DIGITALIS PREPARATIONS 352
Lanoxin - See DIGITALIS PREPARATIONS 352
Lapav - See PAPAVERINE 746
Lardet - See THEOPHYLLINE, EPHEDRINE &
BARBITURATES 960
Lardet Expectorant - See THEOPHYLLINE,
EPHEDRINE, GUAIFENESIN &
BARBITURATES 962
Largactil - See CHLORPROMAZINE 238
Larodopa - See
CARBIDOPA & LEVODOPA 188
LEVODOPA 560
Larotid - See AMOXICILLIN 50
Lasan (topical) - See ANTHRALIN (Topical) 70
Lasan HP (topical) - See ANTHRALIN (Topical) 70

Lasan Promade (topical) - See ANTHRALIN
(Topical) 70
Lasan Unguent (topical) - See ANTHRALIN
(Topical) 70
Lasix - See FUROSEMIDE 464
Lasix Special - See FUROSEMIDE 464
Latropine - See DIPHENOXYLATE & ATROPINE
364
Laudanum - See NARCOTIC ANALGESICS 690
Laud-Iron - See FERROUS FUMARATE 446
Laxagel - See DOCUSATE SODIUM 380
Laxative - See
MAGNESIUM CARBONATE 580
MAGNESIUM HYDROXIDE 584
MAGNESIUM TRISILICATE 588
Laxative (bulk-forming) - See
MALT SOUP EXTRACT 590
METHYLCELLULOSE 640
POLYCARBOPHIL CALCIUM 808
PSYLLIUM 860
Laxative (emollient) - See
DOCUSATE CALCIUM 376
DOCUSATE POTASSIUM 378
DOCUSATE SODIUM 380
POLOXAMER 188 806
Laxative (hyperosmotic) - See
LACTULOSE 554
MAGNESIUM CITRATE 582
MAGNESIUM SULFATE 586
SODIUM PHOSPHATE 920
Laxative (stimulant) - See
CASTOR OIL 202
CASCARA 200
BISACODYL 148
DANTHRON 320
DEHYDROCHOLIC ACID 328
PHENOLPHTHALEIN 782
SENNA 908
SENNOSIDES A & B 910
Laxinate - See DOCUSATE SODIUM 380
Laxinate 100 - See DOCUSATE SODIUM 380
Ledercillin VK - See PENICILLIN V 764
Ledercort - See TRIAMCINOLONE 998
Lederspan - See TRIAMCINOLONE 998
Lemidyne w/Codeine - See
ASPIRIN 112
CAFFEINE 172
Lemtrex - See TETRACYCLINES 958
Lenoltec - See NARCOTIC & ACETAMINOPHEN
688
Lentard - See INSULIN 520
Lente - See INSULIN 520
Lente Iletin I - See INSULIN 520
Lente Iletin II - See INSULIN 520
Lente Insulin - See INSULIN 520
Letter - See THYROXINE (T-4, Levothyroxine) 980
LEUCOVORIN 556
Leukeran - See CHLORAMBUCIL 218
Levamine - See
ATROPINE 116
BUTABARBITAL 166
HYOSCYAMINE 512
SCOPOLAMINE (Hyoscine) 904
Levate - See TRICYCLIC ANTIDEPRESSANTS 1008
Levlen - See CONTRACEPTIVES (Oral) 288
LEVOCARNITINE 558
LEVODOPA 560

Levo-Dromoran - See NARCOTIC ANALGESICS
  690
Levoid - See THYROXINE (T-4, Levothyroxine) 980
Levopa - See LEVODOPA 560
Levorphan - See NARCOTIC ANALGESICS 690
LEVORPHANOL - See NARCOTIC ANALGESICS
  690
Levothroid - See
  THYROID 978
  THYROXINE (T-4, Levothyroxine) 980
Levoxine - See THYROID 978
Levsin - See HYOSCYAMINE 512
Levsin w/Phenobarbital - See
  BELLADONNA ALKALOIDS & BARBITURATES
    130
  PHENOBARBITAL 780
Levsin-PB - See
  BELLADONNA ALKALOIDS & BARBITURATES
    130
  PHENOBARBITAL 780
Levsinex - See HYOSCYAMINE 512
Levsinex Timecaps - See HYOSCYAMINE 512
Levsinex with Phenobarbital Timecaps - See
  BELLADONNA ALKALOIDS & BARBITURATES
    130
Librax - See
  CHLORDIAZEPOXIDE & CLIDINIUM 226
  CLIDINIUM 262
Libritabs - See CHLORDIAZEPOXIDE 222
Librium - See CHLORDIAZEPOXIDE 222
Licetrol (Topical) - See PEDICULOSIDES (Topical)
  756
Lida-Mantle - See ANESTHETICS (Topical) 62
Lidemol - See ADRENOCORTICOIDS (Topical) 18
Lidex - See ADRENOCORTICOIDS (Topical) 18
Lidex-E - See ADRENOCORTICOIDS (Topical) 18
Lidocaine - See ANESTHETICS (Topical) 62
LIDOCAINE (Topical) - See ANESTHETICS,
  DENTAL (Topical) 66
Lidocaine Ointment - See ANESTHETICS (Topical)
  62
Lidox - See CHLORDIAZEPOXIDE & CLIDINIUM
  226
Lifocort - See HYDROCORTISONE (Cortisol) 502
Lignocaine - See ANESTHETICS (Topical) 62
Limbitrol - See CHLORDIAZEPOXIDE &
  AMITRIPTYLINE 224
Limbitrol DS - See CHLORDIAZEPOXIDE &
  AMITRIPTYLINE 224
Limit - See APPETITE SUPPRESSANTS 110
Limitite - See APPETITE SUPPRESSANTS 110
Lincocin - See LINCOMYCIN 562
LINCOMYCIN 562
LINCOMYCIN - See LINCOMYCIN 562
Lioresal - See BACLOFEN 124
LIOTHYRONINE 564
LIOTRIX 566
Lipancreatin - See PANCRELIPASE 742
Lipo Gantrisin - See SULFISOXAZOLE 938
Lipoxide - See CHLORDIAZEPOXIDE 222
Liprinal - See CLOFIBRATE 266
Liquamar - See
  ANTICOAGULANTS (Oral) 86
  PHENPROCOUMON 784
Liqui-Cee - See VITAMIN C (Ascorbic Acid) 1036
Liqui-Doss - See DOCUSATE SODIUM 380

Liquid-Antidose - See CHARCOAL, ACTIVATED 212
Liquid-Pred - See PREDNISONE 826
Liquimat (topical) - See ANTI-ACNE, CLEANSING
  (Topical) 72
Liquimint - See MAGNESIUM CARBONATE 580
Liquiprin - See ACETAMINOPHEN 4
Liquix-C - See
  ACETAMINOPHEN 4
  NARCOTIC ANALGESICS 690
Liquophylline - See XANTHINE
  BRONCHODILATORS 1046
LISINOPRIL 568
Lithane - See LITHIUM 570
LITHIUM 570
Lithizine - See LITHIUM 570
Lithobid - See LITHIUM 570
Lithonate - See LITHIUM 570
Lithostat - See ACETOHYDROXAMIC ACID (AHA) 10
Lithotabs - See LITHIUM 570
Lixaminol - See XANTHINE BRONCHODILATORS 1046
Lixaminol AT - See
  DEXTROMETHORPHAN 336
  XANTHINE BRONCHODILATORS 1046
Lixolin - See XANTHINE BRONCHODILATORS 1046
Lobac - See CHLORZOXAZONE &
  ACETAMINOPHEN 248
Locacorten - See ADRENOCORTICOIDS (Topical)
  18
Locoid - See ADRENOCORTICOIDS (Topical) 18
Lodrane - See XANTHINE BRONCHODILATORS
  1046
Loestrin - See
  CONTRACEPTIVES (Oral) 288
  ETHINYL ESTRADIOL 428
Lofene - See DIPHENOXYLATE & ATROPINE 364
Lomanate - See DIPHENOXYLATE & ATROPINE
  364
Lomine - See DICYCLOMINE 344
Lomotil - See DIPHENOXYLATE & ATROPINE 364
Loniten - See MINOXIDIL 666
Lonox - See DIPHENOXYLATE & ATROPINE 364
Lo-Ovral - See
  CONTRACEPTIVES (Oral) 288
  ETHINYL ESTRADIOL 428
  NORGESTREL 720
LOPERAMIDE 572
Lopid - See GEMFIBROZIL 468
Lopresor - See METOPROLOL 660
Lopressor - See METOPROLOL 660
Lopressor HCT - See BETA-ADRENERGIC
  BLOCKING AGENTS & THIAZIDE DIURETICS
  140
Lopressor SR - See METOPROLOL 660
Lopurin - See ALLOPURINOL 22
Loraz - See LORAZEPAM 574
LORAZEPAM 574
Lorcet - See
  ACETAMINOPHEN 4
  NARCOTIC & ACETAMINOPHEN 688
Lorcet-HD - See NARCOTIC & ACETAMINOPHEN
  688
Lorelco - See PROBUCOL 834
Loroxide - See BENZOYL PEROXIDE 134
Lortab - See NARCOTIC & ACETAMINOPHEN 688
Lortab 5 - See NARCOTIC & ACETAMINOPHEN
  688
Lortab 7 - See NARCOTIC & ACETAMINOPHEN
  688

Marcaine Hydrochloride w/Epinephrine - See
EPINEPHRINE 394
Marcumar - See
ANTICOAGULANTS (Oral) 86
PHENPROCOUMON 784
Marevan - See ANTICOAGULANTS (Oral) 86
Marezine - See CYCLIZINE 298
Marflex - See ORPHENADRINE 726
Marhist - See
CHLORPHENIRAMINE 236
PHENYLEPHRINE 790
Marine - See DIMENHYDRINATE 356
Marinol - See DRONABINOL 384
Marmine - See DIMENHYDRINATE 356
Marnal - See
BUTALBITAL & ASPIRIN (Also contains caffeine)
168
TALBUTAL (Butalbital) 944
Marplan - See MONAMINE OXIDASE (MAO)
INHIBITORS 674
Marzine - See CYCLIZINE 298
MASINDOL - See APPETITE SUPPRESSANTS 110
Maso-Donna - See
ATROPINE 116
HYOSCYAMINE 512
SCOPOLAMINE (Hyoscine) 904
Matropinal - See PHENOBARBITAL 780
Maxamag - See
ALUMINUM HYDROXIDE 28
MAGNESIUM HYDROXIDE 584
Maxeran - See METOCLOPRAMIDE 656
Maxibolin - See ANDROGENS 58
Maxidex - See DEXAMETHASONE 330
Maxidex (ophthalmic) - See ANTI-INFLAMMATORY,
STEROIDAL (Ophthalmic) 102
Maxiflor - See ADRENOCORTICOIDS (Topical) 18
Maxigesic - See NARCOTIC ANALGESICS 690
Maxolon - See METOCLOPRAMIDE 656
Max-Ox 40 - See ALUMINUM HYDROXIDE 28
Maxzide - See
HYDROCHLOROTHIAZIDE 500
TRIAMTERENE 1000
TRIAMTERENE & HYDROCHLOROTHIAZIDE
1002
Maytrex-BID - See TETRACYCLINES 958
Mazanor - See APPETITE SUPPRESSANTS 110
Mazepine - See CARBAMAZEPINE 184
Measurin - See ASPIRIN 112
Mebaral - See MEPHOBARBITAL 608
Mebendacin - See MEBENDAZOLE 594
MEBENDAZOLE 594
Mebutar - See MEBENDAZOLE 594
Meclan (topical) - See ANTIBACTERIALS FOR
ACNE (Topical) 84
MECLIZINE 596
MECLOCYCLINE (topical) - See ANTIBACTERIALS
FOR ACNE (Topical) 84
MECLOFENAMATE 598
Meclomen - See MECLOFENAMATE 598
Meda Cap - See ACETAMINOPHEN 4
Meda Tab - See ACETAMINOPHEN 4
Medicone - See ANESTHETICS (Topical) 62
Medicone Dressing - See ANESTHETICS (Topical)
62
Medicycline - See TETRACYCLINES 958
Medihaler-Epi - See EPINEPHRINE 394
Medihaler-Ergotamine - See ERGOTAMINE 400
Medihaler-Iso - See ISOPROTERENOL 534

Medilium - See CHLORDIAZEPOXIDE 222
Medimet - See METHYLDOPA 642
Medimet-250 - See METHYLDOPA & THIAZIDE
DIURETICS 644
Medipren - See IBUPROFEN 514
Mediquell - See
DEXAMETHASONE 330
DEXTROMETHORPHAN 336
Medi-Spas - See BELLADONNA 128
Medi-Tran - See MEPROBAMATE 610
Medralone - See METHYLPREDNISOLONE 650
Medralone-40 - See METHYLPREDNISOLONE 650
Medralone-80 - See METHYLPREDNISOLONE 650
Medrol - See
ADRENOCORTICOIDS (Topical) 18
METHYLPREDNISOLONE 650
Medrol Enpak - See METHYLPREDNISOLONE 650
Medrone - See METHYLPREDNISOLONE 650
Medrone-80 - See METHYLPREDNISOLONE 650
MEDROXYPROGESTERONE 600
MEDRYSONE (Ophthalmic) - See ANTI-
INFLAMMATORY, STEROIDAL (Ophthalmic) 102
MEFENAMIC ACID 602
Mega-B - See PYRIDOXINE (Vitamin B-6) 864
Megacillin - See PENICILLIN G 762
Megadose - See FERROUS GLUCONATE 444
Megascorb - See VITAMIN C (Ascorbic Acid) 1036
Mejoral without aspirin - See ACETAMINOPHEN 4
Mejoralito - See ACETAMINOPHEN 4
Melfiat - See APPETITE SUPPRESSANTS 110
Melitoxin - See ANTICOAGULANTS (Oral) 86
Mellaril - See THIORIDAZINE 972
Mellaril S - See THIORIDAZINE 972
MELPHALAN (PAM, L-PAM, Phenylalanine
Mustard) 604
Menadiol - See VITAMIN K 1042
Menadione - See VITAMIN K 1042
Menest - See
ESTERIFIED ESTROGENS 412
ESTROGEN 416
Menoject-L.A. - See TESTOSTERONE &
ESTRADIOL 956
Menospasm - See DICYCLOMINE 344
Menotrol - See ESTROGEN 416
Menrium - See
APPETITE SUPPRESSANTS 110
ESTROGEN 416
Mep-E - See MEPROBAMATE 610
Mepergan Fortis - See
NARCOTIC ANALGESICS 690
PROMETHAZINE 848
MEPERIDINE - See NARCOTIC ANALGESICS 690
MEPERIDINE & ACETAMINOPHEN - See
NARCOTIC & ACETAMINOPHEN 688
MEPHENYTOIN 606
MEPHOBARBITAL 608
Mephyton - See VITAMIN K 1042
Mepred-40 - See METHYLPREDNISOLONE 650
Mepriam - See MEPROBAMATE 610
MEPROBAMATE 610
MEPROBAMATE & ASPIRIN 612
Mepro Compound - See
ASPIRIN 112
MEPROBAMATE 610
Meprocon - See MEPROBAMATE 610
Meprogestic Q - See MEPROBAMATE & ASPIRIN
612

Myproic Acid - See VALPROIC ACID
    (Dipropylacetic Acid) 1028
Mysoline - See PRIMIDONE 828
Mysteclin F - See TETRACYCLINES 958
Mytelase - See AMBENONIUM 38
Mytrate - See EPINEPHRINE 394
Mytrate (ophthalmic) - See ANTIGLAUCOMA,
    SHORT-ACTING (Ophthalmic) 98
Mytrex - See
    NYSTATIN 724
    TRIAMCINOLONE 998
Mytrex (topical) - See ANTIBACTERIALS,
    ANTIFUNGALS (Topical) 82

N

NABILONE 676
NADOLOL 678
NADOLOL & BENDROFLUMETHIAZIDE - See
    BETA-ADRENERGIC BLOCKING AGENTS &
    THIAZIDE DIURETICS 140
Nadopen-V - See PENICILLIN V 764
Nadostine - See NYSTATIN 724
Nadostine (topical) - See ANTIFUNGALS (Topical)
    92
Nadostine (vaginal) - See ANTIFUNGALS (Vaginal)
    94
Nadozone - See PHENYLBUTAZONE 788
Nafcil - See NAFCILLIN 680
NAFCILLIN 680
Nafeen - See SODIUM FLUORIDE 918
Nafrine - See XYLOMETAZOLINE 1048
NAFTIDINE - See ANTIBACTERIALS,
    ANTIFUNGALS 82
NAFTIFINE - See ANTIFUNGALS (Topical) 92
Naftin - See ANTIBACTERIALS, ANTIFUNGALS 82
Naftine - See ANTIFUNGALS (Topical) 92
NALBUPHINE - See NARCOTIC ANALGESICS 690
Nalcrom - See CROMOLYN 292
Naldecol - See PHENYLTOLOXAMINE 796
Naldecon - See
    CHLORPHENIRAMINE 236
    GUAIFENESIN 480
    PHENYLEPHRINE 790
    PHENYLPROPANOLAMINE 794
    PHENYLTOLOXAMINE 796
Naldegesic - See
    ACETAMINOPHEN 4
    PSEUDOEPHEDRINE 856
Naldelate - See PHENYLTOLOXAMINE 796
Naldetuss - See CHLORPHENIRAMINE 236
Nalfon - See FENOPROFEN 440
NALIDIXIC ACID 682
Nallpen - See NAFCILLIN 680
NALTREXONE 684
NaMplCIL - See AMPICILLIN 54
NANDROLONE - See ANDROGENS 58
NAPAP - See ACETAMINOPHEN 4
Naphcon (ophthalmic) - See DECONGESTANTS
    (Ophthalmic) 326
Naphcon Forte (ophthalmic) - See
    DECONGESTANTS (Ophthalmic) 326
Napril Plateau - See
    CHLORPHENIRAMINE 236
    PHENYLEPHRINE 790
    PHENYLPROPANOLAMINE 794
    PYRILAMINE 866
NAPROXEN 686
Naprosyn - See NAPROXEN 686

Naptrate - See NITRATES 708
Naqua - See TRICHLORMETHIAZIDE 1006
Naquival - See
    HYDROCHLOROTHIAZIDE 500
    RAUWOLFIA ALKALOIDS 886
    RAUWOLFIA & THIAZIDE DIURETICS 888
    TRICHLORMETHIAZIDE 1006
Narcotic - See
    BUTALBITAL, ASPIRIN & CODEINE (Also
      contains caffeine) 170
    KAOLIN, PECTIN, BELLADONNA & OPIUM 544
    KAOLIN, PECTIN & PAREGORIC 546
    NARCOTIC & ACETAMINOPHEN 688
    NARCOTIC ANALGESICS 690
    NARCOTIC & ASPIRIN 692
    PAREGORIC 752
NARCOTIC & ACETAMINOPHEN 688
NARCOTIC ANALGESICS 690
Narcotic antagonist - See NALTREXONE 684
NARCOTIC & ASPIRIN 692
Nardil - See MONAMINE OXIDASE (MAO)
    INHIBITORS 674
Narine - See SCOPOLAMINE (Hyoscine) 904
Narine Gyrocaps - See
    CHLORPHENIRAMINE 236
    PHENYLEPHRINE 790
Narspan - See
    CHLORPHENIRAMINE 236
    PHENYLEPHRINE 790
    SCOPOLAMINE (Hyoscine) 904
Nasahist - See
    CHLORPHENIRAMINE 236
    PHENYLEPHRINE 790
    PHENYLPROPANOLAMINE 794
Nasahist B - See BROMPHENIRAMINE 156
Nasalcrom - See CROMOLYN 292
Natacomp-FA - See CALCIUM CARBONATE 174
Natacyn - See NATAMYCIN (Ophthalmic) 694
Natalins - See
    CALCIUM CARBONATE 174
    FERROUS FUMARATE 442
NATAMYCIN (Ophthalmic) 694
Natigozine - See DIGITALIS PREPARATIONS 352
National - See MAGNESIUM CITRATE 582
Natrimax - See HYDROCHLOROTHIAZIDE 500
Natulan - See PROCARBAZINE 838
Naturacil - See PSYLLIUM 860
Natural Estrongenic Substance - See ESTRONE 418
Naturetin - See BENDROFLUMETHIAZIDE 132
Nauseatol - See DIMENHYDRINATE 356
Navane - See THIOTHIXENE 974
Naxen - See NAPROXEN 686
N-Caps - See NIACIN (Nicotinic Acid) 700
ND-Stat Revised - See BROMPHENIRAMINE 156
Nebs - See ACETAMINOPHEN 4
Nefrol - See HYDROCHLOROTHIAZIDE 500
NegGram - See NALIDIXIC ACID 682
Nemasol - See PARA-AMINOSALICYLIC ACID (PAS)
    748
Nemasole - See MEBENDAZOLE 594
Nembutal - See PENTOBARBITAL 766
Neo-Barb - See BUTABARBITAL 166
Neo-Betalin - See VITAMIN B-12 (Cyanocobalamin)
    1034
Neobid - See PSEUDOEPHEDRINE 856
Neobiotic - See NEOMYCIN (Oral) 696
Neo-Calglucon - See CALCIUM SUPPLEMENTS 178
Neo-Calme - See DIAZEPAM 338

Nico-400 - See NIACIN (Nicotinic Acid) 700
Nicobid - See NIACIN (Nicotinic Acid) 700
Nicocap - See NIACIN (Nicotinic Acid) 700
Nicolar - See NIACIN (Nicotinic Acid) 700
Nicorette - See NICOTINE RESIN COMPLEX 704
Nico-Span - See NIACIN (Nicotinic Acid) 700
NICOTINE RESIN COMPLEX 704
Nicotinex - See NIACIN (Nicotinic Acid) 700
Nicotinyl alcohol - See NIACIN (Nicotinic Acid) 700
Nicotym - See NIACIN (Nicotinic Acid) 700
NIFEDIPINE 706
Niferex - See IRON-POLYSACCHARIDE 524
Niferex-150 - See IRON-POLYSACCHARIDE 524
Nifuran - See NITROFURANTOIN 710
Nilcol - See CHLORPHENIRAMINE 236
Nilspasm - See
  ATROPINE 116
  BELLADONNA 128
  HYOSCYAMINE 512
  SCOPOLAMINE (Hyoscine) 904
Nilstat - See NYSTATIN 724
Nilstat (topical) - See ANTIFUNGALS (Topical) 92
Nilstat (vaginal) - See ANTIFUNGALS (Vaginal) 94
Niong - See NITRATES 708
NITRATES 708
Nitrex - See NITROFURANTOIN 710
Nitro-Bid - See NITRATES 708
Nitrobon - See NITRATES 708
Nitrocap - See NITRATES 708
Nitrocap T.D. - See NITRATES 708
Nitrocardin - See NITRATES 708
Nitrodan - See NITROFURANTOIN 710
Nitrodisc - See NITRATES 708
Nitro-Dur - See NITRATES 708
Nitro-Dur II - See NITRATES 708
NITROFURANTOIN 710
Nitrogard-SR - See NITRATES 708
NITROGLYCERIN (Glyceryl Trinitrate) - See
  NITRATES 708
Nitroglyn - See NITRATES 708
Nitrol - See NITRATES 708
Nitrolin - See NITRATES 708
Nitrolingual - See NITRATES 708
Nitro-Long - See NITRATES 708
Nitronet - See NITRATES 708
Nitrong - See NITRATES 708
Nitrong SR - See NITRATES 708
Nitrospan - See NITRATES 708
Nitrostablin - See NITRATES 708
Nitrostat - See NITRATES 708
Nitro-Time - See NITRATES 708
NIZATIDINE 712
Nizoral - See KETOCONAZOLE 548
Nobesine - See APPETITE SUPPRESSANTS 110
Nobesine-75 - See APPETITE SUPPRESSANTS 110
Noctec - See CHLORAL HYDRATE 216
Nodaca - See CAFFEINE 172
Nodoz - See CAFFEINE 172
Nolamine - See
  CHLORPHENIRAMINE 236
  PHENYLPROPANOLAMINE 794
Noludar - See METHYPRYLON 652
No-Pred-TBA - See PREDNISOLONE 824
Noradryl - See DIPHENHYDRAMINE 360
Noralac - See
  CALCIUM & MAGNESIUM ANTACIDS 176
  MAGNESIUM CARBONATE 580

Norcet - See NARCOTIC & ACETAMINOPHEN 688
Nordette - See CONTRACEPTIVES (Oral) 288
Nordryl - See DIPHENHYDRAMINE 360
NORETHINDRONE 714
NORETHINDRONE ACETATE 716
Norette - See ETHINYL ESTRADIOL 428
Norflex - See ORPHENADRINE 726
NORFLOXACIN 718
Norgesic - See
  ASPIRIN 112
  ORPHENADRINE, ASPIRIN & CAFFEINE 728
Norgesic Forte - See ORPHENADRINE, ASPIRIN &
  CAFFEINE 728
NORGESTREL 720
Norinyl - See ETHINYL ESTRADIOL 428
Norinyl 1 + 35 - See CONTRACEPTIVES (Oral)
  288
Norinyl 1 + 35 21-Day Tablets - See
  NORETHINDRONE 714
Norinyl 1 + 50 - See CONTRACEPTIVES (Oral)
  288
Norinyl 1 + 80 - See CONTRACEPTIVES (Oral)
  288
Norinyl 2 - See CONTRACEPTIVES (Oral) 288
Norisodrine - See ISOPROTERENOL 534
Norisodrine Aerotrol - See ISOPROTERENOL 534
Norlestrin - See
  CONTRACEPTIVES (Oral) 288
  ETHINYL ESTRADIOL 428
  NORETHINDRONE 714
Norlinyl - See CONTRACEPTIVES (Oral) 288
Norlutate - See
  NORETHINDRONE 714
  NORETHINDRONE ACETATE 716
Norlutate Acetate - See NORETHINDRONE
  ACETATE 716
Norlutin - See
  NORETHINDRONE 714
  NORETHINDRONE ACETATE 716
Nor-Mil - See DIPHENOXYLATE & ATROPINE 364
Normodyne - See LABETALOL 552
Normozide - See BETA-ADRENERGIC BLOCKING
  AGENTS & THIAZIDE DIURETICS 140
Nor-O-D. - See NORETHINDRONE ACETATE 716
Noroxin - See NORFLOXACIN 718
Noroxine - See THYROXINE (T-4, Levothyroxine)
  980
Norpace - See DISOPYRAMIDE 370
Norpace CR - See DISOPYRAMIDE 370
Norpanth - See PROPANTHELINE 850
Norpramin - See TRICYCLIC ANTIDEPRESSANTS
  1008
Nor-Q.D. - See
  CONTRACEPTIVES (Oral) 288
  NORETHINDRONE 714
Norquest - See CONTRACEPTIVES (Oral) 288
Nor-Tet - See TETRACYCLINES 958
NORTRIPTYLINE - See TRICYCLIC
  ANTIDEPRESSANTS 1008
Nortussin - See GUAIFENESIN 480
Norwich Aspirin - See ASPIRIN 112
Norzine - See PROMAZINE 846
Nospaz - See DICYCLOMINE 344
Nostril - See PHENYLEPHRINE 790
Nostrilla - See XYLOMETAZOLINE 1048
Nova-Carpine - See PILOCARPINE 800
Novafed - See PSEUDOEPHEDRINE 856

INDEX

1177

Nu-Iron-V - See
  CALCIUM CARBONATE 174
  PYRIDOXINE (Vitamin B-6) 864
Nulac - See BISACODYL 148
Numa-Dura-Tablets - See
  BUTABARBITAL 166
  EPHEDRINE 392
Numa-Dura-Tabs - See XANTHINE
  BRONCHODILATORS 1046
Numorphan - See NARCOTIC ANALGESICS 690
Nupercainal - See ANESTHETICS (Topical) 62
Nupercainal (rectal) - See ANESTHETICS (Rectal)
  60
Nupercainal Cream - See ANESTHETICS (Topical)
  62
Nupercainal Ointment - See ANESTHETICS
  (Topical) 62
Nupercainal Spray - See ANESTHETICS (Topical)
  62
Nuprin - See IBUPROFEN 514
Nust-Olone - See TRIAMCINOLONE 998
Nutracort - See ADRENOCORTICOIDS (Topical) 18
Nutritional supplement - See LEVOCARNITINE 558
Nyaderm - See NYSTATIN 724
Nyaderm (topical) - See ANTIFUNGALS (Topical) 92
Nydrazid - See ISONIAZID 530
NYLIDRIN 722
Nyquil - See
  DEXTROMETHORPHAN 336
  EPHEDRINE 392
Nystaform - See NYSTATIN 724
NYSTATIN 724
NYSTATIN (Topical) - See ANTIFUNGALS (Topical)
  92
NYSTATIN (Vaginal) - See ANTIFUNGALS (Vaginal)
  94
NYSTATIN, NEOMYCIN, GRAMICIDIN AND
  TRIAMCINOLONE (Topical) - See
  ANTIBACTERIALS, ANTIFUNGALS (Topical) 82
Nystex - See NYSTATIN 724
Nystex (topical) - See ANTIFUNGALS (Topical) 92
Nytilax - See SENNOSIDES A & B 910
Nytol - See DIPHENHYDRAMINE 360
Nytol with DPH - See DIPHENHYDRAMINE 360

O

Oagen - See ESTROGEN 416
Obalan - See APPETITE SUPPRESSANTS 110
Obe-Nil TR - See APPETITE SUPPRESSANTS 110
Obe-Nix - See APPETITE SUPPRESSANTS 110
Obephen - See APPETITE SUPPRESSANTS 110
Obermine - See APPETITE SUPPRESSANTS 110
Obestat - See PHENYLPROPANOLAMINE 794
Obestin - See APPETITE SUPPRESSANTS 110
Obestin-30 - See APPETITE SUPPRESSANTS 110
Obestrol - See APPETITE SUPPRESSANTS 110
Obetrol - See DEXTROAMPHETAMINE 334
Obetrol 10 & 20 - See AMPHETAMINE 52
Obeval - See APPETITE SUPPRESSANTS 110
Obezine - See APPETITE SUPPRESSANTS 110
Obotan - See DEXTROAMPHETAMINE 334
Oby-Trim - See APPETITE SUPPRESSANTS 110
Occlusal (topical) - See ANTI-ACNE (Topical) 74
Octapav - See PAPAVERINE 746
Ocu-Caine (ophthalmic) - See ANESTHETICS,
  LOCAL (Ophthalmic) 68
Ocuclear - See XYLOMETAZOLINE 1048

Ocu-Dex (ophthalmic) - See ANTI-INFLAMMATORY,
  STEROIDAL (Ophthalmic) 102
Ocu-Pred (ophthalmic) - See ANTI-INFLAMMATORY,
  STEROIDAL (Ophthalmic) 102
Ocu-Pred-A (ophthalmic) - See ANTI-
  INFLAMMATORY, STEROIDAL (Ophthalmic)
  102
Ocu-Pred Forte (ophthalmic) - See ANTI-
  INFLAMMATORY, STEROIDAL (Ophthalmic)
  102
Ocusert Pilo - See PILOCARPINE 800
Oestrilin - See ESTROGEN 416
Oestrilin (vaginal) - See ESTROGEN 416
O-Flex - See ORPHENADRINE 726
Ogen - See
  ESTROGEN 416
  ESTRONE 418
  ESTROPIPATE 420
Ogen (vaginal) - See ESTROGEN 416
Omnibel - See
  HYOSCYAMINE 512
  SCOPOLAMINE (HYOSCINE) 904
Omnipen - See AMPICILLIN 54
Omnipen-N - See AMPICILLIN 54
Omni-Tuss - See CHLORPHENIRAMINE 236
Onset - See NITRATES 708
O.p-DDD - See MITOTANE 670
Ophthaine (ophthalmic) - See ANESTHETICS,
  LOCAL (Ophthalmic) 68
Ophthetic (ophthalmic) - See ANESTHETICS,
  LOCAL (Ophthalmic) 68
Ophthochlor - See CHLORAMPHENICOL 220
Ophthocort - See CHLORAMPHENICOL 220
OPIUM - See NARCOTIC ANALGESICS 690
Opium Tincture - See PAREGORIC 752
Opticrom - See CROMOLYN 292
Optimine - See AZATADINE 120
Orabase with Benzocaine - See ANESTHETICS
  (Topical) 62
Orabase with Benzocaine (topical) - See
  ANESTHETICS, DENTAL (Topical) 66
Orabase HCA - See
  ADRENOCORTICOIDS (Topical) 18
  HYDROCORTISONE (Cortisol) 502
Oracit - See CITRATES 258
Oradexon - See DEXAMETHASONE 330
Oradrate - See CHLORAL HYDRATE 216
Oragrafin Calcium - See GALLBLADDER X-RAY
  TEST DRUGS (Cholecystographic Agents) 466
Oragrafin Sodium - See GALLBLADDER X-RAY
  TEST DRUGS (Cholecystographic Agents) 466
Orajel - See ANESTHETICS (Topical) 62
Orajel (topical) - See ANESTHETICS, DENTAL
  (Topical) 66
Oramide - See TOLBUTAMIDE 990
Oraminic - See ISOPROPAMIDE 532
Oraminic II - See BROMPHENIRAMINE 154
Orapav - See PAPAVERINE 746
Oraphen-PD - See ACETAMINOPHEN 4
Orasone - See PREDNISONE 826
Oratestin - See ANDROGENS 58
Ora-Testryl - See ANDROGENS 58
Oratrol - See CARBONIC ANHYDRASE
  INHIBITORS 194
Orbenin - See CLOXACILLIN 278
Orecticyl - See RAUWOLFIA ALKALOIDS 886

INDEX

Palafer - See FERROUS FUMARATE 442
Palaron - See XANTHINE BRONCHODILATORS
 1046
Palbar - See BELLADONNA ALKALOIDS &
 BARBITURATES 130
Palbar No. 2 - See
 ATROPINE 116
 BELLADONNA ALKALOIDS & BARBITURATES
 130
Palmiron - See FERROUS FUMARATE 442
Palohist - See
 CHLORPHENIRAMINE 236
 PHENYLEPHRINE 790
Paltet - See TETRACYCLINES 958
PAMA - See ATROPINE 116
Pama No. 1 - See CALCIUM CARBONATE 174
Pamelor - See TRICYCLIC ANTIDEPRESSANTS
 1008
Pamine - See SCOPOLAMINE (Hyoscine) 904
Pamine PB - See
 PHENOBARBITAL 780
 SCOPOLAMINE (Hyoscine) 904
Pamovin - See PYRVINIUM 870
Pamprin IB - See IBUPROFEN 514
Panadol - See
 ACETAMINOPHEN 4
 PREDNISONE 826
Panasorb - See ACETAMINOPHEN 4
Pan-B-1 - See THIAMINE (Vitamin B-1) 970
Pancrease - See PANCRELIPASE 742
PANCREATIN, PEPSIN, BILE SALTS,
 HYOSCYAMINE, ATROPINE, SCOPOLAMINE &
 PHENOBARBITAL 740
PANCRELIPASE 742
Pandyl - See PYRILAMINE 866
Panectyl - See TRIMEPRAZINE 1016
Panex - See ACETAMINOPHEN 4
Panmycin - See TETRACYCLINES 958
Panolol - See PROPRANOLOL 852
PanOxyl - See BENZOYL PEROXIDE 134
PanOxyl AQ - See BENZOYL PEROXIDE 134
Pantapon - See NARCOTIC ANALGESICS 690
Pantelmin - See MEBENDAZOLE 594
Panthocal A & D - See ANESTHETICS (Topical) 62
Pantholin - See PANTOTHENIC ACID (Vitamin B-5)
 744
PANTOTHENIC ACID (Vitamin B-5) 744
PANTOTHENIC ACID - See PANTOTHENIC ACID
 (Vitamin B-5) 744
Panwarfin - See ANTICOAGULANTS (Oral) 86
PAPAVERINE 746
PARA-AMINOSALICYLIC ACID (PAS) 748
Paracet Forte - See CHLORZOXAZONE &
 ACETAMINOPHEN 248
Paracetamol - See ACETAMINOPHEN 4
Paracort - See PREDNISONE 826
Paradione - See ANTICONVULSANTS, DIONE-TYPE
 88
Paraflex - See CHLORZOXAZONE 246
Parafon Forte - See
 ACETAMINOPHEN 4
 CHLORZOXAZONE & ACETAMINOPHEN 248
Parafon Forte DSC - See CHLORZOXAZONE 246
PARAMETHASONE 750
PARAMETHADIONE - See ANTICONVULSANTS,
 DIONE-TYPE 88
Paraphen - See ACETAMINOPHEN 4

Parasal - See PARA-AMINOSALICYLIC ACID (PAS)
 748
Paraspan - See SCOPOLAMINE (Hyoscine) 904
PAREGORIC 752
PAREGORIC - See NARCOTIC ANALGESICS 690
Parepectolin - See
 KAOLIN & PECTIN 542
 KAOLIN, PECTIN & PAREGORIC 546
 PAREGORIC 752
Pargesic - See NARCOTIC ANALGESICS 690
Pargesic Compound 65 - See
 ASPIRIN 112
 CAFFEINE 172
PARGYLINE - See MONAMINE OXIDASE (MAO)
 INHIBITORS 674
PARGYLINE & METHYCLOTHIAZIDE 754
Parlodel - See BROMOCRIPTINE 152
Par-mag - See ALUMINUM HYDROXIDE 28
Parmine - See APPETITE SUPPRESSANTS 110
Parnate - See MONAMINE OXIDASE (MAO)
 INHIBITORS 674
Parsidol - See ETHOPROPAZINE 430
Parsitan - See ETHOPROPAZINE 430
Partuss T.D. - See
 CHLORPHENIRAMINE 236
 PHENYLPROPANOLAMINE 794
P.A.S. - See PARA-AMINOSALICYLIC ACID (PAS)
 748
P.A.S. Acid - See PARA-AMINOSALICYLIC ACID
 (PAS) 748
Pasna - See PARA-AMINOSALICYLIC ACID (PAS)
 748
Pathibamate - See
 MEPROBAMATE 610
 TRIDIHEXETHYL 1010
Pathilon - See TRIDIHEXETHYL 1010
Pathilon w/Phenobarbital - See PHENOBARBITAL
 780
Pathocil - See DICLOXACILLIN 342
P-A-V - See PAPAVERINE 746
Pavabid - See PAPAVERINE 746
Pavabid HP - See PAPAVERINE 746
Pavacap - See PAPAVERINE 746
Pavacen - See PAPAVERINE 746
Pavadon - See
 ACETAMINOPHEN 4
 NARCOTIC ANALGESICS 690
 PAPAVERINE 746
Pavadur - See PAPAVERINE 746
Pavagen - See PAPAVERINE 746
Pavakey - See PAPAVERINE 746
Pava-Par - See PAPAVERINE 746
Pavased - See PAPAVERINE 746
Pavasule - See PAPAVERINE 746
Pavatest - See PAPAVERINE 746
Pavatine - See PAPAVERINE 746
Pavatran - See PAPAVERINE 746
Pavatym - See PAPAVERINE 746
Paveral - See NARCOTIC ANALGESICS 690
Paverolan - See PAPAVERINE 746
Pax 400 - See MEPROBAMATE 610
Paxipam - See HALAZEPAM 492
Payadur - See PAPAVERINE 746
PBR/12 - See PHENOBARBITAL 780
PBZ - See TRIPELENNAMINE 1022
PBZ-SR - See TRIPELENNAMINE 1022
PCE Dispersatabs - See ERYTHROMYCINS 408
Pecto Kay - See KAOLIN & PECTIN 542

PediaCare - See PSEUDOEPHEDRINE 856
Pedia Care 1 - See
  DEXAMETHASONE 330
  DEXTROMETHORPHAN 336
Pediacof - See
  CHLORPHENIRAMINE 236
  NARCOTIC ANALGESICS 690
  PHENYLEPHRINE 790
Pediaflor - See SODIUM FLUORIDE 918
Pediamycin - See ERYTHROMYCINS 408
Pediapred - See PREDNISOLONE 824
Pediazole - See
  ERYTHROMYCINS 408
  ERYTHROMYCIN & SULFISOXAZOLE 410
  SULFISOXAZOLE 938
Pediculoside - See PEDICULOSIDES (Topical) 756
PEDICULOSIDES (Topical) 756
Pedi-Dent - See SODIUM FLUORIDE 918
Pedric - See ACETAMINOPHEN 4
Peece - See
  ATROPINE 116
  HYOSCYAMINE 512
Peedee Dose Aspirin - See ACETAMINOPHEN 4
Peedee Dose Decongestant - See
    PSEUDOEPHEDRINE 856
Peedee Dose Expectorant - See GUAIFENESIN
    480
Peganone - See ETHOTOIN 434
PEMOLINE 758
Penamox - See AMOXICILLIN 50
Penapar VK - See PENICILLIN V 764
Penbritin - See AMPICILLIN 54
Penderal Pacaps - See APPETITE SUPPRESSANTS
    110
Pendiamycin - See ERYTHROMYCINS 408
Pendramine - See PENICILLAMINE 760
Penecort - See ADRENOCORTICOIDS (Topical) 18
Penglobe - See BACAMPICILLIN 122
PENICILLAMINE 760
PENICILLIN G 762
PENICILLIN V 764
Penioral - See PENICILLIN G 762
PENTAERYTHRITOL TETRANITRATE - See
    NITRATES 708
Pentamycetin - See CHLORAMPHENICOL 220
Pentazine - See
  PROMETHAZINE 848
  TRIFLUOPERAZINE 1012
PENTAZOCINE - See NARCOTIC ANALGESICS
    690
PENTAZOCINE & ACETAMINOPHEN - See
    NARCOTIC & ACETAMINOPHEN 688
PENTAZOCINE & ASPIRIN - See NARCOTIC &
    ASPIRIN 692
Pentestan - See NITRATES 708
Pentids - See PENICILLIN G 762
PENTOBARBITAL 766
Pentogen - See PENTOBARBITAL 766
Pentol - See NITRATES 708
Pentol S.A. - See NITRATES 708
Pentolair (ophthalmic) - See CYCLOPENTOLATE
    (Ophthalmic) 304
PENTOXIFYLLINE 768
Pentraspan - See NITRATES 708
Pentraspan SR - See NITRATES 708
Pentritol - See NITRATES 708
Pentylan - See NITRATES 708
Pen-Vee K - See PENICILLIN V 764

Pepcid - See FAMOTIDINE 438
Pepsogel - See ALUMINUM HYDROXIDE 28
Pepto-Bismol - See BISMUTH SUBSALICYLATE 150
Peptol - See CIMETIDINE 252
Percocet - See NARCOTIC & ACETAMINOPHEN
    688
Percocet-5 - See ACETAMINOPHEN 4
Percocet-Demi - See NARCOTIC &
    ACETAMINOPHEN 688
Percodan - See
  ASPIRIN 112
  CAFFEINE 172
  NARCOTIC ANALGESICS 690
  NARCOTIC & ASPIRIN 692
  PHENACETIN 774
Percodan-Demi - See NARCOTIC & ASPIRIN 692
Percogesic - See
  ACETAMINOPHEN 4
  PHENYLTOLOXAMINE 796
Perdiem Plain - See PSYLLIUM 860
Periactin - See CYPROHEPTADINE 316
Peri-Colace - See
  CASCARA 200
  DOCUSATE SODIUM 380
Peridol - See HALOPERIDOL 494
Perifoam - See ANESTHETICS (Topical) 62
Peritinic - See DOCUSATE SODIUM 380
Peritrate - See NITRATES 708
Peritrate Forte - See NITRATES 708
Peritrate SA - See NITRATES 708
Permapen - See PENICILLIN G 762
Permitil - See FLUPHENAZINE 456
Pernox (topical) - See ANTI-ACNE (Topical) 74
PERPHENAZINE 770
PERPHENAZINE & AMITRIPTYLINE 772
Persadox - See BENZOYL PEROXIDE 134
Persadox HP - See BENZOYL PEROXIDE 134
Persa-Gel - See BENZOYL PEROXIDE 134
Persa-Gel W - See BENZOYL PEROXIDE 134
Persantine - See DIPYRIDAMOLE 368
Persistin - See ASPIRIN 112
Pertofrane - See TRICYCLIC ANTIDEPRESSANTS
    1008
Pertussin 8 Hour Cough Formula - See
  DEXAMETHASONE 330
  DEXTROMETHORPHAN 336
Pervadil - See NYLIDRIN 722
Pethadol - See NARCOTIC ANALGESICS 690
Pethidine - See NARCOTIC ANALGESICS 690
P.E.T.N. - See NITRATES 708
Pevaryl (topical) - See ANTIFUNGALS (Topical) 92
Pfiklor - See POTASSIUM SUPPLEMENTS 816
Pfi-Lithium - See LITHIUM 570
Pfizer-E - See ERYTHROMYCINS 408
Pfizerpen - See PENICILLIN G 762
Pfizerpen-AS - See PENICILLIN G 762
Pfizerpen G - See PENICILLIN G 762
Pfizerpen VK - See PENICILLIN V 764
Pharma-Cort - See ADRENOCORTICOIDS (Topical)
    18
Phazyme - See SIMETHICONE 912
Phazyme 125 - See SIMETHICONE 912
Phebe - See BELLADONNA 128
Phedral - See THEOPHYLLINE, EPHEDRINE &
    BARBITURATES 960
PHENACETIN 774
Phenacol-DM - See CHLORPHENIRAMINE 236
Phenameth - See PROMETHAZINE 848

Phen-Amin - See DIPHENHYDRAMINE 360
Phenaphen - See ACETAMINOPHEN 4
Phenaphen w/Codeine - See
  ACETAMINOPHEN 4
  NARCOTIC & ACETAMINOPHEN 688
  NARCOTIC ANALGESICS 690
Phenate - See
  CHLORPHENIRAMINE 236
  PHENYLEPHRINE 790
  PHENYLPROPANOLAMINE 794
Phenazine - See
  PERPHENAZINE 770
  PROMETHAZINE 848
Phenazine-35 - See APPETITE SUPPRESSANTS
  110
Phen-Azo - See PHENAZOPYRIDINE 776
Phenazodine - See PHENAZOPYRIDINE 776
PHENAZOPYRIDINE 776
Phenbuff - See PHENYLBUTAZONE 788
Phenbutazone - See PHENYLBUTAZONE 788
Phencen-50 - See PROMETHAZINE 848
Phendex - See ACETAMINOPHEN 4
Phendiet - See APPETITE SUPPRESSANTS 110
PHENDIMETRAZINE - See APPETITE
  SUPPRESSANTS 110
PHENELZINE - See MONAMINE OXIDASE (MAO)
  INHIBITORS 674
Phenergan - See
  NARCOTIC ANALGESICS 690
  PROMETHAZINE 848
  PSEUDOEPHEDRINE 856
Phenergan-D - See PSEUDOEPHEDRINE 856
Phenergan Fortis - See PROMETHAZINE 848
Phenergan Plain - See PROMETHAZINE 848
Phenergan VC - See PHENYLEPHRINE 790
Phenergan VC w/Codeine - See PHENYLEPHRINE
  790
Phenerhist - See PROMETHAZINE 848
Phenetron - See CHLORPHENIRAMINE 236
Phenetron Lanacaps - See CHLORPHENIRAMINE
  236
PHENIRAMINE 778
PHENINDIONE - See ANTICOAGULANTS (Oral) 86
PHENMETRAZINE - See APPETITE
  SUPPRESSANTS 110
PHENOBARBITAL 780
Pheno-Bella - See BELLADONNA ALKALOIDS &
  BARBITURATES 130
Phenodyne - See CAFFEINE 172
Phenodyne w/Codeine - See
  ASPIRIN 112
  CAFFEINE 172
Phenoject-50 - See PROMETHAZINE 848
Phenolax - See PHENOLPHTHALEIN 782
PHENOLPHTHALEIN 782
Pheno-o-bel - See BELLADONNA 128
PHENPROCOUMON 784
PHENPROCOUMON - See ANTICOAGULANTS
  (Oral) 86
Phensal - See CAFFEINE 172
PHENSUXIMIDE 786
Phentamine - See APPETITE SUPPRESSANTS 110
PHENTERMINE - See APPETITE SUPPRESSANTS
  110
Phentrol - See APPETITE SUPPRESSANTS 110
Phenylalaline Mustard - See MELPHALAN (PAM, L-
  PAM, Phenylalanine Mustard) 604
PHENYLBUTAZONE 788

PHENYLEPHRINE 790
PHENYLEPHRINE (Ophthalmic) 792
Phenylin - See
  PHENYLPROPANOLAMINE 794
  XANTHINE BRONCHODILATORS 1046
PHENYLPROPANOLAMINE 794
PHENYLTOLOXAMINE 796
PHENYTOIN 798
Phenzine - See APPETITE SUPPRESSANTS 110
Pheryl-E - See VITAMIN E 1040
Phillips Milk of Magnesia - See
  ALUMINUM HYDROXIDE 28
  MAGNESIUM HYDROXIDE 584
PHisoAc BP - See BENZOYL PEROXIDE 134
Phospholine Iodide (ophthalmic) - See
  ANTIGLAUCOMA, LONG-ACTING (Ophthalmic)
  96
Phospho-Soda - See SODIUM PHOSPHATE 920
Phrenilin - See
  ACETAMINOPHEN 4
  CAFFEINE 172
  NARCOTIC ANALGESICS 690
Phyldrox - See
  EPHEDRINE 392
  PHENOBARBITAL 780
  XANTHINE BRONCHODILATORS 1046
Phyllocontin - See XANTHINE
  BRONCHODILATORS 1046
Physeptone - See NARCOTIC ANALGESICS 690
PHYSOSTIGMINE (Ophthalmic) - See
  ANTIGLAUCOMA, SHORT-ACTING
  (Ophthalmic) 98
Physpan - See XANTHINE BRONCHODILATORS 1046
Phytonadione - See VITAMIN K 1042
Pilocar - See PILOCARPINE 800
PILOCARPINE 800
Pilocel - See PILOCARPINE 800
Pilokair - See PILOCARPINE 800
Pilomiotin - See PILOCARPINE 800
Pilopine HS - See PILOCARPINE 800
Piloptic - See PILOCARPINE 800
Pimaricin - See NATAMYCIN (Ophthalmic) 694
PINDOLOL 802
Pindolol - See PINDOLOL 802
PINDOLOL & HYDROCHLOROTHIAZIDE - See
  BETA-ADRENERGIC BLOCKING AGENTS &
  THIAZIDE DIURETICS 140
Piperazine Estrone Sulfate - See ESTROPIPATE 420
Piperazine Estrone Sulfate (vaginal) - See
  ESTROGEN 416
Piracaps - See TETRACYCLINES 958
PIROXICAM 804
Pitrex (topical) - See ANTIFUNGALS (Topical) 92
Placidyl - See ETHCHLORVYNOL 424
Plaquenil - See HYDROXYCHLOROQUINE 508
Plegine - See APPETITE SUPPRESSANTS 110
Plexonal - See TALBUTAL (Butalbital) 944
Plova - See PSYLLIUM 860
PMB - See MEPROBAMATE 610
PMB-200 - See ESTROGEN 416
PMB-400 - See ESTROGEN 416
PMS-Benztropine - See BENZTROPINE 138
PMS-Dimenhydrinate - See DIMENHYDRINATE 356
PMS Dopazide - See
  METHYLDOPA 642
  METHYLDOPA & THIAZIDE DIURETICS 644
PMS Ferrous Sulfate - See FERROUS SULFATE 446
PMS Isoniazid - See ISONIAZID 530

Predair (ophthalmic) - See ANTI-INFLAMMATORY, STEROIDAL (Ophthalmic) 102

Predair-A (ophthalmic) - See ANTI-INFLAMMATORY, STEROIDAL (Ophthalmic) 102

Predair Forte (ophthalmic) - See ANTI-INFLAMMATORY, STEROIDAL (Ophthalmic) 102

Predaject - See PREDNISOLONE 824

Predate - See PREDNISOLONE 824

Predate-S - See PREDNISOLONE 824

Predate-TBA - See PREDNISOLONE 824

Predcor - See PREDNISOLONE 824

Pred Cor-TBA - See PREDNISOLONE 824

Pre-Dep - See METHYLPREDNISOLONE 650

Pred Forte - See PREDNISOLONE 824

Pred Forte (ophthalmic) - See ANTI-INFLAMMATORY, STEROIDAL (Ophthalmic) 102

Pred Mild - See PREDNISOLONE 824

Pred Mild (ophthalmic) - See ANTI-INFLAMMATORY, STEROIDAL (Ophthalmic) 102

Prednicen-M - See PREDNISONE 826

Prednisol TBA - See PREDNISOLONE 824

PREDNISOLONE 824

PREDNISOLONE (Ophthalmic) - See ANTI-INFLAMMATORY, STEROIDAL (Ophthalmic) 102

PREDNISOLONE (Otic) - See ANTI-INFLAMMATORY (Otic) 100

PREDNISONE 826

Predsol (ophthalmic) - See ANTI-INFLAMMATORY, STEROIDAL (Ophthalmic) 102

Predulose - See PREDNISOLONE 824

Prefrin - See PHENYLEPHRINE 790

Prefrin Liquifilm (ophthalmic) - See PHENYLEPHRINE (Ophthalmic) 792

Prelestone - See BETAMETHASONE 142

Prelone - See PREDNISOLONE 824

Prelu-2 - See APPETITE SUPPRESSANTS 110

Preludin - See APPETITE SUPPRESSANTS 110

Premarin - See
CONJUGATED ESTROGENS 286
ESTROGEN 416

Premarin (vaginal) - See ESTROGEN 416

Prenate 90 - See
CALCIUM CARBONATE 174
DOCUSATE SODIUM 380
FERROUS FUMARATE 442

Preparation "H" (rectal) - See ANESTHETICS (Rectal) 60

Presalin - See
ACETAMINOPHEN 4
ACETAMINOPHEN & SALICYLATES 6
ASPIRIN 112
NARCOTIC ANALGESICS 690

Presamine - See TRICYCLIC ANTIDEPRESSANTS 1008

Pre-Sate - See APPETITE SUPPRESSANTS 110

Primatene - See
EPHEDRINE 392
EPINEPHRINE 394

Primatene Mist - See EPINEPHRINE 394

Primatene Mist Solution - See EPINEPHRINE 394

Primatene Mist Suspension - See EPINEPHRINE 394

Primatene, M Formula - See
PYRILAMINE 866
XANTHINE BRONCHODILATORS 1046

Primatene, P Formula - See
PHENOBARBITAL 780
THEOPHYLLINE, EPHEDRINE & BARBITURATES 960
XANTHINE BRONCHODILATORS 1046

PRIMIDONE 828

Principen - See AMPICILLIN 54

Priniril - See LISINOPRIL 568

Prioderm (topical) - See PEDICULOSIDES (Topical) 756

Pro-65 - See NARCOTIC ANALGESICS 690

Probahist - See
CHLORPHENIRAMINE 236
PSEUDOEPHEDRINE 856

Probalan - See PROBENECID 830

Pro-Banthine - See PROPANTHELINE 850

Pro-Banthine w/Phenobarbital - See
PHENOBARBITAL 780
PROPANTHELINE 850

Proben-C - See PROBENECID & COLCHICINE 832

PROBENECID 830

PROBENECID & COLCHICINE 832

Probital - See PHENOBARBITAL 780

PROBUCOL 834

PROCAINAMIDE 836

Pro-Cal-Sof - See
DOCUSATE CALCIUM 376
DOCUSATE POTASSIUM 378

Procamide - See PROCAINAMIDE 836

Procan - See PROCAINAMIDE 836

Procan SR - See PROCAINAMIDE 836

Procapan - See PROCAINAMIDE 836

PROCARBAZINE 838

Procardia - See NIFEDIPINE 706

Prochlor-Iso - See
ISOPROPAMIDE 532
PROCHLORPERAZINE 840

PROCHLORPERAZINE 840

PROCHLORPERAZINE & ISOPROPAMIDE 842

Proctocort - See
ADRENOCORTICOIDS (Topical) 18
HYDROCORTISONE (Cortisol) 502

Proctodon - See ANESTHETICS (Topical) 62

Proctofoam - See ANESTHETICS (Topical) 62

Proctofoam (rectal) - See ANESTHETICS (Rectal) 60

Procyclid - See PROCYCLIDINE 844

PROCYCLIDINE 844

Procytox - See CYCLOPHOSPHAMIDE 306

Pro-Dep-40 - See METHYLPREDNISOLONE 650

Pro-Dep-80 - See METHYLPREDNISOLONE 650

Prodiem - See PSYLLIUM 860

Prodolor - See
ACETAMINOPHEN 4
CAFFEINE 172
NARCOTIC ANALGESICS 690

Profene - See NARCOTIC ANALGESICS 690

Profenid - See KETOPROFEN 550

Progens - See
CONJUGATED ESTROGENS 286
ESTROGEN 416

Progesic - See FENOPROFEN 440

Progesic Compound-65 - See
ASPIRIN 112
CAFFEINE 172

PSORALENS 858
Psorcon - See ADRENOCORTICOIDS (Topical) 18
Psorcon-E - See ADRENOCORTICOIDS (Topical) 18
PSP-IV - See PREDNISOLONE 824
P.S.P.R.X. 1, 2 & 3 - See APPETITE
    SUPPRESSANTS 110
PSYLLIUM 860
Pulmophylline - See XANTHINE
    BRONCHODILATORS 1046
Purge - See CASTOR OIL 202
Purinethol - See MERCAPTOPURINE 614
Purinol - See ALLOPURINOL 22
Purodigin - See DIGITALIS PREPARATIONS 352
P.V. Carpine - See PILOCARPINE 800
P.V. Carpine Liquifilm - See PILOCARPINE 800
P-V-Tussin - See
    CHLORPHENIRAMINE 236
    GUAIFENESIN 480
    PHENYLEPHRINE 790
    PYRILAMINE 866
Pyma - See CHLORPHENIRAMINE 236
Pyma Timed - See PHENYLEPHRINE 790
Pyopen - See CARBENICILLIN 186
Pyracort-D - See PHENYLEPHRINE 790
Pyrdonnal Spansules - See PHENOBARBITAL 780
PYRETHRINS AND PIPERONYL BUTOXIDE
    (Topical) - See PEDICULOSIDES (Topical) 756
Pyribenzamine - See TRIPELENNAMINE 1022
Pyribenzamine w/Ephedrine - See EPHEDRINE 392
Pyridamole - See DIPYRIDAMOLE 368
Pyridiate - See PHENAZOPYRIDINE 776
Pyridium - See PHENAZOPYRIDINE 776
Pyridium Plus - See
    BUTABARBITAL 166
    HYOSCYAMINE 512
    PHENAZOPYRIDINE 776
PYRIDOSTIGMINE 862
PYRIDOXINE (Vitamin B-6) 864
PYRILAMINE 866
PYRILAMINE & PENTOBARBITAL 868
Pyrinyl (topical) - See PEDICULOSIDES (Topical)
    756
PYRITHIONE (Topical) - See ANTISEBORRHEIC
    (Topical) 104
Pyrodine - See PHENAZOPYRIDINE 776
Pyronium - See PHENAZOPYRIDINE 776
Pyroxine - See PYRIDOXINE (Vitamin B-6) 864
Pyr-pam - See PYRVINIUM 870
Pyrroxate - See
    CAFFEINE 172
    CHLORPHENIRAMINE 236
Pyrroxate w/Codeine - See CHLORPHENIRAMINE
    236
PYRVINIUM 870
PZI - See INSULIN 520

Q

Q'Dtet - See TETRACYCLINES 958
Q-Pam - See DIAZEPAM 338
Quadrahist - See
    CHLORPHENIRAMINE 236
    PHENYLPROPANOLAMINE 794
    PHENYLTOLOXAMINE 796
Quadrinal - See
    EPHEDRINE 392
    PHENOBARBITAL 780
    XANTHINE BRONCHODILATORS 1046
Quarzan - See CLIDINIUM 262

Quelidrine - See
    CHLORPHENIRAMINE 236
    EPHEDRINE 392
    PHENYLEPHRINE 790
Queltuss - See
    CHLORPHENIRAMINE 236
    DEXTROMETHORPHAN 336
    GUAIFENESIN 480
Questran - See CHOLESTYRAMINE 250
Quiagel PG - See KAOLIN, PECTIN,
    BELLADONNA & OPIUM 544
Quiagen - See THEOPHYLLINE & GUAIFENESIN
    966
Quibron - See
    GUAIFENESIN 480
    THEOPHYLLINE & GUAIFENESIN 966
    XANTHINE BRONCHODILATORS 1046
Quibron Plus - See
    BUTABARBITAL 166
    EPHEDRINE 392
    THEOPHYLLINE, EPHEDRINE, GUAIFENESIN &
      BARBITURATES 962
    XANTHINE BRONCHODILATORS 1046
Quibron-T - See XANTHINE BRONCHODILATORS
    1046
Quibron-T Dividose - See XANTHINE
    BRONCHODILATORS 1046
Quibron-T/SR Dividose - See XANTHINE
    BRONCHODILATORS 1046
Quick Pep - See CAFFEINE 172
Quiess - See HYDROXYZINE 510
Quietal - See MEPROBAMATE 610
Quinaglute Dura-Tabs - See QUINIDINE 878
Quinalan - See QUINIDINE 878
Quinamm - See QUININE 880
Quinate - See QUINIDINE 878
Quindan - See QUININE 880
QUINACRINE 872
Quine - See QUININE 880
QUINESTROL 874
QUINETHAZONE 876
Quinidex Extentabs - See QUINIDINE 878
QUINIDINE 878
QUININE 880
Quinite - See QUININE 880
Quinobarb - See QUINIDINE 878
Quinsana Plus (topical) - See ANTIFUNGALS
    (Topical) 92
Quless - See PENTOBARBITAL 766
Quotane - See ANESTHETICS (Topical) 62

R

Racet (topical) - See ANTIBACTERIALS,
    ANTIFUNGALS (Topical) 82
Racet-SE - See ADRENOCORTICOIDS (Topical) 18
Radio-pharmaceuticals - See RADIO-
    PHARMACEUTICALS 882
RADIO-PHARMACEUTICALS 882
Radiopaque - See GALLBLADDER X-RAY TEST
    DRUGS (Cholecystographic Agents) 466
Radiostol Forte - See VITAMIN D 1038
Radiostol - See VITAMIN D 1038
Ralabromophen - See BROMPHENIRAMINE 156
RANITIDINE 884
Ratic - See ALUMINUM HYDROXIDE 28
Ratio - See
    CALCIUM CARBONATE 174
    CALCIUM & MAGNESIUM ANTACIDS 176

INDEX

Retin-A - See TRETINOIN (Topical) 996
Retin A (topical) - See ANTI-ACNE (Topical) 74
Retinoic Acid - See TRETINOIN (Topical) 996
Retinoic Acid (topical) - See ANTI-ACNE (Topical) 74
Retrovir - See ZIDOVUDINE (also called AZT,
    Azidothymidine) 1050
Rezamid (topical) - See ANTI-ACNE (Topical) 74
R-HCTZ-H - See RESERPINE, HYDRALAZINE &
    HYDROCHLOROTHIAZIDE 892
Rhinall - See PHENYLEPHRINE 790
Rhindecon - See PHENYLPROPANOLAMINE 794
Rhinex - See
    CHLORPHENIRAMINE 236
    PHENYLEPHRINE 790
Rhinex Ty-Med - See PHENYLPROPANOLAMINE
    794
Rhinidrin - See PHENYLPROPANOLAMINE 794
Rhinocaps - See
    ACETAMINOPHEN 4
    ASPIRIN 112
    PHENYLPROPANOLAMINE 794
Rhinolar - See
    CHLORPHENIRAMINE 236
    PHENYLPROPANOLAMINE 794
Rhinolar-EX - See CHLORPHENIRAMINE 236
Rhulicort - See ADRENOCORTICOIDS (Topical) 18
Rhythmin - See PROCAINAMIDE 836
RIBAVIRIN 894
RIBOFLAVIN (Vitamin B-2) 896
RID (topical) - See PEDICULOSIDES (Topical) 756
Rid-A-Pain - See ANESTHETICS (Topical) 62
Rid-A-Pain Compound - See ACETAMINOPHEN &
    SALICYLATES 6
Ridaura-oral - See GOLD COMPOUNDS 476
Rifadin - See RIFAMPIN 898
Rifamate - See
    ISONIAZID 530
    RIFAMPIN 898
Rifampicin - See RIFAMPIN 898
RIFAMPIN 898
Rifomycin - See RIFAMPIN 898
Rimactane - See RIFAMPIN 898
Rimifon - See ISONIAZID 530
Riobin-50 - See RIBOFLAVIN (Vitamin B-2) 896
Riopan - See
    ALUMINUM HYDROXIDE 28
    ALUMINUM & MAGNESIUM ANTACIDS 30
Riopan Plus - See
    ALUMINUM, MAGNESIUM, MAGALDRATE &
        SIMETHICONE ANTACIDS 32
    SIMETHICONE 912
Riphen-10 - See ASPIRIN 112
Ritalin - See METHYLPHENIDATE 648
Ritalin SR - See METHYLPHENIDATE 648
RITODRINE 900
Rival - See DIAZEPAM 338
RMS Uniserts - See NARCOTIC ANALGESICS 690
Robafen - See GUAIFENESIN 480
Robalate - See ALUMINUM HYDROXIDE 28
Robalyn - See DIPHENHYDRAMINE 360
Robam - See MEPROBAMATE 610
Robamate - See MEPROBAMATE 610
Robamol - See METHOCARBAMOL 632
Robamox - See AMOXICILLIN 50
Robaxin - See METHOCARBAMOL 632
Robaxisal - See METHOCARBAMOL 632
Robicillin VK - See PENICILLIN V 764
Robidex - See DEXTROMETHORPHAN 336

Robidone - See NARCOTIC ANALGESICS 690
Robidrine - See PSEUDOEPHEDRINE 856
Robigesic - See ACETAMINOPHEN 4
Robimycin - See ERYTHROMYCINS 408
Robinul - See GLYCOPYRROLATE 474
Robinul Forte - See GLYCOPYRROLATE 474
Robinul-PH - See PHENOBARBITAL 780
Robitet - See TETRACYCLINES 958
Robitussin - See
    DEXTROMETHORPHAN 336
    GUAIFENESIN 480
Robitussin-AC - See
    NARCOTIC ANALGESICS 690
    PHENIRAMINE 778
Robitussin-CF - See PHENYLPROPANOLAMINE
    794
Robitussin-DAC - See PSEUDOEPHEDRINE 856
Robitussin-DM - See DEXTROMETHORPHAN 336
Rocaltrol - See VITAMIN D 1038
Ro-Cycline - See TETRACYCLINES 958
Rodex - See PYRIDOXINE (Vitamin B-6) 864
Ro-Diet - See APPETITE SUPPRESSANTS 110
Rofact - See RIFAMPIN 898
Ro-Fedrin - See PSEUDOEPHEDRINE 856
Rogaine (topical) - See MINOXIDIL (Topical) 668
Ro-Hist - See TRIPELENNAMINE 1022
Rolabromophen - See
    PHENYLEPHRINE 790
    PHENYLPROPANOLAMINE 794
Rolahist - See PHENYLEPHRINE 790
Rolaids - See
    ALUMINUM HYDROXIDE 28
    SODIUM CARBONATE 916
Rolazine - See HYDRALAZINE 496
Rolidrin - See NYLIDRIN 722
Rolox - See ALUMINUM & MAGNESIUM
    ANTACIDS 30
Romilar - See DEXTROMETHORPHAN 336
Romilar CF - See DEXTROMETHORPHAN 336
Romilar Children's Cough - See
    DEXTROMETHORPHAN 336
Ronase - See TOLAZAMIDE 988
Rondec - See PSEUDOEPHEDRINE 856
Rondomycin - See TETRACYCLINES 958
Ronuvex - See ACETAMINOPHEN 4
Ro-Orphena - See ORPHENADRINE 726
Ropanth - See PROPANTHELINE 850
Ro-Papan - See PAPAVERINE 746
Rosoxol - See SULFISOXAZOLE 938
Ro-Thyronine - See
    LIOTHYRONINE 564
    THYROXINE (T-4, Levothyroxine) 980
Ro Trim - See ATROPINE 116
Roubac - See SULFAMETHOXAZOLE 938
Roucol - See ALLOPURINOL 22
Rounox - See ACETAMINOPHEN 4
Rounox with Codeine - See NARCOTIC &
    ACETAMINOPHEN 688
Rovbac - See TRIMETHOPRIM 1020
Roxanol - See NARCOTIC ANALGESICS 690
Roxanol SR - See NARCOTIC ANALGESICS 690
Roxicet - See NARCOTIC & ACETAMINOPHEN 688
Roxicodone - See NARCOTIC ANALGESICS 690
Roychlor - See POTASSIUM SUPPLEMENTS 816
Roydan - See DANTHRON 320
Roydan Mild - See DANTHRON 320
Royonate - See POTASSIUM SUPPLEMENTS 816
RP-Mycin - See ERYTHROMYCINS 408

Sebasum (topical) - See ANTI-ACNE, CLEANSING
  (Topical) 72
Sebex (topical) - See ANTI-ACNE (Topical) 74
Sebex-T (topical) - See ANTISEBORRHEIC (Topical)
  104
Sebisol (topical) - See ANTI-ACNE (Topical) 74
Sebucare (topical) - See ANTI-ACNE (Topical) 74
Sebulex (topical) - See ANTI-ACNE (Topical) 74
Sebutone (topical) - See ANTISEBORRHEIC
  (Topical) 104
SECOBARBITAL 906
Secogen - See SECOBARBITAL 906
Seconal - See SECOBARBITAL 906
Sectral - See ACEBUTOLOL 2
Sedabamate - See MEPROBAMATE 610
Sedadrops - See PHENOBARBITAL 780
Sedajen - See HYOSCYAMINE 512
Sedamine - See
  ATROPINE 116
  HYOSCYAMINE 512
  SCOPOLAMINE (Hyoscine) 904
Sedapap - See
  ACETAMINOPHEN 4
  NARCOTIC ANALGESICS 690
Sedapar - See
  ATROPINE 116
  BELLADONNA 128
  HYOSCYAMINE 512
  SCOPOLAMINE (Hyoscine) 904
Sedatabs - See ATROPINE 116
Sedative - See
  AMOBARBITAL 48
  BELLADONNA ALKALOIDS & BARBITURATES
    130
  BUTABARBITAL 166
  BUTALBITAL & ASPIRIN (Also contains caffeine)
    168
  ERGOTAMINE, CAFFEINE, BELLADONNA &
    PENTOBARBITAL 406
  ISOMETHAPRINE, DICHLORALPHENAZONE &
    ACETAMINOPHEN 528
  MEPHOBARBITAL 608
  METHARBITAL 626
  PANCREATIN, PEPSIN, BILE SALTS,
    HYOSCYAMINE, ATROPINE, SCOPOLAMINE &
    PHENOBARBITAL 740
  PENTOBARBITAL 766
  PHENOBARBITAL 780
  SECOBARBITAL 906
  TALBUTAL (Butalbital) 944
  THEOPHYLLINE, EPHEDRINE &
    BARBITURATES 960
  THEOPHYLLINE, EPHEDRINE, GUAIFENESIN &
    BARBITURATES 962
Sedative (barbiturate) - See PYRILAMINE &
  PENTOBARBITAL 868
Sedative-hypnotic - See
  ETHINAMATE 426
  METHYPRYLON 662
Sedatromine - See
  BELLADONNA 128
  HYOSCYAMINE 512
Sedatuss - See DEXTROMETHORPHAN 336
Sedralex - See
  ATROPINE 116
  HYOSCYAMINE 512
  SCOPOLAMINE (Hyoscine) 904

Seds - See
  ATROPINE 116
  BELLADONNA ALKALOIDS & BARBITURATES
    130
  HYOSCYAMINE 512
  SCOPOLAMINE (Hyoscine) 904
Seidlitz Powder - See SODIUM BICARBONATE 914
Seldane - See TERFENADINE 952
SELENIUM SULFIDE (Topical) - See
  ANTISEBORRHEIC (Topical) 104
Selenomethionine Se 75 - See RADIO-
  PHARMACEUTICALS 882
Selestoject - See BETAMETHASONE 142
Selsun (topical) - See ANTISEBORRHEIC (Topical)
  104
Selsun Blue (topical) - See ANTISEBORRHEIC
  (Topical) 104
Semilente - See INSULIN 520
Semilente Iletin - See INSULIN 520
Semilente Iletin I - See INSULIN 520
Semitard - See INSULIN 520
Senexon - See SENNA 908
SENNA 908
SENNOSIDES A & B 910
Senokot - See
  SENNA 908
  SENNOSIDES A & B 910
Senokot with Psyllium - See PSYLLIUM 860
Senokot-S - See DOCUSATE SODIUM 380
Senolax - See SENNA 908
Septra - See
  SULFAMETHOXAZOLE 932
  TRIMETHOPRIM 1020
Ser-Ap-Es - See
  HYDRALAZINE 496
  HYDROCHLOROTHIAZIDE 500
  RAUWOLFIA ALKALOIDS 886
  RESERPINE, HYDRALAZINE &
    HYDROCHLOROTHIAZIDE 892
Seral - See SECOBARBITAL 906
Serax - See OXAZEPAM 732
Sereen - See CHLORDIAZEPOXIDE 222
Serenack - See DIAZEPAM 338
Serentil - See MESORIDAZINE 618
Seromycin - See CYCLOSERINE 308
Serophene - See CLOMIPHENE 268
Serpalan - See RAUWOLFIA ALKALOIDS 886
Serpanray - See RAUWOLFIA ALKALOIDS 886
Serpasil - See RAUWOLFIA ALKALOIDS 886
Serpasil-Apresoline - See
  HYDRALAZINE 496
  RESERPINE & HYDRALAZINE 890
  RAUWOLFIA ALKALOIDS 886
Serpasil-Esidrix - See
  HYDROCHLOROTHIAZIDE 500
  RAUWOLFIA ALKALOIDS 886
  RAUWOLFIA & THIAZIDE DIURETICS 888
Serpate - See RAUWOLFIA ALKALOIDS 886
Sertan - See PRIMIDONE 828
Serutan - See PSYLLIUM 860
Serutan Toasted Granules - See PSYLLIUM 860
Sherafed - See PSEUDOEPHEDRINE 856
Siblin - See PSYLLIUM 860
Sidonna - See BUTABARBITAL 166
Silain - See SIMETHICONE 912
Silain-Gel - See
  ALUMINUM, MAGNESIUM, MAGALDRATE &
    SIMETHICONE ANTACIDS 32

INDEX

SK-Probenecid - See PROBENECID 830
SK-Propantheline - See PROPANTHELINE 850
SK-Quinidine Sulfate - See QUINIDINE 878
SK-Reserpine - See RAUWOLFIA ALKALOIDS 886
SK-Soxazole - See SULFISOXAZOLE 938
SK-Terpin Hydrate w/Codeine - See TERPIN
    HYDRATE 954
SK-Tetracycline - See TETRACYCLINES 956
SK-Thioridazine Hydrochloride - See THIORIDAZINE
    972
SK-Tolbutamide - See TOLBUTAMIDE 990
Sleep-Eze - See DIPHENHYDRAMINE 360
Sleep-Eze 3 - See DIPHENHYDRAMINE 360
Sleep inducer (hypnotic) - See ETHCHLORVYNOL
    424
Slim-Tabs - See APPETITE SUPPRESSANTS 110
Slo-bid Gyrocaps - See XANTHINE
    BRONCHODILATORS 1046
Slo-Fedrin A-60 - See EPHEDRINE 392
Slo-Phyllin GG - See
    GUAIFENESIN 480
    THEOPHYLLINE & GUAIFENESIN 966
    XANTHINE BRONCHODILATORS 1046
Slo-Phyllin Gyrocaps - See XANTHINE
    BRONCHODILATORS 1046
Slophyllin - See XANTHINE BRONCHODILATORS
    1046
Slo-Pot - See POTASSIUM SUPPLEMENTS 816
Slow-Fe - See FERROUS SULFATE 446
Slow-K - See POTASSIUM SUPPLEMENTS 816
Slow-trasicor - See OXPRENOLOL 7234
Slynn-LL - See APPETITE SUPPRESSANTS 110
Smooth-muscle relaxant - See FLAVOXATE 448
SMP Atropine - See ATROPINE 116
SMP Atropine (ophthalmic) - See CYCLOPEGIC,
    MYDRIATIC (Ophthalmic) 302
SMZ-TMP - See
    SULFAMETHOXAZOLE 932
    TRIMETHOPRIM 1020
Sobutuss - See DEXTROMETHORPHAN 336
Soda Mint - See SODIUM BICARBONATE 914
SODIUM AUROTHIOMALATE - See GOLD
    COMPOUNDS 476
SODIUM BICARBONATE 914
SODIUM CARBONATE 916
Sodium Chromate Cr 51 - See RADIO-
    PHARMACEUTICALS 882
SODIUM CITRATE & CITRIC ACID - See CITRATES
    258
Sodium Cromoblycate - See CROMOLYN 292
SODIUM FLUORIDE 918
Sodium Iodide I 123 - See RADIO-
    PHARMACEUTICALS 882
Sodium Iodide I 131 - See RADIO-
    PHARMACEUTICALS 882
Sodium Pertechnetate Tc 99m - See RADIO-
    PHARMACEUTICALS 882
SODIUM PHOSPHATE 920
Sodium Phosphate P 32 - See RADIO-
    PHARMACEUTICALS 882
SODIUM SALICYLATE - See SALICYLATES 902
Sofarin - See ANTICOAGULANTS (Oral) 86
Sof-Cil - See PSYLLIUM 860
Soft-N-Soothe - See ANESTHETICS (Topical) 62
Solarcaine - See ANESTHETICS (Topical) 62
Solazine - See TRIFLUOPERAZINE 1012
Solfoton - See PHENOBARBITAL 780

SOLGANAL-injection - See GOLD COMPOUNDS
    476
Solium - See CHLORDIAZEPOXIDE 222
Solu-Cortef - See HYDROCORTISONE (Cortisol)
    502
Solu-Flur - See SODIUM FLUORIDE 918
Solu-Medrol - See METHYLPREDNISOLONE 650
Solu-medrone - See METHYLPREDNISOLONE 650
Solurex - See DEXAMETHASONE 330
Solurex LA - See DEXAMETHASONE 330
Soma - See CARISOPRODOL 196
Soma Compound - See
    ASPIRIN 112
    CARISOPRODOL 196
    PHENACETIN 774
Soma Compound w/Codeine - See
    ASPIRIN 112
    NARCOTIC ANALGESICS 690
Sominex - See
    DIPHENHYDRAMINE 360
    PYRILAMINE 866
Sominex Formula 2 - See DIPHENHYDRAMINE
    360
SominiFere - See DIPHENHYDRAMINE 360
Somnal - See FLURAZEPAM 460
Somnicaps - See PYRILAMINE 866
Somophyllin - See XANTHINE
    BRONCHODILATORS 1046
Somophyllin-12 - See XANTHINE
    BRONCHODILATORS 1046
Somophyllin-CRT - See XANTHINE
    BRONCHODILATORS 1046
Somophyllin-DF - See XANTHINE
    BRONCHODILATORS 1046
Somophyllin-T - See XANTHINE
    BRONCHODILATORS 1046
Som-Pam - See FLURAZEPAM 460
Sopamycetin - See CHLORAMPHENICOL 220
Soprodol - See CARISOPRODOL 196
Sorate - See NITRATES 708
Sorbase - See
    GUAIFENESIN 480
    DEXTROMETHORPHAN 336
Sorbase II - See NARCOTIC ANALGESICS 690
Sorbide - See NITRATES 708
Sorbide T.D. - See NITRATES 708
Sorbitrate - See NITRATES 708
Sorbitrate SA - See NITRATES 708
Sorbutuss - See GUAIFENESIN 480
Sosol - See SULFISOXAZOLE 938
Sotacor - See SOTALOL 922
SOTALOL 922
Soxa - See SULFISOXAZOLE 938
Spabelin - See
    ATROPINE 116
    BELLADONNA 128
    HYOSCYAMINE 512
    SCOPOLAMINE (Hyoscine) 904
Spancap No. 1 - See DEXTROAMPHETAMINE 334
Span-Est-Test - See TESTOSTERONE & ESTRADIOL
    956
Span-FF - See FERROUS FUMARATE 442
Span-Niacin - See NIACIN (Nicotinic Acid) 700
Span-RD - See APPETITE SUPPRESSANTS 110
Sparine - See PROMAZINE 846
Spasaid - See
    ATROPINE 116
    HYOSCYAMINE 512

Sucrets Cough Control - See
    DEXTROMETHORPHAN 336
Sudafed - See PSEUDOEPHEDRINE 856
Sudafed S.A. - See PSEUDOEPHEDRINE 856
Sudagest - See PSEUDOEPHEDRINE 856
Sudahist - See PSEUDOEPHEDRINE 856
Suda-Prol - See PSEUDOEPHEDRINE 856
Sudolin - See
    PSEUDOEPHEDRINE 856
    XANTHINE BRONCHODILATORS 1046
Sudoprin - See ACETAMINOPHEN 4
Sudrin - See PSEUDOEPHEDRINE 856
Sulamyd (ophthalmic) - See ANTIBACTERIALS
    (Ophthalmic) 76
Sul-Blue (topical) - See ANTISEBORRHEIC (Topical)
    104
Sulcrate - See SUCRALFATE 928
Suldiazo - See SULFONAMIDES &
    PHENAZOPYRIDINE 940
Sulfa (sulfonamide) - See
    ERYTHROMYCIN & SULFISOXAZOLE 410
    SULFACYTINE 930
    SULFAMETHOXAZOLE 932
    SULFASALAZINE 934
    SULFISOXAZOLE 938
SULFACYTINE 930
Sulfafurazole - See SULFISOXAZOLE 938
Sulfafurazole (ophthalmic) - See ANTIBACTERIALS
    (Ophthalmic) 76
Sulfafurazole & Phenazopyridine - See
    SULFONAMIDES & PHENAZOPYRIDINE 940
Sulfagen - See SULFISOXAZOLE 938
Sulfamethoprim - See SULFAMETHOXAZOLE 932
SULFAMETHOXAZOLE 932
SULFAMETHOXAZOLE & PHENAZOPYRIDINE -
    See SULFONAMIDES & PHENAZOPYRIDINE
    940
SULFASALAZINE 934
Sulfex (ophthalmic) - See ANTIBACTERIALS
    (Ophthalmic) 76
SULFINPYRAZONE 364
SULFISOXAZOLE 938
SULFISOXAZOLE & PHENAZOPYRIDINE - See
    SULFONAMIDES & PHENAZOPYRIDINE 940
Sulfizin - See SULFISOXAZOLE 938
Sulfizole - See SULFISOXAZOLE 938
Sulfi-10 (ophthalmic) - See ANTIBACTERIALS
    (Ophthalmic) 76
SULFONAMIDES (Ophthalmic) - See
    ANTIBACTERIALS (Ophthalmic) 76
SULFONAMIDES & PHENAZOPYRIDINE 940
Sulfone - See DAPSONE 324
Sulfonurea - See
    ACETOHEXAMIDE 8
    CHLORPROPAMIDE 240
    GLIPIZIDE 470
    GLYBURIDE 472
    TOLAZAMIDE 988
    TOLBUTAMIDE 990
Sulforcin (topical) - See ANTI-ACNE (Topical) 74
SULFUR (topical) - See ANTISEBORRHEIC
    (Topical) 104
SULFURATED LIME (Topical) - See ANTI-ACNE,
    CLEANSING (Topical) 72
SULINDAC 942
Sulmeprim - See SULFAMETHOXAZOLE 932
Sulten-10 (ophthalmic) - See ANTIBACTERIALS
    (Ophthalmic) 76

Summit - See ACETAMINOPHEN 4
Sumox - See AMOXICILLIN 50
Sumycin - See TETRACYCLINES 956
Supac - See
    ACETAMINOPHEN 4
    ACETAMINOPHEN & SALICYLATES 6
    ASPIRIN 112
    CAFFEINE 172
    NARCOTIC ANALGESICS 690
Supasa - See ASPIRIN 112
Supen - See AMPICILLIN 54
Super Anahist - See PHENYLEPHRINE 790
Supeudol - See NARCOTIC ANALGESICS 690
Suplical - See
    CALCIUM CARBONATE 174
    CALCIUM SUPPLEMENTS 178
Suppap - See ACETAMINOPHEN 4
Suprazine - See TRIFLUOPERAZINE 1012
Surfacaine - See ANESTHETICS (Topical) 62
Surfak - See DOCUSATE CALCIUM 376
Surmontil - See TRICYCLIC ANTIDEPRESSANTS
    1008
Susadrin - See NITRATES 708
Susano - See BELLADONNA ALKALOIDS &
    BARBITURATES 130
Sus-phrine - See EPINEPHRINE 394
Sust-A - See VITAMIN A 1032
Sustaire - See XANTHINE BRONCHODILATORS
    1046
Sustaverine - See PAPAVERINE 746
Swiss Kriss - See SENNA 908
Syflex - See NAPROXEN 686
Sylapar - See
    ACETAMINOPHEN 4
    NARCOTIC ANALGESICS 690
Syllact - See PSYLLIUM 860
Symadine - See AMANTADINE 36
Symetra - See APPETITE SUPPRESSANTS 110
Symmetrel - See AMANTADINE 36
Sympathomimetic - See
    ALBUTEROL 20
    EPHEDRINE 392
    EPINEPHRINE 394
    ISOPROTERENOL 534
    ISOPROTERENOL & PHENYLEPHRINE 536
    METAPROTERENOL 620
    METHYLPHENIDATE 648
    XYLOMETAZOLINE 1048
    PHENYLEPHRINE 790
    PHENYLPROPANOLAMINE 794
    PSEUDOEPHEDRINE 856
    TERBUTALINE 950
    THEOPHYLLINE, EPHEDRINE &
        BARBITURATES 960
    THEOPHYLLINE, EPHEDRINE, GUAIFENESIN &
        BARBITURATES 962
    THEOPHYLLINE, EPHEDRINE & HYDROXYZINE
        964
Sympathomimetic (bronchodilator) - See
    ISOETHARINE 526
Symptom 3 - See BROMPHENIRAMINE 156
Symptrol - See
    PHENIRAMINE 778
    SCOPOLAMINE (Hyoscine) 904
Symtrol - See PHENYLPROPANOLAMINE 794
Synacort - See ADRENOCORTICOIDS (Topical) 18
Synalar - See ADRENOCORTICOIDS (Topical) 18

INDEX

Temovate - See ADRENOCORTICOIDS (Topical) 18
Tempra - See ACETAMINOPHEN 4
Tenex - See GUANFACINE 490
Ten K - See POTASSIUM SUPPLEMENTS 816
Tenlap - See ACETAMINOPHEN 4
Tenol - See ACETAMINOPHEN 4
Tenoretic - See
  BETA-ADRENERGIC BLOCKING AGENTS &
    THIAZIDE DIURETICS 140
  CHLORTHALIDONE 244
Tenormin - See ATENOLOL 114
Tenstan - See
  BUTALBITAL & ASPIRIN (Also contains caffeine)
    168
  TALBUTAL (Butalbital) 944
Tenuate - See APPETITE SUPPRESSANTS 110
Tenuate Dospan - See APPETITE SUPPRESSANTS
  110
T-E-P - See
  EPHEDRINE 392
  PHENOBARBITAL 780
  THEOPHYLLINE, EPHEDRINE &
    BARBITURATES 960
Tepanil - See APPETITE SUPPRESSANTS 110
Tepanil Ten-Tab - See APPETITE SUPPRESSANTS 110
Teramine - See APPETITE SUPPRESSANTS 110
Terazol - See ANTIFUNGALS (Vaginal) 94
TERAZOSIN 948
TERBUTALINE 950
TERCONAZOLE - See ANTIFUNGALS (Vaginal) 94
TERFENADINE 952
Terfluzine - See TRIFLUOPERAZINE 1012
Terpin Hydrate w/Codeine - See NARCOTIC
  ANALGESICS 690
Terpin Hydrate and Codeine Syrup - See TERPIN
  HYDRATE 954
Terpin Hydrate Elixir - See TERPIN HYDRATE 954
TERPIN HYDRATE 954
Terramycin - See TETRACYCLINES 958
Terrastatin - See NYSTATIN 724
Tertroxin - See LIOTHYRONINE 564
Tesionate - See ANDROGENS 58
Testa-C - See ANDROGENS 58
Testadiate-Depo - See TESTOSTERONE &
  ESTRADIOL 956
Testaqua - See ANDROGENS 58
Test-Estra-C - See TESTOSTERONE & ESTRADIOL
  956
Test-Estro Cypionates - See TESTOSTERONE &
  ESTRADIOL 956
Testex - See ANDROGENS 58
Testoject - See ANDROGENS 58
Testoject-LA - See ANDROGENS 58
Testolin - See ANDROGENS 58
Testone L.A. - See ANDROGENS 58
TESTOSTERONE - See ANDROGENS 58
TESTOSTERONE CYPIONATE & ESTRADIOL
  CYPIONATE - See TESTOSTERONE &
  ESTRADIOL 956
TESTOSTERONE ENANTHATE & ESTRADIOL
  VALERATE - See TESTOSTERONE &
  ESTRADIOL 956
TESTOSTERONE & ESTRADIOL 956
Testostroval P.A. - See ANDROGENS 58
Testradiol - See TESTOSTERONE & ESTRADIOL
  956
Testradiol L.A. - See TESTOSTERONE &
  ESTRADIOL 956

Testred - See ANDROGENS 58
Testrin P.A. - See ANDROGENS 58
Tet-Cy - See TETRACYCLINES 958
Tetet - See TETRACYCLINES 958
TETRACAINE - See ANESTHETICS (Topical) 62
TETRACAINE (Ophthalmic) - See ANESTHETICS,
  LOCAL (Ophthalmic) 68
TETRACAINE (Rectal) - See ANESTHETICS (Rectal)
  60
TETRACAINE AND MENTHOL (Rectal) - See
  ANESTHETICS (Rectal) 60
Tetrachel - See TETRACYCLINES 958
Tetra-Co - See TETRACYCLINES 958
Tetracrine - See TETRACYCLINES 958
TETRACYCLINE - See TETRACYCLINES 958
TETRACYCLINE (Ophthalmic) - See
  ANTIBACTERIALS (Ophthalmic) 76
TETRACYCLINE (Topical) - See ANTIBACTERIALS
  FOR ACNE (Topical) 84
TETRACYCLINES 958
Tetracyn - See TETRACYCLINES 958
Tetracyrine - See TETRACYCLINES 958
TETRAHYDROZILINE (Ophthalmic) - See
  DECONGESTANTS (Ophthalmic) 326
Tetralean - See TETRACYCLINES 958
Tetram - See TETRACYCLINES 958
Tetramax - See TETRACYCLINES 958
Tetramine - See TETRACYCLINES 958
Tetrastatin (M) - See TETRACYCLINES 958
Tetrex - See TETRACYCLINES 958
Tetrex-S - See TETRACYCLINES 958
Texacort - See
  ADRENOCORTICOIDS (Topical) 18
  HYDROCORTISONE (Cortisol) 502
Tex Six T.R. - See PYRIDOXINE (Vitamin B-6) 864
T-Gesic Forte - See NARCOTIC &
  ACETAMINOPHEN 688
Thalfed - See
  EPHEDRINE 392
  PHENOBARBITAL 780
  THEOPHYLLINE, EPHEDRINE &
    BARBITURATES 960
  XANTHINE BRONCHODILATORS 1046
Thalitone - See CHLORTHALIDONE 244
Thallous Chloride TI 201 - See RADIO-
  PHARMACEUTICALS 882
Theelin - See ESTRONE 418
Theelin Aqueous - See ESTRONE 418
Theo-24 - See XANTHINE BRONCHODILATORS
  1046
Theobid - See XANTHINE BRONCHODILATORS
  1046
Theobid Duracaps - See XANTHINE
  BRONCHODILATORS 1046
Theobid Jr. Duracaps - See XANTHINE
  BRONCHODILATORS 1046
Theochron - See XANTHINE BRONCHODILATORS
  1046
Theoclear - See XANTHINE BRONCHODILATORS
  1046
Theoclear L.A. Cenules - See XANTHINE
  BRONCHODILATORS 1046
Theocolate - See THEOPHYLLINE &
  GUAIFENESIN 966
Theocord - See THEOPHYLLINE, EPHEDRINE &
  BARBITURATES 960
Theodrine - See THEOPHYLLINE, EPHEDRINE &
  BARBITURATES 960

INDEX

1197

Trinsicon - See FERROUS FUMARATE 442
TRIOXSALEN - See PSORALENS 858
Tri-Pain - See ACETAMINOPHEN & SALICYLATES 6
Tripazine - See TRIFLUOPERAZINE 1012
TRIPELENNAMINE 1022
Triphasil - See CONTRACEPTIVES (Oral) 288
Triphed - See PSEUDOEPHEDRINE 856
Tri-Phen-Chlor - See PHENYLTOLOXAMINE 796
Triple X (topical) - See PEDICULOSIDES (Topical)
   756
Tripodrine - See
   PSEUDOEPHEDRINE 856
   TRIPROLIDINE 1024
TRIPROLIDINE 1024
Triptil - See TRICYCLIC ANTIDEPRESSANTS 1008
Triptone - See SCOPOLAMINE (Hyoscine) 904
Trisogel - See MAGNESIUM TRISILICATE 588
Trisohist - See SCOPOLAMINE (Hyoscine) 904
Trisoralen - See PSORALENS 858
Tristoject - See TRIAMCINOLONE 998
Tri-Vi-Flor - See VITAMINS & FLUORIDE 1044
Trocal - See DEXTROMETHORPHAN 336
Tronolane - See ANESTHETICS (Topical) 62
Tronolane (rectal) - See ANESTHETICS (Rectal) 60
Tronothane - See ANESTHETICS (Topical) 62
Tronothane (rectal) - See ANESTHETICS (Rectal) 60
Truphylline - See XANTHINE BRONCHODILATORS
   1046
Trymegen - See CHLORPHENIRAMINE 236
Trymex - See
   ADRENOCORTICOIDS (Topical) 18
   TRIAMCINOLONE 998
T-Serp - See RAUWOLFIA ALKALOIDS 886
T-Star - See ERYTHROMYCINS 408
T-Stat (topical) - See ANTIBACTERIALS FOR ACNE
   (Topical) 84
Tudecon - See PHENYLTOLOXAMINE 796
Tuinal - See
   AMOBARBITAL 48
   SECOBARBITAL 906
Tumol - See METHOCARBAMOL 632
Tums - See
   CALCIUM CARBONATE 174
   CALCIUM SUPPLEMENTS 178
Tums E-X - See
   CALCIUM CARBONATE 174
   CALCIUM SUPPLEMENTS 178
Tusquelin - See CHLORPHENIRAMINE 236
Tuss-Ade - See PHENYLPROPANOLAMINE 794
Tussagesic - See
   DEXTROMETHORPHAN 336
   PHENIRAMINE 778
   PHENYLPROPANOLAMINE 794
Tussaminic - See
   DEXTROMETHORPHAN 336
   PHENIRAMINE 778
   PHENYLPROPANOLAMINE 794
Tussanil - See PYRILAMINE 866
Tussar - See
   CHLORPHENIRAMINE 236
   GUAIFENESIN 480
   NARCOTIC ANALGESICS 690
Tussar DM - See PHENYLEPHRINE 790
Tussend - See
   GUAIFENESIN 480
   NARCOTIC ANALGESICS 690
   PSEUDOEPHEDRINE 856

Tussionex - See PHENYLTOLOXAMINE 796
Tussi-Organidin - See
   CHLORPHENIRAMINE 236
   NARCOTIC ANALGESICS 690
Tussirex - See PHENYLEPHRINE 790
Tussirex Sugar-Free - See PHENIRAMINE 778
Tuss-Ornade - See
   CHLORPHENIRAMINE 236
   PHENYLPROPANOLAMINE 794
Tusstat - See DIPHENHYDRAMINE 360
Twilite - See DIPHENHYDRAMINE 360
Twin-K - See POTASSIUM SUPPLEMENTS 816
Twin-K-Cl - See POTASSIUM SUPPLEMENTS 816
Two-Dyne - See
   ACETAMINOPHEN 4
   CAFFEINE 172
Ty Caplets - See ACETAMINOPHEN 4
Ty Pap - See ACETAMINOPHEN 4
Ty-Tabs - See
   ACETAMINOPHEN 4
   NARCOTIC & ACETAMINOPHEN 688
Tylenol - See ACETAMINOPHEN 4
Tylenol w/Codeine - See
   ACETAMINOPHEN 4
   NARCOTIC & ACETAMINOPHEN 688
   NARCOTIC ANALGESICS 690
Tylenol Maximum Strength Sinus Medicine - See
   PSEUDOEPHEDRINE 856
Tylox - See
   ACETAMINOPHEN 4
   NARCOTIC & ACETAMINOPHEN 688
   NARCOTIC ANALGESICS 690
Tympagesic - See PHENYLEPHRINE 790
TYROPANOATE - See GALLBLADDER X-RAY TEST
   DRUGS (Cholecystographic Agents) 466
Tyrosum (topical) - See ANTI-ACNE, CLEANSING
   (Topical) 72

U

UAA - See ATROPINE, HYOSCYAMINE,
   METHENAMINE, METHYLENE BLUE,
   PHENYLSALICYLATE & BENZOIC ACID 118
Uirspas - See FLAVOXATE 448
Ulo - See CHLOPHEDIANOL 214
Ulone - See CHLOPHEDIANOL 214
Ultabs - See
   BELLADONNA 128
   HYOSCYAMINE 512
Ultracef - See CEFADROXIL 206
Ultralente - See INSULIN 520
Ultralente Iletin I - See INSULIN 520
UltraMOP - See PSORALENS 858
Ultramycin - See TETRACYCLINES 958
Ultratard - See INSULIN 520
Ultra Tears (Ophthalmic) - See PROTECTANT
   (Ophthalmic) 854
UNDECYLENIC ACID (Topical) - See
   ANTIFUNGALS (Topical) 92
Undoquent (topical) - See ANTIFUNGALS (Topical)
   92
Unguentine - See ANESTHETICS (Topical) 62
Unguentine Plus - See ANESTHETICS (Topical) 62
Unguentine Spray - See ANESTHETICS (Topical) 62
Unicelles - See APPETITE SUPPRESSANTS 110
Unicort - See
   ADRENOCORTICOIDS (Topical) 18
   HYDROCORTISONE (Cortisol) 502

VITAMIN B-5 - See PANTOTHENIC ACID (Vitamin B-5) 744
VITAMIN B-6 - See PYRIDOXINE (Vitamin B-6) 864
VITAMIN B-9 - See FOLIC ACID (Vitamin B-9) 462
VITAMIN B-12 (Cyanocobalamin) 1034
VITAMIN C (Ascorbic Acid) 1036
VITAMIN D 1038
VITAMIN E 1040
VITAMIN K 1042
Vitamin supplement - See
 FOLIC ACID (Vitamin B-9) 462
 NIACIN (Nicotinic Acid) 700
 PANTOTHENIC ACID (Vitamin B-5) 744
 PYRIDOXINE (Vitamin B-6) 864
 RIBOFLAVIN (Vitamin B-2) 896
 THIAMINE (Vitamin B-1) 970
 VITAMIN A 1032
 VITAMIN B-12 (Cyanocobalamin) 1034
 VITAMIN C (Ascorbic Acid) 1036
 VITAMIN D 1038
 VITAMIN E 1040
 VITAMIN K 1042
Vitamins - See VITAMINS & FLUORIDE 1044
VITAMINS & FLUORIDE 1044
VITAMINS A, D & C & FLUORIDE - See VITAMINS & FLUORIDE 1044
Viterra E - See VITAMIN E 1040
Vitron C - See FERROUS FUMARATE 442
Vivactil - See TRICYCLIC ANTIDEPRESSANTS 1008
Vivarin - See CAFFEINE 172
Vivol - See DIAZEPAM 338
Vivox - See TETRACYCLINES 958
V-Lax - See PSYLLIUM 860
Vlemasque (topical) - See ANTI-ACNE, CLEANSING (Topical) 72
Vlem-Dome (topical) - See ANTI-ACNE, CLEANSING (Topical) 72
Voltaren - See DICLOFENAC 340
Voltarol - See DICLOFENAC 340
Voltarol Retard - See DICLOFENAC 340
Vontrol - See DIPHENIDOL 362
Voranil - See APPETITE SUPPRESSANTS 110
VoSol HC (otic) - See ANTIBACTERIALS (Otic) 78

W

Wans - See PYRILAMINE & PENTOBARBITAL 868
WARFARIN POTASSIUM - See ANTICOAGULANTS (Oral) 86
WARFARIN SODIUM - See ANTICOAGULANTS (Oral) 86
Warfilone - See ANTICOAGULANTS (Oral) 86
Warnerin - See ANTICOAGULANTS (Oral) 86
Wehamine - See DIMENHYDRINATE 356
Wehgen - See ESTRONE 418
Wehless - See APPETITE SUPPRESSANTS 110
Wehvert - See MECLIZINE 596
Wehydryl - See DIPHENHYDRAMINE 360
Weightrol - See APPETITE SUPPRESSANTS 110
Wellcovorin - See LEUCOVORIN 556
Wesmatic - See EPHEDRINE 392
Wesmatic Forte - See CHLORPHENIRAMINE 236
Wesprin Buffered - See ASPIRIN 112
Westcort - See
 ADRENOCORTICOIDS (Topical) 18
 HYDROCORTISONE (Cortisol) 502
Westrim - See PHENYLPROPANOLAMINE 794

Westrim LA - See PHENYLPROPANOLAMINE 794
Wigraine - See
 BELLADONNA 128
 CAFFEINE 172
 ERGOTAMINE 400
 ERGOTAMINE & CAFFEINE 404
Wigraine-PB - See
 ERGOTAMINE 400
 PENTOBARBITAL 766
Wigrettes - See ERGOTAMINE 400
Wilpowr - See APPETITE SUPPRESSANTS 110
Win Gel - See
 ALUMINUM HYDROXIDE 28
 ALUMINUM & MAGNESIUM ANTACIDS 30
 MAGNESIUM HYDROXIDE 584
Win pred - See PREDNISONE 826
Winstrol - See ANDROGENS 58
Wolfina - See RAUWOLFIA ALKALOIDS 886
Woltac - See BELLADONNA 128
Wyamycin - See ERYTHROMYCINS 408
Wyamycin E - See ERYTHROMYCINS 408
Wyamycin S - See ERYTHROMYCINS 408
Wyanoids - See
 BELLADONNA 128
 EPHEDRINE 392
Wycillin - See PENICILLIN G 762
Wygesic - See
 ACETAMINOPHEN 4
 NARCOTIC & ACETAMINOPHEN 688
 NARCOTIC ANALGESICS 690
Wymox - See AMOXICILLIN 50
Wytensin - See GUANABENZ 482

X

Xanax - See ALPRAZOLAM 24
XANTHINE BRONCHODILATORS 1046
Xenon Xe 127 - See RADIO-PHARMACEUTICALS 882
Xenon Xe 133 - See RADIO-PHARMACEUTICALS 882
Xerac (topical) - See ANTI-ACNE, CLEANSING (Topical) 72
Xerac BP - See BENZOYL PEROXIDE 134
X-Otag - See ORPHENADRINE 726
X-Prep - See SENNOSIDES A & B 910
X-Prep Liquid - See SENNA 908
Xseb (topical) - See ANTI-ACNE (Topical) 74
X-Trozine - See APPETITE SUPPRESSANTS 110
X-Trozine LA - See APPETITE SUPPRESSANTS 110
Xylocaine - See ANESTHETICS (Topical) 62
Xylocaine (topical) - See ANESTHETICSS, DENTAL (Topical) 66
Xylocaine Ointment - See ANESTHETICS (Topical) 62
Xylocaine Viscous - See ANESTHETICS (Topical) 62
Xylocaine viscous (topical) - See ANESTHETICS, DENTAL (Topical) 66
XYLOMETAZOLINE 1048

Y

Yodoxin - See IODOQUINOL 522
Yutopar - See RITODRINE 900

Z

Z-200 Pyrinate (topical) - See PEDICULOSIDES (Topical) 756
Zantac - See RANITIDINE 884
Zapex - See OXAZEPAM 732

Zarontin - See ETHOSUXIMIDE 432
Zaroxolyn - See METOLAZONE 658
Zemarine - See
  ATROPINE 116
  HYOSCYAMINE 512
  SCOPOLAMINE (Hyoscine) 904
Zenate - See
  CALCIUM CARBONATE 174
  FERROUS FUMARATE 442
Zendole - See INDOMETHACIN 518
Zephrex - See
  GUAIFENESIN 480
  PSEUDOEPHEDRINE 856
Zeroxin - See BENZOYL PEROXIDE 134
Zestril - See LISINOPRIL 568
Zide - See HYDROCHLOROTHIAZIDE 500

ZIDOVUDINE (also called AZT, Azidothymidine)
  1050
Zincon (topical) - See ANTISEBORRHEIC (Topical)
  104
ZiPan - See PROMETHAZINE 848
Zorprin - See ASPIRIN 112
Zovirax - See ACYCLOVIR (Oral & Topical) 16
Zovirax Ointment - See ACYCLOVIR (Oral & Topical)
  16
Zoxaphen - See CHLORZOXAZONE &
  ACETAMINOPHEN 248
Zurinol - See ALLOPURINOL 22
Zyloprim - See ALLOPURINOL 22
Zyloric - See ALLOPURINOL 22
Zynol - See SULFINPYRAZONE 936

EMERGENCY GUIDE FOR OVERDOSE VICTIMS

This section lists *basic* steps in recognizing and treating immediate effects of drug overdose. Study the information before you need it. If possible, take a course in first aid and learn external cardiac massage and mouth-to-mouth breathing techniques, called *cardiopulmonary resuscitation* (CPR).

For quick reference, list emergency telephone numbers in the spaces provided on the inside front cover for fire department paramedics, ambulance, poison-control center and your doctor. These numbers, except for doctor, are usually listed on the inside cover of your telephone directory.

IF VICTIM IS UNCONSCIOUS, NOT BREATHING:

1. Yell for help. Don't leave victim.

2. Begin mouth-to-mouth breathing immediately.

3. If there is no heartbeat, give external cardiac massage.

4. Have someone call 0 (operator) or 911 (emergency) for an ambulance or medical help.

5. Don't stop CPR until help arrives.

6. Don't try to make victim vomit.

7. If vomiting occurs, save vomit to take to emergency room for analysis.

8. Take medicine or empty bottles with you to emergency room.

IF VICTIM IS UNCONSCIOUS AND BREATHING:

1. Dial 0 (operator) or 911 (emergency) for an ambulance or medical help.

2. If you can't get help immediately, take victim to the nearest emergency room.

3. Don't try to make victim vomit.

4. If vomiting occurs, save vomit to take to emergency room for analysis.

5. Watch victim carefully on the way to the emergency room. If heart or breathing stops, use cardiac massage and mouth-to-mouth breathing (CPR).

6. Take medicine or empty bottles with you to emergency room.